AF302505

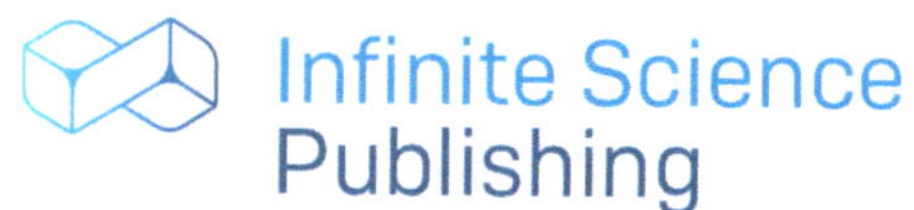

Infinite Science
Publishing

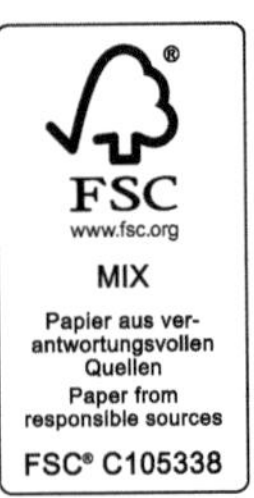

Student Conference Proceedings 2023

12th Conference on Medical Engineering Science
8th   Conference on Medical Informatics
6th   Conference on Biomedical Engineering
5th   Conference on Auditory Technology
3rd   Conference on Biophysics
3rd   Conference on Robotics and Autonomous Systems

Lübeck, March 1-3, 2023

Editors in Chief

T. M. Buzug, H. Handels, C. Hübner, A. Mertins, S. Müller, P. Rostalski

Associate Editors

C. Debbeler, J.-H. Wrage, K. Ehlers, R. Pallenberg, Y.-H. Song, S. Venker

Editors

H. Abbas, M. Ahlborg, E. Barth, P. Bartmann, R. Brinkmann, H. Busch, T. M. Buzug, C. Damiani, J. Ehrhardt, F. Ernst, S. Fudickar, M. Grzegorzek, U. Günther, T. Gutsmann, H. Hamann, H. Handels, M. Heinrich, M. Henke, M. Himstedt, R. Huber, C. Hübner, H. Husstedt, G. Hüttmann, J. Ingenerf, T. Jürgens, S. Karpf, M. Kircher, M. Koch, N. Linz, K. Lohmann, D. Lühmann, E. Maehle, S. Meier, A. Mertins, S. Mulhem, S. Müller, A. Neumann, N. T. Nguyen, J. Obleser, H. Paulsen, M. Rafecas, M. Rahlves, R. Rahmanzadeh, P. Rostalski, G. Schildbach, A. Schrader, F. Spitzenberger, S. Szymczak, J. Tchorz, M. Urban, W.-H. Wang, J. Weil

Student Conference Proceedings 2023

Preface and Acknowledgements

After the great success of the previous meetings from 2012 to 2022, the Student Conference 2023 shows continuing growth both in quality and quantity of scientific contributions. In this year, the 12th Student Conference on Medical Engineering Science is held together with the 8th Student Conference on Medical Informatics, the 6th Student Conference on Biomedical Engineering, the 5th Student Conference on Auditory Technology, the 3rd Student Conference on Biophysics, the 3rd Student Conference on Robotics and Autonomous Systems and the 1st Student Conference on Medical Microtechnology. The organization team has worked to provide an excellent conference, where master students of the campus present their recent research results to a broad public of academics and industry.

The contributions show how new approaches and methods in medical engineering and medical informatics can advance medicine, health, and health care. Moreover, this conference offers a good opportunity for both students and companies to get in touch at the Recruiticon, i.e. a satellite recruiting fair with industrial exhibition. Students from the Life Sciences programs present their results from projects carried out at the laboratories, clinics, and institutes of Lübeck's Universities, in international research facilities, or research-oriented industrial companies. The conference focus has been placed on topics ranging from medical engineering to medical informatics. The interdisciplinary field of medical engineering has been established at the Lübeck University of Applied Sciences for decades, and Medical Engineering Science (Medizinische Ingenieurwissenschaft – MIW) is an important bachelor and master program at the Universität zu Lübeck as well. Both universities jointly offer the international master degree programs Biomedical Engineering (BME) and Auditory Technology (Hörakustik und Audiologische Technik – HAT). Furthermore, in the master program Medical Informatics (Medizinische Informatik – MI) the Student Conference on Medical Informatics is integrated as an important element where project results in the emerging field of digital medicine are presented by the students. These subject areas are widened by the master's programs Robotics and Autonomous Systems (Robotik und Autonome Systeme – RAS) and Biophysics (Biophysik – BP). In 2023, master students of Medical Microtechnology (MMT), an international cooperative degree program offered by the two universities in Lübeck together with the University of Southern Denmark, will participate in the conference for the first time.

As Conference Chairs, we want to thank everybody who worked with enthusiasm and dedication to make the conference a successful event. We want to thank the companies who support the meeting. Moreover, our thanks go to Infinite Science for producing these proceedings and organizing the Recruiticon meeting supporting the Student Conference. Personally, and on behalf of all colleagues of the Student Conference Committee, we especially want to thank Christina Debbeler, Jan-Hinrich Wrage, Silke Venker, René Pallenberg, Kristian Ehlers and Young-Hwa Song. Their in-depth overview of all details of this event is the key to the success of the Student Conference 2023...

Lübeck, March 1-3, 2023

Prof. Dr. Thorsten M. Buzug
Chair of the 12th Student Conference on Medical Engineering Science

Prof. Dr. Heinz Handels
Chair of the 8th Student Conference on Medical Informatics

Prof. Dr.-Ing. Stefan Müller
Chair of the 6th Student Conference on Biomedical Engineering

Prof. Dr.-Ing. Alfred Mertins
Chair of the 5th Student Conference on Auditory Technology

Prof. Dr. Christian Hübner
Chair of the 3rd Student Conference on Biophysics

Prof. Dr.-Ing. Philipp Rostalski
Chair of the 3rd Student Conference on Robotics and Autonomous Systems

Contents

Auditory Technology

Biomedical Engineering

Machine Learning / AI

Signal Processing

Radio Technology and Locating

Sensor Data Analysis

Medical Electronics

E-Health

Medical Imaging

Biochemical Physics

Safety and Quality

Image Processing

Biomedical Optics

1

Auditory Technology

Design and evaluation of a Hearing Aid Demonstrator

Lisa-Marie Simon [1], Florian Denk [2] and Hendrik Husstedt[2]

[1] Auditory Technology, Universität zu Lübeck, lisamarie.simon@student.uni-luebeck.de
[2] German Institute of Hearing Aids, Lübeck, {f.denk, h.husstedt} @dhi-online.de

Abstract

A hearing aid demonstrator is intended to provide an opportunity to increase awareness of hearing aid benefits among hearing impaired people. For this purpose, the demonstrator must fulfil at least comparable performance characteristics as commercial hearing aids, while being easier to use. In this work, electroacoustic measurements were performed on a preliminary version of the demonstrator on an artificial head with different fittings of a hearing aid-like Behind-the-Ear (BTE) headset. Based on the results, it becomes clear that the demonstrator is able to fulfill these requirements. Optimally, effective isolation should be ensured by e.g. closed earmoulds. The significant self-noise of the demonstrator in the high-frequency range can be reduced in the future by using a subsequently programmed expansion plugin. It should be ensured that the measurement room causes as few reflections as possible. A anechoic room would be optimal for the measurements.

1 Introduction

A large number of people suffer from hearing loss. However, they often do not perceive this hearing impairment as requiring treatment. In most cases, progressive hearing loss leads to decreased hearing sensitivity and speech comprehension in noisier situations. For social interaction with other people, hearing impaired people often suffer from higher misunderstandings, increased fatigue and listening effort. This can strongly affect the quality of life. Treatment of hearing loss with a hearing aid can significantly reduce negative consequences, such as social isolation, depression, or increased risk of developing dementia [1, 2, 3]. Despite these positive effects, however, the uptake of a hearing aid treatment is low among many hearing impaired people. Only about 33 % of the hearing impaired (Pure Tone Average (PTA) > 25 dB HL) in Germany are fitted with a hearing aid, in spite of cost coverage by the health insurances.This corresponds to about 3.8 million hearing aid users [4].

For this reason, a hearing aid demonstrator is being developed within the greater scope of this work. It will consist of a portable open-source hearing system and circumaural headphones with integrated microphones. This offers hearing-impaired persons or the general public a simple, hygienic and quickly applicable way to experience the benefit provided by hearing aid processing like frequency dependent amplification. The aim is to increase the awareness of hearing impaired people about the benefits of hearing aid treatment. The demonstrator can be used in clinical settings or at public events. Therefore the demonstrator must fulfill the same requirements and technical performance as commercial hearing systems. Accordingly, the focus of this work is to evaluate the performance characteristics of a preliminary version of the demonstrator with Behind-The-Ear (BTE) headsets comparable to commercial hearing aids. For this purpose, electroacoustic measurements of the maximum output level, the self-noise and the evaluation of the dynamic compression by the percentile analysis were performed based on the standard specifications [5, 6]. In this work, in-situ conditions were simulated by using an artificial head to provide applicability for the final demonstrator based on circumaural headphones.

2 Material and Methods

2.1 Hearing Aid Demonstrator

The hearing aid demonstrator consists of the Portable Hearing Laboratory (PHL), an open-source hearing system. The miniature computer with multi-channel audio board built into the PHL can be combined with various headsets. For this work, a BTE headset with two microphones (TDK ICS 40730 MEMS) on each side was used, as shown in Fig. 1. The headset's receivers are Sonion's RIC-E50D (M earpieces). With six analog input and output audio channels in the PHL, it is possible to implement signal processing (e.g. adaptive directionality) of multiple microphones [7]. For this purpose, the open Master Hearing Aid (openMHA) software is used. The openMHA software is a real-time software specialized in hearing aid signal processing [8]. It consists of a variety of plugins, each representing a hearing aid function (e.g. a plugin for noise reduction). By combining and arranging several plugins in the desired way, the complete signal processing of a hearing aid can be simulated. With a graphical user interface the configurations can be set via a web server. The demonstrator contains several preset gain configurations. In this work, fittings based on the standard audiograms N2 and N3 of DIN EN 60118-15 (2012) were generated using the CAMFIT fitting rationale [9, 10]. The CAMFIT fitting rule is based on a loudness model [10]. In addition to the settings already named, the FOG (Full On Gain) and the linear RTS (Reference Test Setting of the gain control) settings can be selected for the standard measurements. The combination of PHL and openMHA provides this work the opportunity to develop and evaluate a prototype hearing aid demonstrator.

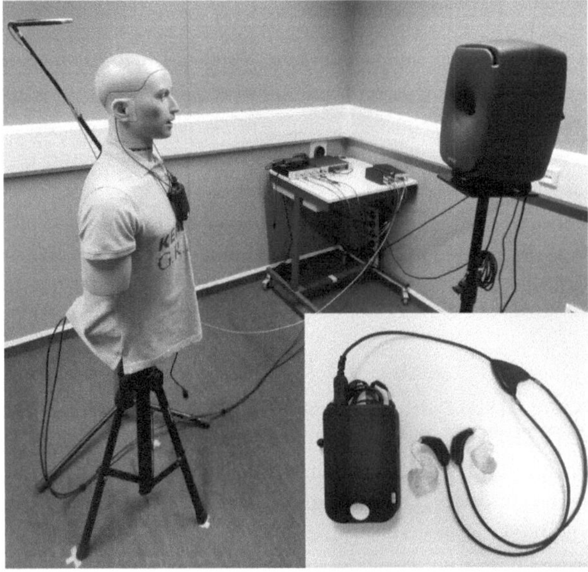

Figure 1: Measurement setup consisting of a loudspeaker at a 0° angle to the KEMAR. The headset of the demonstrator is coupled in the ears of the KEMAR. Bottom right: Prototype of the hearing aid demonstrator with custom earmolds on the headset.

2.2 Setup

The measurements were performed in an acoustically treated room (T20 < 0.1 s) with a background noise level below 30 dB SPL. For this purpose, an artificial head "KEMAR 45BC-1" from G.R.A.S. and a loudspeaker (Genelec 8351A) were positioned in the center of the room. The KEMAR was configured with one ear simulator per side and pinnae. As shown in Fig. 1, the loudspeaker was positioned at a distance of 1 m and at an angle of 0° to the KEMAR. The height of the loudspeaker axis corresponded to the height of the ear canal opening of the artificial head. The headset of the hearing aid demonstrator was coupled to the ears of the KEMAR with the earpieces appropriate for the condition (earmold, open- or power dome). The PHL was placed on the chest of the KEMAR. The measurement was controlled by a laptop with a graphical user interface (GUI) via MATLAB. The parameters (output level, signal length or frequency range) could be set for each measurement in this way. The demonstrator was connected to the

same laptop via network and could be configured via the web browser. All adaptive parameters not investigated in this work were disabled.

2.3 Measurements

In this work, three technical measurements were used. First, the standard measurement according to the DIN EN 60118-0 (2016) specifications was measured with a sine sweep [5]. To determine the maximum values of the output level and gain, the demonstrator was set to maximum gain setting (FOG). All limiting controllers are turned off. The maximum value of the curve and the HFA (High-Frequency Average) are determined. The HFA is the average value at 1, 1.6 and 2.5 kHz. First, the OSPL90 curve (L_{in} = 90 dB, FOG setting) was measured. Followed by the Full-on gain response curve (L_{in} = 50 dB, FOG setting). The basic frequency response curve (L_{in} = 60 dB, RTS setting) measured the output level in the linear range at a typical gain setting and an input level approximately equal to normal speech. The HFA of the basic frequency response curve must be 17 dB below the HFA of the OSPL90. The measurements were performed at KEMAR, therefore the measurements are shown as Real Ear Aided Response (REAR) in decibels SPL [dB SPL] over the frequency range in Hertz [Hz]. The percentile analysis was the second measurement. The International Speech Test Signal (ISTS) was used to verify the amplification in a compressed setting of the demonstrator. Four curves are determined. The 99th and 30th percentiles recreate the dynamics of speech. The 65th percentile and the LTASS (mean long-term speech volume) are used to adjust to the respective target gains [9]. The percentile analysis was measured to provide information about the functioning of the dynamic behaviour of the hearing aid demonstrator. Therefore, all four conditions (earmoulds, open- and power dome) were tested with the N2_CAMFIT fitting rule at 55, 65 and 80 dB and a playback of at least 60 s.

The third measurement is the noise measurement to determine the self-noise of the hearing aid demonstrator. It is detected on the ear simulator without external noise sources. For this purpose, the demonstrator is adjusted to the N2_CAMFIT setting and measured with closed earmolds.

3 Results and Discussion

3.1 Standard measurement

The test results of the response curves from the left side with closed earmould are shown in Fig. 2. These are also representative for the right side. The two top curves are the OSPL90- and the basic frequency response curve. The FOG measurement is also shown in the same figure. It should be noticed that the FOG curve (lowest) shows gain values. For this reason, the measurement is stated as Real Ear Insertion Gain (REIG) in decibels [dB]. The maximum OSPL90 value (125 dB SPL at 2660 Hz) and the HFA-OSPL90 value

(121 dB SPL) were determined from the OSPL90 curve. The OSPL90 curve represents the upper power limit of the demonstrator. The HFA value of the basic frequency response curve should be 17 dB SPL lower than the HFA-OSPL90. The HFA is in tolerance by 104 dB SPL. The frequency range is < 200 Hz and > 8 kHz (HFA-basic frequency response curve - 20 dB SPL: 84 dB SPL).The FOG curve was also calculated with the maximum FOG value (56 dB at 1412 Hz) and the HFA FOG (51 dB).

Strong fluctuations are visible in the two lower standard curves. These are caused by reflections inside the measuring room. With the basic frequency response curve, the distortions become visible due to the linear RTS setting, which amplifies each type of signal equally. Therefore, it would have made more sense to perform the measurements in an anechoic room. A similar problem exists with the FOG measurement. The demonstrator is set to maximum gain, which amplifies the same room acoustic effectS. In addition, the Real Ear measurement of the unaided ear was measured retrospectively for the FOG correction. This could explain the strong fluctuations in the high frequency range. The fluctuations are not visible in the OSPL90 curve, since this curve represents the saturation range (i.e. the performance limit) of the demonstrator. In conclusion, it can nevertheless be said that the results of the performance characteristics test are comparable to the characteristics of commercial hearing systems.

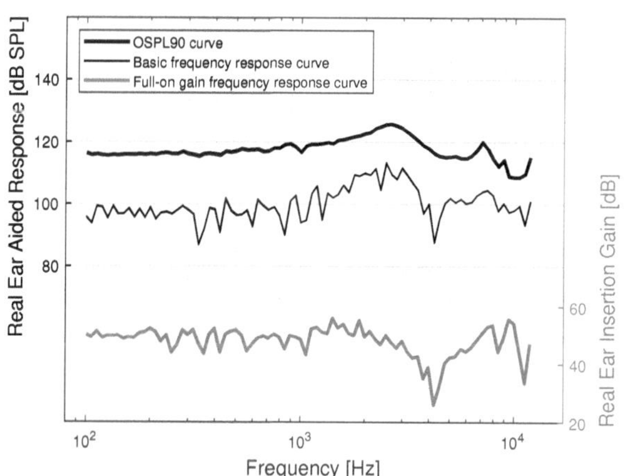

Figure 2: Standard response curves based on DIN EN 60118-0 of the left side of the hearing aid demonstrator. Measured with the closed earmould on the KEMAR.

3.2 Percentile analysis

The 30th, 65th and 99th percentiles were determined at input levels of 50, 65 and 80 dB. The results are shown in Fig. 3. The data are presented as Real Ear Insertion Gain (REIG) in decibels [dB] as a function of frequency in Hertz [Hz]. As expected, the graphs show that the gain values depend on the input level. The amplification values for an input level of 80 dB are significantly lower than for 55 dB. Low level inputs are accordingly amplified more. Furthermore, a lower gain can be seen between the open (bottom left) and

the closed earmould (top left). Similar to commercial hearing aids, an open fitting allows the low frequencies to pass out of the auditory canal. This means that hardly any amplification values can be detected. For the high-frequency range, only low deviations between the conditions can be seen. Because the N2_CAMFIT fitting rule also prescribes significant gain at low frequencies (unlike NAL-NL2), the closed earmould would be the most sensible condition to be able to access the gain. As circumaural headphones are planned for the final hearing aid demonstrator, there should be no problems with occlusion effects. The demonstrator and commercial hearing aids do not differ in the way they connect to the ear.

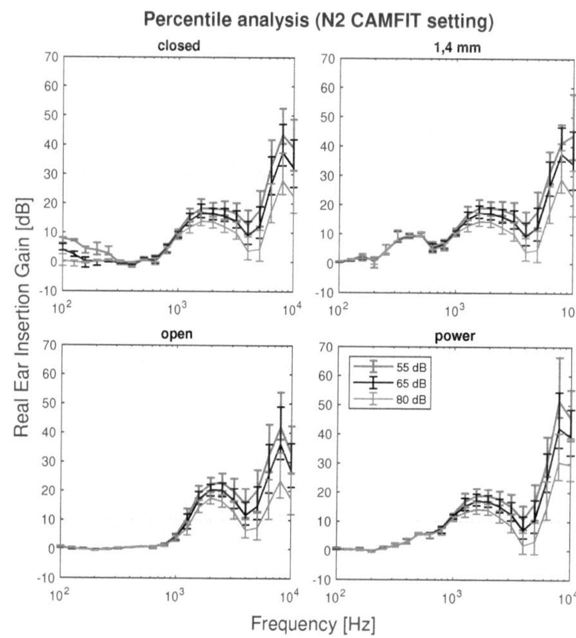

Figure 3: Percentile analysis for the four conditions (closed, 1.4 mm, open and power) as insertion gain values over the frequencies. Shown as the 30th, 65th and 99th percentiles for the output levels 55, 65 and 80 dB.

3.3 Noise measurement

Like other technical devices, hearing aids produce an self-noise that can be audible and annoying to the user. In Fig. 4 the self-noise of the hearing aid demonstrator (left side only) is shown as a function of frequency. The graph shows that the demonstrator, in contrast to the Real Ear reference curve of the unaided ear, has highly increased values in the high-frequency range. This is due to the deposited gain setting of the demonstrator. The high-frequency self-noise can be disturbing to the user, depending on hearing ability. One possibility to suppress the noise would be to implement an expansion plugin in the openMHA software, which was not present at the time of examination. The expansion reduces the amplification of low input levels. The advantage is that people with a mild or low-frequency hearing loss are not disturbed by the noise of the hearing aid and the hearing aid demonstrator itself works more quietly.

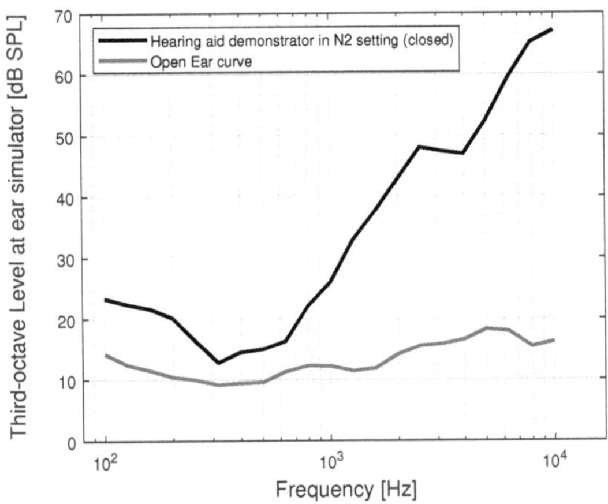

Figure 4: Intrinsic noise of the hearing aid demonstrator in third octave resolution of the left side on the ear simulator. The fitting rule is N2_CAMFIT with closed earmould. The Open Ear curve serves as reference curve.

4 Conclusion

In this work, the hearing aid demonstrator was examined for technical performance characteristics. The measurements were performed on an artificial head based on standardised test methods for hearing systems. It was shown that the demonstrator can fulfil the performance characteristics, but there are still challenges with the coupling and the self-noise. Based on the data of the percentile analysis, it becomes clear that a closed coupling is important. This is the only way to ensure amplification in the low frequency range. For the final hearing aid demonstrator, the circumaural headphone should provide adequate sealing. With the factor of self-noise, it makes sense to integrate an expansion plug-in. People with a mild or low-frequency hearing loss could also use the demonstrator without disturbing noise. All in all, the current hearing aid demonstrator is a good tool to illustrate how commercial hearing aids work.

In the future, the comparison between the final hearing aid demonstrator and a commercial hearing aid with test subjects would be of great interest. Speech intelligibility tests could be used to investigate the subjective speech understanding of hearing impaired people in direct comparison to the hearing system. In addition, other plug-ins could be programmed into the demonstrator that could improve speech perception. The hearing aid demonstrator offers many opportunities for modifications in soft- and hardware to improve the functionality.

Acknowledgement

The work has been conducted and supervised at the German Institute of Hearing Aids GmbH, Lübeck.

Author's Statement

The authors declared no potential conflicts of interest with respect to the research, authorship, and/or publication of this article.

5 References

[1] G. H. Saunders, T. H. Chisolm and M. I. Wallhagen, "Older adults and hearing help-seeking behaviors," *Am J Audiol.*, vol. 21(2), pp. 331–7, 2012.

[2] A. Ciorba, C. Bianchini, S. Pelucchi and A. Pastore, "The impact of hearing loss on the quality of life of elderly adults," *Clin Interv Aging.*, vol. 7, pp. 159–63, 2012.

[3] A. Chern and J. S. Golub, "Age-related Hearing Loss and Dementia. Alzheimer Dis Assoc Disord," *Alzheimer Dis Assoc Disord.*, vol. 33, no. 3, pp. 285–290, 2019.

[4] I. Holube, E. Hoffmann and P. von Gablenz, "Hearing-aid adoption in Northern and Southern Germany," *GMS Z Audiol (Audiol Acoust)*, vol. 1, pp. 1–21, 2019.

[5] DIN EN 60318-0: Akustik - Hörgeräte - Teil 0: Messung der Leistungsmerkmale von Hörgeräten (IEC 601180-0:2015), *Beuth Verlag GmbH*, September, 2016.

[6] DIN EN 60318-8: Akustik - Hörgeräte - Teil 8: Verfahren zur Messung der Übertragungseigenschaften von Hörgeräten unter simulierten In-Situ-Bedingungen (IEC 60118-8:2005), *Beuth Verlag GmbH*, August, 2006.

[7] C. Pavlovic, R. Kassayan, S. Prakash, H. Kayser, V. Hohmann and A. Atamaniuk, "A high-fidelity multi-channel portable platform for development of novel algorithms for assistive listening wearables," *J. Acoust. Soc. Am.*, vol. 146, 2019.

[8] H. Kayser, T. Herzke, P. Maanen, M. Zimmermann, G. Grimm and V. Hohmann, "Open community platform for hearing aid algorithm research: open Master Hearing Aid (openMHA)," *SoftwareX*, vol. 17, 2022.

[9] DIN EN 60118-15: Akustik – Hörgeräte – Teil 15: Methoden zur Charakterisierung der Hörgeräte-Signalverarbeitung (IEC 60118-15:2012), *Beuth Verlag GmbH*, December, 2012.

[10] B. C. J. Moore, J. I. Alcantara, M. A. Stone and B. R. Glasberg, "Use of a loudness model for hearing aid fitting: II. Hearing aids with multi-channel compression," *Brit. J. Audiol.*, vol. 33, pp. 157-170, 1999.

Acoustic Feedback Path of Hearing Aids related to Insertion Gain

Fabian Hettler [1], Florian Denk [2], and Hendrik Husstedt [2]
[1] Auditory Technology, Universität zu Lübeck, fabian.hettler@student.uni-luebeck.de
[2] Deutsches Hörgeräte Institut GmbH, Lübeck, {h.husstedt, f.denk}@dhi-online.de

Abstract

Hearing aids can make inaudible signals of hearing-impaired persons perceptible again by amplification. Depending on the design and the ear coupling of the hearing aid, a certain part of the amplified signal returns to the microphones of the hearing aid. This loop back is the so-called acoustic feedback path. Above a certain gain, a critical feedback condition can occur, which is noticeable as a whistling sound. This article describes a measurement of the feedback path and an estimation of the maximum insertion gain a hearing aid can provide. For validation, this feedback path was measured with a Behind the Ear hearing aid dummy with different couplings at an artificial head. The 'Insertion Gain related Feedback Path', introduced in this article, gives an indication of the frequency-dependent gain a hearing aid can provide, until a critical feedback condition occurs.

1 Introduction

The core feature of hearing aids is the compensation of a hearing loss. For this, the acoustical signal, picked up by the microphones, is amplified depending on the type of hearing loss. Based on the type of hearing aid and the coupling to the ear canal, a part of the outgoing frequency-depend signal $Y(f)$ of the hearing aid loops back from the receiver to the microphones. That feedback signal is added to the input signal $X(f)$ of the hearing aid and gets amplified in a closed-loop condition. The acoustic feedback path is described as a transfer function $H(f)$ from the hearing aid receiver to the microphone and is shown schematically in Figure 1.

In this closed loop condition, the feedback signal gets amplified several times. Depending on the attenuation of the feedback path and the gain of the hearing aid, this can result in a critical feedback condition, which manifests in a whistling sound.

There are different strategies to enable more amplification for the hearing aid without reaching the critical feedback condition, e.g., by maximizing the distance between the microphones and the sound outlet of the hearing aid or by attenuating the loop back signal with a mould in the ear canal. In addition to that, there are different signal processing strategies to enable an added stable gain with feedback suppression algorithms. For instance, there can be added a phase- or frequency-shift in the outgoing signal at critical frequencies in the feedback path [1, 2]. However, there are many factors that influence the acoustic feedback path, like the type of hearing aid or the coupling in the ear canal. Dynamic changes, like a telephone beside the ear, have influence on the feedback path as well [3].

Previously published studies that investigated the acoustic feedback path [3, 4] describe it as a transfer function

$$H(f) = \frac{V_{\mathrm{mic}}(f)}{V_{\mathrm{rec}}(f)} \qquad (1)$$

where $V_{\mathrm{mic}}(f)$ is the voltage of the hearing aid microphone and $V_{\mathrm{rec}}(f)$ the voltage of the receiver.

In some cases, $V_{\mathrm{mic}}(f)$ is presented as a calibrated pressure signal, too [5]. The feedback path can be investigated by measuring the feedback signal in an open loop, so the feedback signal is interrupted after the first loop back. However, by measuring a real hearing aid, a closed loop condition is given. The feedback signal passes the feedback path several times and gets amplified each time.

In the following, a representation of the acoustic feedback path is described, considering the hearing aid response at the eardrum and corrections depending on the hearing aid type and ear canal coupling in an open loop condition. The Insertion Gain related Feedback Path (IFP) shows the frequency-dependent maximum gain the hearing aid can provide, until a critical feedback condition becomes possible. This is shown with three different couplings of a behind-the-ear (BTE) hearing aid dummy with a receiver

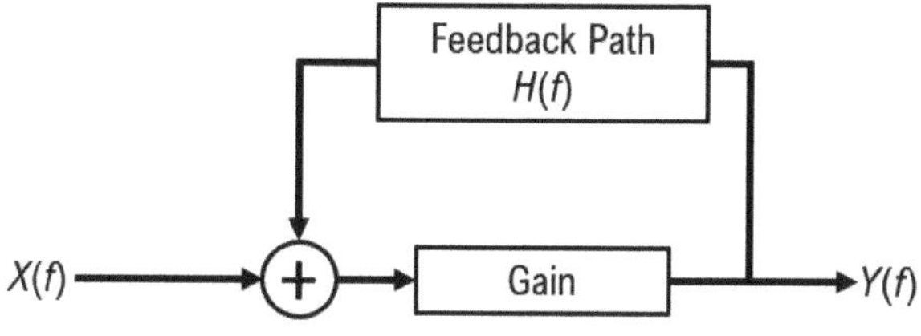

Figure 1: Schematic process of the acoustic feedback path with a hearing aid.

in the ear canal (RIC). The measurement was performed at an artificial head.

2 Material and Methods

2.1 Scenario

A schematic measurement setup and the resulting transfer functions are shown in a cross-section of the ear in Figure 2. For an initial investigation, the IFP was determined on an artificial head (GRAS 45BC KEMAR Head & Torso) with anthropometric pinna (GRAS KB 5001) and ear simulator (GRAS RA0045). Instead of a commercial hearing aid, we used the 'Bat&Cat BTE-RIC' headset [6]. This dummy behind-the-ear hearing aid consists of a hearing aid shell with two 'TDK ICS 40730' MEMS-microphones and a 'Sonion E50D RIC' receiver-in-canal receiver. Its microphones were free field calibrated at 250 Hz. To control the amplitude of the stimulus for the receiver, the voltage output of the sound card was calibrated with a multimeter to 0.32 V (RMS-value of a 1000 Hz sine tone). This is the maximum possible amplitude in which the receiver does not go into saturation. The recordings were performed with Matlab R2022b and a 'RME Fireface 802' sound card.

Three different couplings were measured with the BTE hearing aid dummy: Open dome, power dome and closed mould (tight custom mold for the anthropometric pinna without a venting). The hearing aid dummy was positioned with the coupling at the anthropometric ear. To measure the feedback path, the receiver of the hearing aid dummy was stimulated by a linear sine sweep with a duration of 5 seconds, an amplitude of 0.32 V sound card output and a frequency range from 50 to 20.000 Hz. The microphone of the ear simulator and both microphones of the hearing aid dummy were recording the stimulus.

Both, stimulus and recordings were performed with a sampling frequency of 44100 Hz. Delay generated by the sound card was compensated. Each coupling in the ear canal was measured in ten insertions, each insertion included ten repetitions of the sweep (100 sweeps in total per coupling). After every insertion the hearing aid dummy was removed and reinserted in the ear canal. The resulting spectra in decibel were arithmetically averaged to increase the signal-to-noise-ratio. All measurements took place in a soundproofed room.

The resulting transfer functions describe the path from the receiver to the ear drum (REC2ED) and from the receiver to the hearing aid microphone (REC2HAmic). Both functions present the at the microphones detected sound pressure regarding to the voltage the receiver was stimulated.

2.2 Calculation of the Insertion Gain related Feedback Path

The individual spectra were generated with a DFT-calculation of the measured impulse responses (Matlab's

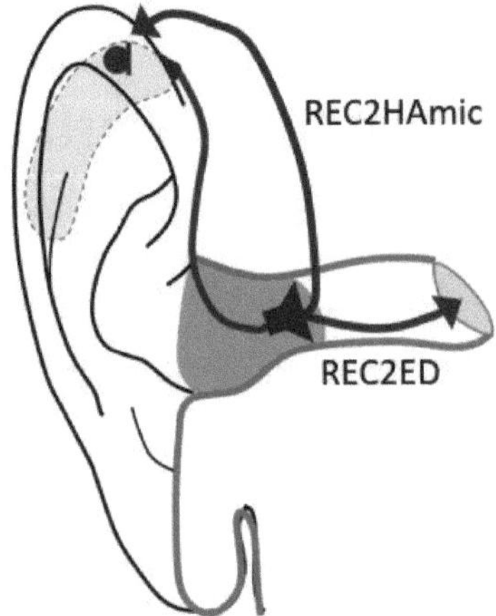

Figure 2: Measurement setup and resulting transfer functions from the receiver to the ear drum (REC2ED) and to the hearing aid microphone (REC2HAmic), shown in a schematic cross-section of the ear.

fft-function). For the presentation all averaged spectra were smoothed with a third octave band resolution as described by [7].

By dividing the REC2ED and REC2HAmic transfer functions, it is possible to calculate the acoustical feedback path. To find the actual maximum gain the hearing aid can generate without reaching a critical feedback condition, there must additionally be considered the Real Ear Unaided Gain (REUG) and the Microphone Location Effect (MLE). The REUG describes the transfer function of the open ear canal and the MLE the effect on the position of a hearing aid's microphone at the ear, both relative to the free field condition. The IEC 60118-8:2005 specifies these transfer functions of the MLE for different hearing aid designs and the REUG at the artificial head [8]. For this calculation, the MLE transfer function for a BTE hearing aid and the REUG are taken from this norm. The IFP can thus be calculated by

$$\begin{aligned} H_{\mathrm{IFP}}(f) = {} & H_{\mathrm{REC2HAmic}}(f) - H_{\mathrm{REC2ED}}(f) \\ & + H_{\mathrm{REUG}}(f) - H_{\mathrm{MLE}}(f) \end{aligned} \quad (2)$$

where all quantities denote the transfer function magnitudes in decibel. The difference of $H_{\mathrm{REC2HAmic}}(f)$ and $H_{\mathrm{REC2ED}}(f)$ gives the attenuation of the feedback path. By adding the $H_{\mathrm{REUG}}(f)$ and subtracting the $H_{\mathrm{MLE}}(f)$, the actual gain of the hearing aid can be calculated [8].

3 Results and Discussion

Figure 3 shows the individual and averaged transfer functions REC2ED and REC2HAmic with the power dome coupling. REUG and MLE function for a BTE hearing device, taken from the IEC 60118-8:2005 [8], and the noise floor, measured at the hearing aid dummy microphone, are shown as well.

Figure 4 shows the IFPs of three measured couplings

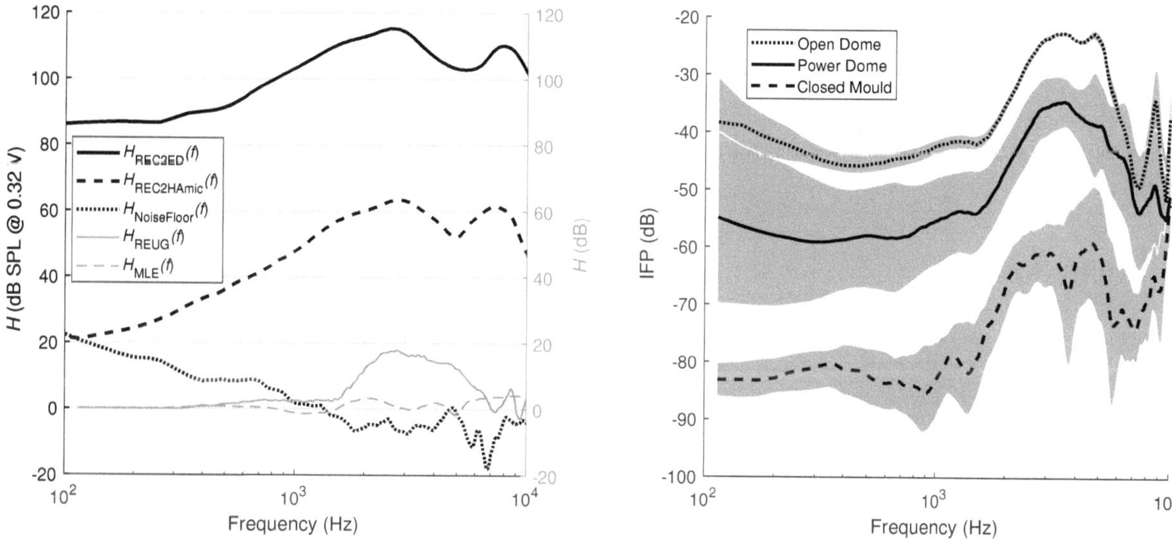

Figure 3: Resulting transfer functions from the speaker to the eardrum (REC2ED) and to the hearing aid front microphone (REC2HAmic) in dB SPL, the Real Ear Unaided Gain (REUG) and the Microphone Location Effect (MLE) with a power dome as coupling in the ear canal in dB. The speaker was stimulated with a linear sine sweep and an amplitude of 0.32 V. Also displayed is the recorded noise floor of the hearing aid dummy front microphone.

Figure 4: Arithmetic average of the Insertion Gain related Feedback Path (IFP) of a BTE-RIC hearing aid dummy with an open dome, power dome and closed mould coupling in the ear canal. The 95% confidence interval of each function is highlighted as gray shading.

with an open dome, a power dome and a closed mould, measured at the left ear of the KEMAR with the BTE-RIC hearing aid dummy, including the 95% confidence intervals (95%-CI). Differences between the transfer functions from the receiver to the front and rear microphone of the hearing aid dummy are negligible. For a better overview, here are only shown the feedback paths regarding to the front microphone.

The IFPs, shown in Figure 4, indicate the frequency-dependent maximum possible gain the hearing aid can provide, until a critical feedback condition can be reached. For instance, the hearing aid can generate about 36 dB of gain at frequencies around 3500 Hz coupled with the power dome until a critical feedback condition can be reached, disregarding the phase shift between the receiver and the hearing aid microphone. With an open dome there is a maximum gain of 25 dB and with the closed mould 60 dB. The more attenuation the coupling in the ear canal ensures, the more gain the hearing aid can provide without reaching a critical feedback condition. A significant shift of the maximum frequency is not visible. In agreement to the experience of hearing aid professions the IFPs display realistic gain values for BTE hearing aids and is confirmed by various measurements (for instance, [9] gives an overview for different couplings).

The attenuation of a power dome in the ear canal changes greatly by a minimal variation of the positioning in fre-

quencies above 600 Hz [10]. Due to the repositioning of the hearing aid dummy ten times per condition, this results in high variations in the coupling, as shown in Figure 4. In frequencies below 600 Hz the IFP scatters by up to 30 dB. The reason for such a high variation could be a strong position-related attenuation. In frequencies around 3000 Hz, which are important for this feedback path, the IFP varies around 10 dB. Using an individual mould reduces the variation of possible positions in the ear canal. This results in less variation of the attenuation (up to 10 dB). However, relevant frequencies for the feedback path show a similar scatter than the power dome. In case of an open dome coupling with almost no attenuation, its position-related influence on the IFP is negligible. When measured on different subjects, this variation is likely to be even wider. By repeating the measurement several times with a repositioning of the hearing aid dummy, a representative IFP can be obtained by averaging for every kind of coupling.

By measuring the closed mould, the signal recorded by the hearing aid microphones is very low due to a high attenuation at the feedback path. This results in a very small signal-to-noise ratio (SNR). Increasing the amplitude of the stimulus would cause distortions of the receiver. Therefore, the noise floor was reduced by arithmetic averaging of ten measurement repetitions, which gives an increase of the SNR by about 10 dB. The resulting noise floor at the hearing aid dummy microphone is shown in Figure 3.

In the IFP the phase is not considered. Depending on the delay generated by the feedback path, the maximum of a phase-corrected IFP with the hearing aid dummy would expected to be slightly weakened and near of the actual measured maximum of the IFP not including the phase.

In case of a real hearing aid with a closed loop condition, a steep phase response is expected, because processing in real hearing aids generates a latency of up to 10 milliseconds [11]. That will also result in a slightly different maximum of the IFP.

4 Conclusion

The Insertion Gain related Feedback Path proposed in this study, shows a procedure to describe the feedback path and an estimation of the maximum insertion gain a hearing aid can provide without reaching a critical feedback condition. For this, the following transfer functions are considered: From the receiver to the ear drum, from the receiver to the hearing aid microphones, the Real Ear Unaided Gain and the Microphone Location Effect (both relative to the free field).

To demonstrate the practical implementation, the Insertion Gain related Feedback Path was measured with a BTE-RIC hearing aid dummy with three different couplings in the ear canal.

It was shown that the Feedback Path Insertion Gain gives a general estimation of the maximal possible insertion gain a hearing aid can provide by a given feedback path, until a critical feedback condition can occur. Since the phase is not considered, the Insertion Gain related Feedback Path in a real hearing aid will not be the same as measured in this study.

For further investigations of the Insertion Gain related Feedback Path, ear moulds with different ventings and In-the-Ear hearings aids should be condidered. The measurement should be performed on real subject ears as well.

Acknowledgement

This study was conducted at the German Institute of Hearing Aids in Lübeck. I would like to thank my supervisors for their great support during this work.

Author's Statement

Conflict of interest: Authors state no conflict of interest.

5 References

[1] A. Spriet, S. Doclo, M. Moonen, and J. Wouters, "Feedback control in hearing aids," in *Springer Handbook of Speech Processing.* Springer, 2008, pp. 979–1000.

[2] J. Chalupper, T. A. Powers, and A. Steinbuss, "Combining phase cancellation, frequency shifting, and acoustic fingerprint for improved feedback suppression," *Hearing review*, vol. 18, no. 1, pp. 24–29, 2011.

[3] T. Sankowsky-Rothe and M. Blau, "Static and dynamic measurements of the acoustic feedback path of hearing aids on human subjects," in *Proceedings of Meetings on Acoustics 173EAA*, vol. 30, no. 1. Acoustical Society of America, 2017, p. 050008.

[4] T. Sankowsky-Rothe, M. Blau, H. Schepker, and S. Doclo, "Reciprocal measurement of acoustic feedback paths in hearing aids," *The Journal of the Acoustical Society of America*, vol. 138, no. 4, pp. EL399–EL404, 2015.

[5] F. Denk and B. Kollmeier, "The hearpiece database of individual transfer functions of an in-the-ear earpiece for hearing device research," Acta Acustica, 2021.

[6] BatAndCat Sound Labs. (January 09, 2023). [Online]. Available: https://batandcat.com/portable-hearing-laboratory-phl.html

[7] P. D. Hatziantoniou and J. N. Mourjopoulos, "Generalized fractional-octave smoothing of audio and acoustic responses," *Journal of the Audio Engineering Society*, vol. 48, no. 4, pp. 259–280, 2000.

[8] German Institute for Standardization e.V., *IEC 60118-8:2005: Verfahren zur Messung der Übertragungseigenschaften von Hörgeräten unter simulierten In-Situ-Bedingungen, Teil 8.* Beuth Verlag, Berlin, 2005.

[9] H. Dillon, "Hearing aids." Hodder Arnold, 2008.

[10] J. Cubick, S. Caporali, D. Lelic, J. Catic, A. V. Damsgaard, S. Rose, T. Ives, and E. Schmidt, "The acoustics of instant ear tips and their implications for hearing-aid fitting," *Ear and Hearing*, vol. 43, no. 6, pp. 1771–1782, 2022.

[11] S. Lansbergen and W. A. Dreschler, "Classification of hearing aids into feature profiles using hierarchical latent class analysis applied to a large dataset of hearing aids," *Ear and hearing*, vol. 41, no. 6, p. 1619, 2020.

How is loudness of amplitude-compressed speech evaluated?
A comparison between the RMS method and Zwicker's algorithm

Iris Borschke [1], Martin Orf [2], and Jonas Obleser [2]

[1] Auditory Technology, Universität zu Lübeck, iris.borschke@student.uni-luebeck.de

[2] Department of Psychology, Universität zu Lübeck, {m.orf, jonas.obleser}@uni-luebeck.de

Abstract

Complex signals such as speech are used more frequently by researchers these days. The calculation of the root mean square (RMS) is a method to match sound pressure levels. To match the perceived loudness a method according to Zwicker's algorithm can be used. Given that RMS matched compressed signals are perceived louder as uncompressed signals, an online experiment will be performed to determine whether Zwicker's algorithm is more suitable to match compressed and uncompressed speech signals. Therefore the loudness of speech signals were rated by 10 subjects. The RMS matched speech signals were rated significantly louder than the uncompressed. No significant difference between the Zwicker matched compressed and the uncompressed speech signals reveal. Hence, the algorithm according to Zwicker is more suitable. Furthermore, level differences of a maximum of 1.2 dB were found, although the question arises whether these are of relevance or negligible, since the human ear perceives level differences from about 1 dB.

1   Introduction

For decades, auditory neuroscience was limited to short, isolated stimuli. While the acoustic environment in which we interact on a daily basis is very complex. Because of advances in computational processing, the field has been able to work on more ecological signals, such as speech. However, complex signals also pose challenges for researchers because they cannot be controlled as precisely, and interactions can confound effects. For example, loudness can have an undesirable and unintended side effect. This is especially important because the perception of loudness is dependent on level intensity and frequency. First of all, a fundamental distinction must be made between volume and perceived loudness. The volume is given in dB SPL and is a unit of measurement for the sound pressure level, this gives the ratio to the hearing threshold at normal pressure. Loudness, in turn, is a psychoacoustic unit and describes the human perception of loudness. The loudness level of sounds varies depending on the sound intensity and the frequency and it is given in the unit phon. Whereby the phon value remains the same for perceived equal loudness. Furthermore, the unit phon can be converted into loudness with the unit sone. 1 sone correlates to 40 phone (1 kHz sinusoidal tone at 40 dB SPL). Unlike the unit phon, the unit sone is ratio scaled and provides information about how much louder a signal is perceived, e.g. a signal with the value of 2 sone is twice as loud as a signal of 1 sone.

Signal compression causes the loudness to be perceived as louder [1]. We regularly encounter compressed signals in everyday life, for example, advertisements on television or radio are often amplitude-compressed to conform to cer-

tain specifications of the broadcasters while increasing the perceived loudness [2]. Another usage where signals are amplitude-compressed is in hearing aids. Amplitude compression is used for hearing-impaired persons, who have limited hearing dynamics, to make quiet signal components audible again, while louder signal components do not become too loud. Amplitude compression alters high and low speech components to different degrees, hence it changes the dynamic range. The ratio of amplitude compression to amplitude deflection before and after compression is the same for all different volumes parts of the signal, but the absolute value is different for high and low sound parts. For the lower sound parts the absolute difference is lower than for higher sound parts. Therefore, the amplitude-compressed speech signal looks different in contrast to the uncompressed, this can be seen in Figure 1.

The compressed speech signals with the same root mean square (RMS) value are perceived louder than uncompressed speech signals [1]. This can be explained by the fact that in the calculation of the RMS value, higher values are weighted more heavily by squaring and therefore over-weighted. A method to evaluate the loudness of speech signals is the method according to Zwicker, which was developed by Eberhard Zwicker in 1965, see "A model of loudness summation" [3].

In order to determine whether Zwickers algorithm method for loudness matching is more suitable for amplitude compressed speech signals than matching the level using the RMS, both methods are compared in this paper. Therefore an online experiment is conducted to investigate the following research questions: First, are the loudness perception of uncompressed and amplitude-compressed speech matched using the RMS rated the same? Second, is the loudness perception of uncompressed and amplitude-compressed speech matched using Zwicker's algorithm rated the same?

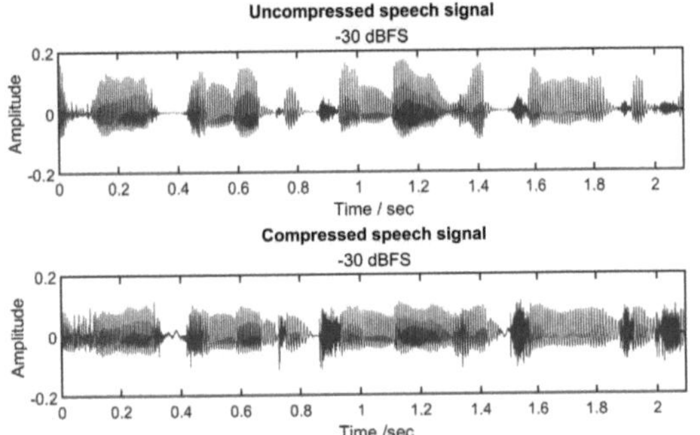

Figure 1: The different amplitude characteristics of an uncompressed and a compressed speech signal over time are shown. The upper signal shows the time domain of an uncompressed speech signal at -30 dBFS. The lower signal in contrast shows this for an amplitude-compressed speech signal (same speech signal and same level).

2 Material and Methods

2.1 Online Experiment

10 subjects (7 female and 3 male) aged 22-32 years participated in this study. All of them reported no hearing impairment and 8 of them were native German speakers. The study was performed online, via a PC with headphones by the participant. For this purpose, the volume on the PC was first set to a level such that a soft speech signal should at least still be heard and a very loud speech signal should not be too loud for the participant. It should be noticed that the volume range was set individually by each participant. In the experiment, the 720 speech signals (40 different speech signals · 3 conditions · 6 volume/loudness levels) previously generated via Matlab were played randomly one after the other. After each presentation, the participants were asked to rate the loudness of the presented speech signal on a number scale from 1 to 9 (soft to loud). The participants were instructed to use the entire scale during the experiment.

	Control – Uncompressed speech signal	RMS matched Compressed speech signal	Zwicker matched Compressed speech signal
RMS [dBFS]	-30	-30	-31.4
Zwicker [sone]	21.5	23.6	21.5

Figure 2: The schematic example shows, for an uncompressed speech signal of -30 dBFS and an associated value of 21.5 sone, which values the same speech signal in a compressed version assumes according to RMS matching and the method according to Zwicker. The arrows indicate to which value the compressed speech signal was matched.

2.2 Stimuli

Two uncompressed audio books ("Basiswissen Beethoven" and "Basiswissen Sophie Scholl") were used for the speech signals. Preprocessing of the audio books was performed using scripts written in Matlab R2022b by MathWorks. First, the audio books were compressed by dynamic range compression with a ratio of 8 (threshold -40 dB, attack time 2 ms, release time 15 ms, sample rate 44100 Hz), following processing strategies used by hearing aid manufacturers [4]. Then, the uncompressed and compressed audio books were limited to 99.95% to prevent clipping. In the next step, the audio signals were split into 2.1 sec long segments, following Moore's study [2], with 3ms fade-in and fade-out each. Furthermore, 20 different signal segments were randomly selected from each audio book (i.e., 40 in total). These signal segments, in uncompressed as well as compressed versions, were then matched to 6 different levels, using the RMS of -36, -33, -30, -27, -24, and -21 dBFS. The different levels were used to generate loudness functions according to the method of Stevens and Marks [5]. Furthermore, the loudness in sone was calculated for the uncompressed speech signals, for each RMS value. Then the compressed audio segments were matched using a Matlab function (acousticloudness) according to ISO 532-1 [6] based on the algorithm developed by Zwicker [3]. A schematic representation for the matching methods and their calculated values for the RMS in dBFS and according to Zwicker's Method in sone is for the example of -30 dBFS shown in Figure 2. The RMS value for the uncompressed and the RMS matched compressed speech signal is the same, while for the Zwicker matched compressed speech signal it is lower. In contrast the calculated loudness value in sone is higher for the RMS matched compressed speech signal, hence it should be evaluated as louder.

2.2.1 RMS and Zwicker's Method

A simple method to calculate the level of a signal is to form the RMS, the amplitude deflections are included in this calculation. The more complex method to calculate the loudness according to Zwicker also weights the frequencies of the signal. It can be used for stationary and dynamic signals, like speech. First, the signal is calibrated to the CalibrationFactor [7] in the time domain. In the next step, the signal is transformed into a 1/3 octave SPL representation using octave band filtering (28 filters between 25 Hz and 12.5 kHz). This representation is in dB and normalized to the reference pressure. According to a fixed weighting table, low-frequency 1/3-octave bands are suppressed and combined into 20 critical bands. The loudness of the 20 critical bands is corrected by the filter bandwidth and the level of the quiet threshold and then converted to the core loudness. This is then converted to the Bark scale (based on human hearing). Then the frequency bandwidth is calculated using a table (level and frequency depending on slopes). Finally, the loudness is calculated as an integral over the specific loudness of the frequency bands, taking into account the frequency bandwidths and slopes [7].

2.3 Statistical Analysis

Statistical analysis is performed via Matlab and Jamovi. The least squares method is used to calculate a linear regression for each condition and subject (including the mean of all subjects) across all loudness levels. Then the dBFS values on the x-axis are mean adjusted, so the zero matches the middle of all used dBFS values. Furthermore, using the calculated linear regression of the mean (slope and intercept), the RMS values for the loudness ratings between 3.5 and 7 are additionally calculated in 0.5 steps for each condition to subsequently calculate level differences. For the results of all conditions, a repeated measures ANOVA and a Bayesian t-test are calculated. The ANOVA is calculated to test if two of all three conditions show differences in mean values. Afterwards the Bayesian paired t-test is calculated to verify if the differences in mean values are significantly different to the control condition (H0: same, H1: different). The Bayesian t-test is also used to get evidence of how strong the null or the alternative hypothesis is accepted.

3 Results and Discussion

In the following section, the research questions of whether the loudness perception of uncompressed and amplitude-compressed matched speech signals using the RMS or Zwicker's algorithm are rated the same is evaluated.
Figure 3 shows the mean values of the different conditions per RMS value (circle) and the resulting linear regression for each subject (dashed line). The linear regressions show a positive slope, i.e., the higher the level, the louder the loudness is perceived, independent of the condition of the speech signal. Furthermore, the mean values over all subjects are shown (square) and as a solid line the regression line over these mean values of all subjects is shown. It is also shown that each subject used almost the same range on the rating scale for all conditions while some preferred the upper and some the lower scale.
In order to be able to compare all conditions the mean rating values were plotted against the mean adjusted dBFS values (Figure 4A). It can be seen that the regression line of the loudness rating for the RMS matched compressed speech signal for all RMS values is above the regression line of the control - uncompressed speech signal and thus this is rated as louder. In contrast, for the Zwicker matched compressed speech signal the regression line is below the control - uncompressed speech signal, at higher levels they are almost on top of each other, or the Zwicker matched compressed speech signal is slightly higher.
Calculated intercepts for all single subjects and also the mean of all are shown in Figure 4B. The results for the calculated ANOVA of all intercepts show a significant difference between two of three conditions ($p < .001$). The Bayesian t-test subsequently performed shows anecdotal evidence ($BF_{10} = 2.709$) that the intercepts of the RMS

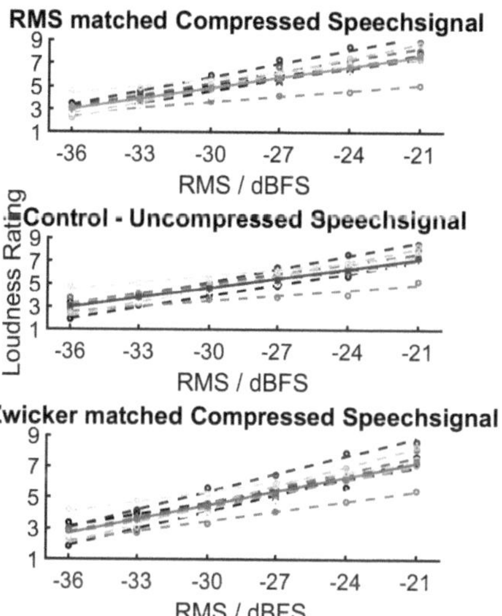

Figure 3: The figure shows the ratings for each level from each single subject (dashed line), split by condition. Furthermore, the mean value over all subjects per condition is shown (solid line).

matched compressed speech signals show differences in mean values to those of the control - uncompressed speech signals (H1). While for the Zwicker matched compressed speech signals this shows an anecdotal evidence ($BF_{10} = 0.814$) that the intercepts show no differences in mean values (H0).

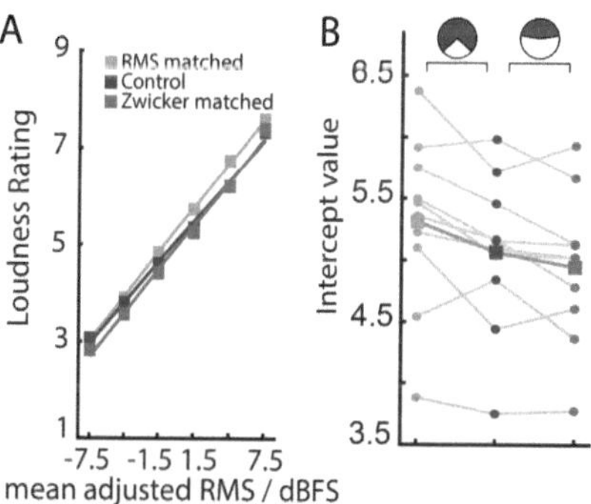

Figure 4: In A, the linear regressions of mean values across all subjects for each condition are shown as a function of the mean-adjusted RMS value. B shows the calculated intercept values of each subject (circle) and mean values across all subjects (square) for mean-adjusted RMS values. Furthermore, the evidence calculated by the Bayes factor is shown in the pie chart above (white = H0 (same), red = H1 (different)).

This shows that based on the calculation of the RMS, it cannot be assumed that speech signals are perceived equally loud when they are in compressed and uncompressed mode. However, the evaluation of the perceived loudness still does not give any information about the differences between conditions. Therefore, for each condition, linear regression is used to determine which RMS value the corresponding value assumes on the rating scale (from 3.5 to 7.5), see Figure 5A. The calculated ANOVA has a p-value of $< .001$, so again there is a significant difference between two of all conditions. The Bayes factor calculated from the Bayesian paired t-test shows extreme evidence ($BF_{10} = 236.19$) that dBFS values associated with the ratings of the RMS matched compressed speech signal show difference in mean values to those of the control - uncompressed speech signal (H1). While for the Zwicker matched compressed speech signal compared to the control - uncompressed speech signal the Bayesian factor shows anecdotal evidence for H1 ($BF_{10} = 2.31$).

The difference between the values of the compressed conditions and the control - uncompressed speech signal indicates how much larger or smaller the RMS value of the control - uncompressed speech signal must be in order to be perceived as equally loud, this can be seen in Figure 5B. The range of differences for the RMS matched compressed speech signal is between 1.2 and 0 dB while for the Zwicker matched compressed speech signal it is between 0 and -1.1 dB. Since the human ear can only perceive volume differences from approx. 1 dB [8], the question arises whether the calculated difference of mostly less than 1 dB is meaningful or negligible for the human ear.

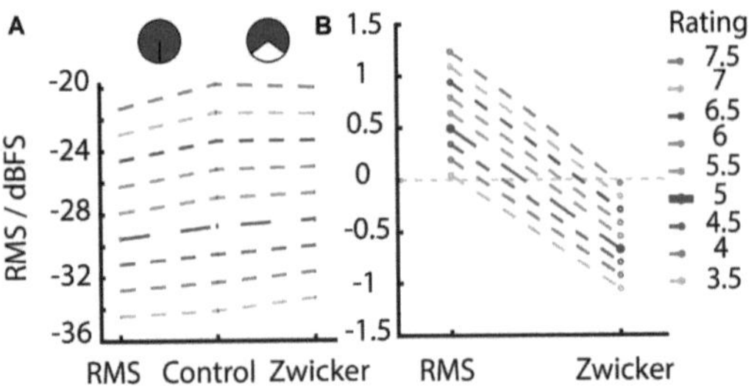

Figure 5: For ratings 3.5 to 7.5, the RMS values were calculated via linear regression of each condition, see A. Also the evidence for the calculated Bayes factor is shown in a pie chart above (white = H0 (same distribution), red = H1 (different distribution)). The difference between the respective compressed conditions and the control - uncompressed condition is shown in B. Furthermore, the zero line is drawn horizontally, representing the control condition.

4   Conclusion

The method of RMS calculation is not suitable for comparing the perceived loudness of compressed and uncompressed speech. It is better to use the method according to Zwicker. However, loudness differences of 3 dB as Moor et al. [2] between compressed and uncompressed speech could not be found. Since this was an online experiment in which the absolute volume at which the speech signals were heard could not be controlled, this may have had an influence. The influence of different loudness levels was not investigated in this study. Further developed methods for loudness calculation may offer a better possibility for the comparison of perceived loudness in the future and avoid loudness differences e.g. in radio or television.

Acknowledgement

The work has been carried out at AG Auditory Cognition, Institute of Psychology, Universität zu Lübeck.

Author's Statement

Conflict of interest: Authors state no conflict of interest. Informed consent: Informed consent has been given by all subjects before participating in the online experiment.

5   References

[1] J. Rennies, I. Holube, and J. Verhey, "Loudness of Speech and Speech-Like Signals," *Acta Acustica united with Acustica*, vol. 99, Mar. 2013.

[2] B. C. J. Moore, B. R. Glasberg, and M. A. Stone, "Why Are Commercials so Loud? ' Perception and Modeling of the Loudness of Amplitude-Compressed Speech*," *Journal of the Audio Engineering Society*, vol. 51, no. 12, pp. 1123–1132, Dec. 2003, publisher: Audio Engineering Society. [Online]. Available: https://www.aes.org/e-lib/browse.cfm?elib=12190

[3] E. Zwicker and B. Scharf, "A MODEL OF LOUDNESS SUMMATION," *Psychological Review*, vol. 72, pp. 3–26, Jan. 1965.

[4] K. Patel and I. M. S. Panahi, "Compression Fitting of Hearing Aids and Implementation," *IEEE Engineering in Medicine and Biology Society. Annual International Conference*, vol. 2020, pp. 968–971, Jul. 2020. [Online]. Available: https://www.ncbi.nlm.nih.gov/pmc/articles/PMC7545261/

[5] J. C. Stevens and L. E. Marks, "Cross-modality matching functions generated by magnitude estimation," *Perception & Psychophysics*, vol. 27, no. 5, pp. 379–389, May 1980.

[6] "DIN 45631/A1:2010-03, Berechnung des Lautstärkepegels und der Lautheit aus dem Geräuschspektrum Verfahren nach E. Änderung: Berechnung der Lautheit zeitvarianter Geräusche; mit CD-ROM," Beuth Verlag GmbH, Tech. Rep. [Online]. Available: https://www.beuth.de/de/-/-/122476084

[7] "Perceived loudness of acoustic signal - MATLAB acousticLoudness - MathWorks Deutschland." [Online]. Available: https://de.mathworks.com/help/audio/ref/acousticloudness.html

[8] S. S. Stevens, J. Volkmann, and E. B. Newman, "A Scale for the Measurement of the Psychological Magnitude Pitch," *The Journal of the Acoustical Society of America*, vol. 8, no. 3, pp. 185–190, Jan. 1937, publisher: Acoustical Society of America. [Online]. Available: https://asa.scitation.org/doi/abs/10.1121/1.1915893

Ocular Biomarkers of Listening Effort in Experienced Hearing Aid Users in Darkness and Light

Jessica Herrmann [1], Lorenz Fiedler [2], Dorothea Wendt [2], Sébastien Santurette [3] and Tim Jürgens [4]

[1] Auditory Technology, Universität zu Lübeck, jessica.herrmann@student.uni-luebeck.de
[2] Eriksholm Research Centre, Snekkersten, Denmark, lfie@eriksholm.com, dowe@eriksholm.com
[3] Centre for Applied Audiology Research, Oticon A/S, Smørum, Denmark, sesn@oticon.com
[4] Institute of Acoustics, University of Applied Sciences Lübeck, tim.juergens@th-luebeck.de

Abstract

Hearing aid users experience higher listening effort due to their hearing impairment. Hearing aid features, e.g. noise reduction (NR) are developed to minimize listening effort. Goal is to explore ocular biomarkers of listening effort in hearing aid users with and without NR in commercial hearing aids. Therefore, pupil diameter was measured during a hearing in noise test, performed in dark and light conditions with NR on and off to isolate sympathetic activity from parasympathetic activity of the autonomic nervous system. Results show no significant effect of NR on pupil dilation in either light or dark. A tendency is observed that in darkness with NR off, there is more sympathetic activity and thus more listening effort compared to NR on. This means on the one hand, pupillometry in darkness may help to investigate listening effort, but on the other that our study has been underpowered or the task has been too difficult.

1 Introduction

People with hearing loss experience higher amounts of listening effort than normal-hearing people especially in situations with more than one talker and background noise [1]. Even with hearing aids listening effort is still a challenge for hearing-impaired people. Listening effort can be measured subjectively with questionnaires, for example by asking the test persons after a listening task how strenuous the task was [1]. However the relationship between self-reported listening effort and physiologically measured listening effort is complex and needs to be further investigated [2]. One way to objectively measure listening effort is to measure pupil diameter. Pupil diameter is under control of the automatic nervous system and reflects the balance of its two main branches: the sympathetic nervous system (SNS) and parasympathetic nervous system (PNS) [3]. Reference [3] describes that the influence of both branches can be investigated by measuring pupil diameter both, in a light and dark room. In the dark room the influence of PNS should be minimal and in the light room both branches contribute to the pupil size. It is assumed that increased listening effort leads to more SNS activity and less PNS activity. However, long-term listening effort leads to fatigue and thus increased PNS activity. In general a larger pupil diameter indicates increased mental effort [2], [3]. Algorithms in hearing aids, e.g. noise reduction (NR) should reduce the listening effort of hearing aid users [4]. The present study investigated whether a difference in pupil size was measurable when performing a listening task with NR on and NR off in a light and a dark room. We expected to see smaller pupil response with NR on compared to NR off because NR should reduce listening effort. Furthermore, we expected to see a smaller difference between NR on and off in light compared to dark, because in darkness the parasympathetic contribution to the pupil size in minimal [3].

2 Material and Methods

2.1 Participants

Eighteen (4 females, 14 male) hearing-impaired adults participated in this study. All participants were native German speakers, experienced hearing aid users and had already attended in another hearing study at the University of Applied Sciences Lübeck. The mean age of the participants was 67.2 years (SD = 5.0). The pure tone average between frequencies of 500 Hz, 1000 Hz, 2000 Hz and 4000 Hz was 48.9 dB hearing level (HL) (SD = 15.1) for the left and 50.0 dB HL (SD = 14.1) for the right ear.

2.2 Hearing Aid Setting

Each participant was fitted with the same hearing aids. The hearing aids were fitted based on the individual audiogram using NAL-NL2 adjustment formula. Using real-ear measurements (REM) the gain curves were verified. Insert ear-tips proposed by the fitting software were used for the acoustic coupling. Two settings were programmed with noise reduction on and off. Otherwise, all signal processing features (e.g. feedback cancellation) were left at default values and did not vary between conditions.

2.3 Auditory stimuli and setup

The test session took place in a room of the University of Applied Sciences in Lübeck. The light in the room was controlled by two lamps (Viltrox VL-500T) placed behind the participant's chair to avoid reflections in the pupils. Three loudspeakers (Genelec 8040A) were positioned around the participant as shown in Fig. 1. As target speech German sentences (male speaker) from the Hearing-in-Noise-Test (HINT) [5] were presented from the loudspeaker positioned in front of the listener at $0°$ with 1.2 m distance. Two different maskers were presented from $\pm100°$. Both maskers consisted of a male speaker mixed with low-level speech-shaped noise. The level of the noise was - 6 dB relative to the running speech level [6]. Each speaker talked about another topic.

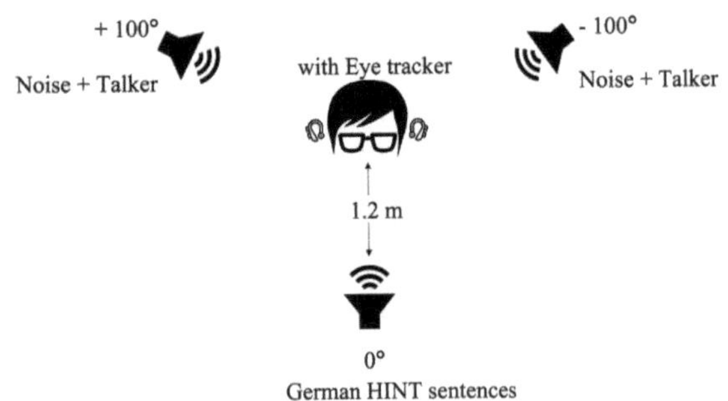

Figure 1: Position of the loudspeakers. Target speech was presented from the front. Masker signals were presented at $\pm100°$

2.4 Speech Reception Threshold Test

First, an adaptive procedure was used to estimate the individual signal-to-noise-ratio (SNR) required for 50 % sentence intelligibility (SRT50) in bright light with NR switched off. A one-up-one-down procedure with SNR adjusted in 2 dB steps were used. The level of the maskers was calibrated so that 65 dB SPL was measured at the participants' ears and the target signal was varied. The SNR was initially set to 0 dB. Participants were asked to repeat the target-sentence words after the sentence was over. Using word-scoring the experimenter marked all words that the participant repeated correctly, then the next sentence was presented. In the subsequent four conditions, the HINT test was conducted at fixed SNR that equals the individual SRT50, recording pupil dilation and additionally speech intelligibility in percent correct.

2.5 Procedure

A luminance measurement with a luxometer (Testo 545) was carried out and the light intensity was adjusted to ensure approximately 370 lux in the light condition and 0 lux in the dark condition. Participants were asked not to wear corrective glasses during the measurement in order to avoid reflexions that may reduce the quality of the pupil size measurements. At first a training run was conducted with NR off, light on using one HINT list with 20 sentences. After that trial the SRT50 was measured with NR off, light on using two HINT lists (40 sentences) (see section 2.4). This was followed by four measurements, each with two HINT lists. HINT lists were randomized across participants and condition using a latin square design. Two conditions in light with NR on and off, and two conditions in darkness with NR on and off.

2.6 Pupillometry

Pupil diameter of both left and right eyes were recorded by Pupil Labs Core eye tracking device (Pupil Labs GmbH, Berlin), with a sampling rate of 200 Hz. For subsequent analysis, only data of one eye per participant was considered which showed lowest amount of failed pupil trackings in the raw data. The following analysis was done with MATLAB R2021a (The MathWorks INC., Natick, Massachusetts, USA). First, a threshold was determined for each data set, setting the 5 % lowest values to values which were not a number. The eye tracking device not only recorded the pupil diameter, but also the confidence that the values reflect the diameter of the pupil. Data with confidence less than or equal to 60 % was discarded, including the time range 35 ms before and 100 ms after their occurrence to minimise artefacts caused by blinks and other noise. Then a linear interpolation was performed to compensate missing samples. The data was smoothed by convolution with a hamming window of 0.5 seconds length. When the pupil data was recorded, timestamps were generated marking the start 2.2 seconds before the sentence onset. In each condition, the first and the last sentence of the total of 40 sentences were discarded. Based on that the pupil diameter was extracted in the time range 4.2 seconds before the annotation and 6 seconds after the annotation. If a sentence had more than 20 % unusable data, it was discarded. As a result of this data processing, 5 out of 18 subjects no longer had valid sentences. The data from these subjects were completely discarded. After visual inspection of the outcome it seemed that the annotations which marked the target onset were set later by the program than the actually time onset. For calculating the baseline pupil diameter (BPD), therefore, the time range between -2 and -1 seconds relative to the annotation was used (Fig. 2). Within this time range the mean pupil size was calculated and subtracted from the pupil size of the whole trial. Fig. 2 shows that the mean pupil dilation (MPD) was defined as the average pupil diameter relative to the trial baseline and were calculated from a 2 second long time window. For each participant and condition MPD values were extracted and averaged from the preprocessed data.

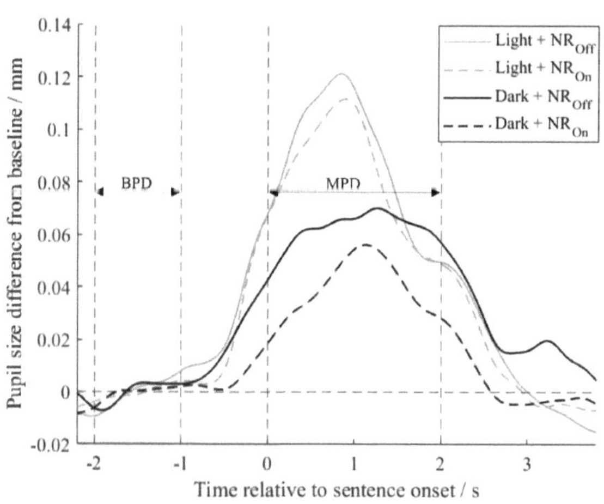

Figure 2: Baseline-corrected pupil response during light and dark measurement with NR on and NR off averaged across all participants and sentences.

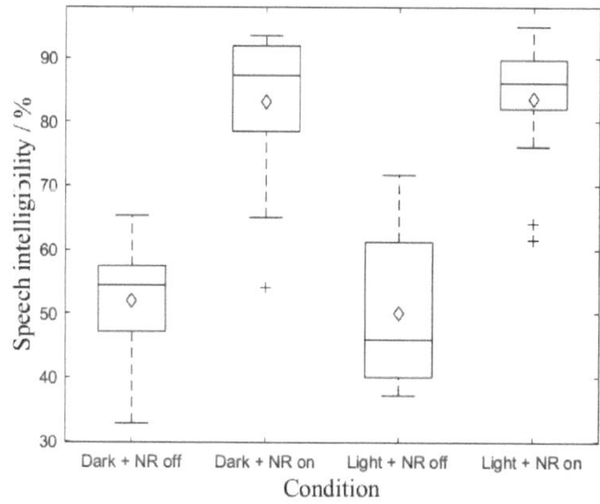

Figure 3: Boxplot showing speech intelligibility in percent for two conditions in darkness with NR off and on and two conditions with light on and NR off and on. Outliers are plotted as a plus and means as a diamond.

2.7 Statistical Analyses

First a descriptive statistical analysis on speech intelligibility and the pupil parameter (MPD) in all conditions was conducted. Next, a 2-by-2 repeated measures analysis of variance (ANOVA) was performed with the independent variables (i.e., factors) luminance (levels: light & dark) and NR (levels: on & off) on the dependent variables MPD and speech intelligibility. Thereby it was investigated whether there is any interaction between luminance and NR on MPD and speech intelligibility. If the result was significant, a post-hoc t-test with a Holm correction was performed.

3 Results

3.1 Speech Intelligibility

Fig. 3 shows the results of the descriptive statistical analysis of the speech intelligibility in percent of each condition as a boxplot. In the dark condition a mean intelligibility of 51.9 % (SD = 9.0 %) with NR off and 83.1 % (SD = 11.8 %) with NR on was achieved. In the light condition the mean intelligibility was 50.1 % (SD = 12.2 %) with NR off and 83.5 % (SD = 10.3 %) with NR on. The repeated-measures ANOVA revealed a significant main effect of NR (F = 77.466, $p < 0.001$, partial η^2 = 0.866). A post-hoc t-test (t(12) = 8.80, $p < 0.001$) confirmed that speech intelligibility was higher with NR on compared to off. There was neither significant main effect of luminance (F(1,12) = 0.177, p = 0.681, partial η^2 = 0.015) nor a significant interaction between luminance and NR (F(1,12) = 0.314, p = 0.585, partial η^2 = 0.026). This means that speech intelligibility was only affected by NR, which was increased when NR was switched on.

3.2 Mean Pupil Dilation

Fig. 4 shows boxplots of MPD in all conditions. The descriptive statistical analysis revealed a mean of the MPD (after baseline correction) in the dark condition of 0.062 mm (SD = 0.051 mm) with NR off and 0.04 mm (SD = 0.044 mm) with NR on. In the light condition, the mean value with NR off was 0.09 mm (SD = 0.048 mm) and with NR on 0.083 mm (SD = 0.054 mm). For MPD the repeated-measures ANOVA revealed a significant main effect of luminance (F = 8.041, p = 0.015, partial η^2 = 0.401). A post-hoc t-test (t(12) = -2.84, p = 0.015) confirmed that MPD was larger in light than in dark. There was neither significant main effect of NR (F(1,12) = 3.750, p = 0.077, partial η^2 = 0.238) nor a significant interaction between luminance and NR (F(1,12) = 0.861, p = 0.372, partial η^2 = 0.067). This means that MPD was only affected by luminance, which led to a higher MPD in light.

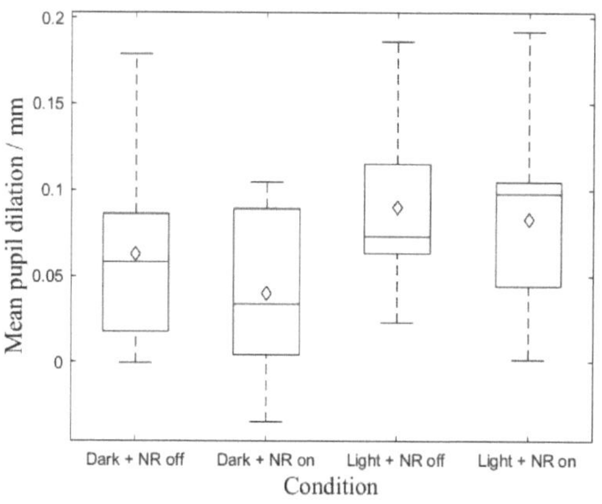

Figure 4: Boxplot showing MPD values for two conditions in darkness with NR off and on and two conditions with light on and NR off and on. Means are plotted as diamonds.

4 Discussion

This study investigated whether there is an interaction between NR and luminance caused by stronger difference between NR on and off in darkness compared to light. For that the results of the speech intelligibility and pupil diameter (MPD) are discussed. The ANOVA showed that speech intelligibility improved significantly for each subject with NR on compared to off in both light and dark conditions. Based on this, it should be expected that NR also reduces listening effort. However, MPD as an ocular biomarker of listening effort was not significantly different with NR on and off. It was expected that the difference of NR on and off in darkness is greater than the difference of NR on and off in the light condition, since SNS activity is isolated in darkness and the influence of the PNS activity on the pupil is not visible [3]. As shown in Fig. 2 there is almost no difference between the pupil dilation curves of NR on and off in the light condition. In darkness Fig. 2 shows that the pupil curve with NR on is always below the pupil curve with NR off. Although the result of the statistical analysis was not significant, there is a tendency of a smaller pupil response with NR on, which suggests higher PNS activity, compared to NR off, because higher PNS activity leads to a smaller pupil dilation. One reason why less listening effort is not evident in the MPD data may be that the study is underpowered. After cleaning the data, 5 out of 18 subjects' data were already discarded and thus only 13 subjects' data were included in the analysis. Another reason may be that the task itself was too difficult for some participants. When the SRT50 was determined, it was measured in light with NR off. Theoretically, the speech intelligibility in percent in Fig. 3 in the condition light + NR off should be distributed around 50 %. However, the box is relatively large, which indicates a scattering of the data. This means that some people in the condition understood less than 50 % of the words and others even more than 50 %. Literature has indicated that below 50 % intelligibility performance there is a risk that participants start to disengage (or give up) which would also lead to a smaller pupil size [7], [8]. If the NR is then switched on and the task becomes easier, it can be expected that the pupil response will not change much in comparison. The pupil dilation is dependent on the SNR in the form of an inverted U-shape due to the give-up effect at about 50 % speech intelligibility and below. Due to this non-linear dependency, the SRT80 should be used instead of the SRT50 for further measurements.

5 Conclusion

This study showed significantly higher speech intelligibility with NR on and larger baseline-corrected pupil response in light than in dark conditions. Against previous expectations, it could not be significantly shown that NR leads to less listening effort. However, the results show a tendency for more SNS activity to be present in the dark with NR off, indicating a higher listening effort.

Acknowledgement

The study has been carried out at the Institute of Acoustics, University of Applied Sciences Lübeck and evaluated and supported by Oticon A/S and Eriksholm Research Centre in Denmark.

Author's Statement

The authors have no conflict of interest to disclose.

References

[1] F. H. Bess and B. W. Hornsby, "Commentary: Listening can be exhausting—fatigue in children and adults with hearing loss," *Ear and hearing*, vol. 35, no. 6, pp. 592–599, 2014.

[2] Y. Wang, G. Naylor, S. E. Kramer, A. A. Zekveld, D. Wendt, B. Ohlenforst, and T. Lunner, "Relations between self-reported daily-life fatigue, hearing status, and pupil dilation during a speech perception in noise task," *Ear and Hearing*, vol. 39, no. 3, pp. 573–581, 2018.

[3] Y. Wang, S. E. Kramer, D. Wendt, G. Naylor, T. Lunner, and A. A. Zekveld, "The pupil dilation response during speech perception in dark and light: The involvement of the parasympathetic nervous system in listening effort," *Trends in Hearing*, vol. 22, pp. 1–11, 2018.

[4] D. Wendt, R. K. Hietkamp, and T. Lunner, "Impact of noise and noise reduction on processing effort: A pupillometry study," *Ear and hearing*, vol. 38, no. 6, pp. 690–700, 2017.

[5] J. Joiko, A. Bohnert, S. Strieth, S. D. Soli, and T. Rader, "The german hearing in noise test," *International Journal of Audiology*, vol. 60, no. 11, pp. 927–933, 2021.

[6] J. Zaar, L. B. Simonsen, T. Behrens, T. Dau, and S. Laugesen, "Investigating the relationship between spectro-temporal modulation detection, aided speech perception, and directional noise reduction preference in hearing-impaired listeners," in *Proceedings of the International Symposium on Auditory and Audiological Research*, vol. 7, pp. 181–188, 2019.

[7] C. M. McMahon, I. Boisvert, P. De Lissa, L. Granger, R. Ibrahim, C. Y. Lo, K. Miles, and P. L. Graham, "Monitoring alpha oscillations and pupil dilation across a performance-intensity function," *Frontiers in Psychology*, vol. 7, pp. 745–757, 2016.

[8] B. Ohlenforst, A. A. Zekveld, T. Lunner, D. Wendt, G. Naylor, Y. Wang, N. J. Versfeld, and S. E. Kramer, "Impact of stimulus-related factors and hearing impairment on listening effort as indicated by pupil dilation," *Hearing Research*, vol. 351, pp. 68–79, 2017.

Evaluating different EEG systems for auditory attention decoding

Pedro Andres Alba Diaz [1], René Pallenberg [2], and Alfred Mertins [3]

[1] Biomedical Engineering, Universität zu Lübeck, pedro.albadiaz@student.uni-luebeck.de
[2] Institute for Signal Processing, Universität zu Lübeck, r.pallenberg@uni-luebeck.de
[3] Institute for Signal Processing, Universität zu Lübeck, alfred.mertins@uni-luebeck.de

Abstract

Human listeners are capable of filtering out individual speakers in a scenario with multiple simultaneously active speakers, described as the "cocktail party problem". Hearing impaired listeners, however, have enormous difficulties in such situations. A possible solution is to use blind source separation algorithms to obtain the individual speech signals and present only one to the listener. However, the problem remains to only present the audio source to which the listener wants to attend to. Such information can be obtained from simultaneously recorded EEG signals. For this purpose, it is necessary to evaluate different EEG signal acquisition setups and to investigate their potential application as input data for auditory attention decoders. The present study evaluates three EEG systems (CGX Quick 32-r, semidry cap and cEGGrid), as well as the implementation of a convolutional neural network to extract auditory attention from neural activity.

1 Introduction

The human auditory system has the ability to focus on one main speaker and ignore other sound sources in multi-talker listening environments. This is called the "cocktail party effect" [1]. However, hearing aid users face great difficulties understanding speech in this scenario. Successful communication can only be achieved in such situations if the listener is aware of the interlocutor and directs his/her attention towards him/her [2]. As a solution, blind source separation algorithms can be used to segregate individual speech signals and expose only the desired one to the listener [3]. To do this, hearing aids would be required to know which speaker the listener wants to focus on, thus constituting an additional obstacle. Nevertheless, auditory attention detection (ADD) can be obtained from neural activity, which can be recorded by electroencephalography (EEG), magnetoencephalography (MEG) or electrocorticography (ECoG), as recent studies have shown [4]. Overall, the approach for ADD is based on reconstructing and decoding the envelope of attended stimuli through EEG signals and correlating them linearly to auditory stimuli [4]. However, this method requires 30 seconds or longer observation periods to decode the information reliably, making it impractical for real applications. Additionally, research has revealed a nonlinear relation between cortical responses and auditory stimuli [5]. In order to address challenges encountered in the aforementioned approach, machine learning techniques can be used to increase accuracy over short observation periods and deal with the nonlinear nature of the auditory system. Convolutional neural networks (CNNs) for EEG-based ADD have been shown to decode the locus of attention within short time decision windows with high accuracy [6], [7].

Most studies focus on ADD from EEG signals, since EEG-based systems provide noninvasive and high-temporal resolution means of recording cortical activity. Classical EEG cap acquisition for ADD has the disadvantage of being impractical for measurements outside the laboratory as it can interfere with the behaviour of the participants due to its poor comfort and numerous electrodes [8]. Ear-centred EEG systems, such as the c-shaped multi-electrode array (cEEGrid), offer a reliable alternative for obtaining EEG signals with greater comfort and mobility [9]. The purpose of this study is to investigate CNNs' potential applications for EEG-based AAD and to try an ear-centred, a semidry/saline-based cap, and a dry headset EEG acquisition setups.

2 Material and Methods

2.1 Participants

One male, middle-aged individual participated in the study with self-reported normal hearing. The participant signed written informed consent before the experiment was conducted.

2.2 Experimental setup

The EEG datasets were recorded using a high-density dry EEG system, *CGX Quick-32r* with 32 electrodes and a *Smarting mobi* amplifier with a semidry/saline-based EEG cap containing 23 channels and a c-shaped multi-electrode array of 18 electrodes, *cEEGrid*, at a sampling rate of 500 Hz as shown in Fig. 1 (a). Electrode impedance of all EEG

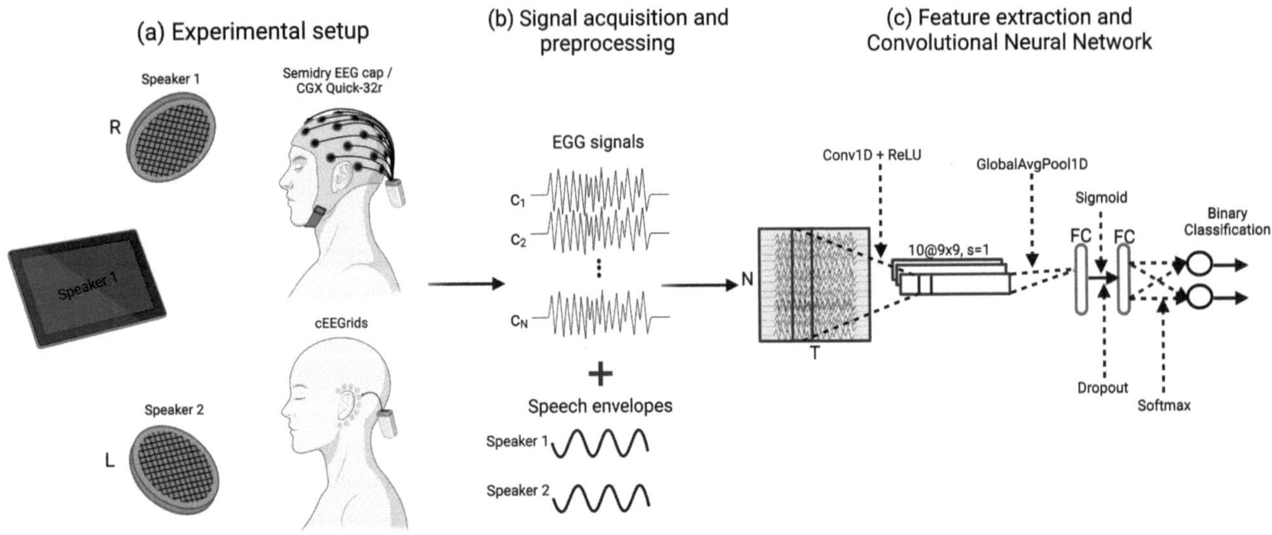

Figure 1: Schematic diagram of the data acquisition and CNN classifier: (a) sound stimuli are presented to the subject and the EEG signal is recorded with different systems; (b) multichannel EEG signals and audio envelopes are prepocessed, down-sampled and standardised; (c) CNN classifier is trained to detect an attended speaker in a dual-speaker scenario from EEG signals and speech envelopes. FC = fully connected, s = stride, N = number of channels, T = number of samples, ReLU = rectifying linear unit, GlobalAvgPool1D = 1D global average pooling, and Conv1D = 1D convolution. Created with BioRender.com.

systems was minimised, as suggested by the manufacturers. The stimuli consisted of two audio books narrated by a female and a male narrator in German, presented to the test subject at 46.5 dB. The loudspeakers were positioned at 90 degrees at 50 centimetres distance from the subject as presented in Fig. 2.

Table 1: Protocol used for presenting auditory stimuli.

Trial	Left stimulus	Right stimulus	Attended ear
1	Female (track 0)	Male (track 0)	Left
2	Male (track 1)	Female (track 1)	Right
3	Male (track 2)	Female (track 2)	Right
4	Female (track 3)	Male (track 3)	Left
5	Female (track 4)	Male (track 4)	Left
6	Male (track 5)	Female (track 5)	Right
7	Female (track 6)	Male (track 6)	Left
8	Female (track 0)	Male (track 0)	Right
9	Male (track 1)	Female (track 1)	Left
10	Male (track 2)	Female (track 2)	Left
11	Female (track 3)	Male (track 3)	Right
12	Female (track 4)	Male (track 4)	Right
13	Male (track 5)	Female (track 5)	Left
14	Female (track 6)	Male (track 6)	Right

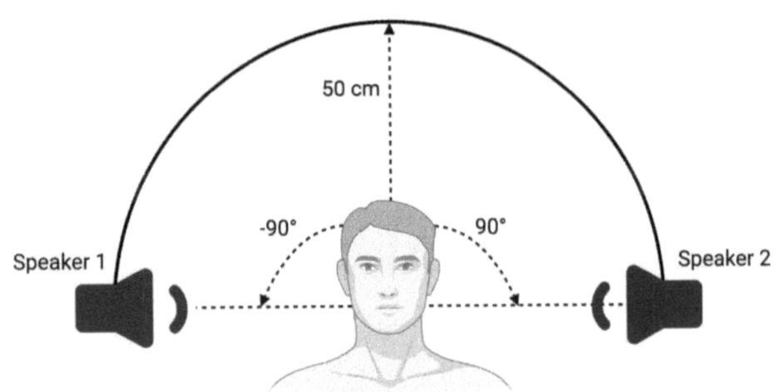

Figure 2: Speakers placement for sound stimuli presentation. Created with BioRender.com

The stimuli presentation was controlled using Psychopy for Python. At the start of the trial, a screen indicated which speaker the subject should attend to by displaying his or her gender. Both stories were of the same loudness and had a duration of 14 minutes, consisting of 14 trials of 1 minute each. To avoid lateralisation, the stimuli were alternated to get an even amount of data per side, as shown in Table 1.

2.3 Data Preprocessing

The EEG datasets were filtered with a Chebyshev bandpass filter of order 2, allowing signals between 1 and 50 Hz to flow. After bandpass filtering, the EEG datasets were downsampled to 128 Hz and standardised. Furthermore, the audio datasets were similarly treated (filtered, downsampled and standardised) to match the EEG data, adding an initial step to extract the speech envelope by a Hilbert transform and computing the absolute value. The preprocessing was chosen based on previous non-linear AAD studies [3]. Afterwards, this data was used to be randomly divided into training (80%) and test (20%) set as shown in Fig. 1 (b). For training, the data was divided into decision windows of 1 second with 0.5 seconds of overlap.

2.4 Convolutional neural network

The proposed CNN presented in Fig. 1 (c) was implemented with TensorFlow. The input was an N by T matrix, where N corresponds to the number of EEG channels plus two audio channels, which differed depending on the acquisition system (CGX Quick-32r $N = 34$, semidry cap $N = 25$, and cEEGrid $N = 20$). T stands for the number of samples in the decision window ($T = 128$). The model started with a convolutional layer. A rectifying linear unit (ReLU) activation function was implemented after ten separate filters of size 9 x 9 and stride, $s = 1$, were applied. Then to reduce the dimensionality, the average of each channel was obtained with an average pool layer. After the pooling step, a 10-neuron fully connected (FC) layer, followed by a sigmoid activation function was used. Lastly, a 2-output-neuron FC layer was connected to a categorical cross-entropy loss function. The CNN consisted of up to 3,202 trainable parameters. The training set was shuffled and partitioned into mini-batches of 120 samples. Adam was used as an optimisation algorithm with a learning rate of $\alpha = 0.001$. The dataset was trained for 100 epochs. To avoid overfitting, dropout regularisation with a probability of 0.5 was used right after the first fully connected layer. All hyperparameters aforementioned were based on the studies done by [6], [7] and [10].

3　Results and Discussion

For the employed model, the speech envelopes were used as input together with the EEG data to contribute to the decision making of the CNN decoder. A decision window length of 1 second was tested with broadband EEG data, as one of the objectives of this study was to make use of a non-linear decoder that required short observation periods for auditory attention decoding. To judge the performance of the model, the *Keras* accuracy class was employed to calculate how often predictions were equal to the labels. Table 2 and Fig. 3 present the accuracies and the value of the loss function obtained with the three EEG acquisition systems. The CNN performed well with all three EEG setups. The best AAD performance was obtained with the CGX Quick-32r input data having a loss value of 0.29 and an accuracy of 92% on the test set, followed by the cEEGrid with a loss value of 0.44 and an accuracy of 80%. The data registered by the semidry EEG device had the poorest performance, getting a loss value of 0.39 and accuracy of 79% on the test set. Electrode impedance in the Smarting mobi amplifier-operated EEG systems was measured prior to testing. Values below $20k\Omega$ and above $10k\Omega$ were obtained for the semi-dry EEG cap and below $7k\Omega$ with the cEEGrid. Since the CGX Quick-32r system allows impedance measurement during the experiments, a mean impedance of $2.05k\Omega$ was recorded.

The lower decoding accuracy of the semidry EEG system can be explained by the fact that at recording time, the cap was not perfectly fitted to the test subject.

Table 2: Loss and metrics values for the CNN models.

EEG system	Loss value	Decoding accuracy (%)
CGX Quick-32r	0.29	92.26
Semidry cap	0.39	79.17
cEEGrid	0.44	80.36

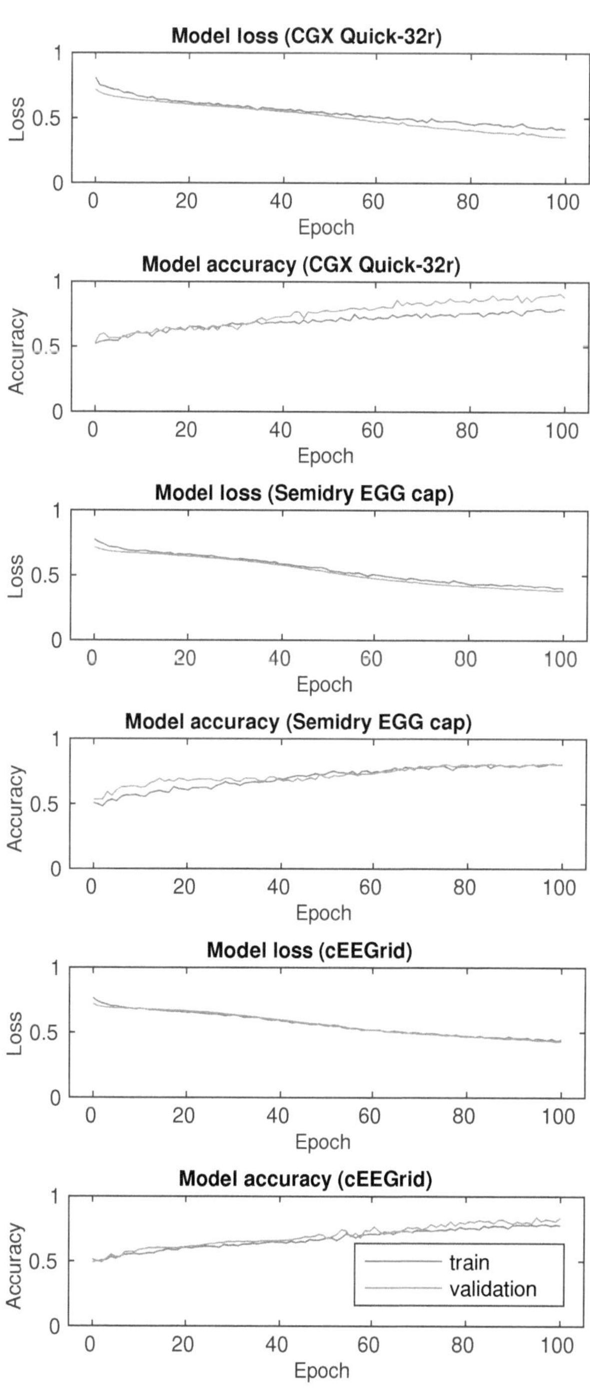

Figure 3: Evolution of accuracy and loss over the epochs in the three EEG acquisition systems evaluated.

Accuracy was used as a metric to assess model performance. AAD using the CGX Quick-32r and cEEGrid systems compared to the semidry EEG cap, validation accuracy outperformed training accuracy. One of the reasons for this was the use of dropout as a method of regulation during training, simplifying the performance of the model. The training ran for 100 epochs, as the model did not benefit from further learning. In Fig. 3, the loss plot shows that the validation error started to flatten out and approach the training error, indicating that the model generalises correctly.

4 Conclusion

Broadband EEG was recorded using three acquisition systems to decode auditory attention. Two speakers were presented simultaneously in a test to record neural activity. With the information obtained, auditory attention was extracted with a CNN. The CNN employed showed considerable success in AAD tasks within a short decision window (1 second), exhibiting potential applications for noise suppression in neuro-steered hearing aids. It was found that, for auditory attention monitoring, all three systems evaluated provide meaningful data for auditory attention detection. The high density dry EEG system (CGX Quick-32r) provided the highest accuracy of the three systems, obtaining 92%. However, this cannot be generalised further as it was implemented on only one subject. Yet, the findings open up the possibility for ongoing experimentation. As future work, testing with more participants and different loudspeaker arrangements can bring potential to improve real-time auditory attention decoding, including noisy backgrounds that resemble out-of-the-lab environments.

Acknowledgement

The work has been carried out and supervised by the Institute for Signal Processing, Universität zu Lübeck.

Author's Statement

Conflict of interest: Authors state no conflict of interest. Informed consent: Informed consent has been obtained from all individuals included in this study.

5 References

[1] E. C. Cherry, *Some Experiments on the Recognition of Speech, with One and with Two Ears*. The Journal of the Acoustical Society of America, vol. 25, no. 5, pp. 975–979, 1953.

[2] N. Marrone, C. R. Mason, and G. Kidd, *Evaluating the Benefit of Hearing Aids in Solving the Cocktail Party Problem*. Trends in Amplification, vol. 12, no. 4, pp. 300–315, 2008.

[3] E. Su, S. Cai, L. Xie, H. Li, and T. Schultz, *STAnet: A Spatiotemporal Attention Network for Decoding Auditory Spatial Attention From EEG*. IEEE Trans. Biomed. Eng., vol. 69, no. 7, pp. 2233–2242, 2022.

[4] J. A. O'Sullivan et al., *Attentional Selection in a Cocktail Party Environment Can Be Decoded from Single-Trial EEG*. Cerebral Cortex, vol. 25, no. 7, pp. 1697–1706, 2015.

[5] M. Keshishian, H. Akbari, B. Khalighinejad, J. L. Herrero, A. D. Mehta, and N. Mesgarani, *Estimating and interpreting nonlinear receptive field of sensory neural responses with deep neural network models*. eLife, vol. 9, p. e53445, 2020.

[6] S. Vandecappelle, L. Deckers, N. Das, A. H. Ansari, A. Bertrand, and T. Francart, *EEG-based detection of the locus of auditory attention with convolutional neural networks*. eLife, vol. 10, p. e56481, 2021.

[7] S. Cai, E. Su, L. Xie, and H. Li, *EEG-Based Auditory Attention Detection via Frequency and Channel Neural Attention*. IEEE Trans. Human-Mach. Syst., vol. 52, no. 2, pp. 256–266, 2022.

[8] M. G. Bleichner, B. Mirkovic, and S. Debener, *Identifying auditory attention with ear-EEG: cEEGrid versus high-density cap-EEG comparison*. J. Neural Eng., vol. 13, no. 6, p. 066004, 2016.

[9] S. Debener, R. Emkes, M. De Vos, and M. Bleichner, *Unobtrusive ambulatory EEG using a smartphone and flexible printed electrodes around the ear*. Sci Rep, vol. 5, no. 1, p. 16743, 2015.

[10] I. Goodfellow, Y. Bengio, and A. Courville, *Deep learning*. Cambridge, Massachusetts: The MIT Press, 2016.

Data-driven analysis of harbour porpoise echolocation clicks

Theresa Hartmann [1], Silke Anders [2] and Jürgen Tchorz [3]

[1] Auditory Technology, Universität zu Lübeck, theresa.hartmann@student.uni-luebeck.de

[2] Social and Affective Neuroscience, Department of Neurology and Center of Brain, Behavior and Metabolism (CBBM), Universität zu Lübeck, silke.anders@neuro.uni-luebeck.de

[3] Institute of Acoustics, Luebeck University of Applied Sciences, juergen.tchorz@th-luebeck.de

Abstract

Harbour porpoises use echolocation clicks with a centre frequency around 130 kHz for orientation and communication. To reduce harbour porpoise bycatch in fishing nets, Porpoise Alarms (PALs) are used. Recorded harbour porpoise sounds from the Baltic Sea thus contain not only the desired harbour porpoise clicks but also those of the PALs and noise. The aim of this work was the detection of harbour porpoise and PAL clicks in noise and their discrimination. This was realized by neural networks with supervised learning. For this purpose, recorded clicks were first analysed using descriptive statistics. Afterwards, the clicks were manually labelled. Next, a neural network was implemented and parameters are adjusted for optimal classification behaviour. Currently, the adjustment of parameters and the final results is under way. Preliminary results suggest an accuracy of the neural network of around 87 % based on 1399 labelled samples.

1 Introduction

Harbour porpoises use echolocation clicks for orientation, hunting and communication. For this, they use sequences of high-frequency clicks, which are called click trains [1]. The main parameters of click trains are frequency, length of the clicks and time lag between single clicks, called Inter-Click-Interval (ICI). Echolocation clicks are used for different reasons, for instance feeding behaviour, which includes hunting, approach behaviour and communication with each other, which also influence the click train parameters [2].

Since harbour porpoises are often victims of fishing because they get entangled in the nets, so-called Porpoise Alarms (PALs) (F^3 Maritime Technology) are attached to the nets. According to manufacturer information, these imitate the frequency of the warning sounds of the animals. The PAL transmitters reduce bycatch in the Baltic Sea by up to 80 % [3]. To study the distribution of harbour porpoises in the Baltic Sea, porpoise detectors (PODs), in this case F-PODs (Chelonia Limited), are used. They are recording the click trains of the harbour porpoises, but also the very similar PAL signals and noise from other whale and dolphin species and passing ships for instance.

The harbour porpoise click trains cannot be detected directly due to the noise. Therefore the recordings from the Baltic Sea have to be preprocessed first. This preprocessing was done by the software of the F-POD manufacturer [4]. However, the analysis is not designed for the detection of PAL signals. Previous studies focussed on the detection of click trains with the help of neural networks. One example is the work of [5], which focuses on detecting harbour porpoise click trains using a neural long-short term memory (LSTM) neural network. The data used in his work originate from the Baltic Sea and he reached a sensitivity of 60 %. His work is not intended for the detection of PAL signals. The aim of this work was to develope an automatic classification of harbour porpoise and PAL click trains by using a neural network with supervised learning.

2 Material and Methods

2.1 Harbour porpoise click trains

Harbour porpoises emit high frequency clicks, which are very narrow-banded. The frequencies of the clicks are mainly around 130 kHz with peaks between 110 to 160 kHz. Thus, harbour porpoise clicks are Narrow Band High Frequency (NHBF) clicks. A single click typically has a length of about 75 μs to 150 μs. Assuming a frequency of 130 kHz, this corresponds to about 10 to 20 cycles-per-click. The level of the clicks ranges from 175 dB to 205 dB re 1 μPa pp (peak-to-peak) @ 1 m. The average ICI is about 60 ms but ICIs can range from less than 10 ms to 120 ms [2].

2.2 Porpoise Alarm

PALs emit clicks similar to harbour porpoise warning calls. The centre frequency of the clicks is around 133 kHz. The maximum level is 145 dB re 1 μPa pp @ 1 m. Click trains emitted by PALs have a fixed length of one second. Randomly between one to three of these click trains are emitted and then repeated at a random rate between 8 to 24 seconds.

PAL click trains range from about 200 to about 1400 clicks per second [3].

2.3 Data

The data were recorded in the Baltic Sea at the coast of Fyns Hoved in Denmark with F-PODs designed to record cetacean sounds. F-PODs record continuously and detect clicks from a frequency of 17 kHz. The FP1 files created by the F-POD were loaded into the software FPOD.exe provided by the manufacturer. The software displays all clicks in different parameters over time. A detection of the click trains with the software is possible via the KERNO-F classifier. A total of 17 F-PODs were used. The approximate arrangement can be taken from the map (Fig. 1). The F-PODs were arranged symmetrically around the gillnet, to which PALs were attached. There are 26 files available, which were recorded in the period from July 20, 2022 to September 08, 2022. On average, the files have a duration of 51d 9h 26m (min. 12d 13h 9m; max. 80d 58m) and contain 171,146,784 clicks (min. 4,878,122 clicks; max. 1,700,998,805 clicks). In total, 4,449,816,388 clicks are available from the 26 files.

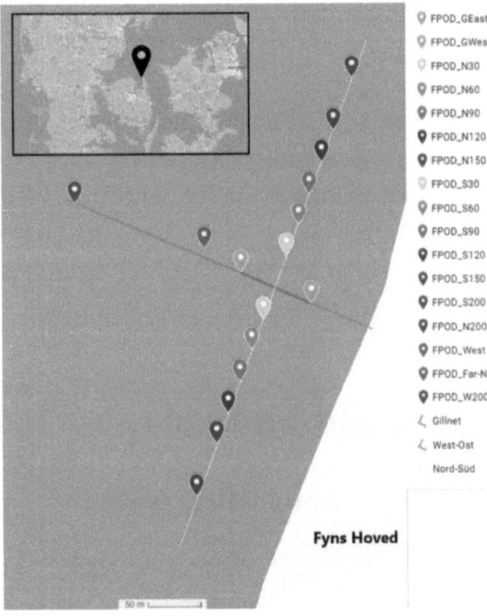

Figure 1: Set-up for watch out for porpoises in Fyns Hoved [6]

Raw data were exported with software provided by the manufacturer [4]. In the exported files each click is described with 24 parameters (primarily in the areas of peak, inter-peak intervals, frequency, bandwidth, cycles) and the time stamp.

2.4 Descriptive analysis

The ICI to the previous click was calculated first, which was not included in the recorded data, but is a crucial parameter for the identification of click trains. For visual inspection, the distribution of each parameter was plotted in a histogram. Additionally, to visualize possible correlations between parameters, selected pairs of parameters were plotted in 3d histograms.

To label the data, the files were windowed into blocks of consecutive 50 clicks. This was realised by an individual graphical user interface (GUI) implemented in Python. In each case, 50 clicks are plotted with centre frequency and ICI over time. This served to identify whether the section contains part of a PAL signal (Label 2), a harbour porpoise click train (Label 1), or noise only (Label 0). The respective label can be selected via three buttons below the plots. Arrow buttons can be used to swipe through the blocks. The data were hand labelled. In total, 1399 samples were labelled ($n_{\text{Label0}} = 768$, $n_{\text{Label1}} = 115$, $n_{\text{Label2}} = 517$).

The 25 parameters (24 exported by the software and the calculated ICI) and the time stamp of each of the 50 clicks within an block were written into a row of the matrix X. The label is written into the corresponding row of the vector y. Subsequently, the dataset was separated into training and test data using the Python function *sklearn.model_selection.train_test_split*. In both datasets, the distribution of the three classes was approximately the same. The training dataset contains 70 % of the labelled samples ($n = 979$, $n_{Label0} = 529$, $n_{Label1} = 82$, $n_{Label2} = 368$), the test data the remaining 30 % ($n = 420$, $n_{Label0} = 238$, $n_{Label1} = 33$, $n_{Label2} = 149$). After that, the datasets were z-standardized ($m_{traindata} = m_{testdata} = 0$; $sd_{traindata} = sd_{testdata} = 0.91$). Afterwards the neural network was trained and validated.

2.5 Neural network analysis

The chosen neural network was a Multi-Layer-Perceptron (MLP). The input layer receives the signal. The output layer makes a decision or prediction based on the input data processed by the MLP. Between the input and the output layer are several hidden layers to process the data. MLPs learn to model the correlations between these inputs and outputs by training on a set of given input-output pairs. During training, the parameters of the model are adjusted to minimize the error [7].

The MLP was implemented in Python by using the library *sklearn.neural_networks*. The default parameter values were used. One hidden layer with 100 units and the function *tanh* was used as activation function for the hidden layer. The chosen solver for weight optimization is *adam*. A constant learning rate with an initialisation of 0.001 was used and the alpha value was 0.0001. The MLP was trained with the train data, shown in subsection 2.4, consisting of 979 samples from three classes.

3 Results and Discussion

Centre frequency, the length of clicks expressed in cycles-per-click, and ICIs are important parameters in the description of click trains. Therefore, the distributions of this parameters over all clicks and over the datasets of the different classes were plotted in histograms.

The distribution of centre frequency over all data shows a high peak around 125 kHz and a lower peak at around 20 kHz. A similar distribution can be seen with Label 1 clicks, while pure noise clicks show a significantly higher peak at 20 kHz. Label 2 clicks are almost exclusively at a centre frequency around 125 kHz (Fig. 2). The peak around 125 kHz corresponds to the centre frequency of both, harbour porpoise clicks and clicks produced by the PALs. An explanation for the much sharper distribution of PAL clicks might be the higher click rate. Accordingly, the 50 clicks of a block contain less noise than the porpoise click trains.

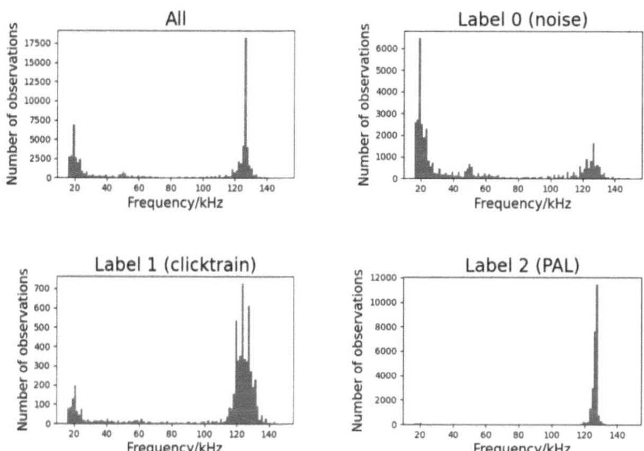

Figure 2: Distribution of centre frequency for all clicks and each label; peaks at around 20 kHz and around 125 kHz.

Some of the harbour porpoise like clicks might be echoes or clicks emitted by echosounders of vessels, which produce clicks with similar acoustic characteristics. The second peak around 20 kHz might reflect passing ships, as well as sounds from the seafloor and sea surface.

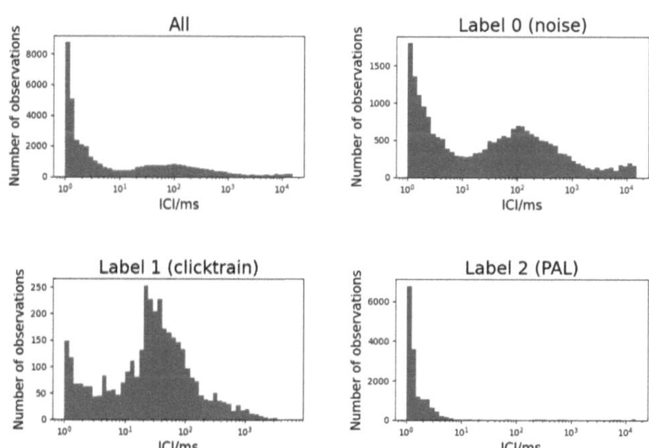

Figure 3: Distribution of inter-click-intervals in ms with logarithmic scale for all clicks and each label; peaks at ICIs under 10 ms and around 100 ms.

In addition to centre frequency, ICIs might also provide important information about whether a recorded click is from a harbour porpoise or not. Typical ICIs of harbour porpoise click trains range from less than 10 ms to 150 ms. The distribution of ICIs across all clicks shows a peak below 10 ms.

Label 0 clicks also show a peak at around 100 ms. On the other hand, clicks with Label 1 show a broad distribution of ICIs with a peak at 20 to 30 ms. Clicks from blocks with PAL signals have a much smaller distribution below 10 ms (Fig. 3). The distribution of ICIs over all clicks shows a peak in ICI that is typical of harbour porpoises, but shows a similarity to the distribution of noise clicks. However, data also include echoes from the sea surface or sea floor, as well as other clutter clicks. For this reason, the amount of harbour porpoise clicks cannot be precisely identified.

The number of cycles per click gives an indication of the length of the click. The clicks of harbour porpoises and PALs usually consist of five to 15 cycles. The distribution of cycles-per-click over all clicks clearly shows that most of the recorded clicks have up to about 20 cycles, Label 0 and Label 1 clicks show a similar distribution. Label 2 clicks show a distribution of cycles-per-click around a peak of about 10 cycles (Fig. 4). Since the distributions of noise and harbour porpoise click trains show a very similar distribution, it is questionable whether the parameter cycles-per-click contributes to the detection of porpoise click trains.

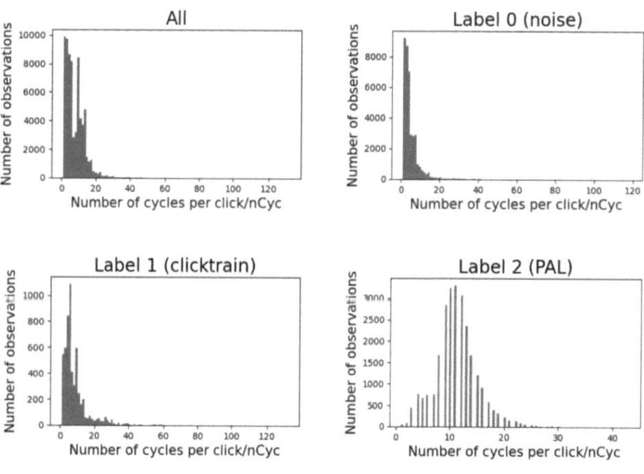

Figure 4: Distribution of the length of the recorded clicks in cycles-per-click for all clicks and each label; number of cycles-per-click mainly under 20.

At the time of the report the accuracy of the neural network was 87.38 %, which means that 367 of the 420 samples in the test data set were correctly recognised. Thus, the accuracy is well above the guess probability of 1/3 for a 3-class problem.

Table 1: Confusion matrix of train data of MLP with three classes (Noise; Harbour Porpoise (HP); PAL).

actual \ pred.	Noise	HP	PAL
Noise	213	9	16
HP	19	12	2
PAL	7	0	142

Table 1 shows the confusion matrix, the rows are the actual labels, the columns are the predicted labels. While the samples of noise and PAL were mostly recognised, harbour porpoise samples were classified as noise several times. A reason for this could be the small number of samples compared to the noise and PAL class. The noise clicks presented in the harbour porpoise samples could also be a reason for this. Positively, no PAL sample was classified as harbour porpoise, which indicates a good distinction between the two classes. Table 2 shows the sensitivity and specificity for all three classes. While the specificity for all three classes is very high, the sensitivity is much more scattered. The sensitivity for the class with harbour porpoise click trains is 36.36 % and thus very close to the guess probability.

Table 2: Specificity and sensitivity of train data of MLP with three classes (Noise; Harbour Porpoise (HP); PAL).

	specificity	sensitivity
Noise	0,8555	0,8875
HP	0,9753	0,3636
PAL	0,9259	0,9530

Limitations are the relatively few labels for the class with harbour porpoise click trains. These do not occur in the data that often and for the identification of some harbour porpoise click trains the software provided by the manufacturer of the F-PODs was used. Also, due to the much shorter click trains, there is more noise in the click blocks of habour porpoise click trains.

Further steps for the project are relabelling and possible labelling by other people (from the German Oceanographic Museum Stralsund) to check the correctness of the labels. For parameter optimisation a gridsearch can be used to improve the accuracy of the MLP. Another step would be to adjust the training data and continue to label more samples so that there is an equal number of samples from each label.

4　Conclusion

The aim of the project was to evaluate a neural network with random sequences of clicks in order to distinguish click sequences of harbour porpoises or PALs. A long-term goal was to develop a classifier that reliably detects harbour porpoise and PAL click sequences in recordings of F-PODs. Based on the distributions of frequencies, ICIs and cycles per click in the data, a presence of harbour porpoises could be assumed. Thus, the data provide a good base for the implementation of the neural network. With the help of the GUI, the data can be labelled. For the implementation of the neural network in this project, an MLP was used. At the time of the report, the number of samples was 1399 and the accuracy of the neural network was 87.38 %. The sensitivity for the harbour porpoise class was 36.36 %, the PAL and noise classes had a much higher sensitivity. The next goals of the work are to obtain a larger data set and to adjust the parameters of the MLP to further improve the accuracy of the MLP and sensitivity of the harbour porpoise class.

Acknowledgement

This work has been carried out and supervised as part of a cooperation of the Institute of Acoustics, Luebeck University of Applied Sciences and the Social and Affective Neuroscience Lab, Center of Brain, Behavior and Metabolism (CBBM), Universität zu Lübeck. I would like to thank my supervisors Jürgen Tchorz and Silke Anders and also Michael Dähne, Ole Meyer-Klaeden and Anja Gallus, Stiftung Deutsches Meeresmuseum Stralsund, for their expertise and for kindly providing the acoustic data.

Author's Statement

Conflict of interest: Authors state no conflict of interest.

5　References

[1] German Oceanographic Museum Stralsund, *Schweins-wale (Phocoenidae)*. https://www.deutsches-meeresmuseum.de/wissenschaft/infothek/artensteckbriefe/schweinswale, [last accessed on 2023-01-05].

[2] Sven Koschinski, Ansgar Diederichs, Mats Amundin, *Click train patterns of free-ranging harbour porpoises acquired using T-PODs may be useful as indicators of their behaviour*. J. Cetacean res. manage, 2008.

[3] Jèrôme Chladek, Boris Culik, Lotte Kindt-Larsen, Christoffer Moesgaard Albertsen, Christian von Dorrien, *Synthetic harbour porpoise (Phocoena phocoena) communication signals emitted by acoustic alerting device (Porpoise ALert, PAL) significantlyreduce their bycatch in western Baltic gillnet fisheries*. Fisheries Research 232 (2020) 105732, doi: 10.1016/j.fishres.2020.105732.

[4] Chelonia Limited Wildlife Acoustic Monitoring, *F-POD*. https://www.chelonia.co.uk/fpod_home_page.htm, [last accessed on 2023-01-05].

[5] Filip Ärlemalm, *Harbour Porpoise Click Train Classification with LSTM Recurrent Neural Networks*. KTH Royal Institute of Technology School of Electrical Engineering, Degree project in electrical engineering, 2017.

[6] Project of German Oceanographic Museum Stralsund (PAL-CE: Pal-Nutzung in deutschen Gewässern), *Set-up Fyns Hoved*. communication with Dipl. Biol. Ole Meyer-Klaeden, map using Google Maps.

[7] C. C. Aggarwal, *Neural Networks and Deep Learning*. Springer International Publishing, Sep. 2018, isbn: 3319944622.

Immediate and Longitudinal Benefit of Unilateral Cochlear Implantation on Spatial Listening

Hannah Meineke [1], Jonas Obleser [2], Malte Wöstmann [2]

[1] Hearing Technology, Universität zu Lübeck, hannah.meineke@student.uni-luebeck.de
[2] Department of Psychology, Universität zu Lübeck, {jonas.obleser, malte.woestmann}@uni-luebeck.de

Abstract

The goal of this study was to evaluate, whether the adaptation to hearing with a Cochlear Implant (CI) is beneficial in spatial listening tasks or can also impede spatial attention. A spatial listening task was conducted with unilaterally implanted CI users with normal or aided contralateral hearing in the first and the seventh month after implantation. Speech reception thresholds (SRTs) were obtained for four different spatial attention conditions. Additionally clinical speech understanding scores and subjective assessment of the CI users' hearing through the Speech, Spatial and Quality of Hearing Questionnaire were collected. The immediate and longitudinal benefit of using the CI was evaluated. A statistically significant immediate CI benefit was confirmed as well as an improvement over time. A detrimental effect of attending to speech on the CI side for the measurement conducted in the seventh month after implantation seems to be supported by the currently available data, but needs confirmation.

1 Introduction

Hearing loss is a widespread health problem which can have debilitating impact on the quality of life for those affected. Especially severe to profound hearing loss can complicate the separation of different sound sources and therefore the differentiation of noise and relevant sounds. This particularly applies if one ear is strongly affected e.g. by single sided deafness or asymetric hearing loss [1]. Profound hearing loss and deafness can be in most cases treated with a Cochlear Implant (CI). But this electrical hearing is degraded in comparison with the acoustic hearing of normal hearing (NH) individuals [2].

Even CI users who perform very well with speech understanding in quiet often have problems with hearing in noisy situations and with multiple talkers (cocktail party scenario). In classical clinical audiological testing, such situations are represented by adding a competing noise to the speech signal which makes up the target sound. This may give information about the patients speech understanding or speech reception threshold (SRT) in stationary noise but fails to represent the more complex situation of a distractor being competing speech or fluctuating noise. But especially those situations are occurring regularly in daily life and can lead to dissatisfaction with the CI.

To enhance relevant sounds and filter out sounds that are not relevant, that is noise or distractor speech, selective attention is needed. A recent study of Kraus et. al (2021) suggests, that there is a neural cost caused by the degraded CI signal [2]. This leads to a delayed differential neural phase-locking to the envelopes of target versus distractor speech.

Whether an adaptation to the degraded signal occurs during adaptation to listening with a CI following activation is not well established. Here, a behavioural experiment with competing talkers from different directions was conducted to investigate the benefit of having one CI to add to the acoustical hearing on the contralateral ear. Additionally the experiment was conducted two times with a time gap of six month to examine longitudinal effects of acclimatization to hearing with a CI.

2 Material and Methods

2.1 Participants

18 native German speakers (age range: 23 to 82 years, *mean age*=61.3 years) unilaterally fitted with a cochlear implant at the *University Hospital Schleswig-Holstein, Campus Lübeck, Germany*, took part in the study. Data of one participant were excluded from this analysis due to implausibly increasing results, which made a reasonable threshold determination impossible.

2.2 Measurement Procedure

Participants completed the same battery of tests once in the first month after activation of the cochlear implant (T1) and once in the seventh month after activation (T2). They all completed the measurements for T1 and nine of the participants have completed T2 at this point in time.
Audiological data in form of pure tone audiogram and speech understanding (German monosyllabic speech test

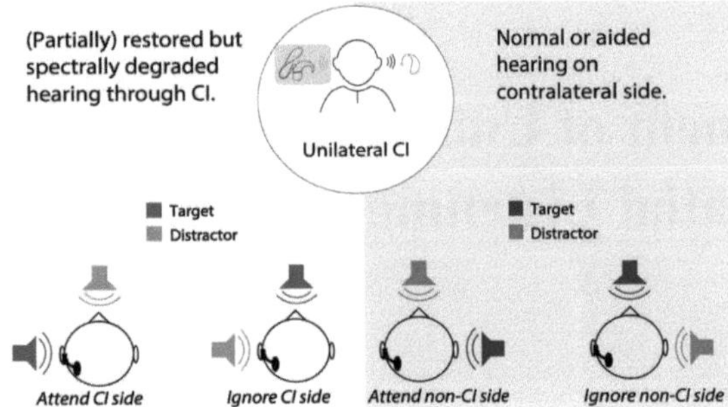

Figure 1: Participants of the study were fitted with a Cochlea Implant (CI) on one side and, if indicated, with a contralateral hearing aid (HA). Spatial listening conditions with target and distractor in front and $\pm 90°$ lateral. Adapted from Wöstmann et al. (2022), Presentation at AuditoryCortex Conference.

"Freiburger Einsilbertest", FE) was provided by the Audiology Department of the *University Hospital Schleswig-Holstein*. The data used were collected in each case prior to implantation, around T1 and T2.

All participants had a pure tone average (PTA; pure tone hearing threshold at 500 Hz, 1, 2 and 4 kHz) hearing loss of at least 60 dB HL (*mean HL*: 89.9 dB HL, *SD*: 15.9 dB HL) in the implanted ear prior to implantation. Hearing loss in the contralateral ear varied from 10 to 93.8 dB HL (*mean HL*: 46.6 dB HL, *SD*: 26.5 dB HL). Participants who were fitted with a hearing aid (HA) in everyday life wore this during measurement (bimodal fitting). The settings of the CI and HA were not changed and therefore correspond to the settings the participants use in every day life.

Participants filled out the short form of the Speech, Spatial and Quality of Hearing Questionnaire (SSQ, German version) at the beginning of each of the two sessions to assess their subjective hearing performance. The SSQ provides a score for the complete questionnaire and each of the three categories. The participants' assessment of their spatial hearing performance was especially interesting given the spatial listening task they performed.

The goal of the main experiment was to assess hearing thresholds for speech stimuli presented in different spatial configurations of target and distractor speech. The behavioral experiment was conducted in a hearing chamber. The participants were sitting in front of a screen which gave instructions during the task. Two loudspeakers at a distance of 0.7 m to the participants' head were used to present the stimuli from the front and lateral from $\pm 90°$, as shown in Fig. 1. The experiments were implemented and controlled via MatLab and PsychToolbox (MathWorks Inc.).

2.3   Stimuli

Spoken numbers from one to nine were presented in random order. Numbers were spoken by a female voice and presented at different sound levels depending on the hearing threshold of the individual participant.

2.4   Threshold Measurement

Before the main experiment, hearing thresholds for different locations (front, left, right) were assessed. The individual hearing threshold for each participant was determined by using a method of limits approach. This threshold was used to set the sound level for each participant and location (front, left, right) individually and for T1 and T2 independently.

2.5   Task Design

For the main task two loudspeakers were used to implement four listening conditions as shown in Fig. 1: One speaker was always located in the front and the other either on the left or right side. In each condition, the target was presented from one speaker position and the distractor from the other. Spoken digits were presented simultaneously (matched for perceptual onset as in [3]) from both loudspeakers participants were instructed to attended to the target and ignore the distractor.

Participants received a visual cue on the display in front of them as to which speech signal should be attended. After the simultaneous presentation of the two speech stimuli from both loudspeakers, participants responded which digit they understood from the target direction. The answer was given via a number pad.

The task adaptively determined the 50% SRT, measured in dB SNR, by adapting the sound level of the stimuli depending on the correctness of the previous answer given. The adaptation was implemented as a one-up-one-down design with 2 dB steps. The task was divided into six blocks, three with the second loudspeaker on the CI side and three on the non CI side. For each block, 25 repetitions of the stimuli per direction were presented leading to 75 repetitions per condition. This whole task was performed first with the *CI on* and thereafter without the CI (*CI off*).

2.6   Behavioral Data Analysis

The mean threshold used to determine the sound level for the main task presentation was calculated as the mean of the last two trials of each threshold determination. The SRT measurements were obtained by averaging over the last 50 trials in each condition. This was done for the measurements with *CI on* and *off* separately as well as for the two sessions.

Statistical analysis was performed using Matlab 2022a. All variables were z-scored beforehand. The development of the self assessment with the SSQ as well as the FE scores from T1 to T2 was analysed using a linear mixed model. To predict the SRT scores, a linear mixed model with restricted maximum likelihood estimation was used.

3 Results and Discussion

3.1 Improvement in Clinical Tests

SSQ scores improved in all three categories (speech, spatial and quality) as a function of duration of CI use. This can also be demonstrated statistically with a linear mixed model which controls for the factors *age, mean threshold* and *FE* (post implantation speech score). For the spatial part of the SSQ questionaire the β of session (T1/T2) is *1.0812* ($p=7.786e^{-17}$). Notably, this is the largest β, also significant are the following factors: mean threshold, FE, session×FE, session×mean threshold×FE. The clinical FE scores similarly improved as a function of duration of CI use, which can be statistically supported (*session*: $\beta=0.4587, p=1.8171e^{-16}$) when using a mixed linear model controlling for age and PTA. It should be noted that the *PTA* also shows a significant influence ($\beta=-0.443, p=6.9249e^{-7}$) as well as the interaction between *session* and *PTA* ($\beta=-0.2263, p=2.8625e^{-10}$). This means a positive impact from T1 to T2 and a negative influence on the speech understanding score stemming from a higher (worse) PTA of the CI ear.

3.2 CI Benefit on Spatial listening

The individual SRTs (T1) contrasted for *CI on* vs. *CI off* for each listening conditions are shown in Fig. 2. The benefit for attending the CI side and ignoring the non CI side seems more prominent. Whether the CI users also benefit from the use of the implant when trying to attend the non CI side or respectively ignore the CI side is not as distinct. There are large interindividual differences in general. This can be attributed to the very diverse group of participants. They have a number of different ethiologies and consequently different durations of (profound) hearing loss and other known contributing factors for CI outcome [4]. For this spatial task in particular the large variability of hearing loss in the contralateral ear, spanning from normal hearing to profound hearing loss, leads to variation in the degree of utilization of the CI to complete the given task successfully. In addition, the "better ear" can also change depending on the spatial setup and individual hearing loss [5].

Additionally the obtained thresholds are plotted, sorted by increasing age of the participants. A trend towards less negative values, which mean less attenuation of the output, can be observed for the older the participant. However, the differences in the contralateral hearing loss must be taken into account because the mean for all three presentation directions is plotted.

Since the study design factors in the individual hearing threshold and adjusts the presentation level of the stimuli accordingly, no strong age differences in distribution can be observed in the SRT data. This is in line with the statistical analysis of the SRT results, where age was not a significant predictor for SRT scores. Only the *mean threshold*, the interaction between *attention* (attend/ignore) and *side* (CI/non CI) and the three-way interaction between *attention*, *side* and *CI status* (on/off) showed significant p-

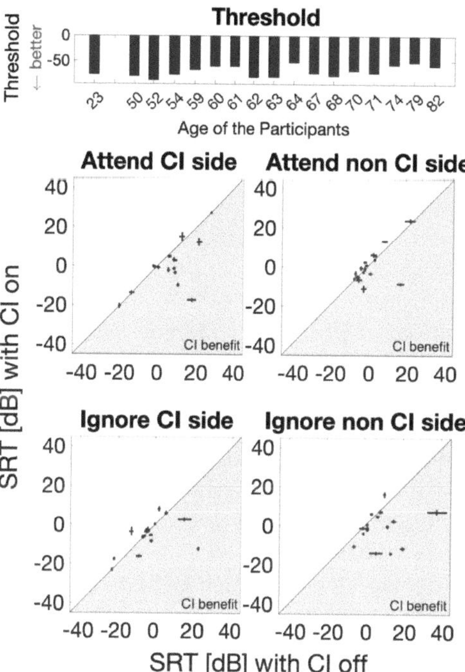

Figure 2: Threshold used for the adjustment of the sound pressure level sorted by age of the participants. For T1: Speech Reception Thresholds (SRT [dB]) with 95% confidence interval error bars. Results with Cochlear Implant (CI) on vs. CI off for the four conditions ignore/attend CI/non CI side for each participants. Negative SRT values are considered "better". Results that fall below the 45° line (darker section) represent a CI benefit.

values as displayed in Tab. 1. The factors *CI status* and *side* were not significant when analysing all data but became significant when the analysis was restricted to T1 (*CI status*: $\beta=-0.3048, p=0.023$, side: $\beta=-0.284, p=0.0339$). The three-way interaction was not significant when limiting the analysis to T1 data but the interaction between *attention* and *side* remained significant ($\beta=0.963, p=0.0004$). The main effect for the factor *session* as well as the effect for *CI status*, limited to T1, is demonstrated in Fig. 3 (A). This visualizes both the longitudinal CI benefit ($\Delta=-3.6$ dB) as indicated also by the SSQ and FE, as well as an immediate CI benefit ($\Delta=-4.6$ dB) due to switching on the implant and is well in line with expected results.

More complex are the interactions between *side* and *attention*, which are visualized in Fig. 3 (B). For the *CI off* condition the ignore non CI task leads to much higher SRTs than the attend non CI task. This side is the, in most cases, better hearing side. In contrast, attending the CI side leads to a higher SRT than ignoring it, which is reasonable considering no input from the CI is given. The same trend can be observed in the *CI off* condition for T2, although there are only 9 data sets as of yet, which is why the results should be interpreted with caution.

The condition *CI on* shows an overall improvement of the SRTs in comparison to the *CI off* condition, most notably for attending the CI side and ignoring the non CI side. This

Table 1: Statistical result from the linear mixed model. Formula: **SRT ~ mean threshold + FE + age + CI status + side + attention + attention×side + attention×side×CI status + (1|Subjects)**

Name	β	$t_{(DF=205)}$	p
CI status	-0.1851	-1.7413	0.0831
side	-0.1168	-1.0984	0.2733
mean threshold	-0.4782	-3.0132	**0.0029**
attention×side	0.5701	2.681	**0.0079**
attention×side×CI status	-1.0989	-2.5846	**0.0104**

difference demonstrates the basis for the immediate CI benefit in the spatial listening task. It helps to hear the stimuli with the CI, not only while attending that side but also in attending the front target and ignoring the lateral distractor on the non CI side.

In contrast to the *CI on* condition in T1 the effect for *side* in T2 seem to reverse. The participants reach higher (worse) SRTs when trying to ignore the CI side, which may indicate a more difficult time ignoring the CI input which is now better processed and understood by the participant. The SRT for attending the CI side gets better in comparison to T1, which is in line with the main effect of a longitudinal CI benefit overall. Also contributing to this main effect are the significantly lower SRTs for the non CI side in both conditions in T2 compared to T1. The CI users are better able to ignore the non CI side and focus on a frontal target but are surprisingly also better able to attend the non CI side. This may indicate a better differentiation between the two different stimuli to identify target and distractor.

One limitation that should be noted is the sequence of the *CI on/off* conditions, where *CI off* was always measured after *CI on*. Due to operational circumstances this could not be avoided. This may confound the shown immediate CI benefit. On the one hand the benefit could be slightly larger, since the hardest and often worst listening situation without the CI are the last tested and the participants may get fatigued. On the other hand there may be an additional benefit from training the same task for a longer time.

4   Conclusion

Overall the results show a strong immediate CI benefit in the spatial attention task as well as a longitudinal CI benefit. The reversal of the interaction between side and attention indicates there may be an acclimatization to hearing with the CI that can be beneficial as well as impeding. This depends on the spatial arrangement of target and distractor.

Acknowledgement

The work has been carried out at the AG Obleser, Department of Psychology, Universität zu Lübeck and was supervised by Malte Wöstmann. This research is supported by Cochlear (Grant to Malte Wöstmann and Jonas Obleser).

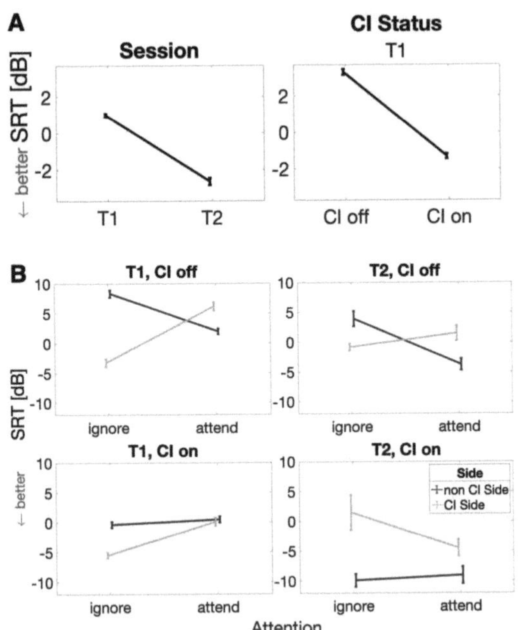

Figure 3: Effects and Interactions calculated from the mean SRTs for all participants. Error estimated as SE. **A** Main effect for *session* and main effect for *CI status* (off/on) for T1. **B** Interactions between *side* (CI/non CI) and *attention* (attend/ignore) for T1 and T2 and *CI off* and *on* respectively.

Author's Statement

Authors state no conflict of interest. Informed consent has been obtained from the participants. They were financially compensated for their participation in the study.

5   References

[1] World Health Organization, "World report on hearing," 2021.

[2] F. Kraus, S. Tune, A. Ruhe, J. Obleser, and M. Wöstmann, "Unilateral acoustic degradation delays attentional separation of competing speech," *Trends in Hearing*, vol. 25, 2021.

[3] M. Wöstmann, B. Herrmann, B. Maess, and J. Obleser, "Spatiotemporal dynamics of auditory attention synchronize with speech," *Proceedings of the National Academy of Sciences*, vol. 113, no. 14, pp. 3873–3878, 2016.

[4] L. K. Holden, C. C. Finley, J. B. Firszt, T. A. Holden, C. Brenner, L. G. Potts *et al.*, "Factors affecting open-set word recognition in adults with cochlear implants," *Ear and hearing*, vol. 34, no. 3, p. 342, 2013.

[5] B. Williges, T. Wesarg, L. Jung, L. I. Geven, A. Radeloff, and T. Jürgens, "Spatial speech-in-noise performance in bimodal and single-sided deaf cochlear implant users," *Trends in Hearing*, vol. 23, 2019.

Design of a multidimensional outcome measure test battery for cochlear implant patients

Kevyn M. Kogel [1], Matthias Hey [2] and Tim Jürgens [3]

[1] Auditory Technology, Universität zu Lübeck, kevyn.kogel@student.uni-luebeck.de
[2] Universitätsklinikum Schleswig-Holstein, Campus Kiel, ENT-clinic, Kiel, Germany matthias.hey@uksh.de
[3] Institut für Akustik, Technische Hochschule Lübeck, Lübeck, Germany, tim.juergens@th-luebeck.de

Abstract

The use of modern cochlear implants (CI) has resulted in well performing CI patients who cannot be adequately characterized by speech intelligibility measurements in quiet alone. The German guideline for CI treatment also calls for monitoring that goes beyond simple measurements of speech in quiet. A test battery describing the full range of CI patients' abilities is therefore needed. This paper reviews several studies in order to find a more comprehensive test battery for patient characterization that is representative for hearing in everyday life. Speech in quiet should be assessed with the measurement of monosyllabic and polysyllabic words not only at 65/70 dB but at lower levels as well. Objective measurements such as electrically evoked compound action potentials and subjective measurements such as questionnaires about life quality as well as about listening effort should be used to characterize the performance. Speech understanding in noise should be tested in fluctuating noise.

1 Introduction

Hearing is one of the most important sensory impressions in humans. If hearing is severely impaired, fitting a cochlear implant (CI) can be a possible form of therapy [1]. Providing people with hearing loss with a CI has proven to be a safe and stable intervention for restoring hearing [2]. The progress of rehabilitation should be documented by audiometric measurements [1]. Especially during the first six months after implantation and fitting of the speech processor, significant improvements can be observed in postlingually deafened adult CI patients. After this time, speech test results become more stable and remain so over years [2]. Ongoing monitoring of patients' performance still remains an important factor in quality management at the clinic for the rest of their lives [1, 3]. Measurements must stay up to date to assess the performance of CI patients their whole life, but the advancing technology of CI components has led to the fact that today's CI users can already achieve much more than just understanding speech in quiet. Measurements in noise or even listening to and enjoying music are possible for today's CI users [2]. The test batteries for evaluating performance have to keep up with the progress achieved in CI technology. Measurements of speech intelligibility in quiet are no longer sufficient to reflect the communication abilities of today's CI patients [2]. The German guideline for cochlear implant fittings also recommends further measurements beyond these basic measurements [3].

The aim of this paper was to design a test battery for the multidimensional characterization of CI patients' abilities in the clinic. Such a test battery can then be used for quality monitoring of CI fittings. To accomplish this, literature was reviewed and both, measurement methods and their outcome in CI patients, were extracted.

2 Methods and Materials

The Studies [2] and [4]-[7] were reviewed to collect the used CI performance measurements. Subsequently, suitable tests were identified, that should reflect the previously described characteristics. The studies were chosen for considering their respective test batteries for determining performance because they aim to capture performance with CI for different motivations. By [2] a cohort of 1005 postlingually deaf adults was retrospectively examined for their long-term performance with CI. The study by [4] investigated performance with the CI532 electrode (Cochlear® Ltd.) in 44 patients. In the retrospective study by [5], 2251 patients were considered. The aim of their work was to identify factors affecting the performance of CI users. The study by [6] was conducted on 100 postlingually deafened or profoundly hearing impaired patients. They were asked about their quality of life before surgery as well as three and six months after surgery with the Nijmegen Cochlear Implant Questionnaire (NCIQ). The questionnaire was evaluated within their study. In the work of [7], 112 adult CI patients were asked about the perceived listening effort in different everyday situations with the Listening Effort Questionnaire (LEQ). The aim was to check whether this questionnaire is also suitable for use with CI patients. After reviewing the studies, the possibility of modification of the respective tests was considered for providing the best possible characterization of the performance of CI patients. An important aspect to consider is that the acoustic environment of CI patients is very complex and consists of situations with speech in quiet as well as speech in noise [8]. The different situations in life should therefore be represented in a modern test battery. Therefore, when considering possible measurements for a test battery, care should also be taken to ensure that the targeted measurement procedures represent various aspects of everyday life [9]. This includes speech tests in quiet at different levels [8] as well as speech measurements in fluctuating noise [9].

Finally, the chosen measurements were evaluated according to the categories "representativeness for everyday life", "simplicity of measurement", "apparatus complexity", "length of measurement" and "usefulness for adjustment of the CI".

3 Results and Discussion

The evaluation of the tests and test setups selected for a possible design of a multidimensional test battery is listed in tables 1 and 2. Advantages, disadvantages and possible modifications will be explained and serve as a foundation for choosing tests for a future test battery. The length of the measurements is an important factor to consider for a test for the test battery, because in clinical practice resources for testing are limited [9].

The Freiburg Numbers Test and the Freiburg Monosyllabic Test are standard clinical tests for measuring speech understanding in quiet. The general representativeness in everyday life of the Freiburg Numbers Test and the Monosyllabic Test are rated rather low, because single word understanding in quiet is not an everyday task. For the Freiburg Monosyllabic Test a more representative measurement could be achieved if the presentation levels used in the measurement reflect, as closely as possible, the speech levels in the listening environment. The study [8] found that speech levels in quiet recorded by CI system data log have in the 50-59 dB level range the highest commonness. Therefore, in order to reflect the performance of CI patients in the best possible way, the measurement levels should not only be at the usual 65/70 dB but also at levels below 60 dB [8]. The simplicity of measurement of the Freiburg Numbers Test and the Monosyllabic Test is high. Most CI patients to date are able to perform both tests. There is not a complex setup needed for the measurements and the length of measurement is also low for both tests. Both tests are useful for fitting the CI. According to [1] the Freiburg Numbers Test and the resulting hearing threshold for speech determined by this test are good indicators for CI microphone sensitivity. The Freiburg Monosyllabic Test is a suitable measurement for documenting speech intelligibility and can provide guidance on the correct setting of C-levels during CI fitting [1]. The Freiburg Numbers Test has been discussed to be limited in assessing modern CI performance. According

to [1], many adults achieve close to 100 % speech understanding on Freiburg Numbers Test already in the first fitting phase at levels between 60 and 85 dB. Therefore for most of the CI patients, discrimination of CI performance is not possible in this level range with the Freiburg Numbers Test. Also the Freiburg Numbers Test is not sensitive enough to show decline in speech understanding at higher speech levels, which should occur when constant stimulation at the C-level causes distortion of speech [1]. As the Freiburg Monosyllabic Test does not show that ceiling effect, it is highly useful for adjustment of CI [1]. For the Freiburg Numbers Test the low level of difficulty indicates nonetheless that it should still be used so that poor performing patients can be monitored by the test battery as well [2]. These reasons and the short length of conducting both tests support the inclusion in the test battery.

Table 1: Evaluation of the Freiburg Numbers Test, the Freiburg Monosyllabic Test, the speech, spatial and quality (SSQ) Questionnaire and the Nijmegen Cochlear Implant Questionnaire (NCIQ), measurement of electrically evoked compound action potentials (ECAPs), and the Listening Effort Questionnaire (LEQ).

	Freiburg Numbers Test	Freiburg Monosyllabic Test	SSQ-Questionnaire and NCIQ	Measurement of ECAPs	LEQ
Representativeness for everyday life	Low	Low	High	Low	High
Simplicity of measurement	High	High	High	High	High
Apparatus complexity	Low	Low	Low	Low	Low
Length of measurement	Low	Low	Low-Moderate	Moderate	Low
Usefulness for adjustment of the CI	High	High	Low	High	Low

The Speech, Spatial, Qualities (SSQ) Questionnaire contains questions about the understanding of speech, the localization of sound and about hearing quality [10]. The focus of the questions in the NCIQ lies on sound perception, speech production, self-esteem and social functioning [6]. The questionnaires have a high representativeness of everyday life, because the questions represent everyday situations. Answering the questionnaires is simple, no complex technology is required and the measurement time is short. The use of questionnaires has the great advantage of a subjective assessment of the performance by the patients themselves. Aspects of hearing capabilities that normally cannot be checked by audiometric measurements, are also assessed. To reflect everyday life in the test battery, a questionnaire about the every day hearing like the SSQ-Questionnaire or the NCIQ should be chosen. Both questionnaires can be used to assess the quality of life with the CI [4], [6].

The measurement of electrically evoked compound action potentials (ECAPs) is an objective method that can provide information about the efficiency of the electrical stimulation of the auditory nerve by the CI. The measurement of ECAPs has no representativeness of everyday life. It is relatively easy to perform the measurement for trained personnel due to automatic threshold determinations. The technology to determine ECAPs is built into today's CI systems as standard, so no additional measurement setup than the programming interface for the CI is needed. For the adjustment of the speech processor, ECAPs provide important information for setting the comfort level (C-level) [4]. As ECAPs examine a feature of CI performance that is not represented by other tests, it is chosen for the test battery. Also ECAP thresholds may show reasons for differences in the performance of CI users [11].

The LEQ, which was used by [7], consists of three categories of questions and is evaluated on the basis of each category individually. Questions in the first category are questions related to the signal-to-noise ratio (SNR). Category 2 consists of questions about signal quality, and the third category relates to situations in quiet and with lip-reading. For all questions the listening effort has to be selected. Compared to the other questionnaires, the LEQ is shorter with only 17 questions and therefore quicker to answer. Understanding speech that is degraded by hearing loss or CI processing involves cognitive work and effort for patients [11]. Therefore the patients' cognitive abilities also affect performance with the CI [11]. Determining listening effort with the LEQ is an appropriate way to evaluate the success of hearing-enhancing interventions and is chosen for the test battery.

Table 2: Evaluation of the different measurement setups for the OLSA.

| | Oldenburg Sentence Test | | | | |
	Fixed Signal to noise ratio S0°N0°	Adaptive stationary noise S0° N0°	Adaptive fluctuating noise S0° N0°	Adaptive fluctuating noise S0° N90°, 180°, 270°	Adaptive fluctuating noise S0° N90°
Representativeness for everyday life	Low	Low	Moderate	High	Moderate
Simplicity of measurement	Moderate	Moderate	Moderate	Moderate	Moderate
Apparatus complexity	Low	Low	Low	High	Moderate
Length of measurement	Moderate	High	High	High	High
Usefulness for adjustment of the CI	High	High	High	High	High

The evaluation of different measurement setups for speech perception tests in noise measured with the widely used Oldenburg Sentence Test (OLSA) is shown in the table 2. For the fixed SNR setup, there is no change in SNR and noise used is stationary. The adaptive setups change the SNR depending on the response behavior and thus are supposed to determine the speech reception threshold. Different loudspeaker positions are also used for the different measurement setups. In the fixed SNR setup as well as in the adaptive stationary noise the signal (S) and the noise (N) both come from the frontal speaker (0°). For the test condition with fluctuating noise there are three different setups. One with signal an noise from the front (S0° N0°), one setup with noise at 90°, 180° and 270° degrees and the speech signal from the front (S0° N90°, 180°, 270°) and one setup with the signal from the front and the noise from the ipsilateral side as the examined CI (S0° N90°).

The everyday representativeness is rather low for the measurement conditions with stationary noise, since stationary noise is relatively rare in everyday life [9]. The measurement conditions in the fluctuating noise, on the other hand, show a higher everyday relevance [9]. The use of more than one loudspeaker, which is the case for the adaptive fluctuating noise in two measurement setups, leads to a higher complexity of the setup than it is the case for the other measurement setups. The time required for measurements with the OLSA is relatively high, since training lists are needed in advance in order to achieve a reliable result [1]. Speech tests in noise can also be used to evaluate noise reduction and directional microphone settings [9]. Therefore usefulness for CI adjustment is high.

As shown in a study by [8] investigating the data log of the CI systems, a large part of the speech signals occurs in environments with background noise. Since today's CI systems support the patient in these situations, a measurement of the performance with the CI must also cover such a situation. Some measurements in noise are also far from a realistic listening situation. Especially the use of a stationary noise has a low representativeness for everyday life, since competing speech signals account much more for difficulties in noise-affected environments: the noise signals in reality are more fluctuating. As a result, a speech test with stationary noise with fixed SNR is not included in the test battery.

As described earlier, OLSA with adaptive stationary noise S0° N0° can be used for evaluating a speech reception threshold in noise and therefore is useful for monitoring CI performance. The use of speech tests in fluctuating noise could bridge the discrepancy of speech tests with stationary noise towards everyday life [9]. Testing OLSA in fluctuating noise with the setup S0° N0° showed results near to the results of stationary noise in the same setup because even the best performers could not show an improvement in fluctuating noise due to the missing property of dip listing in CI patients [12]. Fluctuating noise should be chosen for a S0° N0° setup over stationary noise because possible improvements in dip listening by advancing technology could than be monitored in the future. An experimental setup with S0° N90°, 180°, 270° would be desirable for a reality simulating situation and would be a situation solvable for CI patients [9]. Since such an experimental setup can only be facilitated by a few clinical centers because of the high apparatus complexity, this setup is not included in the test battery. As the setup S0° N90° with moderate apparatus complexity leads to comparable results as the more complex setup with three noise sources [9], it is chosen as part of the test battery.

4 Conclusion

A modern test battery for assessing performance in today's CI patients needs to be much more comprehensive than it was in the past. The use of different measures to capture both objective and subjective performance helps to cover the full range of the outcome potential of today's patients. A mixture of rather simple speech tests in quiet and much more complex audiometric measurements in noise provides both good performing and poor performing CI patients with the opportunity to reflect their performance. The Freiburg Numbers and Monosyllabic Test would be suitable for gaining important information for adjustment of CI and be of low measurement length. The Freiburg Numbers Test is a doable task even for poor performing patients. The measurement levels for the Freiburg Monosyllabic Test used should be the typical 70/65 dB as well as levels lower than 60 dB to use measurement levels oriented to the listening environment.The use of questionnaires helps to determine the personal hearing gain perceived by the patient and to obtain a personal performance assessment. Many aspects of the listening environment can be assessed by questionnaires. Therefore, good questionnaires are a tool that must be used to determine CI outcome. The demands on patients' cognitive resources could be captured by determining listening effort that patients experience with the CI. The use of a subjective questionnaire would represent everyday life and therefore be suitable for this purpose. By measuring ECAP thresholds, the physiological status of the electrode nerve interface can be assessed, which can help to explain differences in the patient's performance. As a more complex task, with a realisable apparatus complexity, the use of the OLSA with adaptive fluctuating noise in the S0° N0° and S0° N90° setup should also be considered.

Acknowledgement

The work has been carried out at Universitätsklinikum Schleswig-Holstein, Campus Kiel and supervised by the Institut für Akustik, Technische Hochschule Lübeck.

Author's Statement

Conflict of interest: Authors state no conflict of interest.

5 References

[1] J. Müller-Deile, *Verfahren zur Anpassung und Evaluation von Cochlear Implant Sprachprozessoren*, 1st ed. Heidelberg: Median Verlag, 2009.

[2] M. Lenarz, H. Sönmez, G. Joseph, A. Büchner, and T. Lenarz, "Long-term performance of cochlear implants in postlingually deafened adults," *Otolaryngology - Head and Neck Surgery (United States)*, vol. 147, no. 1, pp. 112–118, 2012.

[3] Deutsche Gesellschaft für Hals-Nasen-Ohren-Heilkunde Kopf- und Hals-Chirurgie e.V. (DGHNO-KHC), "S2k-Leitlinie Cochlea-Implantat Versorgung," 2020.

[4] M. Hey, T. Wesarg, A. Mewes, S. Helbig, J. Hornung, T. Lenarz et al., "Objective, audiological and quality of life measures with the CI532 slim modiolar electrode," *Cochlear Implants International*, vol. 20, no. 2, pp. 80–90, 2019.

[5] P. Blamey, F. Artieres, D. Başkent, F. Bergeron, A. Beynon, E. Burke et al., "Factors affecting auditory performance of postlinguistically deaf adults using cochlear implants: An update with 2251 patients," *Audiology and Neurotology*, vol. 18, no. 1, pp. 36–47, 2012.

[6] M. Plath, M. Sand, P. S. van de Weyer, K. Baierl, M. Praetorius, P. K. Plinkert et al., "Validity and reliability of the Nijmegen Cochlear Implant Questionnaire in German," *HNO*, vol. 70, no. 6, pp. 422–435, 2022.

[7] A. Illg, S. Pape, and T. Lenarz, "Höranstrengung im Alltag bei erwachsenen Patienten mit Cochlea-Implantat," *22. Jahrestagung der DGA*, pp. 1–3, 2019.

[8] M. Hey, T. Hocke, and P. Ambrosch, "Speech audiometry and data logging in CI patients," *HNO*, vol. 66, no. S1, pp. 22–27, 2018.

[9] M. Hey, A. Mewes, and T. Hocke, "Speech comprehension in noise—considerations for ecologically valid assessment of communication skills ability with cochlear implants," *HNO*, vol. 70, no. 12, pp. 1–9, 2022.

[10] J. Kießling, L. Grugel, H. Meister, and M. Meis, "Übertragung der Fragebögen SADL, ECHO und SSQ ins Deutsche und deren Evaluation," *Zeitschrift für Audiologie*, vol. 50, no. 1, pp. 6–16, 2011.

[11] A. C. Moberly, C. Bates, M. S. Harris, and D. B. Pisoni, "The Enigma of Poor Performance by Adults With Cochlear Implants," *Otology & Neurotology*, vol. 37, no. 10, pp. 1522–1528, 2016.

[12] S. Zirn, D. Polterauer, S. Keller, and W. Hemmert, "The effect of fluctuating maskers on speech understanding of high-performing cochlear implant users," *International Journal of Audiology*, vol. 55, no. 5, pp. 295–304, 2016.

Quality Assurance in Cochlear Implant Rehabilitation
– Development of a Protocol –

Manuel Reinhold [1], Daniela Hollfelder [2] and Jürgen Tchorz [3]

[1] Auditory Technology, Universität zu Lübeck, manuel.reinhold@student.uni-luebeck.de
[2] Department of Otorhinolaryngology, Head and Neck Surgery, Universität zu Lübeck, daniela.hollfelder@uksh.de
[3] Institut of Acoustics, Luebeck University of Applied Sciences, juergen.tchorz@th-luebeck.de

Abstract

Cochlear implant (CI) rehabilitation represents a multidisciplinary complex process which has guidelines but no standardized template to document interdisciplinary diagnosis, planning and cooperation as well as individual benefit of hearing rehabilitation with the CI. In this project work, a protocol was designed in compliance with certain quality parameters of the current guideline *Weißbuch Cochlea Implantat(CI)-Versorgung*. From the resulting protocol, the progress of speech intelligibility and the development of life quality surveyed with questionnaires during hearing rehabilitation can be visualized. It allows near-time conclusions about the outcome quality of CI rehabilitation, identification of possible problems as well as interdisciplinary planning, coordination, and availability of information.

1 Introduction

Cochlear implants (CI) represent an essential option for auditory rehabilitation for people with profound hearing loss, who achieve no sufficient hearing rehabilitation with conventional hearing aids. CIs can improve hearing and speech intelligibility to regain social interaction, and to achieve a higher quality of life [1], [2]. The treatment with a CI requires an individual interdisciplinary cooperation of different disciplines on a high quality level, including ear, nose and throat specialists (ENT), audiologists, neuroradiologists, speech therapists and hearing aid acousticians. The rehabilitation process consists of preoperative diagnosis including evaluation and counseling, implantation, speech and hearing rehabilitation, and lifelong follow-up care [3].

Regionally and internationally, specialists work on quality guidelines for CI rehabilitation in order to set standards for the complex CI therapy that follows a large number of interdisciplinary steps [4]. These include the German *Weißbuch Cochlea Implantat(CI)-Versorgung* (Weißbuch) [5] and the *CI-Register* of the *German Society of Otorhinolaryngology, Head and Neck Surgery* (DGHNO-KHC) [6], the *Guideline CI Care* of the *Association of Scientific Medical Societies* (AWMF) [2] and the *Implant Register Act* (IRegG) [7]. The recommendations for CI rehabilitation formulated in the *Weißbuch*, considering process, structural and outcome quality, form the certification basis for clinics as *Certified Cochlear Implant Providing Institutions* (CIVE) [8]. However, there is no standardized documentation basis and template for clinics, which could serve as evidence for the interdisciplinary diagnosis, planning and follow-up of the individual treatment of CI patients. The aim of this project work is the development of a standardized documentary and working tool, in order to enable interdisciplinary availability while maintaining essential quality parameters. The purpose is to obtain near-time conclusions about the outcome quality of CI rehabilitation, to consider interindividual differences between patients and to identify problems in the rehabilitation process. In addition, it should be possible to make statements about the patients' quality of life and the achievement of their goals.

2 Material and Methods

2.1 Pre- and Postoperative Data Acquisition

The suggested protocol documents information from the preoperative and postoperative status. The information is collected as data sets based on the *Weißbuch*.

In the preoperative phase, differential diagnosis of the hearing disorder and detailed counseling are used to determine the patient's suitability for CI rehabilitation [5]. The data set *diagnostic information* contains information on possible genetic coherence factors and the timeline of the hearing impairment.

In another data set, pre- and postoperative *medical history information* on tinnitus and vertigo is recorded. Relevant parameters for vertigo are the type, attack duration and frequency, time of last attack, and the starting point of vertigo awareness. Tinnitus information includes side-specific data on subjective loudness (loudness scale from 1 to 10), character (f.e. tone or noise), pulse synchrony, tinnitus compensation (yes or no), and since when tinnitus has occurred.

2.1.1 Objective Audiological and Vestibular Diagnosis

Subjective and objective testing procedures are required for the evaluation of the CI patient and the progress documentation of hearing rehabilitation [5]. The objective audiological preoperative tests included in the protocol consist of Brainstem Evoked Response Audiometry (BERA) and stapedius reflex measurements. For BERA, the type of BERA measurement, the averaged hearing threshold in dB and the latencies of wave V are documented for the corresponding ear. For the stapedius reflex measurement, the frequency and level dependent ipsi- and contralateral answer for each ear is documented. To complete the objective diagnosis, the result of a head impulse test is noted for the detection of disorders of the vestibular functions [3].

2.1.2 Subjective Audiological Diagnosis

Pure tone and speech audiograms are carried out pre- and postoperatively as subjective testing procedures [5]. All audiograms are accessible as scanned documents in the protocol to ensure easy availability of relevant information. In addition, relevant measurement values of speech audiometry are documented. In preoperative speech audiometry, the measured values of the unaided ears and the ears fitted with hearing aids obtained via headphones and in free field condition are noted. Therefore, the test material being used, including obligatory word and sentence tests has to be selected in the protocol. If the Freiburg speech test (FST) is selected, the hearing loss in dB and the discrimination loss in percent for both ears are documented in the data set *pure tone/speech audiometry unaided* from the values measured via headphones. The noted free field measurements of the FST with and without hearing aids include the percentage of correctly repeated multi- and monosyllables at levels of 55 dB SPL, 65 dB SPL and 80 dB SPL as well as the monosyllables at 65 dB SPL in noise with a level of 60 dB SPL. Furthermore, the values of a sentence test are measured in free field with and without hearing aids. For example, the 50 % speech reception threshold (SRT 50) in dB recorded with the Oldenburg sentence test (OLSA) in noise is noted for each ear.

The difference in monosyllabic discrimination at a level of 65 dB SPL in free field with and without hearing aids results in a hearing benefit for each ear, which is logged in the data set *pure tone/speech audiometry with hearing aid*. If a CROS or BiCROS system has been tested, the results of the speech audiogram measured in quiet or in noise in free field are additionally documented.

The documentation of the postoperative speech audiometry includes free field measurements of the FST with CI for multi- and monosyllables with levels of 55 dB SPL, 65 dB SPL and 80 dB SPL, as well as the monosyllables at the 65/60 dB SPL signal/noise condition. Moreover, the measurement values of the OLSA are documented. The measurements are carried out preoperatively and 1, 2, 3, 6, 9 and 12 months after the initial activation of the processor. Then, the measurements are taken during annual follow-up visits.

2.1.3 Hearing Aid and CI Processor Information

If the CI patient is fitted with hearing aids prior to implantation or is bimodal CI fitted, the hearing aid fitting must be documented. For this purpose, information such as the aided ear, the hearing aid manufacturer, the model, and the fitting date are stored in the data set *current hearing aid fitting*. Also noted are the basic data of the responsible hearing aid acoustician and since when the patient has been a hearing aid user. The implant data in *implant information* includes site-specific information on the CI manufacturer, implant and the planned CI processor, the implanting clinic, the date and place of initial processor activation and the reason for surgery, such as hearing deterioration. In addition, intraoperative information such as position control, insertion depth and access to the cochlea can be entered.

Up to four weeks after CI implantation, the rehabilitation starts and includes hearing and speech therapy carried out by audiologists and speech therapists. As part of the therapy, free-field pure tone and speech audiometry in quiet and noise is used to verify the progress of rehabilitation with the CI. In general, the therapy is divided into three parts, consisting of the basic therapy with the first setting, the period up to 12 months after implantation (follow-up therapy) and the period from 12 months after implantation (lifelong follow-up care) [5].

Besides the improvement of speech understanding, the assessment of subjective quality of life by questionnaires before and after CI fitting represents another outcome parameter in the evaluation of the CI rehabilitation process [8]. The *Nijmegen Cochlear Implant Questionnaire* (NCIQ) assesses subjective quality of hearing and life and identifies the physical, social and psychological situation of CI patients through 60 questions that are assigned to one of the six subcategories (*basic sound perception* (SPB), *advanced sound perception* (SPA), *speech production* (SP), *self esteem* (SE), *activity limitations* (AL), *social interaction* (SI)). Response options for 55 questions are *never, rarely, sometimes, often,* and *always*. Five of the questions are answered *no, bad, moderately, good,* and *very good*. The NCIQ will be surveyed once preoperatively and then after initial activation at the same intervals as postoperative speech audiometry. For the evaluation, the best possible answer is assigned the value 100 and the worst possible answer is given the value 0. The responses in between are given the values 75, 50, and 25 in descending order. The total score of a subcategory is determined by averaging the assigned values [9].

2.1.4 Medical Imaging

Neuroradiological procedures are necessary to investigate the anatomical requirements for CI implantation. These include, for example, cranial magnetic resonance imaging and computer tomography of the temporal bone [8]. Scanned imaging findings can be visualized in the *radiology* dataset. Specifically for CI fitting, information about the length of the cochlea should be included for implant selection. Therefore, imported data from an otological planning software (Otoplan, Med-EL) for measuring the cochlea and determining the electrode array can also be accessed.

2.1.5 Vaccinations

Patients who have been fitted with a CI have a slightly increased risk of contracting bacterial meningitis. For this reason, preventive vaccination against haemophilus influenzae type B and pneumococcus must have been carried out in children and adults before the surgical procedure [10]. Documentation in the dataset *vaccinations* is required regarding whether and when the vaccinations were given.

2.2 Interdisciplinary Case Conference

An interdisciplinary case conference is implemented in the protocol, in which the planned hearing rehabilitation as well as further questions or problems are formulated on basis of all the audiological parameters, including patient's wishes and goals. The participating interdisciplinary team is documented including the specific discipline. Finally, the interdisciplinary agreement of the conference is formulated and documented.

3 Results and Discussion

3.1 Results

Based on the data acquisition, the progress of NCIQ and speech intelligibility during the CI rehabilitation process can be illustrated. The curve of speech intelligibility displayed in Fig. 1 shows the development of one patient's speech intelligibility measured with the FST in free field in percent at 65 dB SPL. The x-axis displays the measurement time points before CI implantation and 1, 2, 3, 6, 9, 12, 24, and 36 months after initial activation of the processor. Data acquisition starts preoperatively at 0% and follows the described follow-up visits (FU), including all FU at 12, 24 and 36 months. The upper curve displays the SRT of multisylllables at 65 dB SPL in percent, the middle curve the SRT of monosyllables at 65 dB SPL and the lower curve the SRT in the 65/60 dB SPL signal/noise condition. The SRT of the multisyllables displays a maximum of 100 % after 9 months. Data of the monosyllables have a maximum of 70 % after 9 months. Monosyllables in noise show a maximum value of 25 % after 9 months.

The plot of the NCIQ results shown in Fig. 2 illustrates the development of one patient's NCIQ score in percent of each subcategory dependent on the defined FU visits. The lines represent the measurement time points before CI implantation (solid) and 1 (long dashed), 2 (dashed), 3 (short dashed), 6 (dotted line) and 9 (dotted) months after the initial processor activation. Subcategories of NCIQ are shown on the x-axis. The curves represent higher NCIQ scores with increasing distance from the preoperative survey. The subcategories SE, AL and SI depict lower values with a maximum value of 65 % than SPB, SPA and SP.

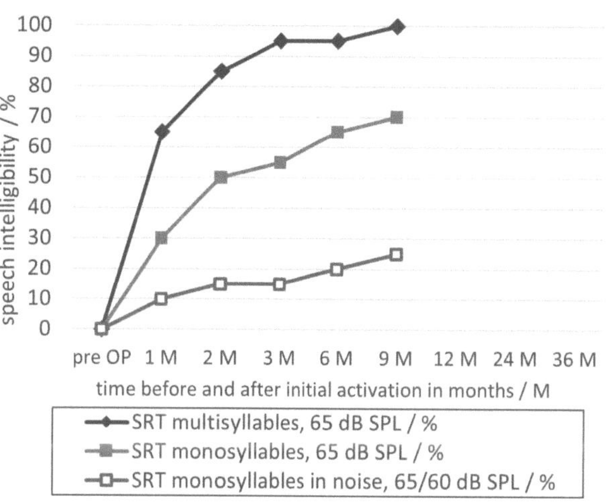

Figure 1: Documentation of speech intelligibility in the FST, SRT for multi- and monosyllables at levels of 65 dB SPL and monosyllables in the 65/60 dB SPL signal/noise condition, before and after initial processor activation at measurement time points preoperative, 1, 2, 3, 6, 9, 12, 24, 36 months.

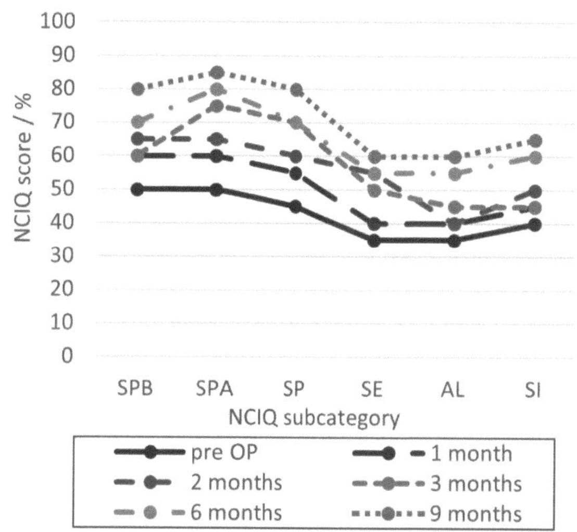

Figure 2: Documentation of the NCIQ results. Represented are the subcategories *basic sound perception* (SPB), *advanced sound perception* (SPA), *speech production* (SP), *self esteem* (SE), *activity limitations* (AL), *social interaction* (SI) at measurement time points preoperative, 1, 2, 3, 6, and 9 months after initial processor activation.

3.2 Discussion

The curve of speech intelligibility before and after implantation clearly visualizes the progress and indicates possible problems in hearing rehabilitation over a long period of time. Deviations in the expected speech intelligibility can be noticed quickly. Consequently, the curve helps to check and permanently secure the achieved hearing improvement. Possible improvements in speech intelligibility with CI can be clearly demonstrated to the CI patient.

The curve of the NCIQ score over time illustrates that the quality of life increases in all subcategories with increasing time interval from the initial activation compared to the preoperative survey. In general, the plot can be used to visualize and document the development in the CI patient's quality of life. It is possible to make statements about the effect of CI rehabilitation on quality of life. During the hearing rehabilitation, a possible intervention regarding audiological, social, and psychological parameters can soon be identified and taken under special consideration in adapting the therapy individually.

A disadvantage is the potentially reduced validity of the NCIQ due to the risk of response bias, as a consequence of answering the questionnaire in noisy, not private environment, including waiting times, and the actual health situation.

Centralizing essential elements of interdisciplinary diagnosis and linking the protocol to imaging findings from Otoplan simplifies access to imaging data and enables personalized CI care and surgery planning.

The interdisciplinary case conference provides and documents the expertise of various disciplines in making pre- and postoperative treatment decisions. The protocol enables a collaborative, coordinated discourse involving the patient's wishes. A team evaluation of findings for or against a CI indication, the appropriate implant choice or complications after surgery can lead to best quality solutions. All persons involved in the CI rehabilitation process have access to each individual protocol to gain information of the rehabilitation process. The goal is to offer each patient best quality in CI rehabilitation.

4 Conclusion

The protocol represents a standardized template to achieve all quality assurance goals in CI rehabilitation process. Conclusions about the outcome quality of CI rehabilitation can be obtained in a near-time period.

It also indicates when patients do not attend follow-up visits on a regular basis. As part of the CI center certification process, the auditor has quick access to all data. The transparency enables both the auditor and responsible professional staff to identify potential problems more easily in the CI rehabilitation process. The protocol could also be used at other clinics due to its universal design.

A disadvantage is the time-consuming realization of the documentation in the daily clinic routine, for which personnel resources are required. Furthermore, modifications during implementation into the patient software system have to be realized, which could limit flexibility.

In the future, the protocol could be adapted to the treatment of patients receiving different hearing implants, such as bone conduction implants or transcutaneous active middle ear implants.

Acknowledgement

The work has been carried out at University Clinical Center Schleswig-Holstein, Section of Otorhinolaryngology and supervised by the Institute of Acoustics, Luebeck University of Applied Sciences.

Author's Statement

Conflict of interest: Authors state no conflict of interest.

5 References

[1] T. R. McRackan, M. Bauschard, J. L. Hatch, E. Franko-Tobin, H. R. Droghini, S. A. Nguyen and J. R. Dubno, *Meta-analysis of quality of life improvement after cochlear implantation and associations with speech recognition abilities.* Laryngoscope, vol. 128, pp. 982–990, 2018.

[2] Deutsche Gesellschaft für Hals-Nasen-Ohren-Heilkunde, Kopf- und Hals-Chirurgie e.V. (DGHNO-KHC), *S2k-Leitlinie Cochlea-Implantat-Versorgung.* AWMF-Register-Nr. 017/071, 2020.

[3] T. Lenarz, A. Büchner and A. Illg, *Cochlea-Implantation: Konzept, Therapieergebnisse und Lebensqualität.* Laryngo-Rhino-Otologie, vol. 101, pp. 36–78, 2022.

[4] A. Loth, C. Vazzana, M. Leinung, D. Guderian, C. Issing, U. Baumann et al., *Quality control in cochlear implant therapy: cinical practice guidelines and registries in european countries.* Eur. Arch. of Otorhinolaryngol., vol. 279, no. 10, pp. 4779—4786, 2022.

[5] Deutsche Gesellschaft für Hals-Nasen-Ohren-Heilkunde, Kopf- und Hals-Chirurgie e.V. (DGHNO-KHC), *Weißbuch Cochlea Implantat (CI)-Versorgung.* no. 2, Bonn, 2021.

[6] *DGHNO Cochlea-Implantat-Register*, https://www.ci-register.de/. Accessed 12.01.2023.

[7] *Gesetz zum Implantateregister Deutschland (Implantateregistergesetz - IRegG)*, http://www.gesetze-im-internet.de/iregg/. Accessed 12.01.2023.

[8] T. Stöver, M. Leinung and A. Loth, *Welche Qualität macht den Unterschied in der Cochlea-Implantat-Versorgung?* Laryngo-Rhino-Otologie, vol. 99, pp. 1–30, 2020.

[9] J. B. Hinderink, P. F. M. Krabbe and P. Van Den Broek, *Development and application of a health-related quality-of-life instrument for adults with cochlear implants: the Nijmegen Cochlear Implant Questionnaire.* Otolaryngology – Head and Neck Surgery, vol. 123, no. 6, pp. 756–765, 2000.

[10] G. O'Donoghue, T. Balkany, N. Cohen, T. Lenarz, L. Lustig and J. Niparko, *Meningitis and cochlear implantation.* Otology & Neurotology, vol. 23, pp.823–824, 2002.

Update of the Freiburg monosyllabic speech test on the basis of word frequency distribution

Maren Harries [1], Larissa Jäger [2], and Hendrik Husstedt [3]

[1] Auditory Technology, Universität zu Lübeck, maren.harries@student.uni-luebeck.de
[2] German Institute of Hearing Aids, Lübeck, {L.Jaeger,H.Husstedt}@dhi-online.de

Abstract

The Freiburg monosyllabic speech test (FMST) was developed by Hahlbrock more than 50 years ago. In German-speaking countries the FMST is frequently used as a standard speech test for audiometry and hearing aid fitting. Obviously not all monosyllabic words are common nowadays, neither in verbal nor written language. Additional to the usage of outdated words, the phonemic and perceptual balance of test lists is subject to critical discussions. To update the FMST, monosyllabic nouns were extracted from six different language corpora and filtered by their word frequency distribution. Furthermore, the phonemic structure was analyzed in order to be able to generate new well-balanced test lists. In this paper, a systematic procedure for erasing outdated and compiling new words with a frequency distribution filter and phoneme analyzer is presented.

1   Introduction

The Freiburg monosyllabic speech test (FMST) is standardized in DIN 45621-1:1995-08 and consists of twenty lists each including twenty monosyllabic nouns, which can be presented via headphones or loudspeaker [1]. Speech reception in quiet or noise is stated as amount of correctly repeated words in percentage. In Germany, the FMST is used for various applications such as testing hearing performance or evaluating benefit of hearing aids. The results of pure tone audiometry and FMST are substantial for the indication of hearing aids and to receive reimbursement from the public health insurance. Considering this, the FMST is the most frequently used test for hearing loss diagnostics and evaluation of hearing aid fittings in Germany.

The speech test dates back to 1969 and has been recorded by the speaker Klaus Wunderlich. Recently, the FMST has been criticized for the use of unpopular and outdated monosyllables [2]. Additionally, it has been stated that there are problems with the phonemic and perceptual balance, contextual issues of test lists and psychological restraints with repeating certain words, e.g. "Sarg" (coffin) [2]. It is important to update and complement words with a higher word frequency and eliminate infrequent and emotional disturbing material regularly because language is under constant change. Due to latest research, test list 5 and 15 of the FMST contained a higher word frequency than most test lists. Despite its higher word frequency, only test list 15 showed a higher speech recognition score, but test list 5 resulted in a lower one compared with other test lists [3]. Phonemic distribution, perceptual references and lexical neighborhood density will most likely have inter-actions with the word frequency distribution for individual speech recognition and should be considered before generating new list compositions [4]. To generate new list compositions, which are close to the phoneme distribution of the German language, it is possible to use literature values of Hahlbrock's distribution scheme [5].

In a previous work by Schwarz et al., monosyllables were extracted from three language corpora "Leipzig corpora collection" (LCC), "Datenbank für gesprochenes Deutsch" (DGD), "Deutsches Referenz Korpus" (DeReKo) and then manually filtered by categories such as regionalisms or anglicisms [6]. The aim of our work was to update and complement a collection of monosyllables by their word frequency from different corpora automatically to increase objectivity, and to reduce processing time and manual errors. On this premise, outdated words should be reduced, and new words analyzed for their phonemic structure to prepare grouping and synthesizing of new lists.

2   Material and Methods

2.1   Selection of corpora

To fulfill the requirements for an updated speech test, it is important to select words from speech out of everyday life. The speech corpora used to update and extend the existing 400 words of the FMST were required to contain current language, to be standard German and to contain a frequency distribution for the occurrence of words in common daily speech. Optimally, the speech corpora should not only include written but also verbal German. Additionally to the speech corpora of Schwarz et al. (DGD,

LCC, DeReKo) [6], "Digitales Wörterbuch der deutschen Sprache" (DWDS), Wikipedia monosyllable corpus [7], and CELEX [8] were used to extract a larger number of mono-syllables. As corpus with spoken language, the speech corpus of the database for verbal German (DGD) was chosen. The LCC, DeReKo, CELEX, DWDS, and the Wikipedia monosyllable corpus were from various corpora of written sources, such as public web, random web pages, and news. Except for the LCC, all of them were created as word rank list to exclude nonexistent words.

2.2   Extraction of monosyllabic nouns

The selection of monosyllabic nouns from all speech corpora was automated with an own script in Matlab R2022b. First all words of six different language corpora were filtered for a capital letter at the beginning, Latin alphabet, spaces, inner majuscules, and special characters. After this first step, monosyllabic nouns were filtered by selecting words with one monophthong, diphthong, or two consecutive monophthongs. The extracted monosyllables were matched, ensuring that each monosyllable appears only once. Those two steps are important to ensure the monosyllabic structure, to filter and reduce the number of words and operational time of the Application Programming Interface (API) categorization for the word frequency filter in the third step [7].

2.3   Selection of frequent monosyllables

The collection of the DWDS corpora for the API word frequency filter contains a total of 35 271 873 584 tokens. Tokens are the number of occurences of a single word or meaningful character in a corpora collection. The DWDS uses four different corpora, the "DWDS-Kernkorpus", "Metakorpus WebXL", "DWDS-Zeitungskorpus (incl. ZDL-Regionalkorpus)", and "Wikipedia-Korpus". Its frequency scale ranges from zero to six and describes the frequency of each word in the German language. The word frequency distribution scale value zero is starting with a minimum of five tokens and ends with a maximum of 35 271 873 584 tokens for the largest scale value six [7].

Beside the fact that it is impossible to make the word material of the speech test equally known for all regions, social classes, educational levels and age groups, these effects should be minimized by considering the word frequency distribution. In case of corpora with spoken language, filler words such as "Ähm" were transcribed occasionally. These tokens sometimes meet the criteria for the first automatic extraction of monosyllabic nouns but are always sorted out by the API word frequency filter. The same holds for expletives, regionalisms, technical language, lyricism, and fantasy words. Numerals were also excluded. This is useful because a related test, the Freiburg multisyllabic speech test, consists of numbers only, which could lead to confusion. Today, also anglicisms are common in the German language and should be included. However, particular words add new phonemes to the speech corpora, e.g. the phoneme /th/ as in "thrill". In general, it is recommended to use foreign phonemes as little as possible but the decision how many of them were taken into the final selection was also done automatically by the API. Only most frequent words in the scale range from value three to six were chosen, therefore uncommon and difficult phonemes could be avoided as well as abbreviations and most misspelled words.

2.4   Phonemic balance and literature reference for Freiburg monosyllabic lists

The words from the FMST and the new monosyllable collections were analyzed for their phoneme distribution and compared to three literature values for German language from Kohler, Meier and Verbmobil. The Freiburg monosyllables and the new collections were phonologically transcribed for structural type groups, such as long and short vowels, voiced and unvoiced fricatives and plosives, and nasal consonants. The three literature phoneme distributions differ from their date of research. The Kohler references are based on the "Kiel Corpus of Read Speech" with a corpus of 23 985 words of read speech in German, which was collected in 1994 [9]. Meier's collection of 7 994 references for spoken German Prosa is the oldest from 1952 [10]. The Verbmobil is the newest but smallest literature collection with 2 500 words from the year 2000. Originally it was developed as a project for a fast automatic language translation [11].

3   Results and Discussion

3.1   Choice of corpora and extraction of monosyllabic nouns

All six corpora represent a total number of 2 109 253 tokens. From the LCC 510 123 tokens, a sum of 6 711 monosyllables were extracted automatically. This huge LCC collection was not representative because most of them were filler or nonsense words and had a wrong spelling of capital letters. The filter for nouns was not able to do a useful selection due to the high number of misspellings. In direct comparison the DWDS resulted in a smaller selection of 1 861 monosyllabic nouns even though the DWDS had the biggest corpus of 1 239 857 tokens. So there is a difference of nearly 5 000 words in the automatic selection. Most corpora had a final list of 1 200-2 200 monosyllabic nouns after using the Matlab filter program. An automatic check for double entries within each of the six corpora and between all corpora lead to a reduction of monosyllabic words from 14 416 to 7 851. An exact overview of all tokens per corpus and filter results can be seen in Table 1. After the analysis of these six corpora, no additional common monosyllables could be found by the individual filter program, and a heterogeneous language corpus can be assumed.

After the selection of speech corpora and the extraction of monosyllabic nouns, the API filtered the selected 7 851 monosyllables by their word frequency into six word frequency scales. As shown in Fig. 1, German monosyllabic

Table 1: List of corpora with number of all tokens and results of extracted monosyllabic nouns selected automatically.

Corpora	Tokens	Filtered nouns
LCC	510 123	6 711
DGD	28 817	1 277
DeReKo	326 950	2 198
Celex	1 386	1 197
DWDS	1 239 857	1 861
Wikipedia	2 120	1 172
Sum	2 109 253	14 416
Sum after doublet filter		7 851

nouns only exist in category zero to five, which can be explained by the fact that monosyllabic nouns are used less frequently than other word groups such as pronouns [7].

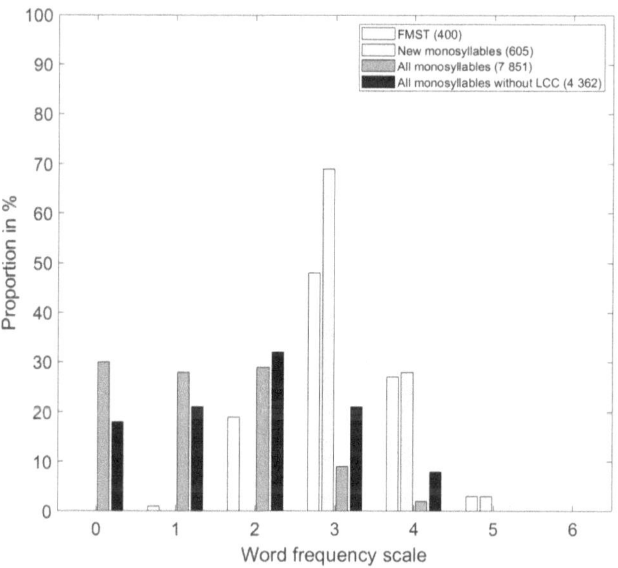

Figure 1: Comparison of word frequency distributions of monosyllables (FMST, new monosyllables, all monosyllables, all monosyllables without LCC).

Considering all monosyllables, the highest proportions can be seen for the categories zero, one, and two. This indicates that there are many unpopular monosyllables in all six corpora. It is known from previous observations, that the LCC includes many misspelled words, which is why all monosyllables were additionally evaluated without the LCC words leading to a lower proportion in category zero and one. For the selection of new monosyllables, uncommon words in the frequency range from zero to two were sorted out. Due to this filter, the highest proportion of new monosyllables can be seen for category three. In category three to five the new monosyllables were similar distributed as the FMST. The API frequency filter for the 7 851 monosyllables resulted in 994 most frequent monosyllabic nouns. The reduced collection was representative for all monosyllables of the word frequency category between three to five, but had to be filtered manually for wrong old German spellings

which led to hidden double entries. Furthermore, the list contained popular names and a few abbreviations, which had to be erased too. Finally, a total of 605 words was selected. In addition, it was possible to identify infrequent words in the FMST as a proof for the existence of outdated words. The analysis resulted in 85 outdated words, for example words from category one like "Grog" (rum toddy) or "Lump" (rogue). So nearly one quarter of the speech material is outdated, as shown in Fig. 1.

3.2 Analysis of phonemic structure

The phonemic distributions in literature are specified in the alphabetic system of the International Phonetic Alphabet (IPA). It is a Latin script based alphabetic system of phonetic notations. For better comparability with literature, the analysis of 7 851 monosyllables, the final word selection of 605 words, and the FMST with 400 words were transcribed in IPA and summarized into seven phoneme groups. The sizes of all corpora and literature references are shown in the legend of Fig. 2. The smallest literature reference

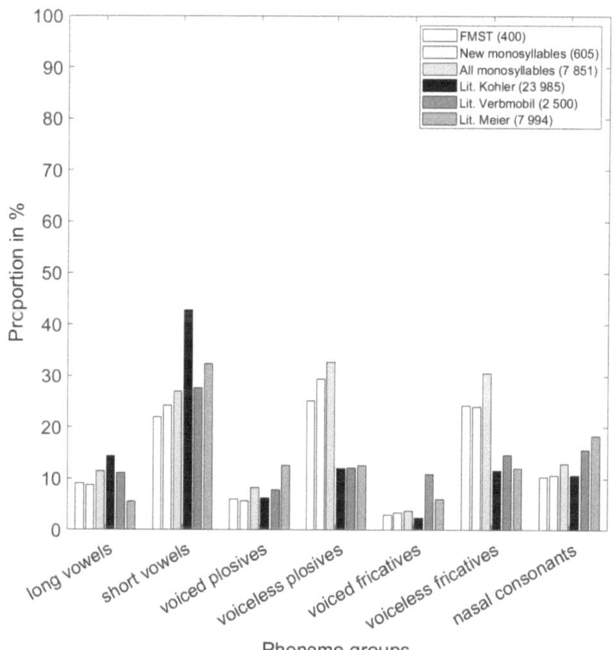

Figure 2: Comparison of phonemic distribution of monosyllables (FMST, new monosyllables, all monosyllables) to literature data (Kohler, Verbmobil, Meier) using phoneme groups.

from the Verbmobil project has the highest similarity with the monosyllabic collections due to its small number of tokens. An important difference is that the groups of voiceless plosives, and fricatives contain a higher amount of words than all of the three literature references. This difference is caused by the typical structure of monosyllables and is independent of the size of monosyllabic corpora. As expected, the phonemic distribution of isolated words, like the FMST and the new monosyllabic collection, deviates from written text of read or spoken language especially in the catrgory of short vowels from the biggest literture collection of Kohler. According to Hahlbrock the difference of the proportion of vowels and consonants between monosyllables and mixed texts with verbal speech is natural [5]. With updated and extended word material of 605 most frequent monosyllables, it is possible to generate new list compositions corresponding to literature values of Hahlbrock's phoneme distribution scheme. The sum of all phonemes in a list has to be 73 phonemes in a distinctive order. Each list of the FMST contains one word with two, seven words with three, ten words with four and two words with five phonemes. The need for one two phoneme monosyllable in each list is a restrictive factor because monosyllabic nouns with two phonemes are rare in the German language. One precondition for the update is to generate 25 updated test lists or more. After the selection of monosyllabic nouns as a basis for the development of new test lists, an examination of psychometric functions is necessary to evaluate the perceptual equivalence of words and lists. This could be a useful way to create new phonetic and perceptual equivalent test lists without using the Hahlbrock scheme. A complete different way to generate more words and lists could also be to lower the cutoff frequency from the value three to two or a token number in-between.

With the new monosyllabic collection of 605 words, it is possible to generate 26 lists of 20 words, if the Hahlbrock phonemic scheme is used without modification. In the further course it can be assumed, that the new collection of 605 monosyllabic nouns should be known throughout the German-speaking area by their high word frequency.

4   Conclusion

The procedure described in this paper is a preparation for an update of the FMST by creating a new monosyllabic collection with an automatic filter for the word frequency distribution. This analysis is done to improve objectivity and processing time, and to extract common monosyllables from different speech corpora. It has not yet been clarified, how many lists can be created, taking into account the requirements of ISO 8253-3:2022 [12] and the criteria which number of tokens or word frequency is the best to choose for getting a well-balanced combination of most frequent words without too much limitation of the total number of monosyllables. The actual results with the Hahlbrock scheme and word frequency distribution from three to five deliver 26 new lists generated from a new 605 monosyllabic nouns corpus. The project is still in progress for research of the best cut-off word frequency value or token number, an improved concept for the list's phonemic compilation and finally a text-to-speech synthesizing. In the end the main goal is to establish an easy, phonemic well-balanced extracting tool for a regular word material update because language and word frequency distribution is under constant change.

Acknowledgement

The project took place at German Institute of Hearing Aids, Lübeck. I would like to thank all my supervisors, who supported me.

Author's Statement

Conflict of interest: Authors state no conflict of interest.

5   References

[1] German Institute for Standardization e.V., *DIN 45621-1:1995-08, Sprache für Gehörprüfung - Teil 1: Ein- und mehrsibige Wörter*. Beuth Verlag GmbH, Berlin, 1995.

[2] S. Hoth, *Der Freiburger Sprachtest*. HNO, Springer Science and Business Media LLC, 2016.

[3] T. Steffens, *Verwendungshäufigkeit der Freiburger Einsilber in der Gegenwartssprache*. HNO, vol. 64, 549-556, 2016.

[4] A. Winkler, I. Holube, R. Carroll, *Impact of Lexical Parameters and Audibility on the Recognition of the Freiburg Monosyllabic Speech Test*. Ear Hear, Ovid Technologies, 2019.

[5] K. -H. Hahlbrock, *Sprachaudiometrie*. Thieme Verlag, Stuttgart, 1970.

[6] T. Schwarz, M. Frenz, A. Bockelmann and H. Husstedt, *Examination of a synthetic voice for the Freiburg Monosyllabic Speech*. GMS Zeitschrift für Audiologie - Audiological Acoustics, vol. 4, 2022.

[7] DWDS, *Digitales Wörterbuch der deutschen Sprache*. hrsg. v. d. Berlin-Brandenburgischen Akademie der Wissenschaften, http://www.dwds.de [last accessed on 10-21-2023].

[8] CELEX, *Lexical databases of German 2.0*. https://catalog.ldc.upenn.edu/topten [last accessed on 01-20-2023].

[9] K. J. Kohler, *Einführung in die Phonetik des Deutschen*. Grundlagen der Germanistik, E. Schmidt, vol. 2, Berlin, 1995.

[10] H. Meier, *Muttersprache*, vol.1, 6-14, 1951.

[11] Bayerisches Archiv für Sprachsignale, *Verbmobil, BAStat*. Ludwig-Maximilians-Universität Müchen, http://www.phonetik.uni-muenchen.de/forschung/Bas [last accessed on 01-10-2023].

[12] International Organization for Standardization, *ISO 8253-3:2022*. Akustik - Audiometrische Prüfverfahren - Teil 3: Sprachaudiometrie (ISO 8253-3:2022); Deutsche Fassung EN ISO 8253-3:2022, Ausgabe 2022-11.

Development of a study environment for school-aged children implanted with cochlearr implants

Sophia Langenbacher [1],

[1] Auditory Technology, Universität zu Lübeck, sophia.langenbacher@student.uni-luebeck.de

Abstract

How to develop a study environment for school-aged children, so they will stay motivated and want to perform the test again and again? Short video games are now an everyday part of children's life. The following paper describes the development of a test-environment for children. The aim of this work is an interactive mini-game developed with python and its toolbox pygame. The mini-game is to be used within a study, where school-aged children perform a simple study test by playing a short video game. The study focuses on school-aged children with normal hearing as well as children implanted with a hearing prothesis (cochlear implant) at an early age. The game will motivate boys and girls with the goal to reach good performing rates within the trials.

1 Introduction

This work is part of a non-disclosure agreement with a company. Therefore, this paper focuses on the development of a computer-based study environment with school-aged children implanted with a cochlear implant and does not give any further details about the study content. The paper focuses on the development of a computer program to be used in the context of a child study. The program is separated into a user interface for the study director and a test interface for the test subjects.

Cochlear implants (CI) are hearing prosthesis which are useful to a person with severe to profound sensorineural hearing loss. A small number of electrodes on the CI stimulate the nerves electrically inside the inner ear. Children born without hearing are indicated to get cochlear implants within 2 years to get the best outcome in their speech intelligibility [1]. Checking further developments within the CI technology and the corresponding hypotheses a child study is implemented. A child study starts with working with children what comes along with understanding the various contexts in which they interact. Child study techniques as observations are necessary to determine the extent to which the program guidelines are being followed [2]. Technology in the form of using technical devices plays an increasingly significant role in children's lives, over the last years. Nowadays, children grow up with smartphones, touch-screen devices and computers at an early age. The extensive use of such devices can be a great opportunity for data collection in the context of clinical trials according to the study of Michael Frank [3]. He describes tablets as a variable method for collecting low-cost, well-controlled data. Another reason for a study environment using a tablet is that the tutor can supervise the children during their task

and make some notes or give instructions while the child performs the test. Moreover, studies that involve interaction with an experimenter may be difficult or impossible to ensure that experimenters are blind to conditions and hypothesis. Although, there are methods for avoiding biased factors. The possibility of eliminating experimenters bias via computerized stimulus presentation is attractive according to Boston's study [4]. Moreover handheld devices with a device-based software programm provide patient-reported outcomes (PRO). PRO are known as important means of evaluating new medical products. One of the reasons is the integrity and accurance of clinical trial data which is why PRO is supported by regulators [5]. Tablet-based experiments can eliminate concerns about bias and uniformity experiments [5]. Developing a child-friendly test-setting, we must understand what motivates children to play video games and what needs the game should meet. Customizing game characters is suggested as making a game more fun because the protagonists can identify with its character [6] . School-aged children have greater motivation when completing tasks within interactive games on a touchscreen or tablet [7] [8] . In one of Leanne Nagels studies the children wanted to play a child-friendly game developed by Etienne Gaudrain again after finishing the test because they were higly motivated. [7]. In the following project a computer-based game environment was developed to keep school-aged children motivated during the study-task. The children will perform a test on a touchscreen whereas the experimenter can supervise the child and interrupt the test at any time with an own (main) computer screen. The aim of the following study project is the development of a child- and user-friendly interface game. The participants, study environment and the software will be described in the following section.

2 Material and Methods

Different programming languages and environments exist as development environments. The programming language Matlab is a very popular in acoustics for evaluations and studies within companies or institutions (e.g universities). Python in contrast, has the advantages of being open source and having a broad internet community to get help with problems. In addition, Python offers the appropriate toolboxes which are necessary for the mini-game and study requirements. The study required a study environment suitable for school-aged children. The aim is to keep the children motivated by the task, so they want to repeat the test, up to three times in a row according to the study requirements.

2.1 Participants

Participants are CI-implanted school children. They should be implanted within their second year. Moreover, they should be acquired by the local clinic. Calling their and their parents' attention for the study should be processed by doctors or the staff of the local rehabilitation centre. The participants are selected due to some specific study criteria which cannot be mentioned (non-disclosure agreement). In total there are four groups, who will participate in the study, one of them are the normal-hearing children and the other groups are CI-implanted children. Normal hearing children will get headphones whereas CI-patients will get the acoustic signal via cable, directly to their speech processor. Before the maintest, the hearing ability of the study participants is determined. Pre-acoustic tests such as BERA and play autometry record the individual hearing thresholds for stimulus reproduction in the main test. Participants and their parents will be informed as to the intent of the research project by a consultation and handing out an information paper which the parents can take home.

2.2 Study environment

The test is performed with a touchscreen tablet, that is placed in front of the children. The participant starts the mini-game by clicking the start-button on the given screen. The window of the game closes if the stimuli list is fully played and the test is finished. During the test, the tutor sits in front of the child and supervises the child and the responses on a own computer screen which is connected to the tablet. Therefore, the tutor can interact at any time if for example the child wishes to stop the test during a trial. Each response is either correct or false. If the response is correct the participant gets a reward to stay motivated. This can help when performing the test multiple times to achieve higher goals next time.

2.3 Software and toolboxes

The programming language Python3 was used. It is open-source and free to use. Another reason is that it comes along with a lot of free toolboxes and a big web-community which offers help for various errors and problems. As programming environment, the group decided to use Spyder because other parts of the team used it before and it was easy to share programming code if help was needed. Spyder comes along with Anaconda and already has some helpful software implemented. Pygame, Pyexcel and PyAudio were installed as toolboxes. The mini-game was written with the help of the toolbox pygame. With pygame it is easy to write small animations and create buttons with a function in the background. Another important toolbox was Pyaudio to add the audio signal to the mini-game with various parameters. The parameters should be changed in order to the participants hearing ability and different testing situations for example pre-test. Another toolbox was pyexcel. It enabled to save the stimuli parameters tested in an excel file which will be saved in the corresponding participant group folder. The code was written according to the file structure.

2.3.1 Requirements

Before starting with the coding in python the requirements were collected. Paper Prototyping was used as a method for manual user tests of surface designs and interaction processes of the program to be developed. The requirements were classified in functional (F) and non-functional requirements (NF). The main requirements are seperated into the a user interface for the study director and a test interface for the children. Collected requirements of the user interface for the study director are: setting stimuli parameters (F), window with check-boxes and text-fields to set the stimuli parameters (NF), code should be able to calculate stimuli on the basis of the given parameters (F) and implementation of a participant ID so that nobody can refer their test results to their personal data (F). The requirements of the user interface for the children are: play a stimulus list in a randomized order (F), interactive game interface with buttons (NF), child-fiendly interface with neutral game character (NF), start the test with a given button on the screen (F), implement motivating feature (e.g. progress bar, collecting points) in order to increase motivation (NF).

2.3.2 Stimulus

First the necessary toolboxes, that enabled to load and to play audio data were implemented to Spyder. Spyder is a open-source environment for scientific programming, using the programming language python. For the reason to develop a user-friendly interface the study tutor should be able to change the stimulus parameters within a user-friendly window. First single stimuli were tested and verified by showing the data plot of the stimulus parameters and checking the visual data of the played stimulus. The audio was tested with headphones by the experimenter. CI-patients will get the stimuli via cable, directly on the implant.

2.3.3 Prototyping mini-game

Animations, Doodle Jump (an endless game, where the playing character "Doodle" jumps from one platform to another and collects points), Puzzle Game or collecting different fruit in a basket were collected as game ideas. The prototype shown in Fig. 1 corresponds to the development version 1.3. It shows a flying bee in front of an endless background by scrolling from right to left window border. At the bottom there are three buttons; one to get the stimulus and two buttons (left and right of the stimulus button) to enter the users' response.

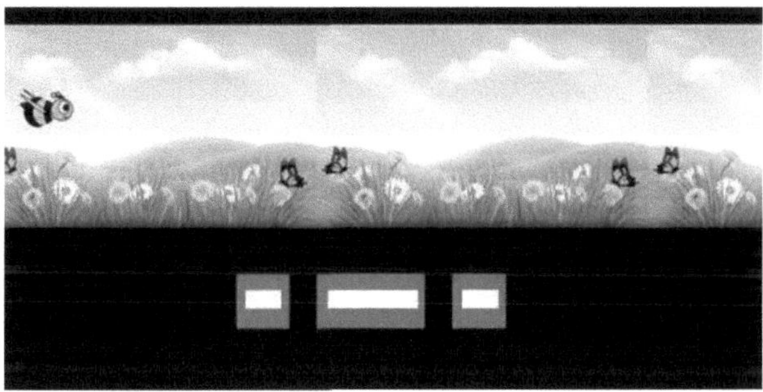

Figure 1: Prototype version 1.3 of the mini-game. The interface contains an animation with a bee as game character, a scrolling background and three interactive buttons. The button in the middle plays the sound. Button left and button right are used to enter the answer by the test person.

The assortment of the responses is shown in table 1. The game has two conditions: false response and a true response. Using the two-alternative-forced-choice (2AFC) method enabled to measure the sensitivity of a person or child. Therefore, the stimuli will be presented in a randomised order. The participant's choice is forced between the two alternatives/ buttons.

Table 1: The given relationship between condition and response is defined in the program code. The user's response is correct if button left was pressed after condition 1 of the stimulus was played.

Response	Condition 1	Condition 2
False	button left	button right
Right	button right	button left

To see if the participants' response was correct and to have a learning outcome, the bee collects points for motivation reasons. Moreover, it is described as a motivation for children to want to play the game again with reaching more points next time. The mini-game will use the stimuli list according to the participants hearing abilities. The list will be load into the game before starting the study-test. The data of the test should be saved in the corresponding folder for later analysing the results. Therefore, a folder structure was implemented where the stimulus parameters used and the corresponding test results will be automatically saved at the right folder with its corresponding file name. For data safety reasons the decision was made to create participants IDs, so that no one can later refer their test results to the personal data of a participant - apart from the head of the study team.

3   Results and Discussion

Before starting the participants test, the individual parameters need to be set by the study director. The user interface window (version 2.0) for the study director is shown in Fig. 2. According to the participants individual hearing ability seen in pre-acoustic-tests the stimulus list generated by filling out the text fields and clicking the submit-button. Pressing the submit button will save the stimulus list in the given test and study-group folder automatically. The title consists of a participant-ID so nobody can refer the testing information to the personal data of a participant. The reason for this are the requirements of the protection of data privacy.

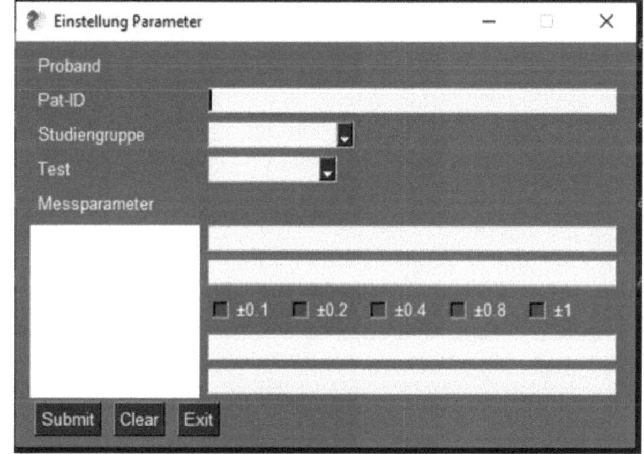

Figure 2: Version 2.0 of the user interface for the experimenter. The window allows entering the test parameters and anonymous assignment to the test person. In this way, an individual test list is created for each test person depending on their hearing ability.

The study tutor can load the corresponding and already prepared stimulus list of the participant before the test starts. The folder structure helps to find the right and already prepared stimulus list for each participant. The mini-game in Fig. 3 shows the version 1.5 of the mini-game.

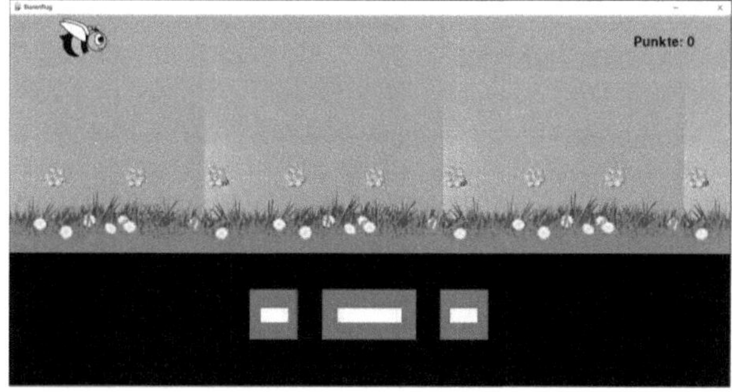

Figure 3: Version 1.5 of the mini-game. It contains a point system for motivating the test subjects by collecting honeycombs. In addition, it further contains the game character, scrolling background and interactive buttons. The final verion of the mini-game is ready to test.

On the left-hand side is the starting position of the game character and on the right-hand side the player can see the points he/she made. If the players answer is correct, the bee flies down to collect one honeycomb, the counter raises one point and the bee flies back to its top position. The stimuli-button is inactive if no answer is given yet. After five seconds it reminds the player to make a submission. After pressing one of the answer-button the stimuli-button is active again. The mini-game window for the participant runs until the test list has been played completely. The test list is presented in randomized order. After playing the last stimulus, the game window will close and the achieved score number is displayed to the study participant participant.

In order to improve the mini-game future developments could be implemented. One of the further development is to add different game characters that can be chosen by the participant due to meet children's individual interests (e.g. dinosaur, butterfly, and more). Another future development is the replacement of the counting points with a loading bar, that visualises the archived number. According to a unknown number of trials the number of reached points can get very high and not known to young children, especially under the age of six. One concern with the developed study design is, that participants with CI might not be able to fulfill the task due to their limited hearing ability. A solution could be the implementation of a just-noticeable-difference (JND) test. The JND-test could be performed as the very first test to detect if the participant is able to perform the main test.

Finally, the mini-game should be tested with normal hearing school-aged children and children with implanted CI. In order to carry out the user test with children, the ethical declaration shall be submitted at the latest before the autumn holidays. Starting the pre-test of the mini-game in the school holidays can simplify the recruitment because the children have free time, and also the testing can be done within one week. Tha aim of testing the study environment is to detect bugs in the programming codes or specify further developments which are nececcary to run the study test without any interruption by the program code or the study participant.

4   Conclusion

Summing up, the mini-game shall be tested to collect the childrens feedback and further improve the program code so the study environment will be ready to use. The programming code still misses specific data, which is necessary for testing the game with CI-participants. In the meantime, the participants - including normal hearing children and children implanted with CI - should be informed and acquired for the study. For finally using the programming code the mini-game should be free of any bugs and works without any problem report.

Acknowledgement

The work has been carried out at the University Hospital Freiburg and supervised by the Implant Centrum Freiburg. I also want to thank my colleagues who provided material for measurement and supported with their expertise.

Author's Statement

I declare that the research was conducted in the absence of any commercial or financial relationships that could be construed as a potential conflict of interest.
The research related to human use complies with all the relevant national regulations, institutional policies and was performed in accordance with the tenets of the Helsinki Declaration, and has been approved by the authors' institutional review board or equivalent committee.

5   References

[1] W. Szyfter, M. Karlik, A. Sekuła, S. Harris, and W. Gawęcki, "Current indications for cochlear implantation in adults and children.," *Otolaryngologia polska = The Polish otolaryngology*, vol. 73 3, pp. 1–5, 2019.

[2] J. King and J. Markant, "Selective attention to lesson-relevant contextual information promotes 3- to 5-year-old children's learning.," *Developmental science*, 2022.

[3] M. C. Frank, E. Sugarman, A. Horowitz, M. L. Lewis, and D. Yurovsky, "Using tablets to collect data from young children," *Journal of Cognition and Development*, vol. 17, pp. 1 – 17, 2016.

[4] J. M. Bosten, L. Álvaro, J. Alvarez, B. J. Meyer, T. Tang, J. Maule, and A. Franklin, "Tablet-based app for screening for cvd in young children," *Journal of Vision*, 2019.

[5] S. J. Coons, S. Eremenco, J. J. Lundy, P. O'Donohoe, H. O'Gorman, and W. Malizia, "Capturing Patient-Reported Outcome (PRO) Data Electronically: The Past, Present, and Promise of ePRO Measurement in Clinical Trials," *The Patient - Patient-Centered Outcomes Research*, vol. 8, pp. 301–309, Aug. 2015.

[6] C. K. Olson, "Children's motivations for video game play in the context of normal development," *Review of General Psychology*, vol. 14, pp. 180 – 187, 2010.

[7] L. Nagels, E. Gaudrain, D. Vickers, P. Hendriks, and D. Başkent, "School-age children benefit from voice gender cue differences for the perception of speech in competing speech," *Journal of the Acoustical Society of America*, vol. 149, pp. 3328 – 3344, May 2021.

[8] L. Nagels, E. Gaudrain, D. Vickers, M. Matos Lopes, P. Hendriks, and D. Başkent, "Development of vocal emotion recognition in school-age children: The EmoHI test for hearing-impaired populations," *PeerJ*, vol. 8, p. e8773, 2020.

Comparison of open and closed test setup for the Göttinger children speech understanding test

Theresa Günther [1], and Siegrid Meier [2]

[1] Auditory Technology, Universität zu Lübeck, theresa.guenther@student.uni-luebeck.de

[2] Akademie für Hörakustik, s.meier@afh-luebeck.de

Abstract

For carrying out a children speech understanding test, some tests are implemented either with provided pictures or as a word repetition task. Because differing implementations rely on different mechanisms, varying results are expected, which could lead to misdiagnosis. This suggestion is confirmed for adults, but not for children. Due to language development processes results might differ. The investigation examined data from nine children tested with closed and open set procedures of the German Göttinger children speech test. The results confirmed the hypothesis that the performance in closed and open set measurement differs. Variations between the tests did not correlate with age, gender, familiarity of words, hearing threshold or order of closed and open set measurement. The results show that the interpretation of the results of children speech understanding tests is of great importance and that a careful documentation of the used procedure is essential to avoid misinterpretations.

1 Introduction

A main task of speech audiometry is to examine speech intelligibility in quiet and in noise. The speech hearing threshold, the speech intelligibility threshold or the number/percentage of correctly understood words is determined [1]. Especially for children in respect of language development, knowing about the status of language development is essential [2]. Problems with the interpretation of tests containing the task of repeating speech can occur in the case of articulation disorders [2]. Apart from phonetic disorders, phonological disorders can also be present in the form of phonematic discrimination weaknesses or expressive disorders. As a variance of changes in articulation are typical for children of young age [3], typically developed, physiologically hearing children could repeat a correctly heard word untypically, so that the result of speech audiometry would mislead with regards to the cause of the test results.

In order to prevent these problems, speech understanding tests can avoid expressive language by a choice of pictures [2]. However, by prescribing answer options by means of pictures, only part of the input has to be discriminated auditorily, which makes the task easier [2].

For both test versions, the familiarity of the used words and pictures plays an important role [2]. If words are not familiar or the layout of a picture is not recognised for what it was supposed to represent, the repetition or choosing of the correct response can be impaired. Therefore material appropriate for the target group has to be chosen (e.g. [4], [5]). The influence of familiarity of vocabulary is

of particular importance for delayed children in respect of language and/or mental development and/or of the multilingual population, as the mental lexicon can differ compared to typically monolingually developed children [1]. Multilingual children growing up with both languages simultaneously perform better, worse or at the same level in terms of phonology compared to monolingual peers [1]. At the same time, the lexicon of only one language is smaller [1]. In respect of test setting, a minor performance in closed setting could be expected for children of small mental lexicon, while good phonological awareness might cause better performance repeating a word without knowing its meaning. This could especially hold true for multilingual children.

Finally, the results are not comparable with the open implementation due to a guessing probability depending on the selection set [2]. When comparing closed and open administration of a test of word comprehension with pictures, it was found that open administration always produced worse results than closed administration for monolingual adults [6]. Furthermore, performance decreased with the number of distractors and their similarity to the target word [6]. According to [6] different processes are involved in recognising what is heard in closed and open tests, so they urge caution when comparing performance. However this finding holds true for adult participants. An assumption about the practises with children are not drawn.

According to the 2013 guideline for peripheral hearing loss in childhood published by the German association for phoniatrics and pediatric audiology, one of the suitable speech understanding tests for children is the Göttinger children speech understanding test (GCST) I and II [2]. Practical expertise as well as research shows that GCST is carried out either with open or closed set (e.g. [4], [7]). Also in the guideline for peripheral hearing loss in childhood, the handling of open or closed procedure is not instructed [2]. For this reasons it should be investigated whether there are discrepancies between different test administrations. Furthermore correlations of possible differences and other factors should be analysed.

2　Material and Methods

2.1　Participants

A post hoc analysis with data from the German Akademie für Hörakustik, which teaches the national wide pediatric hearing professionals training, was conducted. Within the practical training the hearing status of children is tested. As both closed and open set method of speech tests are carried out, these information were used to compare the performance of the children. For further data about language status etc. the anamnesis material, hearing status and word production results of preparing the children for the test were used. The total sum of children participating in the training was 24, whereby only 12 children were old enough for speech audiometry. Due to information out of the documentation three children had to be excluded of the analysis because of refusing to cooperate, a differing method of testing or the use of both GCST I and II. Consequently the data of nine children could be used for further analysis. The age of the analysed children ranged from 3.08 years to 5.75 years (mean: 4.56 years, standard deviation (sd): 1.25 years). The six youngest children were tested using the GCST I, the three older with test II. All children grew up in a monolingual German home. The data of five boys and four girls were evaluated. One child wore bilateral hearing aids. Pure tone average 4 (PTA4) (0.5 kHz, 1 kHz, 2 kHz, 4 kHz) for the child was administered with hearing aids. PTA4 over all children was 11.6 dB HL with a sd of 5.9 dB HL. These levels are rated as typical in respect of the age of the children [2].

2.2　Material

As mentioned, the GCST I and II is an approved tool to test speech understanding for children [2]. GCST I is designed for children between three years and four years, whereas test II is for children of age five years to six years [4], [5]. The items are considered as age-appropriate for the target groups with reference to Kamratowski and Meißner (1971) quoted in [4], [5]. Both tests consist of ten lists each with ten items. Test I contains 20 monosyllabic words, test II 100. For closed set testing a choice of four items is used as visualised in Fig. 1.

The test's concept is to include the same vowel for all four pictures in closed administration [4], [5]. Because for open test setting words need to be repeated orally, an analysis was done to investigate how appropriate items are with respect to children's pronunciation typical for their age. Therefore

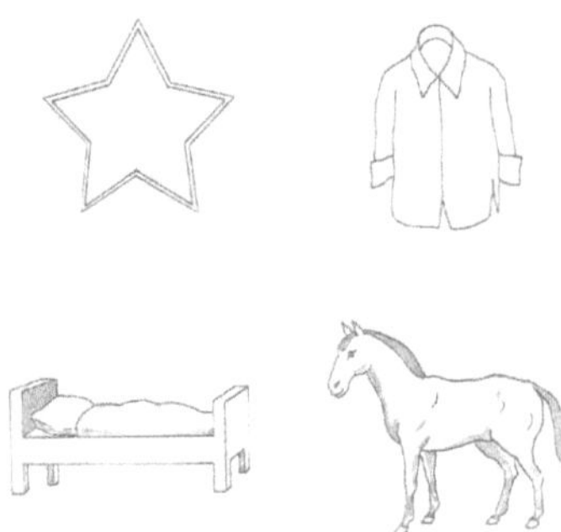

Figure 1: Example for closed set item presentation of GCST I; star, shirt, bed, horse (German: Stern, Hemd, Bett, Pferd

the age of physiological acquisition of the phonemes of the items was determined by using the work of [3]. Subsequently a conclusion was drawn on the percentage of the children at the age of the recommended patients would be expected to articulate the items correctly.

2.3　Procedure

For all testing situations there were two trainees testing one child. Consequently every child was tested by different professionals. Firstly an anamnesis was conducted. Secondly the hearing threshold was elicited by play audiometry. For five children headphones were used (mean PTA4 = 7.38), for four children it was conducted in free field (PTA = 16.88). Thirdly speech audiometry was administered. In the beginning children therefore should name the items to make sure familiarity and to notice pronunciation difficulties for the specific vocabulary. Afterwards either closed or open set administration was tested, followed by the other test setting. Both methods should include at least one list. Mostly this was conducted in free field (8/9). One child was tested wearing head phones. For eight out of nine children the level of 65 dB SPL for both test settings was reported. Optionally objective measures were conducted. Tympanometry was carried out for 6/9 children and distortion product otoacoustic emission for 2/9 children.

2.4　Statistical methods

For statistical measures RStudio 4.1.1 was used. For determining the data's distribution, the Anderson-Darling-test was used. To compare the performance of the children in closed and open set testing the Wilcoxon signed-rank test was chosen as it compares non-parametric paired samples. For the non paired analysis of the test differences of GCST I and II the Wilcoxon-Mann-Whitney-Test was performed. Furthermore the analysis of correlation was conducted. Therefore the rank correlation test by Spearman for non-parametric paired data was used. The correlation between the test differences and age, order of test type, gender, tone hearing level and naming of pictures was calculated.

3   Results and Discussion

3.1   Analysis of the items of GCST I and II

The criterion used by [3] to analyse typical phonological development of children was that children grouped by age (window of half a year) performed two out of three realisations of a phoneme correctly. Consequently information is given, at which age 75 % or 90 % of children realise two out of three of a certain phoneme correctly.

Looking at the items of the GCST I and comparing the speech capability of the youngest target group (beginning with 3 years), the following results appear: 90 % of the youngest children are able to pronounce arm, horse and head (German: Arm, Pferd, Kopf), while only 75 % are expected to perform shoe, table, star and fish (German: Schuh, Tisch, Stern, Fisch) correctly. The remaining 13 words reached the 90 % criterion for all phonemes for children younger than the target group and therefore are expected to be pronounced correctly by more than 90 % of the target group. While for arm, horse and head the 90 % criterion only is reached for the youngest children (3 years to 3.5 years), for shoe, table, star and fish the 90 % criterion is just reached for the oldest children (4.5 years to 5 years). In conclusion for the youngest target group only 75 % of the children are expected to pronounce correctly all the items of GCST I. For GCST II more than 90 % of the children are expected to have acquired all needed phonemes for the used items even in the youngest target group (5 years to 5.5 years). Therefore no hindrance due to typical phonology is expected.

The results from naming pictures beforehand of the speech test show that children, the GCST I had been used for, named 92 % of the words correctly. The documentation showed nevertheless that the majority of 13/14 wrong naming was due to uncertain pictures and lexical difficulties hence not due to phonological problems. The assumption that test items' phonology was too difficult cannot be supported by the data. Nevertheless because of post hoc analysis and not a speech and language therapist documenting, it cannot be made sure that items have been counted correctly when understandable even though wrongly pronounced. This would not be consistent with the test instruction, as already uncertain responses should be counted wrong [4].

The clarity and familiarity of words and pictures should be questioned looking at the results. Also it is questionable, whether items still are suitable as the estimations of applicability by the GCST refers to the year 1971 (Kamratowski and Meißner, 1971, quoted in [4], [5]). Nevertheless analysis showed that only two out of 14 initially wrong named words were incorrectly chosen or repeated in the test. The conclusion could be drawn that unspecific pictures could be introduced well enough before the test, so that there was no clear difficulty recognising the pictures. As the acquisition of words is not always done by only naming a picture once, the difficulties in naming are assumed to be due to uncertain choice of pictures and not because of a minor mental lexicon [9].

The earlier described characteristic of equivalent vowels for each set of four pictures was criticized by [8]. According to [8] vowels do not match correctly, because short and long vowels are well distinguishable. For example items from Fig. 1 include [ɛ] as well as [e] (star: German Stern [ʃtɛrn], shirt: German Hemd [hɛmt], bed: German Bett [bɛt], horse: German Pferd [pfeːɐt]).

3.2   Comparison of open and closed administration of GCST I and II

Fig. 2 shows the results of GCST I and II for closed and open test administration. The Anderson-Darling-test for

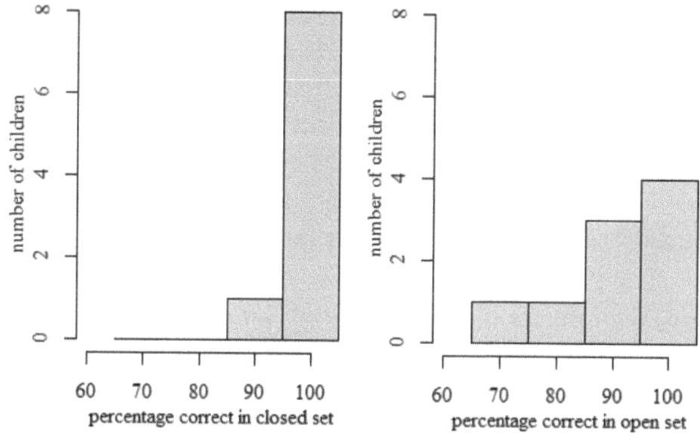

Figure 2: Histograms of the results from GCST of nine children performing closed set (left) and open set (right) implementation

normal distribution was used for the sum of children the GCST I and II had been used for because of the small sample size. It showed that closed and open set results distributions were neglected to be normally distributed (closed: $p < .001$, open: $p = .047$). The same holds true for the calculated differences between closed and open set testing ($p = .009$). In Fig. 2 it can be seen that especially for closed set testing a ceiling effect dominates the distribution. To check for differences between test administrations the Wilcoxon signed-rank test for two-tailed hypothesis was conducted. Again the whole sample of GCST I and II was examined together. A significant better performance in closed set testing was found with a strong effect size ($p = .048$, $r = .95$) [10]. Neither for the data of GCST I ($n = 6$) nor for the data of test II ($n = 3$) alone significant differences between closed and open administration were found (I: $p = .17$, II: $p = .35$). Ultimately the differences between closed and open set were calculated for GCST I and II. These differences were compared using the Wilcoxon-Mann-Whitney-Teste and did not differ significantly between GCST I and II.

Significant differences between closed and open administration confirm the findings of [6]. The suggestion that open set administration could lead to better results than closed set, can not be confirmed. As this suggestion was made especially for multilingual children and no children were found to be multilingual a generalisation of the study's results for this target group could be misleading.

To check for linear correlations the rank correlation test of Spearman was used. All comparisons were conducted to the calculated difference of test results between test administrations. Neither age ($p = .93$), order (first open or closed set) ($p = .17$), gender ($p = .62$), correct naming of the pictures before testing ($p = .97$), nor (aided) hearing level ($p = .2$) correlated significantly with differences between open and closed set testing. Results concerning hearing level can be criticised due to different adminstration methods (headphones or free field) and the high sd (mean: 11.6 dB HL, sd: 5.9 dB HL).

The major critical aspect of this investigation is the small sample size. Calculations only can be carried out with the whole sample size including children who were tested with GCST I and children assessed with GCST II. A separate investigation would have been useful, because beginning with the age of 5 years more than 90 % of the children are expected to pronounce phonemes correctly, the influence of language development is expected to be larger for the GCST I children. Additionally the items differ between the tests so that lexical influence might vary as well.

Another point of criticism is the procedure of a post hoc analysis. As no direct instructions of the trainees by the research team took place and documentation might be incomplete and influenced by subjectivity, missing data might mislead this investigation. Additional support for children by attending parents or trainees cannot be excluded.

Guessing probability impedes the comparison of closed and open set additionally. While in general open set testing of GCST reveals a probability of 25 % for each item to be chosen correctly, open set testing would have a negligible guess probability. For this study guess probability nevertheless might have a minor influence, because all target items had been shown and were to name before the test started. As far as the items were remembered correctly, they could have formed sort of an interior set of possible answers that would have served as a pool for guessing. In that case, for open testing the guess probability would have been 5 % for the first word when remembered all items. For the following words, probability would increase. Guessing probability would not be the same as for closed set, but still be higher than without introducing the items.

4 Conclusion

For monolingual children with normal (aided) hearing threshold better results were found for closed than for open set administration of GCST I and II. Therefore a careful documentation and taking into account the method of testing is essential to avoid misdiagnosis, because better results with closed administration are expected for this target group. Additionally for future testing naming of the pictures before testing is recommended, so that unknown vocabulary or unspecific pictures can be explained and knowledge about the language development is gained. For other target groups such as multilingual, hearing or language impaired children, we recommend further investigations of useful test settings.

Acknowledgement

The work has been carried out and supervised by Akademie für Hörakustik, Germany.

Author's Statement

Authors state no conflict of interest.

5 References

[1] V. Hoffmann and K. Schäfer, *Kindliche Hörstörungen. Diagnostik - Versorgung - Therapie.* Springer, Praxiswissen Logopädie, Berlin, 2020.

[2] Deutsche Gesellschaft für Phoniatrie und Pädaudiologie, *S2k-Leitlinie: Periphere Hörstörungen im Kindesalter. -Langfassung-.* 2013.

[3] A. V. Fox-Boyer, I. Groos and K. SchauSS-Golecki, *Kindliche Aussprachestörungen. Phonologischer ErwerbDifferenzialdiagnostikTherapie.* Schulz-Kirchner Verlag, Idstein, vol. 7, 2016.

[4] R. Chilla, P. Gabriel, P. Kozielski, D. Bänsch and M. Kabas, *Göttinger Kindersprachverständnistest I. Sprachaudiometrie des "Kindergarten"- und retardierten Kindes mit einem Einsilber-Bildtest.* HNO, 24, pp. 342–346, 1976.

[5] P. Gabriel, R. Chilla, C. Kiese, M. Kabas and D. Bänsch, *Göttinger Kindersprachverständnistest II. Sprachaudiometrie des Vorschulkindes mit einem Einsilber-Bildtest.* HNO, 24, pp. 399–402, 1976.

[6] C. G. Clopper, *Effects of open-set and closed-set task demands on spoken word recognition.* Journal of the American academy of audiology, vol. 17, no. 5, pp. 331–349, 2006.

[7] S. Zichner, K. Berger and P. Mir-Salim, *Zusammenhang zwischen Ergebnissen aus Sprachentwicklungs- und sprachaudiometrischen Testverfahren bei hörgeschädigten Kindern.* 18. Multidisziplinäres Kolloquium der GEERS-Stiftung, 21, 2016.

[8] K. Kliem and B. Kollmeier, *Überlegung eines Zweisilber-Kinder-Reimtests für die klinische Audiologie.* Audiologische Akustik, vol. 34, no. 1, pp. 6–10, 1995.

[9] S. Sachse, A.-K. Bockmann and A. Buschmann, *Sprachentwicklung. Entwicklung - Diagnostik - Förderung im Kleinkind- und Vorschulalter.* Springer-Verlag, Berlin, 2020.

[10] J. Cohen, *Statistical power analysis.* Current directions in psychological science, vol. 1, no. 3, pp. 98–101, 1992.

2

Biomedical Engineering

Benchmarking of surgical lights

Ibrahim Alhasan

Medical Engineering Science, Universität zu Lübeck, ibrahim.alhasan@student.uni-luebeck.de

Abstract

Operating theatres and medical equipment have evolved over time to support the surgeons work to help people and save their lives with little risk. Therefore, special hygiene regulations are applied to the operating theatre in accordance with the Infection Protection Act. The medical equipment is placed close to and above the wound, so the system must be easy to clean and disinfect. The surface temperature is important for laminar airflow in the operating room, because the compatibility or ventilation resistance of the operating room lights in relation to the ventilation ceilings for laminar airflow depends on the surface temperature. This paper includes benchmarking and characteristics of ceiling-mounted surgical lights with focus on hygiene and surface temperature, and these characteristics were studied on five different luminaires.

1 Introduction

There are many operating room luminaires companies that offer surgical lights with different designs and features, but do these luminaires meet the requirements of hygiene in the operating room and what more is expected from the luminaires? One of the most common problems in the operating room is that the surgeon does not have enough light in the operating field, so that they have to change the direction of the operating light with their sterilized hands from time to time. Therefore, it is necessary to examine, what problems the surgeon may encounter, when changing the position of the luminaires and what problems may apply to the luminaires when used in the operating room.

Five surgical lights were examined: Polaris 600, marLED® X, HyLED X9, merivaara Q-FLOW and Steris XLED®3.

2 Material and Methods

Surgeries place the highest demands on doctors and medical staff. The supplementary standard IEC 60601-2-41 regulates general safety requirements, tests, and guidelines for surgical and examination lamps. However, the purpose of the standard is to describe basic safety characteristics and tests and give instructions for their application.

To achieve optimal visual acuity for the human eye, the illuminance of the surgical lamp must be high enough to reflect sufficient light despite the high light absorption of the human tissue. An adjustable color temperature between 3,000 and 6,700 K, natural color rendering index more than 90 and high illumination level makes the work of surgeons easier, creates safety and reduces possible sources of error [1].

To ensure high visual performance, the IEC 60601-2-41 lists e.g., the requirements for surgical luminaires to provide 40,000 to 160,000 lux illuminances in the operating field for a high central illuminance at a distance of 1 m [2]. For comparison, the daylight provides 100,000 lux on a sunny day with clear sky.

2.1 Surface temperature measurement

The surface temperature of each light was measured at different points where the medical staff could possibly touch the luminaire during the operation. The luminaires were left in operation for seven hours in order to detect possible heat development of the luminaire body. visual ir thermometer vt02 was used to determine the six hottest spots and the temperature sensors were glued to these six spots: two on the surface, two on the handle and two on the closing glass. The temperature was measured for about four hours (the measurement is started where the temperature has remained constant).

2.2 Hygienic aspects

High hygienic requirements prevail in operating rooms, such as protection against germs, bacteria and dust, not only for personnel, ventilation and air conditioning, but also for the equipment used. The design of the operating room lamp and low surface temperatures are important for hygienic aspects and the laminar air flow in the operating room because a simple design ensures fast and safe disinfection while minimally obstructing the laminar air flow and preventing the spread of airborne bacteria [3]. The following features can help the devices perform well regarding the hygienic aspects of the luminaires:

1. round design without sharp edges and overhangs, smooth surfaces without recesses and niches, because the smooth surface facilitates cleaning, improving hygiene
2. good accessibility of surfaces and covered cable channels
3. Camera behind glass and easy assembly and disassembly of the sterilizable handle

3   Results and Discussion

For a surgical luminaire, several criteria should be taken into account, such as the uniformity of illumination, illuminance, the size of the illuminated area and color temperature. The five surgical lights considered have the following technical characteristics (the date are given at a distance of 1 m) [4] - [7]:

Table 1: Technical characteristics of the five surgical lights

Technical characteristic	Maximal illuminance level	Size of the illuminated area	Color temperature	Color rendering index Ra
Polaris 600	160,000 Lux	190 - 280 mm	3,800 - 5,600 K	95
marLED X	160,000 Lux	140 - 350 mm	3,000 - 5,500 K	99
HyLED	160,000 Lux	140 - 320 mm	3,500 - 5,100 K	97
Q-FLOW	160,000 Lux	200 - 320 mm	3,700 - 5,100 K	98
XLED®3	160,000 Lux	250 - 300 mm	4,400 K	95

3.1   Compare the differences of temperature measurement from the light head

The sensors were glued to the six surfaces mentioned, and connected to a data logger (Almemo 5690-2) for measurement data acquisition. The data logger outputs a measurement every half minute, and based on the measurement data were displayed the following diagrams (Fig. 1 and 2). The diagrams 1 and 2 show the difference in surface temperature between the five luminaires on the middle surface and on the handle. The middle surface area is important for laminar airflow in the operating room. This is because the compatibility and respectively the ventilation resistance of the operating room luminaires in relation to the ventilation ceilings for laminar air flow is mainly dependent on two factors:

The surface temperature and the projection surface in conjunction with the geometry of the luminaire body. The lower the surface temperature, the lower the interference. Therefore, LED technology with low heat generation is preferable.

Regarding the shape of the luminaire, attention should be paid to a geometry that is favorable to flow with an appropriate projection surface.

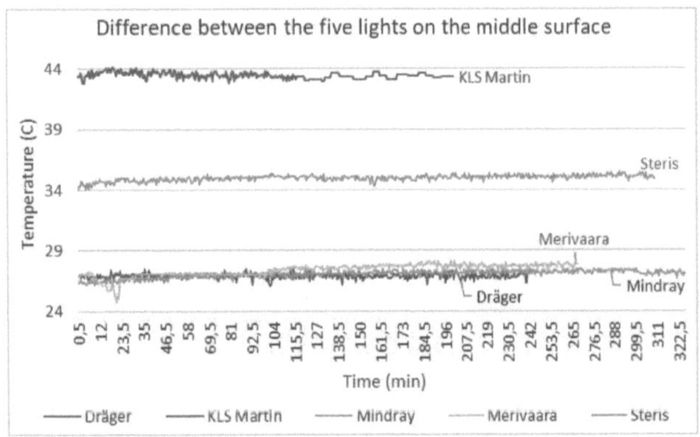

Figure 1: Difference between the five lights on the middle surface

The different design of the luminaire and the aluminum die-cast material leads to different temperatures on the surface. The die-cast aluminum material holds the heat and distributes it through the heat sink, this produces less temperature rise in the working area. To help lower the temperature of the light an increased surface area of the lumiere can increase the heat exchange with the environment. The temperature rises of the surgical lights result from power dissipation during the conversion of electrical energy into ("visible" and "invisible") light. In the process the luminaire body heats up and the radiation is absorbed by the tissues. This causes the exposed tissues (surgical field and surgeon's head) to heat up. A controllable lower heat input of the light can already have a meaningful effect on the temperature of the surgeon's head area, ensuring more comfortable work during long operations.

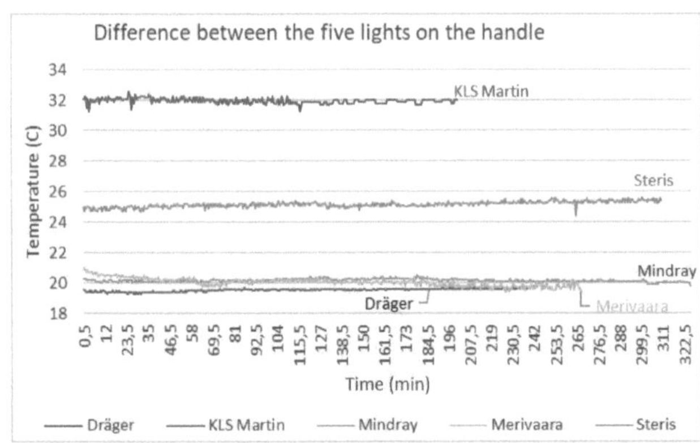

Figure 2: Difference between the five lights on the handle

The handle is very often touched by the surgeon during the operation to change the position of the lamp, therefore a comfortable temperature of the handle ensures a pleasant work.

3.2   Better hygiene and protection types of the luminaire

The luminaires must also meet the high safety and hygiene standards, because nowhere in the hospital is protection against germs and contaminants as important as in the operating room. For easy and hygienic cleaning, luminaires with international protection class IP 42 [1], IP 54 [2] or IP 65 [3] are recommended to protect the luminaires against the ingress of liquids, dust and ensure a thorough disinfection [8]. The five lights have different IP class: Polaris and XLED with IP42, HyLED X9 with IP54 and Q-FLOW with IP65.

In order to increase the hygienic aspects, some well-designed surgical lights, such as Polaris 600 and marLED®X, offer easy operation via a sensor system in the handle. This innovative sensor system in the handle of the luminaire enables the OR staff to position the luminaire body in a sterile manner during surgery and to adjust the light field size as well as the illuminance.

In the figures below (Fig. 3) as can be seen a photo of the Polaris 600, which has a round design without edges and overhangs and Smooth surfaces to make disinfection easier and faster and the other two surgical lights (KLS Martin and Mindray) are also offers a similar design.

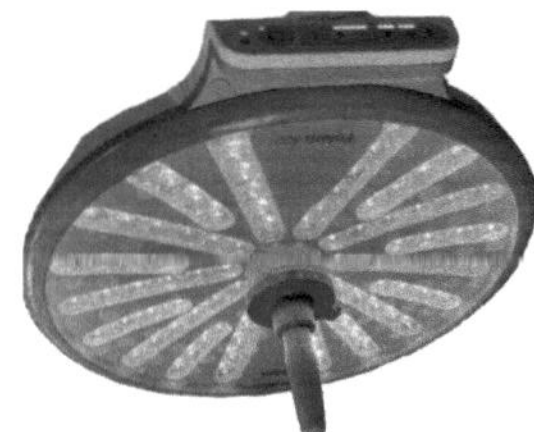

Figure 3: polaris 600

Merivaara has a circular design which sits concentric in the center of a ring shaped luminaire head (Q-FLOW; see Fig. 4) [6]. Steris also offers a similar design (HarmonyAIR). Alternatively they offer a design which consists of two to four luminaire heads mounted side by side (XLED). These designs are optimised for air laminar flow, but this makes cleaning more difficult, because the luminaire have gaps between the heads.

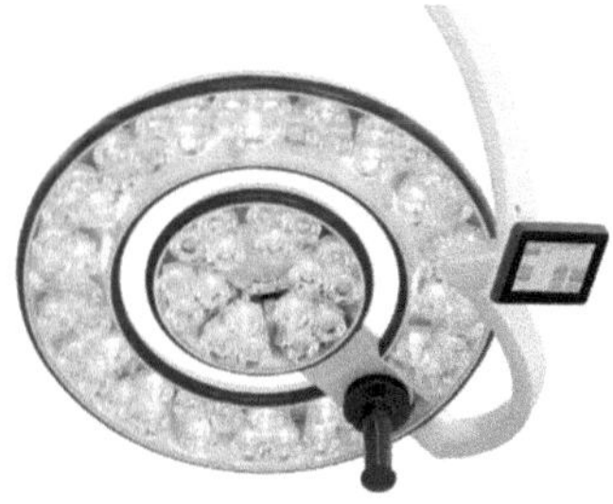

Figure 4: Q-FLOW

The operating lights can have non-sterile and sterile handles that are used to positioning the light. The two of the five available lights (Polaris 600 and marLED X) have a non-sterile handle on the outside of the light head. The handle

was thought in case during the operation the non-sterile staff also wants to adjust the light without violating the hygienic aspects.

The sterilizable handle is located in each operation light in the center of the light head, that the sterile personnel (surgeon) used to adjust the light. The sterilizable handle is the only element of the light head that sterile personnel may touch on the basis of hygienic aspects. It is removed after surgery, cleaned, sterilized and reused. Alternatively, as with the Polaris 600, a sterile disposable surgical handle may be used, which is discarded after surgery.

4 Conclusion

The energy-efficient LED technology and the placement of components for optimal heat distribution within the luminaire can reduce heat generation and power consumption. A surgical light is placed close to and above the wound field, which is a very critical area of the OR.

Therefore, the system must be easy to clean and disinfect. Design criteria for this are: a completely closed housing, no visible screws, smooth surfaces, disinfectant-resistant material, no rough edges and no acute angles. The optimal position of a camera is behind the light glass for easy wipe disinfection without edges to clean.

However, in the case of luminaires used in operating theatres, ribbed surfaces are not permitted, as should be easy to clean and among other things, uncontrollable liquids and dust formation must be avoided. So the operating room light must have an appropriate design for hygiene and temperature.

All of the five luminaires meet the most important requirements, such as illuminance, color temperature and hygienic aspects, in advantage the three luminaires (Polaris 600, Q-FLOW and HyLED X9) show significantly lower temperature than the other two in the six temperature measurements. In terms of hygienic aspects, the Polaris 600 has an easy to clean surface, which is in advantage. The non-sterile handle is also great advantage, so many hygienic aspects would not be violated, due to the lowest measuring temperature and the strongly promoted hygiene, the Polaris 600 is best suited for the operating room.

The next trends of the operating room lights of the future are likely to be with voice control and gesture recognition to simplify the work of surgeons and nurses.

With voice control, a microphone is used as a sound sensor and connected to voice software to replace button or display presses for operations such as changing the light intensity or the light field with voice commands. Multiple sound sensors can be built to increase detection accuracy and response speed, but there are many challenges such as minimizing background noise, eliminating erroneous commands, and coping with accent and dialect.

With gesture recognition, the light can be controlled by hand movement. For testing, a depth camera takes many images to define the optimal lamp position. The lamp position from the depth image can be divided into four steps:
1. Filter the input image

---

[1] A product with IP44 is protected against the ingress of solid foreign bodies larger than 1mm and against splashing water from all directions.

[2] If a product has an IP54 rating, it has full protection against accidental contact, with a small amount of dust entering. In addition, it is protected against splashing water from all directions.

[3] A product with protection class IP65 has full protection against accidental contact. Dust cannot penetrate and it is protected against water jets from any direction.

2. Find the target to be illuminated
3. Calculate an occlusion map
4. Analyze and identify obstacles

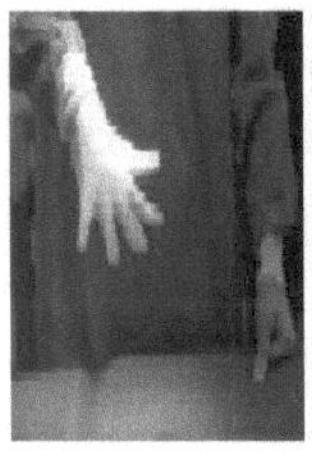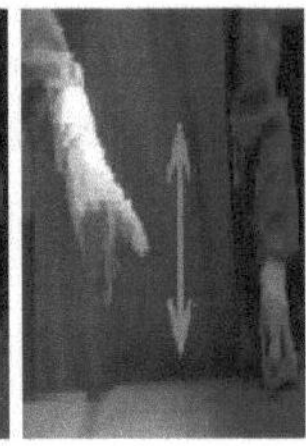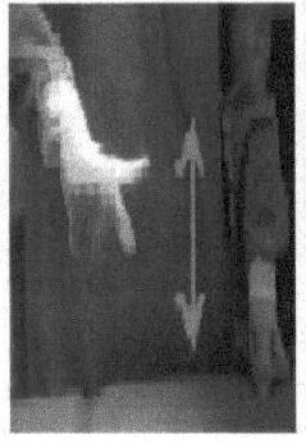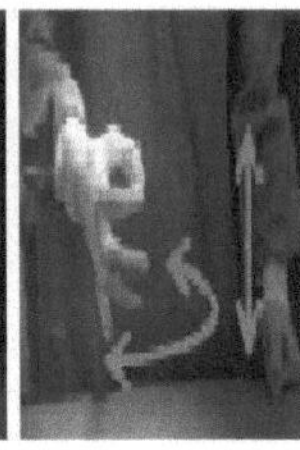

Figure 5: Gesture control of the lamp by hand

The figure 5 shows how this idea of gesture recognition could work, and which commands the system could understand. Gesture and speech recognition are still a research area and are being worked on under the so-called Robotics of the Future [9].

Acknowledgement

The work has been carried out at Drägerwerk AG & Co. KGaA, Lübeck and supervised by Stefanie Hofmann, Head of Medical Lights and Video Systems at Dräger and Prof. Maik Rahlves, Institute of BMO, Universität zu Lübeck. The author is grateful for the reviewer's valuable comments that improved the work.

Author's Statement

Stefanie Hofmann and Prof. Maik Rahlves have supported Ibrahim Alhasan in the work. Conflict of interest: Authors state no conflict of interest.

5   References

[1] Dräger 2022 Lübeck, *Hospital/Medical-Lights*. Available: https://www.draeger.com [last accessed on 2023-01-03].

[2] *Medical electrical equipment - Part 2-41*. In IEC 60601-2-41, 2021.

[3] Külpmann, P. D.-I. *German Society of Hospital Hygiene*. Krankenhaushygienische Leitlinie für die Planung, Ausführung und den Betrieb von Raumlufttechnischen Anlagen in Räumen des Gesundheitswesens. PP. 519 – 525, 2015.

[4] KLS Martin Group, *marLED®X Operating lights*. Available: https://www.klsmartin.com/de/produkte/operationsleuchten/, 2020.

[5] Mindray, *HyLED X9 LED Surgical Lights*. Technical specifications. Available: www.mindray.com, 2019.

[6] Merivaara Q-Flow, *surgical lights*. Technical Specifications Available: www.merivaara.com, 2017.

[7] Steris XLED, *Surgical Lighting*. Available: https://www.steris.com/healthcare/products/surgical-lights-and-examination-lights/surgical-lights.

[8] *Degrees of protection provided by enclosures (IP Code)*. In DIN EN 60529, 2014.

[9] Armin Dietz, Stephan Schröder, Andreas Pösch, Klaus Frank and Eduard Reithmeier *Contactless Surgery Light Control based on 3D*. Institute of Measurement and Automatic Control Leibniz Universität Hannover, Hannover, Germany. PP. 138 – 142, 2016.

Assembly of an Electrochemical Biosensor for the Detection of Tau Protein

Olesya Kostyuk [1], Felismina Moreira [2], and Yuselis Guerrero [3]

[1] Medical Engineering Science, Universität zu Lübeck, olesya.kostyuk@student.uni-luebeck.de
[2] BioMark, Instituto Superior de Engenharia do Porto, ftm@isep.ipp.pt
[3] BioMark, Instituto Superior de Engenharia do Porto, ycastano87@gmail.com

Abstract

Based on the discovery of the correlations between Alzheimer's disease (AD) and atypically phosphorylated Tau protein, a molecularly imprinted polymer (MIP) based electrochemical biosensor was to be developed. MIPs were directly assembled on screen-printed gold electrodes, with L-Cysteine (L-Cys) as the monomer of choice and Tau383 as the target analyte. The cyclic voltammetry (CV) based electropolymerization of L-Cys in the presence of Tau ensured the creation of a polymeric layer, around the Tau. The extraction of the protein with proteinase K, made the polymerized L-Cys serve as a form of plastic antibody, to prevent the use of expensive conventional antibodies. However, the rebinding attempts of the protein with the polymer, were unpromising as the carried out electrochemical impedance spectroscopy and CV-measurements did not show the expected results, since a significant distinction between the MIPs and the non-imprinted polymers (NIPs) was not observed.

1　Introduction

One of the most common neurodegenerative disorders is Alzheimer's disease (AD) causing deficits such as cognitive and functional limitations, accompanied by changes in behavior [1]. Even though the latter clinical symptoms usually do not occur before the age of 65 years, AD can progress asymptomatically decades before the loss of cognitive functions such as memory loss [2]. Therefore an early diagnosis is necessary to provide early treatment.

In this instance, multiple biomarkers have good prerequisites to be used for diagnostic purposes, one of which being phosphorylated Tau protein (p-Tau). Tau protein is atypically phosphorized in the brains of AD patients, causing neuronal dysfunctions, synaptic impairments, and neurofibrillary tangles [3]-[5]. The phosphorization of Tau protein occurs early in the course of the disease. In addition, former studies show promising results in terms of sensitivity and specificity, distinguishing between p-Tau levels for patients with AD and non-AD subjects [6]. Therefore Tau is suitable to be used as a biomarker for the following studies. A suitable apparatus for the detection of such biomarkers are biosensors. To be specific, electrochemical biosensors were used in the course of this work. Electrochemical biosensors produce an electrical signal when the targeted analyte reacts with biological components like antibodies. Depending on the concentration of the analyte, changes in the signal can be observed [7]. In this case, the targeted analyte is Tau protein. Considering the high costs of this method of biological recognition using antibodies, an alternative has to be introduced to ensure a diagnostic technique,

that has promising conditions to be applied in clinical routine [8]. For this instance, the utilization of plastic antibodies based on molecularly imprinted polymers (MIPs), is an auspicious alternative to the use of conventional antibodies. MIPs create a kind of artificial antibody, using a template molecule to assemble around, forming a recognition element specifically for the used molecule. For this purpose the targeted molecules get embedded into a monomer solution, causing the formation of a mantle around the molecules through the initiation of polymerization. By removing the template molecules cavities in the polymer are formed, recognizing only the used molecules. To initiate a successful creation of MIPs, a suitable monomer has to be chosen [9]. In this matter, L-Cysteine was the monomer of choice in this study.

2　Material and Methods

2.1　Equipment and Electrodes

Screen-printed electrodes (SPEs) (Dropsens DRP-250AT) with a gold ink working electrode with a diameter of 4 mm, a platinum auxiliary electrode and a silver reference electrode in a ceramic strip were used in this work. All electrochemical measurements were performed with a Metrohm Autolab potentiostat/ galvanostat and controlled with the software Nova 2.1.5. The connection between the SPEs and the potentiostat/ galvanostat was given by a suitable switch box coupling the electrical contacts of the SPE with the electrical connections of the potentiostat/ galvanostat.

2.2 Reagents

For all purposes, laboratory-grade water was used and all chemicals were of analytical grade. Di-Sodium hydrogen phosphate dihydrate (Na_2HPO_4) and Sodium dihydrogen phosphate dihydrate (NaH_2PO_4) were purchased from Scharlau (Sentmenat, Spain). Kaliumhexacyanoferrat(III) ($K_3[De(CN)_6]$) and Potassium hexacyanoferrate (II) trihydrate ($K_4[Fe(CN)_6]$) were obtained from Riedel-deHaën (Seelze, Germany). L-Cysteiniumchlorid ($C_3H_8ClNO_2S$) was purchased from Merck (Darmstadt, Germany). Proteinase K, Glycerine and DL-dithiothreitol (DTT) from Sigma-Aldrich.

2.3 Solutions

The Phosphate-buffered saline (PBS) at 0.1 M and pH 5.8 was prepared with Sodium phosphate dibasic dihydrate (Na_2HPO_4) and Sodium phosphate monobasic monohydrate (NaH_2PO_4). A solution for electrochemical essays was prepared with 5 mM Potassium hexacyanoferrate II-3-hydrate ($H_4[Fe(CN)_6] * 3H_2O$) and Potassium hexacyanoferrate III ($K_3[Fe(CN)_6]$) at 5 mM in PBS buffer at pH 5.8. A cysteine solution at 1×10^{-2} M was also prepared in PBS buffer at pH 5.8 with 25 % glycerine and 0.004 % DTT.

2.4 Assembly of the Biosensor

Before any modification of the SPE, it has to be cleaned with pure ethanol (99 %) (Fig. 1A), to ensure the elimination of impurities. Imprinting of the protein on the working electrode (Fig. 1B) was done with cyclic voltammetry (CV) based polymerization, with a start potential of -0.2 V and an end-potential of 1.2 V. The scan rate is $50\,mVs^{-1}$ with 5 scan cycles. All three electrodes have to be covered with 80 µl of protein solution containing $0.01\,gL^{-1}$ of Tau and Cysteine with $1 \times 10^{-3}\,molL^{-1}$ in PBS buffer with a pH of 5.6. After the imprinting of the protein, the electrodes get gently washed with distilled water. Following, an incubation with Proteinase K for 2.5 hours takes place.

For this instance, Proteinase K is dissolved in PBS (pH 5.8) with a concentration of $500\,mg/mL$. This results in the removal of the protein as depicted in Fig. 1C. After the incubation time, the electrode must be washed again with distilled water and stored refrigerated until the next day. A stabilization process takes place through the incubation of PBS buffer for 30 minutes on the working electrode. After each incubation CV and Electrochemical impedance spectroscopy (EIS) based control measurements take place to monitor any changes. This process must be repeated until the last two control measurements overlap. Following the rebinding process is initiated (Fig. 1D), which allows the verification of the success of this procedure. It is performed by incubating 5 µl of the standard solutions on the working electrode for respectively 30 minutes, with an increase in the concentration of Tau in each incubation step. The changes between every step were observed by electrical measurements, for which 80 µl of iron solution was pipetted onto the electrodes. In this case EIS and a CV measurements were carried out between each step. All steps were equally carried out for MIPs as well as non-imprinted polymers (NIPs), while the latter was not imprinted with Tau. The amount of Tau in the Cysteine solution was replaced with PBS for the NIP.

2.5 Electrochemical Assays

The effects of the former described assembly of the biosensor were observed through EIS and CV measurements. These measurements were carried out with an iron solution containing $5\,mmol/L$ ($K_3[Fe(CN)_6]$) and $5\,mmol/L$ ($K_4[Fe(CN)_6]$) prepared in PBS buffer with a pH of 5.8. The CV measurements were carried out with a start potential of -0.4 V and an upper potential of 0.6 V. This measurement was performed with the number of scans set to 3 and a scan rate of 0.05 V/s. The EIS measurements were carried out with a first applied frequency of 1×10^5 Hz and the last applied frequency set to 0.1 Hz with 50 logarithmically distributed frequencies. The amplitude is set to 0.01 V with a sinusoidal wave type.

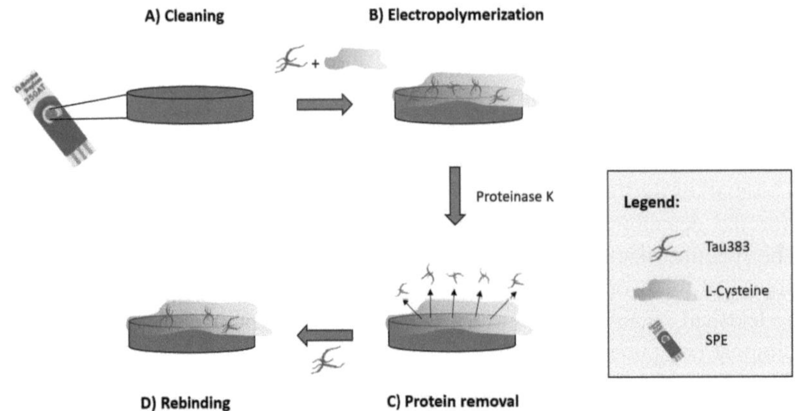

Figure 1: Schematic diagram of the steps in the assembly of a molecularly imprinted polymer based electrochemical biosensor, with Tau protein as the target analyte and L-Cysteine as the monomer of choice.

3 Results and Discussion

3.1 Electropolymerization and Imprinting

Before any modifications take place control measurements for two previously cleaned SPEs, intended to compare NIPs and MIPs, have to be conducted. After initiating the CV-based electropolymerization for 5 scans, a peak at 0.8 V was observed (Fig 2A). The current decreased continuously with every cycle. Higher current was measured for the MIP. Furthermore, an additional wider peak was observed at 1.00 V for the MIP and NIP. This was only the case for the first scan. The formation of these peaks verify the polymerization of the monomer.

Only slight changes in the current in the CV measurements were noticed for MIP and NIP (Fig. 2B) . Nevertheless, a noticeable enlargement of the EIS measurements was observed after electropolymerization (Fig. 2C and 2D). Therefore, a polymeric film must have been created, that increased the resistance of the electrode. Also in these measurements no difference between the NIP and MIP was noticeable. Similar results were observed in comparable experimental trials, with the same procedure. In general, no significant differences could be detected between the NIP and the MIP during the electropolymerization or the following measurements.

3.2 Protein removal

By removing the protein from the polymeric layer the resistance decreases, which was to be expected (Fig. 2C and 2D). The NIP had a higher decrease in resistance than the MIP in this case. However, some comparable procedures showed approximately the same decrease in resistance for NIPs and MIPs. In this matter, a relatively large divergence was observed, which leaves the predictability with a high variance.

3.3 Rebinding of protein

The success or failure of the imprinting was examined, with a stepwise incubation of the Tau standard solution on the working electrode. With every step the concentration of Tau in the solution increased, starting with a concentration of 0.05 ng/ml and a maximum concentration of 500 ng/ml. All steps were carried out for NIPs and MIPs in an equiv-

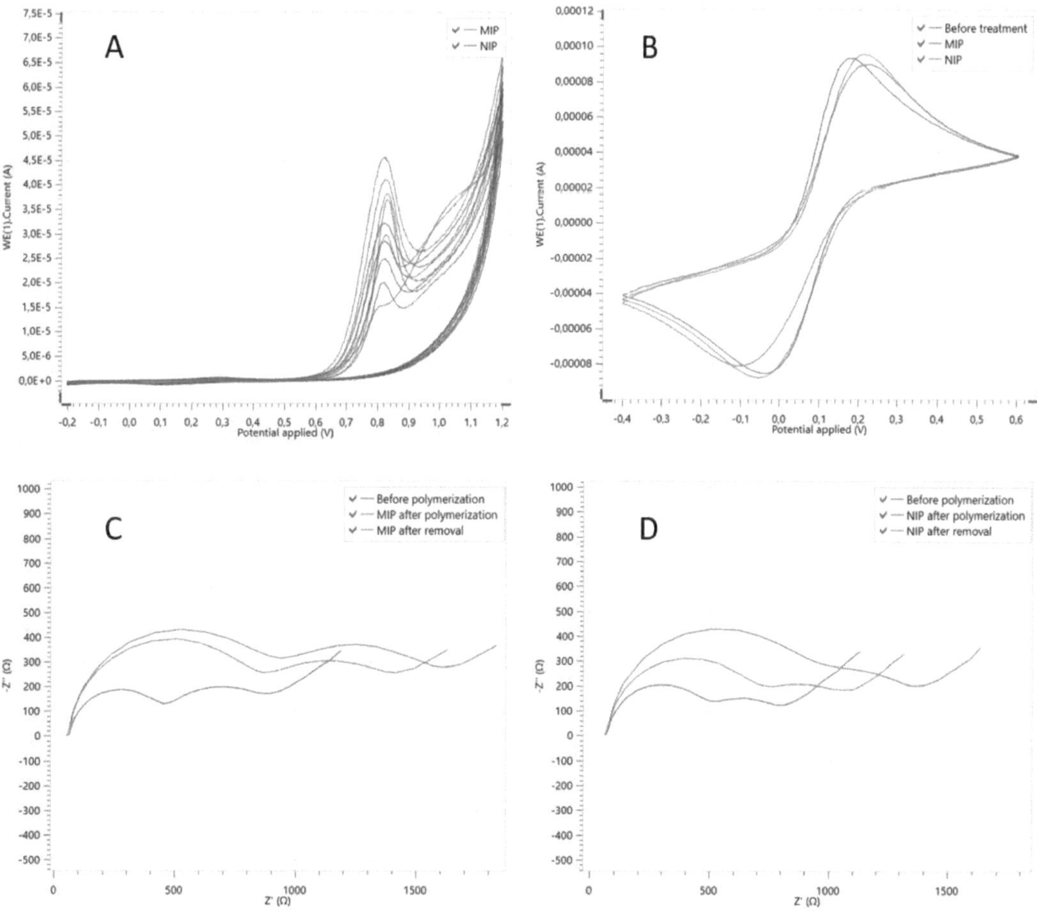

Figure 2: Electropolymerization and following measurements for molecularly imprinted polymer (MIP) and non-imprinted polymer (NIP). (A) Electropolymerization of NIP and MIP for 5 cycles. (B) Cyclic voltammetry measurements for MIP and NIP. (C) EIS measurements MIP. (D) EIS measurements NIP.

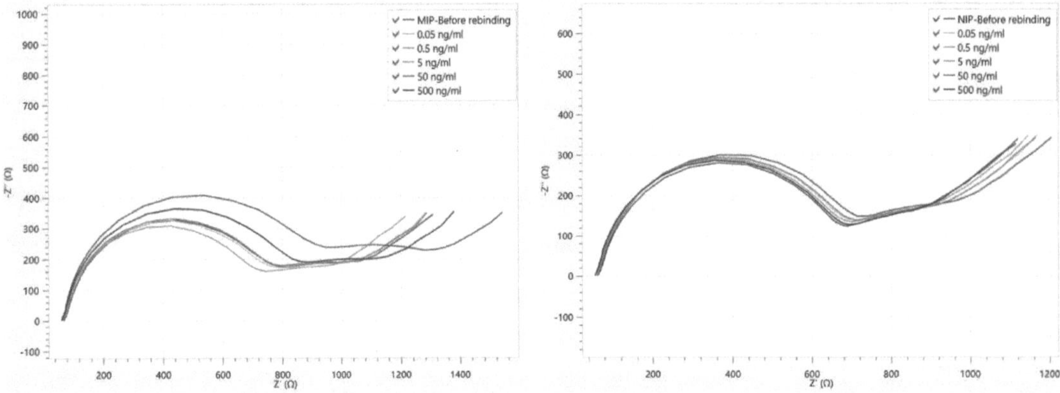

Figure 3: Electrochemical impedance spectroscopy (EIS) measurements of rebinding steps with different concentrations of Tau in probe solution for a molecularly imprinted polymer (left) and a non-imprinted polymer (right).

alent manner, to provide a reasonable comparison between those two. In between every incubation step a CV and EIS reading with iron probe solution took place.

Comparing the measurements of the NIP and MIP, an actual success of the detection of the protein could not be ensured. The changes of resistance were in both cases widely random (Fig.3). A difference between the EIS measurements between the NIP and MIP was observed, but in case of successful rebinding the resistance would have changed in order of the increasing Tau concentration in the standard solution, which was not the case.

4 Conclusion

In the course of this study, a MIP based electrochemical biosensor for the detection of Tau was to be developed, with L-Cysteine as the monomer of choice and a gold ink SPE. Throughout this work, a successful polymerization of the chosen monomer was proven. Nevertheless, multiple steps in this process faced inconsistencies. Especially the disordered arrangement, of the final measurements of the rebinding process, results in an unpromising approach, to constructing a biosensor for the detection of Tau.

Acknowledgment

The work has been carried out at BioMark, Instituto Superior de Engenharia do Porto, and supervised by Dr. Ramtin Rahmanzadeh, Institute of Biomedical Optics, Universität zu Lübeck.

Author's Statement

Conflict of interest: Authors state no conflict of interest.

5 References

[1] L.G. Apostolova *Alzheimer Disease*. Continuum, Minneapolis, 2016

[2] H. Hampel u. a., *The future of Alzheimer's disease: The next 10 years*. Progress in Neurobiology, vol. 95, no. 4, pp. 718–728, 2011

[3] I. Grundke-Iqbal, K. Iqbal,Y. C. Tung, M. Quinlan, H. M. Wisniewski, L. I. Binder, *Abnormal phosphorylation of the microtubule-associated protein τ (tau) in Alzheimer cytoskeletal pathology*. Proceedings of the National Academy of Sciences of the United States of America, vol. 83, no. 13, pp. 4913-4917, 1986

[4] E. Drummond, G. Pires, C. MacMurray, M. Askenazi, S. Nayak, M. Bourdon, J. Safar, B. Ueberheide,T. Wisniewski, *Phosphorylated tau interactome in the human Alzheimer's disease brain*,Brain: A journal of neurology, vol. 143, no.9, pp. 2803-2817, 2020

[5] R. Medeiros, D. Baglietto-Vargas, and Frank M. LaFerla, *The Role of Tau in Alzheimer's Disease and Related Disorders*, CNS neuroscience and therapeutics, vol. 17, no.5, pp. 514-524, 2011

[6] H. Hampel, K. Blennow *CSF tau and β-amyloid as biomarkers for mild cognitive impairment*, Dialogues in Clinical Neuroscience, vol. 6, no. 4, pp. 379-390, 2004

[7] N. J. Ronkainen, H. B. Halsall, and W. R. Heineman, *Electrochemical biosensors*, Chemical Society Reviews, vol. 39, no.5, pp. 1747-1763, 2010

[8] A. Ben Hassine, N. Raouafi, and F. T. C. Moreira. 2021. *Novel Electrochemical Molecularly Imprinted Polymer Based Biosensor for Tau Protein Detection*, Chemosensors, vol. 9, no. 9, 2021

[9] V. Ayerdurai, P. Lach, A. Lis-Cieplak, M. Cieplak, W. Kutner and P. S. Sharma, *An advantageous application of molecularly imprinted polymers in food processing and quality control*, Critical Reviews in Food Science and Nutrition, 2022

Concept development for safe operation of a mobile blood analyzer in harsh environments

Abedalaziz Abdallah [1], Benjamin Kern [2], and Stefan Müller [2]

[1] Biomedical Engineering, Luebeck University of Applied Sciences, Abedalaziz.Abdallah@student.uni-luebeck.de

[2] Medical Sensors and Devices Laboratory, Luebeck University of Applied Sciences, Benjamin.kern@th-luebeck.de, Stephan.mueller@th-luebeck.de

Abstract

Recent advances in technology have made medical devices more accessible and efficient allowing for a growing number of devices to be used outside of traditional medical settings like hospitals and clinics. The objective of this project was to develop concepts for safe operation of a mobile blood analyzer that is intended to be used in harsh environments using computer aided design (CAD) software and three dimensional printing technology. Mechanisms were designed to protect the internal components and to safely remove the test chip that contains the patient's blood after the test complete. The final design was easy to manufacture and includes Polymethyl methacrylate (PMMA) Plastic window attached to a top cover as well as a single torsion spring, and a SIM and microSD connector-style mechanism for removing the test chip.

1   Introduction

Medical devices are a fundamental tool in the healthcare system and play a vital role in the diagnosis, treatment, and management of a wide range of medical conditions [1]. Medical equipment has undergone significant advancements in recent years, with many devices becoming smaller, more portable, and user-friendly. This has facilitated greater accessibility for patients and enabled healthcare providers to offer care in a more efficient and effective manner. The design proficiency of manufacturers is key to the success of the medical device industry, as science and design are closely intertwined in the design process. [2]. Design control is a systematic approach to manage the design of a product or service, from the initial concept phase through development and manufacturing to distribution [3].

In the design of medical devices, many factors must be taken into account such as safety, effectiveness and usability. Patient safety is the top priority in the design of the devices which can be achieved by ensuring that the device is built with materials which are compatible and a simple interaction is required, and that the device has been thoroughly tested to ensure it functionality. Moreover, preventing any infection that could be due to interaction between health provider, patient and device is of a great importance. The second factor is also to ensure that it is effective at achieving its intended purpose. This includes the environment condition in which the device will be used. Finally, the usability must be considered. In essence, the designs of medical devices are crucial as it determine its safety, effectiveness, and usability, and thus plays a key role in success and development of the devices [4].

A blood analyzer is used to diagnose and monitor a wide range of medical conditions in hospitals, clinics, and laboratories [5]. Testing blood is a primary step in emergency department as it is rich of information about functioning of the body. Therefore, the development in medical technology led to establish new and fast blood analysis equipment which called a portable (mobile) blood analysis [6]. These mobile blood analysis devices are often smaller and more portable than traditional laboratory-based blood analysis equipment.

The aim of this paper is to present a concept for safety features that comprises protecting the internal components of a mobile blood analyzer from exposure to fluids in the outside environment, and to identify a mechanism for ejecting the test chip after completion of the blood test.

2   Material and Methods

2.1   Software

SolidWorks (version 2021) is a computer-aided design (CAD) software that was used for planning and drawing the components. SolidWorks software is commonly used to create 3D models for engineering and industrial purposes. It has a wide range of features and tools that aid in creation of desired design in accurate and detailed manner. The draws were imported as stl files to Ultimaker Cura (version 4.12.0) software to generate a gcode for the 3d printer.

2.2   Digital fabrication technology

Digital fabrication technology, often referred to as 3D printing, is a process that involves creating physical 3-dimisional objects from a digital representation such as CAD by adding materials layer by layer which create complex objects in a fast and good manner [7]. The designed components were printed using a 3D printer (Kobra Go, Anycubic version v1.2.9) to perform testing and to make any necessary adjustment in the measurements of the model.

2.3   Polylactic acid bioplastic

Polylactic acid (PLA) is a biodegradable polymer derived from a lactic acid. PLA is commonly used because of its characteristics of having low melting temperatures between 180°C – 230°C. In this project, models were printed using polylactic acid material and assembled to evaluate their fit and functionality. Any necessary adjustments were made to the models based on the results of this testing [8].

2.4   Mechanical springs

In this project, two springs were implemented and employed in order to facilitate the movement of a specific component. It was placed to improve the device functionality and overall design.

The specifications and measurements of the springs that were utilized in the design are listed below:

Table 1: Torsion spring technical data

Coil direction	Left
Leg position	90 degrees
Wire diameter	0.4 mm
Outer coil diameter	2.4 mm
Inner coil diameter	1.6 mm
Length of the spring legs	10.0 mm

Table 2: Compression spring technical data

Coil direction	Right
Wire diameter	0.16 mm
Outer coil diameter	1.36 mm
Inner coil diameter	1.04 mm
Unstressed spring length	9.70 mm
Minimum stressed spring length	4.07 mm

The springs that were used in this project were obtained and procured through the manufacturer "Gutekunst Federn" on their website [9]. They were utilized as they were the appropriate size to fit within the design.

2.5   Design process

The purpose of this project was to make modifications to specific parts of the mobile blood analyzer in order to enhance the safety of internal electrical components and provide flexibility and protection against potential infection risks for users during the removal of test chips.

The main components of the design were:

- Test chip base lower part, Fig. 1(A).
- Test chip base upper cover part, Fig. 1(B).

By assembling the two parts, the sensor head was formed, where sensors and other electrical components were mounted to make it a functional unit.

In order to start working in the design, the process was divided into three phases for the purpose of targeted development and improvements. The aim of this divisions was to work easier and focused on specific sections to achieve the specific design goals. Upon completion of all sections, the designs were consolidated into a cohesive final design for the device. The prototyping process began with the design of the model in SolidWorks, then using the CAD software iteratively, the design was continuously refined and improved until the desired outcome is achieved.

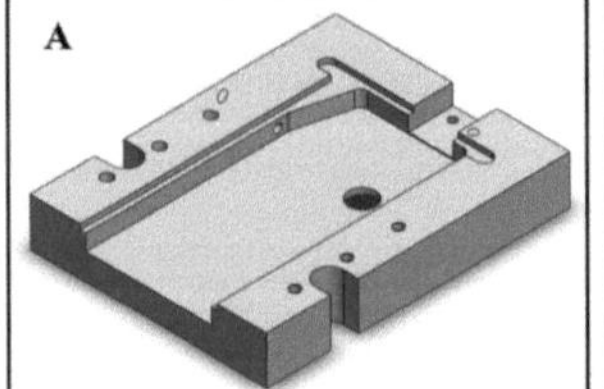
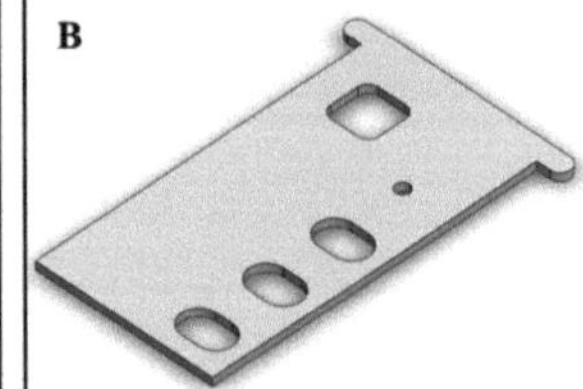

Figure 1: (A) The base of the sensor head with outer dimension 25mm * 58.5mm* 9mm. (B) The top cover.

2.5.1   Primary protection phase

In the first phase of the project, an internal protection was added to protect the upper sensors from external influences, as they were exposed inside the sensor head. Two solutions were proposed for this issue. As a first solution, transparent PMMA windows were incorporated into the top cover for the sensors, while the second solution involved creating a removable slider with transparent PMMA windows. A slider in this method is not attached to the top cover of the sensor head.

2.5.2   Flap mechanism phase

In the second phase of the project, additional protections for the internal parts were added. The concept was to incorporate a flap, similar to the flap on a floppy disk drive, at the opening of the sensor head. This flap open when the test chip is inserted and close when the test chip is removed. The challenge was to find a way to control the flap's opening and closing, either by use of a torsion springs or compression springs.

2.5.3   Ejection mechanism phase

In the final phase of the project, an ejecting mechanism was added to allow safe removal of the test chip without direct contact. Two mechanisms were proposed, one of them based on the push-push mechanism commonly found in SIM and SD card slots of smartphones. The proposed mechanism would feature an external button on the surface of the device. Pressing it will cause the test chip to be released from the sensor head.

The end result of the design was achieved through the use of SolidWorks software, which was utilized to design every separate part. These parts were then printed by a 3D printer and assembled to form the complete design.

3 Results and Discussion

3.1 Primary protection phase

For the first phase of the design, two options were presented. One option was to incorporate PMMA windows that are attached to the top cover, as illustrated in Fig. 2. The other option was to develop a new component referred to as a slider which would feature a PMMA window that can be slid in and out from under the top cover of the sensor head, as shown in Fig. 3.

Both designs in Fig. 2 and Fig. 3 involve adding a PMMA window, each with their own advantages and disadvantages. The slider design is disposable, easily inserted and removed by the medical staff if it damaged or foreign objects were found on it. However, the addition of components can make the overall design more intricate. Additionally, the slider poses a risk of accidental fluid entering the device during removal. The second design, shown in Fig. 2, is safer and simpler as it uses the sensor head's top cover and does not require additional parts, but the medical staff are not able to change the window themselves as it requires removing the top cover.

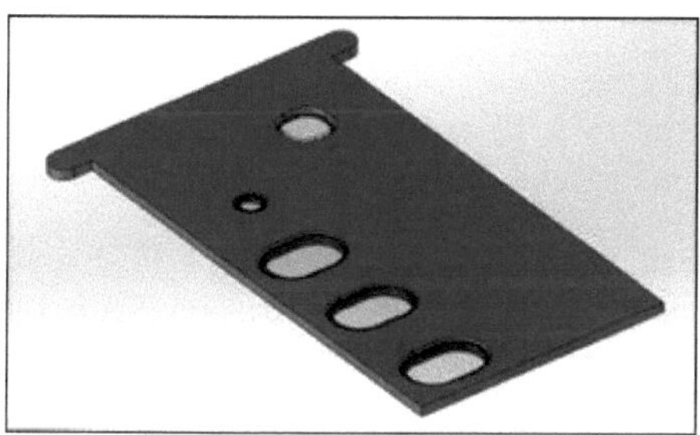

Figure 2: PMMA windows attached to the top cover.

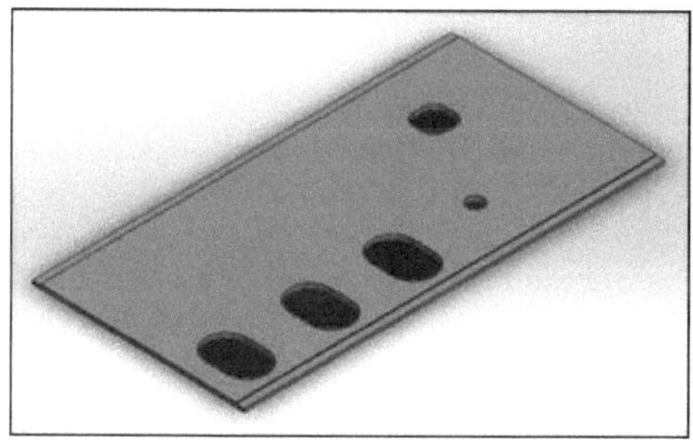

Figure 3: Slider concept contains PMMA windows.

3.2 Flap mechanism phase

In the second phase of development, compression springs or torsion springs were added to the design. A flap with an axis of rotation was fixed in lower base part of the sensor head. For the first concept in this phase, an additional rod and two compression springs were placed on the top and sides of the flap, as depicted in Fig. 4. This design incorporates compression springs to provide additional stability and force to keep the flap closed after the test chip is removed. However,

this design necessitates the use of an additional rod and covers on the sides to hold the springs in place. The surface that comes in contact with the springs must be smooth to avoid friction which may impede the flap's movement. For these reasons, the dimensions of this design are challenging to manufacture. The second design in this phase, shown in fig. 5, involved the use of a single torsion spring connected to the base and flap, and has the same axis of rotation. This design is simple and only requires one spring. Moreover, it can be assembled and disassembled.

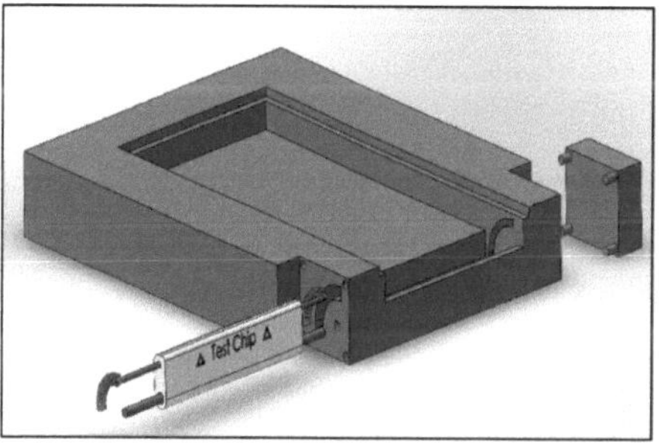

Figure 4: The component of the compression spring model.

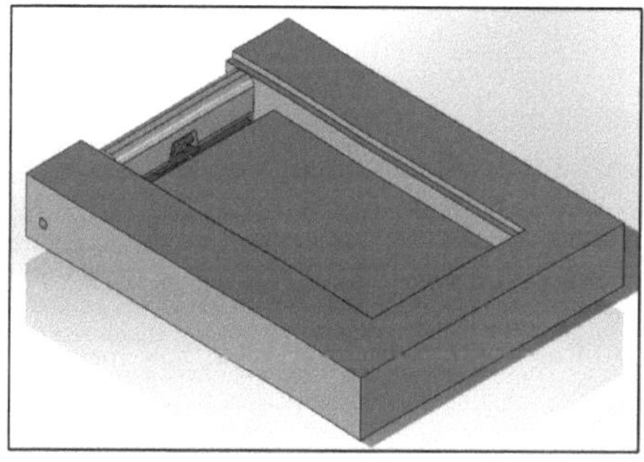

Figure 5: The torsion spring design model.

3.3 Ejection mechanism phase

Two concepts were proposed for the final phase of ejecting the test chip, both of which have almost similar appearance. The first design, illustrated in Fig. 6, uses multiple small components to assist in ejecting the test chip. The device consists of a rod attached to the surface of the device with a button. When the button is pressed, the lock and a pusher component linked to a compression spring are disengaged. However, this method has a complex design with small parts that are difficult to manufacture and requires a high force to be generated in the pusher component by the spring connected to it in order to push the test chip. Additionally, the spring is small and can bend easily, potentially damaging the entire mechanism. The lock system is also connected by an extension spring for opening and closing, adding extra spring to the design. The design concept shown in Fig. 7, which resembled a SIM and microSD card connector slot, was chosen for the final design due to its simplicity. It requires a single compression spring and includes a knob for securing the test chip.

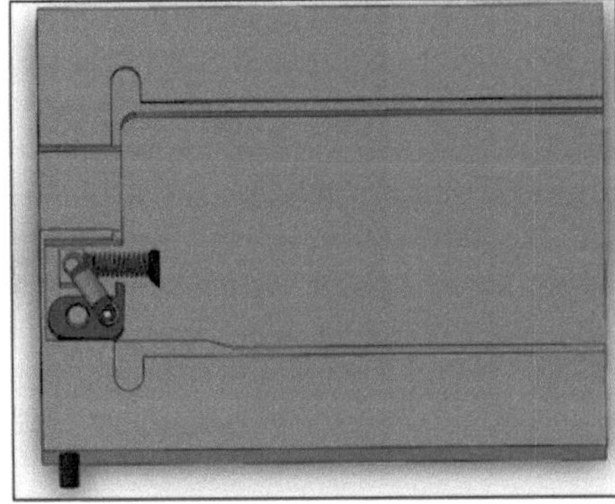

Figure 6: Multicomponent pusher spring model

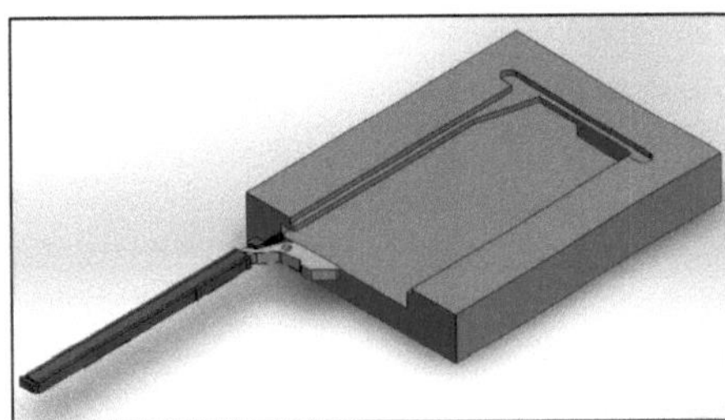

Figure 7: Ejector connector slot design.

After finishing the desired concept, the final design is shown in Fig. 8. The individual components of the design can be forwarded for manufacturing using a Computer Numerical Control (CNC) milling machine with the same dimensions and scales. Each part will be manufactured separately and then assembled afterwards.

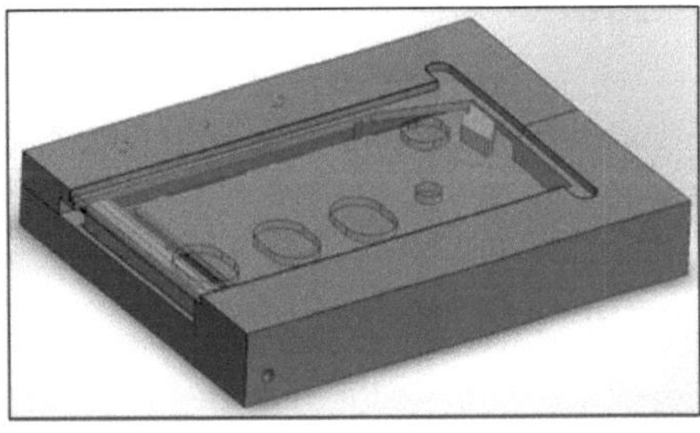

Figure 8: Final design combining the chosen concepts.

4 Conclusion

The aim of this paper was to present a concepts for the safe operation of a mobile blood analyzer in harsh environments. This included protection of the internal components from exposure to foreign substance such as fluids and to identify a mechanism for ejecting the test chip after completion of the blood test. The final design incorporated a PMMA windows attached to the top cover, a single torsion spring, and a SIM and microSD card connector slot-like design for ejecting the test chip. These components were printed individually by the 3D printer and put together afterwards. This design components were chosen due to the simplicity, durability, and ease in manufacture. The flap, PMMA windows

and the robust ejecting mechanism added to the design are able to protect the internal components and to reduce the risk of infection. For further studies the PMMA windows can be tested to determine the effect on the measurements of the sensors.

Acknowledgement

The work has been carried out in the Medical Sensors and Devices Laboratory at Luebeck University of Applied Sciences.

Author's Statement

Conflict of interest: Authors state no conflict of interest.

5 References

[1] World Health Organization, *M*edical devices: managing the mismatch: an outcome of the Priority Medical Devices project, 2010.

[2] M.Tamsin and C.Bach, *T*he Design of Medical Devices, International Journal of Innovation and Scientific Research, 2014.

[3] B. Gilman, J. Brewer, and M. Kroll, *M*edical Device Design Process, IEEE, 2009.

[4] R. Branaghan, E. Hildebrand and L.Foster, *D*esigning for medical device safety, Arizona State University, United States, PP 10–12, 2020.

[5] M. Toner and D. Irimia , *B*lood on a chip, BioMEMS Resource Center, Center for Engineering in Medicine and Surgical Services, Massachusetts General Hospital, Shriners Hospital for Children, and Harvard Medical School, Boston, Massachusetts, 2005.

[6] V. Sands, P. Auerbach , J. Birnbaum and M. Green , *E*valuation of a Portable Clinical B l ood Analyzer in the Emergency Department, 1995.

[7] N. Shahrubudin, T. Lee and R. Ramlan, *A*n Overview on 3D Printing Technology: Technological, Materials, and Application, 2019.

[8] M. Othman, M. Misran and Z. Khamisan, *S*tudy on Mechanical Properties of PLA Printed using 3D Printer, Department of Mechanical Engineering, Politeknik Kuching Sarawak, Malaysa,2019.

[9] Torsion spring and Compression spring *A*vailable: www.federnshop.com/en/products/torsion_springs/t-160011.html

www.federnshop.com/en/products/compression _springs/vd-2065.html

Novel Fabrication of Polymer Based Microfluidic Chips Using Hot Embossing With 3D-Printed Moulds

Bruno Kluwe [1], Kai Mattern [2], Natalia Sandetskaya [3], Maik Rahlves [4] and Dirk Kuhlmeier [5]

[1] Medical Engineering Science, Universität zu Lübeck, bruno.kluwe@student.uni-luebeck.de

[2] Fraunhofer Institute for Cell Therapy and Immunology IZI, kai.mattern@izi.fraunhofer.de

[3] Fraunhofer Institute for Cell Therapy and Immunology IZI, natalia.sandetskaya@izi.fraunhofer.de

[4] Institute of Biomedical Optics, Universität zu Lübeck, maik.rahlves@uni-luebeck.de

[5] Fraunhofer Institute for Cell Therapy and Immunology IZI, dirk.kuhlmeier@izi.fraunhofer.de

Abstract

In this work, 3D-printed moulds are used in hot embossing to fabricate polymer based microfluidic chips. The chips are used in point-of-care diagnostics to perform low cost sensitive assays with small sample volumes. Being able to detect infectious diseases, they have many fields of application. The moulds are produced using stereolithography with photopolymer resin and the microfluidic structures are transferred on polymethyl methacrylate with hot embossing. The moulds have a limited lifetime, which makes them less suitable for mass production. However, they are well suited for rapid prototyping, because they can be produced quickly and cost-effectively allowing major freedom of design and high accuracy. The functionality was shown in fluidic tests and with a simulated sample in a molecular assay integration.

1 Introduction

In the past two decades, microfluidics has become an important part of biomedicine and chemical analysis [1]. The so-called Lab-on-chip- (LOC-) systems represent an important application of microfluidic technologies. These devices are working in the range of micro- to picoliter to control and manipulate fluids in order to perform analysis of biological samples [1]. LOC-Systems have many advantages for a variety of different applications. Typical fields of application are research, analysis or industrial laboratories. Furthermore, non-controlled environments and in-field uses, such as Point-of-care (POC) diagnostics, should be considered [2]. At the clinic or at home, POC diagnostics can produce instant on-site results for rapid diagnosis and monitoring of the patient. Therefore POC devices should be portable, fast, easy-to-use and accurate to guarantee the correct clinical decisions in a short amount of time. As a result, they can contribute to a successful recovery for patients [3]. Microfluidics are essential for POC diagnostics because they are offering robust and sensitive assays at low costs. Furthermore, to perform the assays, only small sample volumes are required. With microfluidics, multiple complex sample-processing steps are combined into one device and, in relation, less reagents are needed [3, 4].

The aim of this work is to design, fabricate and validate a passive microfluidic chip, which is part of a POC-system for infectious diseases. Here, hot embossing with a 3D-printed mould on Polymethyl methacrylate (PMMA) is used as a prototype fabrication technique. First implemented in the 1970s, hot embossing has evolved into one of the most promising processes to replicate micro and nano structures with high precision and quality [6]. With 3D-printed moulds it is possible to produce prototypes with high freedom of design and high accuracy in minimum time. This stands in contrast to the normally long process times and high costs of hot embossing with moulds fabricated using computer numerical control (CNC) milling or microfabrication techniques such as lithography and dry etching [8].

2 Overview and Physical Background

In this work, hot embossing is used to fabricate the microfluidic chips. Hot embossing is a technique for transferring micro-sized structures from a master mould into thermoplastic polymers or other materials like glass [6]. In comparison to other fabrication methods for LOC-devices, it offers a simple cost-effective process with a high replication accuracy [2]. Other advantages include high throughput, compatibility with most thermoplastics and low start-up costs [8].

In order for the POC-device to function properly, the chip must combine various functions. First, the sample has to be purified, otherwise no reliable assay can be performed. Here, the sample purification step is not carried out directly on the chip, but in a sieving device, which is inserted directly into the inlet from above (fig. 1). Second, sample preparation takes place, including DNA amplification. Furthermore, the fluid flow has to be generated and controlled.

The flow is generated by capillary effects and controlled by stop structures in the channel design. At the end the sample is transported to a lateral flow strip where the signal detection takes place.

In general, there are two kinds of microfluidic devices. Active devices need external pumps or power sources to power pumps and actuators on the chip. Passive devices use fluid properties or passive mechanisms to manipulate the fluid flow without the need of any external power sources. The less complex structures in passive devices represent a big advantage in manufacturing and in application [5]. The fluid properties are governed by capillary effects, which depend on the relation between surface tension of a liquid and the channel geometry of the chip. In microfluidics, capillary pressure increases when the microchannel dimensions decreases. This can be shown with the Young-Laplace-Equation which gives the capillary pressure for a rectangular channel [4]:

$$p = -\gamma \left[\frac{cos\phi_t + cos\phi_b}{h} + \frac{cos\phi_l + cos\phi_r}{w} \right] \quad (1)$$

where p stands for the capillary pressure, γ is the surface tension of the liquid in the microchannel and h and w are the channel height and width. The contact angles between liquid and solid are illustrated for each wall of the rectangular duct as ϕ_t for the top wall, ϕ_b for the bottom, ϕ_l for the left and ϕ_r for the right wall [4].

Moreover the surface properties of the channel play an important role. For creating a negative capillary pressure, which presses the fluid into the channel, the surface has to be wettable. The wettability is defined via the contact angle of the liquid with the wettable surface. For angles smaller than 90° the negative pressure pushes the liquid into the channel, for angles greater than 90°, the forces are acting in the opposite direction, the fluid flows out of the channel [4]. As PMMA is used for the fabrication of the LOC-devices, which has a contact angle of 71°, normally a surface treatment is required to guarantee sufficient capillary pressure [4]. For this work no surface treatment is performed, because the chemical coating would interfere with the assay due to a pH shift. Instead additional pressure is generated by pipetting or finger-force pressure through a blister.

3   Material and Methods

3.1   Microfluidic Design Process

For the design process, the commercial computer-aided design (CAD) software *Fusion 360* (Autodesk Inc., San Francisco, California, USA) is used. The chip design consists of four main parts. An input for sample integration, stop structures for controlling the fluid flow, a buffer reservoir to store buffer and a moulding where a lateral flow test (LFT) strip is integrated for signal detection.

Figure 1 shows the two versions of the chip. One design includes an interface for a blister for rinsing (fig. 1b). The inlet is situated in the middle of the chip, which is where

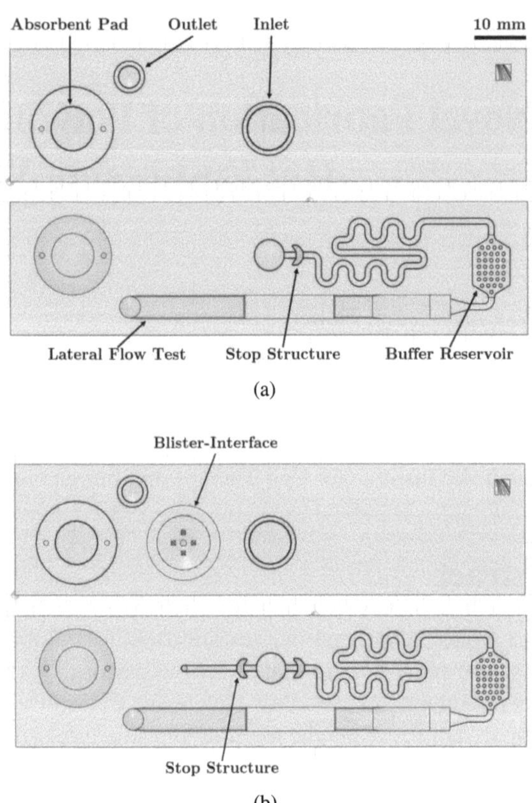

Figure 1: Chipdesign - without Blisterport (a) and with Blisterport (b) (from the top and from the bottom).

the DNA amplification step takes place as well. The sieving device, in which the sample preparation is performed, is inserted in the inlet of the chip. Thus the sample is transferred on chip. For keeping the sample in place, stop structures have been integrated behind the channel entrance. If there is no fluid in the next channel, these passive valves prevent flow of the fluid through the stop structure, by breaking off the capillary forces. At a certain pressure, the fluid overcomes the stop structures and flows into the next channel. After the heating for the amplifcation has taken place, the sample needs to be transported to the LFT. This can either be done by simply adding buffer into the input (chip version in fig. 1a) or by pressing the blister (chip version in fig. 1b). In both cases, the sample is transported towards signal detection. On the left side of the chip a absorbent pad is integrated for the preparation of the sieving device in the first step. Another important design requirement is a positive draft angle in the microchannels, which helps to demould and separate the mould from the chip. Here a draft angle of 12.5° is used, which corresponds to a wall angle of 77.5°.

3.2   Mould fabrication

For the process of hot embossing, a master mould, which has the inverted features of the device structure, is needed. After the design process, a mould is printed with a *Formlabs Form 3B* stereolithographic printer with photopolymer resin *High Temp Resin* (Formlabs, Somerville, MA, USA).

The *Form 3B* uses stereolithography for producing 3D parts by selectively curing a photo polymerizing resin layer by layer. The mould consists of four single chips, showed in fig. 2. Two with an integrated interface for a blister and two without blisterport. At the edge of the mould a channel to capture remaining displaced material and four alignment structures to prevent displacement of the bottom and top of the mould are integrated. After the printing was completed, further steps followed to post-process the mould. First, the mould is removed from the build platform and placed in a bath of isopropyl alcohol where it is washed from both sides. The last step is the curing. First for 120 min at 80 °C and then again for 180 min at 160 °C.

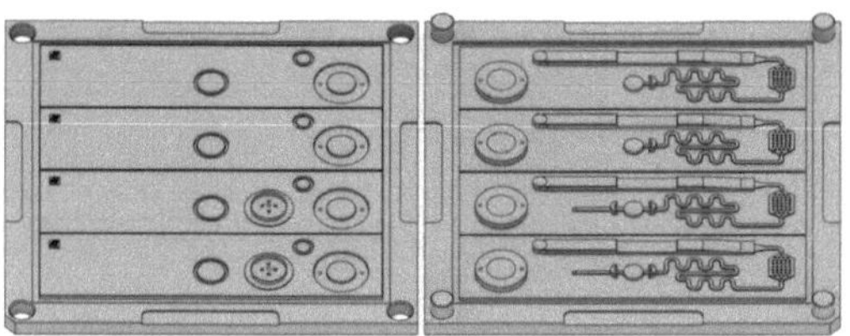

Figure 2: Mould design in Fusion 360. Left: top side of the chip. Right: bottom side of the chip.

3.3 Fabrication process: Hot Embossing

Three main parameters are critical for hot embossing process: glass transition temperature, forming pressure or applied force and holding time. All these parameters depend on the polymer being used [6]. The hot embossing process can be divided into four parts, as shown in fig. 3. First the PMMA substrate is inserted into the mould. Subsequently, it is heated above its glass transition temperature of 105 °C (Step 1). For PMMA the hot embosser is heated to 150 °C. Meanwhile a vacuum is created. Now the master mould is pressed against the polymer with a predefined pressure and time. In the case of PMMA a force of 6750 N is applied for 12 min. This step is repeated three times for receiving a better imprint (Step 2). Finally the mould and the substrate are cooled down to a specific demoulding temperature to 95 °C and separated by opening the tools (Step 3 + 4) [6, 7]. Using a small scraper to move along the edges, the chips are carefully lifted off the mould.

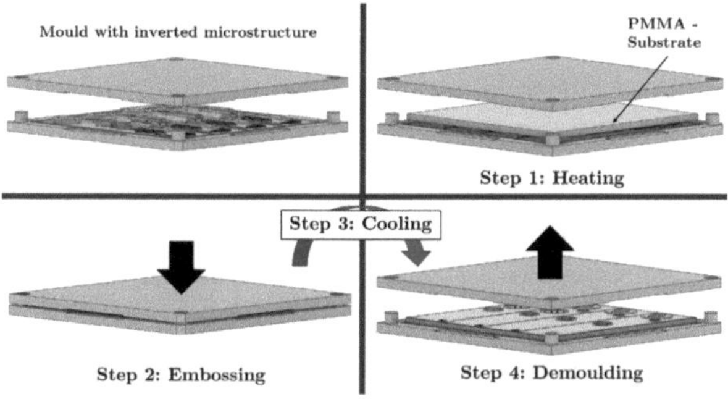

Figure 3: Workflow for hot embossing microstructures in PMMA.

Fig. 4 shows the hot embossing parameters during the process, which takes about 60 min to complete. The embossing force is increased with 650 N/min and during the last embossing cycle the force is applied until the demoulding temperature is reached by cooling the moulds. Several conditions have to be assured for the quality of the manufactured devices. One essential condition is the creation of a vacuum environment which avoids air cavities in the polymer and prevents the polymer from igniting under pressure. Other conditions include uniform temperatures across the mould and low friction between mould and polymer [7].

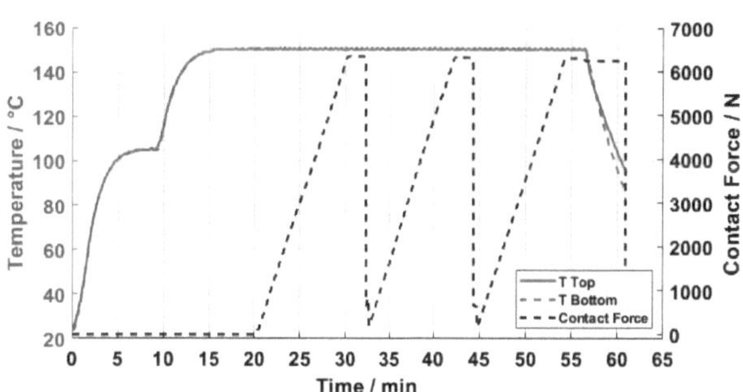

Figure 4: Hot embossing parameters during the process.

The embossing process is performed with the semi-automated hot embossing system *EVG 520HE* (EV Group, St. Florian am Inn, Austria). After demoulding, the chips need to be separated from each other. For this purpose the laser cutter *LaserMAXX-Plott 70* (Lotus Laser Systems, Essex, UK) is used. Parameters are set with 60 % laser power and 40 mm/s traversing speed. The last step is to drill the holes for which a drilling machine is used. To check the working principle of the microfluidic chip, fluidic tests with colored buffer were performed to observe the fluidic behavior. In addition, a molecular assay integration was conducted to show the functionality for a simulated sample.

4 Results and Discussion

4.1 Fabrication Process

The hot embossing process was carried out as described. First, when inserting the PMMA, it should be ensured that it is centered. To remove small dust particles, compressed air is used to clean the PMMA and the mould. Then the moulds are placed on a graphite plate in the press to ensure an uniform transfer of force from the press to the mould. Kapton foil is added to prevent them from sticking together. Now the hot embossing process is performed. To guarantee successful demoulding, the correct temperature has to be selected. If the mould has cooled down too much, it can no longer be removed properly and structures or the mould itself may be damaged. If the mold is still too hot, the entire chip can be deformed. This is particularly important because the planarity of the chip must be ensured for heating processes in the DNA amplification step. After demoulding, the chips are cut with a laser cutter, followed by the drilling of the chips. This has to be done very precisely, otherwise the surrounding flow stop structures can be damaged. The 3D printed moulds made of photopolymer resin have a limited lifetime for approximately 15 uses, because within the demoulding process small parts of the structure can break off and lead to less good results. However, they can be produced quickly and cost-effectively. This is especially important for rapid prototyping, since several iterations are often needed to fulfill all the requirements of the chip. To move to higher production numbers, a more stable mould would be needed. One possibility would be 3D-printed metal moulds, as Lin et al. showed in their work [8]. With longer-lasting moulds, hot embossing with 3D printed moulds could be a promising alternative to traditional microfabrication techniques.

4.2 Fluidic Test

To test the fluidic behaviour of the chip, colored chromatographic buffer was given into the inlet. It was shown, that, on average, 30 seconds after addition, the fluid reaches the LFT. The LFT soaks up the fluid and constant flow through the system is achieved. This shows the function of the chip to transport the sample from the inlet to detection.

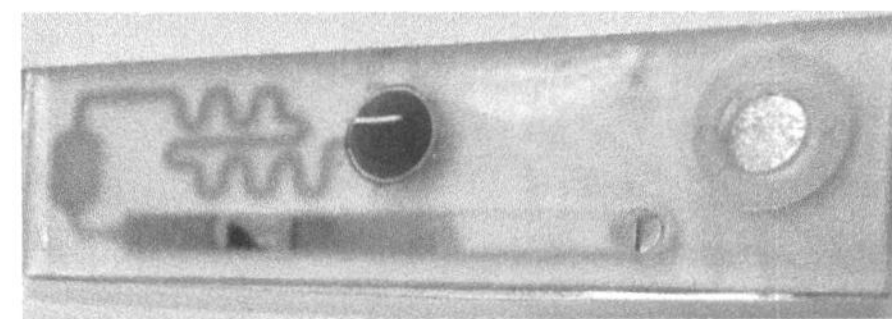

Figure 5: Fluidic test with colored buffer and LFT.

4.3 Assay functionality test

To assess the suitability of the produced chip for the molecular assay integration, a simulated sample (buffer spiked with bacterial DNA) was tested on the chip. Prior the test, the reagents for DNA amplification were deposited in dried form in the dedicated chamber under the sieving device. The sample was applied onto the sieving device to remove undesirable components. Then the purified sample was passively mixed with the dry reagents and the molecular DNA amplification was initiated by placing the chip on a flatbed heating block (65 °C for 40 min). By applying an additional amount of buffer onto the chip the amplified sample was transported to the LFT, where the detection was performed. A successful detection of the amplified DNA was determined visually as a band on LFT. These initial tests have demonstrated the suitability of the described rapid chip prototyping method for the development of LOC devices with an appropriate quality for a primary evaluation of biomolecular tests.

5   Conclusion

This paper describes the successful design, fabrication and validation of a Lab-on-chip device for infectious diseases. Hot embossing with a 3D-printed mould is used for the fabrication of the microfluidic chips. The short durability of the moulds is a disadvantage that makes the process limitedly suitable for mass production. However, the prototypes can be produced cost-effectively within a very short amount of time. In addition, 3D-printed moulds allow high accuracy and major freedom of design. Initial fluidic tests and an assay integration test show the functionality of the chip and prove the quality of the produced devices.

Acknowledgement

The work has been carried out at the Fraunhofer Institute for Cell Therapy and Immunology IZI in Leipzig and supervised by Prof. Dr.-Ing. Maik Rahlves, Institute of Biomedical Optics, Universität zu Lübeck.

Author's Statement

Conflict of interest: Authors state no conflict of interest.

6   References

[1] B. Sharma and A. Sharma, *Microfluidics: recent advances toward Lab-on-Chip applications in bioanalysis.* Advanced Engineering Materials 24.2, 2022.

[2] E. Iannone, *Labs on Chip: principles, design, and technology.* CRC Press, Taylor & Francis Group, Boca Raton, 2015.

[3] S. Hassan et al., *Capillary-driven flow microfluidics combined with smartphone detection: an emerging tool for Point-of-Care diagnostics.* Diagnostics 10.8, 509, 2020.

[4] A. Olanrewaju, M. Beaugrand, M. Yafia and D. Juncker, *Capillary microfluidics in microchannels: from microfluidic networks to capillaric circuits.* Lab on a Chip 18.16, 2323-2347, 2018.

[5] V. Narayanamurthy et al., *Advances in passively driven microfluidics and lab-on-chip devices: a comprehensive literature review and patent analysis.* RSC advances 10.20, 11652-11680, 2020.

[6] L. Peng, Y. Deng, P. Yi and X. Lai, *Micro hot embossing of thermoplastic polymers: a review.* Journal of Micromechanics and Microengineering, 24.1, 013001, 2013.

[7] S.M. Scott and A. Zulfiqur, *Fabrication methods for microfluidic devices: An overview.* Micromachines, 12.3, 2021.

[8] T.Y. Lin, T. Do, P. Kwon and P.B. Lillehoj, *3D printed metal molds for hot embossing plastic microfluidic devices.* Lab on a Chip, 17.2, 241-247, 2017.

Concept study of an adapter for the reprocessing of flexible endoscopes

Frances Binder [1] and Benjamin Ottens [2]

[1] Medical Engineering Science, Universität zu Lübeck, frances.binder@student.uni-luebeck.de
[2] Olympus Surgical Technologies Europe, Olympus Winter & Ibe GmbH, benjamin.ottens@olympus.com

Abstract

Adapters are used to connect the endoscope channels to the washer-disinfector for reprocessing. This ensures the correct inside cleaning of the channels. In this concept study a market and benchmarking analysis of the Olympus Air/Water-Independent-Adapter is performed. The coupling mechanisms of competitors are compared to determine the competitiveness against the same. The used materials and the associated manufacturing processes are explained and opportunities for improvement are revealed. In addition, the requirements for the adapter are revised and evaluated. With the gained knowledge, the previous concept, design and manufacturing process of the adapter shall be optimized with regards to the future viability of the follow-up models, especially focusing on the feasibility of material substitution and production improvements.

1 Introduction

To prevent the transfer of infections between different patients flexible endoscopes need to be reprocessed after every usage [1]. Flexible endoscopes have a channel system to ensure access for tools, water and air. Thus besides the cleaning and disinfection of the outside of the endoscope each of the long and narrow channels needs to be cleaned individually [2]. Therefore the channels are manually connected to the washer-disinfector by using adapters. The adapters with the associated hoses and the adapter plate are the mechanical adaption system between the washer-disinfector and the endoscope to be reprocessed. Via this connection the channels are flushed with rinsing, cleaning and disinfection solution as well as air to dry the endoscope. This ensures the correct reprocessing by controlling each channel separately on connection, flow, pressure and blockage. In the hectical und time-critical work environment of reprocessing, the adapters are under continuous load. They are attached to and removed from endoscopes several times a day by the user. In the washer-disinfector they are also exposed to heat, moisture and processing chemicals. This needs to be considered in the development of new and changes of existing adapters.

2 Material and Methods

This concept study comprises adapters that connect to the air- and the water supply port of Olympus endoscopes. These ports are located at the connector section of the endoscope and during surgery connected to a water bottle. The water bottle is used for supplying water and air to the surgi-

cal site for example to rinse the lens of the endoscope. Due to the small distance between the ports one adapter connects both ports. Usually an adapter is associated with one endoscope port. For this purpose the adapter has two separate channel systems.

To detect improvements of the adapter a market analysis will be performed. Complaints are analyzed in order to draw conclusions about possible problems from customers and users. In a benchmarking analysis it is examined how the connection point works for competitors. If adapters are also used, they should be compared and the advantages and disadvantages of the concepts should be determined. Furthermore, the requirements for the adapter were compiled and examined for improvements. The used materials and the manufacturing process are also significant. Both have the potential to limit design possibilities. Therefore the materials used today as well as possible alternatives are listed and compared. Alternative manufacturing processes depending on the current circumstances are described. The concept, design and manufacturing process of the adapter should be optimized taking into account the knowledge gained.

2.1 Market analysis

To identify improvement points of the current adapter design a market analysis with an evaluation of all received complaints is carried out. The complaints are clustered by the concerning part of the adapter: the endoscope connector, the hose and the connection to the washer-disinfector, see Fig. 1. During this analysis it is shown that 86% of the complaints affect the endoscope connector, 14% concern the hose of the adapter and none of the complaints concern the connection to the washer-disinfector. The complaints regarding the endoscope connector are allocated to two error patterns. Most problems are caused by the material combination of polyether ether ketone (PEEK) and stainless steel. The locking tab of the adapter is made out of stainless steel and is guided by the PEEK-parts of the adapter. If there is a deformation of the tab, the tab deforms and breaks the PEEK-parts. The other problems are lost valve lids and o-rings for sealing. These are presumably levered out of the adapter [3].

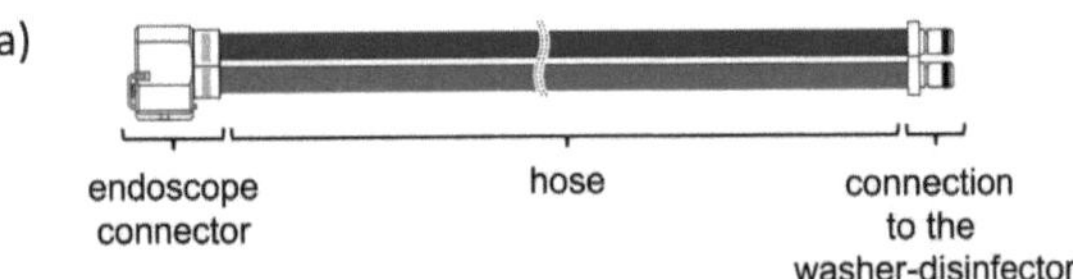

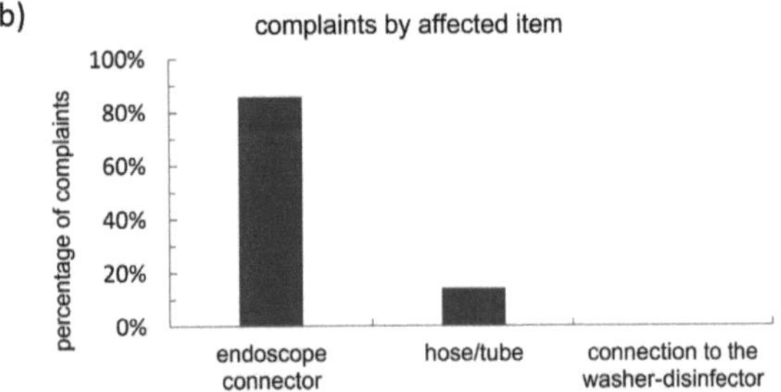

Figure 1: Clustered complaints concerning the Olympus Air/Water-Independent-Adapter, own figure.
a) Composition of an adapter consisting of the endoscope connection, the hose and the connection to the washer-disinfector, b) Number of complaints devided by the affected adapter parts from Figure 1a)

2.2 Benchmarking analysis

The benchmarking analysis compares the Olympus adapter with five corresponding adapters from direct competitors. The aim is to compare the individual adapter concepts and examine how the connection point operates in the washer-disinfector of competitors. The comparison shall be made especially with regards to the use of a double or a single plug, the used materials and the operating principle of the adapters. The advantages and disadvantages of the adapters are listed. The comparison of the different adapters is only possible with restrictions since the design of the adapter depends particularly on the placement of the endoscope in the washer-disinfector.

From the appearance all of the considered adapters are similar and comparable in their measurements. This is attributable to the regulatory standards they have to fulfill and the default space at the connection point to the endoscope. In addition, the used materials are equal. All adapters are made of PEEK, stainless steel or a combination of both materials. All manufacturer use one adapter for both, the air- and the water supply port of the endoscope. This is due to the proximity of the two ports and the fact that both inner endoscope channels converge. Furthermore, it reduces the number of adapters that have to be connected manually by the user. This reduces the working time and the possible error rate of the user.

A feature that distinguishes between the manufacturers is the locking mechanism of the adapters and the related feedback after a successful connection. The simplest adapter is attached and fixed to the endoscope port using sealing rings. Due to this connection mechanism this adapter does not provide any feedback to the user. Other adapters must be plugged onto the endoscope, turned by 180 degree and then plugged further. This mechanism is difficult to recognize and the movement is hard to perform with one hand. Two adapters are very similar in terms of their locking mechanism. However they differ in one point: One adapter can be connected to the endoscope by simply plugging it onto the port due to an integrated mechanism. In contrast when connecting the other adapter the locking tab has to be pressed manually to allow a connection to the endoscope port. This makes the first adapter easier to use since less manual operation is necessary. Due to the requirement of process reliability, manual activities should always be avoided as far as possible or secured separately in order to reduce human error.

2.3 Materials and manufacturing process

The relation between the materials and the manufacturing process results from the need to bring the material into the shape of the component specified by the design using a suitable manufacturing process [4]. The currently used material for the adapter is PEEK. This is a semi-crystalline, thermoplastic high-performance plastic. It has a high temperature and chemical resistance. Therefore it is often used as an alternative to metal as it is similar in terms of resistance but is significantly lighter in weight and does not corrode. However, PEEK is also a very expensive material.

Frequently used alternatives to PEEK are Polyetherimide (PEI) and fiber-reinforced PEEK. PEEK can be reinforced with glass fiber (GF-PEEK) and carbon fiber (CF-PEEK) and therefore adapted to the technical requirements. Carbon fiber reinforced PEEK already exists in a biocompatible form for medical applications. The carbon fiber reinforcement increases the rigidity, the creep strength and the chemical and heat resistance. A disadvantage of the reinforcement with carbon fibers is the possible release of particles. Under usual circumstances the carbon fibers are embedded in the polymer. If the component is damaged for example through cracks, fractures or abrasion carbon fibers could be released. If these remain in the endoscope after reprocessing the fibers could transferred into the patient and lead to complications [5].

A non-plastic alternative to PEEK are metals, especially stainless steel. Metals have the disadvantage that they are more susceptible to corrosion, have a higher density and are therefore heavier. In comparison an adapter made of stainless steel would be around six times heavier than a PEEK adapter of the same size. This must be considered for the usability of the adapter. The benefits of stainless steel are the significantly higher ultimate tensile strength, the modulus of elasticity and the operating temperature. In addition when using stainless steel the concept of the locking tab needs to be considered. Material combinations made of steel tend to release particles when there is friction. Furthermore, the sliding friction of an adapter and a locking tab made out of steel needs to be elaborated since all lubricants are removed during the reprocessing by the process chemicals.

PEEK can be processed by primary shaping processes or machining processes. In primary shaping processes plastic granulate is melted and deformed with a corresponding manufacturing process such as injection molding or extrusion. Because of the high melting point, high processing temperatures need to be selected for these processes. Therefore, these processes are more expensive and only used for producing large quantities because with larger quantities the tool and the equipment costs of the machine are lower for each produced piece. PEEK can also be processed by machining processes such as turning, drilling and milling. Here semi-finished materials are processed by commercial CNC machines until they suit the 3D model. In this separation process the final shape of the component is created by removing material. The advantage towards primary forming processes are the lower tool costs especially for small production series and the faster manufacturing without the time consuming production of specific tools. Unfortunately the material efficiency is lower because the scrap cannot be reused [6], [7]. In medical technology, additive manufacturing processes, such as 3D printing, have great growth potential, as this allows individual special products to be manufactured for each individual patient. PEEK is also suitable for processing with 3D printers. Due to the high processing temperatures that PEEK requires, only a small number of 3D printers are compatible making this processing technique very expensive [8].

2.4 Requirements

Requirements are properties or functionalities that a product must have or fulfill [9]. They include all functions or properties that are intended for the product under development. Requirements form the acceptance criteria for the finished development product. The requirements for the adapter result from the applicable standards and guidelines. Since the adapters are accessories to the washer-disinfectors, they are qualified as a medical product. These include standards for medical products, risk management, usability, labeling and for washer-disinfectors. There are basic requirements for the adapters established by Olympus. These define that the connection and disconnection of the adapter to the endoscope port has to be smooth. When connecting the adapter to the endoscope the user should receive a feedback to ensure that the adapter is firmly connected to the endoscope. The connection between the adapter and the washer-disinfector must be consistent throughout the entire reprocessing cycle. In addition the design and material have to allow a robust, stable and reusable adapter without sharp edges to avoid injuries for example by damaging rubber gloves.

3 Results and Discussion

The purpose of this concept study was to reveal further development potentials of the Olympus Air/Water Independent Adapter. This is intended to optimize the future viability of the adapter for replacement models.

The market analysis revealed various complaints related to the adapter head. There are some difficulties with the locking tab which is often used inevitable roughly. As a result the tab is deformed. In addition to that the holding points of the tab in the adapter are very small so that they cannot provide the necessary stability either. This problem is still amplified by the material combination of stainless steel and PEEK as PEEK ruptures under the force of the stainless steel.

Therefore a reinforcement of the used material with carbon fibers is analyzed. This increases the rigidity, creep strength and chemical and heat resistance of the material. CF-PEEK is also available in a biocompatible form for medical applications. However, there is a risk of a possible release of particles if the surface of the adapter is damaged, which in turn could lead to complications if they are transferred into the patient. This must be carefully considered as part of the risk analysis. As PEEK is an expensive material for cost reducing and strengthening of the material a change to stainless steel would be possible. It is already used in the adapter and therefore tested and approved. Stainless steel has the disadvantage that it is significantly heavier than PEEK due to its higher density. Therefore, the usability of a heavier adapter needs to be considered.

Summarizing currently no design change in the adapter is necessary even though there are some points that could be improved. Some weaknesses of the adapter were identified in this work and possible optimization potentials with regard to the concept, the design and the material were presented.

A consideration of all aspects that need to be taken into account in this optimization cannot be achieved in this analysis. There still remain many unclear aspects that need further clarification. An example are the hygienic aspects. Both, the washer-disinfector and the adapters must create optimal hygienic conditions in order to be able to guarantee a safe reprocessing process. Many different factors have an influence on the hygiene. Most of them cannot be described quantitatively.

When it comes to the design for example it is important to avoid the formation of shadows where inadequate cleaning is taking place due to insufficient flushing fluid. Such areas can hardly be determined theoretically using technical drawings. They can often only be identified through practical tests with prototypes.

The design options that were shown in the benchmarking analysis can only be transferred to a limited extent since each manufacturer has a different adapter concept and endoscopes are positioned differently in the various washer-disinfector. The position of the endoscope has a massive impact on the design possibilities of the adapter.

The fixed positioning of the endoscope and the adapter plate in the Olmpus washer-disinfector, the limited space that is available for the adapter due to the endoscope design and the fixed route of the hoses, limit the design options for the adapter. In a future washer-disinfector these factors need to be considered to allow for improvement of the adapter. As part of the design optimization a relocation of the surface of the locking tab should be aimed in the field of view of the user.

4   Conclusion

The aim of this work is to analyze the current design of the Olympus Air/Water-Independent adapter and reveal optimization possibilities. For this purpose the existing complaints concerning the adapter were analyzed. In order to show concept and design ideas, a benchmarking analysis of companies with corresponding adapters was carried out. To evaluate the possibilities of implementing new concept ideas, the currently used materials and the production processes that can be implemented for them were analyzed. Furthermore, the requirements that form the framework for product development were discussed. This work shows many possibilities for optimization. However, more steps are needed to gain solid insights into these approaches because the results obtained through this work are subject to some limitations. For example, the usage of alternative materials is an entirely theoretical deliberation. To what extent the materials are actually insensitive to the process chemicals used by Olympus in the washer-disinfector needs to be tested in practice. The design optimizations presented must be checked for their implementation and analyzed for advantages and disadvantages. Product and process improvements will be of increasing importance in medical technology and thus also in the development of washer-disinfector in the coming years. To do this, developments in the market have to be followed and the company's own products have to be adapted to the needs of customers consistently.

Acknowledgement

The work has been carried out at Olympus Surgical Technologies Europe, Olympus Winter & Ibe GmbH, Kuehnstraße 61, 22045 Hamburg, Germany and supervised by Prof. Dr. Christian Hübner, Institute of Physics, Universität zu Lübeck.

Author's Statement

Authors state no conflict of interest.

5   References

[1] L. Bader et al., *HYGEA (Hygiene in der Gastroenterologie - Endoskop-Aufbereitung): Studie zur Qualität der Aufbereitung von flexiblen Endoskopen in Klinik und Praxis.* In: Zeitschrift für Gastroenterologie 2002, Georg Thieme Verlag Stuttgart, New York, pp. 157–170, 2002.

[2] Kommission für Krankenhaushygiene und Infektionsprävention (KRINKO), *Anforderungen an die Hygiene bei der Aufbereitung von Medizinprodukten. Empfehlung der Kommission für Krankenhaushygiene und Infektionsprävention (KRINKO) beim Robert Koch-Institut (RKI) und des Bundesinstitutes für Arzneimittel und Medizinprodukte (BfArM).* In: Bundesgesundheitsblatt 2012, Springer Verlag, pp. 1244–1310, 2012.

[3] Olympus, *Designverbesserungen Adapter für ETD Double.* Internal Literature, 2017.

[4] E. Hornbogen, G. Eggeler and E. Werner, *Werkstoffe. Aufbau und Eigenschaften von Keramik-, Metall-, Polymer- und Verbundwerkstoffen.* Springer Vieweg Berlin, Heidelberg, 12. Auflage, 2019.

[5] A. Kalweit, C. Paul, S. Peters and R. Wallbaum, *Handbuch für Technisches Produktdesign. Material und Fertigung, Entscheidungsgrundlagen für Designer und Ingenieure.* Springer Berlin, Heidelberg, 2., bearbeitete Auflage, 2012.

[6] C. Bonten, *Kunststofftechnik. Einführung und Grundlagen.* Carl Hanser Verlag, München, 3., aktualisierte Auflage, 2020.

[7] B. Schröder, *Kunststoffe für Ingenieure. Ein Überblick.* Springer Vieweg, Wiesbaden, 2014.

[8] W. Kaiser, *Kunststoffchemie für Ingenieure. Von der Synthese bis zur Anwendung.* Carl Hanser Verlag, München, 5., neu bearbeitete und erweiterte Auflage, 2021.

[9] Deusches Institut für Normung e.V., *DIN EN ISO 9000:2015-11. Qualitätsmanagementsysteme - Grundlagen und Begriffe (ISO 9000:2015).* Deutsche und Englische Fassung EN ISO 9000:2015, Beuth-Verlag, Berlin, 2015.

Investigation of Cutting Properties of Surgical Scissors in Applications with and without High-Frequency Energy

Lea Sofie Mennerich [1]

[1] Medical Engineering Science, Universität zu Lübeck, lea.mennerich@student.uni-luebeck.de

Abstract

HICURA laparoscopic hand instruments from Olympus are used for various surgical applications. To address the need of different procedures various working inserts exist. In this project, the cutting properties of the Metzenbaum scissors insert were tested. The cutting tests were separated in two sets, with and without high-frequency (HF) energy. In a cold cut scenario - without HF energy - one group of scissors was tested in water and another group of scissors was tested in dry environment. Each of the scissors made 1000 cuts on artificial tissue replacement and the blades were investigated microscopically in regular intervals. Besides that, the closing force was measured and documented. In a second test series 1000 cuts were made on tissue with simultaneous HF energy application. The cutting performance was tested with thread and gauze. It could be shown that the cutting properties remained unchanged under tested conditions with and without HF energy.

1 Introduction

HICURA is a new generation of laparoscopic hand instruments from Olympus. The instruments have various applications in general surgery, gynecology and urology. Besides the mechanical functionality of different inserts, like grasping and cutting, HICURA hand instruments can be used as electrosurgical instrument together with an electrosurgical generator [1]. In this configuration HF energy is able to manipulate tissue thermally for hemostasis, surgical sectioning or tissue sealing. The advantage of using hand instruments with HF energy is the possibility to cut and seal tissue simultaneously. Besides that, through coagulation with HF energy, hemostasis can be reached without using exogenous materials, which leads to a minimization of possible germ carryover [2].

HF surgery can be differentiated in monopolar and bipolar technology. The main difference is the size and position of the neutral electrode. The most common technology for HF surgery is the monopolar type [2]. Monopolar HF surgery requires an active electrode and a neutral electrode which are connected to the electrosurgical generator. The neutral electrode is significantly bigger than the active electrode and is usually placed on the patient's upper arm or thigh. This leads to a large contact area between the patient's skin and the neutral electrode which results in a low current density in order to avoid undesired thermal injuries [3]. The comparably small size of the active electrode leads to a high current density that results in combination with the tissue resistance to the thermal tissue effect at the treatment spot [4].

In this project, test series with the HICURA Metzenbaum scissors insert are conducted. The Metzenbaum scissors and an assembled hand instrument are characterized by a long handle and comparatively short blades [5] and are shown in Fig. 1. Therefore, in one test series it is investigated whether the high current density at the blades has an influence on the cutting properties of the Metzenbaum scissors. In a second test series, the scissors are tested over a long term without the use of HF energy to check whether the cutting performance changes over the application processes.

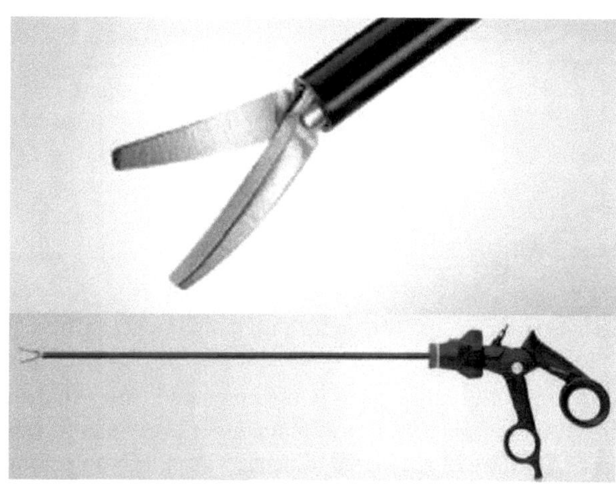

Figure 1: Top: Metzenbaum scissors insert. Bottom: HICURA laparoscopic hand instrument consisting of handle, sheath and insert [1].

2 Material and Methods

To verify the cutting properties test series with and without HF energy were conducted. For cold cutting without HF energy, cutting was done for a defined number of times on artificial tissue replacement. Cutting blades were investigated visually in regular intervals and, in addition, closing force measurements were performed to detect possible changes over the time. For cutting with HF energy, pork tissue was used to simulate a surgery application. As before, the scissors were investigated visually. Both tests imply also cold cuts with either gauze or thread, what is a common test procedure [6].

2.1 Cold Cutting Tests

To test the cutting properties of the scissors over a long term, reproducible test requirements need to be accomplished. For that purpose, a latex resistance band from Theraband® (Akron, Ohio) is used as artificial tissue replacement. Its advantage is the consistent thickness, which leads to invariable requirements. For the tests the Theraband® was cut without being under tension. A test scope of 1000 cuts per scissors was predefined and the scissors were investigated microscopically after every 100 cuts. This led to 10 test cycles in total. 16 Metzenbaum scissors were tested, half of them were tested cutting under water while the other half was tested in dry environment. The test setup for the tests under water is shown in Fig. 2. In the begin-

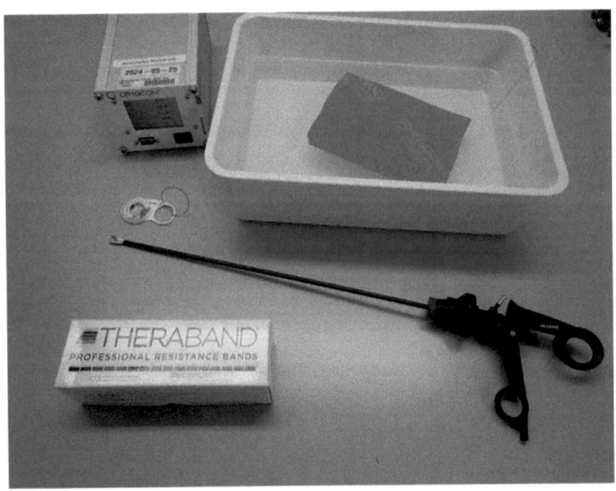

Figure 2: Test setup for the cold cutting tests under water. The temperature of the water was measured with a fiber optic thermometer and was in the range of 20 to 25 °C.

ning the initial situation was documented. After that the first 100 Theraband® cuts were made for every pair of scissors. Additionally, a thread (Coated Vicryl, Ethicon, Johnson & Johnson) was cut twice and the cutting edge was investigated visually to check the cutting property. Besides that, the scissors run a closing force test. For that the testing bench shown in Fig. 3 was developed. The inserts are clamped in the mechanism and the closing force is displayed digitally. To evaluate the attrition of the blades, im-

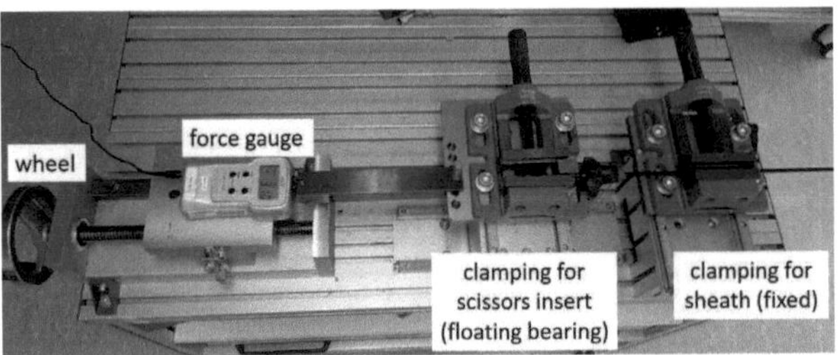

Figure 3: Testing bench for closing force measurements. The blades of the scissors are closed with a rotary wheel and the closing force is displayed on a digital gauge.

ages with the digital microscope DVM6 M (Leica microsystems, Wetzlar, Germany) were recorded with a 79x image magnification. This process was repeated after every 100 cuts.

2.2 HF Cutting Tests

For the HF cutting tests, the hand instrument was connected to the electrosurgical generator ESG-400 (Olympus, Shinjuku, Tokyo, Japan). The electrosurgical generator offers different modes and for investigating changes of the cutting properties, the "PureCut" mode was used because it has a higher output voltage than the coagulation mode and presumably leads to a higher damage to the scissors. Realistic settings for surgery applications (50 W, effect 3) were adjusted. Pork meat was used as tissue which was cut in 5 mm thick slices. The tissue was placed on top of the neutral electrode. Cuts were made in the tissue while HF energy was applied simultaneously. To test the cutting properties of the pair of scissors after cutting the tissue, a thread (Coated Vicryl, Ethicon, Johnson & Johnson) was cut and the cutting edge of the blades was investigated microscopically as in the first test series. The blades were investigated before tissue cutting and after 100, 325, 500, 750 and 1000 cuts. Another requirement for the scissors is the ability to cut gauze. To verify this, an abacterial non-woven compress (Curafit, Budni) is cut after the previously mentioned test iterations. The test setup is shown in Fig. 4.

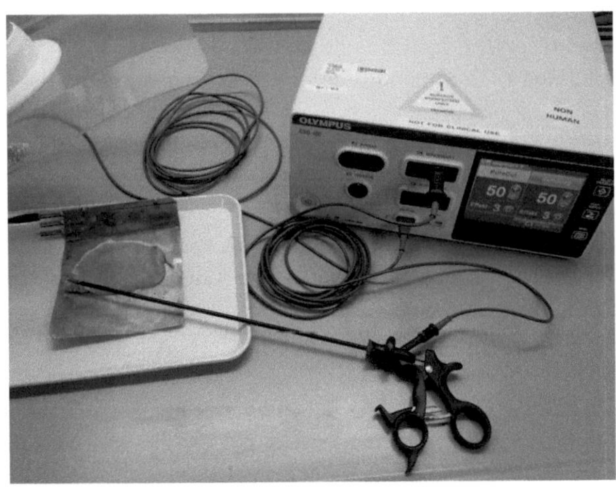

Figure 4: Test setup for the HF cutting tests.

3 Results and Discussion

3.1 Cold Cutting Tests

In Fig. 5 the results of the closing force measurements are summarized. The plot shows the mean values for the two test groups. For the scissors tested without water, the closing force fluctuates around 20 N. For the test group with water, the closing force value is also 20 N, but it decreases over the time. The decrease of the closing force is a result of the attrition of the cutting blades. The more cuts were made, the rounder the cutting blades became, which led to a lower effort for closing the scissors. The closing force values for the test group with water are lower than the values for the scissors tested without water, which can be explained by the fact that water functions as a lubricant.

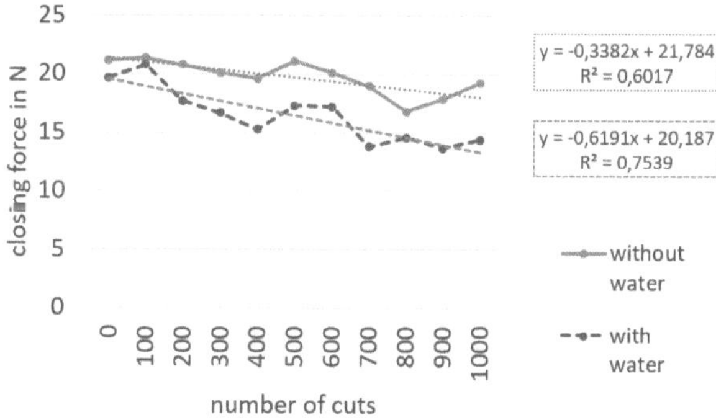

Figure 5: Mean values and regression line of the closing force of the tested scissors groups in water and without water.

Cutting the thread led to a clear cutting edge for every test cycle. Compared to the beginning the cutting performance did not decrease after 1000 cuts were made. Another part of the test series was the visual investigation of the blades. In

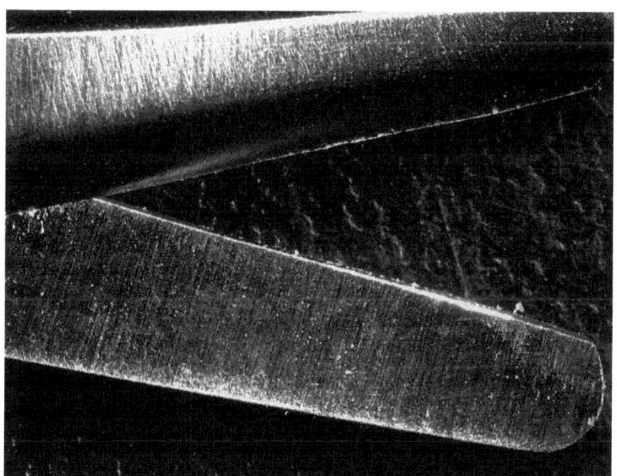

Figure 6: Microscope image of the blades after 100 cuts. The scissors belong to the test group without water.

Fig. 6 a microscope image of the blades of scissors from the test group without water after 100 cuts is shown. The same scissors are shown in Fig. 7 but the image was taken after 1000 cuts. At first sight the images of the blades show no

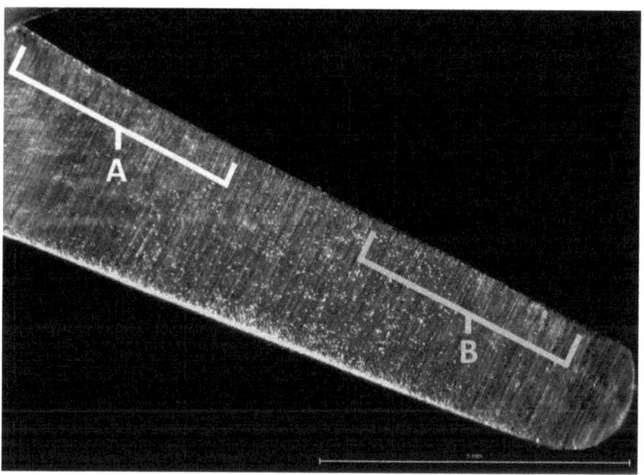

Figure 7: Microscope image of the blades after 1000 cuts. Small attritions visible in the back part (A), unchanged condition in the front area (B). The scissors belong to the test group without water.

remarkable differences. With zooming it becomes visible that the main attrition of the blades is in the back part (A) while the front of the cutting edge (B) is nearly in the same condition after 1000 cuts compared to the beginning. For the group of scissors tested in dry environment, comparable results were obtained. All in all, a small attrition is visible for the scissors from both test groups by cutting the artificial tissue replacement, but the cutting properties do not decrease which can be seen when cutting the thread.

3.2 HF Cutting Tests

In the HF cutting tests the scissors are exposed to a higher stress due to the applied HF energy. In Fig. 8 the microscope image of the blade before cutting is shown. Fig. 9

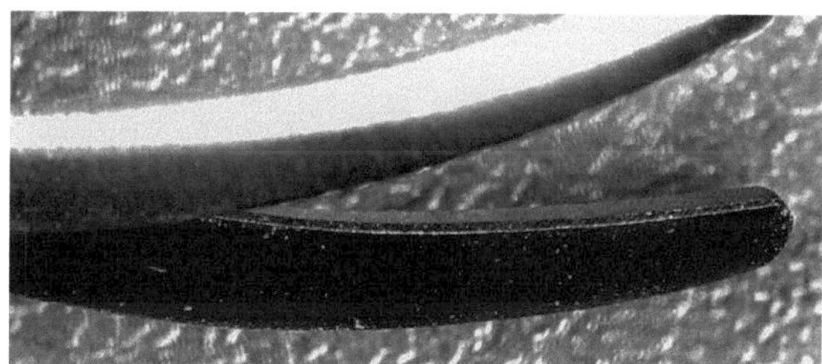

Figure 8: Microscope image of the blades before cutting.

shows the blades after 1000 tissue cuts with the defined settings were made. Both pictures show a clean cutting edge. As it can be seen in Fig. 9 the HF energy leads to a discoloration of the cutting blades (C). In this HF cutting test no or no sufficient cleaning steps were executed, but former tests showed that during reprocessing the residues would be removed. The discoloration has no influence on the cutting performance of the scissors as you can see in Fig. 10, which shows the clean cutting edge of the gauze cut by the scissors after 1000 cuts were made. Besides the gauze, the scissors were able to cut the thread. In Fig. 11 the cutting edges of the thread after different test iterations are compared. After 750 tissue cuts, the cutting edge of the thread was still clean.

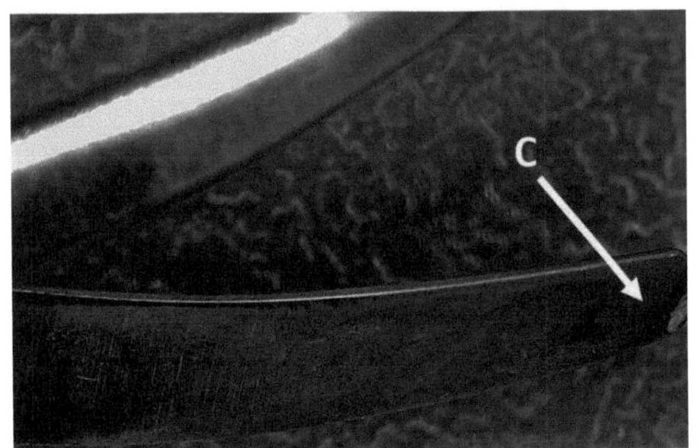

Figure 9: Microscope image of the blades after 1000 tissue cuts with HF energy were made. Discoloration of the cutting blades visible (C).

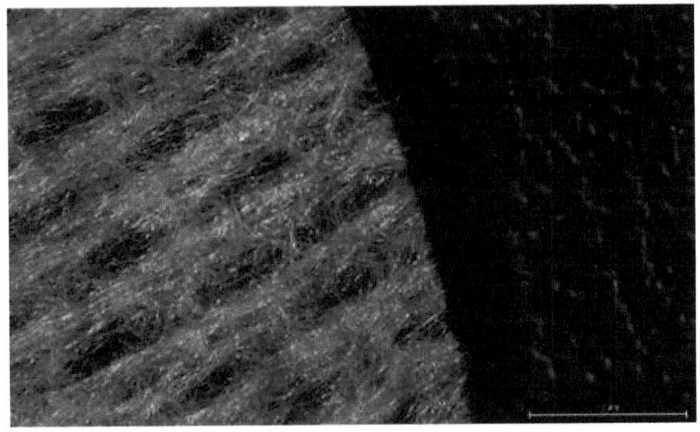

Figure 10: Cutting edge of the gauze after 1000 tissue cuts.

After 1000 cuts it was still possible to separate the thread, but the cutting edge is less clean than before. It can be seen that the discoloration, due to the long-term test and the not performed cleaning and reprocessing, has no influence on the cutting performance. Besides the results that under the

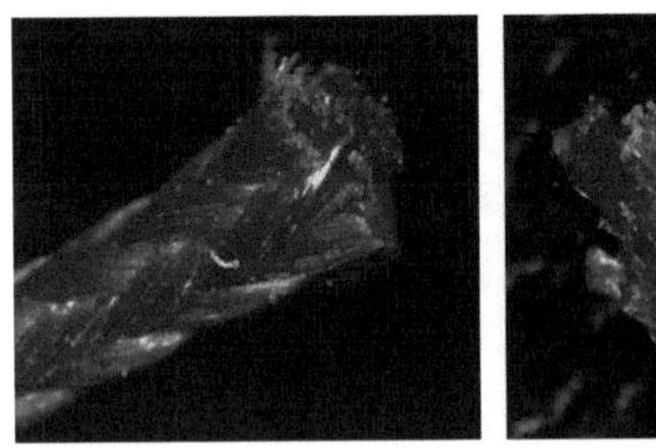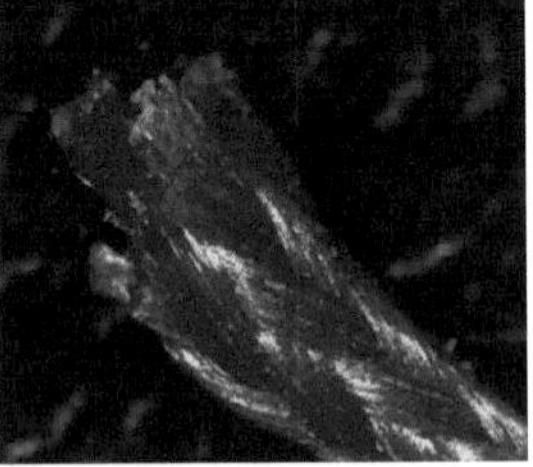

Figure 11: Microscope image of the thread after 750 tissue cuts (left) and after 1000 tissue cuts (right).

given test conditions the scissors still show a good cutting performance after 1000 cuts, it has to be discussed whether the test conditions are realistic. The intended use of the HI-CURA hand instruments does not exclude a simultaneous application of HF energy, but in surgery applications the Metzenbaum scissors are used for mechanical cutting and the HF energy is used for selective coagulation only with the tip of the instruments. This shows that the test conditions represent a worst-case scenario and in real life applications even less damage to the scissors can be expected.

4   Conclusion

Both test series, the cold cutting tests and the HF cutting tests, showed good results for the cutting performance of the scissors over the whole test period. According to the product requirement, the scissors are used for up to 20 cuts per operation and the test scope of 1000 cuts represents the lifetime of 50 cycles. The closing force measurements in the cold cutting test showed consistent or even decreasing values and it can be expected that this trend continues if more than 1000 cuts were made. The HF cutting tests were conducted with realistic parameters and after 1000 cuts no reduction of the cutting performance can be detected. The HF energy led to a discoloration of the blades due to missing reprocessing of the scissors but the cutting properties were not affected. All in all, it could be ensured that the cutting performance of the Metzenbaum scissors remains the same over the lifetime for applications with as well as without the use of HF energy.

Acknowledgement

The work has been carried out at Olympus Surgical Technologies Europe, Hamburg, Germany and supervised by Prof. Dr. C. Hübner, Institute of Physics, Universität zu Lübeck.

Author's Statement

Conflict of interest: Authors state no conflict of interest.

5   References

[1] Olympus, *Hand Instruments - HICURA, HiQ+*. Available: https://www.olympus.de/medical/de/Produkte-und-Lösungen/Produkte/Product/HICURA-Monopolare-und-bipolare-Handinstrumente.html [last accessed on 2023-01-10].

[2] R. Kramme, *Medizintechnik: Verfahren-Systeme-Informationsverarbeitung*. Springer, Heidelberg, 2007.

[3] K. Fastenmeier, *Endoskopische Urologie*. Springer, Berlin, Heidelberg, 2009.

[4] V. Hausmann, *Lagerungstechniken im Operationsbereich*. Springer, Berlin, Heidelberg, 2005.

[5] R. Metson, *Myron F. Metzenbaum, MD: Innovative surgeon, caring physician*. Otolaryngology—Head and Neck Surgery, vol. 110, no. 6, pp. 477–481, 1994.

[6] International Organization for Standardization, *ISO 7741-1986 (E): Instruments for surgery - Scissors and shears - General requirements and test methods*. Beuth, Berlin, 1986.

Fluidic design of a spectroscopic oximetry module

Daniel von Treuenfels [1], Philipp Dominke [2], Sören Scholand [2], and Stefan Müller [3]

[1] Biomedical Engineering, Lübeck University of Applied Sciences; daniel.von.treuenfels@stud.th-luebeck.de
[2] Eschweiler GmbH Co. KG, Kiel; dominke@eschweiler-kiel.de, scholand@eschweiler-kiel.de
[3] Medical Sensors and Devices Laboratory, Lübeck University of Applied Sciences; stefan.mueller@th-luebeck.de

Abstract

This article summarizes a series of laboratory trials, set up to analyze the possibilities, to integrate an oximetry module into an existing blood gas analyzer (BGA), built by the company "Eschweiler GmbH CO. KG." in Kiel. Especially the properties of the fluidic circuit in the device need to fulfill dedicated requirements, to guarantee reliable measurements. The special challenge in this context is, that the blood sample, which is a two phase non-homogeneous system, is not allowed to sediment during the measurement. To prevent sedimentation, which would cause enormous changes in the optical properties of the blood, the trial series is evaluating the possibility, to do measurements while the device is pumping the blood sample thru its fluidic circuit. However, finally it turned out, that completely pausing the pumping procedure for a short period of time will be the favorable solution, because it does not seem to be possible to guarantee steady conditions in all Eschweiler GmbH Co. Kg.'s BGA devices.

1 Introduction

The term blood gas analysis (BGA) is used to address a class of point-of-care-test (POCT) devices, designed to analyze gas concentrations in blood samples. BGA is a frequently used technique to monitor a patient's health condition in intensive or emergency medical care. The measurements are especially useful to evaluate the sufficiency of the respiratory system and balance of electrolytes or acid-base-ratio in the human body [1][2]. To measure various parameters, the BGA device utilizes multiple types of sensors. The ones responsible for analyzing the state of the hemoglobin in the erythrocytes, are called oximeters. They are specially designed spectrometers, set up to detect and separate the hemoglobin molecules, carrying oxygen $(O_2 - Hb)$ from the unloaded $(H - Hb)$ or poisoned ones. Poisoned means transporting carbon monoxide $(CO - Hb)$ or being deformed to methemoglobin $(Met - Hb)$ by oxidization, in this context. An oximetry sensor is also able to determine the overall hemoglobin concentration (Hb). As additional feature the sensor can specify the overall oxygen saturation (SO_2) [3].

Figure 1 shows the specific absorption of different hemoglobin derivates at various wavelengths, visualizing the sensitivity of the measurement method. The way the measurement is done is called spectral decomposition of light or spectroscopy. Whilst there are multiple known variants of spectrometers, oximeters are mostly using absorption spectrometry, i.e., they are detecting and separating fractions of light, sorted by their wavelength, after they passed through a blood sample [5].

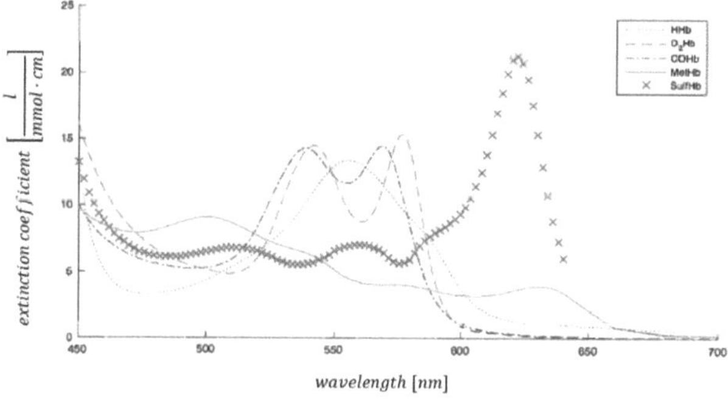

Figure 1: Absorption spectra of various Hb-derivates with respect to the wavelength; based on [4]

All absorption processes in a medium can be estimated using Lambert-Beer's law, denoted in (1). The variables are representing, the Intensity of imminent- I_0 and transmitted light I, as well as the molar concentration c, the extinction coefficient ε and the diameter of the traversed medium d.

$$I = I_0 \cdot e^{-\varepsilon \cdot c \cdot d} \tag{1}$$

As mentioned before, the fluidic properties of blood are very inconsistent, which makes it way more complicated to achieve good measurement results. Due to its consistency, of 55% liquid plasma and its various blood cells, collectively referred to as hematocrit, blood is called a two-phase-system in fluid mechanics [6][7]. While experiencing a high shear-rate, blood behaves like a Newtonian fluid, when the shear is decreasing, it tends to appear non-Newtonian [7]. This is mostly caused by the varying shape, spatial orientation, and rate of aggregation of the erythrocytes. All these factors may affect the reflective and refractive properties of the whole blood [8]. Having this in mind, it is very important to characterize the flow in the measurement-setup, before using it, to verify the data collected during the experiments.

2 Material and Methods

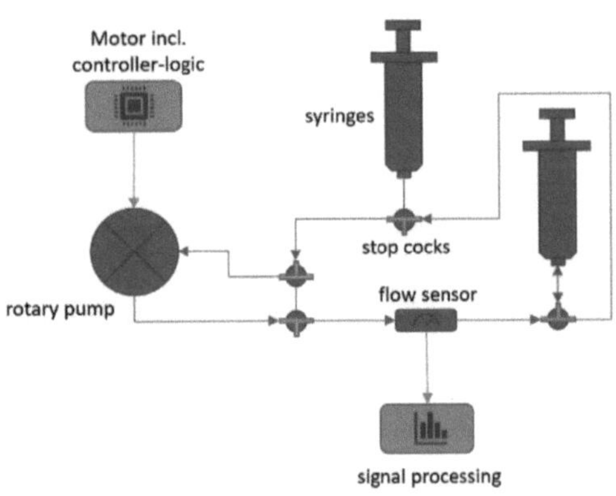

Figure 2: testbench setup for flow characterization

2.1 Fluidic Circuit

In contrast to an actual BGA device, the testbench setup could be set up relatively simple. Because it is the only active component affecting the characteristics of the flow in in the circuit, the pump with the related tubing were the only components extracted from it. The rest of the setup was designed around them. A circular arranged tubing works as fluid source and drain. Additionally, a bypass for the pump was realized, using stopcocks. This bypass can be used to fill the system or test an installed flow sensor. To realize this manual operation, two 50 ml syringes were added to the circuit, also using stopcocks. In addition to this function, the syringes also work as air-traps, extracting air bubbles from the system, using density properties. A schematic of this fluidic circuit can be found in Fig. 2. The setup was changed once during the test series. For the first two tests, a stepper motor was used, to drive a 6-roller rotary pump. The last test was done using a 5-roller rotary pump, powered by a DC-motor. During the tests two variants of fluid have been used.

Table 1: fluidic and electric components of the testbench

purpose	parts mk. 1	parts mk. 2	parts mk. 3	parts mk. 4
sensor	LS32® liquid flow sensor / Sensirion			LS32® liquid flow sensor Sensirion
pump	6-roller peristaltic pump / Eschweiler OEM			5-roller peristaltic pump Eschweiler OEM
motor	42BYG45040-24D - stepper motor / Geeetech			12V DC-motor Eschweiler OEM
motor driver	DRV8825 - stepper driver POLULU	AMIS 30543 - stepper driver POLULU		∅
power supply	E3631A power supply / Hewlett Packard			
microcontroller	UNO rev. 3® - microcontroller / Arduino			∅
tubing	2x Heidelberger® extension line (750mm) / B.Braun			
valves	4x Discofix® - stopcock / B.Braun			
syringes	2x 50ml Perfusor® -syringe / B.Braun			
fluid	100% H$_2$O	100% H$_2$O	55% H$_2$O 45% C$_3$H$_8$O$_3$	55% H$_2$O 45% C$_3$H$_8$O$_3$

As a proof-of-concept stage, the setup has first been filled with distilled water. Later, a 45% to 55% ratio glycerin-water solution was filled in. This mixture is a proper approach to mimic the average viscosity of blood [9]. A detailed list of all used fluidic- and electronic parts can be found in Table 1.

2.2 Data acquisition & Signal processing

To monitor the output generated by the pump, a Sensirion LS32® flow sensor has been integrated into the fluidic circuit. Combined with the respective software "sensor viewer®, the measured flow data can be easily stored in comma-separated files. These files have than been analyzed and visualized, using MathWorks's MATLAB®. There has been no relevant postprocessing of the data. All the tests have been conducted in the same manner. The fluidic circuit was filled with the respective fluid. Following up the tubing was checked for leakages, by applying manual pressure with one of the syringes. After finding no leakages, the system was powered on. Whilst the pump starts to move, the flow was monitored using "sensor viewer®". After a continuous flow pattern has been recognized with a stable amplitude, the flow was logged for a dedicated time. The respective time settings vary according to sensor capabilities and motor setup. The changes in pumping speed, sampling frequency and sampling resolution are reactions to the acquired results and will thus be explained in detail in the next paragraph.

3 Results and Discussion

3.1 Results experiment 1

For this first test, the system was operated at constant rotational speeds of around 0.3 rpm for the pump. It was not possible to increase the flowrate further, because the sensor could not handle high sampling- frequency and -resolution, simultaneously. By choosing this relatively low speeds, the data could be sampled without relevant aliasing problems. A selection of these results can be seen in Fig. 3 and Fig. 4. A reference measurement, to determine the influence of external disturbances to the signal can be found in Fig. 5. This reference data has been acquired for every measurement series. Due to fact, that there are no relevant changes in the one, taken for the next series, only this one is shown as an example. Analyzing the plotted data in Fig. 3 and Fig. 4, the base frequency of the rotating pump-head is clearly visible. The second signal-component, appearing as a continuous high frequency pattern, can be identified as the single motor steps. This theory can be supported by comparing the selected stepper-frequency to the frequency of the oscillation in the graph. Secondly the component is changing its frequency depending on changes in rotational speed of the pump. The slight variation in amplitude can be explained by noise and aliasing effects in that high frequency ranges. It can also be stated, that a fully engaged roller will generate a flow of $0.6 - 0.8$ µl/s, depending on the selected pump settings (see Plateau-phases in Fig. 3 & Fig. 4). In contrast, a single motor step only moves around 0.2 µl of fluid per second, regardless of the rotational speed of the pump. This leads to the conclusion, that the flow, produced by the motor-steps, will vanish, when a higher overall speed is set for the pump, because the flow produce by the engaging rollers will increase drastically, while the influence of the motor's steps will remain on the same level, as in these tests. The expected time for an oximetric measurement will be around 100ms. While moving the pump at an average speed of 30 rpm, which would be the setting in Eschweiler GmbH & Co. Kg.'s devices, the plateau-phase of the flow would take a period of 200ms. Comparing these values leads to the fact, that a measurement can be considered possible, while running the pump, if a reliable synchronization is guaranteed.

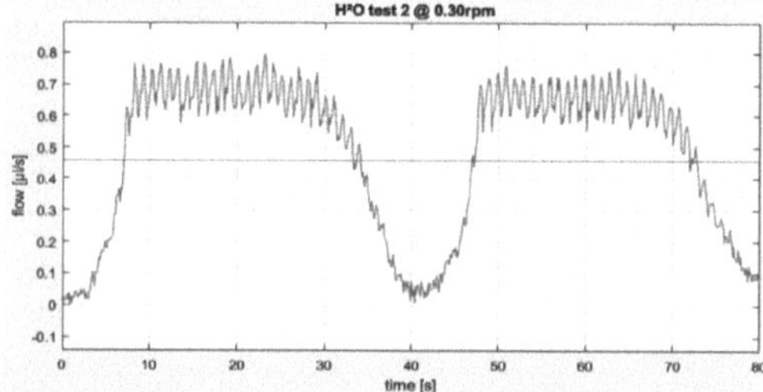

Figure 3: plotted measurement-data at 0.35 rpm, logged during experiment 1

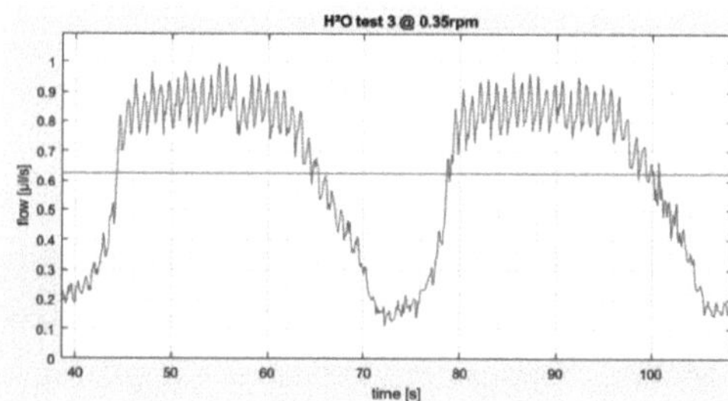

Figure 4: plotted measurement-data at 0.35 rpm, logged during experiment 1

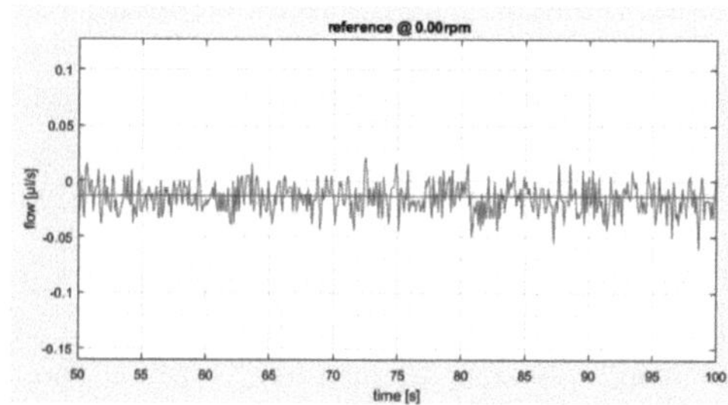

Figure 5: plotted reference-data at 0.00 rpm, logged during experiment 1

3.2   Results experiment 2

Experiment two started the same way as the one before. However, this time, the glycerin/water solution was used to fill the fluidic circuit, instead of water. The previously mixed solution contains around 45% of glycerin and 55% of distilled water. Some logged data can be seen, visualized in Fig. 6. While evaluating the data, there are no eminent differences visible, between this set and the one evaluated before. The average output is slightly higher in this experiment, which might be caused by the fact, that the high viscous fluid is a little less likely to flow back, when the roller clamp of the pump is not completely sealing the tubing of the pump. Overall, this deviation can be considered negligible. These results suggest, that for this pumping technique, the viscosity of the moved fluid is not affecting the pumps output, as long as the tubing is way stiffer than the fluid itself. This result was to be expected but can now be considered proven.

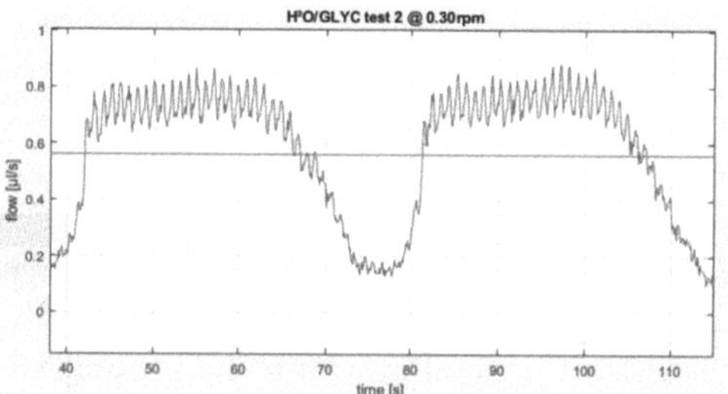

Figure 6: plotted measurement-data at 0.30 rpm, logged during experiment 2

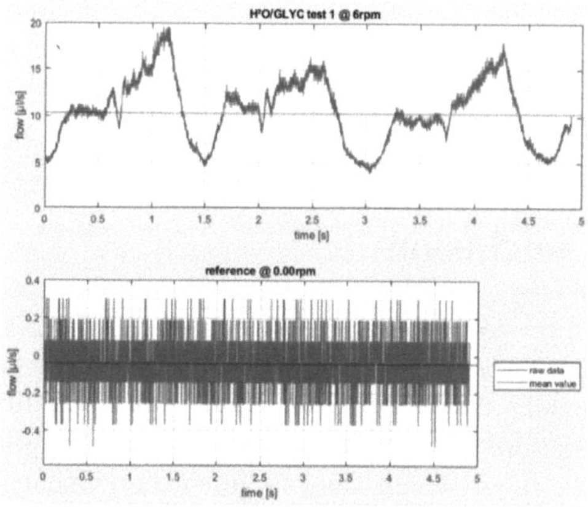

Figure 7: plotted measurement-data, logged during experiment 3

3.3   Results experiment 3

For the last experiment, the stepper-motor-powered pump was replaced by a one, powered by a 12V DC-motor. The initial leakage test was passed without any complaints. To power up the system the motor was supplied with 6V DC resulting in a rotational speed of the pump of 6 rpm. These settings have been a compromise between steady motion of the motor and a sufficient sampling output. As expected, there are no high-frequency components in this signal, because there are no discrete steps, done by the motor. The overall output is also slightly different from the other test because this pump is utilizing a pre-loaded tubing system. In contrast, the one tested first was pressing the tube against a countering-plate. The result of this function principle can be seen in Fig. 7. The exponential increase of flow during the expected plateau phase, is generated by the elastic retraction of the tubing here. Therefore, a plateau-synchronized measurement cannot be accounted feasible.

3.4 Summarizing Discussion

After analyzing all the experiments, it seems feasible to synchronize the measurement-window for the spectrometer with the plateau phase in the pulsation of the flow, i.e., only do measurements while one roller of the pump is engaging. This requires a dedicated monitoring of the pumps position and an almost linear plateau phase. Therefore, this option is only possible using a stepper motor or a DC motor with encoder and a pump setup which is minimizing capacitive behavior of the tubing. An alternative option would be, to stop the pump for a short period of time, i.e. around a second, to make a measurement during steady conditions. This solution could be realized in all systems and is therefore more versatile. The possibility of blood's sedimentation is present but appears to be non-relevant. This is given by the fact, that the period, necessary to do a measurement, is expected to be relatively short, i.e. around 100 ms. Medium viscous blood of a healthy human will sediment at a rate of around 10% of the tubing's height per hour [10], i.e. around 0.03% per second, assuming an exponential decline. This would result in 99.97% non-sedimented blood, at the beginning of the measurement period, after the pump has been stopped.

4 Conclusion

Overall, the tests done can be considered a success. The acquired data is of sufficiently good quality, and the results are matching the expectations. Additional test with better suited sensors or real blood samples could be necessary, if there are inconsistencies in the future measurements. Also, a detailed analysis of the blood's sedimentation character could be necessary if the results of the oximetric measurements, which are planned as a follow up experiment, tend to be inconsistent.

Acknowledgement

The work has been carried out in the Medical Sensors and Devices Laboratory at the Lübeck university of applied sciences. Eschweiler GmbH & Co. KG. was involved, providing fluidic and electronic components. Also, they have been acting as specialist consultants for BGA.

Author's Statement

Conflict of interest: Authors state no conflict of interest.

5 References

[1] K. Dörner, *Klinische Chemie und Hämatologie* (in ger), 8th ed. Stuttgart, New York; Georg Thieme Verlag, 2013.

[2] W. Boehmke, M. O. Krebs and R. Rossaint, "Blutgasanalyse" (in ger), In: *Der Anästhesist*, vol.53, no.5, pp. 471 – 492, July 2004.

[3] P. B. Luppa, *POCT - Patientennahe Labordiagnostik* (in ger), 3rd ed.Berlin, Heidelberg: Springer Berlin / Heidelberg, 2017.

[4] B. Kern (Redmer) and B. Nestler , "Optische Messung von Hämoglobin-Derivaten in nicht hämolysiertem humen Vollblut" (in ger), In: *ImpulsE*, vol.20, pp. 38–40, March 2017. Accessed: Jan. 21, 2023. [Online]. Available: https://www.th-luebeck.de/fileadmin/media_msgt/02_Aktuelles/News/2017/ImpulsE/11_Redmer_Haemoglobindrivate.pdf

[5] M. Löffler-Mang, *Optische Sensorik: Lasertechnik, Experimente, Light Barriers* (in ger), 1st ed. Wiesbaden: Vieweg + Teubner, 2012.

[6] R. Huch and K. D. Jürgens (publ.), *Mensch, Körper, Krankheit: Anatomie, Physiologie, Krankheitsbilder; Lehrbuch und Atlas für die Berufe im Gesundheitswesen* (in ger), 5th ed. München: Elservier Urban & Fischer, 2007.

[7] D. Liepsch, *Biofluidmechanik: Grundlagen und Anwendungen* (in ger), 1st ed. Berlin, Heidelberg: Springer Berlin / Heidelberg, 2022.

[8] A. Roggan, M. Friebel, K. Dörschel, A. Hahn and G. Müller, "Optical Properties of Circulating Human Blood in the Wavelength Range 400 - 2500 nm". In: *Journal of biomedical optics*, vol. 4, no. 1, pp. 36 – 46, January 1999. doi: 10.1117/1.429919 . [Online]. Available: https://pubmed.ncbi.nlm.nih.gov/23015168

[9] M. Y. Yousif, D. W. Holdsworth, and T. L. Poepping, "A blood-mimicking fluid for particle image velocimetry with silicone vascular models". In: *Experiments in Fluids*, vol. 50, no. 3, pp. 769 – 774, March 2011. doi: 10.1007/s00348-010-0958-1 . [Online]. Available: https://link.springer.com/article/10.1007/s00348-010-0958-1

[10] M. A. Taye, "Sedimentation rate of erythrocyte from physics prospective". In: *The European physical journal E, Soft Matter and Biological Physics*, vol. 43, no. 3, p. 19, March 2011. doi: 10.1140/epje/i2020-11943-2 . [Online]. Available: https://pubmed.ncbi.nlm.nih.gov/32201913/

Adjustment and evaluation of a newly designed device to set the reference arm length in swept source OCT

Anneli Dick [1,2], Lars Luft [2] and Carsten Schade[2]

[1] Medical Engineering Science, Universität zu Lübeck, anneli.dick@student.uni-luebeck.de

[2] Heidelberg Engineering GmbH, (anneli.dick,lars.luft,carsten.schade)@heidelbergengineering.com

Abstract

Optical coherence tomography (OCT) is a high-resolution imaging technology which is mainly used in ophthalmology. A newly designed device is presented, which allows a variation of the axial imaging area by changing the reference arm length - the delay line (DL). An optics adjustment concept is presented, using a Shack-Hartmann wavefront sensor and a 4-quadrant diode. In addition, the transmission behaviour of the DL under temperature variation and vibrations is evaluated. The power throughput is invariant against vibrations, but is clearly temperature-dependent as the light transmission deviates by 5.73% at a temperature difference of 27.44°C. A constant signal-to-noise ratio over the axial imaging range is supported, as a power-stable variation of the reference arm length could be realized and the required light transmission of 30% is achieved.

1 Introduction

Optical coherence tomography [1] can be used to generate 2- and 3-dimensional images of scattering tissues. Image generation is based on the measurement of time-of-flight differences of the light waves scattered by the tissue. Since the light frequencies are in the THz range and propagate at the speed of light, interferometric setups are required to measure the time differences. The depth information in swept source (SS) OCT results from the modulation frequencies in the measured interference signal. The larger the path-length difference between the two interferometer arms, the larger the fringe frequency [2]. Due to the limited frequency bandwidth of the signal digitizer, only fringe frequencies from a certain depth range can be resolved. This leads to a limitation of the axial imaging range in OCT [3]. By varying the path-length difference of the interferometer arms with the DL, the axial imaging area can be selected.

The aim of this work is to prove if a stable SNR near the shot noise limit can be supported, using the here presented DL, even under environmental influences.

1.1 SS-OCT and axial imaging range

OCT imaging uses either one of three basic technologies: time domain (TD), spectral domain (SD) and swept source OCT [4]. For this work only SS-OCT is of importance. SS-OCT uses a frequency-tunable light source [5]. The light is split between a reference arm and a sample arm by using a beamsplitter. After reflection at the mirror and scattering at the sample, the light from the two arms is brought together and interferes. If the distance passed by the light in the reference arm and the sample arm is different, the light is recombined with a path-length difference. This creates a modulation frequency in the resulting interference signal [2]:

$$I(t) = I_S + I_R + 2\sqrt{I_S I_R} \; cos(k(t)\Delta z). \qquad (1)$$

I_S is the intensity in the sample arm and I_R is the intensity in the reference arm. $k(t)$ represents the time-dependent wavenumber. Since the light is scattered by several tissue layers at different depths, several fringe frequencies are contained in the interference signal. These can be extracted by a Fourier transformation and thus provide information about the characteristics of the sample [4]. The larger the path-length difference Δz between the two interferometer arms, the larger the fringe frequency contained in the interference signal. Due to the limited frequency bandwidth of the signal digitizer, only a certain axial imaging range of the sample can be digitized [3]. To vary the position of the axial measurement range, an adjustment of the interferometer arm length is needed. In this work this is realized by the integration of the DL in the reference arm. A photodiode is used to detect the interference signal, which converts the light into an electrical current [5].

1.2 SNR in SS-OCT

The optical power in the sample and the reference arm is one factor which affects the signal-to-noise ratio (SNR) of an OCT system. The higher the power in the sample arm, the better the SNR. For the reference arm power there is a sweet spot where the SNR is optimal, in the best case only limited by the signal-to-quantum-noise ratio ($SN_{sh}R$). In

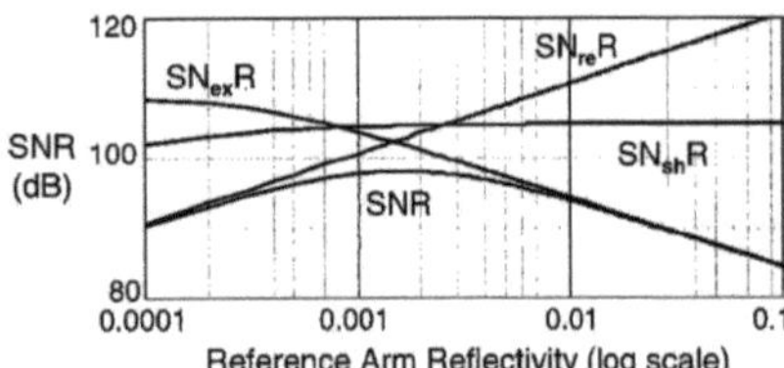

Figure 1: SNR as a function of reference arm reflectivity. Also shown are the signal-to-receiver-noise ratio ($SN_{re}R$), the signal-to-shot-noise ratio ($SN_{sh}R$) and the signal-to-excess-noise ratio [6].

this case the so-called shot noise limit is reached [2], [6]. If the reference arm power is reduced or increased around this sweet spot, either the signal-to-receiver-noise ratio ($SN_{re}R$) or the signal-to-excess-intensity-noise ratio ($SN_{ex}R$) dominates, leading to a decrease in overall SNR [6]. So the reference arm power should be matched to the OCT-system (i.e. to interferometer design and electronics) such that, in the best case, the shot noise limit can be reached. As the DL is located in the reference arm, a constant light transmission is required when varying the reference arm length in order to enable a constant SNR over the axial imaging range. Due to the limited optical power of the light source, used here, the DL must have a certain light transmission to support a SNR near the shot noise limit. For the specific OCT-system, in which the DL will be integrated, a required transmission of 30±5% was calculated.

2 Material and Methods

2.1 Principle and setup of the delay line

The variation of the reference arm length is realized by a collimated free beam that is deflected by a movable 3D glass retroreflector, as shown in Fig.2. Light from the reference arm is collimated by a fiber-coupled collimator (FC). The $1/e^2$ beam diameter is determined to 3.34 mm, measured with a beam profiler (291221, Edmund Optics GmbH, Mainz, Germany). If the beam diameter was smaller, the beam waist would have a noticeable impact on the light transmission of the DL, when moving the retroreflector. If the beam diameter was chosen too large, the angle adjustment of the collimators would be critical. When the beam hits the retroreflector it is directed onto a collimator with an integrated mirror (MC). The retroreflector is attached to a carriage and can be moved along a guide rail by a spindle motor, as shown in Fig.3. This allows a variation of the optical path-length in air by 90 mm, as the retroreflector has a movement range of 45 mm. After the light is being reflected by the MC, it runs the same way backwards and is coupled into the reference arm fiber.

2.2 Adjustment of the optics

To ensure the demands of a power-stable length-variation with an interferometer-compliant power transmission, the

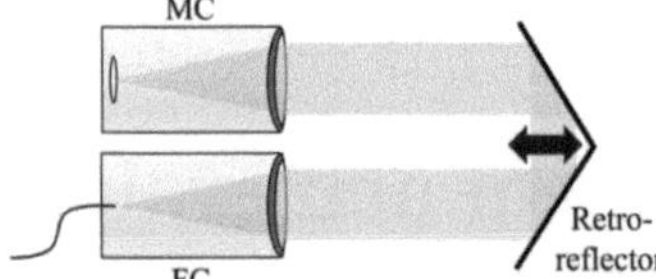

Figure 2: Schematic setup of the delay line basically consisting of a fiber-coupled collimator (FC), a collimator with integrated mirror (MC) and a retroreflector.

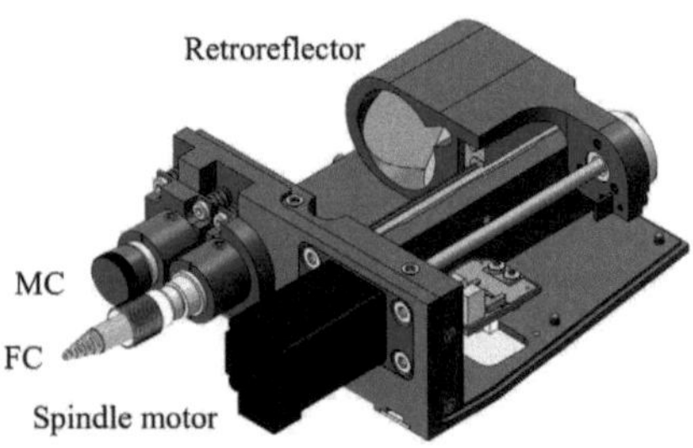

Figure 3: Setup of the delay line consisting of fiber-coupled collimator (FC), a collimator with an integrated mirror (MC), a retroreflector and a spindle motor.

optics of the DL must be adjusted before use. This requires four adjustment steps, which are described below.

2.2.1 Collimation with Shack-Hartmann wavefront sensor

A Shack-Hartmann wavefront sensor (W40150-5C, Thorlabs, Inc., Newton, USA) is used to adjust the fiber-coupled collimator. To create a parallel beam the distance between the lens and the light exit point of the fiber must equal the focal length of the collimator lens. To detect the wavefront, the FC is aligned centrally with the wavefront sensor. By changing the lens position the 5th Zernike polynomial, which corresponds to the defocus, is minimized, which leads to a collimation of the beam.

2.2.2 Beam alignment with position detector

Since the transmitted optical power should remain constant when moving the retroreflector, the optical axis of the beam must coincide with the traverse axis of the retroreflector. Otherwise, the beam travels in the transverse plane and cannot be captured equally well by the collimator lens of the MC. This leads to a fluctuation of the reference arm power, which results in a variation of the SNR. A 4-quadrant diode is used as a position detector to align the optical axis of the light beam. The diode is attached to the position of the MC to align the optical axis. The exit angle of the beam leaving the FC is adjusted while continuously moving the retroreflector, until the position variation of the light spot on the 4-quadrant diode is minimized.

2.2.3 Collimation with beamsplitter setup

For the collimation of the MC, a beamsplitter setup is required, which is realized by a Thorlabs, Inc. 30 mm cage system. Again, the distance between lens and mirror must equal the focal length of the collimator lens. For this purpose, a parallel beam, formed by a FC, is aligned with a beamsplitter cube, reflected at the MC and is deflected by the beamsplitter cube onto a Shack-Hartmann wavefront sensor where the wavefront can be collimated by minimizing the 5th Zernike polynomial (see Fig. 4).

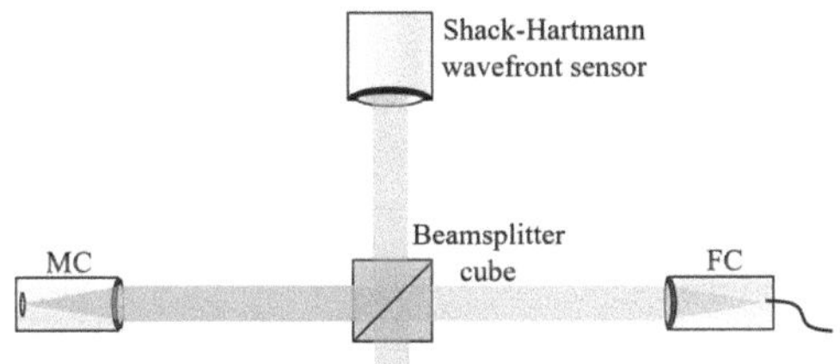

Figure 4: Beamsplitter setup consisting of fiber-coupled collimator (FC), beamsplitter cube, collimator with integrated mirror (MC) and Shack-Hartmann wavefront sensor.

2.2.4 Adjustment with optical powermeter

If the angle of the MC is not adjusted correctly, it can cause a lateral offset of the light beam. As a consequence, there is a loss in light transmission, because the light can not be coupled into the reference arm fiber again. An optical powermeter (7Z01560, Ophir Optronics, Jerusalem, Israel), connected by a 50/50 fiber coupler to the FC, is used to observe the light transmission while adjusting the angle of the MC. The aim is to obtain a light transmission which is $30\pm5\%$.

2.3 Stability and temperature resistance

To evaluate the resistance according to environmental influences, vibration and temperature tests are carried out. To examine the transmission behaviour the change in power throughput is observed, using a powermeter from Ophir Optronics. For the vibration test, the DL is attached to a vibrating plate (700/1-R24, Pferrer GmbH, Zülpich, Germany), which runs at different G-forces. The acceleration is measured by a 3-axis G-force data logger (VB300, Extech Instruments, Nashua, USA). For the temperature test, a temperature cabinet (UN160, Memmert GmbH, Schwabach, Germany) is used to raise the temperature in 10°C steps from room temperature up to 55°C. A thermocouple data logger (492-5105, Pico Technology, Cambrigeshire, UK) is used to detect the temperature. Measurements are recorded at the front (Position 1) and at the back position (Position 2) of the retroreflector.

3 Results and Discussion

3.1 Adjustability

When adjusting the DL, some problems occurred that led to a reduced light transmission. As a consequence, the optimal light transmission of 30% could not be reached completely.

The maximum transmittance achieved here is only 28.28%. So to be closer the optimal transmission value it is desirable to increase the light transmission. The basic findings are discussed in the following.

When performing the second adjustment step, i.e. adjusting the optical axis, it was noticed that one never hits the center of the 4-quadrant diode after adjustment. There is always a lateral offset of up to 500 µm, while the beam diameter is only 3.34 mm. So this offset, caused by inaccuracies in the production process of the DL housing, leads to a reduction of the beam diameter by up to 1 mm, due to aperture trimming by the collimator lenses. To solve this problem, the design of the DL could be extended by an XY-adjustment option of the FC or even the retroreflector.

For the collimation of the MC, a beamsplitter setup was used. It was noticed that an unavoidable reflection by the inside of the beamsplitter cube distorts the wavefront measurement, so that the defocus cannot be adjusted correctly. Since the angular adjustment of the MC reacts very insensitively to tilts, the DL, itself, will be used as adjustment setup in the future. With this adjustment setup, a transmission of up to 34.88% has been achieved so far.

3.2 Evaluation of stability

The results of the vibration test are shown in Fig. 5. The total loss in light transmission is only 0.98% while applying G-forces of up to 5 g. Also, the difference in light transmission between position 1 and position 2 changes very little, which supports a stable SNR over the axial imaging range. A small drift in the transmission can be observed, which could be caused by the increasing acceleration but could also be influenced by other effects, for example due to temperature changes, as the transmission also decreases while no acceleration is applied. Consequently, it can be stated that the DL has a good stability.

If the MC collimator lens was hit more centrally by the light beam, there would be a bigger deadjustment allowance until the light transmission changes remarkably. This could be realized by an XY-adjustment option for the FC/retroreflector, which would lead to an enlargement of the stability.

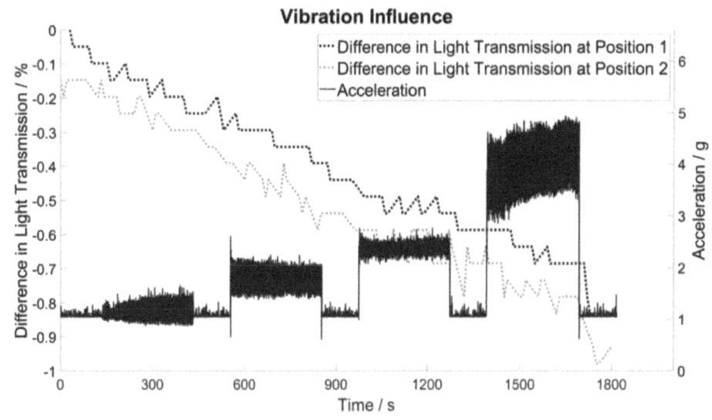

Figure 5: Vibration influence on the light transmission of the delay line measured at the front postion and the back position of the retroreflector.

3.3 Evaluation of temperature resistance

The results of the temperature test are shown in Fig. 6. It is obvious that the power throughput increases as the temperature of the DL housing, which consists of aluminum, rises. The course of the graph shows a hysteresis loop. Since the change in light transmission follows the temperature rise/fall, the structure that causes this effect must need more time to heat up. As the MC collimator lens was not hit centrally by the light beam so far, the increase in transmission could result from a transverse movement of the light beam, caused by thermal expansion of the DL housing. This could have reduced the inaccuracies of the production process, which caused a reduced transmission due to aperture trimming. To test this assumption, the temperature test was repeated using the 4-quadrant diode. The diode was attached to the position of the MC and the movement of the light spot was observed while the measurement. To test the repeatability, the DL was newly adjusted before the test. Indeed, a movement of the light spot towards the center of the 4-quadrant diode, which corresponds to the center of the MC lens, was observed. So in conclusion, the strong temperature dependence seems to be caused by a material expansion of the DL. The sensor for the detection of the housing temperature was positioned at the surface of the housing. To see the expansion effect, also the inner structures of the housing must heat up. This explains the delay of the transmission changes towards the temperature rise/fall.

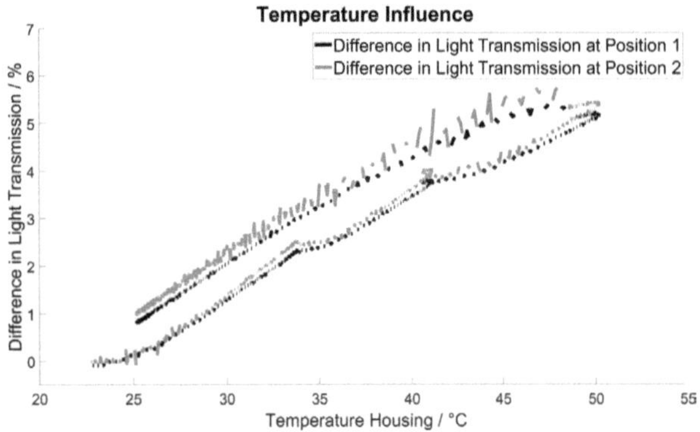

Figure 6: Temperature influence on the light transmission of the delay line measured at the front postion and the back position of the retroreflector.

4 Conclusion

In this work a newly designed device for the variation of the reference arm length is presented and evaluated. A constant power throughput of 28.28% of the DL is realized, which supports a stable and shot noise limited SNR over axial imaging range. However, the power throughput of the DL can be increased further if the design is extended by an XY-adjustment option for the FC/retroreflector. This would also increase the deadjustment allowance and thus the stability. In the future, the DL itself will be used as an adjustment setup for the wavefront collimation of the MC. The DL performed well at the stability test, as the light transmission decreased by only 0.98%, while operating with G-forces of up to 5 g. There was shown a significant temperature dependence of the power throughput, which is assumed to be caused by material expansion of the DL housing and results in a lateral movement of the light beam. The highest increase in light transmission, which is 5.37%, was observed at a temperature rise of 27.44°C, according to the initial temperature. If the inaccuracies in the production process will be corrected in the future, the lateral beam movement while temperature changes would cause a loss in transmission. Consequently, the material the DL consists of should be exchanged by a less temperature dependent material.

Acknowledgement

The work has been carried out at Heidelberg Engineering GmbH, and was supervised by Prof. Dr. rer. nat. Robert Huber, Institute of Biomedical Optics, Universität zu Lübeck.

Author's Statement

Conflict of interest: Authors state no conflict of interest.

5 References

[1] D. Huang, E. A. Swanson, C. P. Lin, J. S. Schuman, W. G. Stinson, W. Chang, M. R. Hee, T. Flotte, K. Gregory, C. A. Puliafito, J. G. Fujimoto, *Optical coherence tomography* Science, Vol. 254, No. 5035, pp. 1178–1181, 1991.

[2] M. A. Choma, M. V. Sarunic, C. Yang und J. A. Izatt *Sensitivity advantage of swept source and Fourier domain optical coherence tomography*. Optics Express, Vol. 11, No. 18, pp. 2183-2189, 2003.

[3] M. Gora, K. Karnowski1, M. Szkulmowski1, B. J. Kaluzny, R. Huber, A. Kowalczyk1, M. Wojtkowsk, *Ultra high-speed swept source OCT imaging of the anterior segment of human eye at 200 kHz with adjustable imaging range*. Optics Express, Vol. 17 No. 17, pp. 14880-14894, 2009

[4] J. A. Izatt and M.A. Choma, *Theory of Optical Coherence Tomography* in Optical Coherence Tomography. Springer Berlin Heidelberg, pp. 47–72, 2008.

[5] Z. Wang, C. Reisman, J. Liu and K. Chan *Introduction to Swept Source OCT* in Atlas of Swept Source Optical Coherence Tomography. Springer, 2017.

[6] Andrew M. Rollins and Joseph A. Izatt, *Optimal interferometer designs for optical coherence tomography*. Optics Letters, Vol. 24, No. 21, November 1999

Automated vessels count algorithm to find novel OCT-based biomarkers for inflammatory skin diseases

Bayan Mustafa [1], Madita Göb [2], Linh Ha-Wissel [3] Jennifer E. Hundt[4], and Robert Huber [5]

[1] Biomedical Engineering, Lübeck University of Applied Sciences, bayan.mustafa@stud.th-luebeck.de

[2] Institute of Biomedical Optics, University of Lübeck, m.goeb@uni-luebeck.de

[3] Department of Dermatology, Allergology and Venereology, University Hospital Schleswig-Holstein, Lübeck (UKSH), linh.ha@uksh.de

[4] Lübeck Institute of Experimental Dermatology (LIED), University of Lübeck, jennifer.hundt@uksh.de.

[5] Institute of Biomedical Optics, University of Lübeck, robert.huber@uni-luebeck.de

Abstract

Novel imaging biomarkers may open new avenues for more precise and objective diagnostics and monitoring of inflammatory skin diseases. Optical coherence tomography (OCT) is a high-resolution imaging tool used in dermatological applications to provide essential biomarkers such as epidermal thickness, vascular density and depth. Implementing a robust and accurate algorithm to integrate vessel count in OCT as new and robust biomarker improves monitoring and therapeutic evaluation of common chronic inflammatory skin diseases such as psoriasis and atopic dermatitis. An automated vessels count (AVC) algorithm was implemented using MATLAB and applied on ten scans for each of psoriasis, atopic dermatitis and healthy skins to accurately detect the skin surface and count the vessels and their elongations at specific depth. The algorithm is able to rapidly provide vessels count by accurately detecting various skin surfaces and subsequent segmentation the vessels and their elongations precisely at different depths.

1 Introduction

The Optical coherence tomography (OCT) is a high resolution, fast and noninvasive cross-sectional imaging technique [1]. The OCT measuring principle is based on Michelson interferometer method which measures the interferometric light reflections from the object. This method provides the location and strength of the reflections, and therefore the depth profile [1] [2]. One of the characteristic parameters provided by OCT is the high axial resolution ranges between 1 and 15 μm [2]. This made the OCT a valuable diagnostic tool in different clinical applications, mainly ophthalmology and dermatology [3].

In dermatology, the OCT method demonstrated a high interest for diagnosis of skin cancer and chronic inflammations especially psoriasis and atopic dermatitis [4]. The introduction of Dynamic OCT (D-OCT) in this field enabled the detection of the blood flow movement, therefore imaging detailed blood vessel network in the inhomogeneous structure of the skin layers that helps in further clinical diagnosis [3][5]. Vascular patterns (dots, lines, coils), density, depth, size, and number of elongated vessels that can be extracted from a top view image in OCT, alongside epidermal thickness measured from a cross-sectional view, are the essential biomarkers to differentiate between healthy and diseased skin as well as to evaluate the disease severity and its therapeutic effectiveness [4]. Skin inflammation leads to higher blood circulation that can originate from a higher count of capillaries as well as higher vascular diameter. As vessel density and diameter might be influenced by internal and external factors therefore they are considered weak biomarkers, a robust imaging biomarker could be the vessel number [4][6].

This work aims to provide an accurate and precise skin surface detection algorithm for D-OCT images that exhibit skin alterations such as hair, wound, scars, and crusts. Integrating the vessels count in D-OCT as a novel biomarker will improve the pathological skin diagnosis and therapeutic evaluation, therefore a second aim of this work is to automatically count the vessels and their elongations, which are a special feature for psoriasis and atopic dermatitis cases, from D-OCT scans at different depths.

2 Material and Methods

2.1 Hardware

The VivoSight (VS) Dx OCT scanner (Michelson Diagnostics, Maidstone, Kent, UK) emits infrared laser light at a central wavelength of 1305 nm. The lateral resolution is less than 7.5 mm and axial resolution less than 5 mm. The field of view is 6 mm x 6 mm. The resulting image can be presented in three forms: vertical B-scans, top-view en-face and three-dimensional (3D) structural and vascular images. The images can be stored as colored DICOM, TIFF or TIFF stack.

Vertical B-scan represents the cross-sectional side of the skin while top-view en-face scan represents the skin layers mapped at the same depth from the surface of the skin. The produced en-face scans are composed of 120 frames with an interslice spacing of 10 mm. Both forms, vertical

B-scans and en-face images, were used as DICOM format in this study.

2.2 Study Data

The analysis was conducted on 30 OCT patients' data stacks (10 psoriasis, 10 atopic dermatitis, and 10 healthy skin).

2.3 Software

MATLAB code was implemented to analyze and evaluate the images as well as to calculate the vessels number at different depths.

The folder path of all images which need to be analyzed was added. For each image, the DICOM data were read providing detailed information about the image including the image type as colored image and size (in pixels) of 460 (height) x 1324 (width) x 120 (frame). The skin surface was then detected using the gray-scaled image volume and binarized with global threshold based on Otsu's method. For each frame, an erosion step was applied on areas of 5000 pixels and less, followed by finding and storing the index of the maximum intensity. Median filter of size 10-by-10 neighborhoods with bilinear interpolation was used and additional filtering steps by detecting the outliers with the nearest non-outlier value and refilling them based on lower and upper percentile threshold of 6% and 100% respectively, were applied on the detected surface. The important step was to straighten the skin surface to provide the en-face view for all depths at constant point. A resize step of 740 x 740 pixels with bilinear interpolation was followed.

After creating the en-face view, a segmentation step for the vessels and their elongations was followed based on simple threshold method. This method started by applying image contrast adjustment with lower and upper limits of 0.20 and 0.75 respectively, then binarization with fixed global threshold of value 0.25 and area opening for sizes less than 4 pixels with 4 connected neighborhoods. Finally, the created white connected components, which represent the vessels, were labeled and counted. For further data evaluation, an excel file including the number of vessels at different depths and their related en-face images was created and saved for all images found in the sub folders. Additional two methods were tested to evaluate the effect of different parameters on accurate vessels and elongations count. The dilation method and the watershed method. In the dilation method, the image intensity was automatically saturated and binarized with variable global threshold, followed by opening the areas of 15 pixels and less, and application of morphological closing mask with disk shape and radius of 2. While in the watershed method, the image contrast was specified at 0.20 and 0.75 for the lower and upper limits respectively, and binarization threshold was fixed at 0.25. Comparing to the dilation method, the opening area size was decreased to 7 pixels and the morphological closing mask remained the same. Finally, it was followed by a watershed step.

3 Results and Discussion

3.1 Surface Detection

Due to the skin surface alterations such as hair, that appear as an outlier and influence the quality of the B-scan images it was challenging to filter them out and detect the surface correctly and precisely. Several parameters affected the detection process as seen in Fig.1 to provide a robust and clear surface.

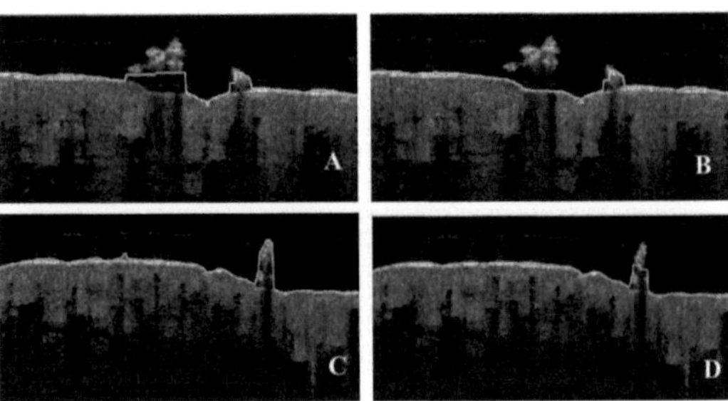

Figure 1: The effect of changing image parameters for the same dataset but different frames. A and B erosion size effect with 1000 and 5000 pixels respectively. C median filter effect. D extra filtering effect.

Binarization of 3D image with global thresholding at 35% of the maximum intensity resulted in more errors and incorrect detection of the surface even if it removed the attached small hair, while changeable global threshold according to each image intensity resulted in more correct detection. The second parameter was the erosion size. Small size of 1000 pixels was able to detect more outliers while 5000 pixels was sufficient to not detect extra and large outliers as shown in Fig. 1 (A) and (B). Increasing the erosion size by more than 5000 pixels did not have an effect due to the large connected area of the skin which represented the area of interest.

The roughness of the surface was strongly varying from patient to patient. For this reason, it was challenging to apply an appropriate smoothing and filtering steps to flatten it. Applying only a median filter of size 10-by-10 neighborhoods, the detected surface included a large attached skin artifacts and therefore was not smoothed enough as illustrated in Fig. 1 (C). Filtering out the remaining outliers from the previous step by detecting them with the nearest non-outlier value and replace them with new values based on lower and upper percentile threshold of 6% and 100% respectively, reduced the skin artifacts presence and was enough for good detection as can be seen in Fig. 1 (D).

The optimal and accurate detected surface used in the AVC algorithm is shown in Fig.2. The detected surface was smoothly preserving the original shape of the surface and neglecting the outlier as illustrated in fig.2. For further evaluation of the detected surface by AVC algorithm, a qualitative comparison step of it with the surface detection algorithm of the VS system was applied and the result is shown in Fig.3. The detected surface with both methods were almost the same. The AVC algorithm detected the sur-

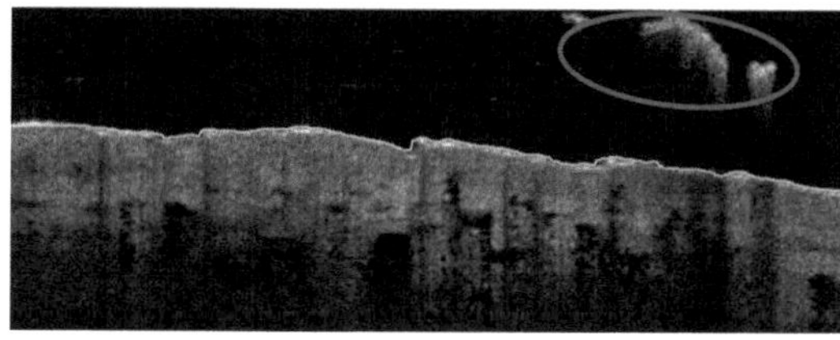

Figure 2: B-scan frame of unhealthy skin acquired by VS with the detected surface (yellow line) by AVC algorithm.

face correctly and preserved the exact shape of it especially around the edges and curves but in some cases it detected some small hairs which were attached closely to the surface and were difficult to filter out, as well as high order of filtration did not improve the detection performance. At the same time, the detected surface of the VS system appeared to be highly smoothed, which could lose some detailed surface information, and in some cases, especially when the surface laid close to the image range edges, the detection algorithm lacks in precision and did not detect the outliers correctly. In general, after applying the surface detection

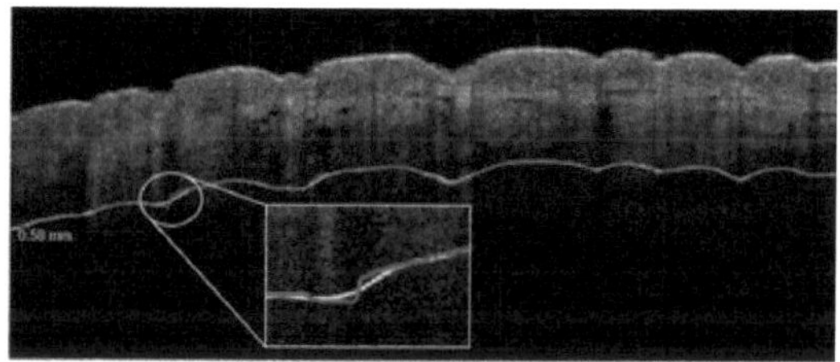

Figure 3: B-scan frame of normal skin taken with VS showing the detected surface (white) at depth 580 μm compared to the detected surface by AVC algorithm (red).

method used in the AVC algorithm on different datasets, it was able to filter out most of the outliers and detect the surface clearly and correctly preserving its detailed structure. The detected surface by AVC algorithm was comparable and good enough to be used for vessels' counts.

3.2   Vessels count

The blood vessels appearance at different depths can vary between dots to linear structures when going deeper. Therefore, the vessels were counted at 150 μm and 360 μm depths to find the most accurate segmentation method at correct depth for further clinical evaluation.

Figures 4 and 5 demonstrate the difference between the three segmentation methods. The dilation method led to an increase in the size of the vessels and overlapped them into each other mainly in deeper skin layers as can be seen in Fig.4 (B) and 5 (B). The watershed method worked perfectly on superficial depths and managed to separate the adjacent vessel dots as illustrated in Fig.4 (C) for the centered vessels, but it did not produce best results in deeper layers due to clustering the single vessel plexus into several parts as shown in Fig.5 (C), and one more drawback of it was the long execution time of 49.72s on all depths. The simple

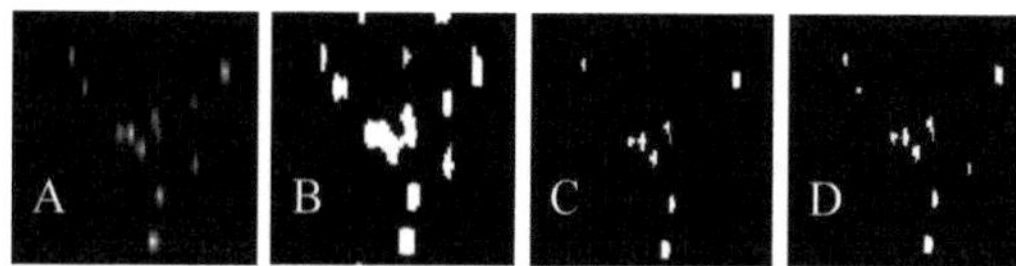

Figure 4: En-face for lesion skin at 150 μm depth. A represents the en-face view read by AVC algorithm. B - D the results of the applied segmentation methods respectively.

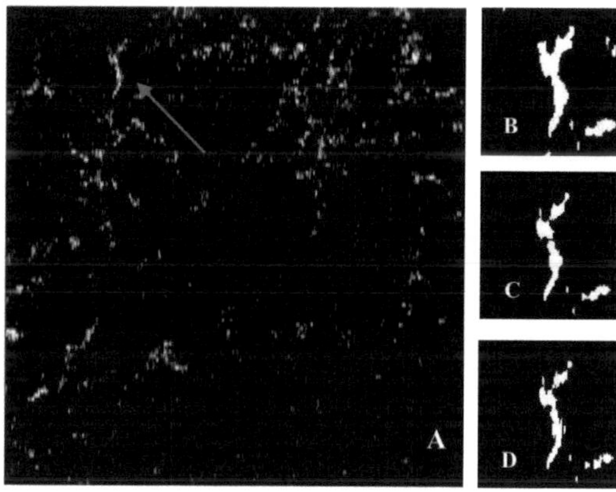

Figure 5: En-face for lesion skin at 360 μm depth. A represents the en-face view read by AVC algorithm. B - D the results of the applied segmentation methods respectively.

threshold method improved the segmentation performance and required only 2s to be executed on all depths. Fig.4 (D) obviously showing the perfect segmentation of small dots distributed at close distances, also a well-defined and organized appearance of the vessels' pattern. Deeper in the dermis, where broader network of vessels exists, was challenging to decide what is related to single vessel elongation and what is not due to the normally intersection of the vessels. However, by the simple threshold, the segmented vessels' elongations were close enough to their shape presented in the en-face view resulted from the AVC algorithm as can be depicted in Fig.5 (D) especially for the elongation indicated by the red arrow in Fig.5 (A).

Comparing the segmentation methods quantitatively was useful to show the difference as indicated in table 1. At

Table 1: Vessels counts resulted from applying the three methods at 150μm and 360μm depths

	General Method	Watershed Method	Simple Threshold
150μm	190	67	87
360μm	249	265	363

the superficial depth of 150 μm, the number of vessels resulted from the dilation method was the highest. While at 360 μm, the dilation and watershed methods resulted close number of vessels and the simple threshold resulted much higher due to the appearance of tiny dots. At both depths, the simple threshold method led to reasonable counting of the vessels and provided more accurate and well-defined segmentation for the vessels' dots and elongations.

3.3 Applying to patients' data

The AVC algorithm was applied on patient's data with psoriasis and atopic dermatitis as well as control healthy skin scans as can be seen in Fig.6.

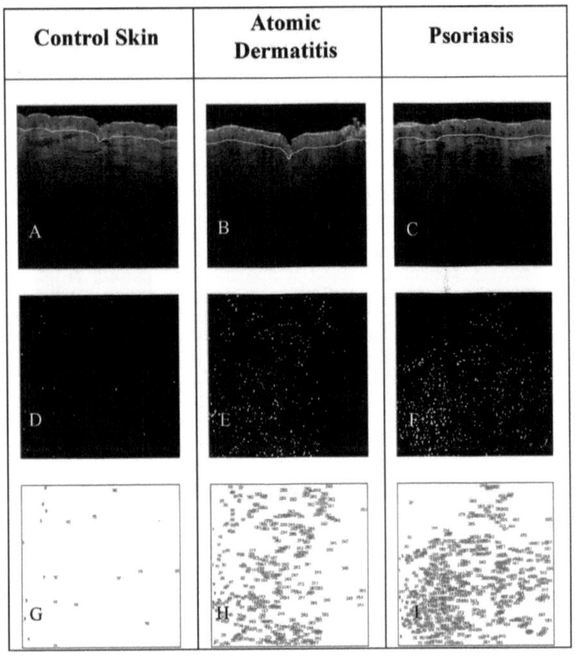

Control Skin	Atomic Dermatitis	Psoriasis

Figure 6: The application of AVC on patients' scans. A, B and C are the B-scan for each patient. D, E and F the counted vessels labeled on en-face scan at 200 μm. G, H and I represent the pinning of each count on to the related vessel.

The surface was detected clearly without outliers and preserved the shape of the curved surface as can be seen clearly in Fig.6(A) and (B) for control skin and atopic dermatitis case. In psoriasis the surface was flat and therefore the detection was done smoothly as shown in Fig. 6(C). The vessels were calculated at depth 200 μm, as illustrated as yellow line in the B-scans in Fig.6, which was expected according to [4] as the appropriate depth for most accurate measurements for the vessel elongations' cross section. In the control skin (Fig.6(D) and (G)) 20 vessels were counted while 353 and 526 vessels in atopic dermatitis (Fig.6(E) and (H)) and psoriasis (Fig.6(F) and (I)) cases respectively. These numbers indicate a normal availability of low vessels counts in normal skin whereas a large increase of the counts could be associated to an inflammatory case which should decrease by applying a specific therapy.

4 Conclusion

D-OCT is a powerful clinical imaging tool for examining blood vessels network in skin layers which provides useful imaging biomarkers such as epidermal thickness, vascular density, diameter, and depth that are of interest to dermatologists. The AVC algorithm was able to rapidly provide vessels count by accurately detecting various skin surfaces as well as segmenting and counting the vessels and their elongations precisely at different depths. Introducing vessels count as a new and novel imaging biomarker in D-OCT will improve dermatological diagnosis and therapeutic evaluation, especially in atopic dermatitis and psoriasis. This novel biomarker will be applied for the development of an inflammation score to guide clinical decisions. Thus, we need to increase the number of test data to evaluate the performance of the algorithm, as it provides a larger sample size to assess the algorithm's generalizability, and stability.

Acknowledgement

This work was carried out in cooperation with the cluster of excellence Precision Medicine in Chronic Inflammation (PMI). The programming script was supported by Sazgar Burhan from the Institute of Biomedical Optics, University of Lübeck.

Author's Statement

Authors state no conflict of interest.

5 References

[1] W. Drexler, U. Morgner, R. K. Ghanta, F. Kärtner, J. Schuman, and J.Fujimoto *U*ltrahigh-resolution ophthalmic optical coherence tomography. Nat. Med, vol.7, PP.502, 2001.

[2] J. Fujimoto, C. Pitris, S. Boppart, and M. Brezinski, *O*ptical Coherence Tomography: An Emerging Technology for Biomedical Imaging and Optical Biopsy, Neoplasia, vol.2, PP.9–25, 2000.

[3] A. F. Fercher, W. Drexler, C. K. Hitzenberger and T. Lasser, *O*ptical coherence tomography - principles and applications, Reports on Progress in Physics, vol.66, PP.239–303, 2003.

[4] L. Ha-Wissel, H. Yasak, R. Huber, D. Zillikens, R. J. Ludwig, D. Thaçi and J. E. Hundt, *C*ase report: Optical coherence tomography for monitoring biologic therapy in psoriasis and atopic dermatitis. Frontiers in Medicine, 2022.

[5] A. S. Aldahan, L. L. Chen, R. M. Fertig, J. Holmes, V. V. Shah, S. Mlacker, V. M. Hsu, K. Nouri and A. Tosti, *V*ascular features of nail psoriasis using dynamic optical coherence tomography. Skin Appendage Disord, vol.2, PP.102--108, 2017.

[6] S. Schuh, J. Holmes, M. Ulrich, L. Themstrup, G. Jemec, N. Carvalho, G. Pellacani, J. Welzel, *I*maging blood vessel morphology in skin: dynamic optical coherence tomography as a novel potential diagnostic tool in dermatology. Dermatol. Ther., vol.7, PP.187--202, 2017.

Wavelength regulation of a 1550 nm Fourier-domain mode-locked laser using a silicon camera

Mahmoud Khalil [1], Tonio Kutscher [2], Stefan Meyer [2], Yannik Kasprzak [3], and Sebastian Karpf [2]

[1] Biomedical Engineering, Luebeck University of Applied Sciences, mahmoud.khalil@stud.th-luebeck.de
[2] Institute of Biomedical Optics, Universität zu Lübeck, {t.kutscher, s.meyer, sebastian.karpf} @uni-luebeck.de
[3] Biophysics, Universität zu Lübeck, yannik.kasprzak@student.uni-luebeck.de

Abstract

Fourier-domain mode-locked (FDML) laser is a relatively new invention used in many applications of the biomedical optics field. FDML lasers emit a swept spectrum of wavelengths. Although this dynamic laser permits various novel high-speed bioimaging applications, the wavelength spectrum can sometimes drift with time, e.g. when the components are affected by thermal drift of the system. This paper discusses the development of a regulation system for a 1550 nm FDML laser system using similar principles used in a previous study. The spectrum of the FDML laser is to be determined using an optical setup with a CMOS camera chip and utilizing the two-photon absorption (TPA) phenomenon. We show that the entire wavelength sweep of the near-infrared FDML at 1550 nm can be detected via TPA and we implement regulation process to control the center wavelength and span of the FDML sweep. The feedback is implemented by controlling the waveform generator that controls the fiber Fabry-Parot tunable filter (FFP-TF). The regulation algorithm is programmed in Python programming language. Overall, a very simple, robust and cheap regulation system could be set up that requires minimal laser power, enabling effective control of many laboratory FDML laser systems.

1 Introduction

Fourier-domain mode-locked (FDML) laser is a relatively new laser system that, instead of operating at a specific wavelength, emits a band of wavelengths [1]. FDML laser systems are used in multiple biomedical applications, including high-speed optical tomography (OCT), high-speed spectroscopy, and two-photon microscopy [2]. Furthermore, Spectro-temporal laser imaging by diffracted excitation, or SLIDE, microscopy especially exploits FDML laser's wavelengths spectrum to achieve high speed microscopy through scanning the x-axis using a grating [3].

However, one of the issues that faces FDML laser systems is the change in the wavelengths spectrum due to thermal and electronic effects. These disturbances can be detrimental to the efficiency and effectiveness of the system and require regular manual readjustment to maintain operation. Further, such manual control requires the constant use of an optical spectrum analyzer (OSA), which is a very expensive laboratory device. Therefore, an automated regulation system was called for to control and maintain FDML systems at the desired center and span values.

In a previous study, a regulation system for an FDML laser in the range of 950 nm to 1000 nm was developed [4]. In this work, the aim is to develop a similar regulation system but for an FDML laser at a center wavelength of 1550 nm and a span of 20 nm. To achieve this goal, the laser output from the FDML system goes from laser fiber to a collimator. Then, the light gets diffracted from an optical grating into a specific, wavelength-dependent angle. Thus, the wavelength sweep of the FDML laser is turned into a line, whose length and center position corresponds to the span and cen-ter of the FDML spectrum, respectively. The diffracted light spectrum is then focused on a CMOS camera chip using a convex lens. By employing a high numerical aperture (NA) focusing condition, the light can be detected on the silicon CMOS camera via two-photon absorption (TPA). The light spectrum is then captured via the camera chip and processed using a Python-based algorithm. After establishing a relationship between the center and span of the laser's spectrum and the captured image from the chip, the Python algorithm can estimate the current center and span of the laser and readjust them accordingly through a waveform generator (Rigol DG1022Z).

2 Material and Methods

2.1 FDML Laser

An FDML laser system was built to help develop and test the regulation system. FDML lasers are narrowband tun-able lasers that can achieve high tuning rates over an optical bandwidth of more than 100 nm. It mainly consists of a resonator, a gain medium, and a tunable bandpass filter with a narrow passband. The function waveform generator controls the fiber Fabry-Parot filter (FFP-TF) and is respon-sible for changing the FDML laser's wavelength spectrum. Fig. 1 below shows a diagram of an FDML laser.

Also, a polarization controller, not shown in Fig. 1, was 3D printed and used to adjust the polarization of light com-ing from single-mode optical fiber (SMF) to polarization maintaining fiber (PM) inside the ring laser system. For the purposes of this study, the SOA used had a range between 1550 nm and 1590 nm.

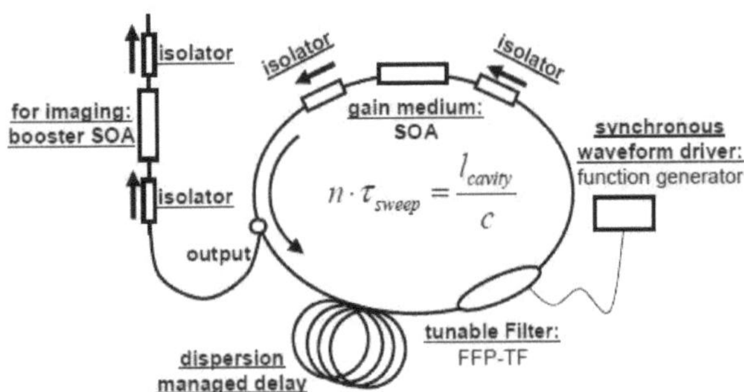

Figure 1: A Schematic diagram of an FDML laser. It consists of a semiconductor optical amplifier (SOA), a fiber Fabry-Parot tunable filter (FFP-TF), optical fiber, a coupler, a delay line, and isolators [1].

2.2 Optics

An optical setup was designed and built to receive the optical output from the FDML laser system, separate the different wavelengths, and focus them onto a camera chip. The output of the FDML laser exits an optical fiber and diverges into a collimating lens. Parallel light rays coming out of the collimator then get diffracted using a blaze grating. The grating diffracts light with different wavelengths into different angles. This property allows to establish a direct relationship between the FDML laser's spectrum and the captured light through the camera. A blaze grating is used such that a high efficiency diffraction into the first grating order is achieved by carefully adjusting the polarization (up to 90 % efficiency).

For the purpose of 1550 nm wavelength, the blaze grating used had a groove density of 600 grooves/mm and a blaze angle of 28.41°. Fig. 2 below shows a schematic of a blaze grating.

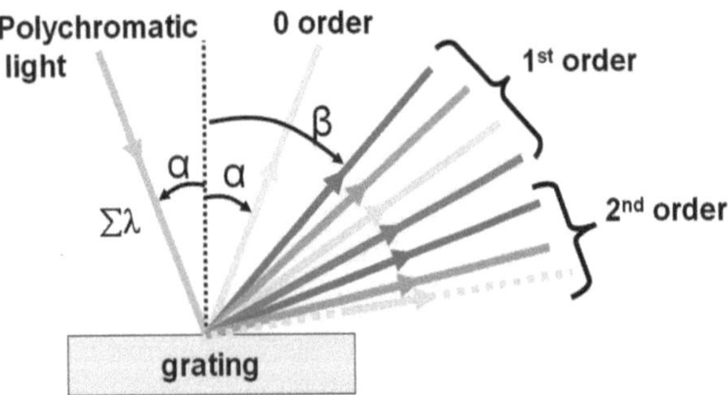

Figure 2: A schematic grating of an optical blaze grating. Polychromatic light is diffracted from the grating at different angles depending on the wavelength and the order [5].

The first order is then focused on the webcam chip using a convex lens. Fig. 3 below shows the layout of the optical setup and the specifications of the components.

Although the CMOS chip of the Logitech C615 webcam used does not have sensitivity for 1550 nm wavelength, it was found that, in this case, the chip was able to capture the spectrum which can be attributed to TPA.

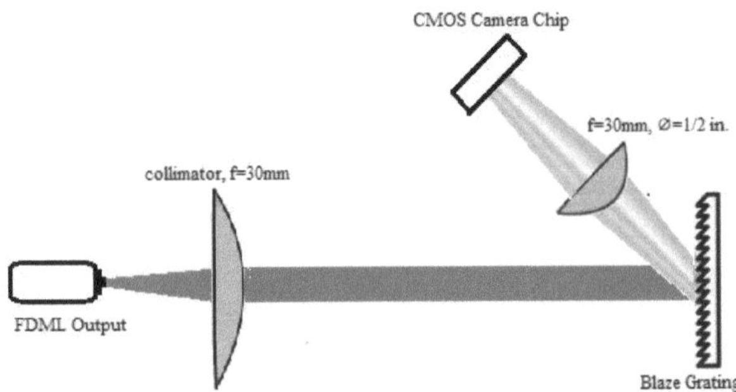

Figure 3: A schematic of the optical layout setup. The distances between the collimator and laser output is 30mm; the distance between the lens and the grating and the camera chip is also 30 mm. Figure is not drawn to scale.

It is important to note that the optical setup had to be within dark environment to prevent the camera chip from being exposed to any external light sources that might intervene with the signal. Therefore, a cardboard box was used to enclose the optical setup. Also, it was important for the power output of the FDML laser used in measurement to be within an acceptable range such that it is neither so weak that it is hard to be captured nor so strong that it over exposes the chip. The acceptable range was found to be between 1 mW and 3 mW. Though, further investigation is required to indicate the exact values.

2.3 Algorithm

After the light signal is received by the camera, the image has to be processed to determine the current center and span of the FDML laser's spectrum and to control the RIGOL waveform generator to adjust the amplitude and offset accordingly to achieve the desired values. Firstly, in order to process the image and calculate the current center wavelength and span, a correlation between the image pixels and the nanometers of the wavelength had to be found. Therefore, 82 samples with different center and span wavelengths were taken to derive this relationship. For each sample, a snapshot of the FDML laser spectrum was taken using the OSA and, at the same moment, an image was captured using the Logitech C615 in the optical setup. Fig. 4 below shows an example of an image captured of the FDML laser spectrum using the webcam chip. The images of the samples were processed to learn the center pixel of the light dash as well as its span in pixels. Using the derived correlations, the measured center pixel of the light dash and its length in pixels can be used to determine the current center and span wavelengths of the laser. Fig. 5 shows a graph of the relationship found between the calculated center pixel and center wavelength in nanometers.

Using the graph from Fig. 5, the equation of the line of best fit was performed as shown in Equation (1):

$$C_p = 10.979 C_w - 16224. \tag{1}$$

where Cp is the center pixel of the light dash and Cw is the center wavelength. Although the derived equation is linear, it is only an approximation that can be used in such a narrow range; the mathematical accurate relationship is known to be a sin-dependent function.

Figure 4: A 1920x1080 image captured using Logitech C615 webcam of the FDML laser light spectrum. The center and span of this spectrum is 1550 nm and 20 nm, respectively.

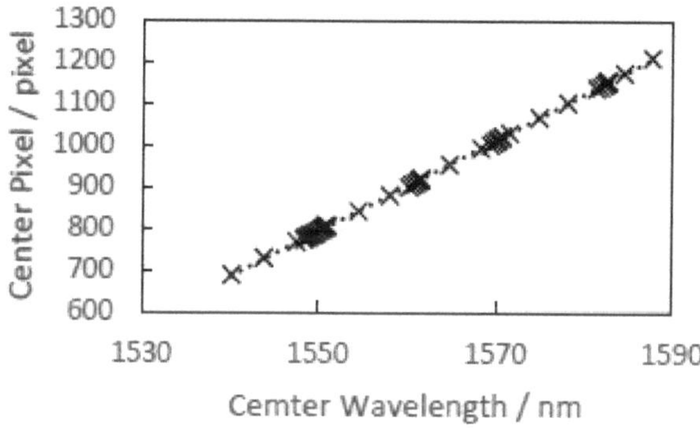

Figure 5: The center of light dash in pixels as a function of the center wavelength.

Similarly, another correlation between the span of the dash in pixels and the span of the wavelengths using the same method was derived. Fig. 6 and Equation (2) below demonstrate the found relationship.

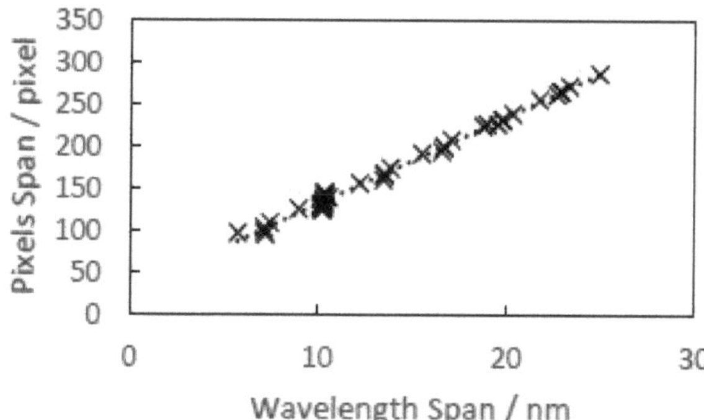

Figure 6: The center of light dash in pixels as a function of the center wavelength.

$$S_p = 10.401 S_w + 27.515. \qquad (2)$$

where Sp is the span of the light dash in pixels and Sw is the wavelength span of the FDML laser spectrum.

Furthermore, the offset and the amplitude of the RIGOL waveform generator were recorded for each of the 82 samples. Using these measurements, the rate of change in center as a function of offset and in span as a function of amplitude was found. These rates can be used to regulate and adjust the waveform accordingly to achieve the desired values.

Finally, an algorithm was coded to control and alter the values of the waveform generator based on the values calculated from the processed images captured in real time.

3   Results and Discussion

3.1   Image Processing

The regulation system was tested to measure its accuracy in calculating the current center and span of FDML laser spectrum. The Python-based regulation algorithm was used to regulate the FDML laser for 30 seconds, after which a reading from the algorithm and the OSA were taken and compared. The highest recorded differences between the calculated and OSA-measured center and span were 0.70 nm and 1.87 nm respectively. Table 1 below summarizes the results of image processing at each center wavelength and span.

Table 1: Percentage errors between code and OSA

center	span	center error	span error
1550 nm	10 nm	0.01%	23.32%
1550 nm	15 nm	0.04%	1.52%
1550 nm	20 nm	0.03%	6.44%
1555 nm	15 nm	0.03%	1.18%
1560 nm	15 nm	0.04%	3.98%
1565 nm	15 nm	0.04%	4.57%
1570 nm	15 nm	0.04%	5.65%
1575 nm	15 bn	0.04%	6.72%
1580 nm	15 nm	0.01%	6.70%
1585 nm	15 nm	0.03%	7.54%
1590 nm	15 nm	0.03%	7.76%

3.2   Regulation

Similarly, the values measured through the OSA after 30 seconds were compared to the target values inputted into the Python program initially to determine how successfully the program achieved the targets. The maximum differences between the target and measured center and span values were 1.33 nm and 0.71 nm, respectively. Table 2 below summarizes the percentage errors between the desired and the measured values.

3.3 Discussion

The regulation system seems to be able to read and regulate the center wavelengths 1550 nm and 1590 nm with a high degree of accuracy. On the other hand, the regulation program appears to be struggling more with calculating and regulating the span of the FDML laser spectrum. However, the span is still within reasonable range.

Table 2: Percentage errors between the target and the measured values

center	span	center error	span error
1550 nm	10 nm	0.00%	19.88%
1550 nm	15 nm	0.00%	3.68%
1550 nm	20 nm	0.01%	4.38%
1555 nm	15 nm	0.04%	1.56%
1560 nm	15 nm	0.09%	2.37%
1565 nm	15 nm	0.07%	1.93%
1570 nm	15 nm	0.00%	2.03%
1575 nm	15 bn	0.08%	3.74%
1580 nm	15 nm	0.01%	3.73%
1585 nm	15 nm	0.05%	3.57%
1590 nm	15 nm	0.02%	3.27%

Through observation, the span seems to be affected by some blurring effect visible in some images captured by the system. This effect could be reduced if lower output power were used from the FDML laser. The blur can be noticed in one of the images in Fig. 7 below. Furthermore, the system is strongly susceptible to external optical noise of any sort. Hence, sealing the optical setup completely to prevent any light from intervening with the system might be a good implementation to increase the efficiency and success of the regulation system.

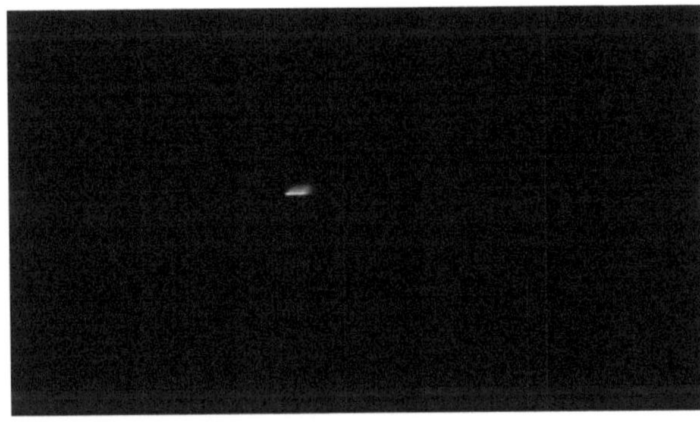

Figure 7: An image of captured light dash with blur noise.

Implementing the mentioned recommendation and further improvements on the Python code for image processing and regulation could further improve the results.

4 Conclusion

The aim of this work was to develop a regulation system for a 1550 nm FDML laser with a 20 nm span. The developed system was mostly successful in performing the required task. Nevertheless, further improvements could still be done to improve the accuracy of regulation, especially for wavelength span. Furthermore, the created program could be made more user-friendly either by transforming it into a desktop application or transferring the Python-based algorithm and the optical setup into a compact device that can be easily used without the need for a computer.

Acknowledgement

The work has been carried out at the Institute of Biomedical Optics, Universität zu Lübeck and supervised by M. Sc. Tonio Kutscher and Prof. Dr. rer. nat. Sebastian Karpf. Earlier work on the system was perfomed by Stefan Meyer and Yannik Kasprzak.

Author's Statement

Conflict of interest: Authors state no conflict of interest.

5 References

[1] R. Huber, M. Wojtkowski, and J. G. Fujimoto, *Fourier Domain Mode Locking (FDML): A new laser operating regime and applications for optical coherence tomography.* Optics Express, vol. 14, no. 8, pp. 3225-3237, 2006.

[2] S. Karpf and B. Jalali, *Fourier-domain mode-locked laser combined master-oscillator power amplifier architecture.* Optics Letters, vol. 44, no 8, pp. 1952-1955, 2019.

[3] S. Karpf, et al., *Spectro-temporal encoded multiphoton microscopy and fluorescence lifetime imaging at kilohertz framerates.* Nature Communications, vol. 11, 2062, 2020.

[4] Y. Kasprzak. *Regelung eines Fourier-domain Mode-locked Lasers mit Hilfe.* [Unpublished undergraduate thesis], 2022.

[5] *All about diffraction gratings.* Edmund Optics. Available: https://www.edmundoptics.eu/knowledge-center/application-notes/optics/all-about-diffraction-gratings/ [last accessed on 2023-02-02].

Evaluation of swept source OCT-based aberrometry measurement

Sathurya Jegatheeswaran [1,2], Michel Wunderlich [2] and Michael Stender [2]

[1] Medical Engineering Science, Universität zu Lübeck, sathurya.jegatheeswaran@student.uni-luebeck.de
[2] Heidelberg Engineering GmbH, {michel.wunderlich, michael.stender}@heidelbergengineering.com

Abstract

Refraction measurements and OCT (optical coherence tomography) technology are widely used techniques in ophthalmology. While OCT is commonly used for imaging of the eye, here the refractive measurement is performed with an OCT-based aberrometer. The recorded phase as well as amplitude of OCT scans are used for the determination of refraction values. The evaluation presented in this paper compares astigmatism angle measurements between clinically approved aberrometry devices and the OCT-based aberrometry setup presented. In-vivo measurements of astigmatism angle showed a mean deviation of 35.02° between the OCT-based aberrometry setup and the reference devices. This result is not satisfactory and further improvements are necessary.

1 Introduction

The use of swept source OCT is planned in an ophthalmic surgical microscope for intraoperative aberrometry measurement in the context of cataract surgery. When using toric intraocular lenses (IOL), which compensate for the astigmatism of the eye, the alignment of the IOL during surgery is essential for the resulting functionality. This alignment is mostly based on preoperative aberrometry measurements and subsequent corneal marking of the insertion direction of the intraocular lens by the surgeon. This procedure suffers from a limited accuracy. The intraoperative toric alignment can lead to an improvement of the correction when using an intraoperative aberrometry measurement [1]. Intraoperative aberrometry measurement can be performed during the surgery to measure the current aberrometry values, in the phakic, aphakic and pseudophakic stages of the eye. An additional advantage of this approach is the integration of the measurement setup into an ophthalmic surgical microscope with an already existing OCT function, without any further technical system modifications.

1.1 OCT System

In the present study, a swept source OCT system is used. In swept source OCT a narrowband, sweepable light source is used. The light source wavelength is tuned. Thus the individual spectral components resulting from the interference between reference and sample arms can be separated in time. A subsequent Fourier transformation of the intensity curve depending on the set wavenumber, results in a complex signal which contains phase and amplitude information for the selected sample depth [2]. A further analysis of this information is used to reconstruct the aberrated wavefront of the eye [3].

1.2 Zernike Polynomials

Zernike polynomials represent the aberration of a wavefront and to what extent a form of aberration is present. The aberrometry setup in this research is used to evaluate the astigmatism angle and therefore only the low order astigmatism Zernike polynomials have to be considered [4]. Furthermore, the first order tilt representations are used in this study.

2 Material and Methods

In this work, the described method is compared with two clinically approved devices. Both of them are based on different operating principles, so that a total of three different operating principles are compared.

2.1 Aberrometry Setup

The digital aberrometry OCT (DAOCT) setup is based on the setup described by Georgiev et al. [3]. It employs a swept source OCT system. An overview of the measurement setup is shown in Fig. 1. An injection beam is reduced to a diameter of 0.5 mm. This reduction of the beam diameter is necessary to ensure that there is no displacement of the individual wavefront due to refraction in form of phase shifts when the injection beam enters the eye and up to the focused point, with a diameter of 60 μm, on the retina. The backscattered light of the retinal plane passes through the eye and is aberrated by the entire visual system, including the lens and cornea. Two adjustable lenses, used for correction of high defocus, are traversed by the wavefront transmitted through the beam splitter. Otherwise, in cases of high defocus, the resulting wavefront cannot be completely coupled into the fiber optic system. The wavefront is sampled in a uniform pattern using two galvanometric mirrors and then coupled into the fiber optic system by the detection collimator. Since the scanner positions are known at each acquisition point, the intensity resulting from the interference of the sample arm wavefront with the light from the reference arm can be processed. This results in phase and amplitude information from the selected sample layer under consideration.

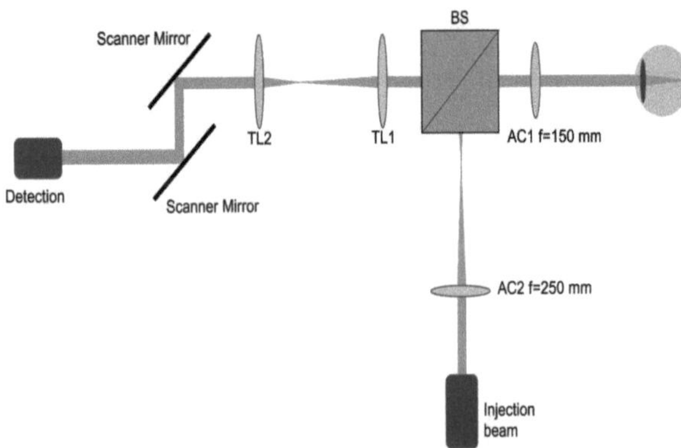

Figure 1: Sample arm of the aberrometry setup, containing the lenses AC_1 and AC_2 for achieving the desired beam diameter of 0.5 mm, the beamsplitter BS and the tunable lenses for correction of high defocus TL 1 and TL 2.

It was shown in an earlier investigation that the astigmatism angle can be determined using the aberrometry measurement setup [5]. This investigation was performed using model eyes. In front of these artificial eyes, a cylindrical lens was inserted and its orientation was varied. With an accuracy of 3.2° and a precision of 1.3° the astigmatism angle was successfully determined. In the artificial eye, the astigmatism angle and the magnitude of measured aberrations is fixed by inserted optical components, when used in the in-vivo environment, reference devices must be used. In this work it is investigated in how far the OCT-based aberrometry setup is useful in a clinical context.

2.2 Reference Devices

In the selection of reference devices, there is no universal gold standard device in clinical use in the context of aberrometry measurement. Two different aberrometry devices were chosen.
The iTrace (Tracey Technologies, Houston, USA) aberrometry device is based on the ray tracing method, where parallel laser beams aligned with the line of sight pass through the pupil [6]. The reflected light is detected by reference sensors and the exact position on the retina from which the reflected light originates is determined. Any local aberrations of the eye that are present on the path of the laser

beam are detected by the measurement of a lateral displacement compared to an emmetropic eye. By sending 256 laser beams through the eye at different locations on the pupil, the absolute wavefront error of the eye is determined. Using iTrace, accommodation influences are considered through the possibility of accommodation at distance and nearby. The iTrace system has a cover that, when opened, allows accommodation into the distance.
The Zywave (Bausch & Lomb, New York, USA) device is based on the functional principle of a Shack-Hartmann sensor for detecting ocular aberrations [7]. An infrared laser beam with a wavelength of 785 nm is focused on the retina. The accommodation influence is considered through an adjustable optical system which compensates the refractive characteristics of a patient and additionally adjusts the accommodation into the distance, by fogging of the fixation image. The backscattered wavefront is detected by a lenslet array in the conjugate pupil plane. The final result is obtained by fitting Zernike polynomials to the backscattered wavefront.

The evaluation and generation of all diagrams was carried out with SpyderIDE 5.1.5 (The Scientific Python Development Environment).

3 Results and Discussion

Besides the comparison between the measured astigmatism angle between the OCT-based aberrometry setup and the reference devices, there were carried out secondary studies. These are to determine the influencing factors and explain the discrepancies or their avoidance. In the comparative study itself as in the secondary investigations, the results have to be put in context of the cylinder magnitude of the measured eye. The measured astigmatism angle is only of high influence if a cylinder magnitude higher than 0.5 diopters is present.

3.1 Comparison Reference Devices

The evaluation of the comparability between the two reference devices is crucial for further investigations. For this secondary comparative study, measurements were taken from 30 subject eyes of healthy volunteers. Ten repeated measurements of angle of astigmatism per eye were recorded with the devices, the mean was calculated. The mean deviation of the measured astigmatism angle between the reference devices is 2.27° and high deviations are seen in cases of low cylinder magnitude (Fig. 2).

3.2 Accommodation

The accommodation ability of the eye has to be taken in account if an accommodation ability of 4 diopters is present [8]. Accommodation leads only to a small change in the low-order Zernike coefficients. Higher-order coefficients are affected by the accommodation ability of younger subjects. The refractive values change with the change in shape

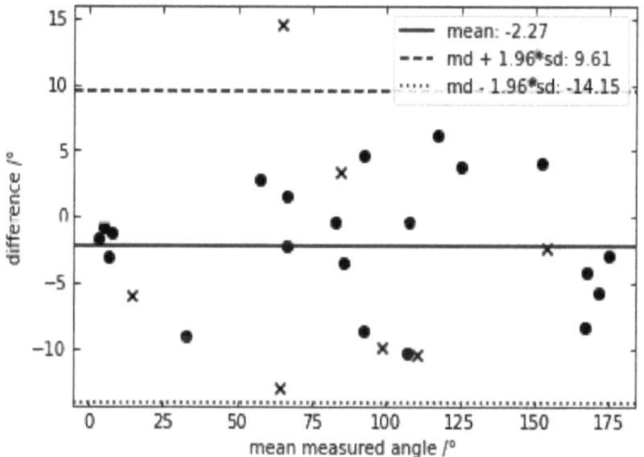

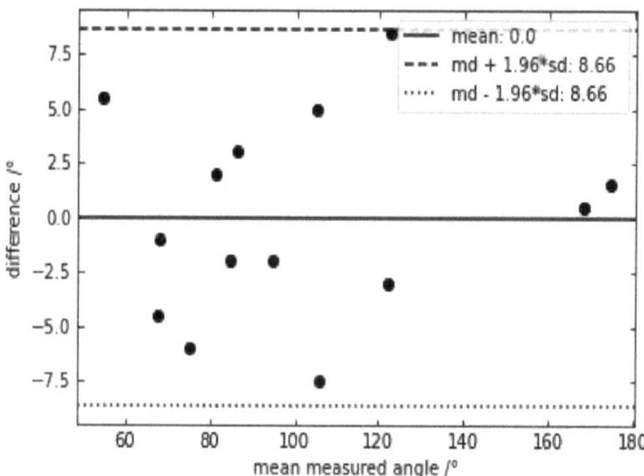

Figure 2: Bland-Altman plot between the two reference aberrometers. The horizontal-axis shows the mean measured angle of the aberrometers, while the vertical-axis represents the difference. The upper and lower limits of agreement are represented by the respective horizontal lines. md stands for the mean deviation and sd for standard deviation. The solid line shows the mean difference between the aberrometer measurements. Measurements with cylinder magnitude higher than 0.5 diopters as measured by both devices are presented as dots.

of the crystalline lens resulting from the accommodative ability. This means that the measured angles should not be influenced by accommodation. The accommodation ability is investigated with the iTrace device using a smaller number of subjects. As expected the deviation between the two measurements at different accommodation setting is low (Fig. 3).

3.3 Pupil Diameter

The measurement setup does not have a pupil camera at the time of this investigation. Accordingly, neither the exact position of the entrance of the injection beam nor the pupil size during the measurement or during the evaluation of the measurement is known. The effect of the pupil size is an important parameter in the evaluation of the refraction values. For this reason, the influence of the pupil diameter was investigated using the iTrace device. The influence of the pupil diameter on the measurement of the astigmatism angle, as seen in Fig. 4, is negligible at this point, since taking into account angle wrappings, a mean absolute difference in astigmatism angle of 5.18° results.

3.4 Measurement Alignment

The alignment of the measurement axis during the measurement procedure is important [9]. To establish a constant measurement alignment, Zernike tilt coefficients were used. It is assumed that when the tilt coefficient for the lateral and horizontal description of the wavefront approaches zero, the injection beam enters the eye centrally through the pupil. Furthermore, the tilt alignment secures a constant value for alignment accuracy for the measurement procedure. As shown in Fig. 5 a mean correction of 15.09 a.u.

Figure 3: Bland-Altman plot for nearby and far accommodation settings, as in Fig. 2.

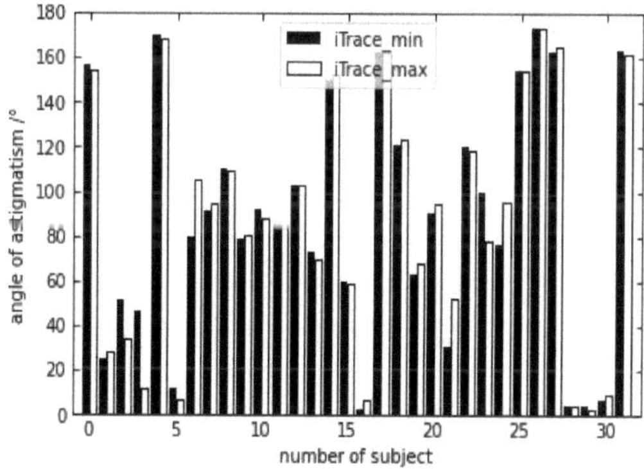

Figure 4: Comparison between measured astigmatism angles at different pupil diameters. Mean pupil diameter for the group of iTrace_min is 2 mm and for the group of iTrace_max 4.22 ± 1.48 mm.

is achieved when readjusting according to the Zernike tilt coefficients was made.

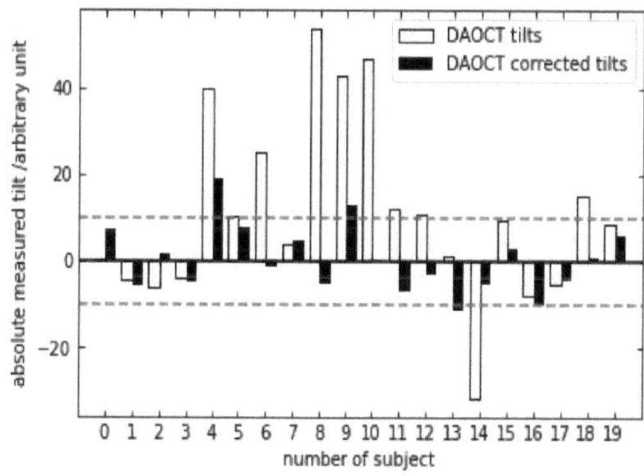

Figure 5: The DAOCT tilts are the tilt coefficients that were recorded without alignment attempts. For the DAOCT corrected tilt measurements the attempt was made to minimize the tilt coefficients in order to achieve a uniform measurement alignment for all exposures with the aberrometry setup. The dashed line is the limit for the tilt coefficients which is understood as an acceptable approximation.

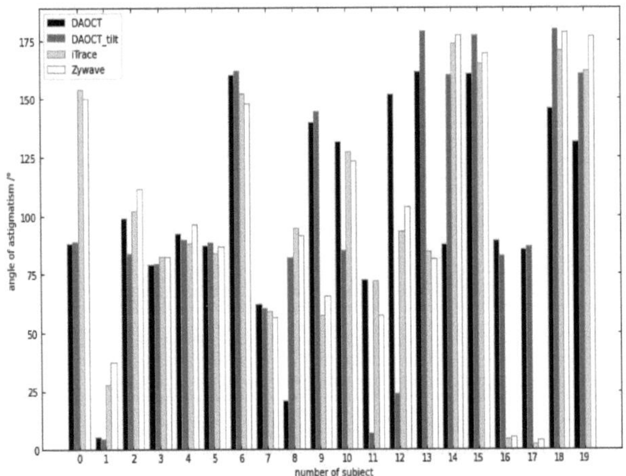

Figure 6: Comparison of the two DAOCT measurement approaches with the reference devices.

3.5 Results Comparison

The setup presented in 2.1 is compared with the reference devices. For this purpose, 20 in-vivo measurements have been compared with each other (Fig. 6). A distinction was made between the tilt alignment and the normal alignment with the measurement setup. For the normal alignment, the mean deviation of astigmatism angle between DAOCT and reference devices is 37.09°. Here, the mean deviation was determined in such a way that the averaged span between the two reference devices was taken as the reference and comparison value. The same comparison was also carried out for the measurements with the tilt alignment; here, the mean deviation of the measured astigmatism angle is 35.02°.

3.6 Discussion

Influencing factors were investigated and each of these influencing factors bring an uncertainty in the comparability of the individual measurements with the respective comparison device. The deviations in 3.5 and shown in Fig. 6 cannot be explained to the same extent on the basis of the secondary investigations in 3. The entire measurement survey must be revised and errors in the data collection and in the processing of these evaluated. The use of a pupil camera could ensure alignment during measurement such as the measurement axis passes through the center of the pupil.

4   Conclusion

In this work the comparability between the aberrometry setup, which is foreseen for the use in an intraoperative setup for the alignment of toric intraocular lenses and clinical approved aberrometers was investigated regarding the astigmatism angle. The accuracy of astigmatism angle determination for in-vivo measurements is with a mean deviation of 35.02° insufficient. Further improvements need to be made to establish a comparable basis between the measurement setup and reference devices.

Acknowledgement

The work has been carried out at Heidelberg Engineering GmbH and supervised by Prof. Dr. rer. nat. Gereon Hüttmann, Universität zu Lübeck.

Authors' Statement

Conflict of interest: Authors state no conflict of interest. Informed consent: Informed consent has been obtained from all individuals included in this study.

5   References

[1] A. H. Elhofi and H. A. Helaly, *Comparison Between Digital and Manual Marking for Toric Intraocular Lenses: A Randomized Trial.* Medicine: 94(38):e.1618, 2015.

[2] W. Drexler and J. G. Fujimoto, *Optical Coherence Tomography: Technology and Applications.* eds.: Springer Berlin, New York, 2008.

[3] S. Georgiev et al., *Digital ocular swept source optical coherence aberrometry.* in: Biomedical Optics Express, vol.12; no.11, 2021.

[4] G. M. Dai, *Wavefront Optics for Vision Correction.* eds.: SPIE Press, Bellingham, Washington USA, 2008.

[5] M. Wunderlich and M. Stender, *Wavefront measurement with swept source OCT for the determination of astigmatism in the eye.* in: Student Conference on Medical Engineering Science 2022, Grin Publishing, München, 2022.

[6] A. Sinha, S. Goel, V. Gupta, D. Kumawat and P. Sahay, *iTrace - A Ray Tracing Aberrometer.* Delhi Journal of Ophthalmology 2019; vol.30; pp.72 – 75, 2019.

[7] M. Dobos, M. Twa, M. Bullimore, *An evaluation of the Bausch & Lomb Zywave aberrometer.* In: Clinical and Experimental Optometry: 92(3), pp. 238 – 45, 2009.

[8] F. Lara-Lacárcel, I. Marín-Franch, V. Fernández-Sánchez, R. Riquelme-Nicolás and N. López-Gil, *Objective changes in astigmatism during accommodation.* Ophthalmic and Physiological Optics, vol. 41; no.5, pp.1069 – 1075, 2021.

[9] S. Arba Mosquera, S. Verma and C. McAlinden, *Centration axis in refractive surgery.* in: Eye and Vision; vol.2, art.-no.4, 2015.

State of the art analysis of medical foot switches for high frequency applications

Gregory Berg [1],
[1] Medical Engineering Science, Universität zu Lübeck, gregory.berg@student.uni-luebeck.de

Abstract

Medical foot switches are the most common tool to activate the instruments of electrosurgical generators. The large variety of generators and suppliers resulted in an overwhelming portfolio of different foot switches that confuse the costumers and strain the life cycle management of these devices. The analysis of modern foot switches presented in this paper is intended to serve as a guideline for general product requirements of these devices and examines the feasibility of a universal foot switch.

1　Introduction

In this paper, an analysis of the state of the art of medical foot switches for high frequency (HF) applications is presented. For this purpose, a function and module analysis of a two-pedal wireless and a two-pedal wired medical foot switch for high frequency applications was carried out independently. The results are used as a basis for product requirements of an up to date medical foot switch. In the field of medical high frequency (HF) application, there is a large variety of electrosurgical generators and therefore, a high variety of foot switches. Most electrosurgical generators have matching foot switches in the field of HF surgery that can be categorised in one-, two-, three-pedal- and four-pedal foot switches that are either wired or wireless. As a result, the number of foot switches in the product portfolio of many medical supply companies grew and, accordingly, the support and effort in the product life cycle. For this purpose, a reduction of the foot switchportfolio is favoured in an economic sense [1]. A state-of-the-art analysis of medical foot switches could conclude in the formulation of general product requirements for a universal foot switch.

2　Material and Methods

For the analysis of modern medical foot switches, a module and interface analysis had to be conducted in order to formulate device requirements and designs. For this purpose, an examination of current foot switches for controlling monopolar or bipolar HF instruments was carried out. The analysis differentiates between wired and wireless foot switches that are compatible with electrosurgical generators. To classify the various components of the foot switch, the datasheets and other available information of different medical foot switchsuppliers was examined. After the components had been assigned to functional groups, their func-

tionality was analysed, and preliminary product requirements were listed. Additionally, the necessary communication components between a medical foot switchand a medical device were identified and formulated. This information is the fundament for creating general product requirements of a universal foot switch for medical high frequency applications. The feasibility of the construction of a universal foot switch will be discussed and solutions for identified difficulties will be presented.

3　Results of the module and interface analysis

3.1　Module analysis

First, the different components of a wired and wireless medical two-pedal foot switch were analysed. To classify the components of the foot switches, the datasheets of various models were examined and compared.

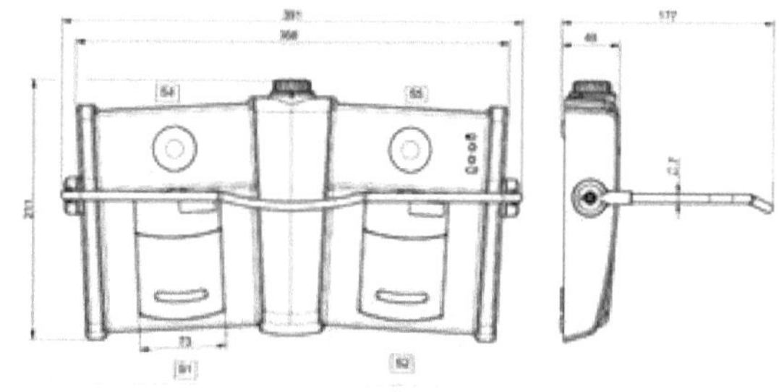

Figure 1: Technical drawing of the wireless foot switch MKF 2 SW2.4LE-MED GP211 by Steute [2]

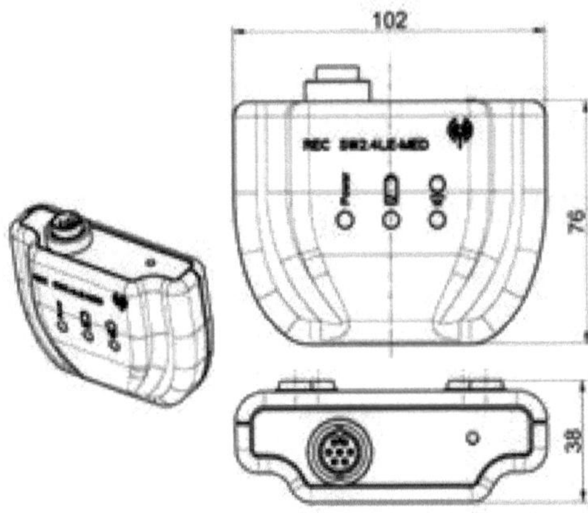

Figure 2: Technical drawing of the wireless foot switch MKF 2 SW2.4LE-MED GP211 by Steute [2]

After the components had been assigned to function groups, their functionality and intended purpose was researched and named. In the following, the determined components and different functionalities of a wireless medical foot switch are listed:

Components:
- Housing
- Power supply
- Pedals and additional switches
- Controlling unit and internal wiring
- Antenna
- Radio module
- Receiver with connection cable

Functionality:
- Power supply
- Functionality and status display
- Signal transmission
- Device recognition
- Actuation functionality
- Electrical safety

Hereinafter, each paragraph deals with a functionality, the involved components and their purpose.

Power supply: The housing serves as a holder for the power supply. Wireless foot switches are usually equipped with rechargeable batteries [2]. A compartment in the housing is needed to be able to replace the power supply. This compartment must be closed with a screw cap (See Fig. 1). The receiver is supplied with power via the cable connection to a generator. The radio module is a component integrated in the wireless foot switch and its receiver and enables the constant communication of the two devices. The radio module is the component with the largest power consumption [2].

Functionality and status display: When using a foot switch for HF applications, it is important that the user receives feedback on the functionality and the status of the foot switch. The functional identification of the pedals of the foot switch is realized by colouring the pedals. Some suppliers add a sign on each pedal, which spells the functionality. The IEC 60601-2-2 norm specifies that the left pedal is for the cutting mode and the right pedal is for the coagulation mode. The standard states that the cutting pedal must be yellow, while the coagulation pedal must be blue [4]. How this colour coding is implemented is not explicitly formulated in the IEC, as well as the colour coding for other functionalities such as ultrasound and high frequency dual applications [5]. In the case of the observed foot switches, the status of the power supply and the connection status to the electrosurgical generator are additionally visually indicated. A transparent material is incorporated into the foot switch housing in two small areas to allow the LED light from the battery and connection status LEDs to penetrate through the housing [2]. The receiver has no normatively specified status indicators according to the IEC [4]. Nevertheless, some receivers have built in LEDs for the indication of the connection status to the HF generator, one indicating the status of the receiver's wireless connection to the foot switch, and one LED indicating the foot switch battery status (See Fig. 2).

Signal transmission: The most important function of the foot switch is the signal transmission during a medical procedure. With a wireless foot switch, information is exchanged between the receiver and the foot switch via a wireless communication. The two defining factors for the quality of the data exchange are the safety of the information and the latency. Modern information exchange between wireless devices is redundant, meaning that the same pieces of data are stored multiple times in a single data package [6]. This communication technique ensures the authenticity and correctness of the received data. The latency describes the amount of time between the actuation of a pedal and the activation of the desired functionality. The receiver transmits the received data via a cable, which is plugged into a suitable electrosurgical generator.

Device recognition: A multitude of electrosurgical generators are capable to automatically recognise the foot switch that is plugged into them. Because wireless foot switches with a different number of pedals are still run with the same receiver [2], it is safe to say that the foot switches can transmit their identity.

Actuation functionality: Medical foot switch are equipped with two categories of switches that can be pressed. The first are the pedals that activate the different modes of the HF application. It was observed that foot switches for electrosurgical applications had one, two, three or four pedals. The transmission of the information about the pedal position is electrically implemented with different switch variants such as reed contacts, micro switches or hall sensors [2]. The other switch-category is the colloquially called "buttons". They are integrated into the housing, allowing the user to cycle through the generator's different modes or HF instruments depending on the procedural protocol. Not every foot switch is equipped with additional buttons. The receiver transmits the different control signals electronically to the generator [2].

Electrical safety: According to the IEC 60529, medical foot switches for high frequency applications must be tested for at least protection class IPX6 and are protected against damage after being immersed in liquids for a brief amount of time [7].

The analysis of wired foot switch models concluded that they can be viewed as a simplified version of wireless foot switches, because the main elements are identical (See Fig. 3).

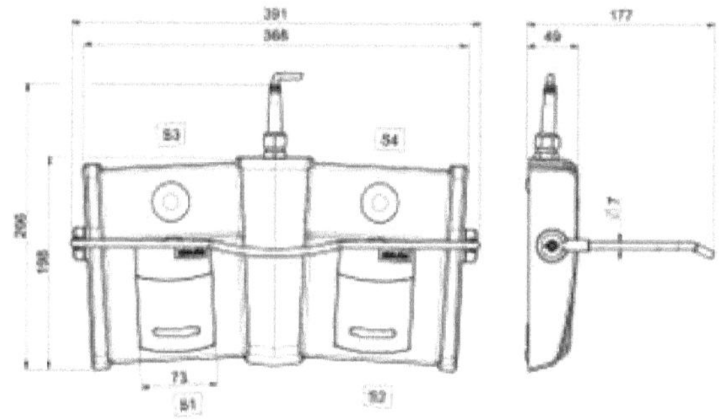

Figure 3: Figure 3: Technical drawing of the wired foot switch MKF 2-MED GP211 by Steute [8]

The communication between a wired foot switch and an electrosurgical generator is the only essential difference and will be explained in the following.
Signal transmission: Since the signal transmission of a wired foot switch takes place via cable, there must be an opening with a thread in the housing. Otherwise, the signal transmission of a wired foot switch with a HF generator is identical to the communication of the receiver of the wireless foot switch with generators.
Device recognition: Wired foot switches must transmit their identity for the same reasons as wireless foot switches, if they are supposed to be automatically recognised and to ensure compatibility. A software solution for the transmission of an identity is the translation of a bit code to an array of digital signals with the use of a microcontroller. Several outputs act as bits and transmit a voltage, which is recognised by the generator as a binary '1', or are grounded, which is read as a binary '0'. A multitude of digital outputs can represent a predefined foot switch identity. The outputs are each connected separately to a pin of the cable of the foot switch and the electrosurgical generator. This allows the identity of the foot switch (e.g. the number of pedals) to be automatically recognised [9].

3.2 Interface and plug analysis

For the interface analysis of a foot switch and its electrosurgical generator, the plug type and number of information channels of the connection cable of various wired two-pedal foot switches was examined. Many foot switches are equipped with round connector plugs. In this case, the number of possible information channels can be read, as each

pin of the connector functions as an information source [2,3 8].
The smallest observed number of pins in a foot switch connector is four, of which two are needed for the power supply and the remaining two are expected to transmit the pedal actuation signal. Further research in the plugs of electrosurgical generators and their foot switches concluded, that foot switches with a different number of pedals still had the same quantity of pins inside their plugs. An electrosurgical generator with two nine pin plugs can be operated with four different foot switches, which have different numbers of pedals and additional buttons. The most pedals and buttons one of these foot switches has, is five. Therefore, it can be assumed, that at least five of the pins are reserved for pedal and switch information, even though not all these foot switches require as many. Two pins must be reserved for the power supply, leaving two free pins. Because every foot switch is automatically recognized by the generator it is safe to assume, that the two free pins transmit the identity of the foot switch. The highest number of pins observed is from the plug of an electrosurgical generator with 14 pins. Because of such a high number of pins, there are most likely additional signals transmitted, for example the state of safety sensors, that could be integrated inside the foot switch. In summary the following transmitted signals could be observed:

- Actuation state of the pedals (one to four pins)
- Actuation state of the additional switches (zero to four pins)
- Identity (zero to two pins)

The signal transmission of wireless foot switches is composed of the wired communication between a receiver and an electrosurgical generator and the wireless transmission of the foot switches state towards the receiver. The content of this information is like the wired foot switches with additional signals. These include the state of the power supply and a signal that indicates the quality of the wireless connection of the foot switch and its receiver [2, 3]. A universal plug should therefore have at least 12 pins to cover for all the information channels named.

4 Requirements for a universal foot switch

The minimal requirements for a universal medical foot switch for HF applications consist of the technical realisation of the default functionality of a medical foot switch, which derived from the module and interface analysis of up-to-date foot switches. The challenges for a realisation of such a device are as follows:

- Unique display of pedal functionality
- Different plug types
- Unique pin assignment
- A market for wired and wireless foot switches

Approaches to solving such problems in operating theatres have already been patented. A temporary solution for the different plugs with different pin assignments could be a universal controlling. It functions as a multipurpose plug adapter and logically decodes the different foot switch signals [10]. With this unit, a universal foot switch could be connected to a multitude of different electrosurgical generators with unique plugs. In the long turn, the connector type and pin assignment should be standardised so that different foot switch and electrosurgical generator suppliers must design their devices to be compatible with any other company's devices. The unique display of functionality results in foot switches with a different number of pedals and a different colouring of them. A compromise would be several universal foot switches, that each represent functionalities that are required for different electrosurgical applications. To avoid the doubling of the foot switch portfolio by differentiation between wired and wireless foot switches, a device that can be used in both ways could be developed.

Conclusion

The investigation of the design and functionality of modern medical foot switches for electrosurgical generators concluded, that their basic construction is similar enough to realise a universal foot switch, apart from their functional display of the foot switch's pedals, their choice of plug type and pin assignment. The fundamental roadblock of plugs with different designs and pin assignments could be solved by means of norms or standards. Short-term solutions, such as a universal medical device control console could already realise, that a large part of the foot switch range is compatible with most electrosurgical generators [10]. The unique medical fields with different functional demands of the electrosurgical generators hinders the conceptualisation of a universal medical foot switch. To work around this problem, an arsenal of universal foot switches could shrink the product portfolio immensely.

Acknowledgement

The work has been supervised by the Institute of Biomedical Optics, Universität zu Lübeck.

Author's Statement

Conflict of interest: Authors state no conflict of interest.

5 References

[1] L.Edquist, *Less Can Be More for Product Portfolios*. BCG Global, Berlin, 2014, August 25. Available: https://www.bcg.com/publications/2014/lean-manufacturing-consumers-products-less-can-be-more-for-product-portfolio-attacking-complexity-while-enhancing-the-value-of-diversity [last accessed on 2023-01-20].

[2] steute Technologies GmbH Co. KG. 2023 *MKF 2 SW2.4LE-MED GP211*. Available: https://www.steute meditec.com/en/products/mkf2-sw24le-med-gp211.html [last accessed on 2023-01-20].

[3] steute Technologies GmbH Co. KG. 2023 *REC SW2.4LE-MED AG43.*. Available: https://www.steute meditec.com/en/products/mkf2-sw24le-med-gp211.html [last accessed on 2023-01-20].

[4] International Electrotechnical Commission, *Medical electrical equipment - Part 2-2: Particular requirements for the basic safety and essential performance of high frequency surgical equipment and high frequency surgical accessories* . IEC, 2018.

[5] G. A. Vilos and C. Rajakumar, *Electrosurgical Generators and Monopolar and Bipolar Electrosurgery.*. In: Journal of Minimally Invasive Gynecology, pp. 279–287, 2013, Available : https://doi.org/10.1016/j.jmig.2013.02.013 [last accessed on 2023-01-20].

[6] Talend, *What is Data Redundancy - Definitions and Drawbacks*. Available : https://www.talend.com/resources/what-is-data-redundancy/ [last accessed on 2023-01-20].

[7] International Electrotechnical Commission, *Degrees of protection provided by enclosures* . IEC, 2013.

[8] steute Technologies GmbH Co. KG. 2023 *MKF 2-MED GP211*. Available: https://www.steute-meditec.com/en/products/mkf-2-sw24le-med-gp211.html [last accessed on 2023-01-20].

[9] R. Keim, *How to Choose a Microcontroller for Digital Signal Processing Applications*. All About CURCUITS, 2019, Available: https://www.allaboutcircuits.com/technical-articles/how-to-choose-a-microcontroller-for-digital-signal-processing-applications/ [last accessed on 2023-01-20].

[10] R.L. Quick, M.V. Shabaz, J.H.Dabney, D. Kussman, F. Louw, P. Lubock *Universal medical device control console.*. SenoRx Inc. 2004, patent identification number : CA2527233C.

Evaluation of the Usability of a Ventilation Test Framework

Emma Bösemann [1], Muhammad Tausif Irshad [2], Hendrik Fischer [3], Marcin Grzegorzek [2]

[1] Medical Informatics, Universität zu Lübeck, emma.boesemann@student.uni-luebeck.de
[2] Institute for Medical Informatics, Universität zu Lübeck, {m.irshad, marcin.grzegorzek}@uni-luebeck.de
[3] Drägerwerk AG & Co. KGaA, Lübeck, Hendrik.Fischer@draeger.com

Abstract

Mechanical ventilators that assist the patient's breathing (respiration) can be found in every hospital. New ventilators are constantly being manufactured and researchers are trying to develop them with even better performance. In the past, a test framework was developed to test ventilators under different conditions to ensure a steady improvement during the development process. To evaluate the usability of the ventilator test framework, a usability test was conducted. A questionnaire was created that focused on the four most important aspects of usability: efficiency, effectiveness, satisfaction, and safety. Four users of the test framework were interviewed. The evaluation confirmed the need for a ventilator testing framework, and the test results provide fundamental insights for ventilator development.

1 Introduction

Breathing is one of the most important processes of the human body. It is executed unconsciously at every minute in life. The inhaled oxygen is transported by the blood to all body parts where it is used to produce adenosine triphosphate which is involved in energy production. A lack of oxygen may lead to severe organ damages. Therefore, ventilation systems are of vital importance for patients with apnea or lung diseases that lead to restricted respiration [1]. A ventilator can either take over the whole respiration or support the respiratory effort of the patient [2]. To provide the best treatment for patients the development of new ventilation systems is pursued constantly by several companies. Especially, the COVID-19 pandemic remarked the importance of ventilators [3]. It is important to regularly test the performance of the device during the process of the development. For all software and hardware changes it must be ensured that the modification yields an improvement to a component of the ventilation and at the same time do not result in a deterioration of another component. For that reason, a test framework was implemented. This framework aims to support the evaluation process of the performance of the ventilation system. The intention is that developer do not need to have specific knowledge of testing, meaning that the framework should be easy to use. To be able to evaluate the usability and merchantability of the framework a questionnaire was prepared to conduct a usability test concentrating on the aspects efficiency, effectiveness, satisfaction and safety. The questionnaire was answered by different users of the test framework in an interview. This paper presents the conduction and results of the usability test.

First, the test framework is described and the structure of the usability test is explained. Afterwards, the results of the usability test are presented and possible future changes are drawn from them.

2 Material and Methods

2.1 Test Framework

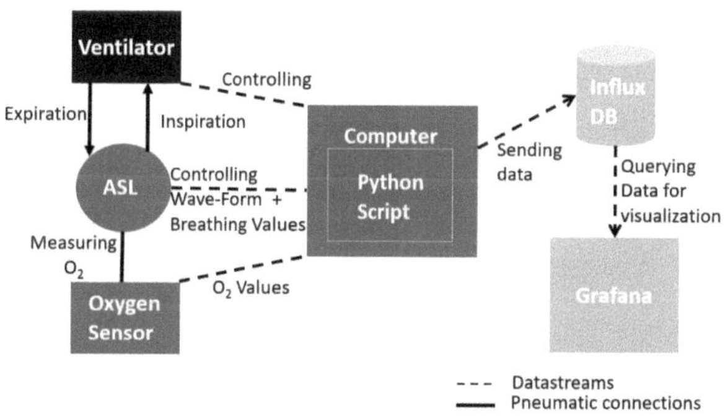

Figure 1: Interaction of the components of the test framework. The black box is the ventilator on test. The dark gray components are involved in the testing process. The light gray components are part of the evaluation process.

The purpose of the test framework is to execute defined test sequences, control the ventilator, record data, and evaluate the performance. The ability to flexibly adapt the tests and evaluation parameters is the biggest advantage of the framework as it gives the opportunity to react on different needs of the ventilation developers. Following, the architecture of the test framework is outlined. The interaction of its components is shown in Fig. 1. The main component is the computer on which the python script of the framework can be executed. Via the computer the ventilator, the active servo lung (ASL) 5000 and the oxygen sensor can be controlled. By starting the python script, the user is first guided through the test setup by different windows of the graphical user interface (GUI). The main window is given in Fig. 2. All information of the device under test including the name, the "FuMu" (a file containing details about hardware components) and the software version must be defined. Further, the choice of how to control the ventilator must be made. The device can either be set by the user manually or the commands for ventilator settings are controlled by the computer via a RS-232 serial connection. In the second part of the main window the test scenarios that should be executed shall be defined. For that, already predefined tests can be chosen by a dropdown menu. Finally, the user must press the start button. The following steps are then executed by the python script on its own. The ASL 5000, a lung simulator by IngMar Medical, is started via the test automation interface (TAI) and the defined lung model file can be set for each test case. The lung model file determines the lung parameters, like the resistance, the compliance and whether the lung works actively or passively. If the framework is in the serial mode, the ventilator is set up by the computer otherwise the ventilator settings must be set manually according to the test definition. If both the ASL and the ventilator are ready, the ventilator can be turned on and the measurements for the first test case are starting. For each test case the breathing parameters and wave form values measured by the ASL are transmitted to the computer. After the execution of the complete set of test cases, the pressure and flow values extracted from the wave form values are examined and predefined performance parameter are calculated. The entire measured and calculated data is sent and saved within a database InfluxDB, specialized for time series data. Grafana is used for visualization purposes. By using the query language Flux, the data can be retrieved from InfluxDB.

2.2 Usage Context

To define a suitable usability test, it is necessary to define the context of use of the test framework. Therefore, the components of the context, namely the user, the tasks, the aim, the resources and the situation of use, must be clarified [4]. There are three different user groups of the test framework. The first one (usage group 1) consists of the engineers and developers of the ventilator in evolution. For them it is important to develop a novel ventilation system that is superior in its performance. After each software or hardware change the test framework should validate changes in performance. The second user group (usage group 2) tries to constantly improve the test framework itself. The developers should be able to implement new functionality while they need to keep the test framework itself in a working condition. The last user group (usage group 3) consists of tester who are building up a dataset for comparing purpose. A novel ventilation system should be enhanced in perfor-

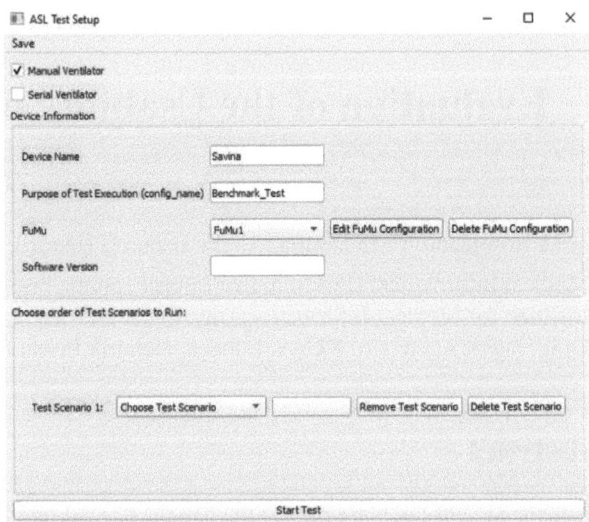

Figure 2: Main window (graphical user interface) of the test framework, where the user can set the device information and the test scenario.

mance compared to other ventilators on the market. For all usage groups the same software and hardware resources, defined in section 2.1, are needed. Each of this resources is reusable. The situation of use is familiar to the users. Therefore, it should not influence the usage. The users do not need to socially interact with any other person. There is only a physical interaction with the computer and the ventilation system during the testing. Depending on the behavior of the ventilator the user has to react.

2.3 Usability Questionnaire

After defining the usage context the questionnaire was made up concentrating on the evaluation of the four main aspects for a positive user experience for medical devices: efficiency, effectiveness, satisfaction and safety [5]. The efficiency is the term of the time spent by the user to reach his goal. The rating of how constructive the path of achieving the aim is, is concluded under the term effectiveness. For a good user satisfaction the user has to be satisfied by the outcome as well as by the procedure. Finally, especial for the usage of medical products, safety for the user and a possible patient has to be ensured.

Before starting the interview with the questionnaire each participant was made aware that the test framework is the subject that should get evaluated and not the participant. This is important to ensure that the participant feels free to critically evaluate the test framework. The first part of the questionnaire collects demographic information of the participants to have an overview on different backgrounds that could lead to contrasting opinions. For example, the amount of experience on ventilation systems is relevant. After this, to start with a smooth opening and to make sure that the subject of the questionnaire is clear, an illustration of the architecture and its components is given together with a scenario of a situation where the participant should describe its course of action for starting a test scenario. A second figure of the main GUI is included as a visual reminder. The main part of the questionnaire is divided into two parts. The first part consist of nine openly raised questions that cannot solely be answered by yes or no, tempting the participant to response detailed. In the second part the participant should answer four assessment questions. One can choose one of the given answers that rate the fulfillment of aspects of the usage of the test framework. The answer choices are: always, often, sometimes, rarely, never. In the end, there is space for further remarks. The questionnaire was fulfilled during a person to person interview. Hence, the interviewer had the possibility to ask for further specifications of given answers.

3 Results and Discussion

3.1 Respondents

The interview has been executed with four different participants. One interview took about 30 minutes and has been conducted at the working station of the test framework. Due to the fact that the test framework is still under development, the conduction of more interviews was not possible as no more persons were familiar with the use of the framework. Nevertheless, it is assumed that the small number of participants can already give helpful insights to this development process. Table 1 displays the demographic information of the respondents. Each usage group is represented by at least one participant. Every user is familiar with the test framework since at least 0.75 years. None of the respondents started the interview unbiased as each has been part of the development process of the framework.

3.2 Assessment Questions

The interviews combined with the questionnaire showed a positive attitude towards the test framework of each respondent. Fig. 3 visualizes the mean of the answers together with error rates and the standard deviation. It can be seen that the most prominent answers are 'often' and 'always' to most of the question indicating an overall satisfaction of the users with the test framework. Independent of the usage group, the test framework aims to aid to achieve the different goals and the users are mostly satisfied with the results. The participant of the usage group 1 stated that the framework is helpful for her engineering work. Important knowledge about the ventilator within a development process can be gained. Especially, the possibility to compare the performance of different time points in the development process is essential to evaluate if hardware or software changes are enhancing the performance. The worst rates are given for the aspect whether the use of the framework is intuitive. None of the respondents stated that in their opinion the test framework is always intuitive. This has also been carried out by the open-asked questions. The main problem is that for starting the test a few settings have to be set and the test

definition has to be formulated by the user. The respondents criticize that, for example in the main GUI given in Fig. 2, there is no explanation on the information that should be filled into the text fields. An appropriate setting is relevant for a correct assignment of the test within Grafana. Furthermore, it is relevant to have at least a basic knowledge about ventilators and the respiratory system.

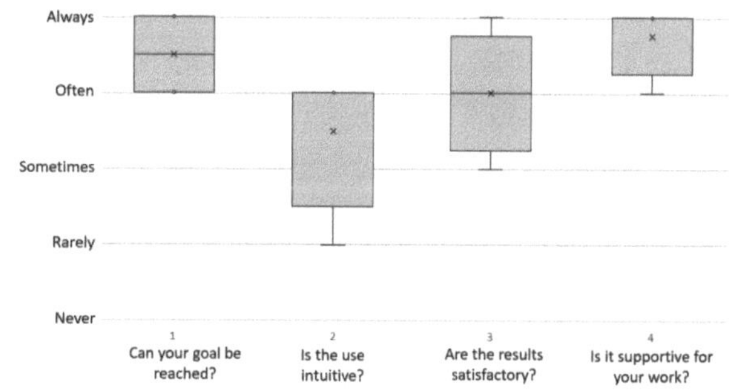

Figure 3: The box plots of the assessment questions are shown.

3.3 Improvement Suggestions

During the interview each participant had the opportunity to suggest improvements for the test framework. Those will be summarized within this section. To make the test setup and its settings more intuitive it was suggested to either insert a pop-up window with an explaining text or text fields within the settings window. Those explanations should include information about the different settings and how they affect the procedure of the test framework. Further, the free text fields for the information of the used device within the main GUI could be replaced by dropdown menus. By this it can be assured that identical devices are defined the same way by each user. An administrator is needed for those dropdown menus that sets up a complete list of devices under test. In that case, the user solely chooses the appropriate device.

The ASL that simulates the patient for the tests provides plenty of settings to imitate different lungs. The test sequences define at the moment only the resistance and the compliance of the lungs and if it is working actively or passively but no further properties of the ASL. A more precise definition of the lung under test could lead to an optimized testing time which is important for the efficiency of the test framework. For example, a functional residual capacity matching the settings of the size of the lung defined by resistance and compliance could decrease the waiting time until the applied oxygen is spread within the whole lung.

It should also be assured that each component of the test framework is working smoothly. For example, the connected oxygen sensor needs often plenty of time to start. Hence, this sensor should be optimized. Further, the test framework lacks the feature to catch errors made by single

Table 1: Demographic Information

Participant ID	A	B	C	D
Gender	w	w	w	w
Age	26	24	44	29
Profession	Student	Student	Senior Engineer	Student
Knowledge about Ventilators (years)	1.5	0.75	11	0.5
Usage Time (years)	0.75	0.75	1	0.75
Usage Frequency	often a week	often a week	every few weeks	often a week
Usage Group	2	2+3	1	2+3

hardware components like the oxygen sensor or the ASL connected to the computer that runs the framework. If errors are unrecognized they can influence the test performance and falsify the results. It must be also possible to execute an emergency stop if unforeseen situations occur.

3.4 Discussion

For the evaluation of the results of the questionnaire, the four aspects of usability within the test framework are examined. The efficiency of the framework is still capable of improvement. Although for the starting procedure of tests, regardless of the problems mentioned for the connected oxygen sensor, it was claimed by each participant that it does not take too long, the tests themselves are not time-optimized. A test case should not last longer than the time needed to reach a sufficient amount of test data. Because of the non-optimized settings of the ASL, the tests include waiting times in addition to the test time, for example, for the settling time of the oxygen.

The effectiveness of the test framework is rated by each respondent positively. Each one is often to always satisfied by the results given by the test framework. Further, this represents a good satisfaction of the user. They claimed that the framework is helpful for their work, which is important to assure repeated use of the test framework. The suggested improvements are mentioned in 3.3, which could increase both effectiveness and satisfaction. These changes could prevent framework errors and reduce the number of tests that have to be repeated due to such errors.

The last aspect is safety. The test framework itself does not yield any risk of safety for the user as one only interacts with a computer and no living patient is part of the testing. An unrevealed misbehaviour of the test framework could lead to mistakes in the development of a ventilator that could follow with potential risks for patients. But such secondary results cannot be evaluated in this usability test. The test framework is not intended as a testing device for the licensing of a medical product but rather solely during the development process.

4   Conclusion

The conducted usability test showed that the test framework is useful for the development of new ventilation systems.

The evaluation parameters of each test can be used to verify whether changes to the hardware or software improve performance. The efficiency of the test framework should be improved to ensure good usability. The test framework itself is still under development. Therefore, the results of usability testing can be used to complete tasks in the development process. After completion of the framework, the usability test should be conducted again with a larger number of participants and with participants who are not involved in the development process of the framework. For this purpose, the created questionnaire can be reused.

Acknowledgement

The work has been carried out at Drägerwerk AG & Co. KGaA, Lübeck and supervised by the Institute of Medical Informatics, Universität zu Lübeck.

Author's Statement

The authors report no conflict of interest.

5   References

[1] SH. Cedar, *Every breath you take: the process of breathing explained.* Nursing Times [online]; 114: 1, 47-50, 2018.

[2] K. Deden, Dräger Medical GmbH, *Beatmungsmodi in der Intensivmedizin.* Broschüre: https://www.draeger.com/Library/Content/ Beatmungsmodi_in_der_Intensivmedizin_nomenklatur-bk-9066354-de.pdf [last accessed on 14/12/2022]

[3] Q. Notz, J. Herrmann, J. Stumpner et al., *Anästhesie- und Intensivbeatmungsgeräte: Unterschiede und Nutzbarkeit bei COVID-19-Patienten.* Anaesthesist 69, 316–322, 2020.

[4] M. Maguire, *Context of Use within usability activities.* Int. J. Human-Computer Studies 55, 453-483, 2001.

[5] International Electrotechnical Commission, *Medical devices — Part 1: Application of usability engineering to medical devices.* (IEC Standard No. 62366-1:2015). https://www.iso.org/standard/63179.html, 2015.

The conception and prototypical development of a valve system for a realistic ventilation management between lung simulator and sleep therapy device

Mohammed Algherbawi [1],

[1] Biomedical Engineering, Luebeck University of Applied Sciences, mohammed.algherbawi@stud.th-luebeck.de

Abstract

The paper presents the design and creation of a valve system that enhances existing lung simulators (e.g. ASL5000) during non-invasive positive pressure ventilation (NIV). The goal was to provide Löwenstein Medical Technology with a tool for further research, testing, and measurement purposes to better monitor apnea events in patients undergoing NIV therapy for Obstructive Sleep Apnea (OSA). The developed valve system offers several benefits, including a high level of accuracy, a wider opening range, and the ability to adjust parameters such as flow rate and resistance. The system is also insensitive to temperature, allowing for precise simulation of obstructive and central apneas. Equipped with a flow sensor and regulator, the system's control over desired flow is more effective. The results indicate that this valve system is a reliable and cost-effective solution for realistic ventilation management between lung simulator and sleep therapy device.

1 Introduction

Non-invasive positive-pressure ventilation (NIV) is the main long-term home treatment for chronic hypercapnic respiratory failure. Unintentional leaks can occur during NIV, affecting its clinical efficacy, reducing tolerance, and compromising device performance [1]. During NIV therapy for Obstructive Sleep Apnea (OSA), two main types of sleep apnea can occur: Obstructive Sleep Apnea (OSA) and Central Sleep Apnea (CSA). OSA is the most prevalent form of sleep apnea and results from a physical blockage of the airway during sleep, caused by the relaxation of the muscles in the throat and tongue [2]. On the other hand, CSA is a less common type of sleep apnea, characterized by a lack of respiratory effort leading to a temporary halt in breathing during sleep [2]. CSA can be linked to medical conditions like heart failure, brainstem disorders, or neurological issues, not physical airway blockage like OSA.[3]. Löwenstein Medical Technology is working on improving its sleep therapy devices. This paper deals with the development of a complementary valve system to simulate obstructive and central events, as well as leaks, to enhance realistic ventilation management between the lung simulator and the sleep therapy device.

2 Material and Methods

The system consists of a mechanical part that blocks the airflow from the therapy device to the artificial lung. This corresponds to the obstructive event in sleep therapy. Another valve, identical to the first, is utilized to simulate leaks. The system also features an electromechanical component, allowing for adjustments to the valve for varying levels of airflow blockage. Finally, an electrical component controls the entire electromechanical system through a PC. The necessary measurements are obtained through various tools. For sleep therapy, the Prisma 25ST and Prisma VENT50 devices (Löwenstein Medical Technology) are utilized. Measuring airflow involves the use of the PF300 and CITREX H4 flow analyzer (IMT Analytics AG). Simulating lungs is carried out with the Active Servo Lung (ASL 5000) (Ing-Mar Medical). The valve utilized is a Gate valve (10 bar, 1 inch) [4]. The electrical component, responsible for controlling the entire system, was designed with an Arduino Uno board, stepper motors, motor driver, heat sink, CNC shield (a board that provides the Arduino microcontroller with the necessary power to operate stepper motors), limit switches for calibration, a 12 V power supply, cables, timing belt pulley, and a timing belt. The results of measurements were evaluated using various software programs, including Flowlab, Somnomat, Matlab, Python, ASL software, and LMT's proprietary software. The software code was created using Arduino IDE. The design process was carried out using CAD software, such as Fusion 360.

- **Determination of the valve characteristic diagram**

To determine the valve's performance, measurements of flow rates and pressure were conducted at varying opening angles. The initial measurement was taken at an opening angle of 0° (when the valve is fully open). At each angle, four readings were taken with motor speeds ranging from 10,000 RPM to 40,000 RPM. The speed was set on the sleep therapy device and the flow values were captured and saved using PF300. It should be noted that the valve still has the ability to open beyond the 360° angle. One full rotation of the valve handwheel ranges from 0° to 360°, while a second turn ranges from 360° to 810° degrees, and so forth. Table 1 shows the different opening levels of the valve depending on the opening angle and Figure 1 shows the experimental setup.

Level	1	2	3	4	5
Angle	0°	90°	180°	270°	360°

6	7	8	9	10	11
450°	540°	630°	720°	810°	900°

12	13	14	15	16	17
990°	1080°	1170°	1260°	1350°	1440°

18	19	20	21	22	23
1530°	1620°	1710°	1800°	1890°	1980°

24	25	26	27	28	29
2070°	2100°	2115°	2130°	2160°	2250°

30
2280°

Table 1: the different opening levels of the valve depending on the opening angle.

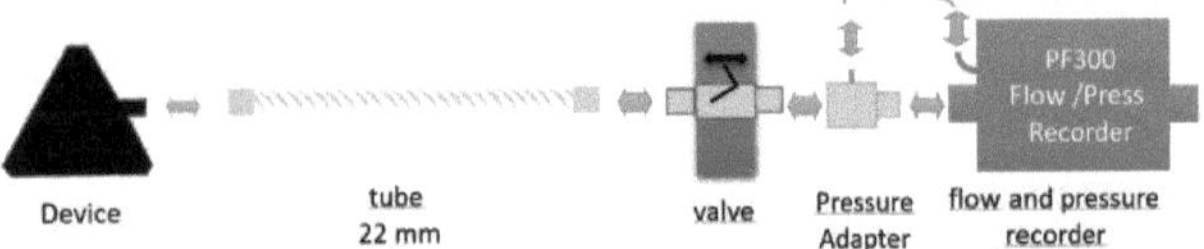

Figure 1: Test setup for measuring the pressure and flow of the valve at different opening levels.

Following the measurements, the results were analyzed to determine the resistances at different pressures and flows. The two different flow models, laminar and turbulent flow, were considered. In laminar flow, the streamlines flow parallel to each other resulting in low resistance. In contrast, in turbulent flow, the air particles move randomly in all directions and collide with many other particles, leading to high resistance. In this paper, the turbulent flow model was utilized and described as follows [5]:

$$R = \frac{\Delta P_{diff}}{\dot{V}_l^2} \tag{1}$$

with:
R: Resistance in $(mbar \times min)/l$
ΔP_{diff}: Pressure difference in air gas in $mbar$
$\dot{V}_l$: the resulting air flow in l/min

The resistances were calculated using Matlab functions and the valve's characteristic map was then generated and plotted using Matlab.
After measuring the valve to be developed, two already developed valve models were measured for comparison.

One is the obstruction valve and the other is the leakage valve. The measurement and evaluation of the two models was carried out in the same way as the measurement and evaluation of the valve to be developed.

- **Valve Testing for Apnoea Detection Using Forced Oscillation Technique (FOT)**

Further measurements on the valve to be developed will focus on detecting central and obstructive apneas. The forced oscillation technique (FOT) will be used for this purpose. The respiratory system will be stimulated by an external pressure signal of high frequency and the reaction of the system will be measured [6]. In the case of obstructive apnoea or hypopnoea, the signal will indicate the obstruction. If the event is caused by a central cause, the oscillation in the respiratory system will continue and then subside [6]. Figure 2 shows the experimental setup:

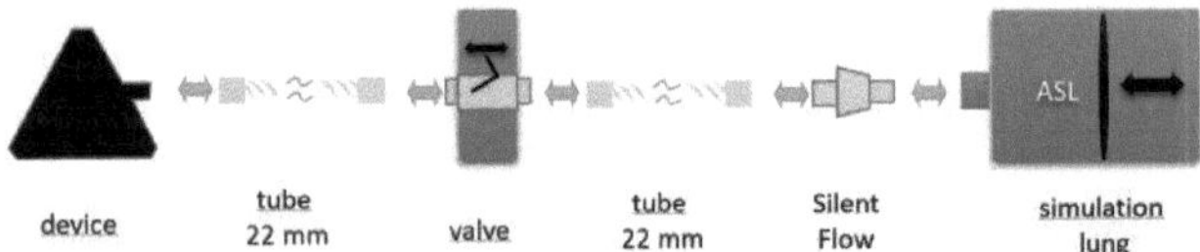

Figure 2: Test setup to check the detection of obstructive and central apnea.

ASL is operated with an expiratory and inspiratory muscle pressure of 16 cmH_2O, a tracheal resistance of 5 $cmH_2O/L/s$, and a compliance of 50 cL/cmH_2O. The prism 25ST is set to 10 hPA. The silent flow is used to prevent rebreathing of the CO_2 exhaled by the patient through the mask. The central apnea detection test is performed as follows after the parameters have been set.

(1) Turning on the ASL and Prism 25ST and waiting for 4-5 minutes.

(2) Setting the expiratory and inspiratory muscle pressures of the ASL to zero, waiting for 20 seconds, and ensuring no more breaths are taken.

(3) Setting the expiratory and inspiratory muscle pressures of the ASL to 16 cmH_2O and waiting for 1-2 minutes.

(4) Turning off the Prism 25ST and stopping the simulation of the ASL. The data stored on the SD card can then be evaluated using the SomnoMat.

To detect obstructive apnoea, the procedure is similar in steps 1 and 4, but steps 2 and 3 change:

(2) Slowly fully close the valve and wait for 20 seconds without turning off the sleep therapy device.

(3) Open the valve completcly again and wait for 1 minute.

- **Initiating the Control System**

After identifying the properties of the valve, the next step was to create a control system that would automatically adjust the valve's opening degree using a stepper motor. The electrical components used for this purpose are shown in

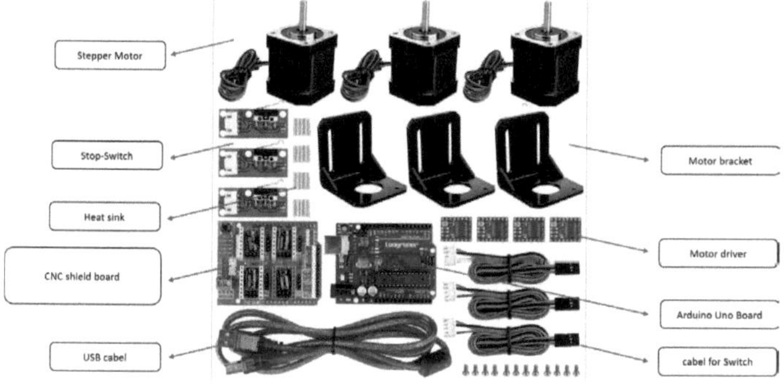

Figure 3: The electrical hardware components

Figure 3.

The CNC expansion board is simply plugged into the Arduino Uno. It requires an additional power supply between 12 V and 36 V. After connecting the motor drivers and stepper motors, the board is ready for use. The Arduino Uno board is connected to the PC via a USB cable and the CNC shield is connected to a mains power supply. The motors can be controlled either through the GRBL software (which doesn't actually stand for anything in particular) or directly through the Arduino library. GRBL is open-source software that can convert G-code into control commands for the CNC output stages. In this work, Instead of using GRBL, a custom script has been written that uses the Arduino library and the AccelStepper library to control the motors. The script also includes functions for clear communication between the user and device, device safety, position setting, API compatibility, and more. The limit switch in the system serves as a safeguard against overloading by preventing the motor from exceeding its limit of movement. It is incorporated into the calibration process and used to define and identify the starting and ending position, as well as the current position of the motor. During calibration, the motor is first positioned at a specific location and then travels until it reaches the limit switch. This marks the zero position or starting point. Next, the motor moves backward until it touches the limit switch again, which determines the end position and the number of possible steps. Once the start and end positions are stored, the motor returns to the zero position and waits for user commands. Before executing a command, the specified value is checked to ensure it falls within the defined range. The system can receive and carry out various instructions from the user, such as moving to a specific position or recalibrating. The commands for moving to positions consist of two letters and a number, where the letters represent the valve and the number indicates the target position. An example command would be "LX 100," where "LX" is the designated valve and "100" is the desired position to be reached. The corresponding flow and resistance for a certain degree of opening or a certain position can be determined from the existing measurement data. This should also be realized in the programming script. There are two possible approaches to this. On the one hand, a linear interpolation method can be used and the lookup tables implemented in the software. This method uses straight-line approximations to estimate the values between two known points and is relatively simple and straightforward. The conversion between flow, resistance, and position can be calculated with a function. On the other hand, the regression-based fitting function method can be used. This method tries to find an appropriate fitting function by finding the best fit between the data points. This approach allows for a more accurate representation of the relationship between the different variables and results in a more precise and reliable outcome. In this work, the regression-based fitting function method was used as it was found to produce more accurate results.

- **Construction and Design of the Valve System Prototype and Installation of a flow sensor**

The valve system was created after finalizing the software. The housing was designed on Fusion 360 and printed on a Flashforge Creator Pro 3D printer. The components were assembled, including toothed belts and pulleys linking the motor, valve, and limit switch. The system was improved with the addition of a flow sensor from Sensirion (model SFM3000-200-C), known for quick measurement speed and high precision. This allows the user to accurately set the desired flow value.

- **Automatic Re-Measurement and Testing of the Valve**

After assembling the entire valve system, automatic measurements were taken on the valve to check the flow values and evaluate its dependence on temperature. The system was operated over a longer period of time and with different commands.

3 Results and Discussion

The valve characteristic diagram refers to the graphical representation of the relationship between the valve's position and the resulting flow, pressure, and resistance. This diagram is used to understand the behavior of the valve system and can be used to predict its performance under different operating conditions. Figure 4 is a 3D representation of the Charasterstic of the valve and describes the relationship between pressure and flow rate and degree of opening. The valve system has 26 distinct opening levels for every 90 degrees of rotation. The flow range that can be achieved is dependent on the motor speed selected on the sleep therapy device. The flow range and opening level of a valve system vary with the motor speed. At a motor speed of 10,000 RPM, the flow range is 0 - 25.3 L/min, with an opening level of 26. With an increase in motor speed to 20,000 RPM, the flow range increases to 0 - 68.2 L/min, while the opening level remains at 26. At 30,000 RPM, the flow range further increases to 0 - 112.9 L/min, with the same opening level of 26. Finally, at a motor speed of 40,000 RPM, the flow range reaches a maximum of 0 - 157.8 L/min, while the opening level remains unchanged at 26. The valve passed the FOT test with the valve fully closed and open with the ASL lung simulator well. The valve can simulate both obstructive and central events well.The test results were evaluated with Somnomat. It measures the degree of airway obstruction,

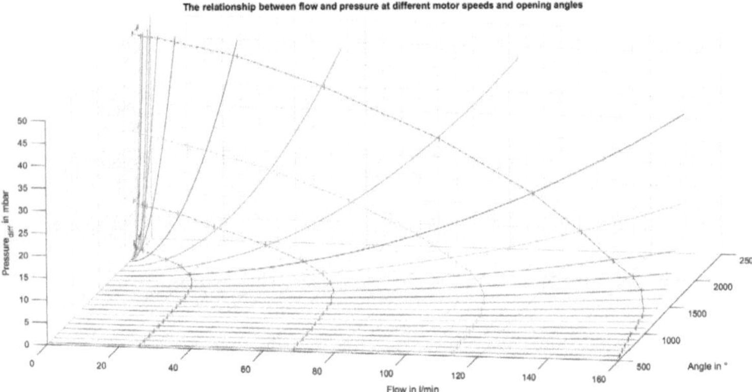

Figure 4: 3D representation of the properties of the valve

ranging from 0 to 100%. Central apnea shows 0% obstruction as expiratory and inspiratory pressures are 0. Obstructive apnea, however, has 100% obstruction with 0 pressures. The software functions have been tested and produced positive results. The system receives and executes commands easily and calibrates automatically when connected to the power source. With a deviation of 1.3% (equivalent to 0-2 l/min) from the table values, the system easily converts between position, flow, and resistance values. The deviation is likely caused by the fitting function, inaccuracies of the flow analyzer, and the valve's low hysteresis. The system is monitored by a flow sensor and controller to maintain the desired flow value and can adjust in 2-3 seconds. The valve system is temperature-insensitive and can be set to exact position, flow, and pressure. The valve system model is shown in Figure 5. It's compact, sturdy, and portable. The valve system can be connected to other devices via tubes on both sides. With this, the valve can now be utilized for future studies and trials. 5.

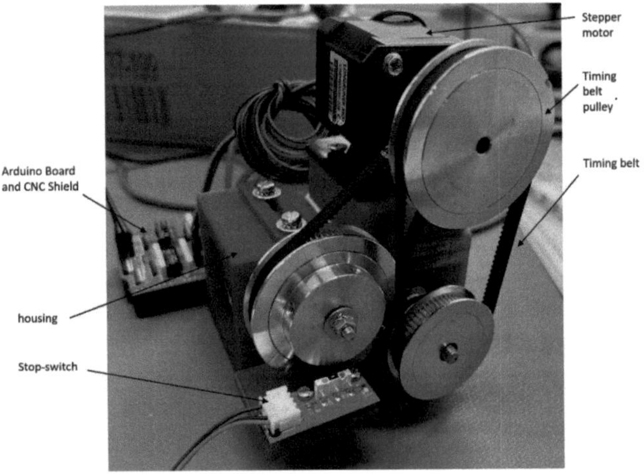

Figure 5: The designed prototype of the valve system

4   Conclusion

The development of sleep therapy devices is a cutting-edge field with numerous challenges. This project aimed to design a prototype valve system for realistic ventilation man-

agement between a lung simulator and a sleep therapy device. The results have shown that the developed valve system offers numerous advantages compared to other valves previously developed at Löwenstein Medical Technology for testing and measurements. The developed valve has a higher resolution and a larger opening range, allowing for precise simulation of obstructive and central apneas. Additionally, it is not temperature dependent, unlike the leakage valve. The valve system's versatility is also a major advantage, as it can be set to specific parameters such as flow rate, position, or resistance, and the built-in flow sensor can monitor and regulate the flow value accordingly. The software of the valve system is compatible with other commands and software of other valves and takes into account system safety and calibration requirements. The precise adjustment of the opening angle by the control system leads to a very accurate achievement of the desired flow rate. In addition, the valve system is sufficiently stable and mobile and can be produced at a low cost.

In summary, the developed valve system has proven to be a reliable and effective solution for realistic ventilation management between lung simulator and sleep therapy and offers several advantages over other existing systems.

Acknowledgement

The work was carried out at Löwenstein Medical Technology, Department of Advanced Development in Karlsruhe, and supervised by Dr. Prof. Stefan Müller, Department of Biomedical Engineering, Lübeck University of Applied Sciences.

Author's Statement

Conflict of interest: Authors state no conflict of interest.

5   References

[1] Teschler, H.; Stampa, J.; Ragette, R.; Konietzko, N.; Berthon-Jones, M., *Effect of mouth leak on effectiveness of nasal bilevel venti-latory assistance and sleep architecture.*, Eur. Respir. J., 1999.

[2] T. Young and P. E. Peppard and D. J. Gottlieb, *Epidemiology of Obstructive Sleep Apnea: a Population Health Perspective.* Band 165(9), American Journal of Respiratory and Critical Care Medicine, 2002.

[3] B. J. Gersh and V. K. Somers and A. S. Shamsuzzaman, *Obstructive Sleep Apnea: Implications for Cardiac and Vascular Disease.* Band 290(14), Jama, 2003.

[4] MCM System, *Gate Valve 10 bar.* Available: https://bit.ly/3YoNawW [last accessed on 2023-01-18].

[5] O., Wolfgang, *Atmen – Atemhilfen.* Georg Thieme Verlag, 2008.

[6] Reisch S, Daniuk J, Steltner H, Rühle KH, Timmer J, Guttmann J., *Detection of sleep apnea with the forced oscillation technique compared to three standard polysomnographic signals..* PubMed, 2000.

TIVA Versus Volatile Anaesthetics
- What Will the Future of Anaesthesia Look Like?

Silja Janßen [1] and Arne Blohm [2]

[1] Medical Engineering Science, Universität zu Lübeck, silja.janssen@student.uni-luebeck.de
[2] Drägerwerk AG & Co. KGaA, Lübeck, arne.blohm@draeger.com

Abstract

Surgical procedures generally require anaesthetic measures to ensure pain relief, unconsciousness and, if desired, relaxation of certain muscles. Anaesthetic substances are mainly either administered intravenously or added to the ventilation air. These two methods differ drastically not just in their application and medical effect, but also in their impact on the environment: volatile anaesthetics, the drugs used for inhalation anaesthesia, are infamous for their high global warming potential. This drawback has promoted the total intravenous anaesthesia (TIVA) using propofol over the last few years. Differences between oral and intravenous anaesthesia concern medical, environmental, practical, and financial aspects. A comparison of these aspects, based on literary research, enables an estimation for the future use of both methods and shows that while intravenous anaesthesia has surpassed the inhalational alternative for several reasons, its use is still stigmatised.

1 Introduction

German doctors conduct approximately 17 million surgical procedures each year [1], which generally require anaesthetic measures to ensure that the patient does not feel pain. The three aspects pain relief, loss of consciousness and muscle relaxation can together be considered the pillars of general anaesthesia.

The anaesthetic substances are mainly applied either intravenously or through inhalation. Volatile anaesthetics, such as sevoflurane, desflurane or isoflurane, can be added to the ventilation air and pass into the respiratory system of the patient. The most popular substance sevoflurane is used in approximately 55 % of all inhalational cases, desflurane in 35 % and isoflurane in 15 % [2]. Total intravenous anaesthesia (TIVA) on the other hand is performed with a direct injection of profopol or another substance into the patient's bloodstream. The largest medical benefit of propofol is its euphoric effect, while volatile anaesthetics have a high global warming potential. These aspects have increased the popularity of TIVA over the past years. In many cases the anaesthesia is initiated with one method and continued with another. Local or regional anaesthesia present alternatives which focus on pain alleviation and do not target the patient's consciousness. While they have gained popularity as well, they will not be mentioned further in this paper. The two main methods for general anaesthesia, TIVA and inhalational anaesthesia, will be compared in the following, leading to an estimate on the necessity of both in the future of medicine.

2 Material and Methods

This work is based on extensive literary research on the topic of intravenous and inhalational anaesthesia. The book "Die Anästhesiologie" [3] provided an overview on the application and medical effect of each method and anaesthetic drug, which was then complemented by several papers covering environmental and financial aspects. There is an abundance of papers especially on the negative impact of volatile anaesthetics on the environment, most of which are based upon the research of M. P. Sulbaek Andersen and colleagues [4, 5]. This complicates the evaluation of the environmental aspect. On the other hand, financial comparisons are difficult firstly due to the difference in purchase prices of machines and drugs from one hospital to the next, especially if a global comparison is desired, and secondly due to a lack of transparency. Thus, this paper focuses on the general cost of substances, devices and infrastructure and the efficiency of each method.

The lack of scientific data, comparisons and overall recommendations leads to an uncertainty for doctors. Studies show that many decisions between intravenous and inhalational anaesthesia are thus based on personal experiences and opinions [6, 7]. This finding was further confirmed in a two-day clinical observation and discussions with local anaesthesists.

2.1 General Anaesthesia

There are two methods to achieve a general anaesthesia: intarvenous or inhalational. For the inhalational method, volatile anaesthetics are used. The three most commonly used substances are desflurane, sevoflurane and isoflurane, which are stored in a vaporiser in their liquid state and vaporised upon leaving the container, originating the term *volatile*. The medical gases are then conducted into the ventilation circuit and enter the patient's respiratory system. They start to have a noticeable effect once they have diffused from the alveoli into the bloodstream after a few minutes. The effect is mostly hypnotic, meaning that inhalational anaesthesia generally requires an additional intravenous access to enable the administration of analgetic and of emergency drugs. Volatile anaesthetics are barely metabolised and instead exhaled unchanged [3]. Another substance used for inhalational anaesthesia is nitrous oxide, which has a relatively high analgetic effect, but it is considered obsolete and almost exclusively used in dentistry and in obstetrics nowadays [3]. The most ideal inhalational anaesthetic is xenon, but its high cost reduces the usage to nearly zero [3].

The most common drug for intravenous anaesthesia is propofol, a substance which promoted the use of TIVA over the last decade due to its positive effects. The drug is injected directly into the patient's bloodstream and shows a hypnotic effect after a few minutes. After a while, it will diffuse into the fatty tissue and musculature, until it is slowly metabolised and eliminated from the patient's body [3]. Additional substances are needed to ensure an adequate analgesia and, if desired, muscle relaxation. TIVA does not require airway access and can be used for light sedations as well, in which case the patient will be present enough to breathe on their own and muscle relaxants are not required. The exact medical effects will be described in the following section.

3 Results and Discussion

3.1 Medical application

Propofol is favoured by many anaesthesists because its hypnotic effect is accompanied by mood enhancement, meaning that patients are content and calm after waking up from anaesthesia [3]. The drawback is that propofol has a risk of addiction and substance abuse [3]. Another risk is propofol infusion syndrome (PRIS), which is characterised by haemodynamic instability, bradycardia, hypotony and respiratory depression, and prohibits a prolonged application of the substance [3]. A more mundane issue is that the intravenous access and the injection of propofol may be frightening, especially for children, as well as painful.

Volatile anaesthetics such as desflurane, sevoflurane and isoflurane have a hypnotic effect during inhalational anaesthesia, with the downside that patients often feel nauseous after waking up. This is described as Postoperative Nausea and Vomiting (PONV) [3]. Volatile anaesthetics are contraindicated if a patient is at risk of malignant hyperthermia, a genetic disease which may lead to a fatal overheating of the body, and caution is also required for patients with a hepatic dysfunction [3]. On the other hand, volatile anaes-

thetics do not act as strongly upon the respiratory and the cardiac system as propofol does, and for this reason they may be especially favoured for vulnerable patients, such as the elderly, or those with respiratory diseases like asthma or COPD [3]. A final advantage is that volatile anaesthetics are exhaled by the patient and the expiration concentration can be measured to estimate the depth of anaesthesia, which is not feasible for TIVA [3]. The disadvantage of this aspect is that all exhaled gases need to be captured in order to minimise the impact of inhalational anaesthetics on the environment. Modern systems are able to achieve this to a high degree and thus prevent clinical staff from side effects. In conclusion, there are nearly no contraindications for a TIVA with propofol, but in some cases an inhalational anaesthesia with volatile anaesthetics may be preferable, such as for vulnerabe or anxious patients. An anaesthesia induction with one method and maintenance with another may work best to ensure the patient's well-being.

3.2 Environmental impact

The major issue with the use of volatile anaesthetics is their impact on the environment. While they are captured by modern scavenging systems to a high degree, some portion of the substance may always escape into the surrounding air and reveal its impact there. Volatile anaesthetics have a high global warming potential (GWP), which can be calculated from their mean lifetime in the atmosphere and from infrared absorption. The calculation of the GWP of a substance x for a 100 year time horizon follows equation (1)

$$GWP_x(100) = \frac{\int_0^{100} F_x exp(-t/\tau_x)dt}{0.676} \qquad (1)$$

where F_x is the radiative forcing and τ_x the response time of the decay curve. The result is divided by the absolute GWP of CO_2, which is 0.676, to provide a more illustrative result [4]. The most commonly cited values are from M. P. Sulbaek Anderson and colleagues and are shown in table 1.

Table 1: Estimated lifetime and 100-year global warming potential (GWP) for inhalational anaesthetics [4, 5, 8].

Substance	Lifetime /years	GWP_{100}
Sevoflurane	1	130
Isoflurane	3 - 6	510
Desflurane	10 - 20	2,540
Nitrous oxide	114	300

Of all modern volatile anaesthetics, desflurane has the highest global warming potential of 2,540, meaning that its impact is 2,540 times as high as the impact of carbon dioxide [4, 5]. This value can be illustrated by a comparison to the environmental impact of a car drive: a 6-hour inhalational anaesthesia with desflurane has approximately the same global warming potential as driving a car for several thousand kilometres [9]. The impact can be reduced by several measures, such as capturing exhaled substances, leading them back into the anaesthetic system and minimising drug expenditure. The modern ventilation systems installed in most clinics are able to practise these measures, but the issue is still prevalent in developing countries.

Nitrous oxide has become obsolete in modern clinical practice not only due to its global warming potential, but also because it is considered an ozone-depleting substance. During its dwell time in the atmosphere it destroys the ozone layer and thus accelerates global warming [8]. The relatively low hypnotic effect renders it inferior to volatile anaesthetics such as sevoflurane, desflurane and isoflurane. The high global warming potential argues against the use of desflurane though, so that only sevoflurane and isoflurane should be considered substances for inhalational anaesthesia.

The TIVA with propofol is not entirely harmless either. It is often associated with high amounts of waste, such as empty ampules, syringes and dressing materials. However, an intravenous access is necessary to enable emergency medication for inhalational as well as for intravenous anaesthesia, so that the amount of waste varies only slightly. In addition, propofol itself may have a toxic impact on the environment when it is not disposed of properly, but there is little research on this subject.

In summary, a TIVA with propofol is to be favoured under the assumption that all waste is minimised and handled responsibly. Inhalational anaesthesia should only be considered with sevoflurane and isoflurane, while desflurane and nitrous oxide are to be avoided. These recommendations ensure a minimal environmental impact.

3.3   Cost and efficiency

Medical and environmental aspects aside, the decision between intravenous and inhalational anaesthesia is often also based on financial reasons. The most inexpensive and simple way to achieve general anaesthesia would be a TIVA with a syringe of propofol. Inhalational anaesthesia requires a few more devices, such as the mechanical ventilator, gas scavenging system and vaporiser unit. These are generally considered standard equipment in modern hospitals, making inhalational anaesthesia an affordable option. A TIVA becomes more expensive when a syringe pump is used instead of a manual syringe, which enables a constant or a model-based automatic administration of propofol or other drugs. The drawback of such a model-based application, apart from its initial cost, is that existing models are not very well-developed and only applicable to standard patients. The most common one was developed by T. W. Schnider in 1998 based on a mere 24 adult patients [10]. In 2014, D. J. Eleveld proposed a model which took 600 patients into account [11], but it is not prevalent. It can be expected that the models for automatic propofol administration will be advanced in the coming years though.

However, TIVA can be considered the less expensive method due to one aspect, which is that patients generally awaken in a better condition and recover more quickly from an intravenous anaesthesia than from an inhalational one [3]. Occupancy and labour in the anaesthetic recovery room are reduced, which in turn minimises costs. In conclusion, this aspect makes TIVA the more affordable option, but specific financial decisions depend on the requirements and premises of each hospital [12].

The efficiency of TIVA and inhalational anaesthesia can be compared further. Inhalational anaesthesia can be considered the easier method, requiring only the ventilator, a vaporiser and a ventilation mask or tube for secure airway access. Drug flow from the vaporiser is controlled by a manual wheel, making it very easy to operate. The administered drug concentration and measured exhalation concentration can be viewed and documented automatically.

Intravenous anaesthesia requires some more effort: after the intravenous access is managed, syringes need to be filled, labeled and kept ready. Syringe pumps are able to operate automatically once the inserted drug and desired concentration are specified, but the intravenous drug concentration can not be measured and the patient and vital parameters need to be observed thoroughly. Manual drug administration is prone to errors and requires additional attention.

While intravenous and inhalational anaesthesia are hard to differentiate from the financial point of view, inhalational anaesthesia can be considered easier to operate. This is countered by the better recovery for TIVA patients, making both methods efficient in their own way.

4   Conclusion

Intravenous and inhalational anaesthesia differ greatly in their effect on the human body and on the environment. This complicates the decision between both methods for any anaesthesist.

A TIVA with propofol is contraindicated if intravenous access is impossible or the patient may react allergic to the drug; an inhalational anaesthesia with volatile anaesthetics is contraindicated if the patient can not be intubated or has a history of malignant hyperthermia. Inhalational anaesthesia may be more beneficial for patients with cardiac or respiratory diseases, and an inhalational induction is favourable for children and other patients who are too frightened to allow for an intravenous access. However, for most patients, TIVA may result in a better clinical outcome and higher satisfaction due to the euphoric effect of propofol.

Another argument in favour of TIVA is the environmental impact, which has been brought to attention especially over the past few years. One measure to reduce the impact is the avoidance of desflurane and nitrous oxide. Inhalational anaesthesia should only be considered with sevoflurane or isoflurane and with a scavenging system for exhaled gases. But while TIVA with propofol is the recommended method with regard to the environment, it requires the reduction of disposable materials and proper waste management to minimise possible toxic effects.

In conclusion, TIVA with propofol should be the preferred method of anaesthesia in many cases. However, this does not coincide with actual clinical practice. It seems that anaesthesists often decide for one or the other method based on a personal preference. Several global studies exist on the

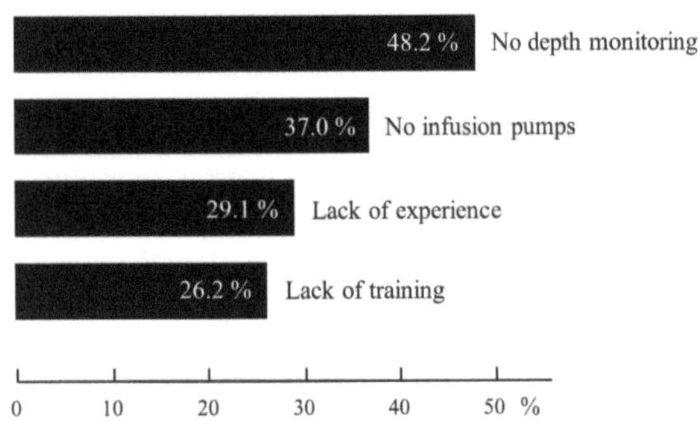

Figure 1: Main limitations for the use of TIVA, as found by a Columbian study [7]

topic of those decisions and mostly identify obstacles that restrict the use of TIVA [6, 7]. Some obstacles are illustrated in figure 1. In summary, one main obstacle is the lack of training or education, another the lack of equipment such as automatic or manual syringe pumps. A distinction must be made here between the clinical standard in more and in less developed countries. Another obstacle associated with TIVA is the uncertainty of anaesthesia depth, since the intravenous drug concentration can not be measured. TIVA further has a reputation for being more complicated to prepare and conduct. While inhalational anaesthesia only requires the turning of a wheel, the preparation of propofol syringes and pumps takes more time.

Many problems may be evaded in the coming years with technological advancement, both for intravenous and for inhalational anaesthesia. Example areas include gas scavenging systems, drug concentration measurement, automated application and anaesthesia depth monitoring. At the same time, synthetic drugs themselves are constantly being refined. This enables ideal anaesthesia for each patient, be it intravenous or inhalational.

Acknowledgement

The work has been carried out at Drägerwerk AG & Co. KGaA, Lübeck and supervised by Philipp Rostalski from the Institute for Electrical Engineering in Medicine, Universität zu Lübeck.

An additional mention goes to Marco Monnig, who has supported this work with his extensive medical knowledge and other resources.

Author's Statement

Conflict of interest: Authors state no conflict of interest.

5   References

[1] Statista, *Operationen und Behandlungsmaßnahmen in deutschen Krankenhäusern bis 2021*. Available: https://de.statista.com/statistik/daten/studie/76889/umfrage/operationen-und-behandlungsmassnahmen-in-deutschen-krankenhaeusern [last accessed on 2023-01-16].

[2] Umweltbundesamt, *CLIMATE CHANGE 17/2015: Implementierung der ab dem Berichtsjahr 2013 gültigen IPCC Guidelines for National Greenhouse Gas Inventories 2006 in die Inventarerhebung fluorierter Treibhausgase (HFKW, FKW, SF6, NF3)*. 2015.

[3] R. Roissant, C. Werner and B. Zwißler, *Die Anästhesiologie*, 4th edition. Springer, 2019.

[4] M. P. Sulbaek Andersen, *Inhalation anaesthetics and climate change*. British Journal Of Anaesthesia, vol. 105, no. 6, 2010.

[5] M. P. Sulbaek Andersen, *Atmospheric Chemistry of Isoflurane, Desflurane and Sevoflurane: Kinetics and Mechanisms of Reactions with Chlorine Atoms and OH Radicals and Global Warming*. The Journal of Physical Chemistry A, vol. 116, no. 24, 2012.

[6] G. T. C. Wong, S. W. Choi, D. H. Tran, H. Kulkarni and M. Irwin, *An international survey evaluating factors influencing the use of total intravenous anaesthesia*. Anaesthesia and Intensive Care, vol. 46, no. 3, 2018.

[7] P. C. Echeverry-Marín, J. Arévalo, P. Pinzón, A. Vanegas-Saavedra and M. Leguizamón, *Use of total intravenous anaesthesia in Colombia: A national survey among active anaesthetists in Colombia*. Colombian Journal of Anesthesiology, vol. 45, no. 2, 2017.

[8] S. Varughese and R. Ahmed, *Environmental and Occupational Considerations of Anesthesia: A Narrative Review and Update*. Anaesthesia & Analgesia, vol. 133, no. 4, 2021.

[9] M. Schuster, H. Richter, S. Pecher, S. Koch and M. Coburn, *Positionspapier mit konkreten Handlungsempfehlungen der DGAI und des BDA: Ökologische Nachhaltigkeit in der Anästhesiologie und Intensivmedizin*. Anästhesiologie & Intensivmedizin, vol. 61, 2020.

[10] T. W. Schnider, *The Influence of Method of Administration and Covariates on the Pharmacokinetics of Propofol in Adult Volunteers*. Anesthesiology, vol. 88, 1998.

[11] D. J. Eleveld, *„A General Purpose Pharmacokinetic Model for Propofol*. International Society for Anaesthetic Pharmacology, vol. 118, no. 6, 2014.

[12] T. Kampmeier, *Cost-Effectiveness of Propofol (Diprivan) Versus Inhalational Anesthetics to Maintain General Anesthesia in Noncardiac Surgery in the United States*. Value Health, vol. 24, no. 7, 2021.

Implementation and validation of a navigation framework for monkey testing of an anesthesia workstation

Tjorven Bahns [1], Stephan Eisenbrand [2] and Dennis Kleinewalter [3]

[1] Biomedical Engineering, Luebeck University of Applied Sciences, tjorven.svea.bahns@stud.th-luebeck.de
[2] Drägerwerk AG & Co. KGaA, Lübeck, stephan.eisenbrand@draeger.com
[3] Drägerwerk AG & Co. KGaA, Lübeck, dennis.kleinewalter@draeger.com

Abstract

Monkey testing is a form of automated testing, randomly interacting with the User Interface (UI) of a device, trying to produce errors. This method requires many interactions to provide a result, making time-efficient navigation on the device critical. This paper aims to modify the navigation on the UI of an anesthesia workstation to use a previously developed utility instead of the slower, already existing protocol, in order to save time for touch interactions and thus for navigation. In order to achieve this goal methods were implemented using a utility for touches and navigation. Afterwards the methods were compared to the currently used one. It was found that using the utility for navigation is about 3,03% to 6,49% faster than without the utility.

1 Introduction

Quality is a development aspect that cannot be compromised on, especially for medical devices that people entrust their lives to. Therefore it is vital that tests can be run as efficiently as possible to ensure this high quality while keeping development times reasonable. For increasingly complex devices automated testing can improve the time needed to execute repeated tests and assure the quality of the device throughout its development. One form of tests used to explore complex User Interfaces (UIs) in all possible states are monkey tests. These monkey tests interact randomly - like a monkey would - with the UI and try to provoke errors. However, it can take many interactions to find such errors. Therefore, a method that improves the time one of these interactions takes can save a lot of time and therefore resources.

The goal of this work was to implement a method used for navigation on the device under test using a utility developed within Dräger. The hypothesis is that this method will perform faster navigation than the currently implemented one. In this paper firstly the basic knowledge needed will be introduced. Then the implementation of the new navigation method and tests used to compare the methods will be explained. Lastly the results will be presented and the hypothesis will be reviewed.

2 Material and Methods

In this section first the needed background knowledge about the development environment shall be given so that the problem of integrating a test utility into an existing framework can be understood and the chosen solution will be explained in the subsequent subsection.

2.1 Automated testing with dumb and smart monkeys

The core principles of agile software development suggest to reach a working state for the developed product as soon as possible and then to continue improving upon this during the development process [1]. As such this software has to be tested continuously. Previously manual testing was utilized as extensive tests were only needed once at the end of the process. The continuous improvement introduced by agile development makes automated testing much more valuable as means to reduce the time of a test cycle [2].
One method established for automated UI testing is the monkey testing method. This subsection will introduce this method and a method derived from this.

The infinite monkey theorem states that if you give an infinite number of monkeys typewriters they will write any book in the libraries of the world [3]. This theorem is believed to be the origin of the term monkey testing [4]. In our case a monkey clicking on the User Interface of a device will eventually, given enough time, find a bug in the UI. There are two general classifications of monkeys in monkey testing as described in [5]: Dumb and smart monkeys. Dumb monkeys have no previous knowledge of the system under test (SUT) and do not know which inputs will lead to an effective interaction. Smart monkeys on the other hand possess a certain knowledge of the system under test. Accordingly a monkey was developed at Dräger which will generate random inputs for the Graphical User Interface of an anesthesia device. Originally this was constructed as a dumb monkey producing random x- and y-coordinates to be touched. As this method is inefficient, producing many non-effective inputs, a smart monkey was developed in a next step:

This smart monkey can utilize the framework used for testing the devices at Dräger. As such it has knowledge of the system states and the objects available to it for interaction. Furthermore, this monkey can use the methods provided by the framework to navigate on the UI and execute touches. For these navigations and touches the framework uses a relatively slow protocol that tends to get slower under load. A possible solution to be tested by this paper is to bypass the protocol with a test utility. This utility was developed at Dräger to perform direct interactions with the SUT. While it was originally designed as a hardware utility it is now available as a software utility, increasing its availability for many devices at once. Due to this increased availability it becomes feasible to use the utility even for slight performance improvements. Such an improvement is anticipated when using the utility to navigate compared to the existing protocol.

The next chapter will explain how usage of this utility was integrated into the framework in order to maintain the system knowledge provided by the framework and gain the speed from the utility.

2.2   Integration of the utility

The goal of this paper is to make the utility accessible via the internal Dräger testing framework. This will allow the usage of the system knowledge provided by the framework in combination with the speed provided by the utility. The main task lies with changing the existing functions for touching and navigation so they use the utility instead of the framework protocol.

The function for touching an object is easily implemented as it only needs to call the navigation, find the corresponding x- and y- coordinates on the UI and then send these coordinates to the utility to touch. The x- and y-coordinates needed are determined by taking the center coordinates of the area the button occupies.

In order to test the general functionality firstly a basic navigation function was developed. This function does not consider whether the system is in the correct system state or if the object is in a selectable state. It will purely check if the given object is visible and if not call itself with the objects navigational parent as the parameter. Next it will determine the object middle's x- and y-coordinates and pass them to the utiltiy to touch. This recursion will then lead to the correct path to the object being taken and eventually the original given object will be touched, provided all objects along the path where in a selectable state.

After confirming that this basic navigation works and indeed provides an improvement of the navigation speed

the advanced navigation was implemented. This advanced navigation provides the same functionality as the navigation function already existing in the framework with the added speed provided by the utility. As the following description of the function will show the advantages compared to the basic navigation lie mainly within its consideration of the current system state, checking of the state of the selected button and verification that the selected button changed states after touching it while it comes with the downside of taking longer.

The advanced navigation will first check if navigation is suppressed by another function. If not it will check if the device is in the correct system state and change if necessary. It will then check if the object is visible and if not try to select its navigation parent. The selection function will first call navigation to the navigation parent, again leading to recursion until a button in the chain is visible. If the button is visible it will then check the state the button is in. The function will take different actions according to the buttons state, ensuring that it is properly selected if possible. After pressing the button it waits for the state of the button to change. This new state will lastly be used to verify that the button now actually is in a selected state.

With these functions implemented they could now be tested as described in the following subsection.

2.3   Testing of the integration

After implementing the functions for navigation and touching using the utility these could now be tested and compared to the currently used touch-method which utilizes the framework-internal protocol. This was done in small, increasingly more complex tests so should time losses occur it could be determined where they most likely stem from.

In a first step only the touch functions themselves where compared. To accomplish this the test navigates to a set menu in the UI via the framework protocol and touches a single button repeatedly. In this case a button in the main therapy settings category was touched 30 times with the utility-based and protocol-based methods and the average time needed per touch (after the initial navigation) measured.

In the next step the navigation functions were compared. For this the test will now use the existing protocol-based as well as the basic and advanced utility-based navigation methods to repeatedly navigate to a set button. In this case the test will navigate to a button which is several interactions away from the start screen 30 times, each time starting on the default start screen. Afterwards the average time needed per navigation will be calculated.

The last test simulates the intended use-case and can give us an estimate on the actual time that can be saved using the utility compared to the existing interface. This test will choose a given number of buttons randomly from the standby-screens available on the device under test. Then these buttons will be navigated to, one after the other, using at first the protocol-based navigation- and touch- functions, then the basic utility-based functions and lastly the advanced utility-based functions, each time starting fresh from the default start screen. Afterwards the total time needed to navigate to all given objects by each method is read out. This test was repeated 3 times with 10, 20 and 50 objects each in order to see if runtime affects the different methods differently.

3 Results and Discussion

In this section the results of the tests described in 2.3 will be presented and discussed.

First the plain touch functions were tested by repeatedly touching the same object. The results can be seen in Table 1:

Table 1: Touch speed by each method

Method	time per touch [s]
Internal protocol	0,799
Utility	0,469

From this data it is clear that the test utility needs only 59% of the time that the internal protocol needs for each touch. This already is promising for those test scenarios that do not need much navigation, for example when many interactions need to be performed in the same sub-menu. As in most cases each navigation touches multiple times this also promises a good improvement of the time needed for navigation.

To see exactly how much time can be saved for an actual navigation command the different navigation functions were tested in the next step. This is done by navigating to a set object multiple times, starting from the standby screen. The results can be seen in Table 2:

Table 2: Navigation speed to the chosen button by each method

Method	time per navigation [s]
Internal protocol	8,453
Utility (basic)	2,732
Utility (advanced)	8,115

From Table 2 it can be seen that the drastic advantage the utility has for each touch does translate to a slight advantage per navigation procedure. While the touches took the utility-based method only 59% of the time the protocol-based method did the actual navigation to the chosen object took 96% of the time. More acutely it can be seen that the basic utility-based navigation has a drastic advantage compared to the methods using the advanced navigation. It took only 32% of the time the protocol-based method did and only 34% of the advanced utility-based method. The advanced methods check for

many factors such as the system state and the original button state and wait for at least one state change to occur for each touch. These added functionalities make the advanced functions more reliable but seem to cause a more significant time delay than what can be gained by using the utility. However, it can still be seen that the utility-based function pulls ahead of the protocol-based function for a single navigation, if only slightly. As for the usage in a monkey test it is to assume that during one test many more navigations will be performed and if each navigation saves 0,3 seconds overall a noticable improvement of the time needed per test can be achieved.

This was investigated in a further test which more closely resembles a monkey test. For this test a list of a given number of random objects available in the standby screen of the device under test is navigated to, one after the other. As can be seen in table 3 this was done three times for each number of objects and method:

Table 3: Total runtime for navigation to a set list of objects by each method

	Number of objects touched	Time needed by method [s]		
		Internal protocol	Utility (basic)	Utility (advanced)
Run 1	10 Obj.	47,77	19,38	43,20
	20 Obj.	99,88	39,58	95,11
	50 Obj.	218,14	94,32	209,61
Run 2	10 Obj.	45,51	18,72	42,17
	20 Obj.	95,42	39,79	89,80
	50 Obj.	235,36	96,83	230,92
Run 3	10 Obj.	45,17	17,89	44,16
	20 Obj.	93,29	36,84	93,77
	50 Obj.	218,17	86,98	210,58
Average time per navigation	10 Obj.	4,62	1,87	4,32
	20 Obj.	4,81	1,94	4,64
	50 Obj.	4,48	1,85	4,34

To make the results more comparable the data was plotted to a boxplot as seen in Fig. 1:

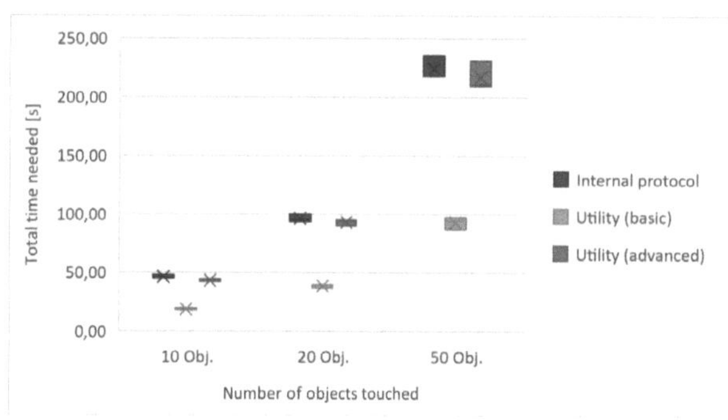

Figure 1: Total runtime for navigation to a set list of objects by each method

The data in Table 3 and Fig. 1 reinforce the findings from the navigation test. While the utility-based method is consistently faster than the protocol-based method for the same list of given objects the most evident time-improvement lies in the basic navigation method. During the test however it was not controlled if each of the objects given was successfully navigated to as this would have cost additional time, possibly distorting the measurements. In some cases a menu opened by a previous navigation might overlap with a needed button. In the check for visibility that all methods perform the needed button would still register as visible because technically the device is on the correct screen for pressing that button. When the x- and y-coordinates are then given for touching that button the touch would possibly happen in an ineffective or wrongly effective area, resulting in no or a false action. This would then result in the program continuing as if the correct navigational parent has been pressed, not further confirming that the navigational child is now actually visible and continuing with further non- or wrongly effective touches. In a similar manner the basic navigation does not check if a button is in a selectable state or needs confirmation, all things that could result in no errors but no correct navigation either.

As can be seen by the average time per navigation in Table 3 there does not seem to be a proportional trend of runtime dependent on the number of objects touched for any of the methods. One thing of note however is that the 20-object average is consistently higher for every method compared to the 10- and 50-object averages. As a new list objects to be touched was generated for each run and each object count one possible explanation of this behavior is that the lists given for the 20-object runs contained on average more objects in succession that are more navigational steps away from the previous one, causing more runs of the recursive methods and thus taking longer on average per navigation.

Still, the utility-based navigation method does in fact increase the speed of navigation. Per single navigation the amount saved ranges from 0,14 to 0,3 seconds with this resulting in a maximum of 8,53 seconds saved in total for the list of 50 objects in Run 1. This translates to the utility-based method being 3,03% to 6,49% faster than the currently used protocol-based navigation.

4 Conclusion

In conclusion it can be said that the goal of this paper of implementing navigation with the utility was achieved. Furthermore, it was proven that the utility-based method for navigation is consistently faster than the protocol-based method. While the time gain does not appear that significant for a single navigation it can add up for the many objects typically touched in automated tests such as monkey tests. As the methods for touching and navigation implemented for this work can be utilized without trouble in further tests this set-up is recommended at least for those devices and tests that likely will perform many navigation operations. While testing for this work no immediate disadvantages of the methods using the utility compared to the established methods were observed. However, introducing an additional utility into the test also opens up another possible point for failure, making error identification more complex.

Future work could involve optimizing more advanced navigation functions. While the significant advantage the basic navigation has compared to the advanced methods can be likely attributed to the checks and waiting times it could possibly be interesting to investigate where specifically the most losses occur and if some checks can be left out if certain conditions are met. If a monkey gets a list of possible objects which are all available in the "operation" state for example, the method does not need to check if it is in the correct system state for every navigation.

Another advantage of the utility compared to the framework-utilized interface is that it performs independent of the load of the SUT. Therefore it might be interesting to perform similar tests as in this work but with the device being under load.

The next steps possible based on this work are the implementation of the navigation and touch methods in an existing monkey and similar tests that could benefit from faster interactions.

Acknowledgement

The work has been carried out at Drägerwerk AG & Co. KGaA, Lübeck and supervised by Professor Stefan Müller, Department of Applied Natural Sciences, Lübeck University of Applied Sciences.

Author's Statement

Conflict of interest: Authors state no conflict of interest.

5 References

[1] M. Glück, *Agile Innovation - Mit neuem Schwung zum Erfolg.* Springer Vieweg, Aalen, pp. 72–74, 2022.

[2] A. Axelrod, *Complete Guide to Test Automation: Techniques, Practices, and Patterns for Building and Maintaining Effective Software Projects.* Apress, Matan, pp. 4–13, 2018.

[3] J. Anderson, *A million monkeys and Shakespeare.* In: Significance, 8, Wiley, Hoboken, pp. 190–192, 2011

[4] C. Haase, *Androids - The Team that Built the Android Operating System.* No Starch Press, San Francisco, p. 95, 2022

[5] B. Hofer, B. Peischl and F. Wotawa, *GUI savvy end-to-end testing with smart monkeys.* In: 2009 ICSE Workshop on Automation of Software Test, Vancouver,2009, pp. 130–137

Evaluation of the temporal response of a lung simulator to a step in FiO$_2$

Salsabeel Alsamna [1], Oliver Garbrecht [2] and Hendrik Fischer [3]

[1] Medical Engineering Science, Universität zu Lübeck, salsabeel.alsamna@student.uni-luebeck.de

[2] Drägerwerk AG & Co. KGaA, Lübeck, Oliver.Garbrecht@draeger.de

[3] Drägerwerk AG & Co. KGaA, Lübeck, Hendrik.Fischer@draeger.de

Abstract

Purpose: The aim of this work is to evaluate the temporal response of the delivery of the required inspiratory oxygen concentration (FiO$_2$) using the ASL Lung simulator as a test device for ventilators at different tidal volumes (VT), e.g., at a small tidal volume (50 ml and 100 ml) compared to a large tidal volume (300 ml and 550 ml). **Methods**: First, an ASL lung simulator was used to evaluate oxygen concentration with a portable gas meter to continuously monitor the concentration FiO$_2$. It measured how the ASL test medium reacts after being flooded with air, i.e. 21% FiO$_2$, and then connected to the ventilator with 100% FiO$_2$. This corresponds to a jump from 21% to 100%. Second, it was investigated whether VT played a role. **Results**: It was observed that there were large differences in the rate of attainment of desired oxygen levels based on tidal volumes in ventilators tested using the ASL and oxygen meter. A problem with low VT was identified and solutions were sought. The first solution could be that a longer test period should be carried out. Flushing the ASL before testing could be a second solution. The third solution could be to reduce the residual ASL volume. **Conclusions**: This study shows that it is possible to improve ASL FiO$_2$ testing at small tidal volumes in the ventilation with the required oxygen levels so that they can be tested more quickly. The best solution is a combination of the first and second solutions. Since an implementation of a flush would be useful for short time and a long test to be sure.

1 Introduction

Breathing is one of the most important processes in human life. Especially in the intensive care unit (ICU), ventilation is an extremely common practice. Because the functional and structural buffering phase occurs after <3 min when O$_2$ supply is interrupted (e.g., during a myocardial infarction), initial brain tissue damage usually occurs after 3 to 5 min, more severe brain damage may occur after 6 to 8 min, and brain death usually occurs after 8 to 10 min [1]. Respiration enriches the blood with oxygen, which is then transported throughout the body by the heart. It is provided to patients with the goal of alleviating respiratory impairment caused by injury or disease by replacing or supporting the functions of natural breathing. Mechanical ventilation is also a core component of medical therapy for various clinical conditions and is used to assist or replace spontaneous breathing when it is inadequate or absent, such as in acute and chronic patients or neonates. Today, it is one of the most modern, technologically advanced and remarkable forms of medicine [10].

The oxygen concentration of a modern ventilator ICU can be adjusted within limits from 21% to 100% of the gas mixture. In diseases with a severe chronic oxygen deficiency, the quality of life and survival time can be improved by long-term, daily oxygen supplementation for several hours or even by inhaling 100% oxygen [3]. Breathing pure oxygen or oxygen-rich air for several hours can cause problems by poisoning the lungs or, if the antioxidant systems are depleted, by oxygen poisoning the central nervous system [3].

To determine the oxygen concentration of a gas more accurately, different measurement methods are used depending on the concentration range to be detected and the accompanying substances. Measuring oxygen does not just depend on the oxygen meter. All components of the system must work perfectly to provide reliable results. Figure 1 shows a problem with oxygen measurement. The problem is more severe with small lungs because the O$_2$ and air valves in a ventilator are not 100% tight, then some gas flow will pass through the membrane even though they are closed. But this would not be a problem in a large lung. For example, if the flow of the oxygen valve is closed, so $\dot{V}_{O_2} = 0$, then it will only pass through the air valve and then FiO$_2$ would be equal to 21%, or for example $\dot{V}_{O_2} = \dot{V}_{Air}$, FiO$_2$ is about with 61,5%. However, because the valve is not tight, the values of FiO$_2$ will be more than 21% or more than 61,5%. Therefore, it is important to measure FiO$_2$ [9].

Another problem is due to the large residual capacity of the ASL of about 2.5 liters, which is a product of the company IngMar Medical [4]. This occurs when the ASL is filled with at FiO$_2$ with small tidal volumes. In comparison, the large VT does not require the same time course. Therefore, it was necessary to measure how long it takes to reach the required FiO_2.

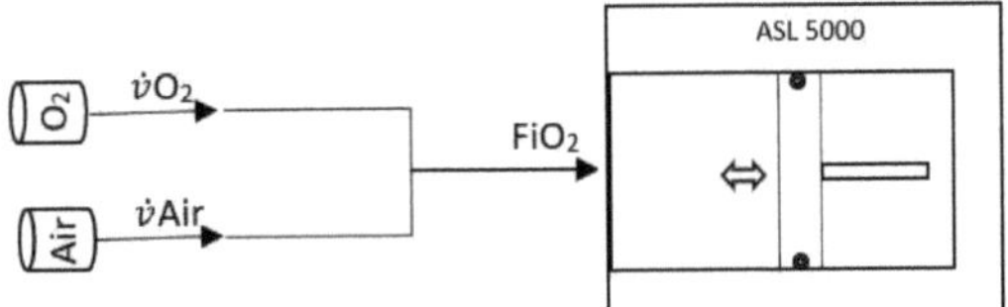

Figure 1: Problem with oxygen measurement. The O_2 and air valves in a ventilator are not 100% tight, then some gas flow will pass through the membrane even though they are closed.

2 Material and Methods

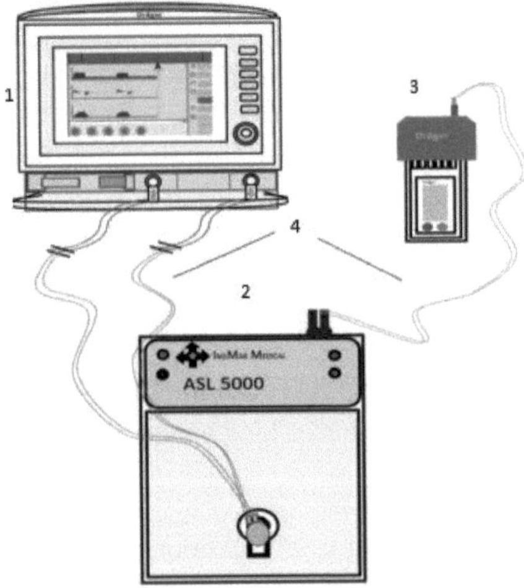

Figure 2: The setup includes the following: 1. Savina 300 respirator, 2. ASL 5000, 3. Dräger X-am 5000 multi-gas detector with DrägerSensor® XXS O_2 100 , 4. Patient hose system and tube to O_2-measurement.

The Savina 300 ventilator, designed for adult and pediatric patients, offers mandatory ventilation modes and ventilation modes to support spontaneous breathing, as well as airway monitoring. As shown in Figures 2 and 3, a system of tubes is used to connect the Savina 300 ventilator to the ASL 5000 testing device. A small tube connects the ASL with the Dräger X-am 5000 Portable gas detector, which reliably measures combustible gases and vapors, as well as oxygen and harmful concentrations of toxic gases, organic vapors, odorant and amines.

Various Dräger-developed sensors, which are characterized by reliability and short response times, can be connected to the gas detector. The DrägerSensor® XXS O_2 100 with X-am detector is used here. The measuring principle of the sensor is based on the measurement of the partial pressure of oxygen; therefore, it is suitable for oxygen monitoring in inert processes and the measuring range is 0-100% vol [5]. The sensitivity of the DrägerSensor® XXS $O_2$100 with the X-am detector is ± 1% of the measured value [8].

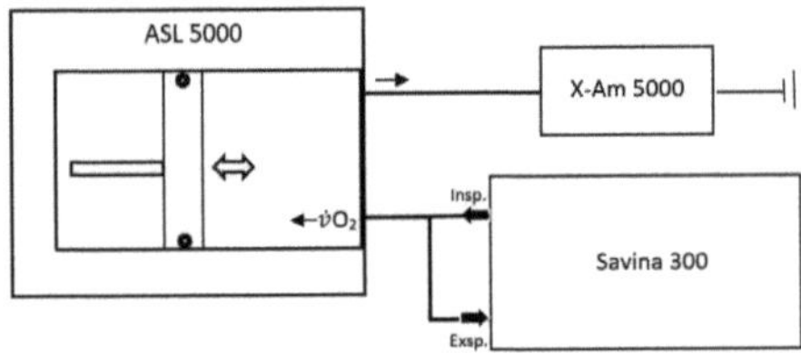

Figure 3: A hose system is used to connect the Savina 300 ventilation system to the Test equipment ASL 5000. Through a small tube is also connected ASL with X-am Portable gas detector.

The ASL 5000 stands for Active Servo Lung. It is a lung simulator for high quality ventilation management training in respiratory, pulmonary, critical care, anesthesia and emergency medicine and can be connected to any ventilator - just like a real patient. The simulators are used for training and continuing education in ventilation management [4]. The ASL 5000 can simulate a lung in both passive and active state. Both an adult and a neonatal lung can be selected, as well as whether the lung should behave like a healthy or a diseased lung [6]. In the experiment, the lungs were simulated in the active state. The type of patient is set to normal neonate. To adjust the different lungs, the lung parameters Compliance (C), which describes the volume-pressure relationship, i.e. the expandability of the lung, and Resistance (R), which on the other hand describes the pressure-flow relationship, i.e. the flow resistance, should be set. In this case, C = 10 ml/mbar and R= 30 mbar/l/sec [7].

A lung simulator consists of at least one resistive element, e.g. a tube, and an elastic element, e.g. a balloon. Mathematically, this is described by the so-called equation of motion, namely as a function of time. It is important to define the functional residual capacity of the lung as a function of and compliance settings and the resulting expected tidal volume. These settings are important for transient times of oxygen. The functional residual capacity is the volume of gas remaining in the lungs after expiration. It therefore also affects the residual oxygen concentration in the lungs [6].

Besides the FiO_2, the most important settings on the ventilator are also the respiratory rate (RR) in breaths per minute and the positive end-expiratory pressure (PEEP) the lower pressure level. Volume-controlled ventilation (VC-Ac) is set as the ventilation mode, which is the most commonly used form of ventilation in emergency care and the operating room [2]. In this mode, the same tidal volume is delivered at a preset constant flow with each mechanical breath "regardless of the inspiratory pressures generated by improving lung compliance" to achieve the set tidal volume (VT). Accurately determining the VT delivered to a patient's lungs is critical during mechanical ventilation of neonates and infants. Given the small VT used in ventilating infants and young children, small inaccuracies in VT determination can result in significant adverse conditions. By setting a specific tidal volume, it is delivered at a constant flow. In the experiment, the jump in FiO_2 from 21% to 100% is monitored with different tidal volumes VT= 50 ml,

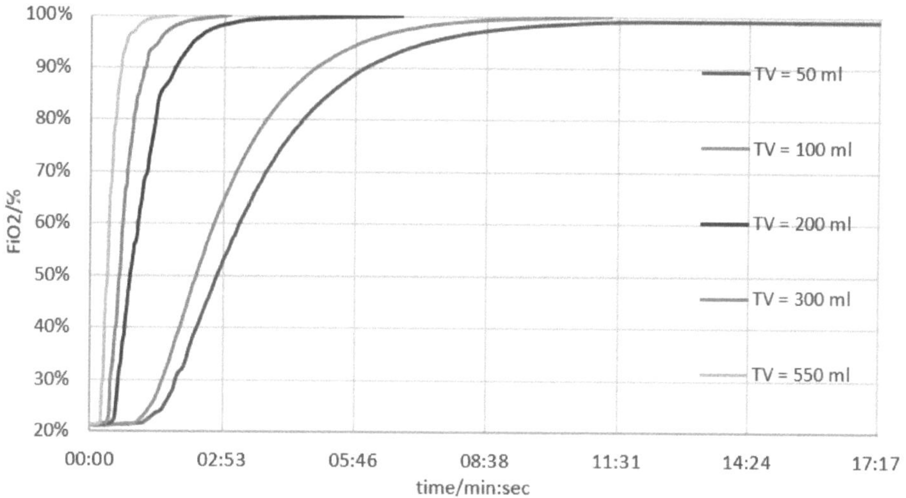

Figure 4: Response to a jump in FiO_2 from 21% to 100%, the graph represents the proportions of the oxygen readings (FiO_2) in percent and time in (min:sec). As can be seen, depending on the volume, it is needed more or less time to reach 100% O_2. At first glance, it is noticeable that the first two curves with the largest tidal volumes (300 ml and 550 ml) between 111 s and 180 s reached the 100% O_2. In contrast, the increase in FiO_2 with the small tidal volumes (50 ml and 100 ml) is very slow, ranging between 679 s and 1509 s to reach 100%.

100 ml, 200 ml, 300 ml and 550 ml during the performance of the experiment. In addition, the respiratory rate (RR) can be set to 12 breaths/min and the inspiration time (TI) to 2 s. The evaluation of the oxygen measurement data recorded by means of the X-am gas detector with an initial FiO_2 of 21% was carried out continuously up to 100% with the DrägerSensor® XXS O_2 100 by reading in the measured value files, further processing and evaluating them after the settings had been made and the information for the test had been defined and selected. Finally, the processed measurement results were displayed graphically and compared with each other.

3   Results

In Figure 4, the graph shows the proportions of oxygen FiO_2 measurements in percent and time in (min:sec). It shows how the ASL test medium reacts to the lung (in principle, the ASL test medium) after initially being flooded with air, i.e. 21% FiO_2, and then being connected to the ventilator at 100% FiO_2. This shows a jump from 21% to 100%. As can be seen, depending on the volume, it will take a greater or lesser amount of time for 100% O_2 to be reached. At first glance, it is noticeable that the first two curves with the largest tidal volumes (300 ml and 550 ml) between 111 s and 180 s have reached the 100% O_2. In contrast, the increase in FiO_2 with the small tidal volumes (50 ml and 100 ml) is very slow, ranging from between 679 s and 1509 s to reach 100%.

4   Discussion

The main finding of this work is that it took time to reach 100% O_2 depending on the volume (ASL and X-am not vol-ume dependent). This leads to the fact that it is possible that a problem with the test agent ASL is particularly affected by small tidal volumes. Since a small volume takes more time to reach 100% O_2. This means that the behavior of the test device does not match what is being tested.

The following is a description of how the scenario runs to understand more. The volume of the ASL is very large 2.5 L initially filled with 21%. However, it is to be filled with 100% O_2 with a small tidal volume, e.g. 50 ml in the ASL. This would take longer than a large tidal volume, e.g. 550 ml, what as can be seen above. But this is problematic and a solution needs to be found. The first solution could be that long testing is carried out. Second Solution could be that the ASL is flushed prior to the test. Flushing simply means that before a test starts, some breathing envelope with a large lung volume is performed at 100%. In Figure 4 it can be seen that a large lung needed about 1 min and 50 sec, which means it will not take long and a fast signal will arrive. Then it could be set with a small tidal volume. It will remain at 100% of O_2, which means that the goal has been reached. The third solution could be to reduce the ASL residual volume. The best solution is a combination of the first and second solutions. Since an implementation of a flush would be useful for short time and a long test to be sure.

But here is a problem for the solution. The scenario is that the ASL test device is flooded with 90%. It is connected to a ventilator that is supposed to deliver 90% FiO_2. But the ventilator is delivering 80% FiO_2. This means that the device has an error of 10% deviation. Therefore, the time then had to be measured in order to see the deviation at all. The graph in Figure 5 shows the ratio of the oxygen values (FiO_2) and the time, if now the oxygen is reduced from 90% to 80%. In the diagram 5 shows that at 550 ml, less than 1 minute had to be tested for it to be sure that the values had changed at all. In comparison, at 50 ml, over 7 minutes

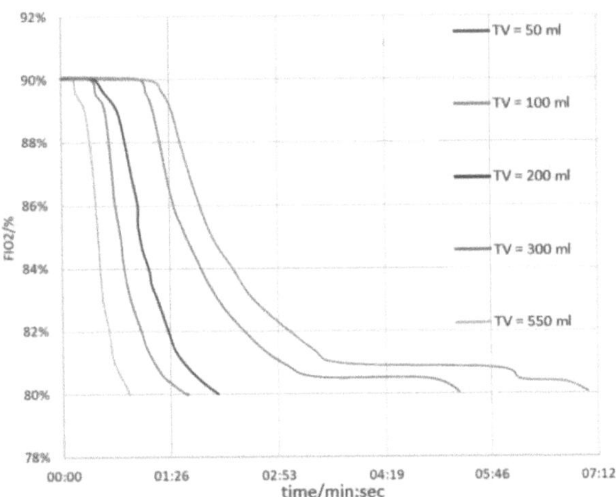

Figure 5: Falling from 90% to 80%, the graph shows the ratio of the oxygen values (FiO_2) and the time when the oxygen is reduced from 90% to 80%. It can be seen that the first two curves with the largest tidal volumes (300 ml and 550 ml) take between 53 s and 99 s to reach 80% of O_2. On the other hand, for the small tidal volumes (50 ml and 100 ml), FiO_2 is very slow and the time required to reach from 90% to 80% of oxygen is between 314 s and 429 s.

would have to be tested for a very long time to even say how much the deviation is. That is the problem with this part. But this is still better than Figure 4, where the wait time for 50 ml would be over 20 minutes. I.e. this is a good method.

Figure 4 shows that it sometimes takes too long to get from 99% FiO_2 to 100% FiO_2, which is not expected. This could be a mistake, one reason for this would be the sensitivity of the DrägerSensor® XXS O_2 100 in X-am, which is ± 1% of the measured value (100% - sensor accuracy%). Measurement error can also occur due to leakage in the connection between the oxygen meter and the ASL, so that not all of the measured inspiratory oxygen concentration FiO_2 reaches the ASL. Leakage may also occur in the connection between the ventilator and the ASL, so that not all of the measured inspiratory flow reaches the ASL. The solution for this leakage could be the use of a hose clamp, but that was not very helpful in this experiment.

5 Conclusion

The ASL was tested as a test device, during volume-controlled ventilation with an oxygen meter. In both neonates and adults, there are large differences in the rate at which desired oxygen levels are achieved as a function of the tidal volume set. Researchers should be aware of these differences, especially when ASLs are used for volume-controlled ventilation with small tidal volumes, which tend to take longer. However, the ASL tested at a small tidal volume with the desired oxygen levels has improved and can be tested more quickly, e.g., by flushing the ASL.

Acknowledgement

The work has been carried out at Dräger, Lübeck in the Advanced Engineering Solution department of the Corporate Technology and Innovation and supervised by the Institute Institute for Electrical Engineering in Medicine, Universität zu Lübeck.

Author's Statement

Conflict of interest: Authors state no conflict of interest. Salsabeel Alsamna designed the protocol, performed the bench testing of the devices, analyzed the collected data, and drafted the manuscript. Dr. Oliver Garbrecht conceived the protocol, realized the evaluation of the devices on the bench test and analyzed the collected data. Dr. Hendrik Fischer contributed to the design of the protocol and analyzed the collected data.

6 References

[1] Prof. Dr.-Ing. Dr. med. Karsten Hiltawsky, University of Lübeck *(2019)*. Beatmung, Physiology of Respiration, © Drägerwerk AG Co. KGaA.

[2] Larsen, R., Ziegenfuß, T. Mathes, A. *(2018)*. Beatmung, Indikationen – Techniken – Krankheitsbilder (6. Aufl.). Springer Berlin Heidelberg.

[3] Bergdohle *(22.12.2022)*. Sauerstoff. Chemie. Available: https://www.chemie.de/lexikon/Sauerstoff.html

[4] (2016). User's Manual ASL 5000, SW. © 2017 IngMar Medical, Ltd. | 11-20. Available: https://www.ingmarmed.com/product/asl-5000-breathing-simulator/

[5] (01.06.2022). *DrägerSensor®- Gasmessgeräte-Handbuch.* © 2022 Dräger Safety AG Co..

[6] (19.10.2016). *ASL 5000 Lungen-Simulator, Laerdal Medical. Laerdal. Link.* Available: https://laerdal.com/de/products/tech/simulation-technology/ASL5000LungSolution/.

[7] Jahnke, Dirk. *Atmung/Beatmung- Resistance und Compliance.* Available: atmungbeatmung.de.

[8] Sensoren, Gebrauchsanweisungen/Datenblätter der verwendeten. Available: Dräger X-am®. www.draeger.com/ifu.

[9] Powers, Kyle A. Dhamoon, Amit S. *(28.01.2022)*. Physiology, Pulmonary Ventilation and Perfusion - StatPearls - NCBI Bookshelf. NCBI. Available: https://www.ncbi.nlm.nih.gov/books/NBK539907/

[10] Pham, T., Brochard, L. J., Slutsky, A. S. *(2017)*. Mechanical Ventilation: State of the Art. Mayo Clinic proceedings, 92(9), 1382–1400. https://doi.org/10.1016/j.mayocp.2017.05.004

Future of Quantum Computing in Healthcare

Sharvari Juvekar [1], and Stefan Müller [2]

[1] Medical Microtechnology, Technische Hochschule Lübeck, sharvari.sanjay.juvekar@stud.th-luebeck.de

[2] Department of Applied Sciences, Technische Hochschule Lübeck, stefan.mueller@th-luebeck.de

Abstract

The research paper deals with the understanding of quantum computing and goes into the depths of application in different fields. The application of quantum computing in the healthcare field is very vast and explained in detail. All the different developments in quantum computing are still not easily available in the market due to the limitations present and the research done to overcome them. The future scope of quantum is very high and can be explored through years to come.

1 Introduction

Quantum computing is a process of computing that uses the fundamentals of quantum theory to analyse a given problem. The theory of quantum mechanics explains the nature and interactions of energy and matter at the quantum (atomic and subatomic) levels. The potential of quantum computing was first recognized in the 1980s but has yet to be realized completely [1]. Quantum computing is the technology of the future and many companies like IBM, Google Quantum AI, Microsoft, and many more have started to implement quantum computers in different applications because of the benefits [10]. All over the world, understanding the Quantum field is still considered paradoxical. The idea of writing this paper was initiated during the internship at Siemens Healthineers AG while understanding different imaging modalities offered by the company like ultrasound, computed tomography (CT), Magnetic Resonance Imaging (MRI), Radiography systems and others. When one of the leading companies in the healthcare sector already got a CT Scanner in the market which uses the fundamentals of quantum mechanics for working, which is the NAEOTOM Alpha (Name of the device) [2]. It created a question then what other marvels will quantum technology possess for the benefit of mankind? This leads to the main aim of the paper is to present the future health technologies involving quantum which would be available say in the next two decades. There is no resource which can state at what rate is the quantum going to develop in the near future. According to a report published in October 2021 by Global Market Insights, a global market research and management consulting company the quantum computing market is expected to grow from USD (United States Dollar) 500 million in 2020 up to USD 28 billion and more by 2028, growing at over 30% CAGR (Compound Annual Growth Rate) from 2021 to 2028. Figure 1 represents the quantum computing market [10].

The paper starts with a brief understanding of quantum, and

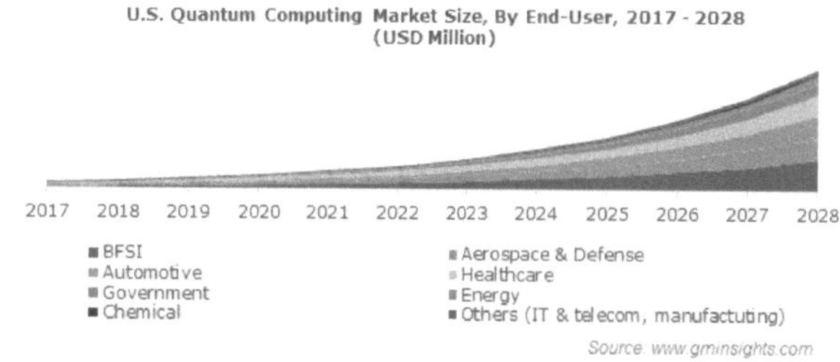

Figure 1: Quantum Computing market growth (Yellow denotes the healthcare market)[10].

its application in different fields and finally focuses on the applications for healthcare. For most of the paper "quantum" word has been used as an abbreviation for "quantum computing" unless specified explicitly, for example, a word like "quantum mechanics". Figure 2 represents the basic differences between classical computing and quantum computing.

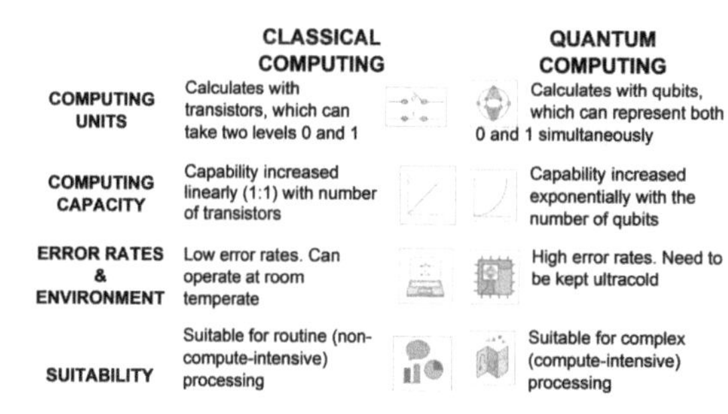

Figure 2: Differences between Classical and Quantum Computing [3].

1.1 Qubit

Quantum computers use a basic unit similar to that of Classical computers known as a qubit (quantum bit), it can be present in two states '0' and '1' or a superposition of the two states. The behaviour of qubits is analogous to that of spinning electrons in an atom around the nucleus. This behaviour creates the fundamental properties of quantum: quantum superposition, quantum entanglement and quantum interference [3]. Qubits are vulnerable entities that can even be damaged by relatively insignificant occurrences involving stray electromagnetic waves, vibrations, changes in temperature, and perhaps cosmic rays.[4].

2 Method

The research paper was written more in the form of a literature review. This is done by going through different research papers and white papers available on the topic. Quantum is one of the recent research fields and there are not many experiments which have already taken place for the application of quantum in healthcare and that is the reason why most of the applications are hypotheses which would come true in future. This research paper mainly presents research fields for healthcare where quantum can be applied in future and these were researched and brainstormed during the internship period. The applications mentioned further are the hypothesis thought and the ones applied in the non-healthcare field are ideations presented by different scientists around the world.

3 Application in the Non-Healthcare Field

Quantum was ideated in different fields like the automotive industry, finance and banking, logistics and others. There are various fields in which quantum computing can be used, explaining all would be out of the scope of this paper, hence some of the sectors worth mentioning are followed further.

3.1 Artificial Intelligence

Artificial Intelligence (AI) has already proven to be a great asset to humankind in different ways, AI models work based on algorithms generated from different datasets available. Researchers use the large datasets available to train the AI models. The integration of AI and quantum has already created a field known as quantum AI [5]. The greater storage capacity provided by the quantum can train AI models in a shorter time and make the whole process faster and more efficient. Quantum has proven to create more efficient machine learning algorithms which are more accurate and tend to have lesser computational time [8].

3.2 Manufacturing and Industrial Design

Manufacturing will benefit from quantum computing in several ways. It helps you optimize your supply chain, analyze software performance, improve cybersecurity, and more [3]. The other use cases for quantum computing include:

- Accelerate prototyping and design development with scenario planning.

- Solve supply chain problems by processing large variables in real-time.

- Improve value stream productivity by dramatically increasing data processing speed.

- Strengthen cybersecurity to reduce the risk of data breaches.

3.3 Agriculture

Numerous sustainability goals are already met by organic farming, and social rather than technological barriers to its widespread adoption now exist [9]. Using quantum concepts in agriculture technology increases input effectiveness and animal welfare while minimizing harmful environmental effects. The developments in this field are likely to have an impact sooner, and the research challenge is to develop new technologies based on wave principles and emerging new technologies in information technology [9]. The technology born out of the merging of different fields is called Quantum Based Agriculture (QBA). A few examples of the implementation of Quantum in Agriculture would come from Wright, Kieft and Diest who noted "QBA holds the potential to address specific challenges in the agricultural sector...existing innovation and technology projects in Europe are already underway although they have not yet been fully documented. These include the use of ultrasound to control blue-green algae (funded by the EU 7th Framework Programme), the use of music based on wine protein and played to vines with beneficial effects, the disinfection of potato and onion from bacteria through ultraviolet light, .., the application of low frequency electro magnetic fields on dairy cow to lower mastitis rates, and treating water with electromagnetic frequencies." [9]

4 Application in Healthcare Sector

Quantum computing will impact different sections of the healthcare sector. It will not only make the process faster and more accurate but also benefit in tackling different diseases which have been a burden to the world for ages. The advancements would not only benefit the patients but also the care providers at different stages of the patient journey.

4.1 Diagnostic Imaging

Quantum Imaging systems will assist in computing more accurate and precise images for the visualization of single molecules at a faster rate. Quantum provides the interpretation and cure of the data acquired through machine learning, while machine learning serves as a tool to identify discrepancies in the body. It is possible to identify the light and dark regions with conventional MRIs, but the radiologist has to interpret and analyze them. Diagnostics can be improved with quantum imaging not only by facilitating tissue classification but also by allowing more detailed analysis and interpretation [6].

4.2 In Silico Clinical Trials

In silico clinical trials refers to the development of patient-specific models to form virtual cohorts for testing the safety and/or efficacy of new drugs and of new medical devices. A virtual set of patients could complement a clinical trial (reducing the number of enrolled patients and improving statistical significance), and/or advise clinical decisions. Experiments are conducted in a completely simulated environment. Quantum can enable the development of virtual settings where experts can examine factors such as skin temperature, bodily fluids, electrolytes, hormones, and metabolism on digital copies of individuals [3].

4.3 Drug Design and Development

The comparison of molecules is the key step in the design and development of new medications. Institutions dealing with drug designing currently use traditional computers to perform millions of comparisons. There is a limitation towards the size of molecules that can be calculated by traditional computers. This can be overcome by the use of quantum as it can promote the comparison of large molecules. As a result, it will facilitate the development of more pharmacological advances and treatments for diverse illnesses. Quantum also makes it possible for medical professionals to model intricate molecular interactions at the atomic level. It will be important for developing new medicines and doing medical research. Therefore, experts will soon be able to recreate every one of the 20,000 human DNA proteins. Additionally, it will start modelling interactions with designs of both new and existing drugs [3].

4.4 Genomics

Genomics is one of the developing fields of biomedical research which deals with the study of an organism's fundamental genetic components. The study involves recombinant DNA, DNA sequencing techniques, and bioinformatics. It includes looking for particular biomarkers and mutations linked to diseases. In the future, quantum is the right approach. Additionally, the data will be more accurate, enabling more accurate diagnoses and customized treatments. A database of genomes will also be developed in future by the scientists to search for mutations and unidentified biomarkers. The use of quantum in genomics will also have an impact on therapy by taking environmental and lifestyle variables into account [6].

4.5 Health Data

Healthcare data is one important piece of information with regard to the security of a patient and it needs to be protected. The biggest threat is from hackers and this can be done by the implementation of quantum. "ID Quantique" is a company which uses the fundamentals of quantum physics to protect data. One of the most useful applications of quantum entanglement is quantum cryptography, which protects the data [6]. Quantum computing is expected to have a large storage capacity which can be linked to health data and provide more structured access to the data with more capacity.

4.6 Precision Medicine

Precision medicine is a relatively new technique developed with an aim to rethink the way we identify, cure and prevent disease. Over the past few years, it has also advanced exponentially, fostering the growth of person-centred medicine. This expansion has been fueled by a number of intricate causes. Some of the significant ones include technological advancements, an ageing population with a higher cancer incidence, a growing market, increased use of big data, and scientific understanding resulting from panomics [3][6]. There has been the implementation of quantum computing for precision medicine which is given in the following case study.

4.6.1 Case study:

The study was conducted on patients with knee osteoarthritis, this is because even though there are a lot of different therapies present in the market for the disease, the effect of the treatment varies from one patient to another. The study team used a Quantum Neural Network (QNN) program to facilitate precise, data-driven clinical judgments for advanced knee osteoarthritis therapy selection. The researchers used 113 patients treated over a 2-year period with a single injection of micro fragmented fat (MFAT) and categorized as responders and non-responders in pain and function at 1 year to train the QNN classifier. The team concluded that Quantum machine learning is a promising technology that has the potential to reduce computational complexity and enhance prognostic performance when applied to data-driven clinical decisions for the individualized treatment of advanced knee osteoarthritis, based on their initial findings from a short validation dataset. To confirm model effectiveness, safety, clinical importance, and significance at the level of public health, the results need to pass through more research validation using bigger, real-world unstructured datasets and clinical validation with an AI clinical trial [7].

5 Limitations

Quantum computing has a higher number of benefits in the healthcare sector. But to get access to these benefits it is important to overcome the limitations that are present in quantum computing. The limitations present make quantum in healthcare unreachable for at least a decade more. The limitations are many like lack of development of quantum algorithms, software and others but noise is one of the biggest limitations as explained further. Noise can be created by various interactions present. The following reasons are responsible for the noise created during the computation:

- Earth's magnetic field

- Local radiation

- Cosmic rays

- Neighbouring qubits

- Signal Control

The processor's isolation and quantum error correction can only overcome the noise. The error correction algorithms have been tested and developed by many companies and institutions, which brings the hope of stabilizing quantum computers.

6   Conclusion

Quantum computing would be a great boon to mankind in all sectors. For the healthcare sector, quantum can facilitate diagnostics by providing more precise measurements along with faster computation time and large storage space needed for the image data. Quantum would make the life of healthcare staff as well as the patient and their caregivers easier by making systems more accessible and precise. Quantum can create possibilities for finding cures to diseases which have been incurable for decades. These all possibilities create motivation for researchers working in the quantum field to develop it to the fullest in near future.

Acknowledgement

The work has been carried out at Siemens Healthineers Innovation Think Tank (ITT) and supervised by the Technische Hochschule Lübeck. I would like to complete the research paper by thanking everyone involved in the creation of the research paper. I would like to express my deepest appreciation towards my supervisors at ITT Prof. Sultan Haider and Mr Schroth Sebastian along with my supervisor at the university Prof. Stefan Müller for their continuous support without whom the paper would not be this big of a success. I am also thankful to Ms Silke Venker for her constant support during the process. I would be remiss in not mentioning all the colleagues of ITT for always contributing towards the paper with small inputs for research.

Author's Statement

The authors state no conflict of interest.

References

[1] Phillip. Kaye, R. Laflamme, and Michele. Mosca, "An introduction to quantum computing." Oxford University Press, 2007.

[2] E. Shanblatt, J. O'doherty, M. Petersilka, P. Wolber, G. Fung, and J. C. Ramirez-Giraldo, "NAEOTOM Alpha with Quantum Technology Whitepaper: The technology behind photon-counting CT How photon-counting works and the benefits it provides.",2022.

[3] R. Ur Rasool, H. Farooq Ahmad, W. Rafiq, and A. Qayyum, "Quantum Computing for Healthcare: A Review."2022.

[4] P. Kumar Sharma and M. Shahbaz Khan, "A Study on Quantum Computing." 2020.

[5] K. N. Sgarbas, "The Road to Quantum Artificial Intelligence," 2007.

[6] F. Flöther, J. Murphy, J. Murtha, and D. Sow, "Exploring quantum computing use cases for healthcare," 2020.

[7] S. Olgiati et al., "A quantum-enhanced precision medicine application to support data-driven clinical decisions for the personalized treatment of advanced knee osteoarthritis: development and preliminary All-internal bone transport View project IJMS special series View project A quantum-enhanced precision medicine application to support data-driven clinical decisions for the personalized treatment of advanced knee osteoarthritis: development and preliminary validation of precisionKNEE QNN,"2021.

[8] Zhang, Y, Ni, Q. Recent advances in quantum machine learning. Quantum Engineering. 2020; 2:e34. https://doi.org/10.1002/que2.34.

[9] Wright, J; Kieft, H. and von Diest, S., "Quantum-Based Agriculture: the Final Frontier." Innovative Research for Organic 3.0 - Volume 1: Proceedings of the Scientific Track at the Organic World Congress 2017, November 9-11 in Delhi India, 2017

[10] Quantum Computing Market Share 2021-2028 Growth Report, October 2020.

Bioprinting 3D anisotropic structures

Nasr M. Ghaleb
Biomedical Engineering, Luebeck University of Applied Sciences, nasr.ghaleb@stud.th-luebeck.de

Abstract

Anisotropic tissues have extraordinarily distinct structural characteristics and functions. Over the past decade, producing anisotropic tissues with mimetic architecture resembling natural tissue has been given a huge effort. Bioprinting is the one technique that has experienced a great concentration in research as a promising and novel strategy in tissue engineering which helps in tissue regeneration and organ replacement. To do so, it requires to create strucures that are mimicing the extracellular matrix and cellular patterns of the specific human tissue. This can be done through different scaffolding methods which can be brought to bioprinting. In this review paper, different types of anisotropic tissues structures are discussed as well as the different bioprinting techniques. In addition, the latest trends in fabrication of such hierarchical(anisotropic) structures through different techniques are introduced.

1 Introduction

There are many types of special structural features in human tissues, Anisotropic structures are one type with unique mechanical and biological functions where they control the growth behavior of cells and tissues regeneration. These structures originate from the extracellular matrix (ECM) or cellular anisotropy seen at different length scales [1]. For example, collagen-oriented fibril and fiber length scales exhibit nanometer- or micrometer-scale anisotropic structures, whereas cell-orientation-dependent structures such as brain and blood vessels skeletal muscle or cardiac and skeletal muscle also exhibit micrometer- or millimeter-scale. Scale anisotropy in complex multilayers Structures such as collagen fibers such as the cornea, bone, or articular cartilage that are heterogeneously and anisotropically organized on length scales from microns to centimeters. To fabricate such native-like tissue structures, many techniques have been used and additive manufacturing techniques,which recently have been developed for cell and biomaterials pattering, considers the best method due to its applicability to construct multi-layered complex structures. These techniques which will be reviewed in this review paper are inkjet-based 3D bioprinting, extrusion-based 3D bioprinting, stereolithographic-based 3D bioprinting , and laser-assisted 3D bioprinting. The applicability of bioprinting strategies has increased significantly, representing a high degree of applicability of additive manufacturing in tissue engineering. 3D bioprinting leads to building tissues or organs structures via layer-by-layer patterns and by harnessing a bottom-to-up approach [7]. The main objective of bioprinting is that, to some extent, to imitate the native-like cellular structure by arranging materials that are including cells (Biomaterials) in a specific pattern which are capable to renovate the ordinary structure and functiony of complex tissues. Bioprinting can be accomplished either in presence of scaffold or scaffold free fabrication manners. In the presence of scaffold mechanism, a biomaterial matrix which can be hydrogels, nanofibers or films are used where the bioink can be patterned. This resulting 3D architecture should imitate the natural ECM microenvironment which permits cell growth, regeneration and proliferation. On the other hand, bioprinting without scaffold deposits cells directly as a spheroid, honeycomb, and cylinder.

2 Anisotropy of different tissues

Most of human tissues have a special structure attributed to the arrangement of the natural ECM which has an decisive role in the functionality of the related tissue. The ECM is formed by fibrous proteins, proteoglycans, polysaccharides, and water. Soft tissues, for example show these anisotropic structures more than hard tissues. These anisotropic structures are direction dependent of physical and chemical properties of the tissue [9].
The tissue anisotropy grants the ECM the ability to optimize its function along the direction of use for the related tissue. The orientation that the anisotropy is dependent on is either arising from ECM fiber orientation or arising from ECM cell orientation. For example, articular cartilage tissue has an anisotropic structure which results from ECM fiber alignment. So, it exhibits three different arrangements in the three different layers. These three layers compose of chondrocytes within distinctly different phenotypes and ECM. The three layers are the superficial layer, middle layer, and the deep layer[10]. These layers are arranged in a way to provide flexibility to move and strength to support load on the joint, as a result, in the superficial layer fibers are oriented horizontally, middle-layer's collagen fibers are oriented randomly , and the deep-layer's fibers are aligned vertically repectively, with respect to the

joint. Also, blood vessels have an anisotropic structure that results from ECM cell alignment. Interestingly, blood vessels consist of two layers, inner layer for lining endothelial cells and the enclosing peripheral layer composes of smooth muscle cells. The anisotropy is found to be aligned longitudinally and circumferentially with respect to the longitudinal axis of the vessel. The arrangement of these two layers has a specific function. Because the inner layer of endothelial cells is longitudinally aligned, it can face mechanical stress (from heartbeat and tissue contraction) and shear stress (from blood streamflow), which are crucial determinants of endothelial cell organization [12] . Whereas the peripheral layer of muscle cells is aligned circumferentially which provides more elasticity.

3   3D bioprinting techniques

Advances in 3D printing, in the form of 3D bioprinting, offer great prospects in the field of tissue and organ regeneration. Currently, 3D bioprinting offers a promising alternative to create cellular and extracellular ordered characteristics found in the original tissues. The main benefit of 3D bioprinting is, that it enables to create anisotropic and/or multi-layered tissue structures that yield better and consistent functional outcomes in patients without the need for mold casting. Use only the recipient's own cells. On one hand, this opens the door to personalized treatment for specific individual patients. On the one hand, the biocompatibility and functionality of printed structures within the body must be met, which is still a challenge. Interestingly, Rapid advances in the field of tissue engineering have resulted in a variety of techniques that are applicable to 3D bioprinting and multiple fabrication approaches for anisotropic tissue architectures have been developed.

3.1   Stereolithographic-based bioprinting

The stereolithographic method of bioprinting is a layer by layer method, precisely by utilizing projection of specific wavelength light as a tool to perform the cross-linking on a photosensitive heat-curable bioink in a plane-by-plane pattern. By employing the light cross-linking method, some bioink must have photocurable moieties. Stereolithography is engaged with some of the clinical imaging modalities, such as CT scan / or MRI, for enhancing the diagnosis approach. Stereolithographic printing falls into two general categories: Single photon and multiphoton methods. In the single-photon method, optical projection systems could execute straightly with laser writing or with usage of physical or digital mask projection systems. The most well-known is the single-photon stereolithography (SLA) apparatus, which uses photons of UV radiation to cross-link UV-sensitive liquid oligomers into networks of gel polymer . Many resins have been used in order to achieve SLA objectives, for instance biodegradable type is used when non-toxicity is on demand, elastomeric type is used when flexibility is desired, and high-strength type is used when mechanical strength is required. Stereolithographic bioprint-

ing has been heavily used in tissue engineering and regenerative medicine to fabricate a biocompatible scaffold in which the cells can proliferate and adhere firmly. One of its applications in tissue engineering is bone ingrowth and regeneration in defective areas by exploiting vinyl ester resin bone regeneration scaffold. Also, the two photon laser scanning photolithography was employed in order to produce 3D liver tissue architecture. However, there are some challenges still open in stereolithographic methods, concerning the fabrication of multiple materials. Fig. 1 depicts the schematic representation of stereolithographic 3D bioprinting.

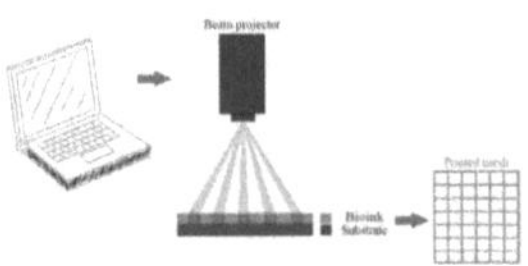

Figure 1: Schematic representation of stereolithographic 3D bioprinting [3].

3.2   Extrusion-based bioprinting

The extrusion-based bioprinting uses bioink which is pushed out of nozzle edge either by pressure, piston, or screw. This mechanism is termed as direct ink writing (DIW). The bioink is ejected analogous to consecutive filament and imprinted layer by layer, resulting in a 3D architecture. Figure 2 shows the three subtype of extrusion-based bioprinting, as shown in Fig. 2.

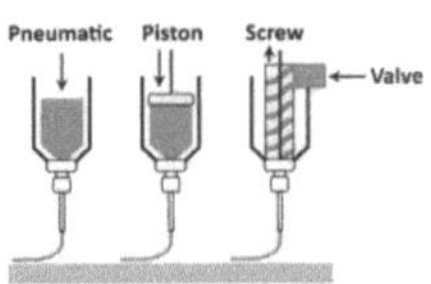

Figure 2: The three sub-types of extrusion-based bioprinting [6].

For easy printing, the material should endure pseudo-plastic behavior to facilitate extrusion through the print nozzle. This means, the printed material must be under a condition with enough shear yield stress in order to assure the extrusion process. Extrusion-based bioprinting is employed in many skin bioprinting relevance. It can also print materials with low to high modulus, thus it supports higher cell densities compared to other bioprinting methods. This method is very versatile due to the variety of nozzle edge designs as well as its applicability with different methods of cross-linking. Polymer resins in extrusion-based bioprinting are commonly blended with fillers. Viscous polymer resins with DIW ranging from a few hundred microns to sub-microns have minimal print resolution, usually determined by the nozzle dimensions. The design as well as optimization of scaffolds using this process is very reliable compared with the other classic scaffolding manners such as electrospinning, salt-leaching and solvent casting where they loss their distinct pore architecture that is acquired from the CAD design before printing. One of its applications is the fabrication of a functional liver construct where rodent hepatocytes are encapsulated in gelatin by using what is called pressure-assisted multi-syringe deposition system.

3.3 Inkjet- based bioprinting

This method uses bioink which is defined as the material intended for bioprinting, which contains cells or other biological materials that can be placed over a hydrogel substrate, culture dish etc. Inkjet-based bioprinting has superiority on the other methods that was brought into bioprinting. It belongs to droplet-based bioprinting methods. Accordingly, this method is a contactless printing technology, where the typography may occur in a fully digital controlled form. Inkjet bioprinting accomplishes in two primary manners, either in a continued manner (continued inkjet) or in a drop on demand (DOD) manner. One application of it is, a successful experiment performed on nude mice where the findings ilustrated that the wounds cured in vivo bioprinting recovered within three weeks compared to the controls where it took five weeks . In comparison with continuous inkjet printing, the DoD experiences a drop-on-demand rather than a continuous stream of drop that is resulting by applied pressure on the bioink extruded from a nozzle, as depicted in Fig. 3.

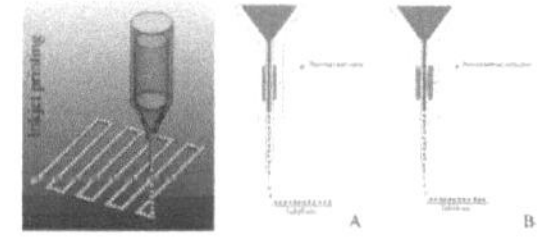

Figure 3: The thermal and piezoelectric methods differ in how the droplet is separated from the ink reservoir [6].

3.4 Laser-assisted bioprinting

A laser beam is exploited in order to deposit the bioink which contains cells onto a substrate. It affords a contactless direct writing process for 3D printing by employing a laser beam for deposition of biomaterials. The volatilization of the heat sensitive bioink is caused by laser beam, where the bioink is enclosed by a quartz target plate to permit the laser beam to pass through. Additionally, as shown in Fig. 4, the substrate where the bioink is to be placed on, is capped with natural polymers, media, or biopolymers to ease the deposition process and ensure cell adhesion and proliferation.

4 Anisotropy with bioprinting

The 3D bioprinting has attracted attention in tissue fabrication over the last decades and being one of the most common technique to solve the limitation of producing anisotropic structures of different tissues. To create

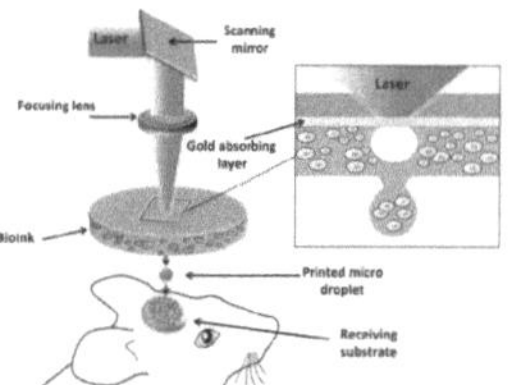

Figure 4: The arrangement of a laser-assisted bioprinter [7].

anisotropic structures that mimic the biological function of the native tissue, enormous tissue engineering scaffolds has been promoted utilizing the alignment of the hydrogel or polymer chains. Here, we reviewed some of the latest trends in fabrication of anisotropic tissue structures by utilizing different alignment methods. In [21] they used real-time magnetically aligned collagen fibers to produce multilayered tissues where a 4D bioprinting is proposed based on real-time matrix remodeling of the structure microarchitecture by magnetism during printing. The collagen fiber is aligned in presence of magnetic field in parallel owing to the unidirectional traveling of the iron nanoparticles blended in the bioink. Also,[22] combined magnetically-and matrix-assisted 3D bioprinting strategies to engineer higher resolution hybrid composites that can mimic the native tissue anisotropy as well as to provide the possibility for remote actuation during tissue construct maturation. In [23], they used an ultrasonic standing bulk acoustic wave (SBAW) to organize cells into controllable anisotropic patterns within viscous bioinks by utilizing SBAW frequency while sustaining the cells viability. To achieve that, hASC-based bioink is used with alginate and GelMA which cross-linked via chemical and photo cross-linking methods. As well as in [24] a vertical 3D extrusion cryo-bioprinting is discussed which is a combination of extrusion 3D bioprinting and ice-templating techniques in order to fabricate high-aspect ratio, vertical, cell laden, hydrogels with anisotropic, gradient microchannel. The bioink used consists of GelMA and CPAs which enable cell encapsulation at higher viability level. The temperature of the substrate ranging from -5 to -20 oC to investigate the effect of this temperature range on the pore size of the scaffold. Here [25], they combine adaptive mesh generation algorithm and greedy search algorithm where a stepped algorithmassisted bioprinting technology is developed in order to design a stable biomimetic anisotropic structure based on natural tissue characteristics and orderly prints.

5 Conclusion

Injuries or defects of most human tissues are difficult to cure unless their unique arrangements in the cellular level are fully understood. This opened door to start fabricating structures that mimic the specific tissue architecture. These structures should be biocompatible as well as no-toxic, So that cells can proliferate and migrant and adhere firmly. Interestingly, with the very and rapid advances of science and technology, a promising solution has been come out to cure the injured tissues minimally invasive. The bioprinting is the one technique that is reliable to create structures that are complex or multi-layered found in the natural tissue structure. In addition, bioprinting is very promising regarding mass production and provide better control over complex structures and cell patterning compared to manual methods of tissue culturing. All of this reflects positively on the tissue engineering and regenerative medicine where it personalizes the medicine and reduces the time and effort of organs donor and tissues regeneration or replacement.

Acknowledgement

The work has been carried out at Leibniz-Instituts für Interaktive Materialien and supervised by Prof. Stefan Müller, medical sensor and device technology laboratory, Technische Hochschule Lübeck.

Author's Statement

Conflict of interest: authors state no conflict of interest.

6   References

[1]Pallab Datta, Veena Vyas, Santanu Dhara, Amit Roy Chowdhury, Ananya Barui *Anisotropy Properties of Tissues: A Basis for Fabrication of Biomimetic Anisotropic Scaffolds for Tissue Engineering* pp. 842-868, 2019

[2]Kroehne V, Heschel I, Schügner F, Lasrich D, Bartsch JW, Jockusch H, *Use of a novel collagen matrix with oriented pore structure for muscle cell differentiation in cell culture and in grafts*, Journal of Cellular and Molecular Medicine, pp. 1582-4934, 2008

[3]Derakhshanfar, S., Mbeleck, R., Xu, K., Zhang, X., Zhong, W., and Xing, M. , *3D bioprinting for biomedical devices and tissue engineering: a review of recent trends and advances*, Bioactive Materials 3, pp. 144–156, 2018

[4]Xiaoxia Le, Wei Lu, Jiawei Zhang,and Tao Chen, *Recent Progress in Biomimetic Anisotropic Hydrogel Actuators*, Advanced Science news 6, pp. 1-14, 2016

[5]Su Ryon Shin, et al., *TAligned Carbon Nanotube–Based Flexible Gel Substrates for Engineering Biohybrid Tissue Actuators*, Advanced Functional Materials, pp. 4486–4495, 2015

[6]Gungor-Ozkerim PS, Inci I, Zhang YS, Khademhosseini A, Dokmeci MR, *Bioinks for 3D Bioprinting: An Overview*, Biomaterials Science 6, pp. 915–946, 2018

[7]Keriquel, et al., *In situ printing of mesenchymal stromal cells, by laser-assisted bioprinting, for in vivo bone regeneration applications*, Scientific Reports, pp. 1-10, 2017

[8]Betsch, M. et al. , *Incorporating 4D into Bioprinting: Real-Time Magnetically Directed Collagen Fiber Alignment for Generating Complex Multilayered Tissues*, Advanced Healthcare Materials 7, pp. 1-9, 2018

[9]Pardo, A. et al *Magnetically Assisted 3D Bioprinting of Anisotropic Tissue-Mimetic Constructs*, Advanced Functional Materials 32, pp. 1-18, 2022

[10]JChansoria, P. and Shirwaiker, R., *3D bioprinting of anisotropic engineered tissue constructs with ultrasonically induced cell patterning*, Additive Manufacturing 32, pp. 1–13, 2020

[11]Zeyu Luo. et al. , *Vertical Extrusion Cryo(bio)printing for Anisotropic Tissue Manufacturing*, Advanced Materials 12, pp. 1-13, 2022

[12]Li, C. et al, *Construction of Biomimetic Tissues with Anisotropic Structures via Stepwise Algorithm-Assisted Bioprinting*, Small 18, pp. 1-10, 2022

3D-printability of composite scaffolds based on PCL and bioactive glass nanoparticles for bone tissue engineering applications

Till Strunk [1], Qaisar Nawaz [2], Christian Damiani [1] and Aldo Boccaccini [2]

[1] Biomedical Engineering, University of Applied Sciences Lübeck
till.strunk@stud.th-luebeck.de, christian.daminani@th-luebeck.de
[2] Institute of Biomaterials, Friedrich-Alexander-University Erlangen-Nürnberg
aldo.boccacini@fau.de, qaisar.nawaz@fau.de

Abstract

In this work, the 3D-printability of Polycaprolactone (PCL) and mesoporous bioactive glass nanoparticles (MBGNs) for bone tissue engineering applications was researched. MBGNs are biodegradable, bioactive and the release of their ions can support bone regeneration. PCL is also a biocompatible material and was used to improve mechanical properties, resulting in a composite material. For this, different techniques were tested among which are Melt-Electrowriting (MEW), Fused deposition modeling (FDM) and dispense plotting. Depending on the application, each technique has its advantages and disadvantages. For bone tissue scaffold, dispense plotting was found to be the preferred technique because of its finely tunable scaffold design, maximum scaffold size, user friendliness and reproducibility. With this, porous PCL and PCL/MBGN scaffolds could be printed. The material investigated can potentially be applied as a bone regenerating scaffold.

1 Introduction

Bioactive materials such as bioglasses are a promising group of materials when developing scaffolds, especially bone scaffolds. Bone scaffolds are of interest in research because although the body's self-healing ability in terms of bone regeneration can repair minor defects (<2.5 cm), larger defects may need healing support [1]. Scaffolds can be of different origin. Today, autologous as well as allogeneic grafts are commonly used in surgery [2]. However, numerous problems arise from the use of these scaffolds, among which are donor site morbidity, scarcity of available donor tissue and rejection of the donated tissue at site of application [3]. Therefore, engineers and scientists try to develop materials and scaffolds which overcome these challenges. Characteristics of a scaffold that should be considered for a successful implementation include porosity and overall microstructure, mechanical properties and osteogenic behavior. Generally, a porous microstructure of 300 µm to 600 µm pore size is considered an optimal size for cells, e.g. osteoblasts, to migrate into the structure [4]. Scaffolds made from bioactive glasses or a bioactive glass composite material are considered one of the most promising approaches [5]. Further, the development and use of additive manufacturing techniques such as 3D-printing has enabled advancements also in the field of (composite) biomaterials. Numerous techniques have been developed and used, each with different positive and negative aspects and fields of application. Murphy et al. [6] describe a PCL and borate-based bioglass composite material by dissolving the polymer in chloroform and mixing the bioglass into the paste. An air pressure controlled 3D printer is then used to print the desired form, a technique termed dispense-plotting. Making a homogeneously composite slurry is possible to achieve but the use of solvents in the process has to be kept in mind. Residues from evaporated solvents can alter aspects like cell viability and growth. Depending on the solvent and later use of the scaffold, a different technique might be preferable. Another approach in additive manufacturing is the Fused Deposition Modeling technique (FDM). For this a filament is combined with a moving nozzle which prints the desired scaffold. Distler and colleagues [7] have printed a porous and osteoinductive PLA/Bioglass composite which was also cytocompatible with pre-osteoblasts (MC3T3E1 cells). An advantage of FDM is the printability without solvents as these have to be taken into account when assessing the characteristics, e.g. biocompatibility. However, a non-homogeneous filament with regard to its diameter and distribution of reinforcement phase can therefore be a source of error. Melt-Electrowriting (MEW) is essentially an extension of dispense-plotting, using the same airpressure controlled nozzle but mounted with an electric field between the nozzle and the printing bed. Following the establishment of an electric field, a so-called Taylor-Cone forms which enables a finer filament than what the nozzle diameter suggests. Abbasi and colleagues [8] showed how PCL scaffolds with a gradient in pore size produced with MEW could close 5 mm large defects in the calvarial (skull) bone of rats. In this work the 3D-printability of PCL and PCL/MBGN composite materials using different techniques shall be assessed. MBGNs is, like its name suggests, a bioactive material and like other bioglasses it has been researched to support a body's self-healing ability in bone regeneration. However, it is rather brittle. PCL is a biodegradable polymer with suitable mechanical characteristics that can help to improve the overall mechanical properties of a scaffold, enable 3D-printability and preserve bioactivity. The printability of PCL/MBGN scaffold was assessed using different 3D-printing techniques and scaffolds of different dimensions were printed. Light microscopy and scanning electron microscopy (SEM) was done to investigate morphological characteristics of the scaffolds. The focus was on FDM and dispense plotting. Because of a limited maximum size in scaffolds, MEW was not in focus for the application of rather larger scale bone scaffolds. Furthermore, stereolithography was tried out, however the choice of material is rather limited because it has to be photocurable. Generally, based on literature research, both MEW and stereolithography are well established and promising techniques of additive manufacturing that should not be neglected when choosing a technique for tissue engineering scaffold production [8].

2 Materials and Methods

2.1 Production of Mesoporous Bioactive Glass Nanoparticles (MBGNs)

The particles were prepared using microemulsion assisted sol-gel approach as described elsewhere [9]. 1.12g Cetrimonium bromide (CTAB) was dissolved in ultrapure water at 37°C for 30 min. Next, 16 ml Ethyl Acetate was added dropwise to form micro-emulsion. The following steps are conducted at room temperature. After 30 min., the basic pH was kept at 9.8 to 10.2 by adding ammonium hydroxide (28% purity). After 15 min. stirring, 6.217 ml Tetraethylorthosilicate (TEOS) was added to the solution. The solution was stirred for 30 min., after which 3 g of calcium nitrate was added. The solution was allowed to react for 4 hours to form MBGNs. Subsequently, the solution is distributed into 50 ml falcon tubes, which are used to wash the nanoparticles. To wash, the tubes are centrifuged (4500 rpm, 5 min) after which the liquid phase on top is discarded. Distilled water is added to fill up the falcon tube and a spatula is used to mix water and the remaining solid phase. This procedure is repeated once again with distilled water and once with pure ethanol followed by drying in a 60°C overnight. Finally, the dried particles are grinded using a mortar and sintered in crucibles at 700°C for 3 hours.

2.2 Filament production and fused deposition modeling approach

For FDM, a filament of the desired polymer is needed, in this case made out of PCL (Mn=45k, Sigma-Aldrich). An extruder (3devo, Netherlands) was used to make such a filament. The temperatures of the heating elements 1-4 were set to 65°C, 90°C, 105°C and 105°C, respectively. The extruding screw was rotating at a speed of approximately 4rpm and once the filament exited the screw, it was cooled by two fans at 100% speed. The filament diameter was set to 2.85 mm. The printing of the scaffolds was then attempted with an Ultimaker S3 printer (Ultimaker, Utrecht, Netherlands). A cubic scaffold of edge length 5 mm was designed

in TinkerCAD (Autodesk, San Rafael, USA) and further processed in Ultimaker Cura 5.2 (Ultimaker). Mostly, the default Cura settings were used but the infill density was changed to 50 %. The printing temperature of the nozzle was set to 105° C while the glass bed was not heated. The nozzle head speed was set to 10 mm/s, and a primal blob as well as a brim around the cube was enabled. The material flow rate was set to 400 % since the material tended to underextrude. The stated values were considered to be the most appropriate, but other values were also tried as stated in Table 1.

2.3 Dispense-plotting using a Gesim 3D printer

Another technique for printing a polymer/glass composite material is called dispense-plotting and uses a temperature controlled pneumatic printing head like in the Bioscaffolder 3.1 (Gesim, Radeberg, Germany). Either pure PCL or a PCL/MBGN composite was filled into a heatable cartridge with a 400 μm nozzle mounted on the bottom.

For a composite material with evenly distributed MBGNs in the PCL matrix, both materials were mixed prior to the melting in the printer cartridge. For this, PCL was dissolved in chloroform (Sigma-Aldrich) at a ratio of 1:1 using a magnetic stirrer and heated stirring plate set to 50°C. Once dissolved, the necessary amount of sintered MBGN powder was added to meet the desired concentration (5 wt % if not stated otherwise). After stirring overnight, the solution was casted into a glass petri dish and left to dry under a fume hood for 2 days. To print a scaffold, the cartridge of the Bioscaffolder was set to a temperature of 85°C (95°C for composites because of higher viscosity) and the polymer was melted for about one hour before the first print to ensure an evenly melted polymer material in the cartridge. The printer was connected to the Gesim Robotics Software (Gesim) and the necessary tool measurements as well as height measurements were conducted. As a base for the scaffolds, a plastic 12 well plate lid was used. A scaffold of the desired dimensions was designed in the Gesim Robotics Software, usually cubicle shaped strands of 10 mm length were printed, unless stated otherwise. After printing two layers alike, the printing direction was rotated by 90° to make a sandwich-like scaffold. To print, the pressure during printing was set to 600 kPa, the strand height and width were set to 400 μm (same as the nozzle), the printing speed was 10 mm/s, nozzle cleaning was enabled before printing of each layer and each strand was ended by enabling the tear-off setting, set to a 60 mm vertical tear-off at maximum speed. To keep strands from melting into each other, the strand distance was set to 1.11 mm, measured between the center of each strand. Additionally, a fan was implemented, which helped to cool down the printed strand more quickly and therefore kept two strand of the same layer from melting into each other. The usage of a fan also enabled the printing of overhang structures which is necessary to print a sandwich-like scaffold.

2.4 Melt-Electrowriting

Melt-Electrowriting (MEW) was carried out using a Gesim Scaffolder 3.1 (Gesim) mounted with a high voltage source. The voltage between nozzle and printing bed was set to 5 kV, while the layer height was set to 100 µm . A pressure of 250 kPa was applied to the nozzle, which contained commercially available PCL beads (Mn = 45k, Sigma-Aldrich) and was heated to 85°C. Before the print of the scaffold was started, it was made sure that the Taylor-cone had successfully formed and that PCL was flowing. The desired scaffold was designed in Gesim Robotics software (Gesim).

3 Results and Discussion

3.1 MBGN synthesis

Successfully producing MBGNs was a core goal of this work as the bioactivity rate of this reinforcement phase is considered to be higher than that of PCL, resulting in faster integration of living tissue. Judging from SEM-Analysis as the Figure 1 suggests, MBGNs could successfully be synthesized using the protocol mentioned in section 2. Their appearance is comparable to that from Nawaz et al. [9]. Energy-dispersive X-ray spectroscopy (EDX) can help in the future to confirm the successful synthesis of MBGNs. These MBGNs can provide a bioactive substrate for bone regeneration and are considered to be more bioactive than the surrounding matrix (PCL) [9]. As the name suggests, their surface can be characterized by pores of a few nanometers which can be loaded with drugs further on.

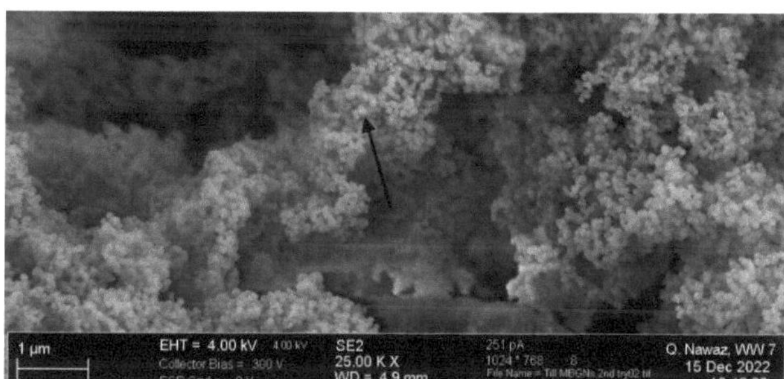

Figure 1: Mesoporous bioactive glass nanoparticles (MBGNs) SEM-image taken using 4 kV. The individual spherical nanoparticles are well visible (exemplarily at black arrow).

3.2 Melt-Electrowriting

MEW with pure PCL produced a scaffold with fine fibers as it can be seen in Figure 2. Thanks to the electric field, designs can be more accurately/finer printed compared to dispense plotting, although it uses the same 3D-printer. The produced scaffold is rather delicate in mechanical appearance compared to a dispense plotted scaffold. Although MEW was not the focus during this work, it should not be disregarded as a potential technique for bone scaffolds all together.

3.3 Printability of fused deposition modeling approach

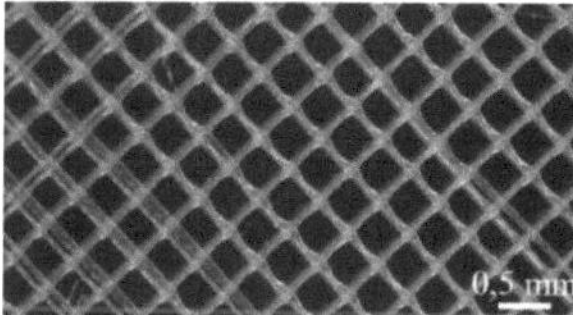

Figure 2: Light microscopy camera image of a PCL scaffold produced using MEW.

The printability using FDM is greatly affected by the used filament, which during the course of this work could successfully be produced with the in parameters mentioned in section 2. Although the filament production was successful by visual means (homogeneous diameter and distribution of MBGNs) the printability using the mentioned Ultimaker S3 printer was not satisfactory. Different parameters were combined in practically all possibilities with different settings as summarized in Table 1. Apart from the printer settings, variables like nozzle contamination from other polymers or deformation of the filament from the printer feeder to an oval shape may have had a significant impact on printability. Often the lack of material extrusion led to

Table 1: Tested parameters for fused deposition modeling

Parameter changed	Value range	Best found value
Nozzle temperature	60°C-200°C	100°C
Material Flow	100%-400%	400%
Bed temperature	RT-60°C	RT
Infill density	10%-90%	40%
Nozzle speed	5 mm/s - 50 mm/s	10 mm/s
Brim printing	0 mm - 7 mm	5 mm

break in material deposition on the printing bed, which is why the material flow was increased to 400%. Furthermore, material was not extruding uniformly which led to agglomeration at the exterior of the nozzle.

Ilyas and colleagues [10] have successfully used Ultimaker 3D printers before to print PCL/Bioglass composite scaffolds, but using the same settings has not worked either. According to this paper and many other in literature, it is shown that FDM can be used and should not be disregarded in future applications.

3.4 Printability of dispense plotting

Dispense plotting using the Gesim printer resulted in scaffolds of satisfactory quality, with a mean pore size of 565 µm (±7 µm), measured from top view light-microscopy images using ImageJ (NIH, USA). The porosity persists in all directions. However, the very bottom layer seems to have slightly smaller pores (445 µm ±7µm) as the initial layer is pushed onto the printing bed by the nozzle with a bit more force to ensure proper hold. Wider strands make tighter pores. A fan was necessary in order to print overhanging structure as in this sandwich-like scaffold. Without a fan, the polymer is too little viscous and flows down the scaffold with gravity, resulting in a hill-and-valley like structure when observed from the side. Sometimes the use of a fan results in thin fibers being blown off to the side of the scaffold. The Figure 3 shows a scaffold of pure PCL and thin blown off fibers. Problems with a PCL/MBGN composite scaffold were persistent but could be resolved by sonicating the MBGNs in ethanol prior to their addition into the

PCL solution. This prevents the agglomeration of MBGNs at the nozzle which would otherwise clog it. Figure 4 shows a closer view of a scaffold containing 5 wt% MBGNs (top view). Regardless of the material used, a scaffold could be produced in approximately nine minutes. Dispense plotting is for this work considered to be the most reproducible technique with a good quality. In future work, the bioactivity, mechanical behavior and other aspects (see section 4) should be investigated. Coating scaffolds with more bioactive layers than the underlying PCL matrix could produce even more promising bone regenerating scaffolds.

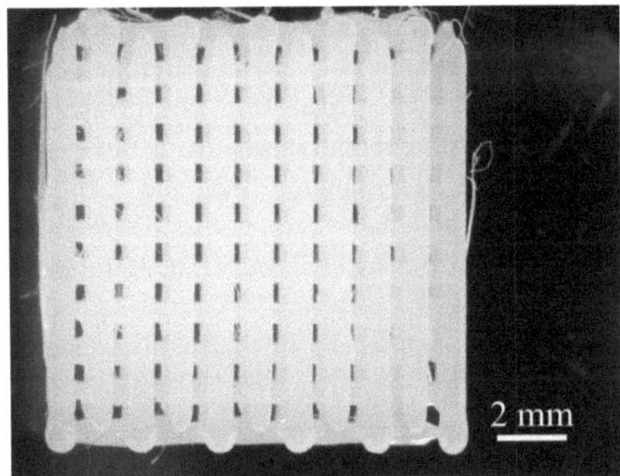

Figure 3: Light microscope camera image (Zeiss Axiocam 105 Color, Carl Zeiss AG, Oberkochen, Germany) of a PCL scaffold. Bottom view.

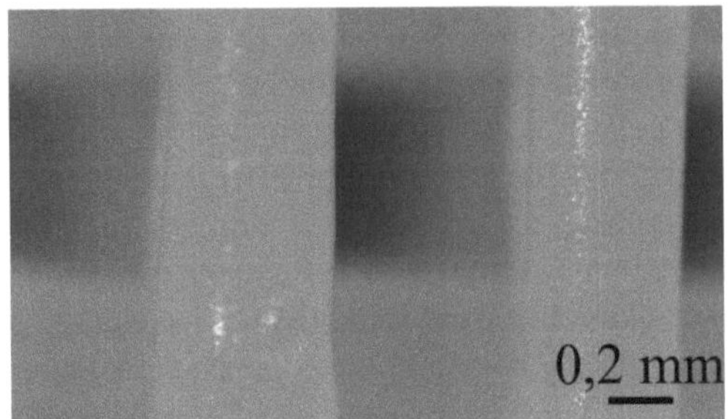

Figure 4: High magnification light microscope camera image (Zeiss Axiocam 105 Color, Carl Zeiss AG) of a PCL/MBGN (5 wt%) scaffold. Top view.

4 Conclusion and Outlook

Four different additive manufacturing techniques for the production of bone scaffolds were tried out and assessed. It was found that dispense plotting using a Gesim 3D-printer yielded the best results, while being quick and easy to handle. At the same time, this technique allowed for a reproducible sample, at a reasonable pace and work effort. Nonetheless, further research should not disregard other techniques. To give an outlook, the produced scaffolds using the dispense plotting technique should be researched in their bioactive capacity, their mechanical characteristics, their porosity and their cytocompatibility. Furthermore, aspects like a time-dependent ion-release rate should be considered that potentially could be achieved by introducing coatings to the scaffold.

Acknowledgements

The work has been carried out at the Biomaterials laboratory of Prof. Dr. Aldo Boccaccini at the University of Erlangen. I thank him and my technical supervisor Dr. Qaisar Nawaz for hosting me and the support during this internship. I further thank Dr. Christian Damiani for being my internship supervisor.

Author's Statement

Conflict of interest: Authors state no conflict of interest.

5 References

[1] A. Nauth, E. Schemitsch, B. Norris, Z. Nollin, and J. T. Watson, "Critical-size bone defects: Is there a consensus for diagnosis and treatment?," *Journal of Orthopaedic Trauma*, vol. 32, pp. S7–S11, 3 2018.

[2] S. Bose, S. Vahabzadeh, and A. Bandyopadhyay, "Bone tissue engineering using 3d printing," 12 2013.

[3] M. J. O'Malley, S. C. Sayres, O. Saleem, D. Levine, M. Roberts, J. T. Deland, and S. Ellis, "Morbidity and complications following percutaneous calcaneal autograft bone harvest," *Foot and Ankle International*, vol. 35, pp. 30–37, 1 2014.

[4] A. Bandyopadhyay, S. Ghosh, A. R. Boccaccini, and S. Bose, "3d printing of biomedical materials and devices," 10 2021.

[5] A. B. Q. C. Ian Thompson, "45s5 bioglass-derived glass-ceramic scaffolds for bone tissue engineering," *Biomaterials*, vol. 27, pp. 2414–2425, 2006.

[6] C. Murphy, K. C. R. Kolan, M. Long, W. Li, M. C. Leu, J. A. Semon, and D. E. Day, "3d printing of a polymer bioactive glass composite for bone repair."

[7] T. Distler, N. Fournier, A. Grünewald, C. Polley, H. Seitz, R. Detsch, and A. R. Boccaccini, "Polymer-bioactive glass composite filaments for 3d scaffold manufacturing by fused deposition modeling: Fabrication and characterization," *Frontiers in Bioengineering and Biotechnology*, vol. 8, 6 2020.

[8] N. Abbasi, R. S. Lee, S. Ivanovski, R. M. Love, and S. Hamlet, "In vivo bone regeneration assessment of offset and gradient melt electrowritten (mew) pcl scaffolds," *Biomaterials Research*, vol. 24, 10 2020.

[9] Q. Nawaz, M. A. U. Rehman, A. Burkovski, J. Schmidt, A. M. Beltrán, A. Shahid, N. K. Alber, W. Peukert, and A. R. Boccaccini, "Synthesis and characterization of manganese containing mesoporous bioactive glass nanoparticles for biomedical applications," *Journal of Materials Science: Materials in Medicine*, vol. 29, 5 2018.

[10] K. Ilyas, M. A. Akhtar, E. B. Ammar, and A. R. Boccaccini, "Surface modification of 3d-printed pcl/bg composite scaffolds via mussel-inspired polydopamine and effective antibacterial coatings for biomedical applications," *Materials*, vol. 15, 12 2022.

Device for Assessment of Quantitative Magnetic Drug Targeting using Magnetic Nanoparticles

Ashong Afotey Albert [1], Patricia Radon [2], Frank Wiekhorst [2],

[1] Biomedical Engineering, University of Applied Sciences-Luebeck, albert.ashong@stud.th-luebeck.de

[2] Metrology for Magnetic Nanoparticle, Physikalisch-Technische Bundesanstalt, Berlin 10587, Germany, {Radon, Wiekhorst}@ptb.de

Abstract

This work describes an artificial artery setup that has been developed to quantitatively assess magnetic drug targeting using magnetic nanoparticles. The setup consists of a pump and a dedicated tubing system with a Y-shaped bifurcation mimicking a human artery. A magnet of a certain dimension and defined magnetic flux density is placed at a specific distance and location of the tubing system to magnetically direct the nanoparticles flowing through the tubing system into one of its tubing branches (region of interest). The device characteristics were determined first, and the targeting behaviour was quantified using magnetic particle spectroscopy, a technique detecting the nonlinear dynamic magnetic susceptibility of MNP. The completed setup was tested with two commercial magnetic nanoparticle systems (FuidMAG and EMG 700).

1 Introduction

The use of magnetic nanoparticles (MNP) as biomarkers in this current era of technology and innovation is something that one must not overlook. Its applications range from the field of medicine to the industry with promising prospects and future. One important application of MNP is its therapeutic application in the treatment and detection of diseases [1]. Drug control and release is an important issue due to the high efficiency of magnetic drug targeting. Due to its efficiency, unwanted side effects can be reduced compared to the systemic administration of drugs [2]. There is also the need to have a look at certain factors that might affect the use of magnetic drug targeting and how much this use of MNP can be quantified. Quantitative measurement of these particles at the desired region of interest will also help to determine the efficiency and efficacy of these nanoparticles. This will enable to extract quantitative parameters for medical and industrial purposes to assess the degree of change relative to the normal [3]. This paper presents a drug targeting setup with defined and controllable parameters (such as tubing diameter, shape, flow, and targeting force) for quantitative measurements of MNP in a dedicated flow model mimicking an aorta with a Y-shaped bifurcation that supplies MNP carrying a drug to the desired targeted body region. With the help of a magnetic field gradient, the flowing MNP shall be directed into one of the branches of the tubing system. The MNP are then collected at the output of branches and subsequently quantified using magnetic particle spectroscopy (MPS) which is a highly sensitive technique for the quantification of MNP [4]. The device and the two used MNP systems are characterized and the general

drug targeting behaviour of the device under the influence of a magnetic targeting force is presented.

2 Material and Methods

2.1 Targeting Device Flow system

As shown in Fig. 1, the dedicated flow setup consists of a reservoir providing a sample volume of up to 50 ml MNP suspension, a peristaltic pump (Ismatec IPC 4), the tubing system with Y-shaped bifurcation with fixed inlet and outlet sampling containers, outlet test tubes, and a strong cube-shaped neodymium magnet (edge length 10 mm).

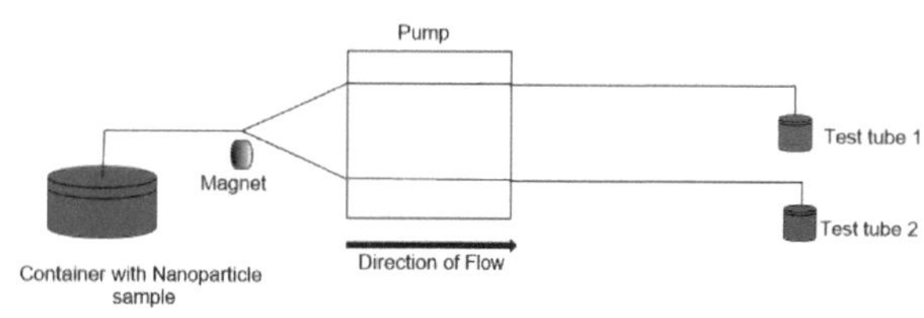

Figure 1: Schematic diagram of the flow setup.

The magnet is applied in front of the bifurcation to provide a magnetic field (gradient) strong enough to (partially) deflect the MNP moving in the flowing suspension medium into the branch selected for targeting (+mag branch) while less MNP material passes through the branch (-mag branch) that is farther away from the magnet.

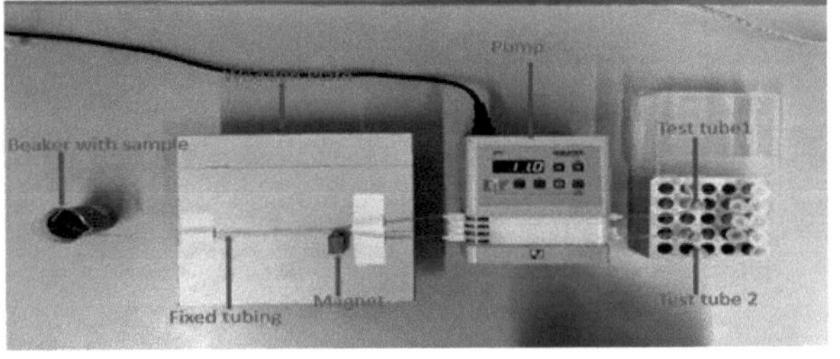

Figure 2: Photograph of the "Y" shape flow model.

The magnetic force experienced by a magnetic particle is given by the formulae:

$$F_{mag} = \mu\mu_0 \partial H / \partial r \qquad (1)$$

where μ is the magnetic moment of the particle (i.e., the huge, collective moment of the atomic moments within the magnetic iron oxide core formed by the exchange interaction), $\mu_0 = 4\pi 10^{-7}$ H/m is the vacuum magnetic permeability constant and $\partial H / \partial r$ is the radial magnetic field gradient [5].

In a flow of velocity v, the MNP experience a drag force F_{drag} moving the MNP with the flow which is proportional to the hydrodynamic diameter d_{hyd} of the particles:

$$F_{drag} = 3\pi\eta d_{hyd}\Delta v \qquad (2)$$

Where η is the viscosity of the carrier fluid, d_{hyd} is the hydrodynamic diameter and Δv is the difference in velocity between particle and medium (in our case of the deflection of flowing MNP into one branch, Δv varies between 0 and v) depending on the strength of the magnetic force F_{mag} that can be adjusted by magnetic field gradient given by the distance of the magnet to the bifurcation [6].

The MNP suspension of defined and adjusted iron concentration c(Fe) was pumped through the silicon tubing system. The tubing system has an inner diameter of 1.42 mm and a total volume capacity of 5 mL. This corresponds to the typical mean size of a normal artery which ranges from 0.1 mm to 10 mm [7].

Close to the bifurcation where the MNP are entering one of the tubing branches, the targeting magnet which was fixed on a wooden slide was placed at a defined distance d between the magnet's front side and the tubing wall. Throughout the experiments, a fixed distance d = 1.6 mm was used. A flow rate of 11 mL/min was set on the pump which corresponds to a mean flow velocity v of 1.02 m/s.

The magnetic field profile of the magnet was determined by hall probe (FM 210 Teslameter, Projekt Electronik) measurements from which a mean magnetic field gradient of -76 T/m at the targeting distance d = 1.6 mm was extracted as shown in Fig. 3. A negative gradient was resulting due to the direction into which the probe was moved. To avoid a complete blockage of the tube by MNP agglomerations the magnet was placed at the chosen moderate distance, while at much larger distances of the magnet, the targeting impact on the MNP was expected to be too low. This is also very important to avoid an increase in resistance in the tubing system.

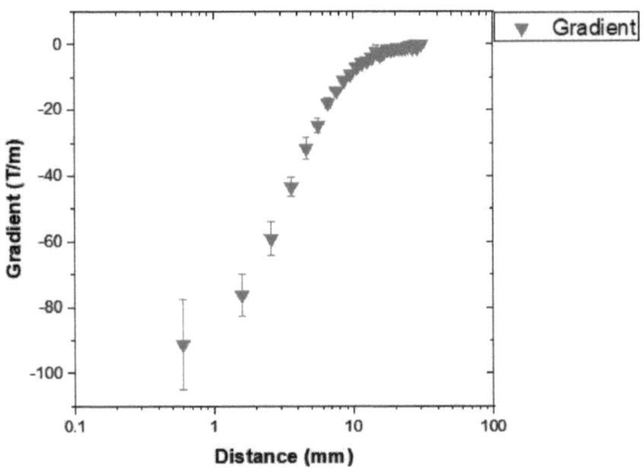

Figure 3: Magnetic field gradient as a function of distance d between magnet surface and targeting site (Hall probe position) extracted from triplicate measurements of the magnetic field profile. This helps in determining the optimal distance at which the magnet was placed and resulting magnetic field gradient determining the targeting force on the MNP. The shown uncertainty was obtained as the standard deviation of triplicate magnetic field profile measurements.

2.2 Magnetic Targeting Procedure

To begin with the experiment, the inlet branch of the "Y" channel was inserted into the MNP reservoir. The MNP suspension was then pumped through the tube system by the peristaltic pump with the magnet placed at the branching of the "Y" channel. For 1 minute the MNP were collected at both outlets and the MNP amount of 10 μL was quantified by magnetic particle spectroscopy (MPS). Due to the attractive force between the magnet and the MNP, the branch of the tube closer to the magnet is expected to have a higher concentration of MNP.

2.3 Magnetic Particle Spectroscopy

To determine the amount m(Fe) and to evaluate the iron concentration c(Fe) of collected sample material, magnetic particle spectroscopy (MPS-3, Bruker BioSpin, Germany) [8] detecting the nonlinear magnetic susceptibility was used. In MPS, a sinusoidal magnetic AC field of frequency f_{exc} = 25 kHz and amplitude B_{ex} = 25 mT is applied to the MNP sample. Due to the non-linearity of the magnetization response of the MNP, the detected signal recorded with a gradiometric induction coil system (to suppress the much higher excitation field in the receive circuit) contains odd higher harmonics (after Fourier transform).

Therefore, the MNP exhibit a characteristic MPS signal spectrum with odd harmonics A_i at $(3_{f0}, 5_{f0}, \dots)$, that is the Fourier transform of the detected time dependent signal. The magnetic nanoparticle quantification uses the amplitude of the third harmonic of the MNP in a sample A_3, sample related to the amplitude of a reference $A_{3,ref}$ with known MNP (iron) amount. Factors that may affect the MPS measurement include the temperature, concentration

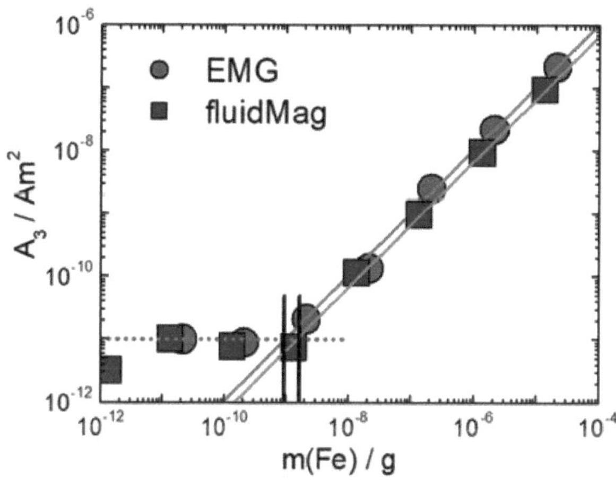

Figure 4: Serial dilutions of the two MNP systems EMG (green circles) and fluidMag (blue square) displaying the measured MPS harmonic A_3 as a function of the nominal iron amount m(Fe) in the sample. From the intersection of the slope A_3 with the background noise level (blue dashed line) the smallest detectable iron amount is extracted.

of MNP suspension and magnetic field strength.

To ensure the linearity between MNP amount and A_3, a serial dilution is carried out as shown in Fig. 4 showing the measured A_3 as a function of the nominal iron amount for the two different MNP systems that were investigated. From this representation, the linearity over several decades of iron amount is confirmed and the specific harmonic amplitude A_3* (which is A_3 normalized to the iron amount, straight lines in Fig. 4) is extracted, i.e., the slope of $A_3(m(Fe))$. For fluidMAG a value $A_3* = 6.86$ Am2/kg(Fe) was determined while for EMG $A_3* = 10.69$ Am2/kg(Fe) was found. Furthermore the detection limit can be estimated as the interception of the slope with the background noise level $A_3, lim = 10^{-11} Am^2$ (obtained by empty sample measurements), For fluidMAG we found 1.5 ng and for EMG 0.9 ng as the smallest detectable MNP iron amount in a sample. This nicely demonstrates the high sensitivity and the huge dynamic range (more than 5 orders of magnitude) of the MPS system.

2.4   Magnetic Nanoparticle

Two different magnetic nanoparticle systems were used, EMG 700 and FluidMAG-D 200. FluidMAG (fluidMAG-D, chemicell, Berlin) is multicore (several smaller particles are combined into a larger one) iron oxide particle system coated with hydroxyethyl starch with a mean hydrodynamic diameter of 200 nm [9]. These MNP are covered with hydrophilic polymers to protect them against aggregation. With a stock concentration of c(Fe) = 0.245 mol/L, they are used for preclinical, biomedical applications such as MRI diagnostics, cell separation, and magnetic drug targeting applications. EMG (EMG 700, FerroTec, USA) is a technical ferrofluid addressing a broad range of industrial applications and is also used for experimentation and application development such as applications where rapid evap-

oration or the ability to mix a nanoparticle into a water-based system is required including domain detection, material separation, and metallic crystallization/fracture analysis [10]. EMG has a stock concentration of c(Fe)= 4.8 mol/L. For serial dilution and adjustment of c(Fe) for magnetic targeting, deionized water was used.

3   Results and Discussion

As expected in magnetic targeting, nanoparticles passing through the "Y" tube will swiftly move through the channel that is closer to the magnet (providing a higher force due to the higher field gradient). Within 1 min (time elapsed to obtain a steady state), more MNP were flowing through the branch closer to the magnet. Fig. 6 shows the quantification by MPS. A significant higher fraction of the MNP is directed through the branch that was closer to the magnet.

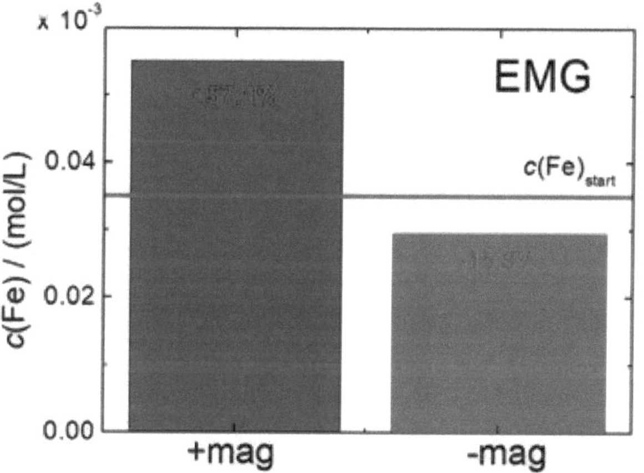

Figure 5: Targeting efficiency of EMG MNP showing the resulting concentration c(Fe) for the Y-branch close to the magnet (+mag), farer away (-mag) together with the original concentration c(Fe)start (grey line) as determined by MPS from 10 μL aliquots by MPS.

The bar graph in Figs. 5 and 6 shows the percentage and the net amount of iron concentration that is flowing in the two branches. For targeting EMG MNP, the concentration in the branch closer to the magnet (+mag) is increased by 57.1% (compared to the starting concentration for the selected targeting and flow parameters). Accordingly, in the other branch (-mag) a reduction of concentration by 15.9% is observed. This demonstrates the influence of external magnetic field gradient on the MNP in the flow, e.g. the magnetic force F_{mag} is strong enough to overcome the drag force and to deflect a fraction of MNP from the -mag to the +mag branch. Likewise, for fluidMAG the same general behavior is observed, here an iron concentration increases of 89.6% is resulting for the +mag branch while the concentration is dropping by 33.1% in the -mag branch as shown in fig. 6.

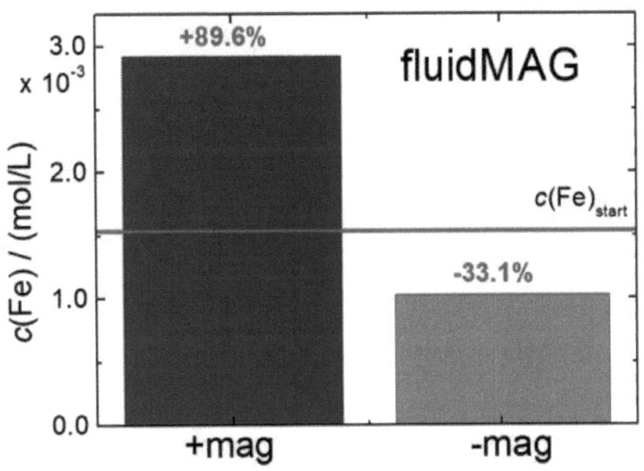

Figure 6: Targeting efficiency of fluidMAG MNP showing the resulting concentration c(Fe) for the Y-branch close to the magnet (+mag), farer away (-mag) together with the original concentration c(Fe)start (grey line) as determined by MPS from 10 µL aliquots by MPS.

4 Conclusion

We developed a device and demonstrated its applicability to study magnetic drug targeting of MNP flowing through a vessel system with a Y-shaped bifurcation. With this setup, the targeting of two commercial MNP systems (fluidMAG-D 200 and EMG 700) was investigated by determining their targeting efficiency using magnetic particle spectroscopy to quantify the MNP amount in a sample. The general operability of the setup was successfully demonstrated and the efficiency of the two commercial MNP types for magnetic drug targeting was verified. By varying the distance d between magnet and bifurcation, by employing different magnet geometries (needle, array of magnets, magnetic field coils, etc.) and by varying flow parameters such as flow rate or tube diameter, a comprehensive experimental analysis of the magnetic drug targeting performance of MNP can be carried out. Even more complex flow geometries such as realistic vessel systems imaged by angiography imaging and generated by additive manufacturing become accessible for drug targeting investigations with the presented approach. This will assist in the selection and optimization of future MNP systems for magnetic drug targeting. To this end, the use of MPS technology for quick and sensitive quantification of the MNP amount is of utmost advantage.

Acknowledgement

This work was carried out at the Physikalisch Technische Bundesantalt. Special thanks to all the staff of PTB, Berlin especially working group 8.23 for their immense support and guidance. A big thanks also goes to Dr. Alexander Neumann from the Institute of Medical Engineering, University of Luebeck for his great supervision.

Author's Statement

Authors state no conflict of interest. Informed consent.

5 References

[1] Q.A. Pankhurst, J. Connolly, S.K. Jones, and J. Dobson, *Applications of magnetic nanoparticles in biomedicine.* Journal of physics D: Applied physics, 36(13), R167, 2003

[2] P. Radon et al, *Magnetic Particle Spectroscopy to Determine the Magnetic Drug Targeting Efficiency of Different Magnetic Nanoparticles in a Flow Phantom.* in IEEE Transactions on Magnetics, vol. 51, no. 2, pp. 1-4, Feb. 2015, Art no. 6000104, doi: 10.1109/TMAG.2014.2326889

[3] A.M. Rauwerdink, and J.B. Weaver, *Measurement of molecular binding using the Brownian motion of magnetic nanoparticle probes.*Applied Physics Letters, 96(3), 033702, 2010

[4] B. Gleich, J. Weizenecker, *Tomographic imaging using the nonlinear response of magnetic particles.* Nature, 435(7046), 1214-1217, 2005

[5] M. Benelmekki et al, *Horizontal low gradient magnetophoresis behaviour of iron oxide nanoclusters at the different steps of the synthesis route.* Journal of Nanoparticle Research 13.8 (2011): 3199-3206.

[6] J. Lim et al, *Magnetophoresis of nanoparticles* Acs Nano 5.1 (2011): 217-226.

[7] E. Matthews,R. Brassington, T .Kuntzer,F. Jichi, A. Manzur, *Corticosteroids for the treatment of Duchenne muscular dystrophy.* The Cochrane Database of Systematic Reviews, 13(5). (2016). https://ncbi.nlm.nih.gov/pubmed/27149418

[8] S.R. Snyder, U. Heinen, *Characterization of magnetic nanoparticles for therapy and diagnostics.*Bruker BioSpin: Ettlingen,Germany, 2010

[9] FluidMAG, *2006-04-06.* Available: https://www.chemicell.com/products/ferrofluid/ferrofluids.html [2022-11-09].

[10] EMG-Series, *2019-10-10.* Available: https://ferrofluid.ferrotec.com/products/ferrofluid-emg/water/emg-700-sp/.[2022-11-16].

3D Tracking and Control of a Magnetic Particle for Automated Lens Emulsification in Cataract Surgery

Max Studt [1]
[1] Medical Engineering Science, Universität zu Lübeck, max.studt@student.uni-luebeck.de

Abstract

This paper presents an approach for automated lens emulsification using magnetic fields during cataract surgery. Here, micro-magnetic objects are inserted into the lens and controlled by an external magnetic field to emulsify the lens nucleus, eliminating the need for a direct and risky mechanical connection between the surgeon and the lens. The magnetic particles are controlled by a position-based control loop. For evaluation purposes, an experimental setup consisting of imaging systems and a magnetic field generator was set up to control the magnets. State-of-the-art imaging systems, including a high-resolution surgical microscope and an OCT device, were used to determine the current positions. The experiments were performed in viscous fluids or in extracted porcine lenses. The experimental results demonstrate the ability to precisely control the magnetic particles and the potential for cataract surgery, but also the challenge of overcoming the rigidity of porcine lenses with limited magnetic force for emulsification.

1 Introduction

The eye represents the sensory organ of the visual system and is thus essential for visual perception. Impairments of the visual system, especially due to cataracts, have a negative impact on visual perception and daily life.

Cataract surgery is the most common surgical procedure in developed countries, while cataracts are the most common cause of blindness in developing countries [1]. Nowadays, ultrasound phacoemulsification (phaco) is the method of choice to remove cataract lenses during surgery. Phaco surgery is a fast procedure that is less traumatic to intraocular structures compared to other cataract surgery techniques, e.g., the Manual Small Incision Cataract Surgery (MSICS). However, phaco surgery is a manual procedure that requires a significant learning curve and carries a risk of lens capsule injury [2]. Automation of the surgical procedure could improve cataract treatment. One possibility to automate lens emulsification and at the same time minimize the risk of complications could be the use of magnetic fields and magnetic particles. The magnetic particle could be steered from the outside through the lens by the external magnetic field to emulsify the lens from the inside. The potential of using magnetic fields to emulsify lenses with potentially lower risk was first recognized by Charles David Kelman [3]. Possible benefits of this method could be fewer complications, a shorter learning curve, as well as partial automation of cataract surgery. Magnetic actuation allows precise exertion of forces in the millinewton range and below. This may reduce or eliminate the risk of capsular ruptures compared to the phaco technique. The magnetic particle could be controlled by the surgeon with a joystick, which may be easier for the surgeon to learn. [2].

This work deals with the scientific question whether an automation of lens emulsification by magnetic actuation can be realized in cataract surgery. The specific task is to design, implement, and evaluate a three-dimensional tracking and control algorithm to steer a small magnetic particle, also called magnobit in the following, through the lens.

2 Materials and Methods

The idea of performing cataract surgery by magnetic actuation is to give the system target positions for the magnobits in order to emulsify the lens automatically or by user input that can be given by the surgeon. For this purpose, a Playstation 3 controller is used as a joystick for user input. State-of-the-art imaging systems are used to determine the actual position of the magnobit: A high-resolution microscope is used to determine the actual position in the xy-plane, while an OCT system provides depth information. Here, the ZEISS Artevo 800 with an integrated OCT system is used. With the current and target positions given, a closed-loop control is implemented to ensure precise movement of the magnetic particle and to prevent so-called *flyouts*, i.e. unintentional puncturing of the capsule bag by the magnet. Based on the localization of the magnobit and a given target trajectory, the controller determines the required magnetic field gradients to be applied to the magnetic field generator used in this project. The system architecture is shown in Fig.1.

The main components of the magnetic field generator system are the Magnebotix MFG-100 coil unit and the Magnebotix ECB-820 power electronics provided by Magnobotix AG, Schlieren, Switzerland. The coils are arranged

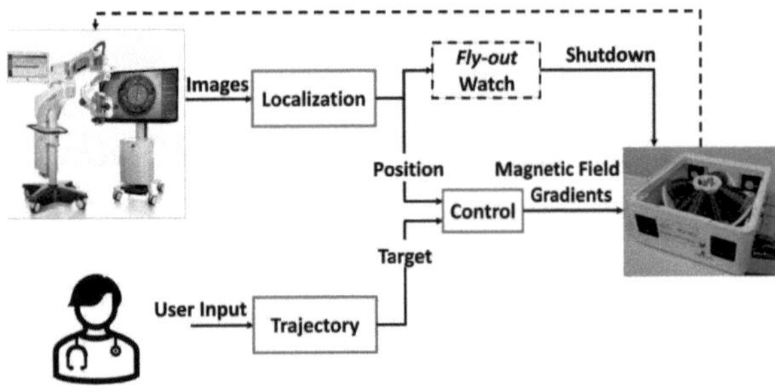

Figure 1: Block diagram of the system architecture. Design and implementation of the framed subsystems are the content of this work.

in a hemisphere to allow easy access for experiments on the coil unit. Each coil is driven by the power electronics through its own channel, which can carry currents of up to 20 A. The magnetic field of the system is limited to 20 mT and the field gradients can reach up to 5 Tm^{-1}. The user can set the magnetic field parameters through the software's graphical user interface (GUI). The software to operate the system is called *MBX_ROS* which is based on ROS, implemented in C++ and runs on Ubuntu. The GUI consists of different panels that also makes it possible to rotate the magnobit around its axes with a maximum frequency of 50 Hz while following a given path. The force F acting on the magnobit is described by

$$\mathbf{F} = v(\mathbf{M} \cdot \nabla)\mathbf{B} \qquad (1)$$

where v is the volume of the magnet, $\mathbf{M}$ the volume magnetization and $\mathbf{B}$ the flux density [4]. Depending on the material and the shape of the magnobits, magnetic forces up to 20 mN can be applied to them. The magnotbits used are listed in Table 1.

Shape	Size	Material
Cube	$a = 1$ mm	NdFeB
Cylinder	$d = 0.8$ mm, $l = 2$ mm	NdFeB
Drill	$d = 1.85$ mm, $l = 3.41$ mm	NdFeB

Table 1: Comparison of the used magnobits.

For the drilling geometry, a cylindrically shaped magnobit was inserted into a self-designed and self-printed drill bit.

2.1 Localization

The x- and y-coordinates can be determined from the camera images and the z-coordinate can be determined from the OCT scans. The information of both sensor modalities then yield the three-dimensional position. To track the magnetic particle in xy-plane, the Channel and Spatial Reliability Tracking algorithm (CSRT) is used. It represents a state-of-the-art tracking algorithm, characterized by a high tracking precision [5]. Compared to machine learning tracking algorithms, the CSRT algorithm does not need to be trained. To initialize the algorithm, an initial bounding box around the magnet is defined by the user and passed to the algorithm.

From this initial bounding box, the algorithm extracts features to detect the magnet in subsequent frames. The estimated camera coordinates are then transformed into the x- and y-coordinates of the reference coordinate system, which is the coordinate system of the magnetic field generator with the origin at the center of the generator. The tracking algorithm was implemented in the ROS environment of the *MBX_ROS* software. For the OCT scans a deep learning tracker has been developed but could not be implemented yet.

2.2 Trajectory

The goal is to emulsify the lens in layers. In other words, to move the magnet in spiral motions from the center to a maximum diameter d_max in total time T and then to move the magnet in z-direction. For this purpose, the time-dependent position of the magnet can be described in polar coordinates (r, ϕ), where r is the radius and ϕ is the angle. With N being whole number of turns, the spiral trajectory can be described by

$$\phi(t) = \frac{2N\pi}{T}t, \quad r(t) = \frac{d_{max}}{T}t. \qquad (2)$$

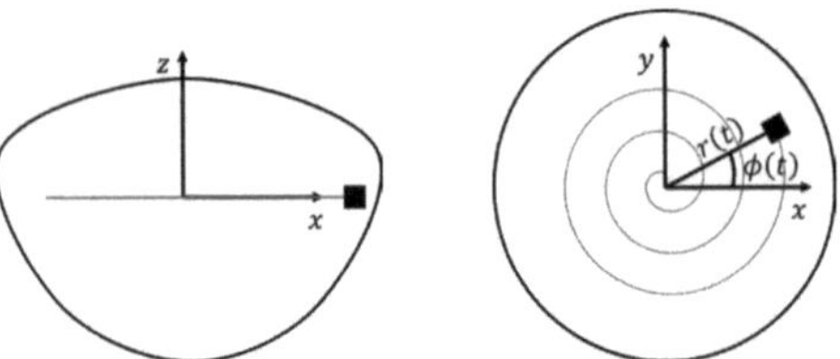

Figure 2: Spiral trajectory from the side view (left) and from the top view (right).

2.3 Control

A combination of feedforward and feedback control is chosen for the control algorithm to achieve fast reference tracking while maintaining good disturbance rejection. The concept of Computed Torque Feedforward control, which is a combination of feedforward and feedback control, is commonly used for motion control in robotics, as described in [6]. The feedforward control calculates the necessary forces to follow the trajectory while the feedback control is essential to minimize the control error caused by external disturbances. This control strategy turned out to be optimal for this project as it yields the best performance. The feedforward control input is described by

$$\mathbf{F}_\text{feedforward} = f(\mathbf{x}_\text{target}, \dot{\mathbf{x}}_\text{target}, \ddot{\mathbf{x}}_\text{target}), \qquad (3)$$

where $\mathbf{F}_\text{feedforward}$ is the computed feedforward control input and $\mathbf{x}_\text{target}$ and the derivatives represent the target states. Instead of using a PID controller, a combination of PI and P controller is used for feedback control. The PI controller represents the position controller and the P controller represents the velocity controller. The reason for excluding the differential controller is the high-frequency and noisy control error signal, which would otherwise be amplified and could lead to control losses. The feedback control input is calculated by

$$\mathbf{F}_{cl} = K_P(\mathbf{x}_{\text{target}} - \mathbf{x}) + K_I \int_{T_0}^{T} (\mathbf{x}_{\text{target}} - \mathbf{x})dt \\ + K_V(\dot{\mathbf{x}}_{\text{target}} - \dot{\mathbf{x}}), \tag{4}$$

where $\mathbf{x}$ represents the current system state, K_P and K_I represent the parameter for the position controller and K_V the parameter of the velocity controller. The heuristic Ziegler-Nichols method was used to set the initial parameters for the controller, but these were further tuned by hand to improve performance as the project progressed [7].

In order to avoid fly-outs, a so-called fly-out watch, which has not yet been implemented, could be implemented in the future as a safeguard. It should only check whether the magnetic particle maintains a minimum distance from the lens capsule. If the distance falls below a given limit, the system should shut down.

3 Results and Discussion

3.1 Evaluation of the Control algorithm

To evaluate the control algorithm, the magnetic actuation is tested in silicone oil. Silicone oil is a clear, colorless and hydrophobic liquid, but less viscous compared to porcine lenses with or without cataract. To evaluate the performance of the control, the magnobit is placed in the sample and the position deviation when the magnet is controlled is compared with the specified trajectory. These experiments were performed only with the cube-shaped magnobit because they were the easiest to control. The error between target and position of the magnobit is calculated in x- and y-direction. From these the euclidean norm is calculated to determine the distance between the target and the actual position. In order to exclude that position errors are calculated, which are caused by lagging or a general time delay of the magnobit, the radial error was calculated. This is a projection of the position error onto the radius of the trajectory. The radial error is particularly interesting because it shows whether the magnet deviates from the trajectory in radial direction and could thus come too close to the capsule bag. The results of the test in silicone oil are represented in Fig. 3.

The errors in x- and y-direction for the PI+P controller did not exceed 150 μm. The euclidean norm of the error shows oscillatory behavior, but remains below a value of 175 μm. The radial error varies between -75 μm and 50 μm, but does not increase significantly over time. All error signals exhibit noise with significant amplitude and low frequency. Overall, the controller can stabilize the magnobit and make it follow the target trajectory.

After obtaining promising results for the control algorithm, the magnetic actuation was tested in porcine lenses. For that, the magnobit was inserted into the lens and the lens was placed on the magnetic field generator. However, the results showed that due to the high resistance of the lens, it was not possible to steer the magnobit through the whole lens with a given trajectory or even with manual control. Therefore, it was only possible to emulsify partial areas of the porcine lenses, which makes an evaluation of the control algorithm based on these experiments not reasonable.

3.2 Forces for Lens Emulsification

Although it was not possible to emulsify the porcine lenses by magnetic actuation, it is of high interest for future work on the project to know what forces would be necessary to emulsify lenses (with or without cataract). To this end, an experimental setup was designed in which magnobits of different shapes are mechanically moved through non-cataract and cataract porcine lenses with a robot arm, in order to measure the required force. Therefor, the lenses were placed on highly sensitive springs and the force could be measured via spring compression. To obtain a continuous measurement of the applied force, a green marker was affixed to the top of the spring and tracked using an RGB tracker. The code for the RGB tracker was written in Python, and the experiments were recorded on a video. The recorded video was then processed by the Python script, which automatically calculated the forces based on the motion of the marker. The experiments assumed that the path along which the magnobit moved through the lens was emulsified. Since pigs do not form cataracts, cataract-like pig lenses were created [8]. For this purpose, fresh pig lenses were extracted from fresh pig eyes and placed in solutions of ethanol and distilled water to harden them. The declaration of the hardness levels is given in Table 2.

Hardness Level	Ethanol Concentration	Insertion Time
I	40%	24 h
II	60%	24 h
III	80%	24 h
IV	100%	24 h

Table 2: Creation of cataract-like porcine lenses

The experiments with non cataract porcine lenses were performed with three different magnobit shapes; with a cube, a cylinder and a drill. The results show that the required force to emulsify non cataract lenses was between 15 mN - 25 mN (see Fig. 4). However, multiple repetitions of the ex-

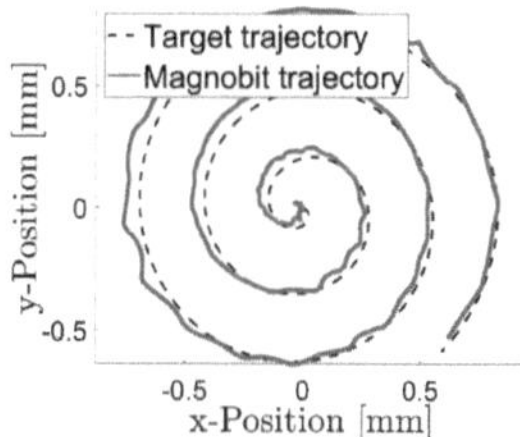

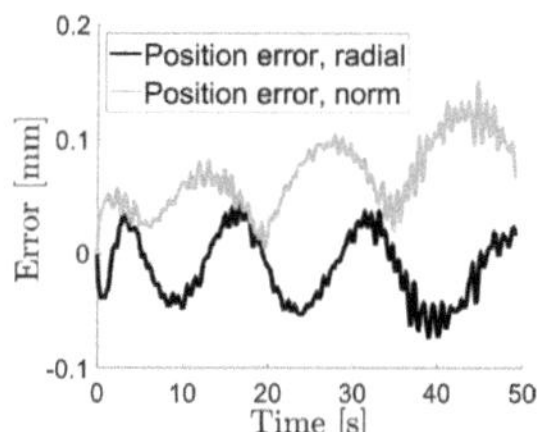

Figure 3: Results of the reference tracking with the cubic magnobit and a given spiral trajectory in silicone oil.

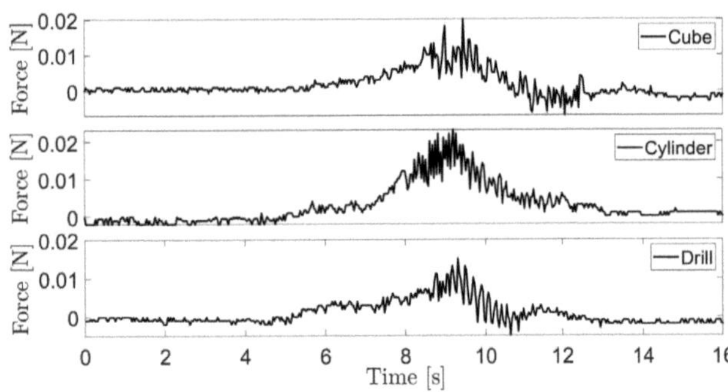

Figure 4: Measured mechanical forces required to emulsify non cataract porcine lenses with different shaped magnobits.

periments have shown that the forces are similar with all geometries, so that no relation between the required force and the shape of the magnobits could be established. Thus, the force measurement on cataract lenses were just performed with the drill shaped magnobits, as they were easiest to use in terms of handling. The results are shown in Fig. 5.

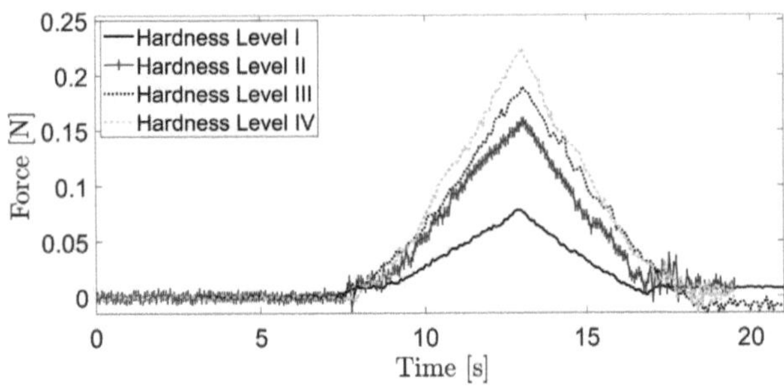

Figure 5: Comparison of the measured forces to emulsify cataract-like porcine lenses with hardening levels **I-IV**.

It can be seen that the forces required to emulsify cataract lenses are 80 mN, 160 mN, 190 mN and 225 mN for hardness levels **I**, **II**, **III** and **IV**, respectively. It perfectly shows the correlation between the hardness levels and the force that must be applied. However, with the fact that only a maximum force of 20 mN can be applied to the magnobits with the selected setup, the force measurements make it clear that emulsification of lenses is not possible at the present time.

4   Conclusion

This study highlights several key achievements and limitations in the application of magnetic actuation for cataract surgery. The first achievement is the demonstration of partial lens emulsification through the movement of a rotating magnobit through the lens using currently available technologies. Additionally, the study shows that automatic closed-loop control of the magnobit is possible in silicone oil. However, it must be noted that the degree of lens emulsification achieved is limited and dependent on the condition of the porcine lenses. Additionally, the movement of

the magnobit inside the lens is slow and non-linear, and frequent shutdowns of the magnetic field generator due to overheating were observed when high magnetic fields were maintained statically.

Despite these limitations, the results of the study confirm the potential advantages of magnetic actuation in terms of automation and learnability. The results also provide important insights into the amount of mechanical force required to emulsify lenses of different cataract stages, which can be used to optimize the experimental setup in the future. This study serves as a starting point for further investigation into the potential of magnetic actuation for cataract surgery and provides a platform for future research.

Acknowledgement

The work has been carried out at Carl Zeiss AG in Karlsruhe, and supervised by Prof. Dr. Philipp Rostalski, Institute for Electrical Engineering in Medicine, Universität zu Lübeck.

Author's Statement

Conflict of interest: Author state no conflict of interest.

5   References

[1] D. Allen, A. Vasavada, *Cataract and surgery for cataract*. BMJ, vol.333, no. 7559, pp.128-132, 2006.

[2] S. Prasad, *Phacoemulsification learning curve: Experience of two junior trainee ophthalmologists*. Journal of Cataract & Refractive Surgery, vol. 24, no. 1, pp. 73-77, 1998.

[3] C. D. Kelman, *The History and Development of Phacoemulsification*. International Ophthalmology Clinics, vol. 34, pp. 1–12, 1994

[4] T. Boyer, *The force on a magnetic dipole*. American Journal of Physics, vol. 56, pp. 688-692, 1988.

[5] A. Lukežic, T. Vojir, L.C. Zajc, J. Matas and M. Kristan, *Discriminative Correlation Filter with Channel and Spatial Reliability*. IEEE Conference on Computer Vision and Pattern Recognition (CVPR), pp. 4847-4856, 2017.

[6] C. An, C. Atkeson, J. Griffiths and J. Hollerbach, *Experimental evaluation of feedforward and computed torque control*. International Conference on Robotics and Automation, vol. 4, pp. 165-168, 1987.

[7] J. Ziegler and N. Nichols, *Optimum Settings for Automatic Controllers*. Journal of Fluids Engneering, 1942.

[8] T. Sugiura et al., *Creating cataract in a pig eye*. Journal of Cataract & Refractive Surgery, vol. 25, no. 5, pp. 615-621, 1999.

Technical Realization of a Medical Assessment of Geriatrics

Lena Hansen [1], Natascha Koch [2], Alfred Mertins [3]

[1] Medizinische Ingenieurwissenschaft, Universität zu Lübeck, lena.hansen@student.uni-luebeck.de
[2] AI in Biomedical Signal Processing, German Research Center for Artificial Intelligence, natascha.koch@dfki.de
[3] Institut for Signal Processing, Universität zu Lübeck, mertins@isip.uni-luebeck.de

Abstract

In clinics geriatric assessments are generally run without much electronic aid. One of these geriatric assessments is the "20-Cent-Test", that is used to measure the progress of patients' fine motor skills during rehab. It is a simple test in which the patients have to place 20 one cent coins in a container, while a medical staff measures the time. The goal of this project was to create a prototype device, that automates the "20-Cent-Test" and measures the time automatically. The project was realized in collaboration with Dr. Dr. Ulrich Kuipers of the Asklepios Klinik Bad Oldesloe. The device was designed with capacitive sensors to detect the fingers picking up the coins and photoelectric sensors to track the presence of the coins.

1   Introduction

For geriatric patients who have problems with fine motor skills, it is important to measure their progress during rehabilitation. There are standardized geriatric assessments [1] that qualitatively and quantitatively assess the resources of older people in terms of significant and relevant functional limitations [3]. They examine different functional levels like: daily living skills and self-help competence, social environment and participation, quality of life, emotion and depression, cognition, locomotion, visual acuity and acusis.

For standardization of the basic geriatric assessment, the so-called AGAST convention was invented in the 1990s in the German-speaking countries of Central Europe (Geriatric Assessment Working Group 1997). Internationally, the interRAI consortium has been promoting further standardization for different areas of application since the 2000s. There are roughly four categories of assessments: Individual tests that measure only one aspect, screeners e.g. geriatric screening according to Lachs, basic assessment like the geriatric assessment according to the AGAST convention and extended assessments e.g. basic assessment extended by a detailed gerontopsychiatric test regarding dementia with SIDAM [4].

One if the individual tests is the "20-Cent-Test. It was first proposed in 2009. In 2015 a study investigating quality criteria for that test was published by Krupp et al. [5]. The test works as follows: 20 one cent coins lie in a circle. The distance between the coins is about the same as the diameter of the coins (16,25 mm). Above the coins is a container with a diameter of at least 8 cm and a maximum height of 4 cm. The task is to place the coins, one by one, in the container, while the therapist or doctor measures the time. Krupp et al. found that there is a correlation between fine motor skill level and task completion time, thus the test is suitable to measure the patient's progress.

In geriatric clinics, geriatric assessments are normally run manually, only with pen, paper and a stopwatch. An electronic device would facilitate the documentation process and could also measure more than a human could, like the time a patient needs to pick up each coin.

The goal of this project is to create a prototype device that automatically measures the time it takes patients to pick up all coins. The device will be developed as an in-house development of the Asklepios Klinik Bad Oldesloe.

2   Material and Methods

The project was planned with Dr. Dr. Ulrich Kuipers of the Asklepios Klinik Bad Oldesloe, who already built a similar test, called the "20 Kugel-Test" (20 ball-test) [6]. It is modeled after the 20-Cent-Test, except patients are required to pick up metal balls weighing 60 g instead of coins. Dr. Dr. Kuipers used heavier objects instead of coins because they can be picked up more easily by capacitive sensors. The device can record the time it takes for each metal ball to be picked up, but cannot detect the fingers of the patient or the placing of the metal balls in a container.

In this paper a prototype device is described that can detect one cent coins and the patients' fingers while they touch the surface of the device for picking up a one cent coin. The device will be operated by medical staff only. A specification sheet detailing the machine's requirements and optional features was created. Multiple possible implementations that meet the given criteria were described and considered.

2.1   Specification sheet

The first requirement is that the device has to work like the manual "20-Cent-Test". The coins may not be significantly heavier than real one cent coins or manipulated in shape. The device should not introduce any bias to the results when compared to the original test. The device should measure the duration of the test from start to finish, capturing the moment the first finger touches the first coin and the moment the last coin is placed in the container. In addition to measuring the duration of the test, the device should also record the duration of finger contact with each coin while it remains on the plate. Further requirements are an easy to clean surface, as it does get in direct contact with every patient, and a sturdy construction, as the individuals might rest their hands on it. Other specifications include the absence of sharp edges, galvanic isolation, and voltage that must be below six volts. The device must be designed with user-friendliness as a priority, especially for elderly people with little technical background.

The optional features are the calculation of variance, median and mean of the duration of the lifting of every coin, further measurements like the arm movement and using a hand tracking tool for hand tracking.

2.2   Implementation options

There are several ways to develop a device that meets these criteria. To meet the first point, the best solution is to find a possibility to use the test with ordinary one cent coins. For the automatic measurement it is possible to connect simple sensors to a micro controller. To detect the coins, a capacitive sensor might not work, but it is easy to use a photoelectric sensor. For finger recognition, a capacitive sensor could be the best choice, as it can easily detect human skin and it allows to shape proximity antennas in any way that is needed and the fingers could be anywhere around the coin, while the patient picks it up. It would be much harder to detect that with a single reflective sensor.

To detect the coins in the container, there are also different possibilities. One could use a scale to measure the weight, but one cent coins are very light (2,3 g), so it must be a very sensitive one. Another possibility is to use a pressure sensor to detect each fall of the coins. An issue arises when patients handle the coins delicately, which may lead to inaccurate measurement. Another possibility is to use a reflective sensor. For this technique to work, the container has to either contain a net of light barriers, or contain a funnel through which coins pass through a tight opening for a single photoelectric sensor.

For hygienic reasons, the surface should be made of plastic or glass and should be made of one piece or different parts that are well sealed. A thin layer of acrylic glass is not stable enough as a cover. Sturdiness can be achieved by another layer of a resilient material underneath the thin top layer.

The next point that has to be addressed is the usability. Touch displays are very intuitive human-mashine interfaces, even for people who use them for the first time. [2] The display should also be large, not only for usability but also because 20 different values have to be displayed at the same time during the test.

3   Results and Discussion

The next step was designing the device in a way that meets all the requirements that were discussed in the chapter before.

3.1   Development of the electronic

The program was run on a ESP32 D1 Mini (Espressif Systems). Infrared (IR)-photoelectric sensors TCRT5000 (Vishay), with a wavelength of 950 nm were used to detect whether or not the coin is lying on the surface and capacitive touch sensors to detect the fingers. So the surface layer has to be IR-permeable for the photoelectric sensors to work and thin enough for the capacitive sensors to work. IR-permeable 1 mm black acrylic glass was used. One additional photoelectric sensor is used for the detection of the coins in the container. Multiplexers route these 20 analog inputs to three input channels before they are fed into the microcontroller. For capacitive input sensing, 20 passive circular proximity antennas are connected to two AT42QT2120-SU controllers (Microchip Technology). The I2C-Bus connects these to the ESP32 D1 Mini. The touch display is directly connected to the controller with a voltage supply of 3.3 volts.

An individual printed circuit board (PCB) that is shown in figure 1 was developed for the system and also the passive circular proximity antennas of the touch sensors were individually designed. They were made of the same material as the board.

For programming the ESP, the application Visual Studio Code with PlatformIO was used. The scripts were written in C_{++}.

During tests, the photoelectric sensors worked perfectly through the acrylic glass, but the proximity antennas had some sensitivity issues. Some of them were too sensitive, and some of them did not work at all. This problem needs further investigation.

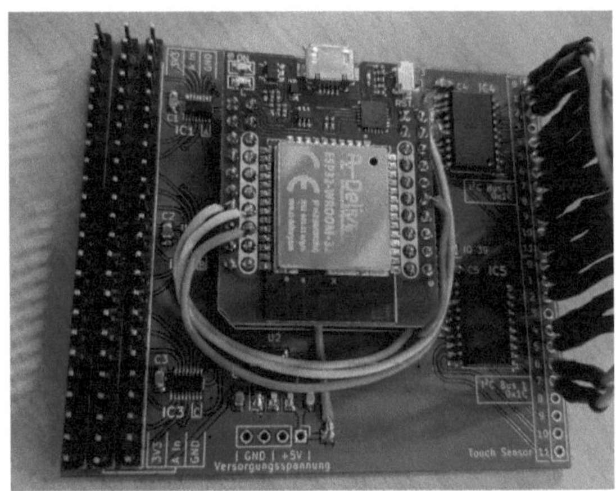

Figure 1: PCB with ESP32 D1 Mini

3.2   Case design

Autodesk Fusion 360 was used for designing the case and the container as shown in figure 2 and 3. For the production, the opportunity was given to use a laser cutter and 3D-printer of the FABLAB Lübeck. The laser cutter can cut through wood and acrylic glass. The case was constructed from thin wood, with the side panels being composed of 5mm-thick white painted MDF. The top panel was composed of two layers of wood, with the lower top panel measuring 3mm in thickness. The circular proximity antennas are put through cut outs in the panel and rest on top of it as shown in figure 4. The upper top panel lies on top of this cover and has cut outs to frame the antennas. It is 2 mm thick, which is enough, so the top layer made of the black acrylic glass can cover it without coming in contact with the proximity antennas, that are 1.6 mm in hight. The covers are screwed into wooden blocks. The height of the case is 4 cm. Sharp edges will be prevented by grinding the edges after assembling the case. To place the coins at the correct position, thin markings will be printed on the acrylic glass.

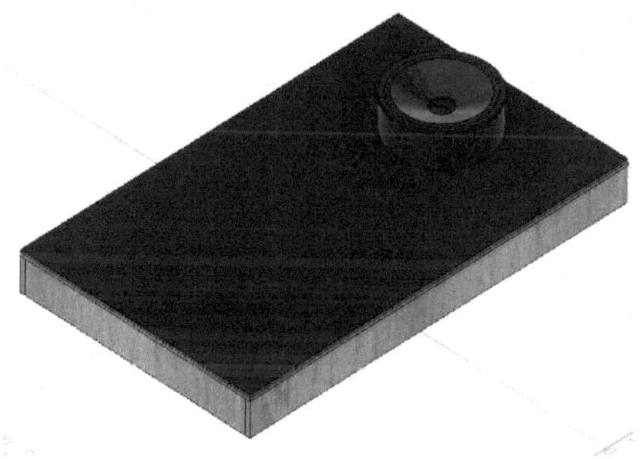

Figure 2: Case with container, designed in Autodesk Fusion 360.

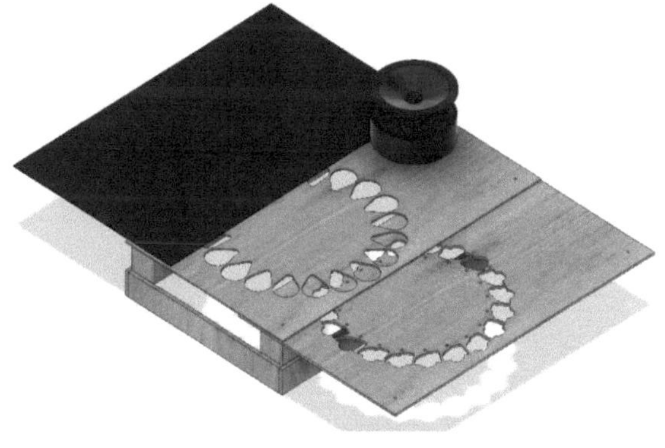

Figure 3: Exploded view of the case with the container

3.3   Design of the container

The container that is shown in figure 5 and 6 is designed with a removable funnel on top, through which the coins

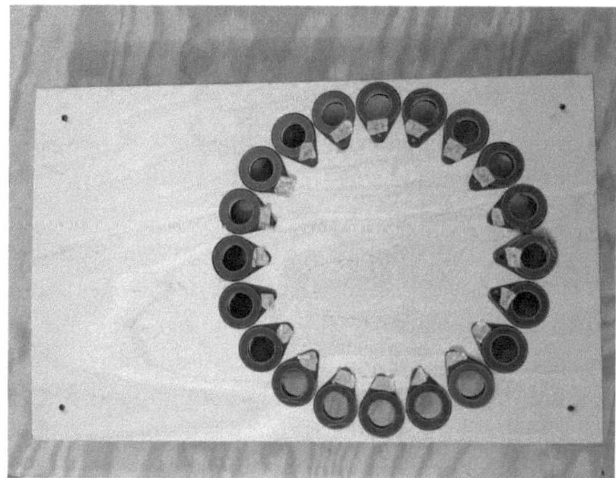

Figure 4: Case with touch sensors, without the acrylic glass top panel.

will fall past a single photoelectric sensor. Autodesk Fusion 360 was used for designing it. The container will be held in place on the case with two magnets, that are placed in the bottom of the container and under the cover of the case. The design preserves the acrylic glass, except for screw holes, making cleaning easier. Another benefit of the magnetic attachment is that the container can be easily detached to empty the coins. The container will be produced by 3D-printing.

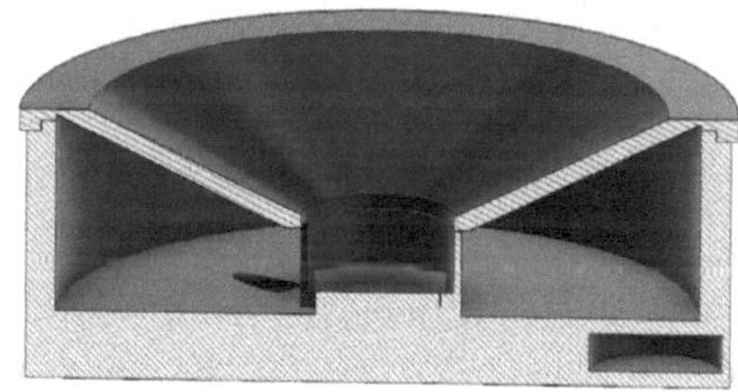

Figure 5: Container (sectional view), the magnet has to be placed in the free space at the bottom of the container during the print.

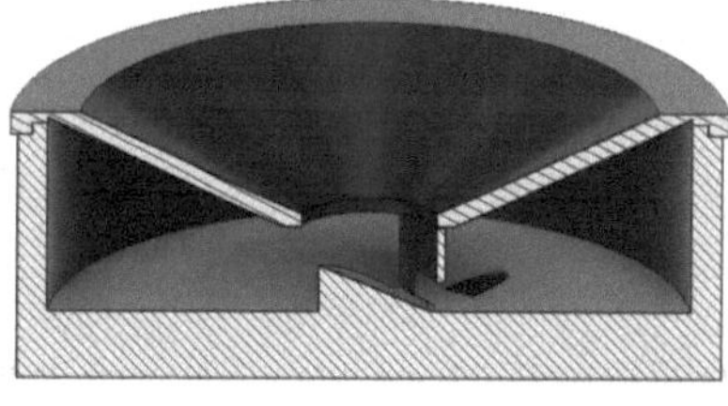

Figure 6: Container (sectional view), the coins fall through the funnel on the slant and slide through an opening in the inner wall. There can be detectet with a single photoelectric sensor, which will be placed behind the slant.

3.4   User interface

The Nextion 7.0" touch display was chosen as a display, because of the size and the fact that it is possible to store a program directly on the display, so it is not necessary to control it completely with the ESP. The user interface should be as intuitive as possible without unnecessary configuration options.

For programming the interface, the programm "Nextion Editor" was used. It is a specialized software designed for that display.

The programm for the device starts by pressing "Starte Test" (start test) as shown in figure 7 on the display. It will then switch to another page, were the 20 coins are depicted as numbers in a circle. When the patient picks up a coin, the number will be highlighted, as long as the fingers touch the surface and disappear, when the coin and fingers no longer have contact to the surface. The individual times and the total duration of the test can be viewed on the next page, if the user presses the button "Ergebnisse anzeigen" (show results). The user can go back to the front page, by pressing "zurück" (back).

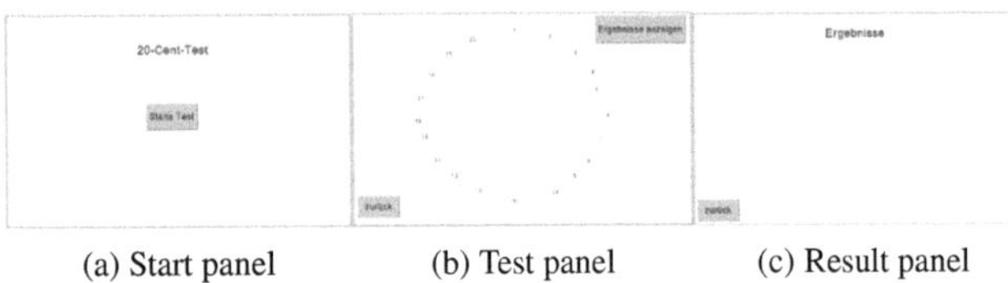

(a) Start panel   (b) Test panel   (c) Result panel

Figure 7: First concept of the user interface, the buttons work, but the display is not yet connected to the ESP

3.5 Current state

At this point, the concept and design of the device have been finalized, but the prototype has not yet been built completely. The touch sensors can detect skin through the acrylic glass, but do not work reliable. The photoelectric sensors are working through the acrylic glass, but are not yet connected to the ESP. Tests have been made with another ESP and single photoelectric sensors. One prototype of the container has been printed, but it is not the final version. There have also been problems with printing the funnel that have to be approached. A test software has been uploaded on the display. The next steps are connecting the photoelectric sensors to the ESP, programming the final software for the ESP and the display and developing a power source.

4 Conclusion

A prototype device that automatically measures the time it takes patients to pick up 20 coins of a flat surface and place them in a container has been designed. A way of measuring the duration of the fingers resting from the surface, while picking up each coin, has also been developed. The detection of one cent coins through a 1 mm layer of acrylic glass works well, however there are still problems with the capacitive sensors that have to be approached. Not all requirements have been implemented in this state of development. The device is not yet galvanically isolated and the case does not meet the safety standards yet.

This device is meant to replace the manual running of the "20-Cent-Test", but this kind of device can also be used for training in form of gamification of the test. The coins can be easily replaced with other objects, without changing the way of tracking them, due to them being detect by simple photoelectric sensors.

Acknowledgement

The work has been carried out by the Institute for Signal Processing at the University of Lübeck. A special thank goes to the FabLab Lübeck e.V. to provide the access to a laser cutter, 3D-printers and soldering equipment.

Author's Statement

Conflict of interest: Authors state no conflict of interest.

References

[1] BfArM. *OPS 8-550 Frührehabilitative und physikalische Therapie - Geriatrische frührehabilitative Komplexbehandlung*. Oct. 16, 2020. URL: `https : / / www . dimdi . de / static / de / klassifikationen / ops / kode - suche / opshtml2021/block-8-55...8-60.htm# code8-550` (visited on 01/21/2023).

[2] A. Britton, R. Setchi, and A. Marsh. "Intuitive interaction with multifunctional mobile interfaces". In: *Journal of King Saud University - Computer and Information Sciences* 25.2 (2013), pp. 187–196. URL: `https : / / www . sciencedirect . com / science / article / pii/S1319157812000420`.

[3] Heinrich Burkhardt. "Geriatrisches Assessment – ein wichtiges Tool für die Therapieselektion in der Onkologie". In: *Geriatrische Onkologie*. Ed. by Matthias Ebert, Nicolai Härtel, and Ulrich Wedding. Berlin, Heidelberg: Springer Berlin Heidelberg, 2018, pp. 37–52. ISBN: 978-3-662-48727-3. DOI: `10 . 1007/978-3-662-48727-3_4`. URL: `https: //doi.org/10.1007/978-3-662-48727- 3_4`.

[4] Sonja Krupp. "Geriatrisches Assessment leitliniengerecht gestalten". In: *Geriatrie-Report* (Nov. 19, 2020). URL: `https : / / doi . org / 10 . 1007 / s42090-020-0634-4`.

[5] Sonja Krupp et al. "Timed up and go test for fingers in the form of the 20 cents test. Psychometric criteria of a simple performance test of fine motor skills". In: *Zeitschrift fur Gerontologie und Geriatrie* 48.2 (2015), pp. 121–127.

[6] Ulrich Kuipers. "e20-ball-test: a new electronic device to explore fine motor skills". In: *Zeitschrift für Gerontologie und Geriatrie* (2022).

Extended Percutaneous MAZE in Combination with Vein of Marshall Ethanol Ablation in Persistent Atrial Fibrillation – EP-AMAZE-IT –

Neha Johny [1], Tolga Agdirlioglu [2], Olaf Krahnefeld [2]

[1] Biomedical Engineering, Technische Hochschule Lübeck, Universität zu Lübeck, neha.johny@stud.th-luebeck.de
[2] Sektion Elektrophysiologie, Sana Kliniken Lübeck, tolga.agdirlioglu@sana.de
[2] Sektion Elektrophysiologie, Sana Kliniken Lübeck, olaf.krahnefeld@sana.de

Abstract

A retrospective single-centre analysis is conducted to evaluate the therapeutic concept in patients with recurrence of Atrial Fibrillation (AF) or Atrial Tachycardia (AT) after successful previous Pulmonary Vein Isolation (PVI). The study was carried out by extracting, collecting, and analyzing the data of the patients who had undergone all four procedures (namely PVI, EIVOM, endo-RF, and LAA-Occlusion). The analysis shows that this hybrid concept consisting of extended endocardial RF-ablation (extended MAZE) preceded by epicardial ethanol ablation of the Vein of Marshall (VOM) and followed by the implantation of an LAA (Left Atrial Appendage) occluder is a highly safe treatment in patients with AF or AT recurrence when all four veins are isolated.

1 Introduction

Over the years, there has been an increase in the number of patients with recurrence of Atrial Fibrillation (AF) or Atrial Tachycardia (AT) after Pulmonary Vein Isolation (PVI) who show persistent isolation of all four pulmonary veins (PV) during re-procedure.

Left atrial (LA) low-voltage areas (LVAs) may trigger atrial fibrillation in these patients. A recent study by Bordignon consisted of a percutaneous MAZE procedure including isolation of the LVAs on the LA anterior wall along with electrical isolation of the Left Atrial Appendage (LAA) with subsequent implantation of an LAA-occlusion device for stroke prevention. Freedom from AF or AT has been achieved in 65% of these patients. However, it was associated with a slightly higher complication rate of 7%, mainly pericardial tamponade or effusion, compared to PVI-only procedures [1].

Moreover, the scientific literature data support ethanol-ablation of the VOM as an add-on therapy in patients with persistent AF, besides other complex LA procedures. After the ethanol-ablation of the VOM was performed, the patients with persistent AF were observed to be very often in sinus rhythm (SR) during the follow-up. The electrical blocking of the lateral mitral isthmus has been achieved several times by using comparatively lower RF energy after a previous ethanol-ablation of the VOM, which was illustrated already in other studies [2], [3], [4]. Furthermore, the electrical isolation of the LAA might result in a better long-term outcome if LAA isolation was performed by ostial but not linear (remote-line) isolation, which further avoided the recurrence of AT probably originating from the reconnection of the ablation lines.

In this retrospective single-centre study, EP-AMAZE-IT, the objective is to investigate the safety and outcome of a treatment combination of the ablation strategies- mentioned above with a more extensive percutaneous MAZE ablation. Besides, the study evaluates whether these methods are associated with increased complication rates due to performing three consecutive procedures in a single patient. Here, it is hypothesized that the ethanol ablation of VOM leads to a better outcome for the electrical isolation of a substantial proportion of the anterior wall, including the LAA. Additionally, the isolation of the posterior wall instead of a roofline is less dangerous and more effective in the era of the CLOSE protocol.

2 Material and Methods

The patients who suffer from recurrence of persistent AF after PVI outside the blanking period of 3 months were identified as candidates for EP-AMAZE-IT. As a part of the re-ablation, an extensive percutaneous MAZE procedure in combination with the ethanol ablation of the VOM was done in cases of persistent AF. The patients were informed about the procedures (EIVOM, endo-RF, and LAA-Occlusion) and the potential risks. Written informed consent was also obtained from each patient.

Pulmonary Vein Isolation (PVI):
The prerequisite was the persistent isolation of all four PVs after PVI was done according to CLOSE protocol.

Ethanol Infusion of Vein of Marshall (EIVOM):
The ethanol infusion or ablation of the Vein of Marshall was performed as previously described in the paper [4].

Endocardial Radio-Frequency Ablation (endo-RF):
After 3-6 weeks, an endocardial RF ablation procedure was performed. If the patients had all four PVs isolated, however, with the presence of an LVA in the LA that was not due to ethanol ablation, the following endocardial ablation was done.

The ablation line set in the endocardial procedure (endo MAZE) is as follows:

- A lateral mitral isthmus line from the mitral annulus to the left inferior pulmonary vein.
- A posterior wall line from the left inferior vein to the right inferior vein.
- An anterior wall line from the carina between the right superior and right inferior pulmonary vein to the superior part of the mitral annulus.
- Isolation of the anterior wall, posterior wall, and LAA was proven with high-density mapping acquired during sinus rhythm of the isolated area.
- An ablation protocol according to the CLOSE protocol.
- After the successful isolation of anterior and posterior walls, the induction protocol was performed. All mappable tachycardia were mapped and ablated. An RA (right atrial) CTI (cavotricuspid isthmus) block was created if typical RA flutter was inducible, and SVC (superior vena cava) isolation was performed if rapid non-mappable AT was still inducible.

The approach used for the re-ablation procedure also consisted of the following: ultrasound-guided vascular access of the femoral veins, uninterrupted (phenprocoumon, rivaroxaban, edoxaban) or ultrashort (dabigatran, apixaban) interrupted oral anticoagulation, intraprocedural anticoagulation with heparin (target ACT- activated clotting time>300s), mechanical ventilation during the procedure, real-time esophageal temperature monitoring, invasive monitoring of the arterial blood pressure, blood gas samples every 30 minutes, partial antagonization of the heparin effect with protamine at the end of the procedure, vascular closure with Z (also called Figure of 8) suture, and transthoracic echo.

Implantation of LAA occlusion device:
3-6 weeks after the endo-RF procedure, the implantation of the LAA occlusion device was performed as described in the paper [5]. The LAA closure device used was WATCHMAN FLX™ or WATCHMAN™ *(Boston Scientific Corporation)*.

Inclusion criteria:

- Age >18 years
- Previous PVI with invasively demonstrated isolation of all four PVs.
- Persistent recurrence of AF or AT.

Exclusion criteria:

- No low-voltage zones in the LA (except for the area of ethanol ablation).
- The patient is neither willing nor a candidate for subsequent implantation of the LAA occluder.

This retrospective analysis included relevant data corresponding to all the patients who had undergone PVI from November 2019 to August 2021 at the Electrophysiology Unit of Sana Kliniken Lübeck. The necessary data were obtained from *E&L, MCC, Carto, and Sensis*. Further data, such as Holter-ECG(electrocardiogram) reports, were collected through follow-ups and others through telephone interviews. Ablation energy and RF time employed for the interventions, post-procedural complications, and follow-up data were considered crucial parameters for the analysis. All the data were pseudonymized and stored in an Excel spreadsheet. *Tableau 2021* was used to create the graphs for analysis.

3 Results and Discussion

Of the 399 patients identified with PVI, 298 had undergone only the standard PVI procedure following the CLOSE protocol. However, another 90 had a recurrence of AF, even with all four PVs isolated, and had undergone EIVOM. Among them, there were 41 EP-AMAZE-IT candidates chosen based on the criteria discussed. Of these, 5 cases were found to have no LAA occluder implanted during the study period. Additionally, there was one patient who received an occluder before PVI.

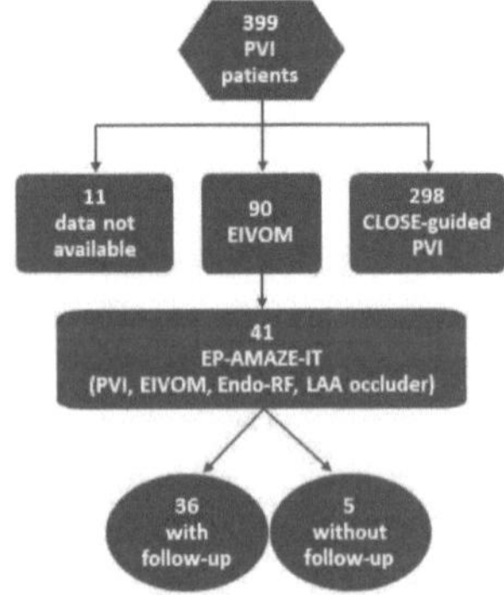

Figure 1: Flow chart showing the patient extraction

3.1 Baseline Patient Characteristics

Table 1 illustrates the baseline characteristics of the 90 patients. In the echocardiography, the LA diameter was dilated in 65 patients. It was dilated heavily in one and slightly in 15 other patients. The left ventricular (LV) function was preserved in 79 patients. Around 11 patients had mildly to severely reduced LV function.

Table 1: Baseline Characteristics

Characteristics	$N = 90$
Age, mean±SD	69.90 ± 10.27
Males, n (%)	39 (43.33)
Females, n (%)	51 (56.67)
BMI, mean±SD	28.44 ± 4.81
CVRF, n (%)	81 (90)
Hypertension, n (%)	68 (75.55)
Nicotine, n (%)	18 (20)
Dyslipidemia, n (%)	18 (20)
Family history vascular disease, n (%)	12 (13.33)
Diabetes mellitus, n (%)	15 (16.67)
Sleep apnoea, n (%)	2 (2.22)
Hyperuricemia, n (%)	4 (4.44)
Impaired Glucose Tolerance, n (%)	4 (4.44)
Hypercholesterolemia, n (%)	17 (18.89)
GFR before EIVOM (mL/min/1.m²) $n = 77$, mean±SD	66.77 ± 20.29
GFR after EIVOM (mL/min/1.m²) $n = 85$, mean±SD	70.62 ± 18.95
CHA2DS2-VASc score $\geq$ 3, n (%)	57 (63.33)
HAS-BLED score (0 or not available), n (%)	43 (47.78)
HAS-BLED score $\geq$ 1, n (%)	47 (52.22)
EHRA score $\geq$ 2, n (%)	86 (95.55)
LAA velocity (cm/s) $n = 84$, mean+SD	41.63 ± 22.18
Undergone previous procedures (PVI, CTI, etc), n (%)	88 (97.78)

BMI=Body Mass Index, CVRF=Cardio Vascular Risk Factors, SD=Standard deviation, GFR=Glomerular Filtration Rate, EHRA=European Heart Rhythm Association

The CHA2DS2-VASc score helps to determine the annual thromboembolic or stroke risk for patients with AF. The HAS-BLED score is a similar approach which estimates the risk for major bleeding in patients with AF taking anticoagulants. In both cases, a higher score implies a higher risk.

3.1.1 Medications

Monitoring the medicine intake is an essential part of the planning and treatment of AF. The drug intake after the endo-RF procedure was documented. The drugs prescribed to the patients after EIVOM were recorded if the list of medications after endo-RF was unavailable.

Of the 90 patients mentioned earlier, around 80 consumed oral anticoagulants (OAC) and beta-blockers (BB) after EIVOM or endo-RF. More than half of the patients took angiotensin convertase inhibitors (ACEI) or angiotensin receptor-1 blockers (AT1B). Roughly 15 patients were on antiarrhythmic drugs (AAD) and aldosterone antagonists. Nearly half of the patients were on the drug TAH (Telmisartan, Amlodipine, and Hydrochlorothiazide). Around 40% of the patients took diuretics, and another 10% were on phenprocoumon or Marcumar.

Filtering out the EP-AMAZE-IT patients, it was clear that over 85% patients were on medications such as OAC, TAH, BB, and AT1B/ ACEI after the endo-RF procedure. Over 43% still took diuretics, and nearly 15-20% were on Marcumar and AAD.

3.2 PVI and EP-AMAZE-IT

In every individual treatment or intervention, all applicable information corresponding to the parameters such as fluoroscopy time, radiation dosage, need for mechanical ventilation, amount of the contrast fluid, procedure duration, heart rhythm at the start and end of the procedure, LAA velocity before and after the ablation, and the volume of ethanol used was recorded. The data analysis showed that the number of CLOSE-protocol ablation points, averages of LA volume, ablation temperature, impedance during ablation, and ablation index used for PVI were 98, 128.8 ml, 24°C, 130 Ω, and 507, respectively, and that for EP-AMAZE-IT were 116, 152.2 ml, 24°C, 123 Ω, and 507 respectively. The following sections describe the further inferences that were made.

The average ablation energies used for the PVI and the EP-AMAZE-IT procedures were analyzed. The energy used on the anterior wall, posterior wall, and that for the whole ablation procedure were compared. Fig.2 elucidates that the ablation energy employed for EP-AMAZE-IT is slightly greater than that for the standard PVI. However, it is noteworthy that the energy difference is not so huge, provided the extensive MAZE ablation performed in the patient. Similarly, the average time taken for the RF abla-

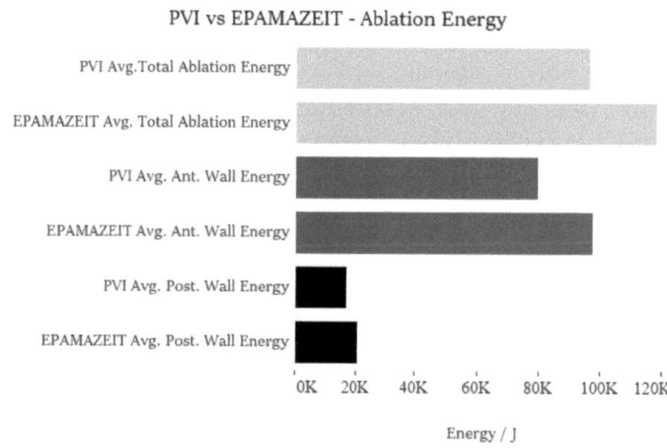

Figure 2: A comparison of the ablation energies used in PVI and EP-AMAZE-IT.

tion in the standard PVI and the EP-AMAZE-IT procedures were compared. Fig.3 depicts that the RF exposure time for the entire ablation procedure and that of the posterior wall of the heart were quite comparable in both the PVI and the

EP-AMAZE-IT. Therefore, it is evident that the ablation energy and RF time used for the EP-AMAZE-IT protocol is as safe as the standard PVI procedure.

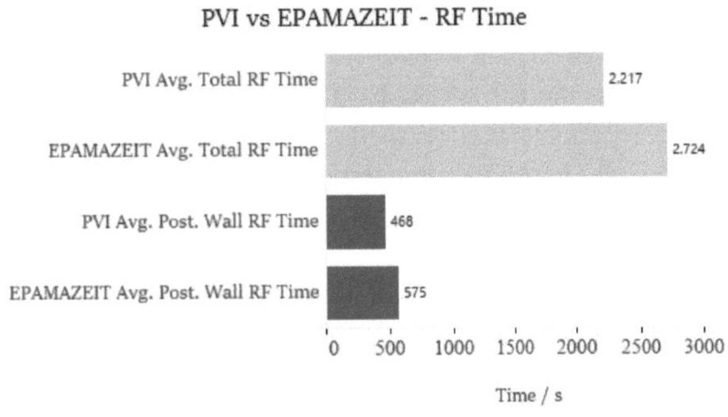

Figure 3: A comparison of the RF times taken for PVI and EP-AMAZE-IT.

3.3 Complications

Some primary risks of the patients undergoing ablation treatments for AF comprise pericardial tamponade or effusion, apoplexy, TIA (transient ischaemic attack or stroke), AV (arteriovenous) fistula, thermal esophageal lesions, hematoma, and death. Among these, stroke, apoplexy, AV fistula, and death were entirely ruled out in all the EP-AMAZE-IT candidates. On the contrary, one patient (2.78%) suffered from pericardial tamponade, and three patients (8.33%) had thermal lesions in the esophagus after the endo-RF procedure. Another three (8.33%) and two patients (5.55%) had hematoma after endo-RF and LAA occlusion procedures, respectively. 89% of the EP-AMAZE-IT patients underwent cardioversion before EIVOM or after PVI. However, none of these patients had cardioversion during the blanking time or after the endo-RF ablation.

3.4 Follow-ups

The follow-ups of 36 EP-AMAZE-IT patients were carried out as the remaining five candidates were unavailable. The follow-up data were collected after a minimum of three months to a maximum possible duration of 21 months. One key follow-up parameter was ECG. During the 24-hour Holter monitoring, 34 patients, i.e., 94.44%, and 20 patients, i.e., 55.55% among the 36 patients, were in SR(sinus rhythm) after 6 and 12 months of EIVOM, respectively. Again, 28 patients, i.e., 77.77%, and 16 patients, i.e., 44.44% of the 36, were in SR after 6 and 12 months of endo-RF, respectively. The follow-up data suggest that these patients often attained freedom from the recurrence of persistent AF at one-year follow-up.

4   Conclusion

Based on the results, it can be deduced that the patients who underwent all the procedures according to the EP-AMAZE-IT protocol were often free from recurrence of persistent AF at one-year follow-up. The EP-AMAZE-IT patients suffered only from a few post-procedural complications despite performing three consecutive interventions in the same patient. The ablation energy and RF time employed for the ablation strategies are also acceptable or justifiable. However, the study has some limitations despite the meticulousness given to the investigation. One of the downsides is the small number of subjects involved in the study. Another drawback is the short time frame for the follow-up and collecting enough post-procedural information. Nevertheless, the study indicates the high safety of the hybrid treatment protocol for treating persistent AF, besides giving an outcome comparable to the treatment strategies or studies previously conducted. There is future scope- the study presents a possibility for performing the investigation further on a large scale for patients diagnosed with persistent AF.

Acknowledgement

The work has been carried out at the Sana Kliniken Lübeck GmbH and was supervised by Prof. Dr. med. Joachim Weil, Universität zu Lübeck and Sana Kliniken Lübeck GmbH.

Author's Statement

Neha Johny has received a research grant from Boston Scientific for this work. All other authors state no conflict of interest.

5   References

[1] S. Bordignon, L. Perrotta, et al., (2017). *Electrical isolation of the Left Atrial Appendage by maze-like catheter substrate modification: A reproducible strategy for pulmonary vein isolation nonresponders?* Journal of Cardiovascular Electrophysiology.

[2] M. Valderrábano, L. E. Peterson, et al., (2020). *Effect of catheter ablation With Vein of Marshall ethanol infusion vs catheter ablation alone on persistent atrial fibrillation.*, JAMA, 324(16), 1620–.

[3] X. Liu, M. Valderrábano, et al., (2009). *Ethanol infusion in the vein of Marshall: Adjunctive effects during ablation of atrial fibrillation.*, 6(11), 1552–1558.

[4] M. Takigawa, K. Vlachos, et al., *Acute and mid-term outcome of ethanol infusion of vein of Marshall for the treatment of perimitral flutter.*, EP Europace, Volume 22, Issue 8, August 2020, Pages 1252–1260.

[5] M. Glikson, R. Wolff, et al., (2019) *EHRA/EAPCI expert consensus statement on catheter-based left atrial appendage occlusion – an update*, EP Europace, Volume 22, Issue 2, February 2020, Page 184.

Determination and Evaluation of the Connection Process and Speed of the Communication Protocols UART, I²C and SPI for a given Ultra-Low Power Hardware with Limited CPU Power

Andreas Wolf [1], Jasper Schöler [2], Thomas Graßl [3], Max Urban [4]

[1] Biomedical Engineering, Lübeck University of Applied Sciences, andreas.wolf@stud.th-luebeck.de
[2] Mechatronik, Hamburg University of Applied Sciences, jasper.schoeler@haw-hamburg.de
[3] BU HCA, Drägerwerk AG Co. KGaA, Lübeck, thomas.grassl@draeger.com
[4] Department of Applied Natural Sciences, Lübeck University of Applied Sciences, max.urban@th-luebeck.de

Abstract

The new standard *Service-oriented Device Connectivity* (SDC) is supposed to be utilized by developing a hub. This hub is supposed to collect the digitized and SDC-compliant data from multiple sensors and provide it to a hospital network. The digitization and conversion into an SDC-compliant format is done via an ultra-low power and limited CPU performance TI MSP430 microcontroller. To investigate which of the three communication protocols I²C, UART and SPI are the best suited for the described tasks, the data string of a simulated measurement was used and transmitted between two corresponding MSP430s. The transmissions were then measured using a logic analyzer. Of interest were mainly the effective data rate and the behavior of the protocols in dependence to the distance of the data transmission. Finally, SPI was found to have the highest bit rate and a low variance depending on the connection length. Combined with the native support of addressing multiple devices, this protocol turned out to be the most promising for the project.

1 Introduction

Monitoring patients' vital signs is a common procedure in hospitals. This monitoring is often done by sensors of different manufacturers which require their own monitoring system. This is hindering the interoperability of the devices, which is of importance to reduce errors and adverse events in a hospital environment [1].

To ease the interoperability, the standard IEEE 11073 SDC [2] was developed. It defines the communication of devices used in a medical context and allows the bi-directional, encrypted communication of devices from different manufacturers. Additionally, SDC defines the provision of the collected data to a hospital network, so that it can be accessed and processed remotely [3]. The hub project is using this standard to enable the interoperability of different sensors. Besides the described digitization and provision of the data into a network, the goal of the project is to ease the usage of different sensors and to reduce unnecessary cables which are of high priority for medical professionals [4].

The first prototype of the system is currently running according to the principle shown in Fig. 1. A sensor is connected to a TI MSP430 microcontroller (μC) which is attached to a PCB. This specific μC was mainly chosen for its Universal Serial Communication Interface (USCI) module which allows for easy alternation of communication interfaces and its ultra-low power consumption, which would allow the sensors to be also used with battery powered de-

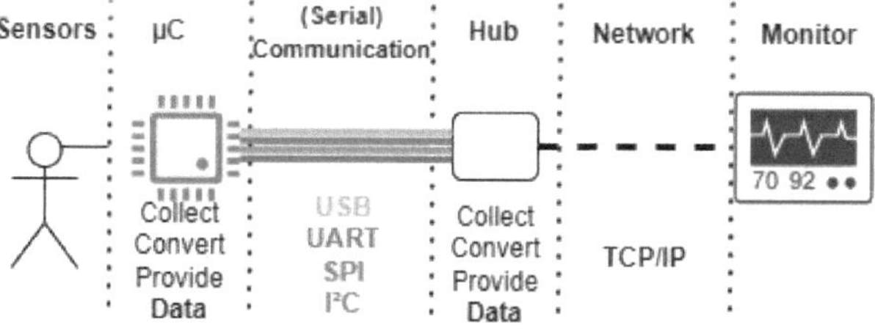

Figure 1: Concept of the hub

vices such as the portable monitor Dräger M540. The μC converts the signal into a specific .xml format and sends it via USB-CDC towards a development computer which functions as the hub. The computer provides the data via SDC so that it is accessible from any compatible monitor which is part of the network. Currently, three types of sensors are implemented to operate alone in this system. There are plans to add more sensors to the hub system. The aim is to combine and even daisy-chain them via an extension-hub that is also currently developed. This requires a high control over the bus, as well as the highest possible bandwidths in communication. The USB-CDC protocol, albeit working, is relatively restrictive in its control over the bus. Due to bulk transfers, it is not real-time capable. Therefore, other communication alternatives are to be found. For their speed properties, serial communication protocols were selected as the most promising. In order to decide which protocol is the best suited for the future plans of the project, the restrictions in terms of bandwidth and other protocol-dependent restrictions are to be determined, especially considering the hardware limitation of the microcontroller.

The eligible serial communication protocols are Inter-Integrated Circuit (I²C), Serial Peripheral Interface (SPI) and Universal Asynchronous Receiver Transmitter (UART).

1.1 Theoretical Background

For I²C to work, two wires are needed. Serial Dataline (SDA) and Serial Clockline (SCL) of at least one master have to be wired to the corresponding slave's inputs, as is depicted in Fig. 2. Each I²C device has an address, allowing for multiple slaves to be easily attached and the network is thus expanded. The main advantage of I²C is the need of only two wires for multiple slave devices. To address the individual slaves, I²C uses a dedicated address for each slave. However the often hard-coded addresses in I²C devices may lead to address overlapping when combining sensors of different manufacturers.

Each transmission frame begins with a start condition from the master to the slaves, followed by the address byte. Only then the actual payload bytes are delivered. Between each sent byte, an acknowledgement bit from the receiving device (i.e. the device with the matching address) must be sent, or else the communication is aborted. These additionally transmitted bits and bytes lead to lower effective data rates when using I²C. Depending on their rating, devices can reach anywhere from *up to* 100 kbit/s (standard mode) to *up to* 3.2 Mbit/s (high speed). The used microcontroller theoretically supports speeds of *up to* 400 kbit/s [5], [6], [7].

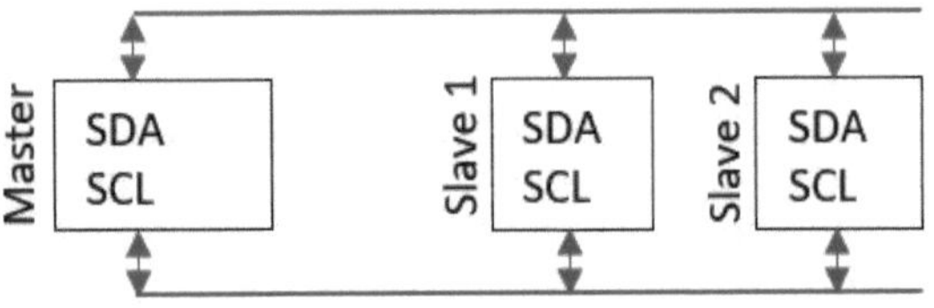

Figure 2: Principle function of I²C. SDA and SCL are shared by all participants

As depicted in Fig. 3, SPI needs at least 4 wires, namely *Serial Clock* (SCLK); *Master Output, Slave Input* (MOSI); *Master Input, Slave Output* (MISO) and *Chip Select* (CS). The master chooses which slave to access, by setting the corresponding CS wire to high. This means that a *separate* CS wire is required for *each* additional sensor connected to the hub. This circumstance quickly leads to complex cabling requirements inside the hub. By addressing each slave by their own wire, no additional addressing or framing bits or bytes are necessary, resulting in a higher effective bit rate. The synchronisation is done via the SCLK line from the master [5], [6], [7].

UART is atypical compared to the other two protocols, as it natively only connects *two* devices. In order to support the communication between multiple devices, as is the case

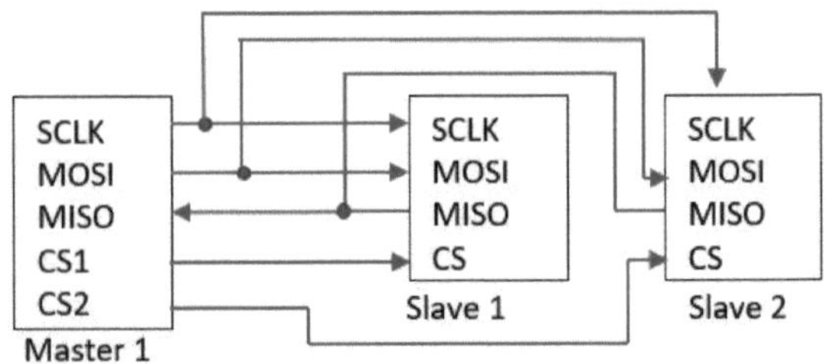

Figure 3: Principle function of SPI. SCLK, MOSI and MISO are shared. One additional separate CS line is necessary per slave.

with SPI and I²C, another software-layer would have to be implemented in the firmware of the various devices.

Like I²C, UART only requires two wires. Here, a connection between the Transmit (Tx) output of one device to the Receive (Rx) input of the other device and vice versa has to be realized. As there is no clock signal, the frequency of communication has to be arranged beforehand. The receiving device's baud rate must match the one of the transmitting device. A parity bit allows for a verification of the correctness of the transmission, but is not mandatory. A UART transmission data package usually consists of one start bit, a payload of eight bits (including one parity bit) as well as a stop bit. Afterwards, a new transmission is started [5], [6], [7].

2 Material and Methods

The test bench on which the measurements were taken consists of two TI MSP-TS430 socket target boards, each equipped with a MSP430 microcontroller (μC). Both devices are interconnected via wires. Additionally, an Arduino UNO R3 Board was used for debugging. The wiring was done using conventional jumper cables of a combined length of 40 cm, respectively an additional 1 m long ribbon cable which extended the connection length between the μCs to 140 cm. For each mentioned communication protocol, a C-code example of TI was taken and adjusted, so that it fitted the respective registers and requirements of the MSP430. The coding was done using the IDE Code Composer Studio, Version 12.1.0. Debugging, measurement and verification of the communication were done using an eight channel, 24 MHz logic analyzer from AZDelivery coupled with the software Logic (2.4.2) from Saleae. The logic analyzer was interposed between the two μCs, and was run at a sample rate of 4 MHz, as this proved to be a good compromise between a high sample frequency as well as low system-loading. The software allows for a real-time interpretation of the sent or received data. Fig. 4 shows the capture of the UART transmission of the numbers *3* and *6*. In order to process and provide the data of a sensor to an SDC network, it first has to be converted into an SDC compatible *.xml* format. The MSP takes the sensor data and combines it with the current time, which is provided to it by the hub. The following 157 byte data string: "<sen-

sor><deviceID>sensr</deviceID><timestamp>2023,01 ,13,09,58,36</timestamp> <measures>Body Temperature</measures><unit>°C</unit><value>36.84</value> </sensor>" was captured from the measurement of a temperature sensor, as it was transmitted to the hub and further to the network. Strings in C are Null-terminated. This means an additional \0 byte is added to the string, making it 158 bytes long. Because this string simulates the actual size, format and value of such a transmission and allows to control the correctness of such a transmission, this string was used in order to test the three communication protocols. The frame of each protocol differs. For each UART package, one start and one stop bit is required. No parity bit was used, and no addressing byte has to be sent. One package therefore has a length of 10 bit, with 8 bit being the payload. For the 158 character long message, 1580 bits are sent, which adds up to 198 bytes per transmission. One transmission sent via I²C, has a total size of 1432 bits or 179 bytes. This includes an 8-bit address byte, as well as an additional *Acknowledge* bit attached to every byte. These bits accumulate to additional 168 bits or 21 bytes, which -if subtracted from the total transmission size, equals the size of the simulated string. However for SPI, no additional bits are needed. The communication takes place as soon as the CS line is pulled high. All transmitted bits and bytes are therefore the pure payload. The measured duration for each character therefore is also the duration per byte. As previously described, each protocol is transmitting data differently. However, the procedure of measurement is mostly similar across the protocols and is elaborated in the following paragraph for all protocols, using UART as an example. First, the highest possible internal clock source *Sub Main Clock* (SMCLK = 1.045 MHz) was chosen. Via alternation of the baud rate and clock registers, the baud rate and the byte sending frequency can be set. Starting from a low baud rate and a low byte sending frequency, the transmission was sent and then recorded and measured using the logic analyzer. After confirming that the transmission was error free, both sending parameters were increased and the transmission measured again. This was repeated until the highest, error free, transmission rates were reached. To also test for possible connection length dependencies, this procedure was repeated only this time with an additional 100 cm long ribbon cable that was inserted between the two μCs, so that the total connection length was 140 cm.

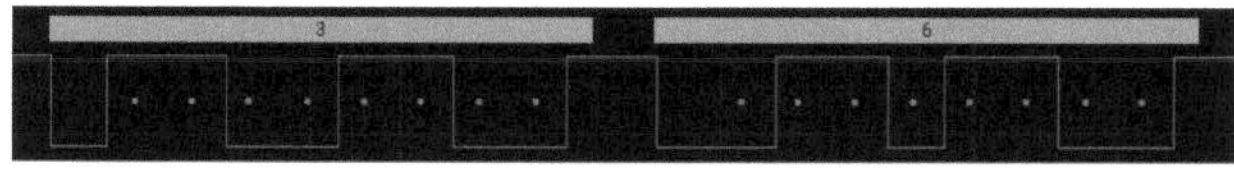

Figure 4: Captured UART transmission of the numbers 3 and 6 at a baud rate of 115200 Bd and a character frequency of 74kHz, as displayed in the software *Logic 2.4.2* from Saleae.

3   Results and Discussion

Each of the following statements concerning the time and frequency of the connection, were made by analyzing and comparing the mean of 1000 measured values. Table 1 shows the fastest achieved parameters for the two measured connection lengths of 40 cm and 140 cm when using I²C.

Table 1: Transmission parameters I²C

Conn. Length	Clovk	Duration/Char	rel. SD
40 cm	108.1 kHz	76.96 μs	11.02 %
140 cm	88.279 kHz	90.38 μs	11.06 %

It can be seen that I²C is dependant on the length of the connection between its corresponding devices. The maximum achievable clock frequency for the connection length of 40 cm was 108.1 kHz, which was reduced by approximately 18 % to 88.279 kHz when increasing the connection length by 1 m. The higher clock rate of the shorter connection, led to a shorter time per char of 76.96 μs as compared to 90.38 μs in the longer connection length. The whole transmission of the mentioned string takes 12.16 ms for the shorter, and 14.28 ms for the longer connection. The bit rate of the shorter connection is calculated to be 119.06 kbit/s. For the longer connection it is reduced to 101.39 kbit/s. With the short connection length of 40 cm a value can be sent 82 times per second. This number is reduced to 70 times per second, when the μC are connected via the 140 cm long wire. The standard deviations of the measured transmission durations are over 11 %, regardless of the connection length or the set connection parameters. Therefore, the connection length does not seem to influence the uniformity of the transmission timing.

For UART, using only the internal crystals to generate the baud rate, the highest baud rate to achieve (while still receiving/sending readable values) was 115200 Bd. The results showed no difference between the transmission using the shorter connection length as compared to the longer connection length. The results of the fastest possible connections are shown in Table 2.

Table 2: Transmission parameters UART

Conn. Length	Clock	Duration/ Char	rel. SD
40 cm	115200 Bd	82 μs	0.00 %
140 cm	115200 Bd	82 μs	0.00 %

At a duration of 82 μs per character and 158 chars per transmission, the total duration of one transmission was 12.956 ms.

The results for the SPI based transmissions are shown in Table 3.

Table 3: Transmission parameters SPI

Conn. Length	Clock	Duration/Char	SD
40 cm	1 MHz	37,69 μs	14.64 %
140 cm	1 MHz	38,20 μs	14.03 %

A whole transmission of 158 bytes took 5.96 ms for the 40 cm connection, and 6.04 ms for the 140 cm connection. Even though the standard deviation of around 14 % is considerably high, the transmissions showed no errors. This however changes at slightly higher clock rates of around 1.05 MHz. The high standard deviation does not seem to be connected to greater connection lengths. At 5.96 ms and 6.04 ms per transmission, a value can be sent 168 or 166 times every second, respectively. The calculated bit rate was 212.217 kbit/s for the shorter, and 209.41 kbit/s for the longer distance.

3.1   Discussion

Out of the compared protocols, I²C was the slowest one. Distances of greater than 40 cm are to be expected. Therefore, its high sensitivity to longer distances, with a 18 % drop of the clock by increasing the communication distance by 1 m, poses a problem. This negatively outweighs the protocol's possibility of simple connection of slaves to the master. UART was completely insensitive to distance changes within the measured range and had a slightly higher bit rate than the I²C implementation used here. However, to use it as desired, another software-layer must be implemented which allows the addressing of different slaves. Aside from a certain programming effort (in the master as well as in the slave) to achieve this functionality, the additional software layer will most likely result in a reduced effective bit rate. However, since only the internal SMCLK (which clocks with 1.045 MHz) was used here, the baud rate is limited to 115200 Bd. According to the TI data sheet (see [5]), an external 16 MHz clock allows a baud rate of 460800 Bd and should compensate for the expected reduced bit rate. SPI showed the highest bit rate with only a minor distance-dependent reduction of approx. 1.4 %. While clocking at 1 MHz, the limiting factor of the transmission speed was, that the transmission frequency of the individual packages could not be brought below 32 μs. It is not clear what triggers this limitation, and whether it can be removed. By reducing the transmission frequency, the achievable bit rate could be further increased. Due to each additional sensor needing its on CS line, the cabling is expected to be quite complex. A double assignment of one address, as is possible with I²C, is however excluded.

4   Conclusion

A serial communication protocol was sought that would allow a limited amount of data to be transferred quickly from different sensors to a common hub where it would be processed further. UART, I²C and SPI were to be investigated. While UART works distance independent, it cannot natively address multiple slaves. This would have to be solved by an additional layer in the software. The limited bit rate of 122.26 kbit/s could be increased by attaching an external clock to compensate the expected reduction of the bit rate by the additional software implementation. I²C natively allows to address multiple slaves, but the bit rate is the lowest

with only 119 kbit/s at 40 cm distance and 101.39 kbit/s at 140 cm distance. Since I²C seems to be quite sensitive to larger distances, it is not ideally suited for this purpose. SPI has the highest bit rate of 212.22 kbit/s for 40 cm, and 209.41 kbit/s for 140 cm distance. It can potentially reach even higher bit rates and natively supports the addressing of multiple attached sensors. The dedicated CS line per sensor, would eliminate the risk of accidentally addressing multiple sensors simultaneously as may be the case for I²C addressed sensors. It is expected that with SPI the best results will be achieved with the least effort. Therefore, it is recommended to continue the project hub, with the protocol SPI.

Acknowledgement

The work has been carried out at Drägerwerk AG Co. KGaA, Hospital Consumables and Accessories and supervised by the Department of Applied Natural Sciences, University of Applied Sciences Lübeck.

Author's Statement

Conflict of interest: Authors state no conflict of interest.

5   References

[1] FDA, *Medical Device Interoperability*. Available: https://www.fda.gov/medical-devices/digital-health-center-excellence/medical-device-interoperability, [last accessed on 2023-02-05].

[2] "DIN EN ISO 11073-20701:2020-07, Medizinische Informatik_- Geräteinteroperabilität_- Teil_20701: Kommunikation patientennaher medizinischer Geräte_- Service-orientierte Architektur und Protokoll für Medizingeräte-Kommunikation;," tech. rep., Beuth Verlag GmbH.

[3] Dräger, *Dräger SDC*. Available: https://www.draeger.com/en_sea/Hospital/Service-Oriented-Device-Connectivity, [last accessed on 2023-02-05].

[4] A.-S. Poncette, L. Mosch, C. Spies, M. Schmieding, F. Schiefenhövel, H. Krampe, and F. Balzer, *Improvements in Patient Monitoring in the Intensive Care Unit: Survey Study*, vol. 22. June 2020.

[5] T. Instruments, *MSP430FG662x, MSP430FG642x Mixed-Signal Microcontrollers datasheet (Rev. B)*.

[6] D. Dawoud and P. Dawoud, *Serial Communication Protocols and Standards*. River Publishers, 2022.

[7] K. Wüst, *Mikroprozessortechnik: Grundlagen, Architekturen, Schaltungstechnik und Betrieb von Mikroprozessoren und Mikrocontrollern*. Mikroprozessortechnik, Wiesbaden: Vieweg+Teubner Verlag, 2011.

Implementation of process validation for the application of gel wax phantom manufacturing process

Andreea Răileanu [1], Ledia Lilaj [2], and Shauna Coen [3]
[1] Biomedical Engineering, Luebeck University of Applied Sciences, andreea.raileanu@stud.th-luebeck.de
[2] iThera Medical GmbH, ledia.lilaj@ithera-medical.com
[3] iThera Medical GmbH, shauna.coen@ithera-medical.com

Abstract

The purpose of this paper was to implement product validation in iThera Medical GmbH to enable quality control when non-destructive testing is not possible. For that, gel wax samples were produced, and their reflectance and transmittance were measured using double integrating sphere system (DIS) to assure reproducibility and replicability of results. The measurements were converted to optical absorption and scattering using inverse adding-doubling (IAD). The measurements were then used to set up the process characterization using design of experiments (DOE). DOE analysis showed that both reflectance and transmittance were significantly influenced by the temperature set for the vacuum oven. The residual plots for reflectance and transmittance indicated that the normality assumption and equal variance were not violated. Though the results show the manufacturing process of gel wax phantoms can be established with process characterization, the ideal result could not be predicted, needing additional research.

1 Introduction

Photoacoustic imaging (PAI), also known as optoacoustic imaging (OAI), is a relatively recent in vivo and noninvasive medical imaging modality that uses optical excitation and acoustic detection to generate images of tissue structures [1]. PAI has now developed into early clinical trials for indications ranging from oncology to inflammatory disease. Phantoms are essential, as they replicate important biological tissue properties to provide a more clinically realistic imaging environment [2], enabling device design comparison, optimization, calibration, constancy testing, and regulatory decision-making [3].

An ideal tissue-mimicking material for PAI phantoms would possess optical and acoustic properties that are both tunable and biologically relevant [3], mechanically robust, stable over time, and simple, as well as highly reproducible to manufacture. The phantom should be flexible in geometry and architecture, made with non-toxic ingredients that are widely available and affordable. Unfortunately, a widely used phantom that satisfies all of these criteria is not currently available to the PAI industry [4]. The most relevant optical properties of a PAI phantom are optical absorption and reduced scattering coefficients [2], but, since optical characterization has not been defined by standards, the factors that are affecting phantom production need to be studied.

To ensure that the gel wax phantom manufacturing process can work effectively, process validation needs to be implemented. Process validation is the documented evidence that a process can work effectively and reproducibly [5]. The process validation lifecycle is covered by a risk-based approach. One of the critical steps in the process validation lifecycle is process characterization. Process characterization represents the methods used to determine the critical unit operations or processing steps and their process variables, which usually affect the quality and consistency of the product outcomes or product attributes [6].

2 Material and Methods

2.1 Fabrication of gel wax

To produce gel wax, the following components were required: mineral oil (Sigma Aldrich-330779-1L), low-density polyethylene (LDPE - Alfa Aesar 43949.30), butylated hydroxytoluene (BHT - Sigma Aldrich W218405-1KG-K), polystyrene-block-poly(ethylene-ran-butylene)-block-polystyrene (SEBS - Sigma Aldrich 200557-250G), and silicon oil for oil bath (Sigma Aldrich 85409-1L) where mineral oil served as the base, SEBS allowed the oil to set into a soft gel, LDPE increased the base material's mechanical stability, and BHT served as an antioxidant to increase the stability of the material and prevent discoloration of SEBS at high temperatures.

In suitable glassware, an oil bath using silicone oil was prepared and placed on a hotplate. A small magnetic stir bar was positioned in the oil bath, and the temperature and revolutions per minute were set. The aforementioned components were weighed while the oil bath was warming up. The beaker containing the mineral oil was added to the oil bath and heated to the specified temperature once the oil bath had reached the predetermined temperature. To measure the temperature, a thermometer was added to the mineral oil beaker. After the mineral oil reached the temperature, the rest of the components were added to the mineral oil beaker in the specified order and stirred. The beaker was then transferred into the vacuum oven that was preheated, and the vacuum pump was set to low to degas the solution in the beaker, and the timer to an hour. The procedure was repeated for 8 samples at different weights and temperatures.

The exact values cannot be released directly to the public research community due to the confidentiality between the researcher and the company.

2.2   Optical characterization

Reflectance and transmittance were measured using the DIS [7], which consists of two spheres with a rectangular sample with a thickness ranging from 2.89 to 3.54 mm placed between them, as shown in Fig. 1. Each sample was measured in a wavelength range of 400-1000 nm in 25 data points, with 5 data points in each position: the samples were measured in 5 data points in the same position to assure replicability with DIS, and in 5 positions to ensure the results' reproducibility with DIS.

The measurement of the reflectance and transmittance allowed the determination of the optical absorption and reduced scattering coefficients by recording and entering the raw data obtained with DIS into a format for analysis using inverse adding-doubling (IAD) [8]. The IAD iteratively searched for a solution to the radiative transfer equation by assuming layered samples with homogeneous optical properties and uniform light illumination [4].

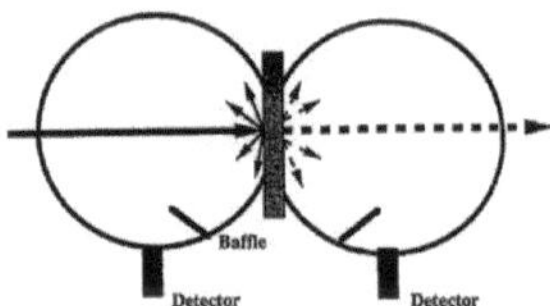

Figure 1: Two integrating spheres with a sample in between make up the experimental setup, and the unscattered collimated transmitted light is permitted to leave the system [7].

2.3   Process Characterization

Subsequently, process characterization was established to determine the relationship between the factors shown in Table 1 affecting the gel wax phantom manufacturing process and the outputs (the optical reflectance and transmittance properties from DIS) of this process and test the stability of the protocol. For conducting and analyzing the study, the tool design of experiments (DOE) in Minitab was used to identify the significant variation factors and their interactions, that impact process performance, product performance, and quality. The parameters deemed to have minor

influence (such as beaker heating time in oven vacuuming, or without vacuum) were excluded from the categorization. For the DOE, two levels were assigned to each factor (low and high values). A 2^k (where k is the number of factors) fractional factorial design was used to create a designed experiment to study the effects of the factors and identify the important factors and interactions. A 24-full factorial design would entail 16 experiments. That is not an efficient approach. According to the sparsity of effects principle, main effects (factors) and lower-order interactions are likely to have a dominant influence on a process' response. In general, the higher-order interactions are not very significant [9]. Therefore, the selected design for this study is 1/2 fraction of a 24 design, which means 8 experiments.

In the analysis, the Pareto chart was analyzed to display the absolute values of the standardized effects from the largest effect to the smallest for each response, while the model summary was used to determine the R-squared which measured how close the data are to the fitted regression line. The residual plots for each response were used to assess the goodness-of-fit in regression and the Analysis of Variance (ANOVA). The normal probability plots of residuals verify the assumption that the residuals are normally distributed. The histogram of residuals was used to determine whether the data are skewed or whether outliers exist in the data. The versus fits was used to verify the assumption that the residuals have a constant variance, while the residuals versus order of data was used to verify the assumptions that the residuals are uncorrelated with each other.

Table 1: Factor name and Factors

Factor name	Factors
A	Vacuum oven set temperature
B	Quantity of mineral oil
C	Quantity of Low-density-polyetylene (LDPE)
D	Quantity of polystyrene-block-poly(ethylene-ran-butylene)-block-polystyrene (SEBS)

3   Results and Discussion

The average of reflectance (a), transmittance (b), absorption coefficient (c), and reduced scattering coefficient (d), obtained by the IAD algorithm, are plotted in Fig. 2. Reflectance slowly decreased as the wavelength increases with some minimal changes, while the transmittance increased with the wavelength. The optical absorption coefficients stayed approximately constant, with small variation at 670-700 nm with the lowest peak at 0.05 mm^{-1} and between 900-950 nm, where the peak reached 0.09 mm^{-1}, the optical absorption was shown as being inversely proportional to reflectance. The reduced scattering coefficients decreased continually in the visible spectrum at longer wavelengths starting at 0.25 mm^{-1} and ending at 0.1 mm^{-1} in the range

400-800 nm. Towards the near-infrared, the reduced scattering coefficients continually decreased to 0.07 mm^{-1} at 930 nm with a small increase to 0.9 mm^{-1} at 1000 nm. The standard deviation of reflectance, transmittance, optical absorption, and reduced scattering was 1.10% for reflectance, 2.44% for transmittance, 4.20% for optical absorption coefficients, and 4.22% for reduced scattering, indicating that the values tend to be close to the mean of the set. These results showed that the DIS can reproduce and replicate the results, thus the results could be further used for process characterization.

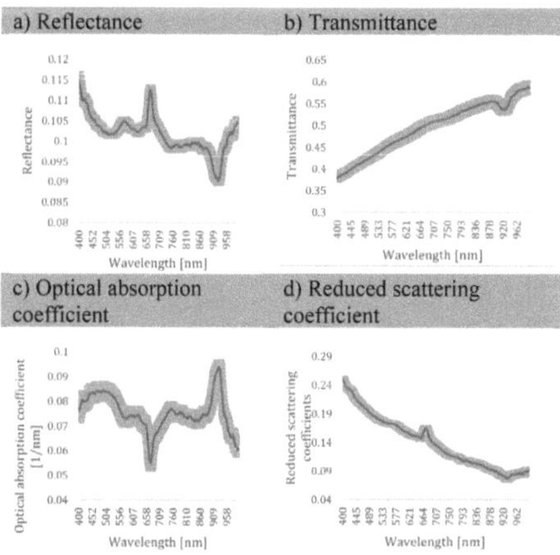

Figure 2: Average of a) reflectance, b) transmittance, c) optical absorption coefficients, and d) reduced scattering coefficients versus wavelength for all 25 data points; Error bars show the standard deviation.

Because the optical properties were measured between 400-1000 nm, the responses of interest were noted at the wavelength of 800 nm for the design of experiments. Table 2 displays the factor combinations for a 24 design, The low values are represented by -1, whereas the high values by +1.

Table 2: Combinations

Vacuum oven temperature	Mineral oil	LDPE	SEBS
-1	-1	-1	-1
+1	-1	-1	+1
-1	+1	-1	+1
+1	+1	-1	-1
-1	-1	-1	-1
-1	-1	+1	+1
+1	-1	+1	-1
-1	+1	+1	-1
+1	+1	+1	+1

The results from DIS were further used to complete process characterization in Minitab. The plots in Fig. 3, respectively Fig. 4 revealed that the vacuum oven's temperature had a significant impact on both reflectance and transmittance at wavelengths of 800 nm. The interaction between vacuum oven temperature and mineral oil had the least significant effect on reflectance, while SEBS had the least influence on transmittance.

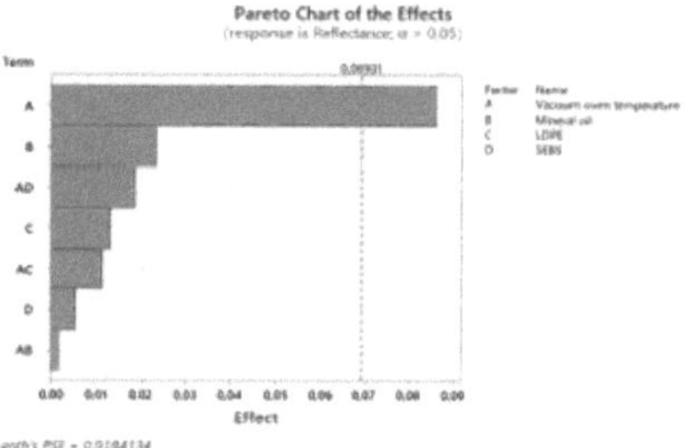

Figure 3: Pareto chart of the standardized effects for reflectance.

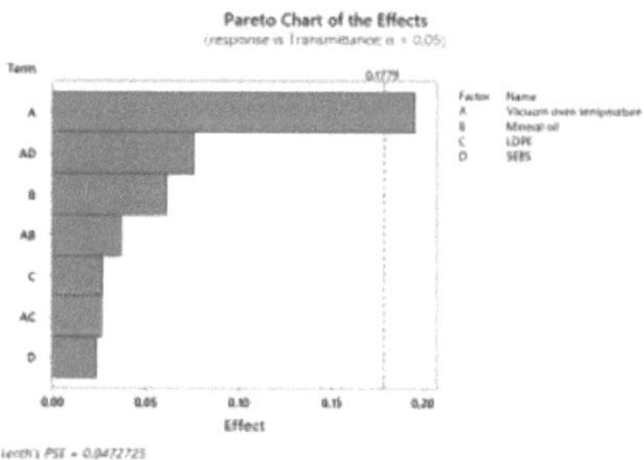

Figure 4: Pareto chart of the Standardized effects for transmittance.

As shown in Table 3, the model summary displays R-squared values of 94.14% for reflectance and 83.52% for transmittance, which indicate that the reflectance and transmittance variables can be explained without error by the predictor variable. The adjusted R-squared values were 89.74% for reflectance, and 71.16% for transmittance, which could mean that the results are difficult to predict.

Table 3: Model summary

S	R-sq	R-sq(adj)
Reflectance		
0.0040101	94.14%	89.74%
Transmittance		
0.0367836	83.52%	71.16%

Furthermore, ANOVA modeled the relationship between the factors and the responses, as shown in Fig. 5 for reflectance and Fig. 6 for transmittance. It is observed that the normality probability plots in both analyses show the residuals lie on a straight line in the normality probability plot, which indicates that the normality assumption is not violated with this data set. The histogram confirms normality for the reflectance, but for transmittance, the long bars on the right in the histogram plot might indicate skewness, which could mean that the data may not be normally distributed. This can occur when there aren't enough data points in the histogram to reliably display skewness or outliers. The residuals versus fits plots show that the distribution of the residuals is generally indicating equal variance, which indicates that the equal variance assumption is not violated. Moreover, the residuals versus order plot show in both cases a stable and capable process.

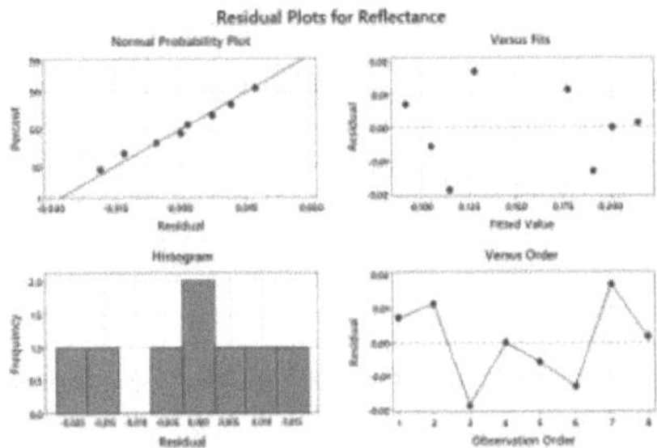

Figure 5: Residual plots for reflectance.

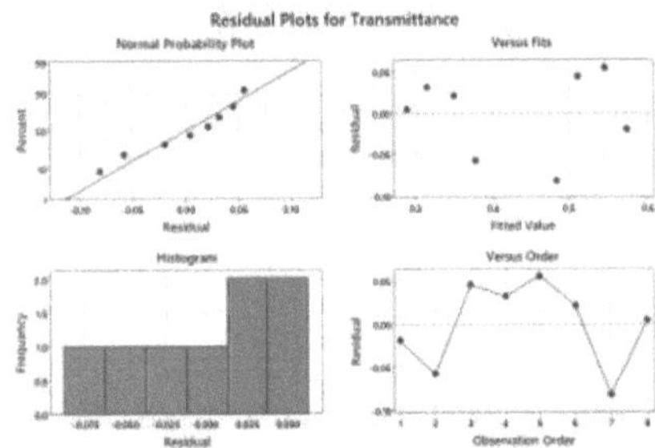

Figure 6: Residual plots for transmittance.

4   Conclusion

This experiment established that DIS could be used for process characterization, since the reflectance and transmittance of the gel wax samples could be replicated and reproduced. This led to converting the measurements to optical absorption and reduced scattering coefficients for the process and evaluation of tissue-mimicking properties that can be improved or used for different applications.

The process characterization results revealed that, while SEBS had the least effect on the transmittance and the interaction between vacuum oven temperature and mineral oil on reflectance, the temperature of the vacuum had the highest influence in both cases. This result aided in adjusting the factor levels; it indicated that the elements with the least impact on the outcome are set to an economical level, meaning that the values of the factors are set to a minimal value to minimize waste.

Furthermore, ANOVA indicated that the residuals against order plot showed a steady and capable process in both situations, and the residuals are independent of one another, indicating that no systematic influence exists. The residuals versus fits plots reveal that the residuals have a generally equal variance distribution. Although the results were positive, the R-squared values indicated that they were difficult to predict. Therefore, while there is adequate evidence to consider process characterization for

establishing a good protocol to ensure quality control and waste reduction throughout the manufacturing process of gel wax phantoms, the ideal result could not be predicted in this study necessitating additional research.

Acknowledgement

The work has been carried out at iThera Medical GmbH and supervised by Technische Hochschule Lübeck and Prof. Dr.-Ing. Wen-Huan Wang, Department of Applied Sciences.

Author's Statement

Conflict of interest: Authors state no conflict of interest.

5   References

[1] M. W. Schellenberg, H. K. Hunt, *Hand-held optoacoustic imaging: A review*, Photoacoustics 11, pp. 14–27, 2018.

[2] J. R. Cook, R. R. Bouchard, S. Y. Emelianov, *Tissue-mimicking phantoms for photoacoustic and ultrasonic imaging*, Biomedical optics express 2, pp. 3193–3206, 2011.

[3] J. Palma-Chavez, K. A. Wear, Y. Mantri, J. V. Jokerst, W. C. Vogt, *Photoacoustic imaging phantoms for assessment of object detectability and boundary buildup artifacts*, Photoacoustics 26, pp. 100348, 2022.

[4] L. Hacker, J. Joseph, A. M. Ivory, M. O. Saed, B. Zeqiri, S. Rajagopal, S. E. Bohndiek, *A Copolymer-in-Oil Tissue-Mimicking Material With Tuneable Acoustic and Optical Characteristics for Photoacoustic Imaging Phantoms*, IEEE transactions on medical imaging 40, pp. 3593–3603, 2021.

[5] M. A. Durivage, B. Mehta, *Practical process validation*, ASQ Quality Press, Milwaukee, Wisconsin, 2016.

[6] I. R. Berry, R. A. Nash, *Pharmaceutical process validation* Marcel Dekker, New York, 2003.

[7] J. W. Pickering, S. A. Prahl, N. van Wieringen, J. F. Beek, H. J. Sterenborg, M. J. van Gemert, *Double-integrating-sphere system for measuring the optical properties of tissue*, Applied optics 32, pp. 399–410, 1993.

[8] S.A. Prahl, *Everything I think you should know about Inverse Adding-Doubling*. Available: https://omlc.org/software/iad/manual.pdf [last accessed on 2023-02-06] 2011.

[9] A. Dean, D. Draguljić, D. Voss, *Design and Analysis of Experiments*, Springer International Publishing; Imprint: Springer, Cham, 2017.

Development of an in-vitro model mimicking mechanical properties of brain cortex tissue

Nisha Neupane [1], Kara Krajeswki [2] Christian Damiani [3],

[1] Biomedical Engineering, Luebeck University of Applied Sciences, neupane.nisha@stud.th-luebeck.de

[2] Altonaer Children's Hospital, KaraLeigh.Krajewski@kinderkrankenhaus.net [3] Department of medical sensors and devices (MSGT lab), Luebeck University of Applied Sciences, christian.damiani@th-luebeck.de (corresponding author)

Abstract

This study investigates manufacturing of the brain cortex mimicking phantoms. Several water-based materials including agar, gelatin, polyvinyl alcohol have been used to produce brain tissue mimicking phantoms. However, the stability of water based materials degrade over time and they require special storage conditions. We aim at producing a stable tissue mimicking phantom from Room Temperature Vulcanizing Silicone mixed with silicone oil. Silicone samples were mixed with 25%, 30%, 40%, 50% vol. of silicone oil. Compression relaxation testing was done initially to calculate the relaxation modulus of the samples. An experimental setup was used to measure the applied force and track deformation of the samples. Furthermore, semi-quantitative feedback during simulated surgical procedure was collected. The results showed that the stiffness of silicone decreased as expected with an increasing concentration of silicone oil. Sample with 40% vol. of oil were found to best resemble the mechanical properties of the brain cortex tissue.

1 Introduction

Mammalian brain is a complex heterogeneous structure composed of the cortex, basal ganglia, corona radiata and corpus callosum [1]. The cerebral cortex is an outer layer of gray matter comprising of cell bodies, dendrites and unmyelinated axons [2]. Stiffness of the brain depends on the factors like age, regions of brain, post-mortem times and preconditioning [3]. Currently, Magnetic Resonance Elastography (MRE) is the only approach to test the mechanical properties of the brain in-vivo [3]. However, this technique is not able to derive mechanical values directly. Previous works [2, 4] showed that, the elastic modulus of gray matter varies between 0.59 ± 0.19 kPa to 1.389 ± 0.289kPa.

Different materials mimicking the mechanical properties of the brain have been proposed previously and hydrogels, polyvinyl alcohol, gelatin/ agarose are the most widely used materials for soft tissue mimicking phantoms [5]. Unfortunately, these materials are not stable in the long-term and needs to be stored in a special storage conditions [6]. Development of a stable phantom material that could mimic mechanical properties of the brain cortex tissue is an initial area of interest of our project. Silicone is a major type of chemically synthesized polymer (CSP) with wide range of mechanical properties and long-term stability. They do not have the problems of evaporation and bacterial growth [7]. In this study, we evaluated the mechanical properties of Room Temperature Vulcanizing (RTV) silicone with different volume of silicone oil. Furthermore, an experimental set-up was used to measure the applied force and track the

deformation under simulated surgical procedure [8].

2 Material and Methods

2.1 Manufacture of Silicone-Based phantom

RTV silicone (ZA00) with the shore hardness of 0 ShA was purchased from polymerschmiede, GmbH. RTV silicone comprised of the base (0 ShA) and catalysator (0 ShA). Silicone oil (SF-V50) was added to adjust the mechanical properties of the prepared samples. Five different samples with varying concentration of RTV silicone and silicone oil were prepared in the metal container as illustrated in Table. 1. Metal containers made from corrosion resistant tinplate was bought from Goodma DE through Amazon. Each container has a capacity of 62ml and a height of 2.5 cm. At first, universal mold release (Smooth-On Inc.) was sprayed in the container and brushed uniformly over the surface.

For the first sample, 31ml of silicone base was poured into the clean glass beaker. The same volume of catalysator was mixed with the base for 15 minutes with wooden spatula. Then the mixture was allowed to rest for 10 minutes to avoid the formation of bubbles. In the mean time, second coating of mold release was sprayed on the metal container. The mixture was then transferred to the container and finally allowed to polymerize for 24 hours at room temperature as shown in Fig. 1. The rest of the samples were prepared by mixing varying concentration of base and silicone oil as shown in Table. 1 in a clean glass beaker for 10 minutes. Then, catalysator was added into the mixture and further mixed for 10 minutes. The mixture was then transferred into the metal containers and allowed to polymerize for 24 hours.

Table 1: Samples prepared from silicone and oil

Sample No.	Vol. of base (ml)	Vol. of catalysator (ml)	Vol. of oil (ml)	Conc. of oil (%)
1	31	31	0	0
2	23.25	23.25	15.5	25
3	21.7	21.7	18.6	30
4	18.6	18.6	24.8	40
5	15.5	15.5	31	50

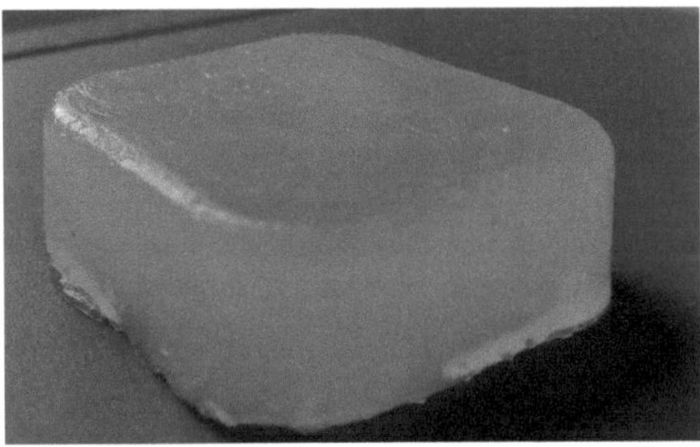

Figure 1: Prepared silicone sample

2.2 Mechanical testing

Unconfined compression- relaxation tests were performed to calculate the relaxation modulus of prepared specimens. The experimental setup is shown in Figure. 2. The setup comprised of two vertical metal stands acting as a support to the metal load. Two flat metal plates of 2 mm thickness were placed on the top of each stand. Silicone sample was placed on the top of load measuring scale (PCE-BSH 1000, PCE instruments, Germany) with an accuracy of ± 0.6 g, at resolution of 0.2 gram, a recording frequency of 1 sec and connected to a PC computer for data acquisition through the serial port. Cylindrical plane indenter of 5 mm diameter was placed on the top of metal stands and the measuring scale was adjusted so that the indenter just touched the sample. A metal load was placed on the top of indenter. Initial load was set to zero in the measuring scale and then the metal plates were carefully removed so that the metal load remains on the top of indenter applying the load during measurement. The test was performed on all of the prepared samples with constant deformation and holding time of 120 seconds.

The calculation of the relaxation modulus was performed by the equation [9]:

$$E = \frac{\Delta P(1 - n^2)}{D_i nd \cdot h \cdot k}. \tag{1}$$

Where, E= relaxation modulus in kPa, ΔP= Load in Newton, $n^2 = 0.5$ is the Poisson's Ratio of viscoelastic specimen,

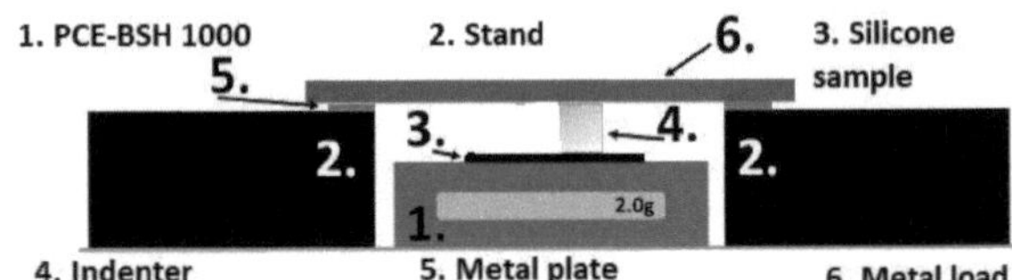

Figure 2: Experimental setup for compression-relaxation testing

$D_i ndent$= 5 mm is the diameter of indenter , h= 2 mm is the displacement of indenter, k= 1.172 is the coefficient value for the plane-cylindrical indenter calculated by the ratio of radius of indenter to the height of specimen.

2.3 Setup for monitoring force and deformation during simulated surgical condition

To monitor force and deformation in simulated surgical conditions, an experimental setup was used as shown in Figure. 3. The detailed description of the setup is given in separate publication for this student conference [8]. Blinded samples were placed in the sample holder and the samples were displayed in random order to the neurosurgeons as shown in Table. 2. Two neurosurgeons were asked to press on the sample using neurosurgical instruments. The surgeons were asked to apply similar force as done during the brain surgeries. The surgeons could press on the samples as many times they require to provide a semi-quantitative feedback of the samples regarding their resemblance to brain cortex tissue or resemblance to the previously tested samples.

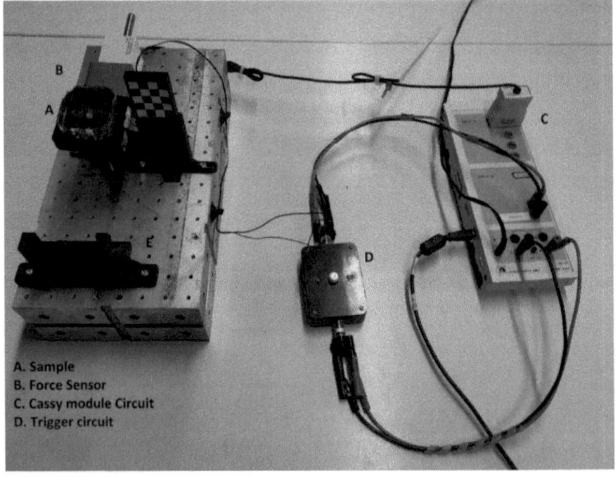

Figure 3: Experimental setup for force and deformation

2.4 Resection tests

One of the surgeons was asked to select two samples out of the displayed samples that felt similar to the cerebral cortex for resection tests. The aim of the test was to assess if the samples felt similar to real brain tissue when dissected by a dissector. Sample no. 3 (30%. vol. of oil) and 4 (40% vol. of oil) were selected by the surgeons and quantitative

Table 2: Order of sample display in simulated surgical conditions

Position	Sample No.	Concentration of oil (%)
1	1	0
2	3	30
3	4	40
4	2	25
5	5	50

overview in terms of resistance of the samples to dissection was given.

3 Results and Discussion

3.1 Mechanical Characterization of the prepared samples

Relaxation modulus obtained from the compression- relaxation testing is illustrated in the Table. 3. Highest relaxation modulus was obtained for 0% vol. of silicone (3.29 kPa) and lowest for 50% vol.of silicone oil (0.98 kPa). Sample 3 and 4 showed resemblance with the brain tissue [2, 4]. Fig 4. shows the relaxation curve obtained for all of the samples. The obtained curve for 0% vol. of oil was stiffer and it took longer time to reach in steady position making the relaxation time higher compared to the other samples. The sample with 50% vol. of oil obtained a steady relaxation within 40 seconds of the measurement time.

Table 3: Obtained relaxation modulus of silicone samples

Sample no	Vol. of oil (%)	Relaxation modulus (KPa)
1	0	3.29
2	25	2.59
3	30	1.83
4	40	1.26
5	50	0.98

3.2 Test under simulated surgical conditions

The result of silicone sample with 40% vol. of oil from the simulated surgical condition is shown in Figure. 5. Negative peaks in the curve signified compression applied during the test. The deformation peak appeared before the force peak due to compliance of the sensor and inertia of the samples during testing.

3.3 Semi quantitative feedback

The results of semi-quantitative feedback from the surgeons by pressing various samples through surgical instruments as done in real brain surgery are illustrated in the Table. 4 and 5. The feedback given by both the surgeons were almost similar, except for the sample no. 4. For one of the surgeons

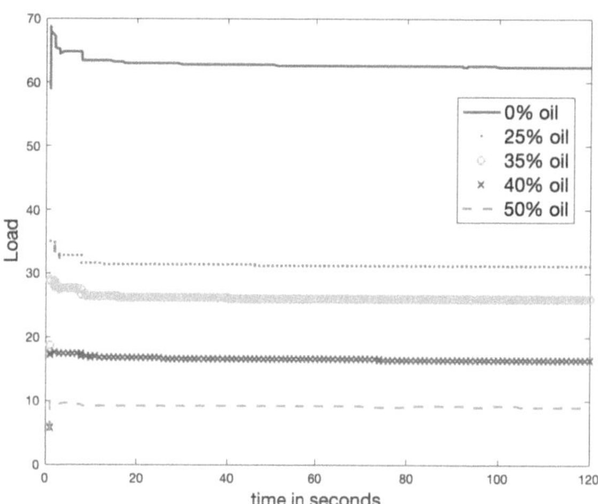

Figure 4: Compression-relaxation test of samples

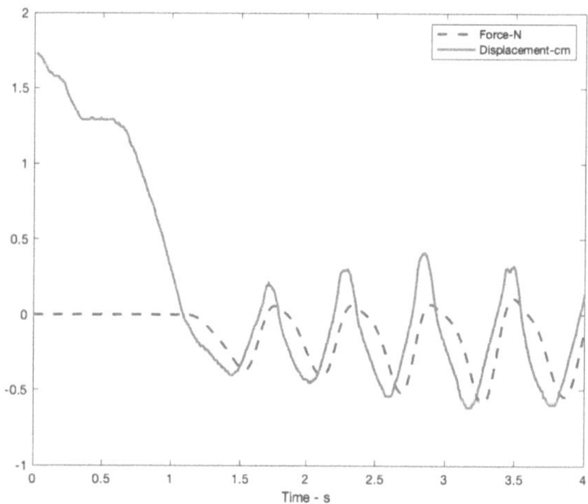

Figure 5: Force - Deformation Curve

it felt like cerebellum and for the other it felt like cerebral cortex.

3.4 Resection tests

According to the surgeons, sample 4 closely resembled the behaviour of brain cortex tissue. Though sample 3 also felt similar to the brain cortex during the test but it required higher effort during the dissection. The lateral resistance of the specimen was higher than the brain cortex making it stiffer and harder to cut than the brain cortex.

4 Conclusion

We were able to manufacture silicone samples with similar mechanical properties to the brain cortex tissue. Preliminary tactile test under simulated surgical conditions was successfully performed and semi quantitative feedback from the surgeons were taken. Further goal of the project

Table 4: Semi-quantitative feedback by surgeon 1

Sample No.	Stiffness compared to brain cortex	Stiffness compared to previous sample	Resemblance with brain	Region of brain
1	Higher		No	None
3	Higher	Lower	Yes	Stiff glioma
4	similar	Lower	Yes	Cortex
2	Higher	Higher	No	None
5	Lower	Lower	Yes	Cerebellum

Table 5: Semi-quantitative feedback by surgeon 2

Sample No.	Stiffness compared to brain cortex	Stiffness compared to previous sample	Resemblance with brain	Region of brain
1	Higher		No	None
3	Higher	Lower	Yes	Cortex
4	similar	Lower	Yes	Cerebellum
2	Higher	Higher	No	None
5	Lower	Lower	Yes	Cerebellum

will be to develop a setup that could obtain elastic modulus of the brain cortex in real time. Communication between the surgeons during tactile test would completely be restricted to avoid any kind of human influence during the experiments and more quantitative data could be obtained. It was also observed that the surgeons applied higher force to the samples that felt stiffer compared to the brain cortex. Samples from different materials with similar elasticity will be synthesized and the behaviour of the surgeons during dissection will be observed.

Acknowledgement

The work has been carried out at the Department of medical sensors and devices lab, Lübeck university of Applied Sciences. We thank Dr. Michael Worsch, Altonaer Children's Hospital, Hamburg for participating in the surgical simulation and semi-quantitative feedback of the measurements.

Author's Statement

Authors state no conflict of interest.

5 References

[1] S. Budday, G. Sommer, C. Birkl., C. Langkammer, J. Haybaeck, J. Kohnert, M. Bauer, F. Paulsen, P. Steinmann, E. Kuhl, and G.A. Holzapfel, *Mechanical characterization of human brain tissue.* Acta biomaterialia, vol.48, pp. 319-340, 2017.

[2] S. Budday, R. Nay, R. de Rooij, P. Steinmann, T. Wyrobek, T.C. Ovaert, and E. Kuhl, *Mechanical properties of gray and white matter brain tissue by indentation.* Journal of the mechanical behavior of biomedical materials, vol. 46, pp. 318-330, 2015.

[3] S. Budday, T.C. Ovaert., G.A. Holzapfel, P. Steinmann. and E. Kuhl, *Fifty shades of brain: a review on the mechanical testing and modeling of brain tissue.* Archives of Computational Methods in Engineering, vol. 27, no. 4, pp.1187-1230 , 2020.

[4] J. Weickenmeier, R. de Rooij, S. Budday, S. Steinmann, S. Steinmann, P. Ovaert and E. Kuhl, *Brain stiffness increases with myelin content.* Acta Biomate- rialia, vol. 42, pp. 265–272, 2016

[5] Y. Cao, G.Y. Li, X. Zhang, and Y.L. Liu, *Tissue-mimicking materials for elastography phantoms: A review.* Extreme Mechanics Letters, vol. 17, pp. 62-70, 2017.

[6] J. Oudry, C. Bastard, V. Miette, R. Willinger and L. Sandrin, *Copolymer-in-oil phantom materials for elastography.* Ultrasound in medicine biology, vol. 35, no. 7, pp. 1185-1197, 2009.

[7] Y. Wang, B.LTai, H. Yu, and A.J.Shih, *Silicone-based tissue-mimicking phantom for needle insertion simulation.* Journal of Medical Devices, vol. 8, no. 2, 2014.

[8] R. Catena, K. Krajeswki, C. Damiani, *Experimental setup for the investigation of forces and displacement during brain surgery using medical phantoms .* Luebeck student conference, 2023.

[9] W.C. Hayes, L.M. Keer, G. Herrmann, and L.F. Mockros, *A mathematical analysis for indentation tests of articular cartilage.* Journal of biomechanics, vol. 5, no. 5, pp. 541-551,1972.

Experimental setup for the investigation of forces and displacements during brain surgery using medical phantoms

Riccardo Catena [1], Kara Leigh Krajewski [2], Christian Damiani [3]

[1] Biomedical Engineering, Luebeck University of Applied Sciences, riccardo.catena@stud.th-luebeck.de

[2] Altonaer Children's Hospital Hamburg, KaraLeigh.Krajewski@kinderkrankenhaus.net

[3] Department of medical sensors and devices (MSGT), Luebeck University of Applied Sciences, christian.damiani@th-luebeck.de

Abstract

The assessment of brain mechanical properties is of increasing importance. In-vivo methods could provide novel metrics useful for trauma and disease evaluation. Currently, the only method employable in-vivo is magnetic resonance elastography (MRE), which is not a gold standard and cannot be employed during surgery. A tactile approach may be used as an alternative, but first typical forces and displacements during surgery need to be estimated. This information can be used to design a tactile surgical device. During this work an experimental setup was designed and tested to estimate these parameters under simulated surgical conditions on silicone phantoms. Manual indentation tests performed by surgeons showed an offset between the load and displacement peaks, deformation preceding the applied force. This could be caused by excessive force sensor compliance and inertia of the samples during cyclic motion. Further research is needed to obtain reliable force-displacement data for the design of tactile devices.

1 Introduction

The mechanical characterization of the brain tissue has been a topic of interest in the past years. As reported by Budday et al. [1], obtaining mechanical parameters of the brain tissue is useful for several reasons: 1) it would allow for better computational models to understand injury and disease development; 2) it would improve the planning of surgical procedures, and the development of new therapeutic methods. Obtaining reliable in-vivo mechanical data during surgical operations may also provide objective measures for assessment of brain trauma or other pathological conditions associated to a change in mechanical properties.

In [1] the authors also summarize the experimental results in the field of brain mechanical characterization, along with the state-of-the-art methods. Several key facts can be listed: 1) drainage conditions impact on the mechanical properties of the tissue; 2) The stress-strain relationship of brain tissue is not linear; 3) brain tissue displays hysteresis when being loaded and unloaded; 4) brain stiffness increases with the strain rate when being loaded, but no data is available for indentation speeds higher than 150 $\mu m/s$); 5) brain tissue softens after a stress has been applied (preconditioning) and slowly returns to the previous stiffness; 6) brain stiffness seems to be constant in the physiological body temperature range.

Different methods can be used to obtain stiffness data of soft tissues, as indicated by several reviews [2–6]. However, as indicated by Budday et al. [1], magnetic resonance elastography (MRE) is currently the only viable method for in-vivo mechanical characterization of brain tissue. MRE has its limitations, and it is currently not reliable enough to be defined as a gold standard [1]. Furthermore, it cannot be used to assess the stiffness of the brain tissue during surgical operations.

A tactile approach can be used to provide a novel device for measurement of tissue stiffness, also applicable during surgery. In order to design such a device, the right sensors need to be selected or built depending on the range of forces and deformations which are applied on the tissue in surgical settings.

This paper aims at: 1) presenting an experimental setup to evaluate the range of forces and deformations applied on the brain during surgery, employing a brain-mimicking material; 2) discuss initial results of tactile tests performed by a neurosurgeon on a silicone sample.

Further test results using this setup can be found in a publication by Neupane et al. [7].

2 Material and Methods

2.1 Materials

Sample preparation

Similarly as what is seen in Neupane et al. [7], room-temperature-vulcanizing silicone ZA00 base and catalyst were bought from Polymerschmiede GmbH. Both had shore hardness of 0 ShA. The samples were obtained first combining the 23.25 ml of base with 15.5 ml of silicone oil (SV-V50). Base and silicon oil were mixed for 5 minutes and then 23.25 ml of catalyst was added. A corrosion resistant tinplate container obtained from Goodma DE was brushed with mold release spray from Smooth-On Inc. The container measured 5.5 x 5.5 x 2.5 cm and had a capacity of 62 ml. The components were mixed for 10 minutes and the liquid was poured into the container. After resting for 24 hours at room temperature the sample was ready to be extracted from the container and used to test the setup.

Experimental setup

Fig. 1,2 illustrate the experimental setup. Fig. 1 shows the force sensor (A), the sample holder and the sample (B), the iPhone holder (C), the calibration grid (D) and the LED (E). Fig. 2 shows the Sensor-Cassy (F) and a plastic case containing the trigger circuit (G). The Sensor-Cassy converts the analog force signal into digital, and is made of three components: 1) input port A (Fa), connected to the force sensor with a plug (Ff); 2) input port B (Fb), connected to the output port of the the trigger circuit; 3) bottom port, used to power the Sensor-Cassy (Fc) and output a 5V voltage to power the trigger circuit (Fd). The usb cable at the left side of the Sensor-Cassy connects it to a computer (Fe). The small cables coming from the left side of the trigger circuit are used to power the LED. The switch to trigger the force measurement is located at the center of the circuit's plastic case. A pair of ERBE 20195-547 bipolar forceps and an AESCULAP FF301R dissector, as shown in Fig. 3 were employed to deform the sample and test the setup. Stickers were applied next to the tips as markers, in order to track the displacement of the tool and the deformation of the sample. Fig. 4 shows the forceps applying the load onto the sample.

The measurement of the applied force was done by a LEYBOLD® 524 060 uniaxial force sensor, connected to the input port A of a LEYBOLD® 524010 Sensor-CASSY. A holder was designed and 3D printed to place the samples on top of the force sensor. The Sensor-CASSY was connected to a computer with CASSY LAB software installed (version 2.27). The measurement of the force was triggered by a voltage signal coming into the port B of the Sensor-CASSY from the trigger circuit. The trigger circuit consists of a LED in series with a 220 Ω resistor and an on-off switch. The voltage between the LED and the switch was 5V, taken from the voltage output port of the Sensor-Cassy. The voltage between the ends of the resistor was taken from the trigger circuit and input into the port B of the Sensor-Cassy to be used as trigger signal. The force sampling interval was set to 2 ms and the total measuring interval was set to 10 seconds. The threshold value to start the measurement was set as +1V in the CASSY LAB software. When activated with a button, the triggering circuit outputs a voltage of 2.7V, going above the threshold and triggering the measurement from the force sensor. An iPhone 12 mini was used to record high speed videos (182.79 fps) of the sample being deformed. A

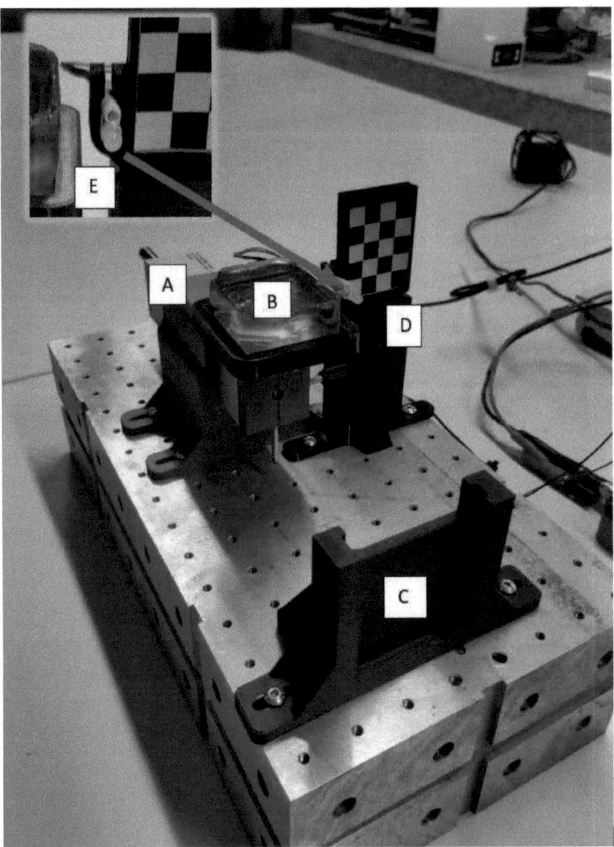

Figure 1: First part of the experimental setup: force sensor(A), sample holder with sample (B), phone holder (C), calibration grid (D) and LED light (E)

calibration grid was placed next to the sample to track the deformation of the samples from the recorded footage. To allow the synchronization of force and motion data from the video footage, the trigger circuit's LED was placed in the video frame. When pressed, the trigger switch not only starts the data acquisition from the force sensor but also turns the LED on. The software "Kinovea" (version 0.95) was used to analyze the footage and extract the motion data.

2.2   Methods

To test the set up and obtain the first initial data, the sample was put onto the holder. The output value of the force sensor was offset to 0 to remove systematic error due to the weight of the sample and the sample holder. The iPhone was inserted in its holder and then set to start recording at a frame rate of 182.79 fps.
The trigger circuit was activated pressing the button on the case. A neurosurgeon was then asked to repetitively tap on the sample using one of the surgical instruments, until the end of the recording. The subject was asked to apply a similar force and deformations as those taking place while testing the brain tissue during surgery. The force data was saved and the recordings were imported in the Kinovea software. A 2D coordinate frame with horizontal axis co-

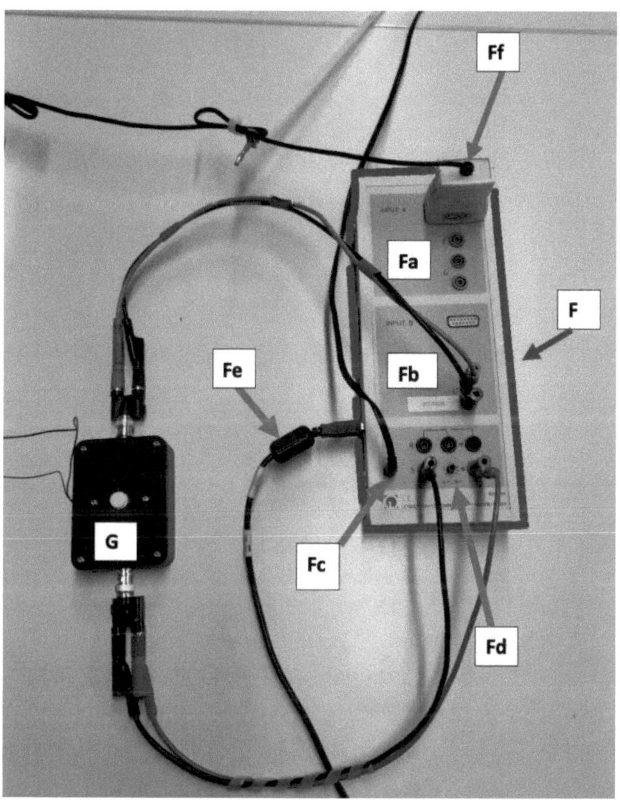

Figure 2: Second part of the experimental setup: Sensor-Cassy (F); trigger circuit (G); Input port A of Sensor-Cassy (Fa); Input port B of Sensor-Cassy (Fb); 12V power supply cable (Fc); Voltage output port with cables to power trigger circuit (Fd); Usb cable for connection to computer (Fe); Plug to connect the force sensor to the Sensor-Cassy (Ff).

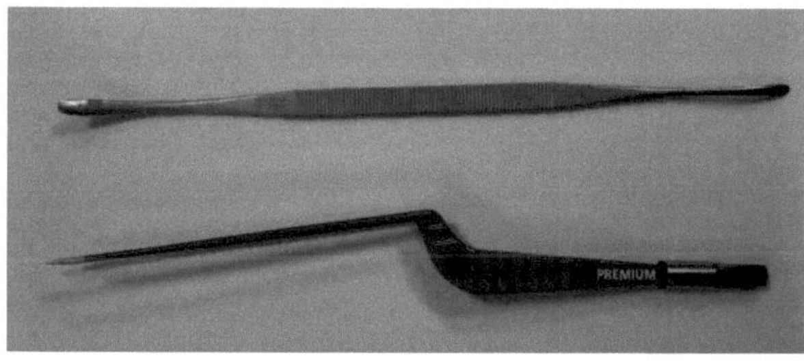

Figure 3: Dissector (top) and forceps (bottom) used to perform the compression test and test the setup

incident to the top surface of the sample was set, and the calibration grid was used to set the scale. This allowed to track the vertical motion of the tool tip and obtain the deformation of the sample during the measurement period. Both deformation data and force data were imported into Matlab (Mathworks®, R2021b). The two measurement series were synchronized and plotted against time.

3   Results and Discussion

Fig. 5 shows vertical displacement of the tool tip and force values recorded during the same measurement period. Neg-

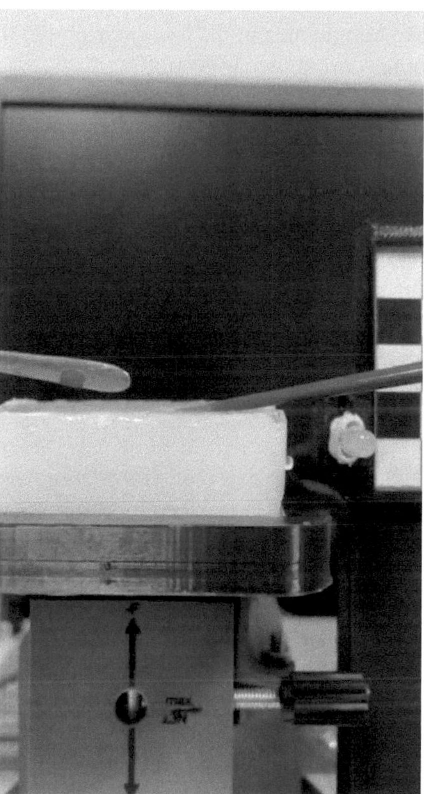

Figure 4: Forceps applying the load onto the sample.

ative peaks of the displacement signal correspond to a compression and deformation of the sample. Positive values of displacement indicate that the tip of the tool is not touching the sample. Sample indentation depths were in the range 0-2.97 mm. Negative values of force were used to indicate compression of the sample. Compressive force values were in the range 0-1.063 N.

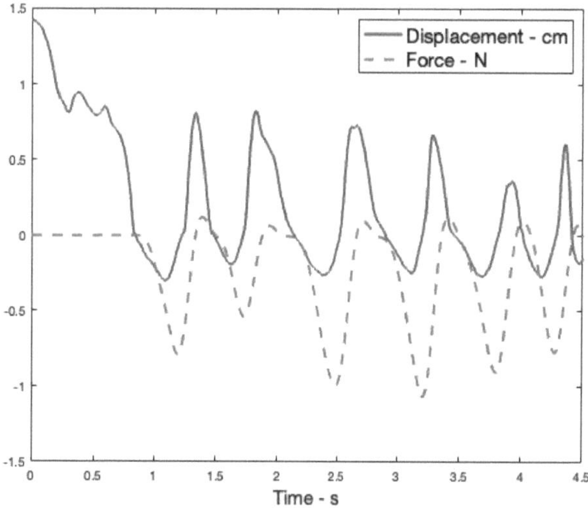

Figure 5: Displacement and force

It is possible to observe that the deformation peaks precede the force peaks by approximately 0.1 s. This may be due to an excessive compliance of the force sensor and the inertia of the samples during the cyclic motion.

The force signal also presents positive peaks indicating adhesion between the sample and the surgical tool during the upwards motion.

4   Conclusion

This paper aimed at 1) presenting an in-vitro experimental setup for the evaluation of forces and deformations of brain tissue during surgery; 2) analyze some initial measurements to validate the setup.

The deformation peaks always anticipate the measured force peaks. The exact cause of this phenomenon is still unclear, even though it is reasonable to think it is due to the compliance of the sensor and the inertia of the sample under test. Further experiments need to be performed with different sensors or different indentation speeds to confirm this hypothesis.

Due to the lack of data, the force and displacement ranges presented in this paper cannot be considered reliable enough to be used for the design of a tactile device. Additional experiments with different setups and more participants are needed to obtain reliable range values. Further work is needed for the design of a device to be used in-vivo during surgery.

Acknowledgement

This work has been carried out at the department of medical sensors and devices (MSGT), Technische Hochschule Luebeck and supervised by the department of medical sensors and devices (MSGT), Technische Hochschule Luebeck
We thank Dr. Michael Worsch, Altonaer Children's Hospital for participating in the simulated surgical tests.
We also thank Karan Iqbal Singh Grewal and Max Ramien for the help during the 3D printing of the components.

Author's Statement

Conflict of interest: Authors state no conflict of interest.

5   References

[1] S. Budday, T. C. Ovaert, G. A. Holzapfel, P. Steinmann, and E. Kuhl, "Fifty Shades of Brain: A Review on the Mechanical Testing and Modeling of Brain Tissue," *Archives of Computational Methods in Engineering*, vol. 27, pp. 1187–1230, Sept. 2020.

[2] J. Konstantinova, A. Jiang, K. Althoefer, P. Dasgupta, and T. Nanayakkara, "Implementation of Tactile Sensing for Palpation in Robot-Assisted Minimally Invasive Surgery: A Review," *IEEE Sensors Journal*, vol. 14, pp. 2490–2501, Aug. 2014.

[3] E. Afshari, M. Rostami, and F. Farahmand, "Review on different experimental techniques developed for recording force-deformation behaviour of soft tissues; with a view to surgery simulation applications," *Journal of Medical Engineering & Technology*, vol. 41, pp. 257–274, May 2017.

[4] A. B., S. Rao, and H. J. Pandya, "Engineering approaches for characterizing soft tissue mechanical properties: A review," *Clinical Biomechanics*, vol. 69, pp. 127–140, Oct. 2019.

[5] N. Bandari, J. Dargahi, and M. Packirisamy, "Tactile Sensors for Minimally Invasive Surgery: A Review of the State-of-the-Art, Applications, and Perspectives," *IEEE Access*, vol. 8, pp. 7682–7708, 2020.

[6] W. Othman, Z.-H. A. Lai, C. Abril, J. S. Barajas-Gamboa, R. Corcelles, M. Kroh, and M. A. Qasaimeh, "Tactile Sensing for Minimally Invasive Surgery: Conventional Methods and Potential Emerging Tactile Technologies," *Frontiers in Robotics and AI*, vol. 8, p. 705662, Jan. 2022.

[7] N. Neupane, K.L. Krajewski, and C. Damiani, "Development of a in-vitro model mimicking mechanical properties of brain cortex tissue," *Luebeck Student conference 2023*.

Generation of an average brain template conditioned on age

Andrei Tiurin [1], Jan Ehrhardt [2]

[1] Biomedical Engineering, Luebeck University of Applied Sciences, andrei.tiurin@stud.th-luebeck.de

[2] Institute of Medical Informatics, University of Luebeck, jan.ehrhardt@uni-luebeck.de

Abstract

This paper presents a bidirectional approach for modeling healthy brain aging in neuroimaging. The motivation for this research is the need for more precise and accurate methods for detecting and understanding neurodegenerative diseases such as Alzheimer's and Parkinson's. The proposed approach combines age-conditioned brain morphology template generation and brain age prediction into a single model. The method used an invertible normalizing flow architecture to learn the probability distribution of 3D brain morphology conditioned on age. The proposed method was evaluated on a MR images dataset and results showed that it generates realistic age-specific brain morphology templates, predicts brain age, can be utilized for subject-specific brain aging simulation, and provides interpretability through visual explanations. The proposed bidirectional model offers a powerful tool for studying healthy brain aging and its potential applications in the diagnosis, monitoring and understanding of neurodegenerative diseases.

1   Introduction

In neuroimaging, brain morphology from MR images is often used for clinical analysis. As the brain ages, the loss of neurons leads to notable morphological changes that can be observed in T1-weighted structural MR images. These changes include a decrease in overall brain volume, as well as an increase in the size of ventricular spaces. Furthermore, age is an important covariate for many age-associated neurodegenerative diseases, such as Alzheimer's or Parkinson's, which accelerate these neuronal loss effects [1].

So, the morphology of an individual patient can be compared to normal brain morphology at the patient age, to detect a neurodegenerative process. With non-linear diffeomorphic image registration, the difference between the actual patient MR image and the normal brain results in a velocity field, showing the morphology changes relative to the template.

The utilization of universal template seems to be promising solution, but it does not provide precise image for specific age group. The conditioned generation of the template image, based on age, would allow to get more precise morphology template for the patient.

Machine learning and deep learning techniques are commonly used for generative modeling tasks, such as estimating template MR images of the brain for specific populations. Traditional approach would be usage of Generative Adversarial Networks [2] or Variational Autoencoders [3]. However, these methods are difficult to train, and do not provide enough explainability or interpretability.

In this work, we will focus on usage of normalizing flow method [4]. The method provides the direct estimation of invertible functions between complicated probability distributions and simple priors, direct training through maximum likelihood optimization, efficient data sampling, and the exact inverse of both directions. The single model jointly trains in both directions between brain morphology and age value, results in multi-purpose, explainable, and interpretable model. The invertibility of the model allows to predict brain age and it can simulate brain aging for the patient, as additional features.

2   Material and Methods

2.1   Methods

The whole approach consist of three steps: diffeomorphic image registration, principal components analysis (PCA) and normalizing flow. The steps and main architecture of the solution were inspired by [5].

Overview of the whole process is presented on the Fig. 1.

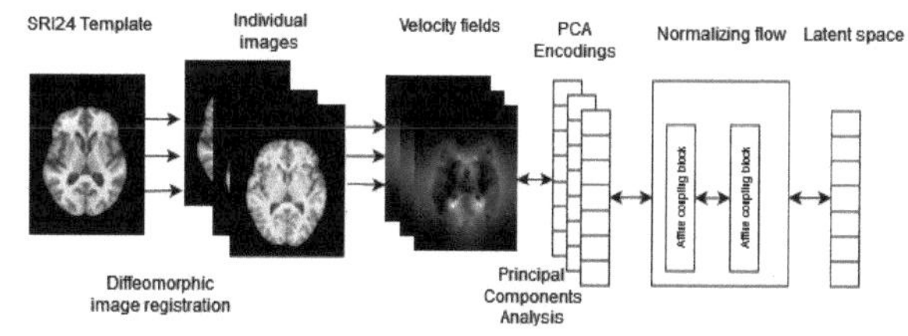

Figure 1: Overview of proposed approach. MR images are registered to a global template, producing velocity fields. Velocity fields are encoded to low-dimensional PCA vectors. PCA vectors are feeded into normalizing flow model and mapped into a latent space.

First, we apply image registration, to obtain mappings between individual MR images and a predefined atlas image.

We used the open-access SRI24 brain image template [6], as a reference for registration. These mappings are non-linear diffeomorphic deformations, parametrized by velocity fields, which describe morphology of the brain relative to the atlas. This process computes a mapping function from image space to velocity field space $v_i : \mathbb{R}^3 \to \mathbb{R}^3$. This is done before the main training process, so the velocity fields are stored and then loaded during further steps.

Processing of 3D MR image scans requires a lot of computational and memory resources, so to overcome this problem, PCA encodings of deformation fields are used. PCA encodings respresent high-dimensional 3D data in a low-dimensional space. Velocity fields are used as the input of PCA, as they represent 3D deformation vectors for each scan, with respect to the reference atlas. We sample every voxel of deformation field v_i to form a vector $\boldsymbol{v_i} \in V \subset \mathbb{R}^{3n}$, where n is the number of image voxels. This high-dimensional vector is used for PCA encoding process : $g : V \to Q$, where $Q \subset \mathbb{R}^{n_{pca}}$ is a low-dimensional PCA encoding and $n_{pca} = 128$ in our method. As principal component analysis is an invertible operation, the backward function can be written as $g^{-1} : Q \to V$. The model for PCA encodings was trained separately, providing encoded vectors of each input velocity field for the training process of normalizing flows. We will not go into details of PCA model training in this paper.

Part with normalizing flows takes PCA vectors as an input and transform it to a latent space encoding. It can be written as $h(\cdot, \theta) : Q \to Z$, where $Z \subset \mathbb{R}^{n_{pca}}$ is a latent encoding vector and θ are the learnable parameters of the normalizing flow.

One of the main features of normalizing flows is invertibility, so the inverse $h^{-1}(\cdot, \theta) : Z \to U$ can be easily computed. Normalizing flow consist of chain of functions - affine coupling layers [7] and can be stacked together: $q = h_1^{-1}(\cdot, \theta) \circ h_2^{-1}(\cdot, \theta) \circ ... \circ h_{n_{layer}}^{-1}(\cdot, \theta), q \in Q$.

Each layer $h(\cdot, \theta)$ performs element-wise affine transformation (1). The input vector for each layer is split into two parts $z_{1:j}, z_{j+1:n_{pca}}$, where one of the parts $z_{1:j}$ is used for conditioning of the transformation functions, and another one $z_{j+1:n_{pca}}$ is transformed. Normalizing flow in our method consists of 16 of such layers, performing swapping the halves of the output vector, to provide interaction between all latent variables.

$$z'_{j+1:n_{pca}} = t(z_{1:j}, \theta) + exp(s(z_{1:j}, \theta)) \odot z_{j+1:n_{pca}} \quad (1)$$

$s(\cdot, \theta)$ and $t(\cdot, \theta)$ in (1) represent neural networks, which take latent vector as an input and produce scaling or translation factors as an output. In our method, these networks consist of 4 fully connected layers with hidden size = 8, and ReLU activation functions. For the implementation of the whole neural network, we used FrEIA library [8], based on Pytorch.

First dimension of the latent encoding $z \in Z$ represents the age of the subject, where the rest represent subject-specific encodings: $z = [a, \tilde{z}]$. The whole normalizing flow is trained through maximum likelihood optimization, with

loss function as in (2), with predicted latent components $\hat{a}$ and $\hat{z}$. The first term in the function use a zero-centered Gaussian distribution as a prior for $\tilde{z}$ and ensures that it will follow Gaussian prior. The second term is a mean squared error for a ensures disentanglement of the age component in the latent vector and provides age prediction. The third term is logarithm of Jacobian determinant, which controls density deformation of distribution between the latent space and input space [4].

$$\mathcal{L}(\theta) = 1/n \sum_{i=1}^{n} 1/2 \|\hat{z}\|_2^2 + \|\hat{a} - a\|_2^2 - log|det(J)|) \quad (2)$$

After training the model, we can generate brain images by setting the age a and latent vector $\tilde{z}$ as shown in Fig. 2. Here, the initial SRI24 atlas is deformed by velocity fields generated from $g^{-1}(h^{-1}([a, \tilde{z}], \phi))$. As we can see, the method is able to generate wide range of images with different morphology and age, while preserving the specific age-related properties of the brain, such as the ventricle size. Also, it should be noted, that images have the same intensities, because we use the same reference MR image template and only the brain shape changes in diffeomorphic transformations. These MR images also can be used to train neural networks for other tasks, such as segmentation or object detection.

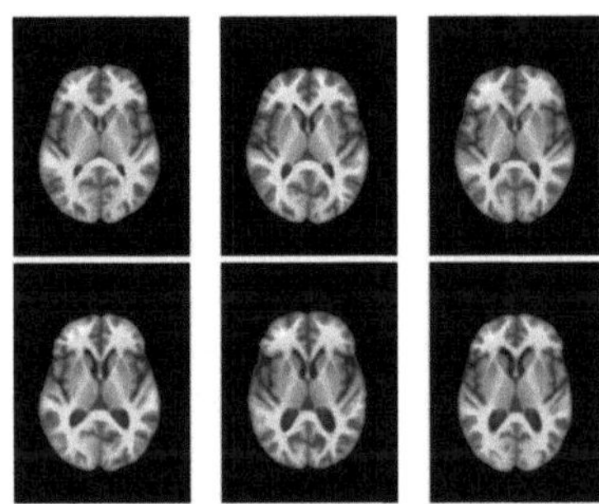

Figure 2: Randomly deformed template image conditioned on age=35 (upper row) and age=75 (lower row) and with latent vectors $\tilde{z} \sim \mathcal{N}(0, 1)$

2.2 Application

2.2.1 Age prediction

To predict the brain age $a \subset \mathbb{R}$ of a subject's 3D brain image scan I, we start with image registration to the SRI24 atlas, which results to a velocity field $V : I \to V$. Velocity field then transformed to a PCA encoding $q : q = g(\boldsymbol{v})$. After that, PCA encoding q is feeded into normalizing flow model, resulting into latent space vector: $z = h(q, \theta)$. From latent space vector the first element indicates the age of the subject: $z = [\hat{a}, \hat{z}]$.

Additionally, it is possible to produce attribution map for a specific subject, which can explain which part of brain is used for specific estimation. Because $\boldsymbol{v} = g^{-1}(h^{-1}([\hat{a}, \hat{z}], \phi))$ we can compute derivatives of $\boldsymbol{v}$ with respect to the age. For that, we need to take vector z after age estimation, and then produce two images and calculate derivative of velocity field with respect to a by finite difference approximation of $\frac{\partial v}{\partial a}$.

After that, this partial derivative can be visualized after calculating a magnitude of each point of the field (see Fig. 3).

2.2.2 Age-conditioned average brain template generation

As the main idea of generative task to produce age-conditioned template, first of all, we need to set age a for the latent vector Z, which will be used further to feed the normalizing flow model. The rest of the latent vector should be set to the mean value of latent vector $\tilde{z} = 0$, this way it will produce an average brain morphology for the specific age. After setting the latent vector z, the velocity field of the template can be easily generated through the inverse functions of the model: $v = g^{-1}(h^{-1}([a, \mathbf{0}], \theta))$. The final template brain image can be produced by applying inverted velocity field to the global brain reference template, which was used in image registration.

2.2.3 Subject-specific brain image generation

Additionally, to conditioned template generation, the model can be used to generate random brain images, conditioned on age as well. For that, the age-unrelated part of the latent vector $\tilde{z}$ should be sampled from a zero-centered normal distribution $\tilde{z} \sim \mathcal{N}(0, 1)$, Fig. 2. After that, the same backward process should be applied.

For the subject-specific brain aging simulation, the z latent vector should be sampled from the age estimation task: $[\hat{a}, \hat{z}] = h(g(v), \theta)$. $\hat{z}$ will contain subject-specific anatomy latent encoding, which describes uniquely the brain image scan. By varying $\hat{a}$ with fixed $\hat{z}$, it will produce subject-specific brain images for different ages: $v = g^{-1}(h^{-1}([\hat{a} + \tau, \hat{z}], \theta))$.

2.3 Materials

We trained our model on approximately 1500 T1-weighted healthy brain MR images with age range from 20 to 90 years old. 4 different open datasets were used, IXI database [9], SALD (Southwest University Adult Lifespan Dataset) [10], DLBS (Dallas Lifespan Brain Study) [11], ADNI (Alzheimer's Disease Neuroimaging Initiative) [12], all scans were acquired from different scanners. All datasets, except ADNI contains scans of healthy subjects. For ADNI dataset, we filtered the dataset, keeping for training only subjects with normal cognitive function.

3 Results and Discussion

3.1 Age prediction

We evaluated age prediction ability on a left-out part of dataset and we got mean absolute error (MAE) of 6.6 years.

To compare, [5] reported MAE of 4.5 years. We explain the difference between reported metrics because of the smaller training dataset in our study and PCA-space encoding size. So, in case of more MR brain images available, we expect to get better metrics. However, it's difficult to compare results with other studies, as results largely depend on the size and the age distribution of the used train and test datasets.

In contrast to pure regression approach, normalizing flow model allows to provide insight into its predictions and demonstrate it through the use of attribution map, as shown in Fig. 3. The map is generated by application of finite difference approximation of a image, with fixed $\tilde{z}$-encoding and a step = 0.1 year. This map illustrate that the model primarily uses information from the ventricles, but also takes into account the shape of other brain structures such as gyri and sulci. This highlights the transparency and interpretability of the proposed model's predictions.

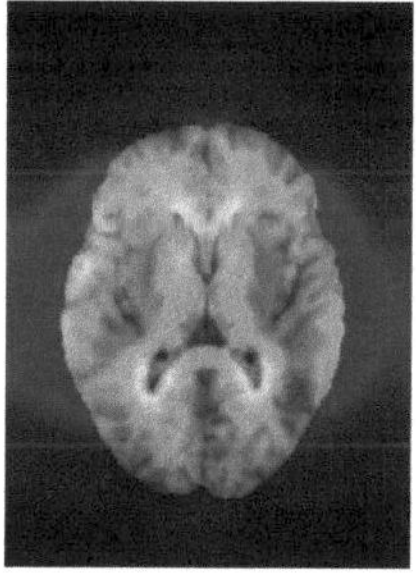

Figure 3: Attribution map of age prediction. Predicted age $a = 51$.

3.2 Age-conditioned average brain template generation

For the template generation task, age-conditioned brain templates generated by the model are shown in the Fig. 4. The results demonstrate that our model effectively captures the typical pattern of healthy brain aging, such as the increase in ventricular volume as age progresses.

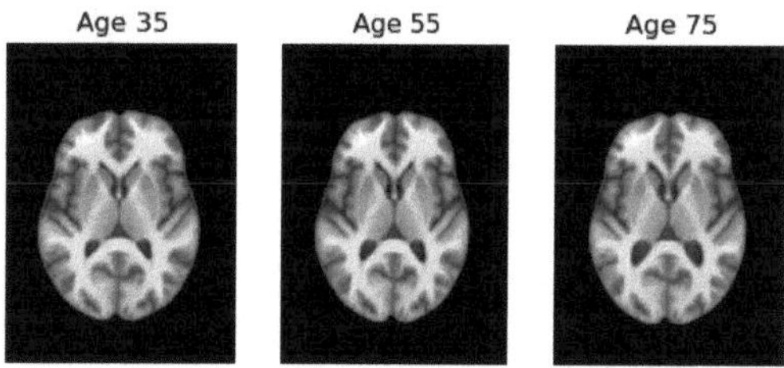

Figure 4: Generated average brain templates conditioned on age.

3.3 Aging simulation

Additionally, images generated by the model provide a visual representation of the model's focus on the ventricular structures and its ability to predict changes in brain structure with age. It can be seen by the increase in ventricular size in patient's images with older age. The results of the subject-specific aging simulation using our bidirectional model are illustrated in Fig. 5. The simulated images shows the typical changes in brain morphology associated with aging, while maintaining subject-specific characteristics.

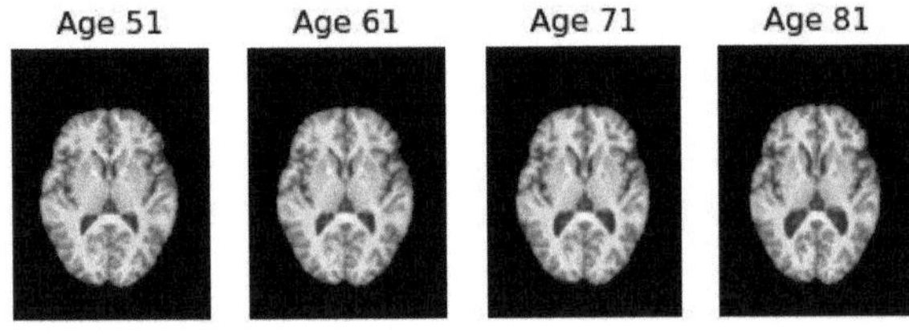

Figure 5: Simulation of aging for a specific patient. Original age = 51.

4   Conclusion

In this study, we present a bidirectional modeling approach that combines regression and generative modeling in neuroimaging. We use normalizing flow to learn a population-based distribution of 3D brain morphology conditioned on age, as the variable of interest.

Our method encodes variations in brain morphology using diffeomorphic deformations. Additionally, we limit the brain image to a low-dimensional vector in order to effectively process high-resolution 3D imaging data.

Model can be used for several task: age prediction, age-conditioned average brain template generation and subject-specific aging simulation.

Additionally for age prediction, we can produce attribution maps, which can explain model's decisions. The morphology deformations look quite realistic, as the typical healthy brain would have - change in size of ventricles.

For the brain image generation, results also show realistic changes in brain structures for every average brain image for specific age. As an additional feature, such changes can be visualized for patient's brain image, simulating healthy aging of the brain.

For further work, the model can be parametrized by more variables of interest, such as a disease. Also, as we use one common reference atlas for all images in registration process, we can utilize atlas segmentation to analyze morphological changes in brain structures, and how they change over the age.

Acknowledgement

The work was carried out at Institute of Medical Informatics, University of Lübeck and supervised by Dr. rer. nat. Jan Ehrhardt, Institute of Medical Informatics, University of Lübeck.

Author's Statement

Authors state no conflict of interest.

5   References

[1] P. Coupé, , J.V. Manjón, , E. Lanuza, and G. Catheline, *Lifespan Changes of the Human Brain In Alzheimer's Disease*. Sci Rep 9, 3998, 2019.

[2] T. Xia, A. Chartsias, C. Wang, S. Tsaftaris, *Learning to synthesise the ageing brain without longitudinal data*. Medical Image Analysis, vol. 73, 2021.

[3] P. Mouches et al., *Unifying Brain Age Prediction and Age-Conditioned Template Generation with a Deterministic Autoencoder*. Proceedings of Machine Learning Research, vol. 143, pp. 497-506, 2021.

[4] I. Kobyzev, S. Prince, and M. Brubaker, *Normalizing flows: An introduction and review of current methods*. IEEE Transactions on Pattern Analysis and Machine Intelligence, vol. 43, pp. 3964-3979, 2020.

[5] M. Wilms et al., *Invertible Modeling of Bidirectional Relationships in Neuroimaging with Normalizing Flows: Application to Brain Aging*. IEEE Transactions on Medical Imaging, vol. 41(9), pp. 2331-2347, 2022.

[6] T. Rohlfing, N.M. Zahr, E.V. Sullivan, and A. Pfefferbaum, *The sri24 multichannel atlas of normal adult human brain structure*. Hum Brain Mapp, vol. 31(5), pp. 798–819, 2010.

[7] L. Dinh, J. Sohl-Dickstein, and S. Bengio, *Density estimation using Real NVP*. arXiv preprint arXiv:1605.08803, 2016.

[8] Ardizzone et al., *Framework for Easily Invertible Architectures (FrEIA)*. Available: https://github.com/vislearn/FrEIA [last accessed on 2023-01-15]

[9] Biomedical Image Analysis Group, Imperial College London, *IXI Dataset*. Available: https://brain-development.org/ixi-dataset/ [last accessed on 2023-01-15]

[10] D. Wei et al., *Structural and functional mri from a cross-sectional southwest university adult lifespan dataset (sald)*. BioRxiv, p. 177279, 2017.

[11] Iternational Neuroimaging Data-sharing Initiative, *Dallas Lifespan Brain Study*. Available: http://fcon_1000.projects.nitrc.org/indi/retro/dlbs.html [last accessed on 2023-01-15]

[12] ADNI, *Alzheimer's Disease Neuroimaging Initiative*. Available: https://adni.loni.usc.edu [last accessed on 2023-01-15]

Regulatory strategy for market introduction of an IoT-based laboratory sample tracking system for Access to the United Kingdom market

Catalina Avendaño Mejía [1], Yannick Timo Böge [2]

[1] Biomedical Engineering, Universität zu Lübeck, catalina.avendano@stud.th-luebeck.de

[2] Regulatory Department, Smart4Diagnostics GmbH, timo.boege@s4dx.com

Abstract

This paper describes the regulatory research made for SmartDiagnostics GmbH (S4DX) in order to access to the United Kingdom market. More than 70 percentage of all medical decisions are based on diagnostic results. S4DX aims at closing the preanalytical gap between blood collection and laboratory analysis in medical diagnostics, which consist of a preanalytical ecosystem for biological samples to assure the quality of samples. The purpose of this paper is to determine which regulations and designated standards S4DX needs to follow to achieve market access in Great Britain. Firstly, an extensive analysis of the hardware products and its technical specifications was done. Secondly, a regulatory analysis of potentially applicable regulations was performed. The conclusion is that S4DX hardware products do not fall under the medical device regulations but fall under the classification as radio frequency equipment. Therefore, S4DX need to follow the radio equipment regulations and its corresponding designated standards.

1 Introduction

S4DX is a company based in Munich, Germany, which offers solutions to the preanalytical phase of clinical laboratories. S4DX had created a system, which starts from the biological sample ordering at the doctor's office until the sample arrival to the laboratory for analysis. S4DX products consist of a hardware system as well as a software system (Fig 1). This study has a focus on the S4DX hardware system. As a result, the software products will not be detailed out in this paper. Moreover, it is important to understand that the data collected and processed by S4DX is not intended for use in any clinical, therapeutic, analytical, or diagnostic purposes and only serve to manage the preanalytical sample workflow processes.

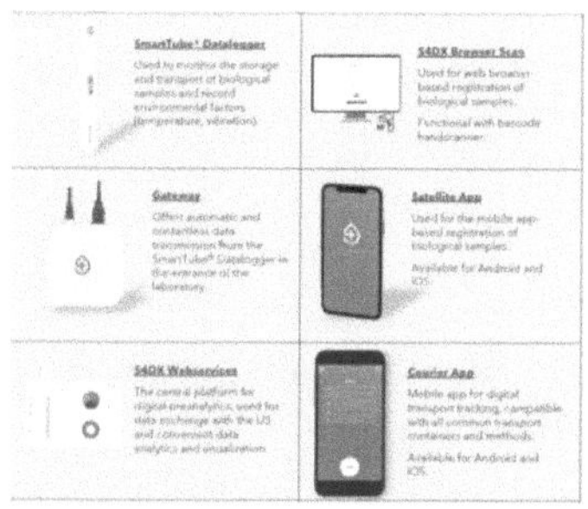

Figure 1: Components of S4DX system

2 Material and Methods

The focus of this regulatory analysis is the hardware products. The S4DX hardware products consist of SmartTubes and Gateways and are described as follows.

2.1 Gateway

The Gateway consists of a Raspberry Pi 4 Model B. The Raspberry Pi 4 is a low cost tiny dual-display, desktop computer, which its main function is to communicate with the SmartTube via Bluetooth 5.0, BLE communication protocol in the frequency band of 2.4GHz . In order to receive, track, monitor and transfer data. These data will be automatically sent to the S4DX Web Services via Wi-fi. Where all the information of the SmartTubes can be tracked and shown to process the information. The Gateway has a Polypropylene (PP) case designed for S4DX.

According with the manufacturer: "The Raspberry Pi 4 has undergone extensive compliance testing and meets a number of regional and international standards." [7].

2.2 SmartTube

The intelligent sample tube "SmartTube" was created with the purpose of impulse the digitalization and automation of the preanalytical supply chain. The SmartTubes are datalogger in the shape and in the dimension of a conventional blood tube and are transported next to the biological samples from the collection site (doctor's office/clinic) to the delivery site (analysis laboratory) where the analysis of the sample will take place. The SmartTube contain sensors to continuously monitor and collect data over environmental factors that could affect the sample integrity. The Smart-Tubes are digitally linked to a specific number of biological samples traveling with the same temperature conditions. The SmartTubes track temperature, physical shocks, and time stamps until it is wirelessly read out at the delivery site by the S4DX Gateway, which is located at the laboratory entrance. The SmartTube case is also made of (PP) SmartTube hardware is compose of a Sensor Unit (Fig 2) and a Battery Unit, which consist of two 1.5 Volts alkaline batteries connected in series with a combined capacity of 1700mAh.

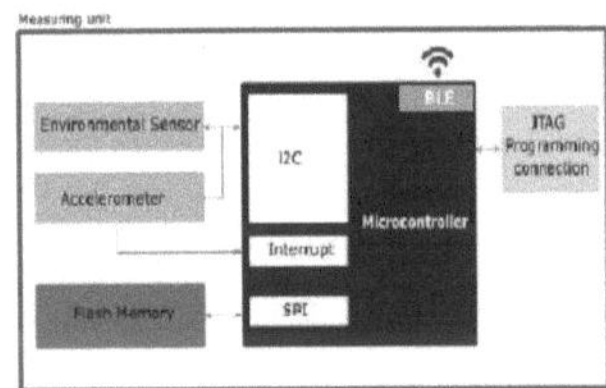

Figure 2: Sensor Unit SmartTube

The Sensor Unit consists of 2 type of sensors which are: the environmental sensor, which monitor the temperature from the biological samples and the accelerometer, which register if the biological samples had fell down in a manner that could affect the quality of the sample due to the shock-induced burst of blood cells and thus the future analysis of the sample. Both sensors communicate with the microcontroller using Inter-Integrated Circuit (I2C) communication protocol. Moreover, an external flash memory is used to storage the data collected and communicates with the Microcontroller using SPI communication protocol. The Microcontroller used in the SmartTubes is the BGM13S32F512N, which is an MCU that contains a radio transceiver which supports Bluetooth® low energy protocol. The modulation type used for the MCU Bluetooth is the Gaussian Frequency Shift Keying (GFSK). For the SmartTube PCB design the values of resistors and capacitors were chosen following the MCU and sensors datasheets suggestions. According with the MCU manufacturer, the MCU is in conformity with the essential requirements and other relevant requirements of the Radio Equipment Directive. However, according to EN 301 4 89-1 designated standard, for every application using the BGM13S22 an EMC test will need to be performed on the end product.

2.3   UKCA and CE marking

Due to the fact that UK were part of the European Union, the product marking to place products in GB used to be the CE marking. Where the CE marking is the product marking use for placing products in the European Union. As a result of the Brexit, the UKCA marking was created to place products in the Great Britain market (GB), this marking applies

just for England, Scotland and Wales. The UKCA have been operating since 1 January 2021. However, in order to provide businesses flexibility, the UK government will allow the recognition of the CE marking for most goods which are already placed on the market, or the ones that will be place on the marked before 11pm on 31 December 2024. After this date only UKCA marking will be accepted for the GB market [1]. For being compliance with the UKCA marking, the UK relevant regulations needed to be consulted. The entity responsible of regulating medical devices in UK is the Medicines and Healthcare products Regulatory Agency (MHRA). All medical devices as well as Invitro Medical Devices placed in UK needs to be registered with the MHRA. The first analysis was to evaluate if the S4DX hardware products falls under the regulatory definition as "medical device". The second analysis was to review some applicable regulations for electronic devices.

3   Results and Discussion

3.1   Regulatory Evaluation according to Medical Device Regulations

3.1.1   Scenario "Medical Device"

The S4DX system does not full fill the definition of "medical device" according to the UK Medical Device Regulations (UKMDR). Reference [2] shows the concept of "medical device". The analysis can be seen in Table 1.

Table 1: Medical Device scenario analysis

SmartTube	Gateway
The SmartTube function is to collect environmental parameters such as temperature and movement (shock events) in the sample transportation process. Which means that it does not diagnostic, monitoring or treat any disease, injury or handicap neither perform any investigation, modification, or replacement of any physiological Process.	The Gateway function is to register the Smart-Tubes arriving to the delivery site and collect the data recorded by these SmartTubes and send this information collected to a Browser Scan service which is part of the Software products. As a result, neither the SmartTube nor the Gateway full fill the definition of medical device from the UKMDR.

3.1.2   Scenario "In Vitro Diagnostic Medical Device" (IVDMD)

The S4DX system does not neither fall under the IVDMD classification. Reference [2] shows the concept of "In Vitro Diagnostic Medical Device". The corresponding analysis can be seen in Table 2 [2], [10].

Table 2: IVDMD scenario analysis

SmartTube	Gateway
The SmartTube function is to collect environmental parameters such as temperature and movement (shock events) in the sample transportation process. Which means that it does not diagnostic, monitoring or treat any disease, injury or handicap neither perform any investigation, modification, or replacement of any physiological Process.	The Gateway function is to register the SmartTubes arriving to the delivery site and collect the data recorded by these SmartTubes and send this information collected to a Browser Scan service which is part of the Software products. As a result, neither the SmartTube nor the Gateway full fill the definition of medical device from the UKMDR.

3.1.3 Scenario "Specimen Receptacles"

The blood collection tubes are considered as so-called specimen receptacles. However, S4DX is not a producer of blood collection tubes. In the case of the SmartTube its function is just to monitor the Specimen Receptables during its transportation but not contain or preserve the specimens derived from the human body. As a result, S4DX system does not fall under this category [2], [10].

3.1.4 Scenario "IVD accessory"

It could be though that S4DX system falls into this category. Because of the fact that it is an article intended to be used together with an In Vitro Diagnostic Medical Device, which are the specimen receptacles. (An extend concept of IVD accessory can be found in references [2] and [10]). However, as it was previously explained S4DX is not a producer of specimen receptables, therefore any part of the S4DX system could be considered as an accessory of an IVDMD [2], [10].

3.2 Regulatory Evaluation according to Technical Specifications

Both hardware products Gateway and SmartTube are electronic devices. Therefore, the regulations under the classification of "electrical and electronic products" had to be reviewed. Those regulations are: "The Electrical Equipment (safety) Regulations", "Electromagnetic Compatibility Regulations" and "The Radio Equipment Regulations" [1]. After reviewing the previously mentioned regulations it can be neglected "The Electrical Equipment (safety) Regulations" because this regulation applies to electrical equipment designed for use with a voltage between 50 and 1000V A.C and between 75 and 1500V D.C, which is out of the operating voltage of the SmartTube and Gateway [6].

3.2.1 Scenario "Radio Frequency Equipment"

Table 3: Radio Frequency Equipment analysis

SmartTube	Gateway
The SmartTube is an electronic product which uses Bluetooth communication protocol to communicate with the Gateway. Therefore, the SmartTube falls into this category due to the fact, that it is an electronic product which emits radio waves for the purpose of communication. Therefore, it could be implied that the SmartTube needs to at least follow the same legislations than the Gateway to be in conformity with the UKCA marking.	According with the UK regulations, the Raspberry Pi falls under the category as Radio Frequency Equipment. The manufacturer of the Raspberry Pi 4 Model B had claim on his declaration of conformity that the Raspberry Pi 4 Model B is in conformity with The Radio Equipment Regulations (RE) and with the Restriction of Hazardous Substance (RoHs).

3.3 Conformity Assessment

As it was previously mentioned, the Gateway consists of a commercially available small computer "Raspberry Pi 4 model B" in a polypropylene case designed for S4DX. Where its declaration of conformity states that the conformity assessment procedure that the Raspberry Pi Ltd had followed was the "Internal Production Control" [7]. Therefore, the conformity assessment procedure that S4DX had followed to place the Gateway on the European market. i.e., for the CE marking is also the Internal Production Control. In the case of the SmartTube, S4DX had followed the conformity assessment procedure of the internal production control as well for the CE marking to place the SmartTube in the European Market. UK allows the same conformity assessment procedure. As a result, the same "Internal Production Control" will be followed for both hardware products (Gateway and SmartTube) to access to the UK market.

3.4 Designated Standards

Designated Standards are a list of standards that manufactures can use to show that their products and services comply with the GB law. By Following the applicable designated standards, which depends on the product that you want to place in the UK market, manufactures can claim "presumption of conformity" with the corresponding essential requirements. [8], [9]. The analysis of the designated standards that S4DX hardware products must follow is described in Table 4. This analysis is done by reviewing the electric and electronic engineering designated standards categories, which are: "electromagnetic compatibility

(EMC)", "low voltage equipment (LV)", "radio equipment (RE)", and "restriction of the use of certain hazardous substances (RoHS)". The designated standards that the Gateway must follow are those described in the "Raspberry Pi 4 model B" declaration of conformity and which are applicable for S4DX application. Due to the use of the propylene case an additional "Electromagnetic Compatibility (EMC)" test needs to be done. In the case of the SmartTube, in order to determine the designated standards that the SmartTube must follow an extensive analysis of the technical specifications of the SmartTube, and electronic components needed to be done.

Due to the Polypropylene case and its potential impact on the electromagnetic behaviour The same conformity assessment procedure performed to affix the CE marking can be use to affix the UKCA marking on both hardware products Gateway and SmartTube.

If a so-called Self-Declaration of Conformity was performed for CE marking, the UKCA marking also allows a Self-Declaration of Conformity. However, these two declarations of Conformity need to be done in two separate documents.

Under the UK legislation for RoHS compliance, it is not necessary to perform a test report.

Table 4: Designated Standards for presumption of conformity

Gateway	SmartTube
EN 300 328 V2.2 (Radio spectrum access (2,4GHz)) (RE)	EN 300 328 V2.2 (Radio spectrum access (2,4GHz)) (RE)
ETSI EN 301 893 V2.1.1: 2017 (Radio spectrum access (5GHz)) (RE)	EN 300 440 V2.1.1 (Short Range Devices (SDR) in the frequency range (1 GHz to 40GHz)) (RE)
ETSI EN 301 489-1 V2.2.3: 2019 (For radio equipment and services.) (EMC)	EN 61326-1:2013 (Electrical equipment for measurement, control and laboratory use.) (EMC)
ETSI EN 301 489-17 V3.1.1: 2017(For radio equipment and services.) (EMC)	EN 61326-2-1:2013 (For EMC unprotected applications)
IEC EN 62368-1: 2018 (Electrical safety)	EN 61326-2-3:2013 For transducers (EMC)
IECEN 63000: 2018 (RoHS)	EN IEC 63000:2018 (RoHS)

4 Conclusion

During the regulatory analysis of S4DX hardware products, it was concluded that neither the SmartTube nor the Gateway are considered as medical device or IVDMD under the scope of UK regulations.

The Gateway as well as the SmartTube fall into the classification as Radio frequency Equipment. Therefore, the applicable legislation (The Radio Equipment Regulations 2017) must be followed.

The Gateway consists of a Raspberry Pi 4 model B in a propylene case designed for S4DX. The UK declaration of conformity performed by Raspberry Pi Ltd for its Raspberry Pi 4 model B had been taken as reference for analyse which designated standards need to be followed by S4DX for its Gateway UK declaration of conformity. Moreover, reviewing the designated standards requirements it was concluded that additional EMC test to the ones performed by Raspberry Pi Ltd are needed for compliance.

Acknowledgement

The work has been carried out at the start-up company Smart4Diagnostic GmbH.

Author's Statement

Conflict of interest: Authors state no conflict of interest.

5 References

[1] E. . I. S. Department for Business,guidance Placing manufactured products on the market in Great Britain,2022.

[2] U. S. I. The Secretary of State UK Government,The Medical Devices Regulations,UK,2002.

[3] U. S. I. The Secretary of State UK Government,The Radio Equipment Regulations, UK, 2017.

[4] U. S. I. The Secretary of State UK Government,The Electromagnetic Compatibility Regulations,UK, 2016.

[5] U. S. I. The Secretary of State UK Government,The Restriction of the Use of Certain Hazardous Substances in Electrical and Electronic Equipment Regulations,UK,2012.

[6] U. S. I. The Secretary of State UK Government,The Electrical Equipment (Safety) Regulations,UK, 2016.

[7] R. P. Ltd, «U.K. Declaration of Conformity Raspberry Pi 4 Model B, » Cambridge, 2022.

[8] O. f. p. s. a. standards,Designated standards: EMC,UK, 2022.

[9] e. a. i. S. Office of product safety and Standards and department for business, «Designated standards: radio equipment,UK, 2022.

[10] D. o. f. t. EU,Directive 98/79/EC of the European Parliament and of the Council,UK, 1998.

3

Machine Learning / AI

Autonomous locomotion of a quasi-omnidirectional rover

Franek Stark [1,2], Levin Gerdes [2,3], and Georg Schildbach [4]

[1] Robotics and Autonomous Systems, Universität zu Lübeck, franek.stark@student.uni-luebeck.de
[2] Automation and Robotics Section, ESA, Noordwijk, The Netherlands, {franek.stark, levin.gerdes}@ext.esa.int
[3] Department of Systems Engineering and Automation, University of Málaga, Málaga, Spain, gerdes@uma.es
[4] Institute for Electrical Engineering in Medicine, Universität zu Lübeck, georg.schildbach@uni-luebeck.de

Abstract

This work introduces a ROS2-based software stack for a six wheeled rover with quasi-omnidirectional locomotion system. It includes a generic Ackermann locomotion to perfom any planar rigid body twist with the rover, while taking into account the motor constraints. To improve autonomous path tracking, the existing pure pursuit controller is extended to exploit the omnidirectionallity. The improved trajectory controller was evaluated in both simulation and on the rover. It was found to minimize lateral and heading error, but requires more steering movements. Moreover the results indicate that this extension can also be used as a stand-alone omnidirectional path tracking controller.

1 Introduction

European Space Agency (ESA)'s Planetary Robotics Lab (PRL) developed multiple planetary rover prototypes to support flight missions and industry R&D activities. One of the newest developments is the Martian Rover Testbed for Autonomy (MaRTA) (Fig. 1), which is designed as a 1:2 scale model of the ExoMars rover Rosalind Franklin. It is the lab's first rover to feature an omnidirectional locomotion system, as the older rovers cannot steer their middle axle wheels. Lately, the PRL took the decision to use ROS2 on their rovers. Therefore, this work integrates the locomotion system into ROS2 and furthermore improves the autonomous path tracking by using the omnidirectionality.

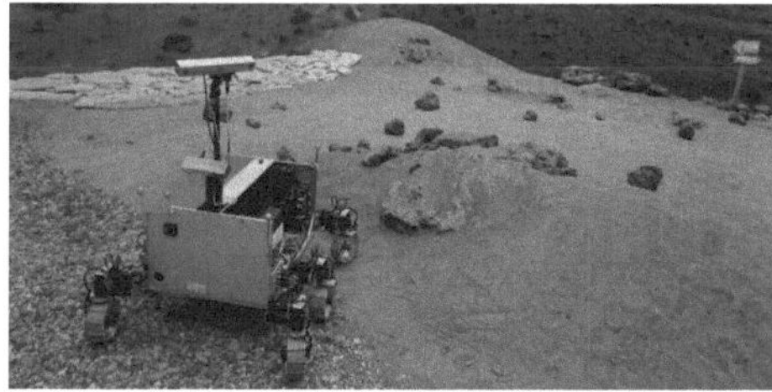

Figure 1: MaRTA in PRL

2 Material and Methods

2.1 Quasi-omnidirectional rover platform

MaRTA features a triple-bogie passive suspension with six wheels. Each wheel has a driving and steering motor and is mounted on a leg which has a deployment motor. The latter is to unfold its respective leg after landing [1]. The driving motor's velocity limit is $1.9 \frac{\text{rad}}{\text{s}}$, resulting in $\approx 12 \frac{\text{cm}}{\text{s}}$ as max rover velocity. MaRTA requires wheel repositioning, with a steering motor velocity up to $0.38 \frac{\text{rad}}{\text{s}}$, before changing its movement and the steering joint limit is $\pm 100°$. Hence, it is considered a quasi-omnidirectional robot [2].

2.2 ROS2 with Nav2

ROS2 is an open source robotics framework that offers tools to implement and analyze communication between processes running on a robot. It comes with a C++ and Python client library and helpful tools for interaction and visualization [3]. An extension is the Nav2 project, which provides a software architecture and algorithmic implementations to autonomously drive the robot [4]. This is realized by several nodes, which work together in a hierarchy to tackle the problem on different levels of abstraction. The nodes are called servers as they can host different implementations for the respective problem by using the ROS2 plugin mechanism. For example, there exist different, dynamically exchangeable, plugins which represent different algorithms to track a given path. The Nav2 project can be extended by implementing new plugins [4].

2.3 Locomotion modes

On the lowest level, Nav2 outputs a rigid body twist, which the rover needs to perform via appropriate control of the hardware actuators. In the case of MaRTA, any planar twist can be achieved by a respective wheel configuration, which is discussed in section 2.4. Moreover, MaRTA is able to use the deployment motors to *walk* on its wheels [5]. This requires the distinction between different *locomotion modes*. To optimally integrate this into the existing system, this work introduces a ROS2 locomotion package that follows the Nav2 concept. Fig. 2 shows the overall architecture, which contains the locomotion server as the central node. It receives the desired robot twist from the Nav2 controller and the current robot state. Analog to Nav2, it uses different locomotion plugins. Periodically, it calls the active plugin to map the twist to motor control commands. These plugins implement the different locomotion concepts. A ROS2 service handles the selection of the active locomotion mode.

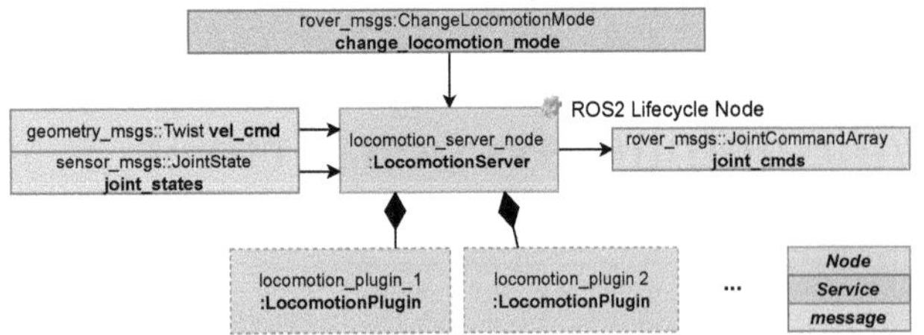

Figure 2: Locomotion package to switch locomotion modes

2.4 Generic Ackermann locomotion

The generic Ackermann locomotion mode was introduced in earlier works and completed here. It is used to perform any planar rigid body twist with MaRTA. From the kinematics for the rigid body, the equations for each wheel's longitudinal (1) and lateral (2) velocity can be derived. The rover's twist in body coordinates is $\dot{\xi}_b = \left[\dot{x}_b, \dot{y}_b, \dot{\theta}_b\right]^T$, β_i is the steering angle, and $h_{x,i}, h_{y,i}$ the location of the ith wheel in body coordinates, as sketched in Fig. 3.

$$
\begin{aligned}
v_{ti} =&\cos(\beta_i) \cdot \dot{x}_b + \sin(\beta_i) \cdot \dot{y}_b \\
&+[-h_{yi} \cdot \cos(\beta_i) + h_{xi} \cdot \sin(\beta_i)] \cdot \dot{\theta}_b \quad (1)
\end{aligned}
$$

$$
\begin{aligned}
v_{ni} =&-\sin(\beta_i) \cdot \dot{x}_b + \cos(\beta_i) \cdot \dot{y}_b \\
&+[h_{xi} \cdot \cos(\beta_i) + h_{yi} \cdot \sin(\beta_i)] \cdot \dot{\theta}_b \quad (2)
\end{aligned}
$$

Assuming no lateral tire skid ($v_{ni} = 0$) and rolling without slip ($v_{ti} = r_w \dot{\phi}_i$, with r_w wheel radius and $\dot{\phi}_i$ wheel velocity) the desired steering angle β_i and velocity $\dot{\phi}_i$ for each wheel i can be derived [2]:

$$
\beta_i = \tan^{-1}\left(\frac{\dot{y}_b + h_{xi}\dot{\theta}_b}{\dot{x}_b - h_{yi}\dot{\theta}_b}\right) \quad (3)
$$

$$
\dot{\phi}_i = \frac{v_{ti}}{r_w} \quad (4)
$$

Note, that every rover twist can also be interpreted as a rotation around the Instantaneous Center of Rotation (ICR). This work extends this concept to respect the velocity and position limits of the rover's steering and driving motors.

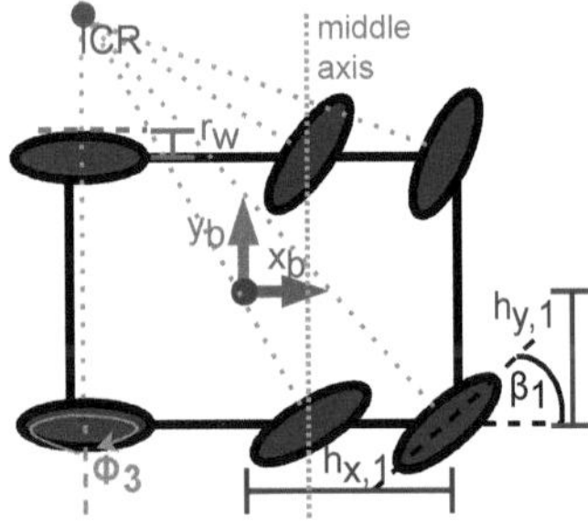

Figure 3: Schematics of 6-wheeled rover

2.4.1 Driving velocity constraints

The wheel velocities (4) are scaled down by λ, if a desired twist exceeds at least one wheel's maximum velocity:

$$
\dot{\phi}_i = \lambda\frac{v_{ti}}{r_w}, \quad (5)
$$

$$
\lambda = \begin{cases} \max_i \left|\frac{r_w}{v_{ti}}\right| \dot{\phi}_{max}, & \text{if } \max_i \left|\frac{v_{ti}}{r_w}\right| \geq \dot{\phi}_{max} \\ 1, & \text{otherwise} \end{cases} \quad (6)
$$

It can be shown that applying the scaling factor will not affect the location of the ICR, but only the velocity of the rotation around the ICR. Therefore, the desired movement of the rover is slowed down while preserving its shape.

2.4.2 Steering velocity constraints

The maximum velocity of the steering motors constrains the twist's changing rate. Additionally, when a wheel is close to its joint limit, it might be necessary to turn the respective wheel by $180°$. In that case, the rover must be stopped, as the kinematic constraints would be violated. As the used path tracking controller or a person who manually controls the rover might not be aware of this, the locomotion mode must handle abrupt changes of the desired twist. This work introduces a simple, yet effective, steering angle threshold. If a new desired twist for at least one wheel results in a change in steering angle above this threshold, the rover is stopped until the desired wheel configuration is reached.

2.5 Trajectory controller

The PRL uses an adapted version of the Pure Pursuit (PP) algorithm as the main path tracking controller. This algorithm is described in [6] and is implemented as a Nav2 controller plugin. As in planetary robotics the rover velocity is slow and a fast and exact path convergence is the main goal, it extends the original PP algorithm by an adaptive look ahead distance reduction [6]. Also, the controller distinguishes between two *control modes*. In the normal PP mode, also called *double Ackermann* mode, twists are commanded which lead to a curve whose ICR lies on the middle axis line but outside the rover body (see Fig. 3). For turns that are too sharp, the controller changes into *point turn* mode, where the ICR lays in the exact center of the middle axis [6]. The controller thus constraints the ICR onto the middle axis to be compatible with the old rovers. In this work, an extension is introduced to exploit MaRTA's omnidirectionality. The modification is designed as an additional control mode, being active when the rover is on a nearly straight path(-segment). The situation is shown in Fig. 4. The rover has a small lateral deviation ϵ and a small difference, lower than θ_{thresh}, between the rover heading and the desired heading θ_{lh} at the lookahead point. The idea is that in such a situation, it might be faster and easier to move diagonally (vec$_{lh}$) instead of steering the PP arc (arc$_{turn}$).

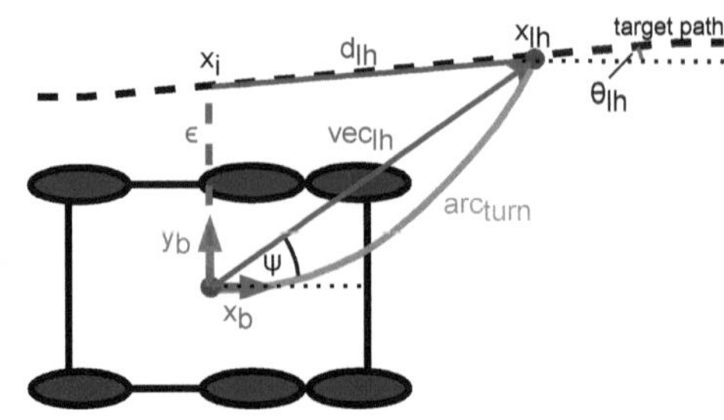

Figure 4: Look-ahead point x_{lh}. Circular arc$_{turn}$ would be commanded by PP-algorithm. Instead, a diagonal movement following vec$_{lh}$ is commanded.

2.5.1 Lateral path alignment

The linear part of the rover's twist (7, 8) is a movement vector pointing towards the lookahead point with the desired rover velocity v_{lon} as length. It is constructed from the angle ψ between the rover's heading and $\mathrm{vec}_{\mathrm{lh}}$ (see Fig. 4). To speed up the alignment, the vector can be rotated by increasing ψ, which is done in (9) via the proportional gain K_p^{pos}. To prevent oscillations, gain K_d^{pos} controls the damping.

$$\dot{x}_b = v_{\mathrm{lon}} \cdot cos(\widehat{\psi}) \quad (7)$$

$$\dot{y}_b = v_{\mathrm{lon}} \cdot sin(\widehat{\psi}) \quad (8) \qquad \widehat{\psi} = K_p^{\mathrm{pos}} \cdot \psi + K_d^{\mathrm{pos}} \cdot \dot{\psi} \quad (9)$$

2.5.2 Orientational path alignment

To keep the rover heading aligned, a PID controller (10) controls the angular component of the rover's twist. It acts on the difference between the current rover heading and the desired heading θ_{lh} at the lookahead point (see Fig. 4).

$$\dot{\theta}_b = K_p^{\mathrm{head}} \cdot \theta_{lh} + K_i^{\mathrm{head}} \cdot \int_0^t \theta_{lh} d\tau + K_d^{\mathrm{head}} \cdot \dot{\theta}_{lh} \quad (10)$$

Thus, the orientational alignment is independent of the minimization of the lateral deviation. Whereas in the PP algorithm the lateral error is minimized by changing the orientation, here the desired orientation can be maintained.

2.6 Experiments

The implemented features have been tested on the Gazebo simulator and with MaRTA at PRL. The driven trajectories are recorded by the simulation or with the tracking system available at PRL. The desired heading is always straight ahead on the path. To compare the controller's performance, the Mean Absolute Error (MAE) for position and heading is calculated. To evaluate how many steering maneuvers are needed, the total steering angle over all wheels is calculated. Moreover, the total time the rover stops to reconfigure its wheels is measured. A path close to a hill is selected, leading to sections with a bank angle of up to $14°$.

3 Results and Discussion

3.1 Generic Ackerman locomotion

With the presented adaptions the rover performs a kinematically feasible movement even for twists that would exceed the motors' velocity limits. The threshold for which steering angles the rover stops must be set depending on the desired behavior. For low thresholds, the rover will often stop, with the advantage that the exact desired twist is performed. For high values, the rover movement looks smoother at the expense of accuracy and increased mechanical stress on the wheels. The threshold should also be upper-bounded, such that the rover stops in case the desired wheel configuration can only be achieved by significantly breaking a kinematic constraint on the way to it (e.g., when hitting the steering limit). During the tests, a threshold up to $60°$ achieves smooth but accurate enough results.

3.2 Trajectory controller

The PP controller was tuned as described in [6], which leads to a lookahead distance d_{lh} of 0.4 m. The introduced omni-

		$d_{\mathrm{lh}}/$ m	K_p^{pos}	K_d^{pos}	K_p^{head}	K_i^{head}	K_d^{head}
comb-	sim	0.4	1.0 / 2.0	0.6	0.2	0.02	0.05
ined	lab		2.0	0.6	0.2	0.06	0.05
omni-	sim	0.1	2.0	0.6	0.2	0.02	0.05
dir.	lab		1.5	0.5	0.12	0.03	0.03

Table 1: Controller parameters

directional control mode became active for θ_{thresh} of $15°$. In the following, this control strategy is referred to as the *combined* controller. The introduced control mode can also be used as a stand-alone *omnidirectional* controller by setting θ_{thresh} to $180°$, together with a reduced d_{lh} of around 0.1 m, to avoid cutting corners. Tests done without the modifications are referred to as the *original PP* controller.

3.2.1 Test in simulation

Table 2 shows the simulation results. The controller settings are shown in Table 1. Already, setting K_p^{pos} to 1.0 reduces the lateral error ϵ and the heading error ψ by 0.03 m and $4.0°$. Fig. 5 shows the resulting trajectories. After sharp

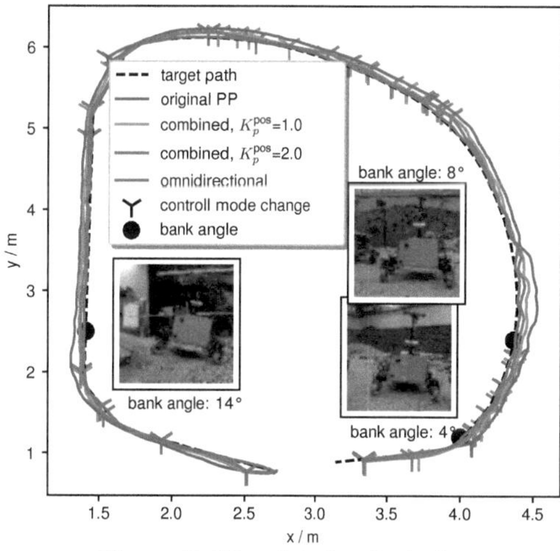

Figure 5: Simulated trajectories

turns done in PP mode, there remains a lateral deviation. The omnidirectional mode quickly reduces the lateral error while maintaining the heading. For the parts of the path that have a bank angle (marked in plots), the PP controller needs to change the rover's heading to reduce the lateral error. In contrast, the omnidirectional alignment mode can maintain the desired rover heading while reducing lateral error. To minimize the error, additional control movements are required, increasing the total steering movements by $1500°$. The additional steering movements are small, such that the rover had to stop for a negligibly longer time. With a higher K_p^{pos}, the lateral error is further reduced by 0.05 m. Compared to original PP, this is an improvement of $60\,\%$, but then steering movements and stop time are almost doubled. When using the mode as a stand-alone omnidirectional controller, during sharp curves, the high orientation error leads

controller	MAE		Σ steer / °	reconf. time / s
	ϵ / m	ψ/°		
$K_p^{\text{pos}} = 1.0$	0.042	3.039	4837	1.4
$K_p^{\text{pos}} = 2.0$	0.028	3.011	5808	2.4
omnid.	0.009	3.479	10 908	2.9
PP	0.075	7.605	3390	1.2

Table 2: Simulation results

the ICR to jump between or close to the rover's wheels. Therefore, the rover needs to stop to reconfigure its wheels. This leads to an increased stop time and more than triple the steering movements, but also reduces the lateral error by 85 % compared to original PP. A trade-off between accuracy and smooth movement has to be found. During turning, with decreasing heading error, the ICR slowly moves from the rover's center to infinity. Here, the controller must be tuned carefully, since close to the wheels even small movements of the ICR have a large effect on the steering angle and therefore lead to a start-stop behavior of the rover.

3.2.2   Tests on MaRTA in PRL

controller	MAE		Σ steer / °	reconf. time / s
	ϵ / m	ψ/°		
combined	0.012	6.054	8264	9.2
omnid.	0.007	7.527	8992	12.5
PP	0.031	6.613	5225	13.0

Table 3: Lab results

The simulation, especially the complicated wheel terrain interaction, does not perfectly model reality. It leads to increased rover slippage in the simulation, which is why MaRTA shows slightly different behavior. Table 3 shows the results for the tests done on MaRTA. The resulting trajectory is shown in Fig. 6. The original PP controller here used point turns for some sharp turns. This decreases the errors of the PP controller compared to the simulated results. However, it increases the stop time due to configuration changes. The combined controller decreases this time by 30 % while also decreasing the lateral error by 60 % (see Table 3). To prevent the ICR from being too close to the wheels in wide curves, for the omnidirectional controller,

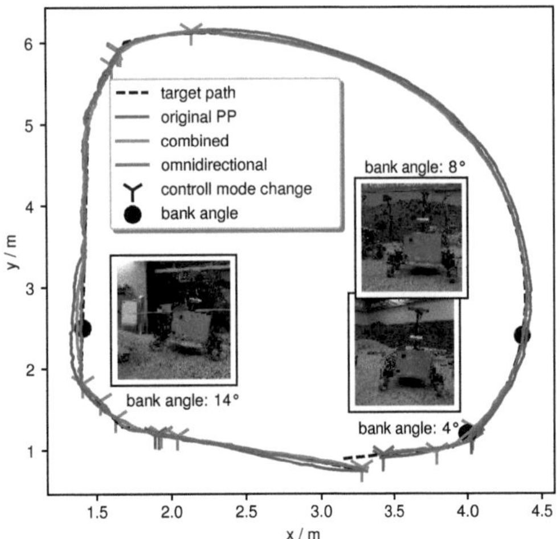

Figure 6: Trajectories driven by MaRTA in PRL

K_p^{head} has been decreased as shown in Table 1. Therefore, the heading error is slightly worse. However, the lateral error is reduced by 0.024 m which is 75 %. It should be noted that this is a fully functional omnidirectional controller, which theoretically allows any orientation of the rover along the path. Depending on the chosen parameters, a very precise path tracking with higher steering costs (energy consumption, material wear, stop time), or a rather smooth but less precise result can be achieved.

4   Conclusion

The above work presents the software stack based on ROS2 to use the quasi-omnidirectional locomotion system of six wheeled rovers, which respects the hardware constraints of the motors and better exploits its capabilities. It is shown that autonomous path tracking can be improved by commanding diagonal movements instead of curves in certain situations at the cost of more steering movements. Furthermore, this concept can also be used as a stand-alone omnidirectional controller, which must be tuned carefully, but then can compete with the original PP controller.

Acknowledgement

The work has been carried out at the European Space Research and Technology Centre (ESTEC) under supervision of ESA's PRL in collaboration with the Institute for Electrical Engineering in Medicine, Universität zu Lübeck.

Author's Statement

Conflict of interest: Authors state no conflict of interest.

5   References

[1] M. Azkarate *et al.*, "Design, testing, and evolution of mars rover testbeds: European space agency planetary exploration," *IEEE Robotics & Automation Magazine*, vol. 29, 2022.

[2] M. Sorour, A. Cherubini, R. Passama, and P. Fraisse, "Kinematic modeling and singularity treatment of steerable wheeled mobile robots with joint acceleration limits," in *IEEE International Conference on Robotics and Automation (ICRA)*, 2016.

[3] S. Macenski, T. Foote, B. Gerkey, C. Lalancette, and W. Woodall, "Robotoperatingsystem2: Design, architecture, and uses in the wild," *ScienceRobotics*, vol. 7, no. 66, 2022.

[4] S. Macenski, F. Martin, R. White, and J. G. Clavero, "The marathon 2: A navigation system," in *2020 IEEE International Conference on Intelligent Robots and Systems*, 2020.

[5] M. Azkarate *et al.*, "First experimental investigations on wheel-walking for improving triple-bogie rover locomotion performances," *Proceedings Advanced Space Technologies for Robotics and Automation (ASTRA). Noordwijk, The Netherlands: ESA*, 2015.

[6] J. Filip, M. Azkarate, and G. Visentin, "Trajectory control for autonomous planetary rovers," in *14th Symposium on Advanced Space Technologies in Robotics and Automation (ASTRA)*, 2017.

Development of Machine Learning Model for Image Segmentation in Solder Joints

Mahmoud Maan [1] Abhilaash Ajith Kumar [2]

[1] Robotics and Autonomous Systems, Universität zu Lübeck, mahmoud.mohamedmaanhemidaelhendawi@student.uni-luebeck.de

[2] Automotive Electronics/Engineering Assembly and Interconnect Technology (AE/EAI), Robert Bosch GmbH, Robert-Bosch Straße 2 - 71701 Schwieberdingen, Germany, Abhilaash.AjithKumar@de.bosch.com

Abstract

Poorly soldered joints in automotive electronics can lead to problems such as intermittent connections, short circuits, and complete failure of the component, which can negatively impact the performance and efficiency of the automotive electronic control units (ECU). In this research, we aim to develop a machine learning model for automated image segmentation of specific regions of interest (ROI) in solder joints. Two machine learning methods for ROI segmentation are utilized. The first method *(method A)* involves using an encoder-decoder convolutional neural network (CNN) architecture. The second method *(method B)* involves a similar structure of *method A*, but with a modified pre-trained version of the encoder. The models are trained and tested on a dataset of cross-section microscopy images. The results demonstrate that *method B* significantly outperformes *method A*, which achieved 13% improvement in intersection over union (IoU) score on testing dataset.

1 Introduction

In the field of automotive electronics, reliability is crucial for ensuring the safety of vehicles. Faulty or defective electronic components in safety-critical applications, such as the brakes, steering, and airbags can cause a variety of problems. This may potentially result in accidents or other safety hazards. Consequently, ensuring good quality solder joint is a crucial aspect in reliability improvement.

The soldering system *(system A)* used in this study leads to the formation of two layers, ROI 1 and ROI 2 [1]. Fig. 1 shows the two ROI layers in *system A*. The thickness of the ROI layers is a key factor in determining the risk of failure of solder joints and it can have a significant impact on the strength and reliability of the solder joint. The ROI layers thickness can be affected by various processing and service conditions, such as temperature and time of soldering. Calculating ROIs thickness is important to ensure that they are thick enough to provide a strong, reliable joint, but not so thick that they cause the joint to become brittle and prone to failure.

Developing an automated method for image segmentation helps to analyze an extensive image dataset in order to create a robust modelling of the system. In this study, we are particularly interested in segmenting ROI 1 and ROI 2 layers separately as they are the primary regions of interest as shown in Fig. 1.

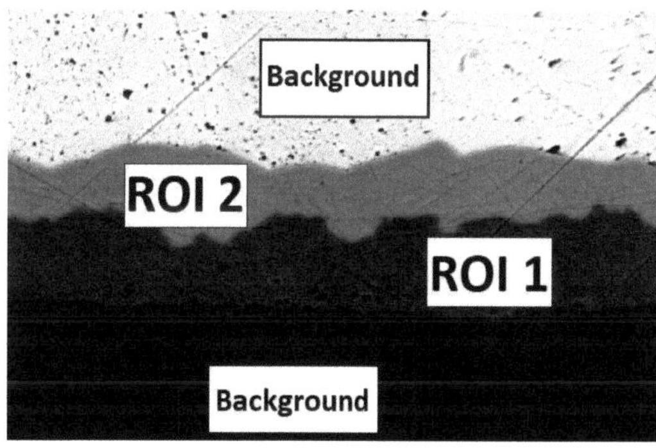

Figure 1: ROI 1 and ROI 2 layers in soldering *system A* [1].

In terms of calculating the thickness of ROI layers, image segmentation [2] could potentially be used to automatically identify and separate the two ROI layers irrespective of the changes in imaging conditions, or image artifacts, etc. This could be done by training a deep neural network model to recognize their features and segment them from the background materials. After segmenting the ROI layers in the images, any standard image processing software can be used to calculate their thickness.

2 Material and Methods

This section covers the dataset and the segmentation framework utilized in the study, as well as the metrics used to evaluate the results.

2.1 Dataset

In this study, we utilized a dataset of images of various *system A* samples with different processing conditions. These different processing conditions have a direct impact on the shape and thickness of the ROI layers. During *system A* samples preparation, some preparation artifacts can occur. The artifacts include scratches and particles, which may exist in the final output images. Additionally, the user and image acquisition settings can affect the image properties, especially the brightness, contrast, and how smooth the transition in color is between the two ROI layers.

As a result of all these factors, we encountered a variety of different and diverse images, containing various shapes and thickness of ROI layers, scratches, particle artifacts, and varying image properties. As shown in Fig. 2, two images from the dataset are presented. Fig. 2a has a high quality and is free of scratches or particles. Additionally, the boundary between the two ROI layers is clearly distinguishable. Fig. 2b on the other hand, contains scratches and particles. Furthermore, the boundary between the two ROI layers is not clearly visible, making it challenging to distinguish. The images dataset was carefully labeled and annotated into three classes: class 0 for ROI 1, class 1 for ROI 2, and class 2 for the background, to reflect the ground truth for image segmentation.

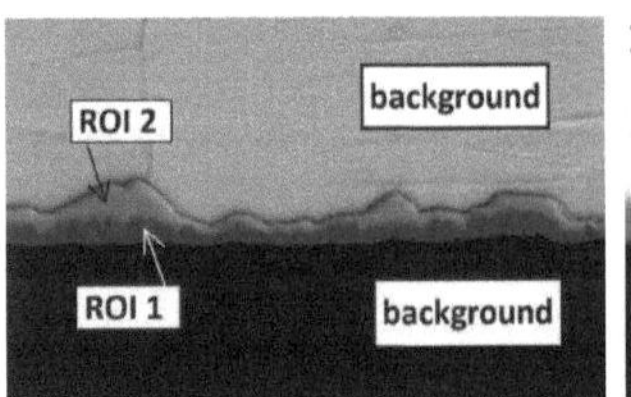

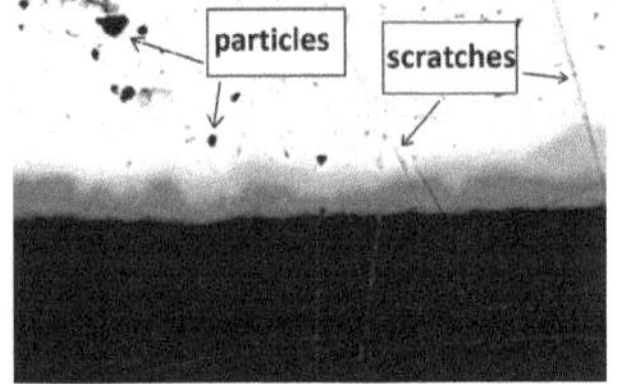

(a) High quality image sample without artifacts.

(b) Image sample with scratches and particles artifacts.

Figure 2: Two samples from the dataset.

2.1.1 Data Preprocessing

To ensure the best results for training the model, a comprehensive pre-processing of the dataset is performed. The first step is data cleaning, where any images with poor quality, potential noise or irrelevant content were eliminated. The data cleaning process resulted in three categories of images, namely valid, partially valid, and invalid images. The partially valid and invalid images were used after the training to test the model robustness.

One limitation of the dataset is its size, as it consists of only a limited number of annotated images. Additionally, the network needed to be able to handle the change in brightness, contrast, shifts, flips, shears, and zooms in this dataset. Consequently, data augmentation techniques are applied [3]. After data augmentation, the dataset significantly increased by nearly 400%, which provided the model with

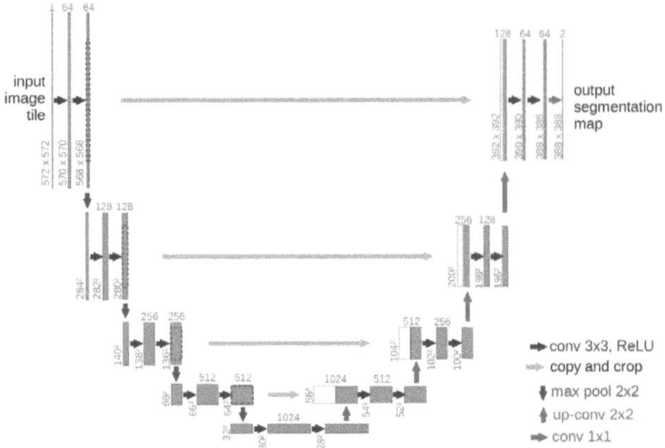

Figure 3: Example of an encoder-decoder network architecture [4].

more diverse data to learn from. Additionally, a data split strategy is applied to the dataset. It is divided into training, validation and testing sets, with a ratio of 70%, 15%, and 15% respectively. This step is important to evaluate the model's performance on unseen data. The validation set is used to tune the model's hyperparameters and to monitor the training process to avoid overfitting.

2.2 Segmentation Framework

As previously discussed in Dataset section, the images contain a wide range of properties and features. This complexity poses a challenge for traditional image segmentation techniques, such as thresholding and active contours, which may not be able to accurately segment these images. While these methods may perform well on certain images, such as those with simple and clear shapes, they may not be suitable for images with more complex shapes or artifacts, such as Fig. 2b. Therefore, it becomes necessary to employ modern deep learning-based methods to overcome these limitations and achieve good segmentation results.

The present study employs deep learning-based methods for image segmentation. In the following section, we describe in details the specific methods utilized, as well as the post-processing steps applied.

2.2.1 Network Architecture

The study employed an encoder-decoder CNN as the base architecture as shown in Fig. 3. In this research, two methods were employed: *method A* utilized the encoder-decoder CNN [4], while *method B* involved the same structure of *method A*, but with a modified pre-trained version of the encoder [5]. *Method B* network consists of 22 convolutional layers with varying filter numbers, ranging from 64 to 512, a kernel size of 3x3, a stride of 2, and 'same' padding. The activation function used was ReLU, and the optimizer used was Adam with 0.001 learning rate. The batch size used in training was 16, and the model was trained for 25 epochs. Furthermore, the model included 5 dropout layers, primarily located in the decoder, with a dropout rate of 0.3. The utilization of the pre-trained encoder in *method B* allowed for the leverage of its powerful feature extraction capabilities, thus improving the model performance.

2.2.2 Transfer Learning

The study employed transfer learning [5]. By using a pre-trained model, the data and computation requirements for training are reduced, resulting in faster training time and improved performance. In *method B*, the pre-trained parameters of the encoder are frozen, meaning that its weights would not be updated during training. The total number of parameters in the network is 25,854,787, out of which 14,714,688 are frozen and the remaining 11,140,099 are trainable. Freezing the encoder parameters, which account for more than half of the total parameters, positively impacted the training performance and time.

2.2.3 Post-processing

After segmenting the regions of interest in the images, post-processing techniques are applied to *method B* to improve the quality of the segmentation masks. The first technique is filling holes in the segmented regions, which can occur due to incomplete segmentation or noise in the input image. A hole filling algorithm is used [6]. It utilizes a flooding method where a point within the hole is chosen and the surrounding area is filled with foreground pixels until the hole is entirely filled. Later, a noise reduction technique is applied to eliminate isolated pixels that do not belong to the ROI layers. A connected component analysis method is employed. This method identifies and removes connected components that do not meet a certain size threshold.

However, there are some limitations to these postprocessing techniques. For example, the hole filling algorithm is not sufficiently effective for filling very large or irregularly shaped holes. Additionally, the size threshold used in noise reduction technique may need to be adjusted for different types of images and segmentation tasks.

2.3 Performance Metrics

In order to evaluate the effectiveness and accuracy of the machine learning models in our study, two commonly-used performance metrics for segmentation tasks were employed: Intersection over Union (IoU) and Dice coefficient. IoU, as defined in equation (1), is a measure of the overlap between the predicted segmentation mask (A) and the ground truth mask (B).

$$IoU = \frac{A \cap B}{A \cup B} \tag{1}$$

The Dice coefficient in equation (2) is another measure of the overlap between the predicted (A) and ground truth (B) masks.

$$Dice\ Coefficient = \frac{2 * (A \cap B)}{|A| + |B|} \tag{2}$$

3 Results and Discussion

In this section, the results of this study are presented. The aim is to compare the performance of the two different methods that were discussed for the segmentation task.

Method	IoU	Dice coefficient
Method A	0.76	0.71
Method B	0.89	0.85

Table 1: Evaluation results for *method A* and *method B* on testing dataset.

The results of the two models evaluation on testing dataset are summarized in Table 1. *Method A* achieved an average Intersection over Union (IoU) score of 0.76 and an average Dice coefficient of 0.71. *Method B*, on the other hand, achieved an average IoU score of 0.89 and an average Dice coefficient of 0.85.

Visual results of both methods and the post-processing step are presented in Fig. 4. As seen, *method A* could segment the images, but with various defects. In Fig. 4a, there is a separate region that is segmented, despite not being part of ROI 2. This is likely due to heavy scratches in the lighter background. Furthermore, the edges and borders of both ROI 1 and 2 segmented masks in *method A* exhibit a high level of smoothness. For example, in Fig. 4a and Fig. 4b, the edges and borders of both ROI layers are not as sharp as those in the ground truth. Similar failure is shown in Fig. 4c, where the edges are not sharply identified. Despite this weakness, *method A* could identify a larger portion of the extreme peak compared to *method B*.

The limitations of *method A* are addressed by *method B*. As seen in Fig. 4a, the segmented mask produced by *method B* is free of any irrelevant regions in the background and is nearly similar to the ground truth. In Fig. 4b, there are some noisy regions in the background and some holes inside ROI 2. Most likely, this is due to the extreme change in pixels values between the background and both ROI. Regarding the edges and borders of both ROI, *method B* is able to accurately identify them, as they are almost as sharp as those in the ground truth. However, the border of ROI 1 in Fig. 4c is not easily noticeable to the human eye, even though *method B* is able to segment it. In some of test images such as Fig. 4c, a limitation of *method B* is observed, as the model fails to detect the extreme peaks features. This is likely due to a lack of training data, as the model was not exposed to a sufficient number of images that contained such features.

The post-processing step is applied to the segmented masks produced by *method B*. As seen in Fig. 4b and Fig. 4c, the post-processing step is able to remove all the noisy regions in the background and fill in the holes inside ROI 2. Overall, the post-processing step is able to overcome some of the limitations of *method B*, resulting in more high quality segmentation masks.

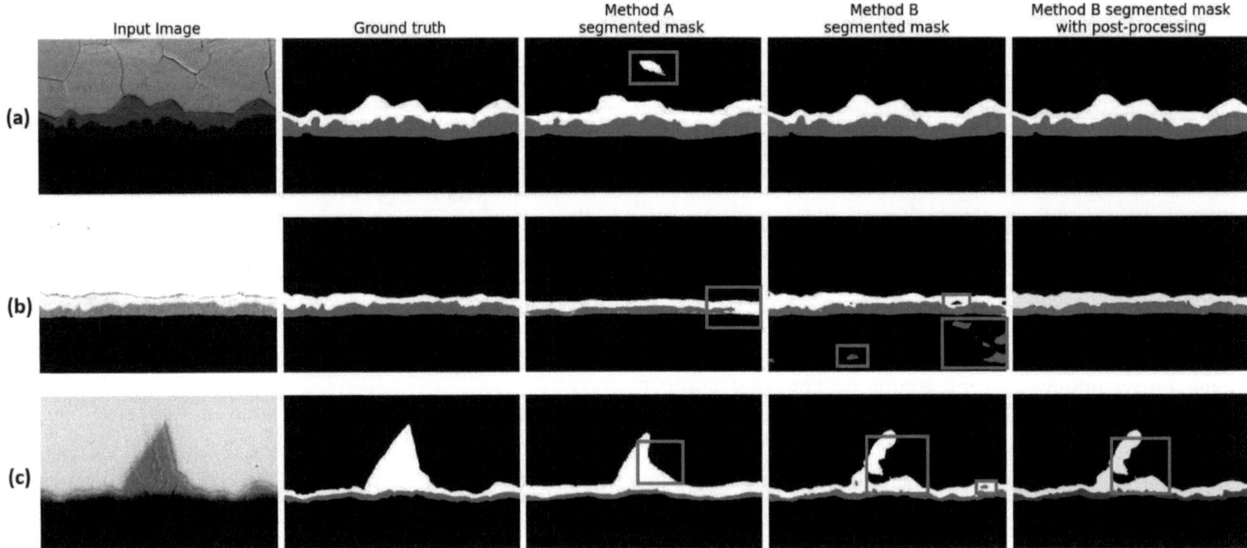

Figure 4: Comparison of 3 different samples (a-c) from *system A* dataset between the ground truth and the segmented masks from *method A* and *method B*, as well as the segmented mask from *method B* after applying post-processing techniques. Green boxes highlight the defects on the segmented masks. The lower layer (ROI 1) is in gray, the upper layer (ROI 2) is in white, and the background is in black.

4 Conclusion

This study highlights using deep neural networks for image segmentation of solder joint microscopy images. The segmentation performance of two methods involving standard encoder-decoder CNN network without pre-trained parameters (*method A*) and another CNN with pre-trained encoder parameters (*method B*) is compared. The results demonstrate that *method B* with post-processing step are able to overcome the limitations of *method A*, which achieved 13% improvement in IoU score, resulting in more accurate segmentation of testing dataset. It is worth noting that there are a limited number of *system A* images, which is a constraint in this research work. Training on a more diverse dataset, including the use of elastic deformation as a data augmentation technique is a solution to address the weakness in *method B*'s ability to identify extreme peaks in ROI layers. Future work includes exploring other state-of-the-art architectures and post-processing techniques to further improve the accuracy of the segmentation results.

Acknowledgement

The work has been carried out and supervised at Robert Bosch GmbH, Automotive Electronics/Engineering Assembly and Interconnect Technology department and the Institut für Neuro- und Bioinformatik, Universität zu Lübeck.

Author's Statement

The authors declare that they have no conflicts of interest.

5 References

[1] T.-T. Luu, A. Duan, K. Aasmundtveit, and N. Hoivik, "Optimized cu-sn wafer-level bonding using intermetallic phase characterization," *Journal of Electronic Materials*, vol. 42, 12 2013.

[2] S. Minaee, Y. Boykov, F. Porikli, A. Plaza, N. Kehtarnavaz, and D. Terzopoulos, "Image segmentation using deep learning: A survey," *CoRR*, vol. abs/2001.05566, 2020. [Online]. Available: https://arxiv.org/abs/2001.05566

[3] A. Buslaev, V. I. Iglovikov, E. Khvedchenya, A. Parinov, M. Druzhinin, and A. A. Kalinin, "Albumentations: Fast and flexible image augmentations," *Information*, vol. 11, no. 2, 2020. [Online]. Available: https://www.mdpi.com/2078-2489/11/2/125

[4] O. Ronneberger, P.Fischer, and T. Brox, "U-net: Convolutional networks for biomedical image segmentation," in *Medical Image Computing and Computer-Assisted Intervention (MICCAI)*, ser. LNCS, vol. 9351. Springer, 2015, pp. 234–241, (available on arXiv:1505.04597 [cs.CV]). [Online]. Available: http://lmb.informatik.uni-freiburg.de/Publications/2015/RFB15a

[5] D. Cheng and E. Y. Lam, "Transfer learning u-net deep learning for lung ultrasound segmentation," 2021. [Online]. Available: https://arxiv.org/abs/2110.02196

[6] Y. He, T. Hu, and D. Zeng, "Scan-flood fill(scaff): an efficient automatic precise region filling algorithm for complicated regions," *CoRR*, vol. abs/1906.03366, 2019. [Online]. Available: http://arxiv.org/abs/1906.03366

The Optimal Crowd Machine
for multi-omics data integration

Marina Bleskina [1], Silke Szymczak [2]

[1] Medizinische Informatik, Universität zu Lübeck, m.bleskina@student.uni-luebeck.de
[2] Institut für Medizinische Biometrie und Statistik, Universität zu Lübeck, silke.szymczak@uni-luebeck.de

Abstract

The optimal crowd machine (OCM) for combining several classifiers is adapted to the task of integrating multi-omics data where data of single omics levels can be missing for some individuals. An implementation as R package is provided. Using experimental multi-omics data from The Cancer Genome Atlas we show that despite missing values in data, prediction of OCM is at least as good as the best single classifier used, assuming the number of missing values in data set is not high.

1 Introduction

In biomedical research omics data is used to identify and to predict specific diseases. Omics data are the result from high-throughput biochemical assay analysis of biological samples [1]. Examples for this kind of data set are genomics, transcriptomics, proteomics and metabolomics. To overcome the lack of good prediction models for complex diseases, the information of multiple omics data sets is often combined. This is then called a multi-omics data set.

The collection of samples for the different omics types is complex and often expensive, so that not each omics type is available for each observation. However, most of the integration methods assume that all omics types have been measured. This greatly reduces the sample size und thus statistical power. It is therefore important to examine integration approaches that can deal with missing values.

In this work we propose to use the so-called optimal crowd machine (OCM) to predict classes from multi-omics data sets with missing values. OCM integrates classification outcomes from several classifiers to provide a final classification [2]. In their work Battogtokh et al. showed that OCM is optimal in the sense, that the prediction is at least as good as the best single classifier used. If a classifier exists that minimizes the prediction error, so does the OCM [2]. To test our suggested approach, we first implemented an R package, that provides an optimal crowd machine adopted to missing values. This implementation is then tested by applying it to a real-world multi-omics data set.

2 Material and Methods

2.1 Optimal crowd machine

The OCM integrates classification predictions from several classifiers to provide a final classification.
In order to adapt the OCM to the problem of missing measurements in multi-omics data sets, we have implemented

the R package "ocm" in such a way that the two classes of the binary outcome are extended by a class NA. This value is used for observations that can not be classified otherwise, for example, due to missing measurements.

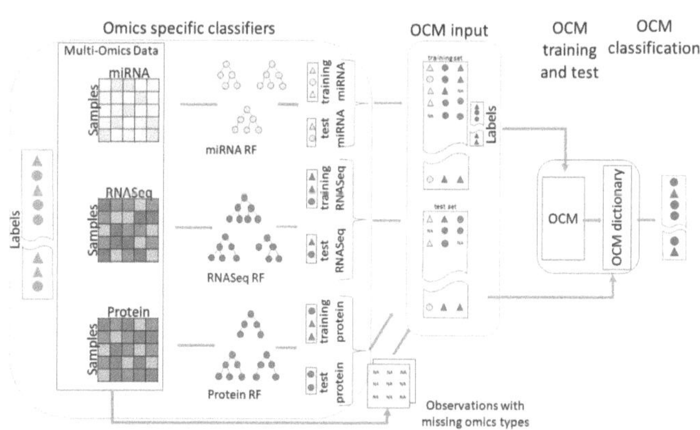

Figure 1: OCM-based integration of multi-omics data set

The OCM workflow can be summarized by the following steps (Fig. 1):

1. Omics specific classifiers
   The training process is carried out by several classifiers, so several predictions for each observation are obtained. Different classifiers can be applied to the same data set. However, we trained a separate classifier for each omics type separately. If classification of an observation is not possible due to missing measurements, this observation is not used for training but is assigned to the NA class.

2. OCM input
   The predicted class of each classifier is used as input for the OCM. If one of the omics data sets is not available for a specific observation, the prediction is class NA.

3. OCM training

   The OCM training process is a mapping process. In doing so, a dictionary of all possible classification combinations across classifiers, i.e. omics, is generated from the OCM training data set (Fig. 2). For each combination, the true class labels of the training observations with this particular combination are saved.

4. OCM test

   Each test observation of the OCM test data set is assigned to the classification combination of the dictionary that has the same combination. True class labels corresponding to dictionary combinations are averaged and the majority class is assigned to the test observation.

   If several classification combinations from the dictionary are equally similar to the test observation, the corresponding training labels are merged and averaged to obtain the final classification.

   In the referenced paper, Euclidean distance was used as a similarity measure. We used the Simple Matching Coefficient that calculates the ratio of the number of voting classes to the number of total classes.

5. OCM classification output

   Final classification is delivered.

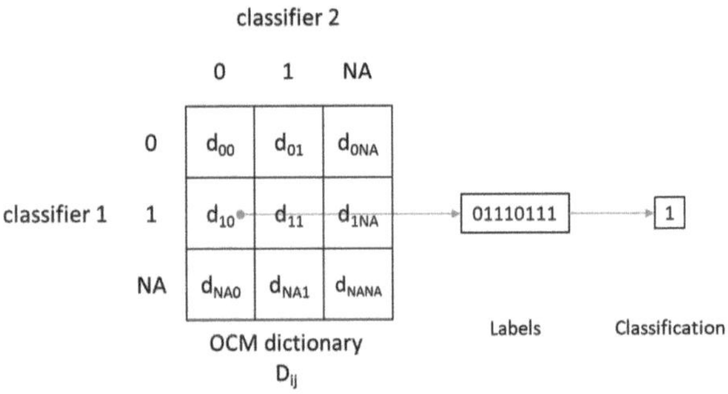

Figure 2: Suppose we have two classifiers. The possible classes are 0, 1 and NA. Classifier 1 predicted class 1 for the test observation, classifier 2 predicted class 0. Thus, the test observation is assigned to cell d_{10} of dictionary D_{ij}. The corresponding training labels to this cell are averaged. The test observation is assigned to class 1, since the majority decides.

2.2   Multi-omics data sets

To apply the "ocm" R package to multi-omics data, we used publicly available data from The Cancer Genome Atlas (TCGA) project. The omics types along with the clinical data are stored as R objects ("MultiAssayExperiment") [3] in the Bioconductor package "curatedTCGAData" [4].

We selected 17 cancer types for which RNA-Seq, miRNA-Seq and protein data are available and we performed the following additional filtering steps: 1) Restrict to primary tumor, 2) Remove replicates (keep first one), 3) Keep only basic clinical information, 4) Remove proteins with missing values.

We have selected appropriate outcomes from the available clinical data based on the following criteria: 1) Binary, 2) At least 40 patients, 3) Balanced (minor class maximal 40 %), 4) Not gender or information about availability of specific data types.

Table 1 shows the characteristics of the final 17 data sets.

Table 1: Overview of the multi-omics data sets

Cancer type	Outcome	Cl1 / Cl2	No. obs.	No. var. RNASeq	No. var. miRNA	No. var. Protein
ACC	C1A.C1B	43 / 35	78	20502	1047	193
BLCA	vital_status	230 / 182	412	20502	1047	196
BRCA	radiation_therapy	446 / 556	1002	20502	1047	217
BRCA	Node.Coded	385 / 405	790	20502	1047	217
HNSC	vital_status	304 / 224	528	20502	1047	161
LGG	Grade	216 / 241	457	20502	1047	182
LUSC	vital_status	284 / 220	504	20502	1047	196
OV	vital_status	225 / 325	550	20502	706	196
THCA	multifocality	227 / 266	493	20502	1047	176
UCEC	radiation_therapy	278 / 224	502	20502	1047	196
KICH	laterality	30 / 36	66	20502	1047	194
LGG	TERT.promoter.status	130 / 162	292	20502	1047	182
LGG	TERT.expression.status	224 / 289	513	20502	1047	182
PRAD	ERG_status	152 / 181	333	20502	1047	187
STAD	TP53.mutation	152 / 137	289	20502	1047	187
STAD	Copy.Number.Cluster	159 / 134	293	20502	1047	187
COAD	hystory_of_colon_polyps	70 / 67	137	20502	706	197

The first column contains cancer types, the second contains outcome variables, the third shows the distribution of classes 1 and 0 in the data set. The fourth column gives the number of observation and the last three columns gives the number of variables.

2.3   OCM on TCGA multi-omics data sets

Each of the data sets was used to obtain predictions for each of three omics types by training random forest models [5] using 5-fold cross validation with 200 trees and otherwise default parameter settings of the R package "ranger" [6]. The aim of training the three classifiers was not to find the best prediction model, but to create an input for the OCM. Prediction performance of each classifier, the OCM and the majority vote (MV) across the omics specific classifiers was evaluated using overall prediction error.

2.4   Performance of OCM under different types of missingness

The aim is to determine how different types of missing values affect the classification performance of the OCM.

For each of the three complete omics data sets five data sets were generated.

For each of these data sets with missings were generated as follows:

1. Random selection of individuals

   Seven data sets were generated by randomly setting some of the observations to missing. The proportion of missingness (15, 20, 30, 40, 50, 60 or 70 %) was varied.

2. Random selection of individuals based on outcome

   In total 49 (7 x 7) data sets were generated by randomly setting some of the observations to missing, accounting for the distribution of outcome classes. The proportion of missingness for each of the classes was varied separately (15, 20, 30, 40, 50, 60 or 70 %).

Training and evaluation of classifiers was performed as described in the previous section.

3 Results and Discussion

3.1 R package ocm

To predict classes despite missing values in multi-omics data, we implemented the R package "ocm". The original algorithm implemented in Python was re-implemented in R and the binary case was extended by a third class to store the information about missingness (Fig. 2).

3.2 OCM on TCGA multi-omics data sets

We refer the random forest classifier (RF) for RNA-Seq data as classifier 1, for miRNA-Seq data as classifier 2 and for protein data as classifier 3. Prediction error of these three classifiers, OCM and MV for each of the 17 TCGA data sets are given in Table 2. Here, OCM is 1 percentage points (pp) worse than the MV if the prediction errors of classifiers 1 and 2 are similar and that of classifier 3 is higher, or if the classifiers 1, 2 and 3 have similarly high errors (see ACC and LUSC data sets). OCM shows similar or 1 - 3 pp better results than MV when the three omics classifiers have similarly high prediction errors. This can be seen in data sets LGG - THCA. The COAD data set has no values at all in the miRNA data, here prediction error of OCM is 5 pp better. The OCM error of the bottom six data sets (PRAD - KICH) is less than that of MV. Here classifier 1 consistently shows better results compared to the other two omics classifiers. OCM's prediction error is better than the best of the three omics classifiers for the BLCA, HNSC, OV, UCEC, LGG (result: TERT.promoter.status) and COAD data sets.

Table 2: Prediction error of the different classifiers on each of the TCGA data sets

Data set	Outcome	RF for RNASeq	RF for miRNA	RF for protein	OCM	MV
ACC	C1A.C1B	0.0641	0.0633	0.1477	0.0766	0.0633
LUSC	vital_status	0.4332	0.4526	0.4259	0.4445	0.4344
LGG	Grade	0.3064	0.3359	0.3733	0.3218	0.3305
HNSC	vital_status	0.3828	0.3946	0.3674	0.3465	0.3692
OV	vital_status	0.4334	0.3840	0.3833	0.3672	0.3963
BLCA	vital_status	0.4063	0.3934	0.4412	0.3882	0.40
COAD	hystory_of_colon_polyps	0.55	-	0.4934	0.4304	0.4814
BRCA	radiation_therapy	0.4289	0.4868	0.4307	0.4401	0.4401
UCEC	radiation_therapy	0.5116	0.4624	0.4927	0.4563	0.4561
BRCA	Node.Coded	0.4421	0.4952	0.4670	0.4594	0.4658
THCA	multifocality	0.4525	0.4795	0.5105	0.4746	0.4847
PRAD	ERG_status	0.0450	0.2061	0.2641	0.0450	0.1261
LGG	TERT.promoter.status	0.0755	0.1406	0.1815	0.0721	0.0891
LGG	TERT.expression.status	0.0916	0.1531	0.2025	0.0975	0.1209
STAD	Copy.Number.Cluster	0.0983	0.2542	0.2747	0.1125	0.1601
STAD	TP53.mutation	0.2255	0.4034	0.4264	0.2733	0.3387
KICH	laterality	0.4846	0.5780	0.6346	0.4989	0.5758

3.3 Performance of OCM under different types of missingness

To analyze the impact of missing values on the OCM prediction performance, we focus on two exemplary scenarios: a data set with a similarly high error on the three classifiers (Fig. 3 and 5) and a data set with low error on only one classifier (Fig. 4 and 6). The BLCA data set was used for Fig. 3 and 5, the LGG (outcome: TERT.promoter.status) data set was used for Fig. 4 and 6, missing values were assigned to all three classifiers.

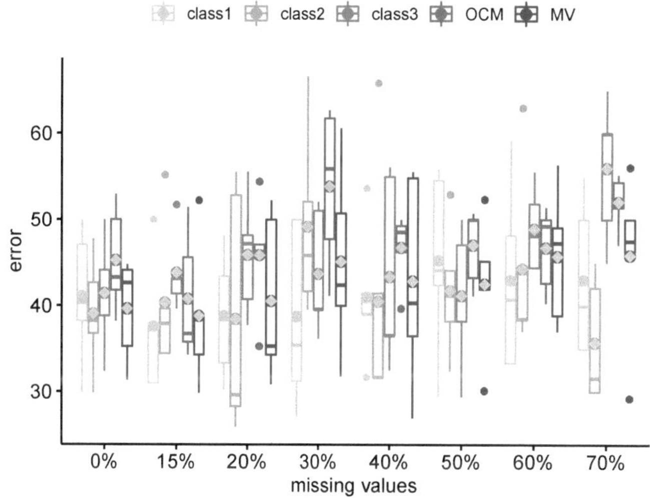

Figure 3: Prediction error of the different classifiers across varying levels of missingness in a data set. All omics classifiers have similarly high errors.

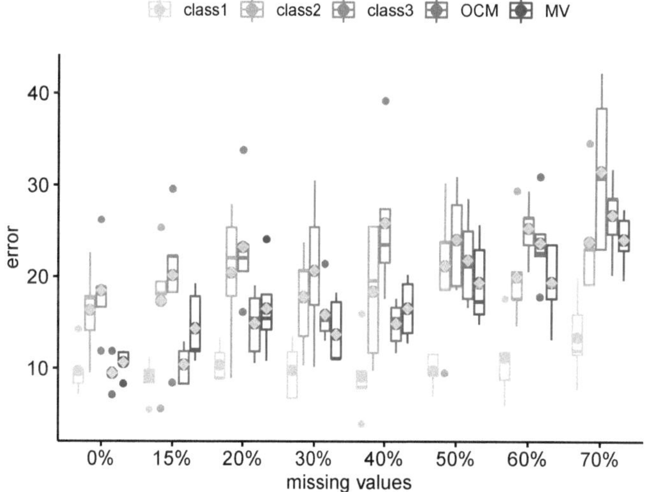

Figure 4: Prediction error of the different classifiers across varying levels of missingness in a data set. One omics classifier has a low error.

1. Random selection of individuals

   Fig. 3 shows the prediction error for all five classifiers when all omics classifiers have high errors. The OCM shows slightly worse prediction errors than the MV across the different levels of missingness, as well as for the complete data set.

   The results are different, if one of the classifiers has a low error (Fig. 4). As the missing values in the data set increase, the error of classifier 1 remains constantly low, the errors of classifiers 2 and 3 grow very slowly. Only with complete data and 15% missing values is the OCM as good as classifier 1. MV is worse than the best classifier, but still good. From 15% missing values errors of the OCM and the MV increase. The errors of classifiers 2 and 3 grow very slowly as the missing values increase. For large freqeuncies of missingness, MV becomes better than OCM. This can be explained by the fact that OCM always returns a classification even if the predictions of the three classifiers are missing. These are taken into account in the OCM result and displayed in the graphics. In such cases, MV does not return any predictions and their error cannot be graphed.

2. Random selection of individuals based on outcomes
   Fig. 5 shows the results for the setting when the probability of missingness depends on the outcome and omics specific classifiers have high errors. Here the error of MV is lower than the one of OCM for low frequencies of missingness but the error of OCM drops substantially for large frequencies when class imbalance increases.
   Fig. 6 shows the results for the setting when the probability of missingness depends on the outcome and one of the classifiers has a low error. While errors of classifiers 2 and 3 as well as MV increase with higher class imbalance, error of classifier 1 and OCM decreases at lower frequencies of missingness and stays constant at higher frequencies.

4   Conclusion

From the results it can be concluded, that despite missing values in the omics data, OCM performs as well or better than the best classifier in the family, assuming the number of missing values is not high. In the data sets with imbalanced classes in outcomes, the OCM's prediction error is small if the error of any of the classifiers is small.

With similar prediction errors of all classifiers, OCM is as good or worse than alternative methods (e.g. MV) and is not recommended because of computational cost. Howerever, in this case with highly imbalanced classes in outcome OCM shows a good prediction performance.

Acknowledgement

The work has been carried out and supervised by the Institut für Medizinische Biometrie und Statistik, Universität zu Lübeck. The results published here are in whole or part based upon data generated by the TCGA Research Network: https://www.cancer.gov/tcga.

Author's Statement

Authors state no conflict of interest.

5   References

[1] A. Conesa and S. Beck, *Making multi-omics data set accessible to researchers.* Scientific Data, vol. 6, no. 1, 2019, Art. no. 251.

[2] B. Battogtokh, M. Mojirsheibani and J. Malley, *The optimal crowd learning machine.* BioData Mining, vol. 10, 2017, Art. no. 16.

[3] M. Ramos, L. Schiffer, A. Re, R. Azhar, A. Basunia, CR. Cabrera, T. Chan, P. Chapman, S. Davis, D. Gomez-Cabrero, AC. Culhane, B. Haibe-Kains, K. Hansen, H. Kodali, MS. Louis, AS. Mer, M. Reister, M. Morgan, V. Carey and L. Waldron, *Software For The Integration Of Multi-Omics Experiments In Bioconductor.* Cancer Research, vol. 77, no. 21, pp. e39-e42, 2017.

[4] M. Ramos, L. Geistlinger, S. Oh, L. Schiffer, R. Azhar, H. Kodali, I. de Bruijn, J. Gao, V.J. Carey, M. Morgan and L. Waldron, *Multiomic Integration of Public Oncology Databases in Bioconductor.* JCO Clinical Cancer Informatics, vol. 4, pp. 958-971, 2020.

[5] L. Breiman, *Random Forests.* Machine Learning, vol. 45, no. 1, pp. 5-32, 2001.

[6] M. N. Wright and A. Ziegler, *ranger: A fast implementation of random forests for high dimensional data set in C++ and R.* Journal of Statistical Software, vol. 77, no. 1, pp. 1-17, 2017.

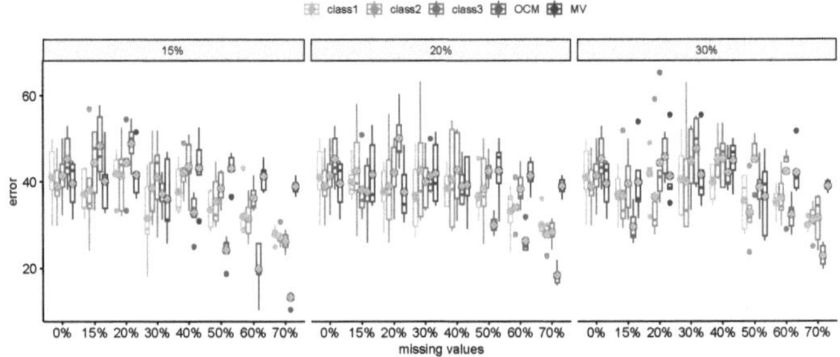

Figure 5: Prediction error of the different classifiers, when the probability of missingness in a data set depends on the outcome and omics specific classifiers have high errors. The proportion of missingness for class 0: 15, 20 or 30%, for class 1: 15, 20, 30, 40, 50, 60 or 70 %.

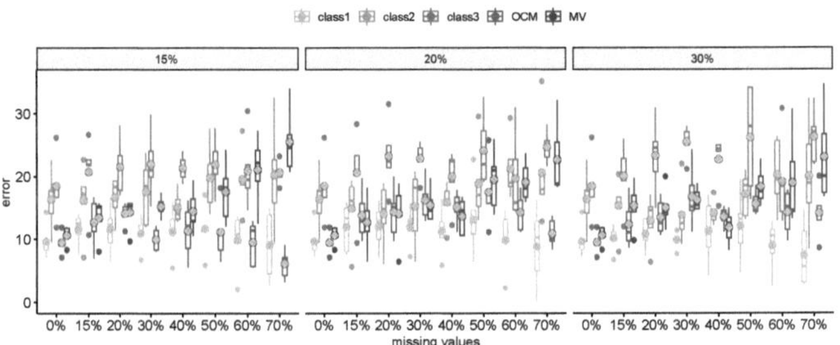

Figure 6: Prediction error of the different classifiers, when the probability of missingness in a data set depends on the outcome and one classifier has a low error. The proportion of missingness for class 0: 15, 20 or 30%, for class 1: 15, 20, 30, 40, 50, 60 or 70 %.

Autonomous Mapping of Rumex in Grassland with a Mobile Robot

Niklas Kompe [1], Ngoc Thinh Nguyen [2]
[1] Robotics and Autonomous Systems, University of Lübeck, niklas.kompe@student.uni-luebeck.de
[2] Institute for Robotics and Cognitive Systems, University of Lübeck, nguyen@rob.uni-luebeck.de

Abstract

A key task in agriculture is the control and monitoring of weeds. For those purposes, we present a prototypical system for the small mobile robot Jackal, which is equipped with a LIDAR sensor and a stereo camera. First, an area can be selected in the program window on a map of the field. Second, the robot explores the selected area while navigating with the standard ROS navigation tool and building an obstacle map with *GMapping*. After planning a simple path for rumex mapping, the reference is followed using the Monte Carlo localization algorithm *amcl*. Meanwhile, rumex plants are detected using a YOLOv4 object detector and tracked through frames of the camera. The position of the robot, the obstacle map, the planned path, and the positions of detected rumex plants are plotted live in the program window. The whole process is validated under simulation in realistic agricultural environments in Gazebo.

1 Introduction

Noxious weeds can reduce the quality and quantity of crops in agriculture and cause problems during harvest [1]. Rumex obtusifolius is referred to as the most problematic weed on permanent pasture [2]. It spreads fast, displaces forage grasses, is very resistant and has a lower energy density. Moreover, no really economical solution for the control of rumex is available. Especially in ecological agriculture without the use of herbicides, this is a very labour-consuming task. State-of-the-art high-technology solutions for monitoring and control of weeds are mostly not economically viable for smaller farms. Furthermore, the growing demand of biomass in addition to foodstuffs and feedingstuff is enhanced further due to the transition to renewable energy sources [2]. Thus, the control of rumex among others is essential for an efficient usage.

Therefore, the goal of the this project is to acquire knowledge for further research projects by implementing a prototypical system for mapping rumex plants in grassland by use of a small mobile robot.

The Jackal mobile robot is a customizable, easy-to-use research platform for field robotics from Clearpath Robotics shown in Fig. 1 [3]. Its main PC contains a Nvidia GTX 1050 GPU and runs on Ubuntu 18.04 with ROS Melodic installed, which provides a structured communications layer. Additionally, a ZED stereo camera and an Ouster 3D LIDAR sensor are added. The difference to state-of-the-art weed-control systems for large farms is the small size and the use of off-the-shelf components. Also, the Jackal is versatile and could be used for further applications as well. This results in a comparably low price, which would make an investment for smaller farms economically viable.

The program is implemented as a ROS package in python. A program window is used to select the area, and visualize results during exploration and mapping. For initial tests, the ROS integrated simulation software Gazebo is used. When using the Jackal in the real world, the frames of the program window are sent wirelessly to a different PC with a monitor.

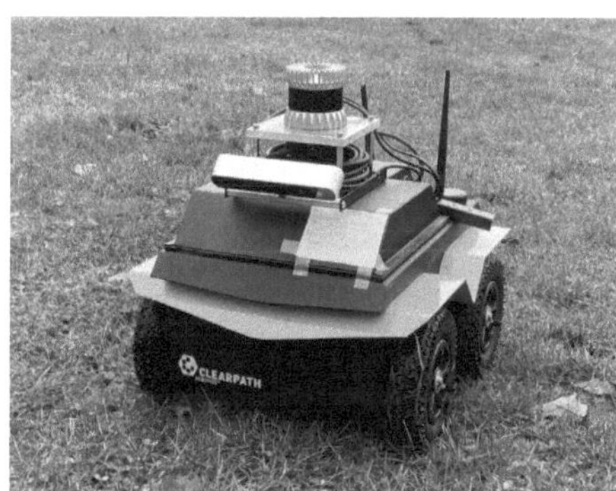

Figure 1: The Jackal mobile robot with dimensions of 51 × 43 × 25 cm, a ZED stereo camera in front and the Ouster LIDAR on top.

2 Material and Methods

2.1 Program Behaviour

In the following, the program is explained starting with the initial map and the process of selecting the area, and followed by the exploration and finally the rumex mapping phase.

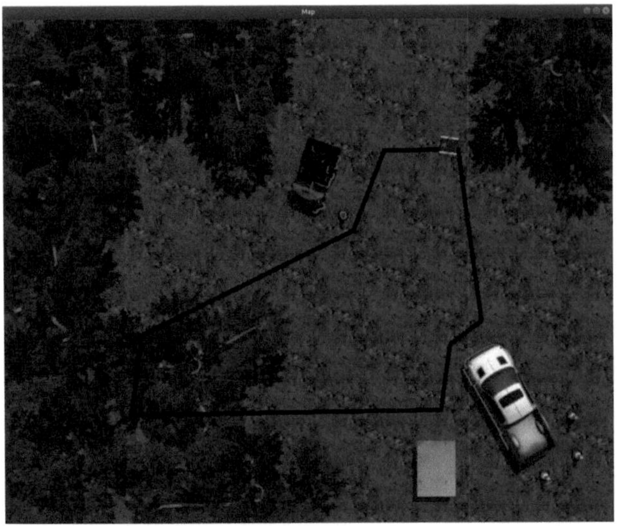

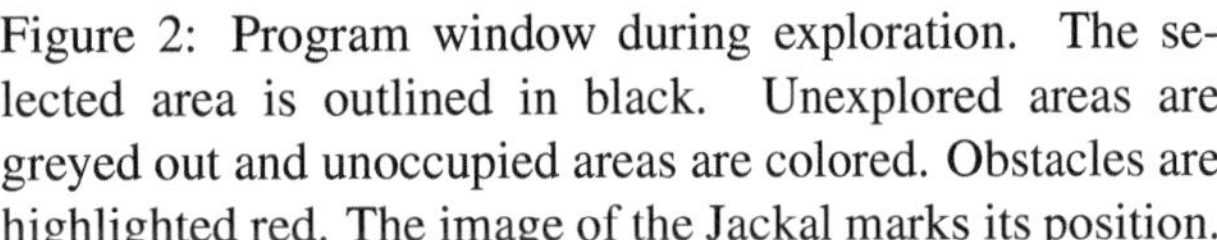

Figure 2: Program window during exploration. The selected area is outlined in black. Unexplored areas are greyed out and unoccupied areas are colored. Obstacles are highlighted red. The image of the Jackal marks its position.

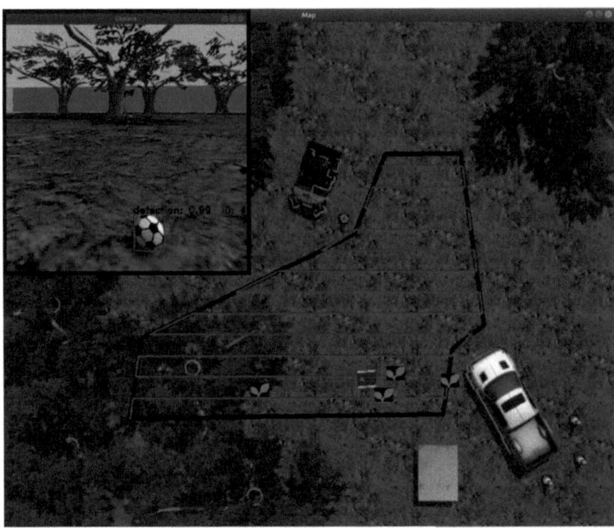

Figure 3: Program window during rumex mapping. The planned path is highlighted in blue. Additionally, the camera view with the detections is displayed overlaying the program window. Plants are marked by the green leaf symbol.

In the program window, a map of the field is displayed. The map has to be provided by the user. It should be an image of the ground of the field in a top-down view. In the simulation, a screenshot of the field can be used and in the real world, a satellite map cutout of the field is recommended. A simple sketch would be sufficient as well. In addition, the relative size of the map must be specified in meters. Also, the starting position of the robot has to be entered.

After starting the program, the user can specify the area which shall be explored by selecting its corner points with the left click on the map of the field shown in the program window. A right click on a corner point removes the point. When the area is selected, the user can click on the "finish" button, then, a polygon whose vertices are the selected points is shown, indicating the area to be explored.

The first phase is the exploration of the area. Thereby, an occupancy grid map of the obstacles is created, which is used for localization during the rumex mapping phase. The robot moves to all corner points of the area in sequence. For navigation, the standard ROS navigation package *move_base* [4] is used. It utilizes a global and local planner to navigate to a goal while avoiding obstacles. This allows to navigate without a global map, solely based on odometry and the obstacles detected by the LIDAR at the current time. While navigating the area, an occupancy grid map is constructed by the ROS *GMapping* package [5]. *GMapping* is a laser-based SLAM (simultaneous localization and mapping) package to create a 2D occupancy grid map. On the Jackal, the 3D LIDAR point cloud is converted by a ROS node into a 2D scan for compatibility with *GMapping*. The occupancy map, the selected area and the last position of the Jackal is saved in files and loaded during the rumex mapping phase. During exploration, the position of the robot and the current obstacle map are displayed onto the map in the program window. As can be seen in Fig. 2.

The previously selected area is outlined in black. Boundaries of mapped obstacles are plotted in red, the unoccupied area is indicated by the colored map and unexplored parts of the map are greyed out. The transformation of the robot frame to the map in the program window can be performed easily with the prior knowledge about the starting position in the map and the size of the map.

The second phase is the mapping of rumex plants in the area based on the previously constructed obstacle map. The path for rumex exploration is planned with a simple lawn mowing pattern as shown in Fig. 3 (blue path). The pattern is constructed by creating the parallel lines first. Then, the intersections of the lines with the boundary of the area are calculated. The points of intersection are connected to form a continuous path. The path is followed by sequentially navigating to its corner points in the map by use of the *move_base* package. The navigation is based on the robot's position in the previously constructed occupancy grid map, which is estimated with the *amcl* package [6]. *Amcl* is a probabilistic localization method in form of the adaptive Monte Carlo localization approach. The user can start this rumex mapping phase right after the aforementioned exploration phase and in that case, the last position has been automatically saved. Otherwise, if a predefined map is selected, the user needs to provide the initial position as required by *amcl*. The planned path and encountered rumex plants are plotted in the program window. As can be seen in Fig. 3. The image published by the camera is displayed in the upper left corner overlaying the program window. The detections of the object detector are drawn onto the image. In the simulation, a model trained to detect sport balls is used instead of the one detecting rumex plants. In this way, it is possible to test the procedures of the system in the simulation without rumex plants. The object detector is explained in the next section.

2.2 Rumex Detection

For the detection of rumex plants in the RGB-images of the ZED camera feed, the YOLOv4 (You Only Look Once) [7] object detector is used. YOLOv4 has proven to reach a good average precision and is developed with broad usability in mind and optimized for conventional single-GPU systems. This makes YOLOv4 suitable for this project. The YOLOv4 object detector was implemented on the Jackal during the bachelor thesis of the author and is further described in [7]-[10] and explained in the following paragraphs.

YOLOv4 is a real-time one-stage CNN-based object detector consisting of a backbone, neck and head. The backbone is a CSPDarknet53 and extracts features from the input image. It consists of 53 convolutional layers with skip-connections. The neck pre-processes the extracted features from the backbone by use of path aggregation and spatial pyramid pooling.

The head receives the output of the neck and predicts object bounding boxes by use of a dense prediction network. This is performed in a single stage without a separate region proposal and in an anchor-based manner as described in the following. A set of anchor boxes with different shapes is learned during training. The feature map is subdivided by a grid. Every grid cell holds a set of anchor boxes. For each box, class probabilities and an offset to the anchor box are calculated by the prediction process. These predictions are performed on feature maps of three different backbone levels. The resulting predictions are summarized by use of non-maximum suppression.

Forward propagation of an image through the network results in bounding box predictions as described above. During training, a loss function is used to calculate an error by comparing the predictions with the ground-truth object boxes. An optimizer adjusts the weights in order to minimize the loss. This is done by use of the gradient of the loss function in respect to the weights propagated back through the network. Further methods are utilized by YOLOv4 to improve the training process. Notably, genetic algorithms to find optimal hyper-parameters and different data augmentation methods to enhance robustness and reduce overfitting.

During training, transfer learning is applied by using weights pre-trained on the COCO dataset[1] as a starting point. The dataset for subsequent training for rumex detection is recorded with the Jackal on a field with rumex plants by driving around [10]. It contains 2455 images for training and 547 for testing/validation combined. All are labeled with ground-truth bounding boxes. Successive frames are not split into different sets. To put the dataset in context, 0.9 rumex plants are visible in an image on average. An example image of the testing/validation set is shown in Fig. 4 with the corresponding ground-truth boxes and the predictions of the trained model. The model is based on the weights with the highest mAP (mean average precision) on the validation set during training, however, training is continued until a significant trend of overfitting is observed.

---

[1] https://cocodataset.org

Object tracking is necessary to identify the same plant in different frames of the camera feed. This is accomplished by a simple center-based tracking approach, which compares the distance of predicted objects in successive frames to conclude which plants where already seen in the prior frame. In the simulation, the position of the robot is saved as the plant position when the tracked plant disappears under the robot. For the real robot, the precise plant position relative to the robot can be determined through the depth-image of the stereo camera. The camera feed with detections can be watched live.

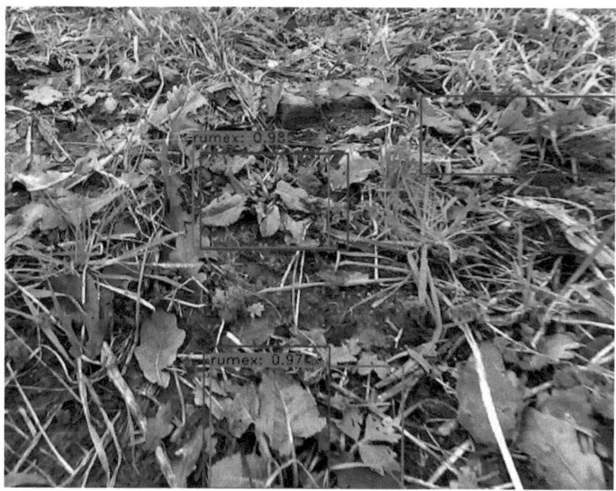

Figure 4: The predicted rumex bounding boxes in red with their score on an image of the test dataset. The blue bounding boxes are the ground-truth boxes.

3 Results and Discussion

3.1 User Interface

Because the system is still in a prototypical stage, there is room for improvement in different areas. The program windows are a great way to input data, illustrate what the robot perceives and present the results after mapping the plants in a user-friendly way.

Additional information could be displayed like the current path planned by the path planner. In addition, more information of the detected plants would be helpful for future application. For example, it would be useful for the farmer to be able to click on the position of a detected rumex plant and get an image of the plant displayed.

3.2 Mapping and Navigation

The navigation and mapping packages have proven reliable during tests in different simulated worlds with a multitude of obstacles. However, further tests of the navigation and mapping methods on a real field are necessary. Especially, the localization performance could be problematic. The odometry might become inaccurate due to more tire slip on uneven soil or damp grass. Additionally, the map-based localization might become incorrect with less obstacles on a field to estimate the relative position of the robot. GMapping based on a 2D LIDAR scan has shown to be error-prone for obstacles smaller than the LIDAR height. More accurate mapping approaches utilising the 3D LIDAR would make sense. For example, the Google Cartographer should be investigated. The rumex search pattern is sufficient, however, the benefit of more advanced patterns could be investigated. In some cases, the planned path is not ideal. Especially, if the selected area is branched out.

3.3   Rumex Detection

The detection of rumex plants using the YOLOv4 object detector reaches a mAP of 52% on the test dataset with a precision of 78% [10]. Generally speaking, larger and older rumex plants are getting detected more reliable than smaller younger plants. Frequently, rumex plants are only detected when appearing closer to the camera after the robot moves in its direction. This observation is supported by a recall of only 46%. However, according to these observations, most of the relevant rumex plants are getting detected at one point or another.

Further tests of the trained network have shown the robustness of the model. Despite a changing environment compared to its training dataset, the quality of detections is still acceptable. Tests of the model on the Jackal were conducted in a different season, on different fields with different light conditions and slightly different-looking rumex species in different growth stages. Despite these sufficient results, more training data with a higher versatility would benefit the detection accuracy and, especially, prevent false positives in new environments. Consequently, test and validation sets could be separated in case of a larger dataset. Also, switching to a newer version of YOLO could be considered. The tracking method can be improved by implementing feature-based tracking and taking the position of the robot into account to prevent plotting an already plotted rumex plant in the map when it is passed for a second time.

4   Conclusion

Monitoring of weeds is an important but time-consuming task in agriculture and, thus, holds an opportunity to be automated. Therefore, a prototypical system based on a small mobile robot equipped with a LIDAR sensor and a stereo camera is presented.

A user-friendly program window is used to select an area on the map of a field. The area is explored using the ROS *move_base* package and an occupancy grid map is constructed with *GMapping*. Further evaluation on fields outside of the simulation is required to assess whether a more advanced localization and mapping algorithm is required. Rumex plants are mapped while following a lawn mowing pattern. Therefore, navigation in the map is based on the position of the robot estimated with *amcl*. For the detection of rumex plants, an implementation of the YOLOv4 object detector is used. The model has proven to be robust and able to detect most rumex plants. The current position of the Jackal, the path for rumex mapping, the positions of detected plants and obstacles in the map are displayed in the program window onto the map of the field.

In conclusion, the prototypical system shows that the detection of weeds on grassland is possible on a small mobile robot. However, further evaluation of the system is necessary.

Acknowledgement

The work has been carried out at the Institute for Robotics and Cognitive Systems, University of Lübeck. We would like to thank many of our colleagues for fruitful discussions during the project.

Author's Statement

Conflict of interest: Authors state no conflict of interest.

5   References

[1] B. Liu, R. Bruch, *Weed Detection for Selective Spraying: a Review.* Current Robotics Reports vol. 1, pp. 19–26, 2020.

[2] T. Schulz, *Rumex obtusifolius L. im Wirtschaftsgrünland.* Humboldt-Universität zu Berlin, Landwirtschaftlich-Gärtnerische Fakultät, 2013.

[3] Clearpath Robotics Inc., *Clearpath Jackal Robot.* https://clearpathrobotics.com/jackal-small-unmanned-ground-vehicle [last accessed on 2023-01-18]

[4] *ROS move_base package.* https://github.com/ros-planning/navigation/tree/noetic-devel/move_base [last accessed on 2023-01-18]

[5] *ROS gmapping package.* https://github.com/ros-perception/slam_gmapping [last accessed on 2023-01-18]

[6] *ROS amcl package.* https://github.com/ros-planning/navigation/tree/noetic-devel/amcl [last accessed on 2023-01-18]

[7] A. Bochkovskiy, C.-Y. Wang, and H. M. Liao. *Yolov4: Optimal speed and accuracy of object detection,* 2020.

[8] J. Redmon and A. Farhadi. *Yolov3: An incremental improvement,* 2018.

[9] J. Redmon, S. Divvala, R. Girshick, and A. Farhadi. *You only look once: Unified, real-time object detection,* 2016.

[10] N. Kompe. *Implementation of a neural network for detection of rumex with a mobile robot,* 2021.

A Decentralized Multi-Robot Warehouse Picking Mechanism with High Scalability, Robustness and Low Wear

Robin Luckey [1], Kristian Ehlers [2] Heiko Hamann [3]

[1] Robotics and Autonomous Systems, Universität zu Lübeck, robin.luckey@student.uni-luebeck.de
[2] Institute of Computer Engineering, Universität zu Lübeck, kristian.ehlers@uni-luebeck.de
[3] Department of Computer and Information Science, Universität Konstanz, heiko.hamann@uni-konstanz.de

Abstract

The logistic industries require innovative and efficient solutions for the ever growing number of shipments in warehouses. Pocketsorters are widely used due to their high throughput and modularity. A new pocket sorting solution is being developed by EMHS that introduces the flexibility of swarm robotics and uses local sensing for collision avoidance and a central approach to remove goods. In order to further exploit the advantages of swarm robotics, improve robustness and scalability and reduce wear and operational costs, we developed a decentralized withdrawal of goods procedure. It uses neighbor communication to gather information and coordinate robot movements and requires minimal back-end communication.

1 Introduction

Efficient warehouse logistics, that is the movement and storage of goods within ever growing storage facilities, is a critical aspect of modern supply chain management. According to a recent report, the global logistics market, including warehouse logistics, is expected to have grown at around 8.5% in 2022 [1]. There has been an increasing interest in using swarm robotics for warehouse logistics in recent years. Swarm robotics involves the use of large numbers of simple, autonomous mobile robots that can work together as a team to achieve a common goal. Decentralized robot groups have several advantages over traditional central fleets, including increased robustness and scalability. [2] These properties are crucial for keeping up with the current growth of the market.

Pocket Sorters are highly versatile and efficient sorting systems. Capabilities of handling up to 700,000 items per day have been reported. [3] These sorters can handle hanging, lying, or any types of goods that fit into a grocery bag. Each bag in the pocket sorter system serves as a single shelf location and is moved along a guide rail by a dragging chain. To identify the goods in the bags, RFID tags or barcodes are used. The system's high modularity allows for efficient use of space and is commonly used for picking, storage, and buffer systems. [4]

AFLE is a German abbreviation for Autonomous Driving Storage Units. These units are developed by EMHS GmbH as low-cost, autonomous agents that in unison form a storage system. The work featured in this paper was developed based on this system. This warehouse system addresses common problems of traditional pocket sorters by using a swarm of AFLE instead of a dragging chain. An AFLE and the bag it is carrying form a storage unit together. The robots hang on a rail grid that also powers them. The approach has the potential advantages of being more flexible because it reduces the interdependence of storage units that were literally chained together before. This allows for the optimization of operational processes through software updates without having to modify the hardware. Furthermore, the robots are estimated to run at estimated speeds of up to 4 m/s while chain approaches thus far only reach up 2 m/s. By dividing the warehouse into independent segments the system can potentially scale indefinitely.

A previously developed simulator for this system was implemented by Fister and Hamann [5]. It features a hybrid removal of goods approach with central path planning and decentralized, reactive behavior for collision avoidance. We extend this simulator with direct messaging between robots and implement a picking mechanism that uses local communication to improve scalability, robustness and reduce wear on the robots.

1.1 Related work

Currently there is only a small number of fully autonomous warehouse systems including Amazon Robotics, the System of the Ocado Group, and Exotec. The Amazon robotics solution uses flat, earthbound, driving robots that carry entire shelves to the picking station [6]. The Ocado group uses 3000 per warehouse robots that are centrally controlled by an AI. [7] These Omnidirectional robots move along a grid and can quickly collect grocery items [8]. Exotec uses a modular warehouse of stacked crates. Their fleet of au-

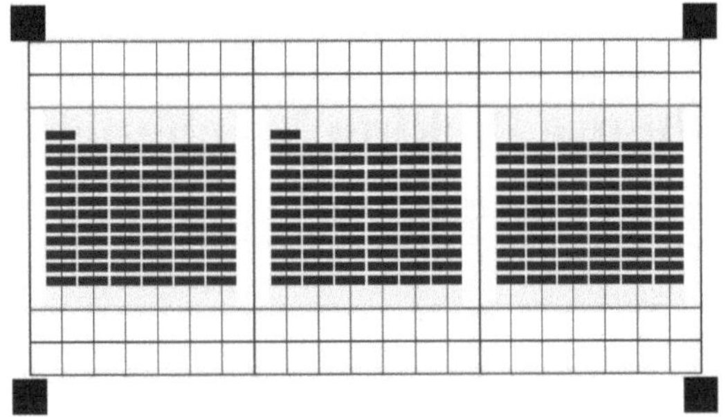

Figure 1: In our simulation we divide a warehouse into three subgrids (yellow background) Each subgrid contains six vertical storage rails where 200 AFLE are stored (dark green). Horizontal bufferrails (red) connecting the storage rails provide space for manoeuvring. One-way high-speed tracks (light blue) lead to the elevators (dark blue squares) and thereafter to the picking station.

tonomous robots drive to the shelf and move vertically to collect a bin containing goods [9].

2   Approach

Our approach is based on a modular warehouse comprising multiple subgrids see Fig. 1. The segments are connected by high-speed rails that lead to pick up zones via elevators. Each segment contains rails that form a grid. AFLE carrying goods are stored in parallel storage rails at the center of each segment. The storage rails are interconnected by buffer rails on both ends. Robots located at the end of the storage rails can simply drive to the exit. However, when robots are extracted from the middle of a storage rail with other robots blocking on each side, collective movement patterns must be applied to allow the demanded robot to leave (Fig. 2).

2.1   Circling

Circling is a central extraction method implemented in previous works [5]. It was implemented in a central way due to the small amount of communication needed and the simplicity of central algorithms. When extracting a robot, two neighboring storage rails together with the connecting buffer rails form a roundabout. All robots on both storage rails are exchanged (see Fig. 2a). They drive around the roundabout until they reach a predefined point on the neighboring rail, passing by the buffer rails. However, when reaching the buffer rail, the robot being extracted does not enter the neighboring rail but leaves towards the highway instead.

2.2   Buffering

Buffering is our novel alternative extraction method based on local communication using Bluetooth (see Fig. 2b).

Only a single request by the back-end, carrying only the information which robot should leave, is needed. This is important since the system's global wireless communication could otherwise limit scalability. The extracting robot starts a daisy chain informing a blocking neighbor on the sides that is closer to the end of the rail, that it needs to make way. The neighboring robot passes on the message. On each hop, the robots add their width, which depends on the product they are storing, to the message. When a robot located at the end of a storage rail receives the information, it can determine how far it must drive onto the buffer rail in order to make enough room for all following robots. It then starts a second communication chain telling all robots involved to follow it. As soon as all blocking robots are buffered, the extracting robot can drive past them and subsequently start a third message chain telling all buffered robots to return to the storage rail. Sometimes, robots that have previously been requested by the back-end but have not yet received clearance (see "mutual exclusion" below) are asked to make way. In these cases, the robots will be extracted along with the initiator of the current Buffer. While Buffering could be implemented in a central way, we chose a decentralized approach due to wireless communication restrictions caused by the high number and high density of robots in this system.

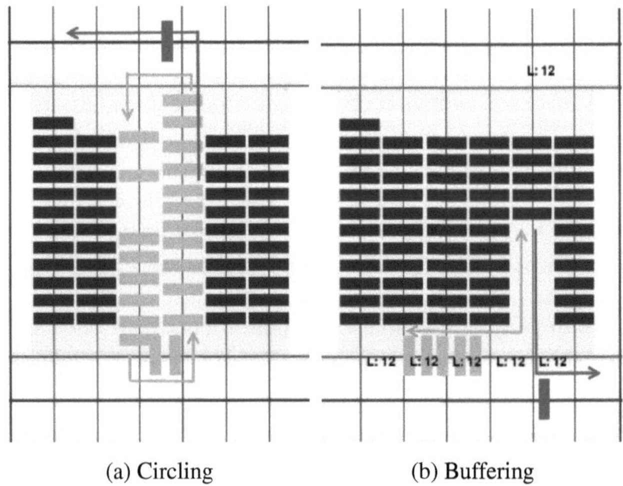

(a) Circling   (b) Buffering

Figure 2: Comparison of extraction methods. Left: Buffering, the magenta colored AFLE is extracting, the yellow AFLE makes way and return to the storage rail afterwards. "L: 12" at the top indicates that AFLE with ID 12 is locking a storage rail and the "L:12"s at the bottom mark the segments of a buffer rail currently locked by ID 12. Right: Circling, the yellow AFLE on two neighboring rails exchange positions, clearing the way for the magenta AFLE in the process.

2.3   Mutual exclusion

Mutual exclusion based on [10] is used to prevent deadlocks. We use a semi-central approach because decentralized mutual exclusion requires a lot of communication and introduces high complexity due to the ever changing communication partners involved when robots come and leave the subgrids. We still achieve scalability by adding a simple arbitration instance to every subgrid that manages the robots in its subgrid via Bluetooth. A robot can request two different types of locks: At first, it needs a rail lock to prevent run conditions with other robots on the same storage rail, then it can initiate the Buffer. And a second that locks segments on the buffer rail. Only when the first message chain has reached the AFLE at the end of the storage rail, the information on how much space is needed on the buffer rail is available. This information is needed by the arbitrator, which tries to find sufficient consecutive unused buffer rail segments on either side of the storage rail. If the second lock cannot be acquired after 10 tries, the first lock is lifted, and the initiating robot sets a timeout before starting over. To prevent deadlocks during the acquisition of locks, the robots use random timeouts in between requests. Furthermore, to reduce wireless communication traffic, we implemented a capped Exponential Backoff [10]. It increases the maximum random waiting time on each attempt exponentially until a maximum is reached.

2.4 Comparing Circling & Buffering

The two methods differ in two essential aspects: the movement pattern and the communication pattern. We mainly concentrate on comparing the movement patterns since both methods could be implemented with either central or decentral communication. When using Circling there is no need for coordination except for collision avoidance during the process which can be solved in a reactive manner. This also means that robots can be extracted from all storage rails at the same time. The main drawbacks from Circling arise when only a small number of robots are extracted per storage rail at a time. Circling always moves all robots on at least two entire storage rails and can cause high wear and energy costs. Robustness is also a challenge, a single failing robot on a rail makes Circling on that rail impossible. Buffering addresses these issues by attempting to only move those robots that are blocking the way. However, an optimal solution depends on information that is not locally available to the robots. For example, which direction is more advantageous for leaving the storage rail in terms of number of robots blocking on each side. The main disadvantage of Buffering besides its complexity is the need of several simultaneous instances to often share a buffer rail which can become a bottleneck.

3 Results and Discussion

The simulation runs were performed using three warehouse subgrids storing a total of 200 AFLE. For each run a fixed number of AFLE were chosen randomly. Each run was repeated 50 times. The AFLE were extracted simultaneously, simulating the extraction of a customer order with multiple goods.

Extraction times are an important metric that determines

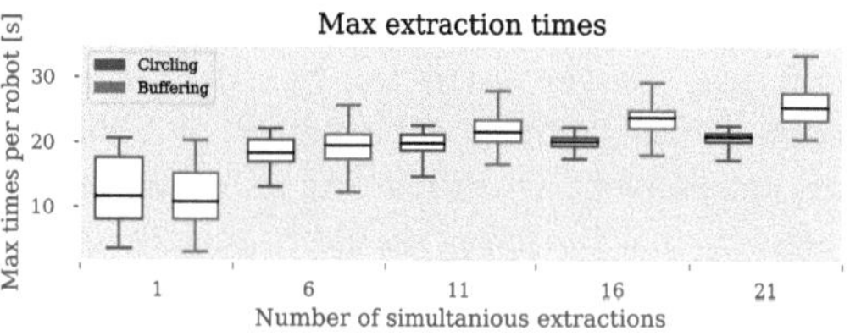

Figure 3: With increasing shipping volumes and demand for quick delivery times, extraction times are an important metric. All robots are extracted concurrently, for this reason the robot with the slowest extraction time determines how fast a method can extract an order comprised of multiple goods. When extracting small orders, both the Circling and Buffering methods showed similar performance. However, when extracting large orders, the Circling method was faster.

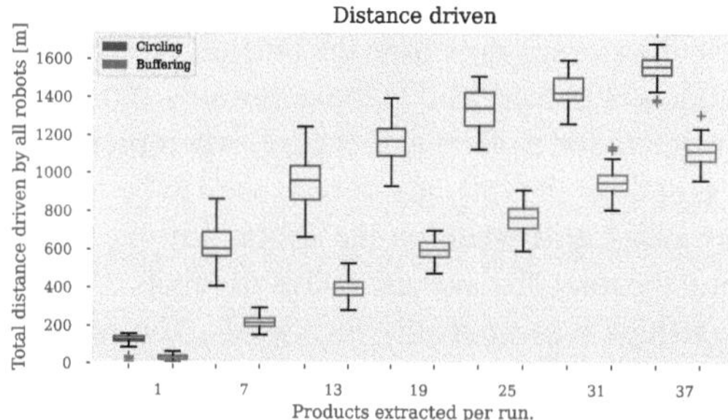

Figure 4: Energy consumption and wear on robots are important cost factors. Buffering can reduce the distance the fleet needs to cover to fulfill orders and thus reduce operational costs and wear.

Table 1: Locking attempts and wait times (max.)

Num. extractions	20	30
Without Backoff	19.5 (98.3)	31.0 (143.8)
Maximum exponent 5	6.2 (34.2)	10.57 (64.6)
Maximum exponent 9	4.33 (13.2)	5.82 (20.58)
Wait time, no Backoff [s]	1.82 (7.49)	2.82 (10.81)
Wait time, exponent 5 [s]	1.92 (7.53)	2.82 (10.87)
Wait time, exponent 9 [s]	2.03 (8.21)	2.95 (11.57)

In order to achieve scalability it is crucial to reduce wireless communication traffic. With an increasing number of simultaneous extractions, the wait time and therefore the amount of communications also increases. The table shows the amount of requests that where send per robot and the average waiting time before a rail lock could be acquired. Exponential Backoff prolongs the timeout in between attempts exponentially with every request the robot sends until a maximum is reached. It shows a good reduction of messages of up to 77% without raising the wait time significantly.

whether a method is suitable in practice. The results are shown in Fig. 3. We found that for small orders Buffering and Circling were both fast with mean maximum extraction times of 18.37 seconds for Circling and 19.4 seconds for Buffering. Larger orders can be extracted with mean maximum extraction times, for example, of 20.68 and 25.5 seconds respectively, when fetching 21 different products. This suggests that Buffering should be mainly applied during low load of the warehouse. The actual load in practice is difficult to predict and depends on the use case. However, 20 simultaneous extractions already equal 10% of the stock being extracted at once. There are many aspects that might influence the performance in practice that have to be studied. These include the robustness of the system. Faults can quickly block entire storage rails when using Circling, causing a reduction in throughput. Moreover, the shape of the warehouse and speed of the picking stations play an important role. The performance also depends on the sorting of the goods stored. We assumed a well-mixed order of all products resulting in an equal probability for each order to be picked. However, if incoming products are always added to the storage rails from the outside, products that are not frequently picked tend to move inwards. This would be advantageous for Buffering, because, when picking orders near the ends of the rails less robots need to be moved.

Energy costs and wear on the robots can be reduced by lowering the total distance driven by all robots. The number of extractions was gradually increased. The results show a reduction in the total distances driven by the entire fleet when using Buffering (see Fig. 4). As with extraction time the size of the orders also influence the efficiency. The more items need to be fetched from a rail the more efficient Circling becomes.

Optimization of communication, that is keeping wireless traffic to a minimum, is important to ensure scalability and allow for dense setups with hundreds of thousands of robots in a warehouse. The use of exponential Backoff was assessed. We varied the number of simultaneous extractions in three steps with 10, 20 or 30 extractions. The base waiting time used was 100 ms seconds, an estimate that accounts for two-way Bluetooth communication and computing time. We then varied the maximum exponent from 0, meaning no exponential Backoff, to 9 resulting in a maximum waiting time of 100×2^9 ms $= 51.2$ seconds. For tests with 20 robots, the mean number of attempts was reduced by up to 77% when using exponential Backoff, while the maximum extraction times hardly deteriorated (see Table 1). The results also show that with an increasing number of simultaneous extractions the coordination overhead increases.

4   Conclusion and Outlook

A continuous stream of small orders in quick succession could be efficiently fulfilled using Buffering and thereby spreading the load over time at other parts of the warehouse. Collecting several orders over times and then fulfilling them using Circling might also be a suitable approach but might cause bottlenecks at other parts of the warehouse. For larger orders in slow successions, Circling seems to be the method of choice. Here the coordination overhead in Buffering becomes larger, while Buffering is more robust against single robot faults. It still has a great potential for improvements. Better scheduling algorithms in the arbitrator could reduce waiting times and increase the number of robots that are extracted with each Buffer. The flexibility that arises from using swarm robots enables a seamless combination of both methods and switching during live operation. In conclusion Buffering is a promising new approach well suited to supplement Circling and we hope this new method can serve as a means of improving scalability, robustness and reducing wear and energy costs in future warehouse systems.

Acknowledgement

The work has been carried out at EMHS GmbH, efficient material handling solutions and supervised by Kristian Ehlers, Institute of Computer Engineering, Universität zu Lübeck and Heiko Hamann, Department of Computer and Information Science, Universität Konstanz.

Author's Statement

Conflict of interest: Authors state no conflict of interest.

5   References

[1] Zusammenfassung der Ergebnisse Herbstgipfel, http://www.logistikweisen.de, 23.09.2022 [accessed on 2022-12-26].

[2] Hamann, Heiko. Swarm robotics: A formal approach. Vol. 221. Berlin: Springer, 2018.

[3] https://www.mm-logistik.vogel.de/steckt-alles-andre-in-die-tasche-a-1020729/ [accessed 02 Jan 2023]

[4] Wehking, Karl Heinz, and Wolfgang Albrecht. Technisches Handbuch Logistik. Springer Vieweg, 2020.

[5] Pfister, Kai, Hamann, Heiko, Decentralized Multi-Robot Movement for Warehouses with high Scalability Goals, Universität zu Lübeck, 2021

[6] J.-t. Li and H.-j. Liu, "Design optimization of Amazon robotics," Automation, Control and Intelligent Systems, vol. 4, no. 2, p. 48–52, 2016.

[7] M. Davis. (2021) 3,000 robots working in Ocado's automated warehouse for faster online grocery.

[8] Dale, M. (2018) 'Automating grocery shopping', Imaging and Machine Vision Europe, (85), 16+

[9] https://www.exotec.com/de/ [accessed on 2023-01-02]

[10] Tay, Y. C., Kyle Jamieson, and Hari Balakrishnan. "Collision-minimizing CSMA and its applications to wireless sensor networks." IEEE Journal on selected areas in Communications 22.6 (2004): 1048-1057

Flood Detection using Optical and SAR Satellite Data

Candice Bomane [1]

[1] Robotics and Autonomous Systems, Universität zu Lübeck, candice.bomane@student.uni-luebeck.de

Abstract

Climate change such as ice melting and warmer temperatures has intensified heavy rain in the last few years. In addition to urban development, strong precipitation rise flood risk, a phenomenon that is coming more frequent and more intensive in the next years. To warn road users and show them the actual risk, this work has been done with the goal to detect water and flooding areas. Different threshold methods are used, one simple and one more complex with the help of different satellite imagery based on Optical and Synthetic Aperture Radar (SAR). The first method is thresholding, which is based on classifying each pixel in an image. A second method is a learning-based approach obtained from a deep neural network. They help to visualize flooded regions, observe changes before and after the flood event, and aim to identify vulnerable regions. For the evaluation, all threshold methods are compared. The results show that they all have the capability to estimate water content.

1   Introduction

Over time, the coastal urban area has been more exposed to flood due to the sea level rise and strongest precipitations. In the last few years, many applications for flood detection have been created especially in the field of Artificial Intelligence (AI) with the development of multiple earth observation techniques and the huge amount of available data. Flooding is a phenomenon that can occur at any time, everywhere without warning. This is what happened, on July 2021. Heavy rainfall overhung the region of west Germany causing an overflow in the Rhine river submerging multiple cities for some weeks. The one which was the most affected was the city of Ahrweiler [1]. This catastrophe ruined a high number of infrastructures, buildings and ravaged agriculture. It impacted the economy, the environment but also cost the life of many people. The inundation was so large that it could be detected with satellites. Satellite imagery is used for mapping floods and detecting significant changes in water, and can serve to warn the population of the risk they face. It can detect the electromagnetic radiation reflected back from the earth's surface and can provide high-resolution data for land monitoring, climate change, or disaster detection. There are different satellite technologies including remote sensing as optical and Synthetic Aperture Radar (SAR) applicable for water detection. Optical remote sensing provides multispectral bands for a variety of applications. With a frequent revisit time of the same area, the satellite is able to give a variety of information and monitor changes on land. The data can be collected fast and easily and require simple data processing but with the inconvenience to be affected by atmospheric conditions, such as clouds or haze, which can reduce image quality. The other sensor commonly used is radar such as SAR imaging which emits active electromagnetic radiation and measures the amount of energy returned to the satellite with the advantage to penetrate the clouds and give measures during nighttime conditions. The objective of this study is to extract the flood event and to evaluate the effectiveness of flood detection using two different kinds of satellite data, optical images from Sentinel-2 satellite and SAR data from Sentinel-1 satellite performed in different regions where inundation was huge.

2   Material and Methods

2.1   Sentinel-2

To perform water detection, high-resolution optical images is adopted. The program Copernicus Mission of the European Space Agency (ESA) is composed of different missions gathering different satellites from Sentinel-1 to Sentinel-6 and delivering open-source satellite data from the whole world. Satellite-2 provides optical images in 13 spectral bands in the range from visible and near-infrared to shortwave infrared with different high resolutions: 10 m, 20 m, and, 60 m according to the band. It is also composed of five levels: level-0, level-1A, level-1B, level-1C, and level-2A which provide different orthorectified reflectance, radiometric and geometric corrections. The level-2A is the most used because it contains more information about the earth's surface and it has a superior image quality. It has the particularity to have three more bands including one called Scene Classification Layer (SCL). The SCL is a classification algorithm able to distinguish different cloud types, snow, and water pixels. It is accessible in the last processed band in Sentinel-2.

The data are collected from the Copernicus Hub platform at

different periods of time [2]. An illustration of the Sentinel-2 can be seen in Figure 1 on the RGB band from level-2A image.

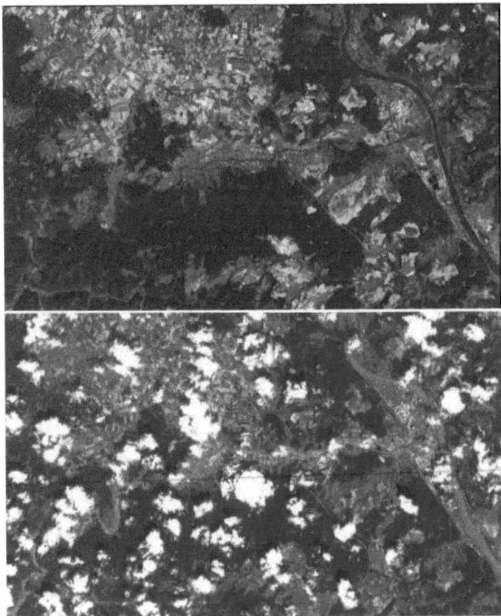

Figure 1: Raw image on RGB band from Sentinel-2 level-2A. Top: Ahrweiler city before flood. Bottom: Ahrweiler city during flood.

During the flood period, clouds are often predominant and reduce the quality of the image making complicating the observation. Thus, they are masked by using a cloud mask from the SCL band where clouds are turned to black pixels but in most cases, rivers situated under clouds were hidden by the mask. The SCL provides also a water mask able to detect water. The first approach to detect water bodies is to select the band containing the water mask in the SCL and mask rivers. However, the water mask was not very accurate, and considered roads as water pixels.

2.2 Sentinel-1

Due to the large cloud image covering, in most cases, the flood was not observable on Sentinel-2 by using a water mask from SCL. The focus is then made on another satellite that carries the Synthetic Aperture Radar (SAR) sensor[3]. Radar sensors utilize longer wavelengths from centimeters to meter scale with the ability to see through clouds and can provide good quality images even in bad weather and at night. It is an active sensor that can emit a signal and record the amount of energy reflected after interaction with the earth. Composed of one band, the C-band, the radar signal can interact with the ground surface and detect changes in the water extension. It provides 10 m high-resolution images and it is constituted of two main polarizations used in this paper for land monitoring, vertical transmission vertical reception (VV) and vertical transmission horizontal reception (VH). Figure 2 shows a raw image from Sentinel-1 of Ahrweiler city during the flood on the band VV. The observation of the water and the localization of the river in raw images is challenging which is why some preprocessing steps are necessary.

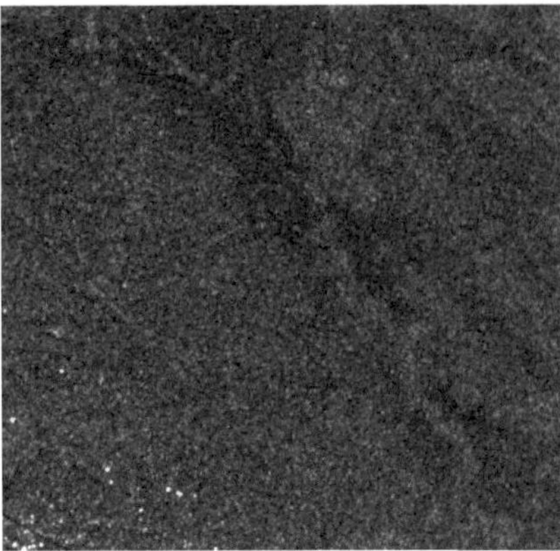

Figure 2: Raw image from Sentinel-1 from the VV band in Ahrweiler during flood.

2.3 Binary threshold technique

Binary threshold consists of finding an optimal value capable to differentiate water from the ground. The first approach used is the Normalized Difference Water Index (NDWI) on Sentinel-2 data. The NDWI in eq. 1 returns an index in the range [-1, 1].

$$NDWI = \frac{GreenBand - NIRBand}{GreenBand + NIRBand} \qquad (1)$$

The propriety of the range of values is to estimate the quantity of water present in an image. Pixel values between [-1, 0] mean that the soil is dry and values higher than 0 mean sufficient water surface is observable [8]. This index is followed by a threshold defined empirically to separate the water body from the landscape. Pixel values below -0.2 are considered as non-water and above as water. Multiple thresholds were applied to find the optimal one. An example is visible in the Figure 3.

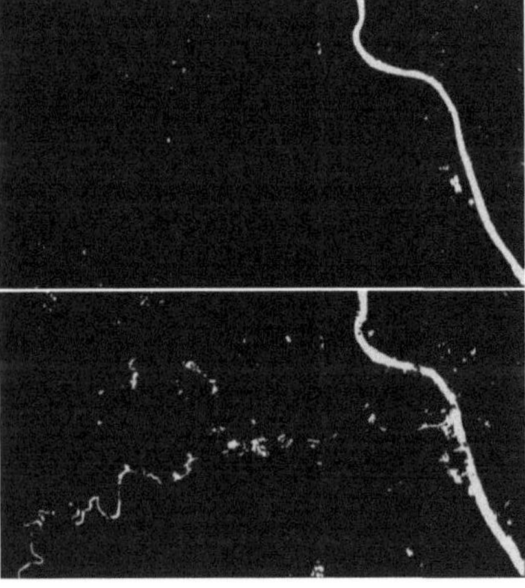

Figure 3: Water mask colored in yellow performed with the NDWI threshold value of -0.2 on Sentinel 2 level-2A. Top: Ahrweiler city before the flood. Bottom: Ahrweiler city during flood.

A binary threshold is also tested on SAR images. SAR images are collected from the Wekeo platform and are first preprocessed with an application called ESA SNAP. The processing steps are based on radiometric correction, calibration, speckle noise removal, and correction of terrain. From the preprocessing steps, noise is generated. Therefore, a gaussian filter is applied to remove it. The raw images provided by Sentinel-1 have pixel values in the range between 0 and 1. A threshold is applied manually to extract the water body. Figure 4 shows a water mask on SAR image with a binary threshold during the flood period. The flood is observable but, some noise is still visible, and after the processing of the image some pixel values were considered as no data which appeared in black pixels.

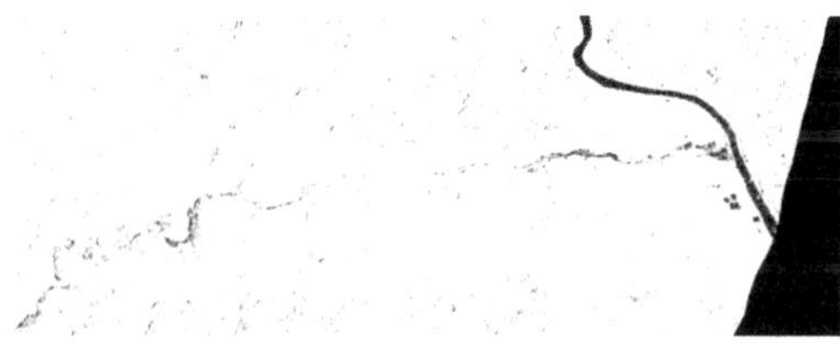

Figure 4: Water mask on Sentinel-1 during flood period. Black pixels represent water and white pixels represent the ground. However, on the right side, black pixels represent no data.

2.4 U-net

To find the optimal threshold, a learning-based method is applied. It aims to automatically determine the optimal threshold value for each image and improve the accuracy. An open-source project ML4Floods [5] is selected to perform flood segmentation on Sentinel-2. The project contains a dataset composed of 422 images from different regions in the world, where huge inundation happened. The images are of the size of 256×256 pixels and they are segmented labeled with water and no water mask. For this dataset a pre-trained model is used where a U-Net network is implemented. A U-net is a fully convolutional neural network (FCN) architecture used for segmentation tasks. It operates symmetrically by downsampling and upsampling images with a sequence of convolutional layers wich leads to capture fine details [7].

In the same way, a U-Net network is trained on Sentinel-1. Another dataset is used from the platform Radiant ML-Hub containing SAR images and labels from two areas in the United States and Bangladesh [4]. The data are divided into training, validation, and test. The model parameters are trained on data with a batch size of 8, a learning rate of 0.1 on 30 epochs. The dataset is composed of 52 images but it presents less diversity. Therefore, a data augmentation technique is used to increase the size and the variety of the dataset. Flip, rotation, shearing, and Gaussian blurring is applied to the trained model so it leads to better performance. Then, the images are normalized between 0 and 255 and divided into patches and inferred in the U-net. A Binary Focal Loss is chosen as an optimization criterion. The output is a segmented image where each pixel is classified into two classes water and ground. In figure 5 the water mask

prediction is observable on Sentinel-1.

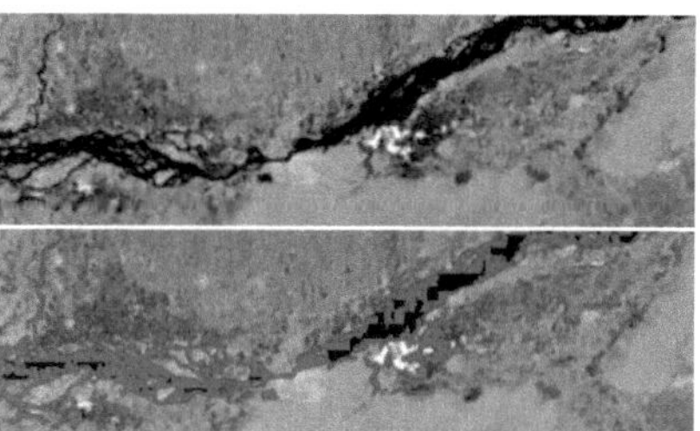

Figure 5: Top: Raw image in Bangladesh from Sentinel-1 of a flooding area. Bottom: Water mask prediction colored in red obtained after using a U-Net.

3 Results & Discussion

Four different methods have been implemented on optical and SAR images to detect water bodies before and during flooding. A metric has been determined for each method with the Intersection over Union (IoU).

$$IoU = \frac{\text{target} \cup \text{prediction}}{\text{target} \cap \text{prediction}} \qquad (2)$$

The results are summarized in Table 1 and shows a lower IoU on Sentinel-2 in comparison to Sentinel-1. Training a network on Sentinel-1 shows the highest performance ending up with an Iou = 0.305. However, on Sentinel-2, using a deep network performed better than the binary method whereas on Sentinel-1 the binary threshold gave a better result. An example of the results is observable in Figure 6. The binary threshold on Sentinel-1 performed 28% better than the other methods. The water pixel predictions are the closest one compared to the other method but lot of noise is visible.

Table 1: Comparison different methods on Sentinel-2 and Sentinel-1

Satellite	Method	IoU
Sentinel-2A	NDWI + threshold pt	0.018
Sentinel-21C	U-Net	0.016
Sentinel-1	threshold	0.021
Sentinel-1	U-Net	0.305

Comparing the different methods in flood detection is complex because of multiple parameters. Using optical images has the advantages to be multispectral and to extract lots of information from the data but can face the problem of cloud covering. In general, during floods, the weather is rainy which complicates visualizing the ground due to clouds. Even if clouds can be removed from the band SCL with the cloud mask, the region of interest is still not visible. Applying a binary threshold shows a good ability to extract water bodies but with more difficulty when it is mixed with sedimentation. Moreover, the threshold is specific to a region, and an optimal one will change with the area so it can

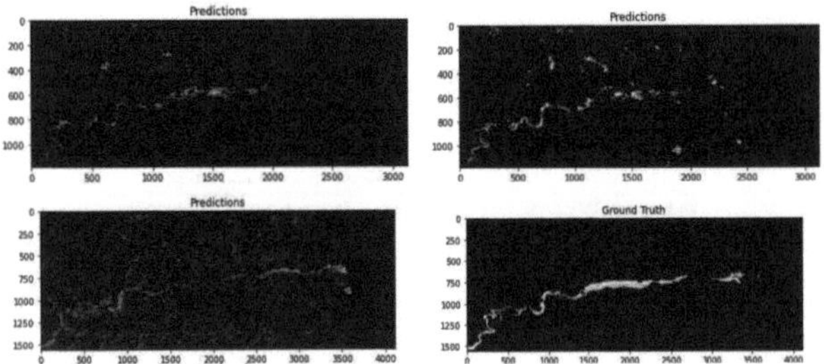

Figure 6: Comparison of different methods on Ahrweiler during the flood. The above images are the predictions and the one below represents the same ground truth of the Ahr river. Top left: Binary threshold on Sentinel-2. Top right: U-net on Sentinel-2. Bottom left: Binary threshold on Sentinel-1. Bottom right: Ground truth

be time-consuming to look at each optimal threshold manually. Using an adaptative threshold by training a deep neural network on the Senintel-2 appears with the lowest performance. The dataset provided contained too few images which impacted the training and resulted in a low IoU value even by using data augmentation. Moreover, the ground truth images contained only flood pixels whereas in the predictions made from the U-net, they are based on permanent and flood water, resulting in false interpretation.

SAR has the advantage to generate images in all weather. Applying a binary threshold gives generally good results and was efficient to extract the water body. SAR always has to be preprocessed to be able to work with the data. But the preprocessing steps on the images are very tedious and require lots of effort. Even by trying different preprocessing steps, output images were still noisy, which is a phenomenon that regularly happens. The noise in the images was not easy to remove after the implementation of the binary threshold where noise and water were seen both as black pixels and making it difficult to differentiate them. The trained model on SAR images from the MLHub project shows the best performance. Nevertheless, the authors of this project did not provide enough information on the preprocessing steps leading to confusion on the preprocessed data on Ahrweiler.

All different methods were able to extract the water body, however, each technology provided some issues. Sentinel-1 data on the U-net showed the best metrics but the images were tested on a small dataset only in two different areas.

4   Conclusion

This study presented four different techniques for flood detection using optical satellite data from Sentinel-2 and SAR satellite images from Sentinel-1. The binary threshold, used as the first approach, was able to recognize the main rivers during the flood period. However, it can perform poorly due to the spectral profile of water which varies due to the presence of debris, vegetation, or sedimentation and has to be adapted to each environment. A pre-trained model with the ML4Flood package can produce similar results but with

the drawback of cloud obstruction. SAR images can overcome this problem but with their own challenges, such as preprocessing and dark areas. Generally, training a model was difficult due to the lack of data. Overall, the use of Sentinel-1 showed good results in water and flood detection. This application might be useful for providing early warning to people in a flood area, allowing them to take the necessary steps to protect themselves and their property. Additionally, it may provide valuable data to help improve flood prevention.

Acknowledgement

The work has been carried out at Bareways company and supervised by the Institute for Robotics and Cognitive Systems, Universität zu Lübeck.

Author's Statement

Conflict of interest: Authors state no conflict of interest.

5   References

[1] *Hope following the catastrophe* https://www.deutschland.de/en/topic/environment/ catastrophic-flooding-in-germany-rebuilding-in-the-ahr-valley [last accessed on: 2021-12-18]

[2] K. Fletcher, *Sentinel-2: ESA's Optical High-Resolution Mission for GMES Operational Services*. Esa Communications, 2012, vol. 1, pp. 11-20.

[3] S. Xinyi, D. Wang. and M. Emmanouil *Inundation Extent Mapping by Synthetic Aperture Radar*. Institute of remote sensing, Peking, pp. 2, 2019, doi:10.3390/rs11070879.

[4] S. Gahlot, I. Gurung and A. Molthan, *Flood Extent Data for Machine Learning*, 2021, pp. 3, doi:10.34911/rdnt.ebk43x, 2021.

[5] ESA *ML4Floods* https://github.com/spaceml-org/ml4floods [last accessed on: 2022-02-21 20:53]

[6] D. Duque-Arias, S. Velasco-Forero, J.E. Deschaud, *On power Jaccard losses for semantic segmentation*. 16th International Conference on Computer Vision Theory and Applications, Vienne, 2021, pp. 4, doi:10.5220/0010304005610568.

[7] I. Kotaridis, M. Lazaridou *Semantic segmentation using a U-net architecture on sentinel-2 data*. Aristotle University of Thessalonik, 2022, vol. 63, pp. 4, doi:10.5194/isprs-archives-XLIII-B3-2022-119-2022.

[8] W. Jiang, J. Ni, Z. Pang, X. Li, H. Ju, G. He, J. Lv, K. Yang, J. Fu, X. Qin*An Effective Water Body Extraction Method with New Water Index for Sentinel-2 Imagery*, 2021, pp. 7, doi:10.3390/w13121647.

Reinforcement Learning Algorithms for Lateral Vehicle Control in ROS

Abby Kandathil Abraham [1], Tobias Dentler [2], Elena Sapozhnikova [3]

[1] Robotics and Autonomous Systems, Universität zu Lübeck, abby.kandathilabraham@student.uni-luebeck.de
[2] AI System & Control (DISA1), ZF Friedrichshafen AG, tobias.dentler@zf.com
[3] AI System & Control (DISA1), ZF Friedrichshafen AG, elena.sapozhnikova@zf.com

Abstract

The application of reinforcement learning (RL) to robotics and autonomous vehicles is gaining increasing attention in recent years because of its high potential to enhance safety and performance. This research aims to apply a state-of-the-art RL algorithms to lateral vehicle control. A custom OpenAI gym environment was created to train and test agents created from proximal policy optimization (PPO) with residual policy learning (RPL) and soft actor-critic (SAC) RL algorithms. To simulate dynamic systems such as electronic control units, and mechatronic systems in a vehicle, a functional mock-up unit (FMU) was used. Robot operating system (ROS) serves as middleware for the entire simulation. By comparing the error of the baseline controller and RL agents, promising results were shown by the PPO algorithm as it resulted in a much more stable agent with course angle error and cross-track error in an acceptable range and also with a minimal oscillating steering angle.

1 Introduction

Technological advancements in autonomous vehicles have dominated the automotive industry over the past decade. Self-driving vehicles feature lateral control as one of their most significant and challenging functions. The lateral controller in a vehicle entails adjusting the steering angle in order for the vehicle to follow the reference path. The controller minimizes the distance between the existing position of the vehicle and the reference path. Lateral control requires information such as lateral error, yaw rate, and steering angle in order to maintain a vehicle's intended course. A reference path or a baseline acts as a standard in such a control measure. A common control approach adopted by manufacturers is model predictive control (MPC) and proportional-integral-derivative (PID) [1].

In response to the popularity of RL-based algorithms in different control tasks in robotics, a current trend has emerged to replicate these methods for autonomous driving [2], [1]. In this paper, we present a study based on RL algorithms to solve the problem of lateral control in vehicles. Instead of perception data, coordinates were used as input for creating the tracks. The task was accomplished with model-free algorithms such as PPO (on-policy) and SAC (off-policy). Due to the fact that testing a real vehicle would be dangerous, we used the ROS framework and FMU to simulate the agent. The results show that the PPO's error signals were well within the acceptable limits, and it performed equally well or better than the baseline.

As for the remainder of the paper, it follows this structure: Section 2 provides a brief overview of PPO, SAC, and functional mock-up interface (FMI) as well as an implementation of the RL algorithms. Section 3 presents the simulation results and a discussion of the graph plotted, and the final section concludes the work and discusses the next phase of the study.

2 Material and Methods

An overview of the RL algorithms tested for lateral vehicle control and the training process carried out as part of the research are presented in this section.

2.1 Proximal Policy Optimization

PPO is a reinforcement learning algorithm using a typical policy gradient method that is used to optimize a surrogate objective function by employing stochastic gradient ascent. This method switches between sampling data through interacting with the environment [3]. It incorporates excellent performance, scalability, and a steady training procedure [4]. As opposed to other popular Deep RL algorithms, such as Deep Q-Learning, PPO learns online i.e., the agent learns directly from the environment rather than storing past data (experiences) in a replay buffer. The policy gradient loss can be expressed as

$$L^{PG}(\theta) = \hat{\mathbb{E}}_t \left[\log \pi_\theta(a_t|s_t) \hat{A}_t \right] \tag{1}$$

where $\hat{\mathbb{E}}$ represents the expectation, π_θ represents the stochastic policy for the policy parameter θ, $\hat{A}$ is the advantage function, a and s are the action and state at timestep t. An input to the policy is observed states from the environment, and output is suggested actions. The advantage function estimates the relative value of a selected action in a given state. Furthermore, it illustrates how much better the action taken is based on what would have normally happened in the current situation [5]. Multiplying the log probability of the policy actions by the advantage function yields the objective function for policy gradient optimization. Moreover, PPO uses trust region optimization from the policy optimization algorithm (TRPO) [6] to clip the gradient size and perform multiple stochastic gradient ascent epochs for each policy update [7]. The objective function of TRPO is

$$\underset{\theta}{\text{maximize}} \quad \hat{\mathbb{E}}_t \left[r_t(\theta)\hat{A}_t \right] \tag{2}$$

$$\text{subject to} \quad \hat{\mathbb{E}}_t[\text{KL}[\pi_{\theta_{old}}(\cdot|s_t), \pi_\theta(\cdot|s_t)]] \leq \delta \tag{3}$$

where $r_t(\theta) = \frac{\pi_\theta(a_t|s_t)}{\pi_{\theta_{old}}(a_t|s_t)}$ i.e., the probability ratio between the new policy and old policy and θ_{old} is the policy parameter vector before the update. The Kullback-Leibler (KL) constraint ensures that the new updated policy remains as close as possible to its predecessor. The main objective function in PPO is expressed as

$$L^{CLIP}(\theta) = \hat{\mathbb{E}}_t \left[\min(r_t(\theta)\hat{A}_t, \text{clip}(r_t(\theta), 1 - \epsilon, 1 + \epsilon)\hat{A}_t) \right] \tag{4}$$

where the objective function is composed of two parts, of which $r_t(\theta)\hat{A}_t$ is a normal policy gradient that helps policy to select the actions with better performance over the baseline. And the second part which is a clipped version of the normal policy gradient, a clipping operation is performed between $1 - \epsilon$ and $1 + \epsilon$. ϵ is a hyperparameter that indicates how far the new policy can deviate from the old one [3].

To make PPO more data efficient and for executing longer horizon events RPL is used [8]. The main idea behind this approach is to use the initial policy π and residual f_θ to make an improved policy. Here the initial policy's output determines the residual in RPL. Hence the improved policy is given by,

$$\pi_\theta(s) = \pi(s) + f_\theta(s) \tag{5}$$

2.2 Soft Actor-Critic

SAC is used when continuous actions are involved in RL tasks. As opposed to just maximizing rewards, SAC aims to maximize the policy's entropy as well. A policy with a high entropy favors exploration and assigns the same probability to actions that have similar or nearly equal action values. Moreover, it ensures that high probabilities are not assigned to a range of actions. The SAC involves three networks: a state value function V with ψ as its parameter, a soft Q-function Q with θ as its parameter, and a policy function π with ϕ as its parameter.

The objective function is expressed as,

$$J_\pi(\phi) = \mathbb{E}_{s_t \sim \mathcal{D}, \epsilon_t \sim \mathcal{N}} \left[\log\pi_\phi(a_t|s_t) - Q_\theta(s_t, a_t) \right] \tag{6}$$

$$\text{where } a_t = f_\phi(\epsilon_t; s_t)$$

Here a and s are the action and state at timestep t, $\mathcal{D}$ is the distribution of previous states and actions, $\pi_\phi(a_t|s_t)$ is tractable policy, Q_θ represents the soft Q-function, and ϵ_t is the input noise vector [9].

2.3 Functional Mock-up Interface

FMI is a standard that facilitates the exchange and co-simulation of dynamic models [10]. The generated dynamic models are saved as a functional mock-up unit (FMU) which is a software module that represents a functional aspect of a physical system. It can be used in a model-based development process to test, simulate, and integrate the functional aspects. Through the FMI interface, FMU accesses a shared file containing all relevant model information. In addition, the FMU archive contains an XML file containing information about the model, such as names of input and output variables, parameters, and values related to the constants used [11]. For our implementation co-simulation FMU was used. Since the FMU module was created by a different team, further description is out of the scope of this paper.

2.4 Training Process

The ROS noetic version and open-source operating system Ubuntu 20.04 were used to perform the RL algorithms. Stable baselines3, an improved version of OpenAI baselines, provide a simple approach to training the PPO model. The training was done in a custom environment with a pre-recorded track as shown in Fig. 1. For loading and executing the FMU model a python package called PyFMI was installed.

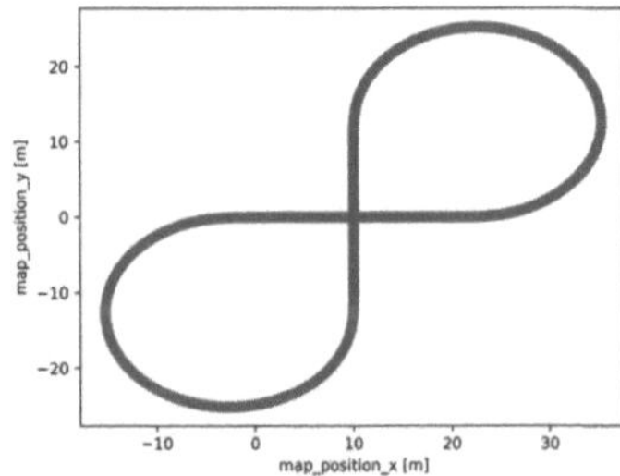

Figure 1: The infinity track used for training RL algorithms.

The FMU provided values for setting up the initial parameters such as starting course angle, starting velocity, and x and y positions required for the simulation. The action to be taken is the front steering angle with input being the current state. The state is an array consisting of cross-track error, course angle error, longitudinal acceleration, longitudinal velocity, actual angle, yaw rate, and target curvature. The reward R is calculated as R = 1 - cross-track error - course angle error. The cross-track error is the distance between the vehicle's reference point and the closest point on the trajectory at each timestep. This shows how close the vehicle is to the desired trajectory. Using the reference point along the trajectory as a reference, the course angle error represents the difference between the path heading and the vehicle heading. In other words, it is a measure of whether a vehicle is aligned with the trajectory and moving in the right direction.

3 million timesteps were designated for training the agent. Once training has been initiated, the model begins to learn and the trained agent is saved. The architecture for testing the algorithms consists of two main software blocks i.e., OpenAI gym and ROS. The environment created in gym interacts with the ROS node *ppo_testing_node*. In order to test the trained agent, first the infinity track was chosen, and then a simulation time of 150 seconds was set for each episode. An episode is considered complete when testing on the track completes a loop and it continues until the set number of episodes is reached. As part of the training process, the *evaluate_policy* function from stable baselines3 was called to test the trained agent in the custom environment. Since the SAC agent was trained by another team member, a detailed description is not included in this paper.

3 Results and Discussion

This section describes the studies conducted using a PPO with RPL and a SAC agent, as well as the most significant findings of our research. In our trials, we demonstrated the necessity of picking the most effective agent. The baseline error plot generated after the simulation of FMU serves as a reference for comparing the performance of different agents. As a result of the baseline error, acceptable error limits were determined.

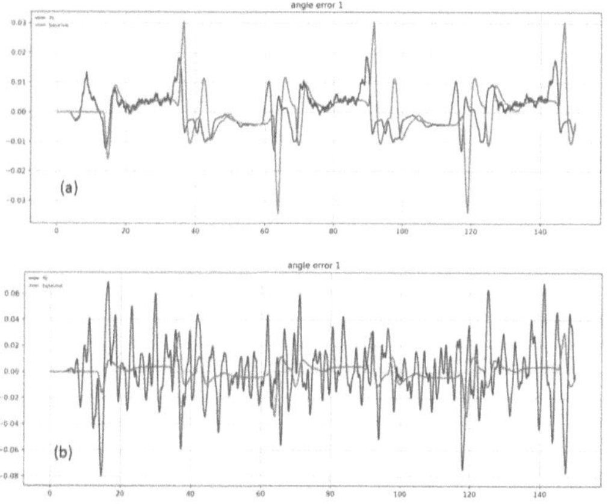

Figure 2: Course angle error obtained while testing the PPO (a) and SAC (b) agents are plotted over time.

Test results focused primarily on the effectiveness with which PPO and SAC agents managed to change the steering angle in order to solve the lateral control problem i.e.,

minimize the offset to the reference track. The agent's performance was evaluated based on the course angle error and cross-track error of the vehicle.

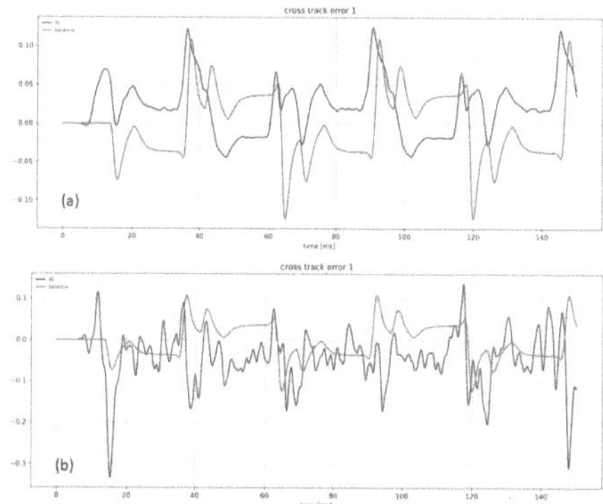

Figure 3: Cross-track error obtained while testing the PPO (a) and SAC (b) agents are plotted over time.

Fig. 2 shows the course angle error attained after performing the simulation with PPO (Fig. 2(a)) and SAC (Fig. 2(b)) agents. By comparing the graph plotted between the RL agents PPO and SAC and the baseline, it is clear that our PPO agent has performed well by keeping itself between the error limits. In Fig. 2(a) the baseline error was between -0.035 radians and +0.030 radians and the PPO agent stayed between -0.012 radians and +0.018 radians. Between the first 20 ms, the course angle error shoot up a little but for the later part of the track it performed well. Fig. 2(b) shows the graph plotted between the SAC agent and the baseline. It exhibits that our agent has not performed well as compared to the PPO agent. The baseline error was between -0.035 radians and +0.030 radians and the course angle error of the RL agent stayed between -0.080 radians and +0.070 radians. The course angle error shoots up more frequently and comes close to the baseline readings at times.

Fig. 3 illustrates the cross-track error plot generated from the simulation of the RL agents PPO (Fig. 3(a)) and SAC (Fig. 3(b)). The cross-track error limit was set between -1m and +1m. The comparison shows that the PPO agent has been close to the baseline most of the time. Fig. 3(b) illustrates the cross-track error plot generated from the simulation of the SAC agent. The cross-track error limit was set as same as before and it is evident from the comparison that the SAC agent has been deviating too far from the baseline most of the time.

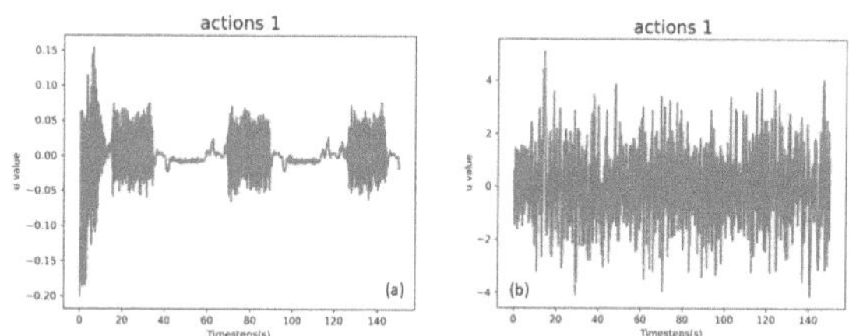

Figure 4: Oscillation of Steering angle for each action with PPO (a) and SAC (b) agents over time.

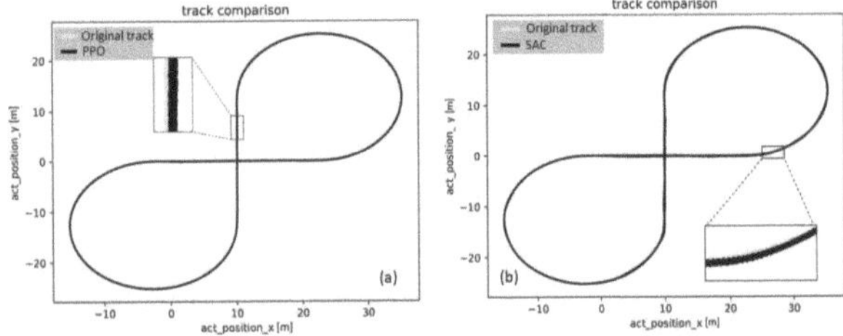

Figure 5: A comparison between the plot generated after testing the PPO and SAC agents with the original track.

Fig. 4 represents the steering angle initiated by PPO (Fig. 4(a)) and SAC (Fig. 4(b)) agents for each timestep. In PPO, for the starting few seconds the steering angle seems to oscillate too much but later on, it recovers well and for SAC, it appears that the steering angle oscillates too much and doesn't show any sign of recovery. A comparison of the trajectory or path taken by the PPO agent (Fig. 5(a)) and SAC agent (Fig. 5(b)) with respect to the original track is shown. In the case of PPO, a slight deviation was visible in certain areas, especially at the beginning of the track. And with SAC, a deviation could clearly be seen in most areas.

4   Conclusion and Future Work

This paper aimed to examine lateral vehicle control with RL algorithms. Out of the two selected algorithms, PPO with RPL performed significantly better than SAC. Intriguingly, both the cross-track error and course angle error were within the acceptable range, and the results were equivalent to or better than the baseline. Despite the fact that the work presented in this research yields good outcomes, various improvements are also necessary. To see if the cross-track error may be reduced further, hyperparameter tuning should be performed. In order to evaluate the agent's resilience and generalizing capability, it is also necessary to test the agent on multiple simulation tracks. Other on-policy and off-policy RL algorithms should also be tested to evaluate the performance.

Future works include a plan for tests that will be conducted on a prototype car to determine the algorithm's accuracy. Actuators will be controlled by MicroAutobox in a real scenario.

Acknowledgement

The work has been carried out at ZF Friedrichshafen AG and supervised by Prof. Dr. Georg Schildbach of the Institute for Electrical Engineering in Medicine, Universität zu Lübeck.

Author's Statement

Conflict of interest: Authors state no conflict of interest.

5   References

[1] B. Arifin, B. Y. Suprapto, S. A. D. Prasetyowati, and Z. Nawawi, "The lateral control of autonomous vehicles: A review," in *2019 International Conference on Electrical Engineering and Computer Science (ICECOS)*, IEEE, oct 2019.

[2] O. M. Andrychowicz, B. Baker, M. Chociej, R. Jozefowicz, B. McGrew, J. Pachocki, A. Petron, M. Plappert, G. Powell, A. Ray, *et al.*, "Learning dexterous in-hand manipulation," *Int. j. rob. res.*, vol. 39, no. 1, pp. 3–20, 2020.

[3] J. Schulman, F. Wolski, P. Dhariwal, A. Radford, and O. Klimov, "Proximal policy optimization algorithms," *arXiv preprint arXiv:1707.06347*, 2017.

[4] J. Zhang, Z. Zhang, S. Han, and S. Lü, "Proximal policy optimization via enhanced exploration efficiency," *Inf. Sci.*, vol. 609, pp. 750–765, 2022.

[5] J.-S. Byun, B. Kim, and H. Wang, "Proximal policy gradient: Ppo with policy gradient," *arXiv preprint arXiv:2010.09933*, 2020.

[6] J. Schulman, S. Levine, P. Abbeel, M. Jordan, and P. Moritz, "Trust region policy optimization," in *Proceedings of the 32nd International Conference on Machine Learning* (F. Bach and D. Blei, eds.), vol. 37 of *Proc. Mach. Learn. Res.*, (Lille, France), pp. 1889–1897, PMLR, 07–09 Jul 2015.

[7] A. Zhang, Y. Wu, and J. Pineau, "Natural environment benchmarks for reinforcement learning," *arXiv preprint arXiv:1811.06032*, 2018.

[8] T. Silver, K. Allen, J. Tenenbaum, and L. Kaelbling, "Residual policy learning," *arXiv preprint arXiv:1812.06298*, 2018.

[9] T. Haarnoja, A. Zhou, P. Abbeel, and S. Levine, "Soft actor-critic: Off-policy maximum entropy deep reinforcement learning with a stochastic actor," in *International conference on machine learning*, pp. 1861–1870, PMLR, 2018.

[10] R. Lange, S. Traversaro, O. Lenord, and C. Bertsch, *Integrating the Functional Mock-Up Interface with ROS and Gazebo*, pp. 187–231. Cham: Springer International Publishing, 2021.

[11] C. Andersson, J. Åkesson, and C. Führer, *Pyfmi: A python package for simulation of coupled dynamic models with the functional mock-up interface.* Centre for Mathematical Sciences, Lund University Lund, Sweden, 2016.

NN-MPC - Replacing a First Principles Model with a Neural Network

Moritz Friedrich Gerwin [1], Sahar Zeinali [2], and Georg Schildbach [2]

[1] Robotics and Autonomous Systems, Universität zu Lübeck, moritz.gerwin@student.uni-luebeck.de

[2] Institute of Electrical Engineering in Medicine, Universität zu Lübeck, {sahar.zeinali, georg.schildbach}@uni-luebeck.de

Abstract

In this paper, a learning-based model predictive control (MPC) method is proposed for the longitudinal control of autonomous vehicles. In order to take into account uncertain longitudinal models in real applications, neural networks (NNs) are utilized to learn the system dynamics based on its input-output data. The resulting NN model is used in the MPC optimization problem for speed tracking purpose. This controller is compared to another MPC, utilizing a physical model with uncertainties to simulate the inaccuracies of real systems. As a proof of concept, four NNs with different architectures are trained to recreate a physical model of the vehicles longitudinal dynamics. The results show that the trained NNs can simulate the real model. Moreover, the closed-loop response of the system shows that the learning-based MPC performs well in following the desired speed. However, due to high computational demand, the method could be improved for real world applications.

1 Introduction

Model Predictive Control (MPC) has grown in popularity over the last years in the area of automated driving for different applications such as Adaptive Cruise Control (ACC) [1] or tracking a predefined path [2]. Similar to classical controllers such as PID, the MPC is based on a model of the controlled system. The complexity and uncertainty of this model may vary and can therefore have an impact on the performance of the closed-loop system. The best performance is usually achieved, if the model is as close to the real system as possible [3]. This leads to a trade-off between accuracy of the model and computation time, since more complex models usually take more time to be evaluated. However, even the most complex models can be inaccurate if some parameters are unknown or the model is time-variant. Here the idea of learning based models can be introduced. Instead of a model that has been formulated based on the physical relations of the system, a model is trained using input-output data of the system to recreate its dynamics [4]. Neural networks (NNs) are a powerful tool to learn the behaviour of the dynamical system. In one approach, MPC is completely substituted with a NN [5]. That way no online optimization is needed as input-output data of the controller is determined beforehand that is then used to train the network. One more approach to utilizing NNs is presented in [6], where they are trained to negate the residual error from a simple physical model.

In this paper we used another approach in which the whole uncertain model of the system is substituted by the NN. As a proof of concept, a simple model of the longitudinal dynamics of a vehicle is created using a feed-forward NN. For validation, the NN-MPC is compared against a classical MPC using a first principles model with added noise as the uncertainty in different ACC scenarios. The uncertainty is introduced to replicate any inaccuracies that might occur when modelling a physical system in real world applications.

2 Material and Methods

2.1 Vehicle Model

The reference model of the vehicle is a simple exclusively longitudinal model. The lateral movement of the vehicle is neglected for the purpose of this paper. By applying Newton's second law in the longitudinal direction, the following model is obtained

$$\dot{x} = v \tag{1a}$$

$$\dot{v} = \frac{Tj\eta}{mr} - \frac{1}{2m}\rho S c_x v^2 - g\mu \cos(\alpha(x)) - g\sin(\alpha(x)) \tag{1b}$$

where x is the vehicle's longitudinal position and v is its velocity. The current torque applied from the engine is represented by T. This torque is translated to the wheels by multiplying it with the active gear ratio j, consisting of the gearbox ratio and the static ratio of the differential. $\alpha(x)$ represents the slope angle of the road as a function of the current vehicles position x. The rest of equation (1b) consists of vehicle and environment specific parameters. Namely, the vehicles mass m, its drag coefficient c_x, the drivetrain efficiency η, the tire radius r and the vehicles reference area S. Environmental parameters include the tire road friction coefficient μ, the density of the air ρ and earth's gravitational acceleration g. The equation is made up of four parts. The first term is representing the engines accelerating force at the wheels, the second term is a drag force caused by the air resistance. The third term is accounting for the friction between the tire and the road. In the final term the drag force caused by the roads slope angle. A similar model is used in [7]. While this exact model is used for the training of the NN, Gaussian noise is introduced to ρ, μ and α for the reference controller to simulate the uncertainty of estimating these parameters in the real world.

2.2   Neural Network

A neural network consists of multiple layers that have multiple neurons each. In each neuron, except for the inputs, a weighted sum of the neurons from the previous layer is calculated. An additional bias is added in each neuron. Then an activation function is applied to the resulting sum. The result of this is then treated as the input for the next layers. Fig. 1 shows the structure of a singular neuron.

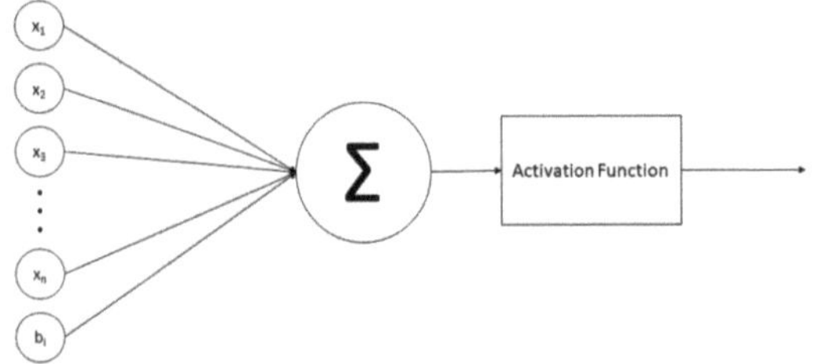

Figure 1: Structure of a singular neuron within a neural network

The proposed network maps the velocity, torque and current gear number to the acceleration of the vehicle according to (1b). The data for the training phase of the network is acquired by precalculating equidistant data points with labels $(v, T, i) \mapsto (\dot{v})$, where i is the number of the selected gear. Due to the physical limitations of the vehicle, it is not necessary to train the network on the complete $\mathcal{R}^3 \mapsto \mathcal{R}$. The points are generated on the intervals $v \in [v_{min}, v_{max}]$, $T \in [T_{min}, T_{max}]$ and $i \in \{1, 6\}$. The torque and velocity intervals are divided in steps of 1 leading to roughly 60.000 data points. In total, four different networks are trained that differ in the number of hidden layers as well as the number of hidden neurons. The used configurations are listed below that can be read as number of neurons in each layer. This also includes the input and output layers:

I	3-50-1
II	3-25-25-25-1
III	3-50-50-50-1
IV	3-128-256-128-1

The input and hidden layers are utilizing a ReLU activation function, while the output layer is using a linear activation function. For the training phase the ADAM optimizer is used with an exponential learning rate scheduler. The initial learning rate is 0.01 with a decay rate of 0.9. All networks are trained for 100 epochs. The implementations are done using TensorFlow 1.15.5 in Python 3.6.9.

2.3   MPC Controller

The objective of the controller is the tracking of a desired velocity as ACC. It is built following the standard MPC scheme with a time horizon of 0.5 s and a discretization of 0.05 s. All relevant physical limitations of the vehicle, such as torque output of the engine and top speed of the vehicle are taken into consideration. This leads to the optimal control problem

$$\min_{T} \sum_{k=1}^{N} w_0 \cdot (v_k - v_{ref})^2 + w_1 \cdot \Delta T^2 + w_2 \cdot T^2 \quad (2a)$$

$$\dot{v} = f(v, T, i) \quad (2b)$$

$$v_{min} \leq v \leq v_{max} \quad (2c)$$

$$T_{min} \leq T \leq T_{max} \quad . \quad (2d)$$

Objective function (2a) consists of a speed tracking error term and control input efforts of the torque value and the change in its value. Here w_0, w_1 and w_2 are weights for different cost terms, respectively. There is no terminal cost included since the application of the ACC is a continuous task and the terminal cost is not needed. This Optimal Control Problem (OCP) is solved by the IPOPT solver. The implementations for the OCP formulation and the solver interface are done using CasADi 3.5.5.

2.4   Test Setups

In the first step, the trained networks are tested against the vehicle model in a discretized velocity simulation. The update steps are calculated as

$$v(k + 1) = v(k) + dt \cdot f(v, T, i) \quad (3)$$

where the discretization time $dt = 0.05s$. The function that determines the acceleration is subsequently substituted by the vehicle model or one of the networks. The simulation is determined for a total of 2400 steps, resulting in a total simulation time of 120 s. For the duration of the simulation, the input torque and the gear number are kept constant, since the purpose of this test is only the accuracy of the trained models. All models are evaluated in two different scenarios. In one scenario the initial condition is set to $0\frac{m}{s}$ and a constant torque of $20Nm$ is applied for the whole duration of the simulation. In the other scenario, the initial condition is set to $15\frac{m}{s}$ and a constant torque of $-10Nm$ is applied. As a metric, the mean squared error (MSE) between the networks and the models response is calculated.

Additionally the resulting controllers are tested in three different scenarios on the same discretized simulation used before. To this end an initial (v_0) and a desired (v_{ref}) speed are defined. The closed loop simulations are performed for a total time of 10 s. The controllers are tuned with the same weights to isolate the effect of the different models. The test scenarios are listed in Table 1.

Table 1: Test scenarios for the controllers

Test scenario	$v_0\left[\frac{m}{s}\right]$	$v_{ref}\left[\frac{m}{s}\right]$
1	0	10
2	10	8
3	35	40

3   Results and Discussion

3.1   Network

In the first step, the trained networks are compared to the vehicle model as described above. The resulting trajectories of the velocity are depicted in Fig. 2.

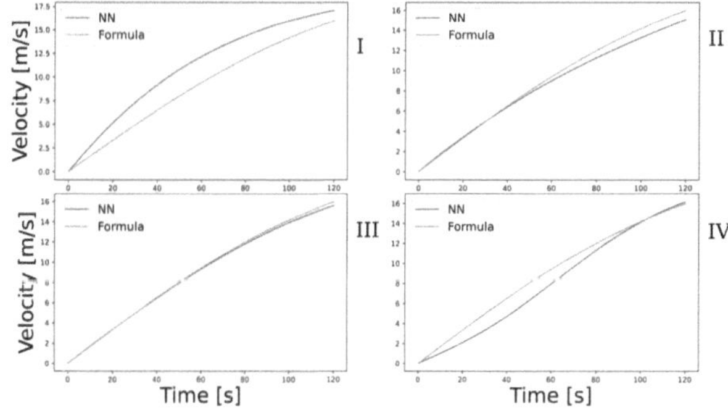

Figure 2: First test scenario, $v_0 = 0\frac{m}{s}$, $T = 10Nm$

It can be observed that the networks with more than one hidden layer outperform the smallest network with only one hidden layer. However, it can also be seen that the largest, most complex network performs worse than networks II and III for this scenario. The results of the second scenario, shown in Fig. 3, does not show any major differences as the first one. Here it seems that all networks are more or less performing equally well, with some minor fluctuations.

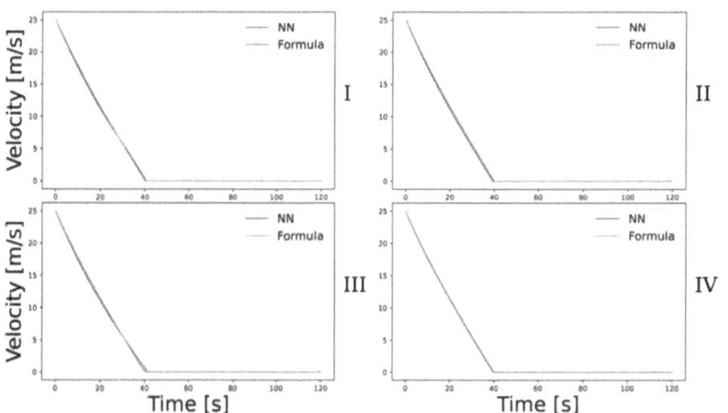

Figure 3: Second test scenario, $v_0 = 25\frac{m}{s}$, $T = -10Nm$

Table 2 shows the MSE between the networks and the model's response. It can be seen that the networks II and III are the best performing ones overall. Networks I and IV are performing rather poorly in the first scenario, while all networks are performing similarly in the second scenario.

Table 2: MSE between the networks and the model's response for two test scenarios

Network	Scenario 1	Scenario 2
I	4.642	0.027
II	0.330	0.040
III	0.029	0.038
IV	1.234	0.005

It can be concluded that some complexity is required for the network to replicate the vehicle model, however, adding arbitrary many neurons may not be necessary or might even perform worse than the mid-size networks. It is also worth to note that for an MPC controller computation time is an important factor. For this reason, only network II with good enough performance and less complexity will be used in the closed-loop simulation study.

3.2   Closed-loop simulation

Fig. 4 shows the results of the closed loop simulation for scenario 1. The velocity profiles of the reference controller are on the left and the proposed controller on the right. Below the velocity profiles, the corresponding input torques are presented.

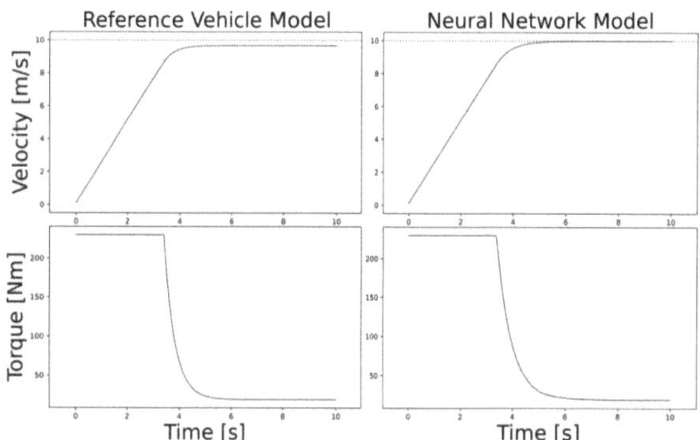

Figure 4: First test scenario, $v_0 = 0\frac{m}{s}$, $v_{ref} = 10\frac{m}{s}$

It can be observed that the vehicle is quickly accelerating until the desired reference velocity is reached. While both controllers are showing a smooth input profile, the network controller is reaching the desired velocity more closely. A similar behaviour can be observed in scenario 2, shown in Fig. 5. The network controller decelerates the vehicle quickly to the desired speed, while keeping a smooth input profile. It can also be seen that the reference model actually performs worse again.

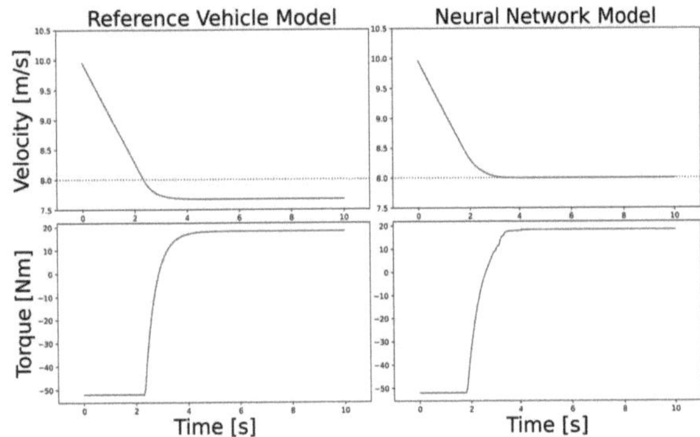

Figure 5: Second test scenario, $v_0 = 10\frac{m}{s}$, $v_{ref} = 8\frac{m}{s}$

The third scenario, shown in Fig. 6, is chosen deliberately close to the physical limit of the vehicle's speed. As a consequence it can be observed that both controllers struggle to reach the desired velocity. This is the case because the data the model is trained on is also limited to the vehicles limits. This could be prevented by adding data to the training set that goes beyond the physical limits.

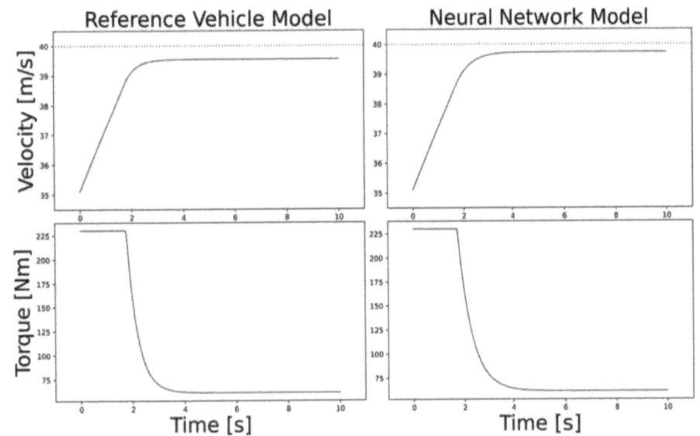

Figure 6: Third controller test scenario, $v_0 = 35\frac{m}{s}$, $v_{ref} = 40\frac{m}{s}$

It can be concluded from the simulation results, that the controller with a NN model is working better than a physical model that is introduced to uncertainties, that could very well occur in a real vehicle. This shows that utilizing input-output data to train a model can be beneficial over a model derived from physical relations.

4 Conclusion

In this work, a NN-based MPC has been designed for speed following purpose in autonomous driving applications. The main idea is to use the NN to learn the behaviour of the real system and to overcome the uncertainties in the physical model. The simulation results show that the NN can approximate a dynamic model very well. However, the choice of the network size is non-trivial since the relation between model-complexity and performance is highly non-linear. The proposed controller performed better than the one with an uncertain physical vehicle model. This could open up the possibility of utilizing neural networks in a model identification process from real world data and get

a better model for the real vehicle. Though, computation time for MPC controller is crucial for it to be usable in a real application. This is especially true in safety related applications, like autonomous driving. Taking this into consideration it can be said that while the concept works, the proposed method could further be improved for real applications.

Acknowledgement

The work has been carried out and supervised by the Institute of Electrical Engineering in Medicine, Universität zu Lübeck.

Author's Statement

Conflict of interest: Authors state no conflict of interest.

5 References

[1] J. Matute, M. Marcano, A. Zubizarreta, and J. Pérez, "Longitudinal model predictive control with comfortable speed planner," 04 2018, pp. 60–64.

[2] J. Kong, M. Pfeiffer, G. Schildbach, and F. Borrelli, "Autonomous driving using model predictive control and a kinematicbicycle vehicle model," in *2015 American Control Conference*, 2014.

[3] N. Resalat, J. E. Youssef, R. Reddy, and P. G. Jacobs, "Evaluation of model complexity in model predictive control within an exercise-enabled artificial pancreas," *IFAC-PapersOnLine*, vol. 50, no. 1, pp. 7756–7761, 2017, 20th IFAC World Congress. [Online]. Available: https://www.sciencedirect.com/science/article/pii/S2405896317330732

[4] J. Langford, R. Salakhutdinov, and T. Zhang, "Learning nonlinear dynamic models," *CoRR*, vol. abs/0905.3369, 2009. [Online]. Available: http://arxiv.org/abs/0905.3369

[5] M. L. C. Vianna, E. Goubault, and S. Putot, "Neural network based model predictive control for an autonomous vehicle," *CoRR*, vol. abs/2107.14573, 2021. [Online]. Available: https://arxiv.org/abs/2107.14573

[6] T. Salzmann, E. Kaufmann, J. Arrizabalaga, M. Pavone, D. Scaramuzza, and M. Ryll, "Real-time neural-mpc: Deep learning model predictive control for quadrotors and agile robotic platforms," 2022. [Online]. Available: https://arxiv.org/abs/2203.07747

[7] C. Pan, A. Huang, J. Wang, L. Chen, J. Liang, W. Zhou, L. Wang, and J. Yang, "Energy-optimal adaptive cruise control strategy for electric vehicles based on model predictive control," *Energy*, vol. 241, p. 122793, 2022. [Online]. Available: https://www.sciencedirect.com/science/article/pii/S0360544221030425

Using Systolic Arrays and SystemC for Hardware Optimization of Deep Neural Networks

Tavia Plattenteich [1],

[1] Robotics and Autonomous Systems, Universität zu Lübeck, tavia.plattenteich@student.uni-luebeck.de

Abstract

Artificial intelligence, specifically deep neural networks (DNNs), has been becoming a tool in an increasing amount of applications. Optimization if only considered in software is limited. Systolic arrays are specialized hardware architectures for matrix multiplication. They present one method of incorporating hardware optimization for DNN acceleration. In this work, we implemented systolic arrays in SystemC on different abstraction levels. The tested use-cases were matrix multiplication and convolution. Additionally, we added certain restrictions to further explore the possibilities and limitations of systolic arrays. Results show the effect of limitations on performance in the case of matrix multiplication and the overhead of unnecessary calculations in the case of convolution. Further work could include testing the implementation at a bigger scale and with an actual DNN or convolutional neural network.

1 Introduction

The utilization of DNNs has been rapidly increasing in various fields of application in recent years. While DNNs are typically considered a software architecture, it is important to note that optimization of DNNs is limited when solely utilizing general purpose processors such as CPUs. To overcome these limitations, specialized hardware that accelerates DNN specific operations such as matrix multiplication and convolution can greatly enhance DNN performance [1]. These specialized hardware devices are able to perform simple mathematical calculations in parallel, such as multiplication and accumulation. One specific approach for accelerating matrix multiplication for DNNs is through the use of systolic arrays. For the modeling of these systolic arrays, the use of SystemC, a system-level modeling language, is commonly employed.

1.1 Hardware design

As the complexity of software systems increases and the need to consider the underlying hardware becomes more crucial, the importance of hardware-software co-design has become increasingly apparent. One approach to achieve this is through the use of the double roof model, as illustrated in Fig. 1. This model comprises of two distinct components: the software components, such as the system's functions and processes, and the hardware components, including the system architecture and functionality at the register transfer level. The double roof model features various levels of abstraction, represented by the dotted horizontal lines. The green line indicates the desired behavior for each level. The yellow line, on the other hand, represents the

structure for the implementation at each level. The model is set up in a cascading manner, where the requirements are defined at the system level and then iteratively handed down to lower levels for realization.

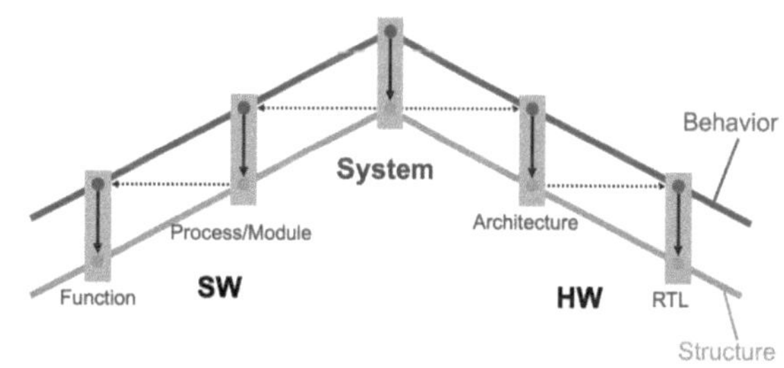

Figure 1: Double roof model. Left and right side describe the software and hardware respectively. The upper line represents the desired behavior for each level and the lower line corresponding implementation. Graphics adapted from [2]

1.2 SystemC

Hardware Description Languages (HDLs), such as VHDL and Verilog, are commonly utilized for hardware modeling at the register-transfer and behavioral level. However, they face difficulties in modeling at the system level design. Additionally, hardware-software co-design is typically less efficient when utilizing HDLs, due to limitations in simulating hardware and software together within a system. To overcome these limitations, SystemC, a C++ library, can be used for hardware modeling at various abstraction levels, including register-transfer levels, behavioral levels, and system levels [3]. Being a C++ library, advantages include

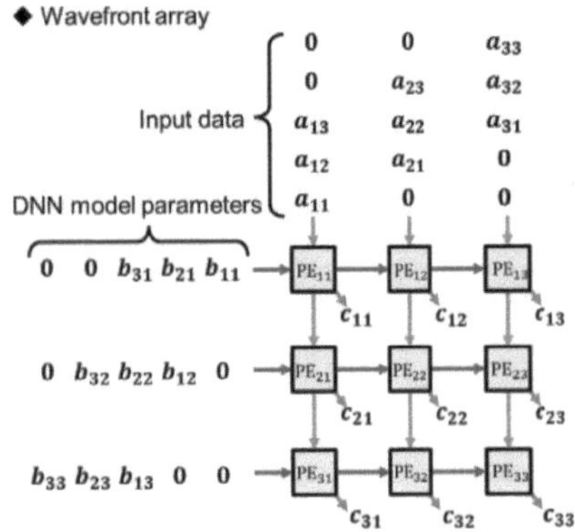
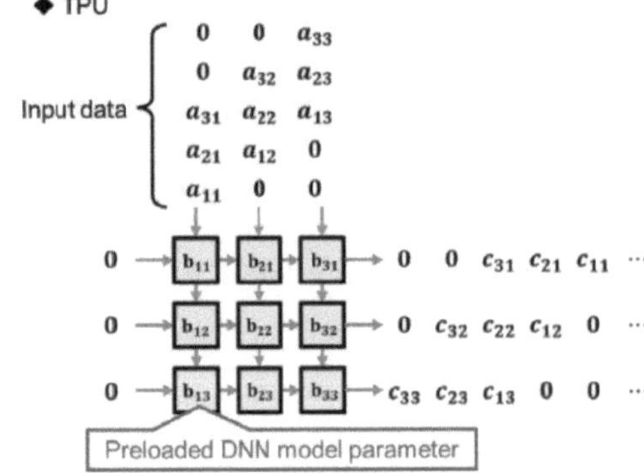

Figure 2: Comparison of wavefront array on the left and TPU systolic array on the right. Graphics adapted from [4]

data abstraction, modularity, and object-oriented programming.

SystemC, as a hardware modeling language that is based on C++ libraries, models, and tools, can be used for hardware-software co-design. The use of SystemC allows for the creation of a test bench that can evaluate performance and correctness at all levels of abstraction, without the need for separate test benches for each level. This approach enables a more efficient hardware-software co-design process.

1.3 Systolic Arrays

Systolic arrays are specialized hardware architectures designed to accelerate artificial intelligence (AI) calculations by efficiently performing matrix multiplication with low power consumption. They primarily focus on the dot product of matrices A and B. Two popular types of systolic arrays are the wavefront array, proposed by Kung [5], and the tensor processing unit (TPU), proposed by Jouppi et al. [6]. The main difference between the two is that in TPUs, one matrix is pre-loaded into the systolic array, while in wavefront arrays, both matrices are shifted in simultaneously, as illustrated in Fig. 2. In this discussion, we will focus specifically on TPUs. A systolic array is composed of tiles, which are further made up of Processing Elements (PEs) arranged in a grid pattern. Each PE comprises of accumulators and multipliers, with at least two inputs and two outputs. The inputs are used to load the components of each matrix, while the outputs are utilized to pass the inputs to the right and lower PEs. In the case of TPUs, the components of matrix B are pre-loaded and stored as weights in each PE. The upper input is then multiplied with the weight and added to the input from the left PE. The result is passed on to the right PE, which then adds it to its own calculation until the result is shifted out of the tile. The rows of the result matrix are not shifted out all at once but each with one clock cycle delay more than the previous. This results a total of $2 * n - 1$ clock cycles, with n being the dimension, for the complete calculation. Because of this offset, a controller is required to rearrange the matrix in its correct order and shape. The controller is also responsible for loading the matrices into the tile and adding an offset to the components if necessary.

2 Methods and implementations

In this section, the methods used for the implementation of the different abstraction levels are covered. This includes low-level and high-level implementation of a systolic array as well as using it for convolution.

2.1 Low-Level Implementation

In the initial stage of the design process, a single processing element (PE) and a 2x2 tile consisting of said PEs is developed at a low-level implementation. The inspiration for this design is shown in Figure 3. The biggest restriction is the limitation of memory. In hardware there is a limited amount of limited-sized registers. Therefore, all inputs and outputs have to be processed immediately. A multiplexer is utilized to distinguish between pre-loading and saving the weights and incorporating the result from the adjacent PE into the multiplication outcome. For the very left PEs, the left input is set to zero after the pre-loading of the weights. Inputs from the top are multiplied with the weight and then given to the lower PE. Results are given to the right PE.

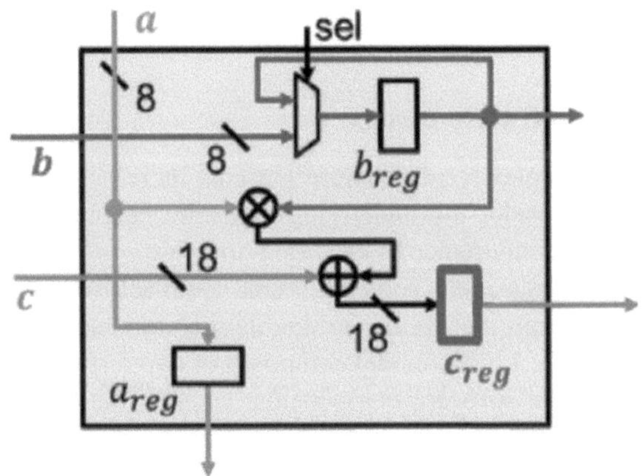

Figure 3: A TPU based PE in hardware. Graphics adapted from [4].

2.2 High-Level Implementation

At the next level of abstraction, we designed a tile which internally did not consist of individual PEs. The functionality and timing, meaning at which clock step the result is shifted out of the tile, remained consistent with the low-level representation. Additionally, the tile size was made variable. In an optimal scenario, the tiles at hand have the exact same size as the matrices used for the calculation. However, this is not always the case. In real application, the matrices size increments the higher the complexity of the DNN. Hardware has size limitations and may not be custom built for the application. Thus, we also explored loop nest optimization (LNO) approaches. LNO is used for the reduction of memory access latency, reduction of the cache bandwidth or for parallelization. These approaches work with block sizes smaller than the matrix dimensions. Preferably, the block sizes are a natural divisor of the matrices themselves to avoid the necessity of clean up due to the overlap of calculations. To realize this with a systolic array, the controller takes on more responsibility. It has to properly divide the matrices to fit into the limited sized tiles, as well as later accumulate the partial results of the tiles to get the correct result of the whole matrix multiplication. Fig. 4 shows how the matrices could be divided.

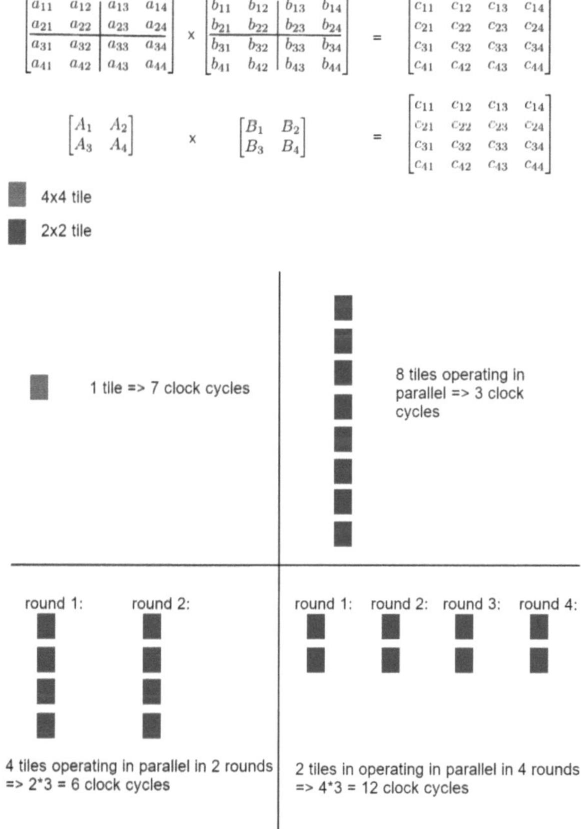

Figure 4: An example of the loop nest optimization (LNO) approach demonstrated through a 4x4 matrix multiplication in four different scenarios. The 4x4 matrices can be divided into 2x2 blocks and fed into 2x2 tiles individually.

In this example, the 4x4 matrices are divided into four 2x2 matrices. The smaller matrices can then be multiplied with each other. Additionally, three different possible scenarios of LNO and their clock time are compared with a tile with the accurate size. In the initial realization of this, the amount of tiles was sufficient for the calculation processes to all run in parallel. Parallelization is a big advantage in terms of clock cycles. It takes less then half compared to the 4x4 tile. The next step is to take into consideration that not only the size of the tiles may be limited but the amount of the tiles as well. In this scenario, the calculations cannot all be done in parallel, but must be executed sequentially, which again requires more coordination from the controller entity. The process of deciding how and when the matrices are given to the tiles in a sequential order is called scheduling. For this, we need information about the amount of tiles at our disposal, and then calculate the number of turns it takes for all the calculations to be completed. We only focused on well-posed problems, meaning that the block sizes were an even divisor of the matrix. The controller would then perform the partial calculations sequentially, while the controller would perform the accumulations. Fig. 4 shows two cases of this, one with half and one with a fourth of the required tiles. In this representation, only the the four round version is slower than the 4x4 matrix. This may look promising but it should be noted that first, for complex DNNs, the amount of tiles is most likely considerably bigger which also would result in possibly more necessary rounds, and second, the the complexity of the controller increases.

2.3 Convolution

In addition to matrix multiplication, systolic arrays can also be used to perform convolution. Convolutional neural networks are mainly used with image recognition which is a big part in most AI applications. Therefore the acceleration of convolutional calculations is a big part in accelerating AI. Opposed to matrix multiplication, convolution is not per se a matrix multiplication. The kernel, in our case matrix B, is flipped twice, once alongside the rows and once alongside the columns. The actual calculation then is only an element-wise multiplication with blocks of matrix A of the same size as the kernel. Therefore, we were able to utilize the basic principles of the LNO approach and only needed to adjust the functionality of the controller. One difference, however, is that the inputs, as opposed to the LNO matrix multiplication approach, are not separate parts of the matrix, but overlapping regions, see Fig. 5. To compute the convolution with a systolic array, one more change is needed. The already flipped kernel needs to be transposed so that partial results of the matrix multiplication can be used for the convolution result. Fig. 5 portrays the calculations done in the multiplication process and which partial results are required for the convolution result.

$$\left[\begin{array}{cccc} \boxed{a_{11}} & \boxed{a_{12}} & a_{13} & a_{14} \\ a_{21} & a_{22} & a_{23} & a_{24} \\ a_{31} & a_{32} & a_{33} & a_{34} \\ a_{41} & a_{42} & a_{43} & a_{44} \end{array}\right] * \left[\begin{array}{cc} b_{11} & b_{12} \\ b_{21} & b_{22} \end{array}\right] = \left[\begin{array}{ccc} \boxed{c_{11}} & \boxed{c_{12}} & c_{13} \\ c_{21} & c_{22} & c_{23} \\ c_{31} & c_{32} & c_{33} \end{array}\right]$$

$$\left[\begin{array}{cc} a_{11} & a_{12} \\ a_{21} & a_{22} \end{array}\right] \times \left[\begin{array}{cc} b_{22} & b_{12} \\ b_{21} & b_{11} \end{array}\right] = \left[\begin{array}{cc} d_{11} & d_{12} \\ d_{21} & d_{22} \end{array}\right]$$

$$d_{11} = a_{11}b_{22} + a_{12}b_{21}$$
$$d_{12} = a_{11}b_{12} + a_{12}b_{11}$$
$$d_{21} = a_{21}b_{22} + a_{22}b_{21}$$
$$d_{22} = a_{21}b_{12} + a_{22}b_{11}$$
$$c_1 = a_{11}b_{22} + a_{12}b_{21} + a_{21}b_{12} + a_{22}b_{11} = d_{11} + d_{22}$$

Figure 5: Convolution translated into matrix multiplication.

3 Results and Discussion

The abstraction of hardware in SystemC is simpler compared to other HDLs. As it is a C++ library, it shares all components and features of high-level programming languages, which are more familiar to many people. This is true regardless of the level of abstraction, but especially for higher levels of abstraction. SystemC code resembles less a hardware description and more any other software code. The implementation of systolic arrays for matrix multiplication has various advantages. When considering the two types of abstraction, we observed that the behavior in functionality as well as concerning the clock was the same. In an optimal scenario, where there is enough tiles or even tiles big enough, the calculation is considerably fast. Parallelization of tiles can further increase the performance speed. One disadvantage in case of matrix multiplication is the delay with which the result is shifted out of the systolic array. The bigger the tile size, the bigger said delay. Another disadvantage is that for DNN applications and their considerably big matrices the restrictions affect the performance speed more. It is still, however, a useful tool. Looking at other applications for systolic arrays, the difference in performance compared to matrix multiplication is notable. Convolution is possible with systolic arrays, however, there is a significant overhead as the systolic array performs more calculations than necessary. This results in longer cycles than if done directly and unnecessary calls for values as well as calculations.

4 Conclusion

In conclusion, systolic arrays are a valuable tool in accelerating DNNs. They are particularly useful for efficiently performing matrix multiplication with low power consumption. However, it is important to note that there are certain limitations to their applicability. The use of specialized hardware, such as systolic arrays, can greatly enhance DNN performance, especially for large scale matrices. Additionally, SystemC, a system-level modeling language, can be a useful tool for creating virtual prototypes and for validation of systolic arrays design and implementation. It makes the abstraction of hardware straightforward and can be an efficient way to model systolic arrays for DNN acceleration. For future work, it would be interesting to look at the implementation of the systolic array abstraction at a bigger scale and use it for an actual DNN or convolutional neural network. This could be done in combination with a virtual prototype.

Acknowledgement

The work has been carried out at Institute of Computer Engineering, Universität zu Lübeck and supervised by Andrija Neskovic and Saleh Mulhem.

Author's Statement

Conflict of interest: Authors state no conflict of interest.

5 References

[1] H. Genc et al., *Gemmini: Enabling Systematic Deep-Learning Architecture Evaluation via Full-Stack Integration*, 58th ACM/IEEE Design Automation Conference (DAC), San Francisco, CA, USA, 2021.

[2] Mladen Berekovic, *Hardware/Software Co-Design, Chapter 5*, Universität zu Lübeck, 2022.

[3] P. R. Panda, *SystemC - a modeling platform supporting multiple design abstractions*, International Symposium on System Synthesis, Montreal, QC, Canada, 2001.

[4] Yoshida, Kota et al. *Model Reverse-Engineering Attack against Systolic-Array-Based DNN Accelerator Using Correlation Power Analysis*. IEICE Trans. Fundam. Electron. Commun. Comput. 2021.

[5] Kung, *Why systolic architectures?*, Computer vol. 15, 1982.

[6] N. P. Jouppi et al., *In-Datacenter Performance Analysis of a Tensor Processing Unit*, CoRR, 2017.

Deep feature learning for fidgety movement detection using inertial measurement unit data

Falco Lentzsch [1], Frédéric Li [1], Friederike Pagel [2], Margot Lau [2], Karen Otte [4], Hanna Marie Röhling [4], Anne Stein [4], Adeel Nisar [1], Leopold Zieser [5], Sebastian Glende [5], Nico Kaartinen [3], Sebastian Mansow-Model [4], Ute Thyen [2], Marcin Grzegorzek [1]

[1] Institut for Medical Informatics (IMI), University of Lübeck, Germany, falco.lentzsch@student.uni-luebeck.de
[2] Sozialpädiatrisches Zentrum (SPZ), UKSH Lübeck, Germany
[3] KAASA solution GmbH, Düsseldorf, Germany
[4] Motognosis GmbH, Berlin, Germany
[5] YOUSE GmbH, Berlin, Germany

Abstract

Fidgety Movements (FM) are subtle involuntary movements seen in infants less than 20-week of age that play an important role in early childhood development. Their absence suggests a high chance for a future neurological disorder such as cerebral palsy. Since the severity of the outcome strongly depends on the time of detection, it is necessary to detect the absence of these movements as early as possible to initiate therapy. Current approaches mostly use either video data, or Inertial Measurement Unit (IMU) data of the limbs from which features are extracted by hand. These features are often not abstract enough to detect and describe FM. To overcome these limitations, we developed a multi-branch convolutional architecture that can detect FM based on raw IMU limb data. This model is then used to detect the presence or absence of FMs in an infant, and classify the latter between normal or at risk with a simple threshold-based rule. Our approach yielded subject-independent accuracies of 79.98% and 85.93% for the FM and infant classification respectively on a dataset of 19 subjects.

1 Introduction

Between 9 and 12 weeks post-term, early infantile movement patterns occur. These movements, also referred to as *General Movements* (GM), usually last until the end of the first year of life [1]. During the development of the child, GMs change in amplitude, speed and acceleration. If abnormal movement patterns occur, this usually indicates a neurological disorder. GMs can be divided into different categories depending on the developmental stage of the child. The most important of them from the clinical perspective are *Fidgety Movements* (FM). The latter are involuntary multidirectional movements characterized by a small amplitude and a medium speed. They usually start around 9-12 weeks postpartum and last from 6 to 12 months postpartum. FMs occur with an alternating acceleration on the neck, trunk and extremities. They also account for the majority of movements at this age stage. FMs being completely absent or having an abnormal amplitude is often a sign of neurological diseases occurring, whose most common prognosis is infantile Cerebral Palsy [1]. It is therefore important to detect possible neurological issues by the examination of FMs as early as possible so that appropriate treatment can be provided with maximum efficiency. The examination of each child - also referred to as *screening process* - is however a very time-consuming process because FMs are not trivial to recognize and require specifically trained medical personnel. Obtaining an automated screening system using machine learning would thus be valuable.

Therefore, our goal is to proceed with a two-stage classification approach: deep learning models are firstly trained to learn features for the detection of FMs in 1-second-long data windows of raw IMU data from the limbs. The estimations of the trained model are then analyzed over a time-period of 1 minute to classify the infant as normal or at risk.

2 Materials and methods

2.1 *Partici ants*

103 children between 3-5 months of age were recruited in the Kinderklinik in UKSH Lübeck, of which 19 were provided with FM annotations by experts at the time of writing. For each child, both video data and IMU data were recorded over a period of 5 to 15 minutes. All parents signed a consent form. For data recording, the children were first placed in a bed on their back, and kept away from any external interaction. 2 RGB-Depth cameras were placed above them to acquire video data during the examination and 4 IMUs were placed on the shoulders and hips of the infant, as shown in Figure 1.

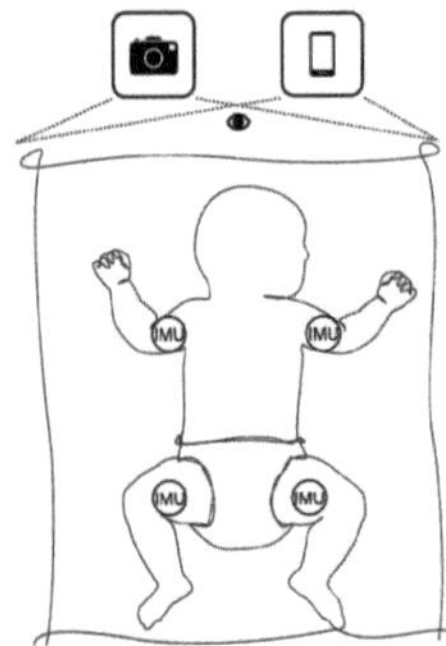

Figure 1: Placement of the IMUs and cameras.

2.2   *Sensor ecording*

We used 4 *Movesense HR+* IMUs which were attached at the level of the shoulders and the hips on each side as shown in Figure 1. *Movesense HR+* contains a 3-axis accelerometer and gyroscope. We used a sampling frequency of 52 Hz. In this work, only IMU data were used, since the RGB-Depth video processing was performed by a *ScreenFM* partner, Motognosis GmbH (Berlin).

2.3   *Video ecording*

For the video data, we used two devices: one Iphone 12 pro and one Kinect Azure 3D camera. Cameras were mounted on a support and pointed downwards to have the whole child in the frame. Motognosis GmbH computed some features from the literature on tracked body parts obtained after applying Google's *MediaPipe* tracking algorithm [2]. To ensure that both sensor and video data are recorded synchronously, an app from KAASA solution GmbH (Düsseldorf) was used to control the entire recording process. Because the video features were not available at the time of writing, they were not used in this study. In addition, the RGB video streams were used by clinicians in UKSH Lübeck to annotate the data with FM-related information. Two independent experts had the possibility to assign 3 different labels to time intervals while watching the video stream using a tool developed by KAASA solution GmbH: FM present, FM absent or invalid data (e.g. person between the infant and camera, infant crying, etc.). Due to the high heterogeneity of the invalid class, the latter was not considered in the FM classification problem.

2.4   *Pre rocessing   Segmentation*

For each of the 19 subjects used in this study, a CSV file containing the time-series data acquired from the 4 IMUs during the examination was obtained. Each file contained 6 columns that are corresponding to the 3 channels of the 3D accelerometer and the 3 channels of the 3D gyroscope. The CSV data files were first processed to separate the data from each IMU, and synchronise the 6 channels to a target frequency of 100Hz using linear interpolation. The data streams were then segmented into windows of 1 second using a non-overlapping sliding window approach to generate data arrays of size 100×6 for each IMU. To generate the

corresponding labels, we used the annotations of the clinicians provided for the part of the video stream corresponding to the 1-second data array. A single label corresponding to the majority annotation was attributed to the data array. A threshold to put the majority at 60% was used to discard arrays with potentially ambiguous annotations (e.g. right between FM and no FM).

2.5   *classifier architecture*

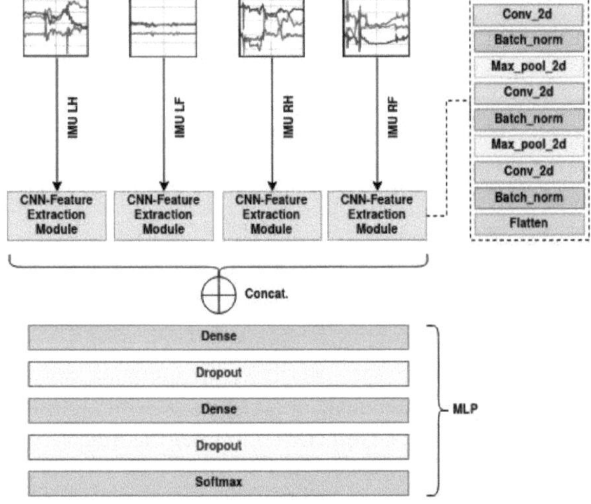

Figure 2:   Architecture of the Multi Branch-CNN (LH = left_shoulder, RH = right_shoulder, LF = left_hip, RF = right_hip)

After testing several deep neural networks, we decided to use a *Multi-Branch Convolutional Neural Network* (mCNN) that takes 4 different inputs, one for each IMU, as shown in Figure 2. Each input is then processed by a CNN feature extraction block which returns 288 features as output for each of the 4 inputs. The output of each feature block is then concatenated to a 1152 dimensional feature vector and further processed by a multi-layer perceptron. Dropout was used between the layers to achieve a better generalization. The output of the network consists of two probabilities, one for each of the 'FM' and 'no FM' classes.

To achieve a better generalization of the selected features, regularization was used in the CNN feature blocks in addition to the layers shown in the figure. The model was trained with a loss L defined by Equation 1:

$$L = L_{SCC} + \lambda_1 \sum_{j=1}^{m} \sum_{i=1}^{n^{(j)}} |w_i^{(j)}| + \lambda_2 \sum_{j=1}^{m} \sum_{i=1}^{n^{(j)}} w_i^{(j)2} \quad (1)$$

where L_{SCC} refers to the Sparse Categorical Cross-Entropy, $\lambda_1, \lambda_2 > 0$ are weighting factors, $w_i^{(j)}$ designates the weights of the layer, $n^{(j)}$ the number of weights per layer and m the layers on which we applied regularization. The second term of the loss is a L1 regularization which has the effect that some features become 0 and our solution gets more sparse. A L2 regularization was also used as indicated by the last term of Equation 1, which results in smaller weights. As weighting factors we used $\lambda_1 = \lambda_2 = 0.01$.

Subject_Id	Accuracy (%)	F1-Score (%)	Subject_ID	Accuracy (%)	F1-Score (%)
31	94.67	48.63	41	79.33	44.24
32	97.13	49.27	42	89.85	47.33
33	91.02	47.65	43	67.88	50.37
34	57.56	55.61	44	69.18	52.87
35	97.05	49.25	45	63.49	49.69
36	85.00	74.03	46	62.09	46.68
37	87.13	46.56	47	96.25	49.04
38	57.25	57.25	48	100	50.00
39	81.25	44.53	49	66.03	40.42
40	76.60	44.24			
Average	79.98 ±14.56	49.89 ±7.05			

Table 1: Test-Accuracy & F1-score for the FM classification

2.6 *odel Training and Evaluation*

For the training of our network we use a leave one subject out (LOSO) cross-validator. Data arrays annotated as invalid were first excluded from the dataset. Subsequently, the aforementioned network was trained 19 times. 18 infants served as training dataset, one infant as testing dataset, and the process was repeated so that each infant was used in the testing set once. The evaluation was done based on the network with the highest test accuracy after each training.

For the evaluation of the FM classifier we used again our testing dataset. We compared the predictions of the networks to the ground truth labels to generate accuracy, Average F1-Score (AF1) and confusion matrices. It is worth to mention that the testing set in our LOSO cross validation is highly imbalanced due to infants beings either mostly fidgety or non-fidgety. This can introduce a bias in the test evaluation metrics, including the accuracy and AF1 we used in our study.

2.7 *n ant Classification*

Our final objective is to classify whether children are at risk or not at risk. Clinicians use the following rule: the more FM, the more normal the infant is likely to be. Therefore, we adapted our decision rule to the one used by the experts and designed a simple threshold criterion. The output of our FM classifier gives us a prediction for every second. We aggregated this second-by-second prediction over a time horizon of 1 minute. If the proportion of seconds considered as FM is above a certain threshold, the 1-minute segment is classified as normal. Otherwise, it is considered as at risk. We tried various thresholds in the range from 10% to 90% with a step size of 10%. In order to be as close as possible to a real scenario, we re-included the invalid data for the infant classification. This way, that we had no discontinuous 1-minute segments.

3 Results

3.1 *Classification*

For the classification of FMs, we achieved a mean testing accuracy of 79.98% with a standard deviation of ±14.56% across all folds of the LOSO, as shown in Table 1. The same procedure was used for the calculation of the mean F1-score also shown in Table 1. Here we achieved a mean value of 49.89 ±7.05%.

3.2 *n ant Classification*

The classification results are provided in Table 2, where 3 numbers are computed for each infant and threshold: number of 1-minute segments correctly classified (#cc), total number of 1-min segments (#total), number of 1-min segments with at least 50% invalid data (#invalid).

threshold	10	20	30	40	50	60	70	80	90
31 = at risk	(4, 4, 2)	(4, 4, 2)	(4, 4, 2)	(4, 4, 2)	(4, 4, 2)	(4, 4, 2)	(4, 4, 2)	(4, 4, 2)	(4, 4, 2)
32 = normal	(7, 7, 0)	(7, 7, 0)	(7, 7, 0)	(7, 7, 0)	(7, 7, 0)	(7, 7, 0)	(7, 7, 0)	(7, 7, 0)	(7, 7, 0)
33 = normal	(5, 5, 0)	(5, 5, 0)	(5, 5, 0)	(5, 5, 0)	(5, 5, 0)	(5, 5, 0)	(5, 5, 0)	(5, 5, 0)	(5, 5, 0)
34 = at risk	(1, 7, 0)	(1, 7, 0)	(2, 7, 0)	(4, 7, 0)	(6, 7, 0)	(7, 7, 0)	(7, 7, 0)	(7, 7, 0)	(7, 7, 0)
35 = normal	(6, 6, 0)	(6, 6, 0)	(6, 6, 0)	(6, 6, 0)	(6, 6, 0)	(6, 6, 0)	(6, 6, 0)	(6, 6, 0)	(6, 6, 0)
36 = normal	(6, 6, 5)	(6, 6, 5)	(6, 6, 5)	(6, 6, 5)	(6, 6, 5)	(6, 6, 5)	(6, 6, 5)	(6, 6, 5)	(6, 6, 5)
37 = normal	(15, 15, 9)	(15, 15, 9)	(15, 15, 9)	(15, 15, 9)	(15, 15, 9)	(15, 15, 9)	(15, 15, 9)	(15, 15, 9)	(15, 15, 9)
38 = normal	(9, 9, 0)	(9, 9, 0)	(9, 9, 0)	(9, 9, 0)	(4, 9, 0)	(2, 9, 0)	(0, 9, 0)	(0, 9, 0)	(0, 9, 0)
39 = normal	(9, 9, 0)	(9, 9, 0)	(9, 9, 0)	(9, 9, 0)	(9, 9, 0)	(9, 9, 0)	(9, 9, 0)	(9, 9, 0)	(9, 9, 0)
40 = normal	(8, 8, 0)	(8, 8, 0)	(8, 8, 0)	(8, 8, 0)	(8, 8, 0)	(8, 8, 0)	(8, 8, 0)	(8, 8, 0)	(8, 8, 0)
41 = at risk	(6, 6, 0)	(6, 6, 0)	(6, 6, 0)	(6, 6, 0)	(6, 6, 0)	(6, 6, 0)	(6, 6, 0)	(6, 6, 0)	(6, 6, 0)
42 = at risk	(5, 7, 0)	(7, 7, 0)	(7, 7, 0)	(7, 7, 0)	(7, 7, 0)	(7, 7, 0)	(7, 7, 0)	(7, 7, 0)	(7, 7, 0)
43= normal	(8, 8, 0)	(7, 8, 0)	(2, 8, 0)	(0, 8, 0)	(0, 8, 0)	(0, 8, 0)	(0, 8, 0)	(0, 8, 0)	(0, 8, 0)
44 = at risk	(0, 7, 0)	(0, 7, 0)	(0, 7, 0)	(0, 7, 0)	(0, 7, 0)	(0, 7, 0)	(0, 7, 0)	(0, 7, 0)	(1, 7, 0)
45 = normal	(6, 6, 0)	(6, 6, 0)	(6, 6, 0)	(6, 6, 0)	(6, 6, 0)	(6, 6, 0)	(6, 6, 0)	(6, 6, 0)	(4, 6, 0)
46 = at risk	(0, 5, 0)	(0, 5, 0)	(0, 5, 0)	(0, 5, 0)	(0, 5, 0)	(0, 5, 0)	(0, 5, 0)	(0, 5, 0)	(1, 5, 0)
47 = normal	(6, 6, 0)	(6, 6, 0)	(6, 6, 0)	(6, 6, 0)	(6, 6, 0)	(6, 6, 0)	(6, 6, 0)	(6, 6, 0)	(6, 6, 0)
48 = at risk	(7, 7, 0)	(7, 7, 0)	(7, 7, 0)	(7, 7, 0)	(7, 7, 0)	(7, 7, 0)	(7, 7, 0)	(7, 7, 0)	(7, 7, 0)
49 = normal	(7, 7, 0)	(7, 7, 0)	(7, 7, 0)	(7, 7, 0)	(7, 7, 0)	(7, 7, 0)	(7, 7, 0)	(7, 7, 0)	(7, 7, 0)
#_correct	(115, 135)	(116, 135)	(112, 135)	(112, 135)	(109, 135)	(108, 135)	(106, 135)	(106, 135)	(106, 135)
%_correct	85.19	85.93	82.96	82.96	80.74	80.00	78.52	78.52	78.52
#_invalid	16	16	16	16	16	16	16	16	16

Table 2: Classification result on infant level.
(#cc, #total, #invalid)

For the evaluation of the infant classification, labels of the clinicians were available. Infants could be labeled either as at risk or normal. These annotations are provided in Table 2. For each threshold a ratio between cc and total was computed. We achieved the best result with a threshold of 20%. Here, 116 of 135 1-minute time windows were correctly classified, which corresponds to an accuracy of 85.93%. In general, thresholds <50% gave better results than high thresholds. In total, 16 of the 135 time intervals were marked as invalid. Table 2 also shows that the classifier produced very poor results for certain subjects. For example, for subjects 34, 44 and 46, almost all 60 second time intervals were incorrectly classified. This is likely due to the poor FM classification accuracy (below 65%) for these 3 subjects, as shown in Table 1.

4 Discussion

The results we obtained are very promising. We managed to perform a correct classification for more than 85% of all 1-minute time intervals. Children are usually classified by the clinicians as 'normal' when a small number of FMs are present. This statement seems to be in line with our results showing that lower thresholds on the proportion of detected FMs in one minute provide better performances for the infant classification.

A similar study was carried out beforehand at IMI using simple statistical hand-crafted features like in Li et al. [3], instead of learning them with a mCNN. Afterwards a Random Forest Classifier was trained with these features.

Statistical handcrafted features (HCF) have shown to provide fairly good results in the time-series classification literature, despite their simplicity. Unfortunately, this was not verified on the ScreenFM data set. The results when using HCFs were very poor as shown in Table 4. One reason might be the fact that the computed HCFs are not generalising well enough across multiple infants, due to their sim-

	mCNN	HCF
Accuracy (%)	79.98 ±14.56	47.10 ±18.12
F1-Score (%)	49.89 ±7.05	32.73 ±10.12

Table 3: FM Classification: mCNN vs. HCF

plicity. Because of their poor FM recognition performance, HCFs also did not perform well for infant classification as shown in Table 4.

threshold	cc - mCNN (%)	cc - HCF (%)
10 (%)	85.19 (115, 135)	**56.59 (73, 129)**
20 (%)	**85.93 (116, 135)**	48.84 (63, 129)
30 (%)	82.96 (112, 135)	41.86 (54, 129)
40 (%)	82.96 (112, 135)	34.88 (45, 129)
50 (%)	80.74 (109, 135)	32.56 (42, 129)
60 (%)	80.00 (108, 135)	32.56 (42, 129)
70 (%)	78.52 (106, 135)	34.88 (45, 129)
80 (%)	78.52 (106, 135)	33.33 (43, 129)
90 (%)	78.52 (106, 135)	32.56 (42, 129)

Table 4: Infant Classification: mCNN vs. HCF

In general, all evaluation metrics for FM classification - including the accuracy and AF1 - have to be carefully interpreted in this study. Most subjects are either fidgety or not fidgety, which leads to a strong class imbalance in the LOSO test sets, and therefore induces a strong bias in the evaluation metrics. Future studies will use a stratified k-fold cross validation instead when more subject annotations become available to address this issue.

5 Conclusion

A machine learning method using IMU data in combination with a mCNN to detect FMs in infants less than 20 weeks of age was presented, and used to estimate whether children are at risk of an abnormal neurological development (e.g. Cerebral Palsy). Very promising results were obtained on a dataset of 19 subjects (7 at risk, 12 normal) whose data were acquired in the Kinderklinik in UKSH Lübeck. But the study still has several limitations. One of the biggest was the relatively small size of the dataset, which meant that the network had to be strongly regularized in order not to overfit. Another problem of the dataset is the high class unbalance, since most infants either provided a lot of FM data, or no FM data at all. We hope to be able to increase the size of our dataset in the future by obtaining new annotations from the clinicians in UKSH Lübeck. This would allow us to use a stratified k-fold cross validation making sure that all folds contain approximately equal numbers of samples of both classes while keeping the evaluation setup subject-independent by having different subjects in each fold. This could also help to produce more meaningful metrics. We would also like to add more information during the training of our network. During the labeling process, experts not only did tell when FMs occur, but also on which part of the body they were seen. FMs often only occur on one part

of the body at the time, for example the left arm. However, our network is currently trained with the assumption that all IMUs should be able to detect a FM occurring on any part of the body, which is likely not true (e.g. the IMU located on the right hip will probably not detect any FM occurring in the left hand). Therefore, we would like to integrate the information about the position of FM into the training process. This could be done by using a modified loss inspired from supervised contrastive learning [4] to add constraints on the branches of the mCNN depending on whether the IMU processed by the branch was meant to see a FM or not. Finally, another very promising approach would be to merge the IMU features with the RGB-Depth video features extracted by Motognosis GmbH when they become available [5].

Acknowledgement

The work was carried out at the University of Lübeck in the Medical Data Science. I would like to thank Jasmin Walter and Svenja Neumann, who supervised the data acquisition process.

Author's Statement

The authors declare no conflict of interest. Parents of the subjects in this study provided informed consent.

6 References

[1] H. F. Prechtl, "State of the art of a new functional assessment of the young nervous system. an early predictor of cerebral palsy," *Early Human Development*, vol. 50, no. 1, pp. 1–11, 1997.

[2] C. Lugaresi, J. Tang, H. Nash, C. McClanahan, E. Uboweja, M. Hays, F. Zhang, C. Chang, M. G. Yong, J. Lee, W. Chang, W. Hua, M. Georg, and M. Grundmann, "Mediapipe: A framework for building perception pipelines," *CoRR*, vol. abs/1906.08172, 2019.

[3] F. Li, K. Shirahama, M. A. Nisar, L. Köping, and M. Grzegorzek, "Comparison of feature learning methods for human activity recognition using wearable sensors," *Sensors*, vol. 18, no. 2, 2018.

[4] P. Khosla, P. Teterwak, C. Wang, A. Sarna, Y. Tian, P. Isola, A. Maschinot, C. Liu, and D. Krishnan, "Supervised contrastive learning," *CoRR*, vol. abs/2004.11362, 2020.

[5] A. Machireddy, J. van Santen, J. L. Wilson, J. Myers, M. Hadders-Algra, and X. Song, "A video/imu hybrid system for movement estimation in infants," *IEEE EMBC*, pp. 730–733, 2017.

Evaluation of Estimated Substance Compositions by AI-based Classification of Optical Absorption Spectra

Tom Kruse [1], Ole Sellhorn [2] and Horst Hellbrück [3]

[1] Applied Information Technology, TH Lübeck, tom.kruse@stud.th-luebeck.de
[2] Department of Electrical Engineering and Computer Science, TH Lübeck, ole.sellhorn@th-luebeck.de
[3] Department of Electrical Engineering and Computer Science, TH Lübeck, horst.hellbrueck@th-luebeck.de

Abstract

AI-based classification of substance compositions is a major challenge. While it is possible to predict absorption spectra based on given compositions, it is difficult to classify the substance based on given spectra. This work uses deep and machine learning classifiers to determine real spectra of substance compositions in form of images. The training is done with synthetic data generated from real data. The deep learning classifiers achieve an accuracy of 62.5 % and a brier score of 0.44, whereas the machine learning classifiers achieve an accuracy of 50 % with a brier score of 0.83. The results show that the deep learning classifiers reached a higher accuracy and solve the given problem.

1 Introduction

The analysis of chemical substance compositions is still a versatile field of research. While it is already possible to predict the optical absorption spectra from different compositions, it is still difficult to reliably determine the composition based on a given spectra. In addition, AI-based methods are gaining in popularity besides conventional analytical methods such as chromatography [1].

This work uses synthesized spectra of benzene-water compositions with different concentration values (c-values) and water types for binary and multi-class classification of real spectra. This is realized by applying different machine learning classifiers (MLCs) like Support Vector Machines (SVMs) and Random Forest Classifiers (RFCs) and deep learning classifiers (DLCs) like Convolutional Neural Networks (CNNs). They are trained and evaluated in comparison. Usually, MLCs are very suitable for binary classification, but they are only taken for multi-class classification. The CNNs are used for both binary and multi-class classification. With regard to the CNNs, we investigate whether the results differ when both water types, as well as c-values, are classified at once or in two steps. Therefore we have a binary classification for the water types and two subsequent multi-class classifications for the c-values.

The available data is given in form of images. The CNN is particularly suitable for image classification [2]. In the field of machine learning, SVMs are very popular for image classification as well as RFCs [3].

Mozaffari et al. use CNNs to perform a multi-label classification of chemical mixtures to distinguish the components they contain. For this purpose, Raman spectra are used. The test data contains several hundred synthesized data sets, which are classified with an accuracy of 100 % [4]. The difference is that we use synthesized training data to predict real test data.

Li et al. investigated the classification of various substance compositions with the help of chromatogram images. A CNN was also used here. The substances were classified with an average accuracy of 98 % [5].

Both works investigated a classification of different substance compositions with special spectra for feature extraction and reaches a high accuracy score for the test data. In contrast, we investigate the classification of the optical absorption spectra with a few amount of synthesized training data.

Section 2 explains which data is used for the training of the classifiers, how it is synthesized and preprocessed. Furthermore, it contains the implementation and training of the classifiers as well as the optimization of selected hyperparameters. In section 3, the results of the classifiers are evaluated and discussed in terms of accuracy and probability metrics. Finally, section 4 summarizes the results and gives an outlook for future work.

2 Material and Methods

This section covers the procedure for data processing and the use of the classifiers. It also gives information about the database as well as the evaluation metrics.

2.1 Data Set

We produced synthesized training data featuring the optical absorption spectra shown in Fig. 1. The x-axis displays the wavelength and the y-axis shows the absorption unit. The legend identifies the water types - distilled water (DW) and

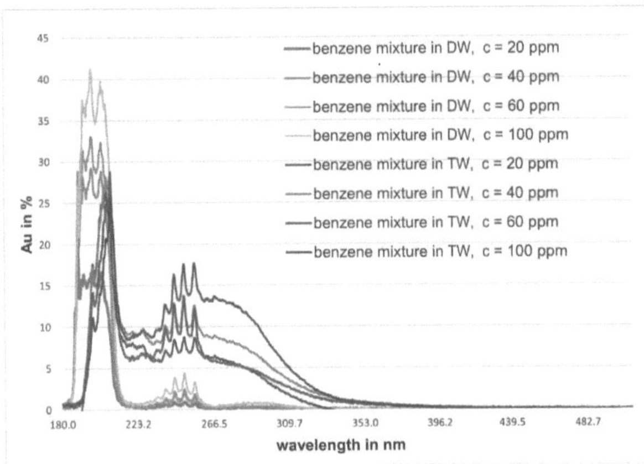

Figure 1: Spectra of the real benzene-water compositions

tap water (TW) - and their corresponding c-values in parts per million (ppm). We generated 200 synthesized training data with the help of another neural network. This given training data set contains 100 for distilled water (DW) and 100 for tap water (TW), each with c-values ranging from 1 to 100. The training data set comes in the form of portable network graphics (png) with 640x480 pixels. Fig. 2 shows an example image of the synthesized data.

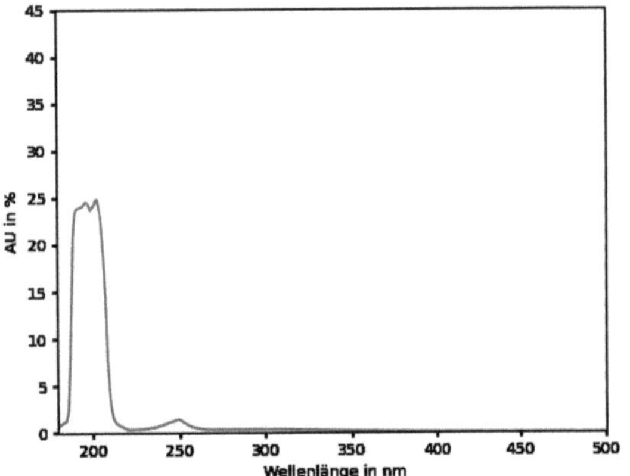

Figure 2: Synthesized data: example image, TW with c-value 34

2.2 Image Preprocessing

The images are not well suited as input for the classifiers, both in scale and color format. For the extraction of the axes and their labeling, morphological operations are performed using the image processing library OpenCV. Therefore, the images are converted into binary images. Then the extraction of the horizontal and vertical lines is done as described in the following documentation for "Extract horizontal and vertical lines by using morphological operations" [6]. The image area without axes is then defined and cropped so that the axes and their labeling are removed. In addition, the images are resized to a dimension of 256x256 pixels to reduce the amount of data.

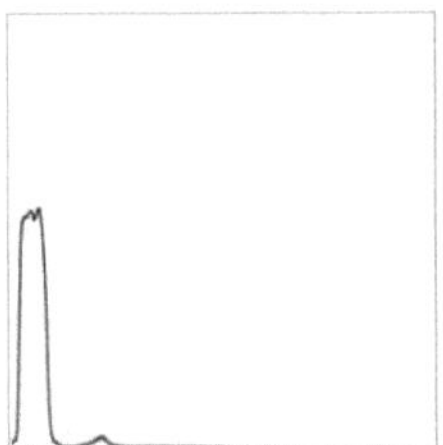

Figure 3: Example image after applying all operations; The gray frame is for presentation purposes and does not exist inside the data in use.

As a final step, the algorithm converts the images from RGB to grayscale color format. This transformation reduces complexity, improves the classification results, and increases the range of use, as the images become one-dimensional and the original color becomes irrelevant [7]. Fig. 3 shows the result for Fig. 2 after applying all operations.

2.3 Data splitting and classes

To improve the training of classifiers with the limited 200 image dataset, we divided the images into groups of 5. This group size remains meaningful and the 40 resulting classes (20 for DW and 20 for TW) are arranged in ascending order of their c-values. For example, the first group has c-values from one to five, the second group from six to ten, and so on. Especially for the deep learning part, it is necessary to split the existing estimated data into training and validation data. Therefore, one data is taken from each class for the validation data. This results in a split of 80 % training data to 20 % validation data for both binary and multi-class classification. The machine learning part uses all estimated data for the training. We use the eight spectra from Fig. 1 as test data in the end.

2.4 Convolutional Neural Networks

For the implementation of the CNNs, TensorFlow and Keras are used in Python. A total of four CNNs, one for the classification of all classes at once (CNN all) and three for the classification in two steps (CNNs two steps) were developed. Two steps state the binary classification based on the water type and the multi-class classification based on the c-value ranges for distilled and tap water, respectively.

Table 1: Structure of the CNNs

layer	types	filters/ kernel size	pool size
input	Conv2D	32/ (3, 3)	
	MaxPooling2D		(2, 2)
	Dropout		
hidden	Conv2D	64/ (3, 3)	
	MaxPooling2D		(2, 2)
	Dropout		
hidden	Conv2D	128/ (3, 3)	
	MaxPooling2D		(2, 2)
flatten	Flatten	Units	
	Dense	128	
output	Dense	40, 20, 2	

Table 1 shows the structure of the CNNs. Three units are

specified for the output layer. This is due to the different allocation into binary and multi-classes. Subsequently, tuning hyperparameters is realized by using Talos. In total, 48 combinations of the hyperparameters are tested for each of the CNNs except the CNN for binary classification, which is trained successfully with the first combination regarding the validation accuracy and loss.

2.5 Machine Learning Classifiers

The library scikit-learn is used to implement the MLCs. As a rule, SVMs do support binary classification by computing the slice between two data sets which separates them maximally. Multi-classes are split into smaller binary subclasses which enables the possibility for multi-class classification. For this case, the "one-vs-one" method is applied using the SVM from sklearn. Therefore, a hyperplane separates two classes disregarding the points of the third class. This means that only the points of the two classes in the current split are considered in the separation [8]. The RFCs work with decision trees for each class and merge them together in the end [9]. That is why they are also suitable for multiclass classification. The hyperparameters are tuned with GridSearchCV. For the SVMs 80 combinations of hyperparameters and 60 combinations for the RFCs are reached.

2.6 Evaluation Metrics

The accuracy (acc) indicates how many predictions are correct. It is calculated by dividing the sum of the correct predictions - true-positive (TP) and true-negative (TN) - by the number of all predictions, plus false-negative (FN) and false-positive (FP) [10]. Equation(1) shows the calculation in percentage:

$$acc = \frac{TP + TN}{TP + TN + FN + FP} * 100 \tag{1}$$

In addition, the F1 Score ($F1$) is faced in the evaluation. It represents the harmonic mean between recall and precision in a range of 0 to 1. The best possible result is 1. The precision indicates the ratio of true positive results that were correctly predicted. The recall tells how well the classifier identifies positive results [10]. Below is the calculation of $F1$ using $precision$ and $recall$ in (2), (3) and (4):

$$precision = \frac{TP}{TP + FP} \tag{2}$$

$$recall = \frac{TP}{TP + FN} \tag{3}$$

$$F1 = 2 * \frac{precision * recall}{precision + recall} \tag{4}$$

We do have balanced test data (one per given class), but not all classes are available. This means looking at $F1$ alone is not quite sufficient.[10].

At least, the prediction probability p in % is included for the evaluation in combination with the brier score (BS). It measures the accuracy of probabilistic predictions and the actual outcome in a range of 0 to 2. The smaller the brier

score, the better. Since we have multi classes we apply (5) for the calculation:

$$BS = \frac{1}{N} \sum_{t=1}^{N} \sum_{i=1}^{R} (f_{t,i} - o_{t,i})^2 \tag{5}$$

The number of test classes is described by N, while R is the number of possible classes. The predicted probabilities for class i are represented by $f_{t,i}$ while $o_{t,i}$ is 1 if the true class has the index t,i. Otherwise, it is 0 [10].

3 Results and Discussion

Table 2: Classification results for the given test data

Classifiers	acc	BS	F1
SVM	50	0.83	0.33
RFC	50	0.84	0.33
CNN all	62.5	0.61	0.44
CNNs two steps	62.5	0.44	0.44

Table 2 shows the results of the classifiers for accuracy, brier and F1 score. The classification of substance compositions based on optical absorption spectra using DLCs is performed with an accuracy of 62.5 %. The MLCs achieved an accuracy of 50 %. Here it is noticeable that $F1$ between the MLCs is equal as well as for the DLCs because the number of correctly predicted test data is the same.

In general, the number of test data is very low and influences the result with regard to the significance. Here, a classification of more than 8 test data is interesting to check whether the accuracy varies over all classes, remains in a similar range, improves or even becomes worse.

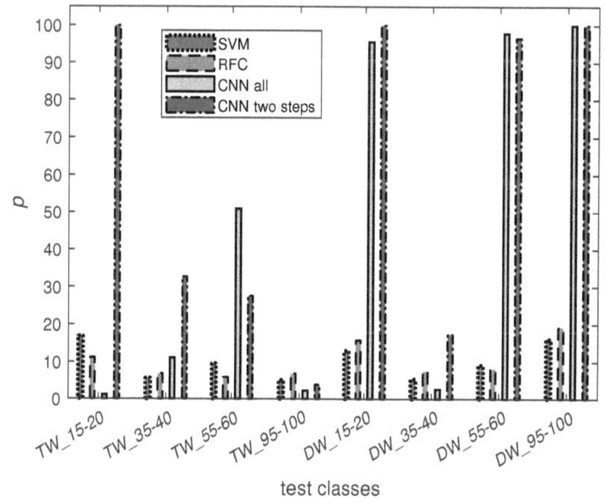

Figure 4: Prediction probabilities p of the test classes

While $F1$ differ in a small range of 0.11 for the MLCs and DLCs, there are large differences of up to 0.4 for BS. The reason is the lower prediction probabilities of the MLCs. Fig. 4 shows the prediction probabilities p with which the classifiers determine the test classes. The test class names are composed of the water type with the respective c-value range. Here, the maximum confidence of the MLCs is 19.23 % while the DLCs reach 99.99 % for the correct class in some cases. This is explained by the different ways of learning. Due to the fact that SVMs aim for a linear separation of the test data with each possible class by the one-vs-one method, there are clearly larger intersections. A similar problem exists with the RFCs, except that decision trees instead of linear separation handle the problem. In addition, some of the predicted classes differ by one class, because the real data represent the boundaries between them. Therefore, the confidence according to p is significantly higher for CNNs, which are optimal for image classification.

With a closer look at the CNNs, the stepwise classification using multiple CNNs is more complex overall, but also more robust compared to the use of only one CNN for all classes. This is also confirmed by the BS at a difference of 0.17. The reason is that we split the classification problem and reduced the complexity of the data. Important to say is that the training data is created based on the test data so the result may be additionally biased. In the future, training should already be carried out with a larger amount of real data only supplemented with synthesized data. Another important point is that the test data must always have the same scaling, otherwise the classifiers will fail. Also for this purpose, additional methods like data augmentation could be applied, which bypass a fixed scaling of the data.

4 Conclusion

The classification of substance compositions is still difficult. Within this work, optical absorption spectra of benzene-water compositions with different concentration values are classified with an accuracy up to 62.5 % and a brier score of 0.44 using machine and deep learning classifiers. Synthesized data is chosen for the training of the classifiers. The confidence of the prediction probability of the deep learning classifiers is significantly higher than for the machine learning classifiers, which is explained by the way of learning. In the future, it is reasonable to investigate data regardless of scaling. Furthermore, it makes sense to use noticeably larger amounts of real data only supplemented by synthesized data for a higher significance.

Acknowledgement

This publication is a result of the research of the Center of Excellence CoSA and funded by the Federal Ministry of Education & Research of the Federal Republic of Germany (Id [LPW-E/1.2.1/1631], [Innovationsorientiertes Netzwerk KI-Transfer-Hub Schleswig-Holstein – KI-Know-how für KMU durch Hochschulkompetenz]). Horst Hellbrück is adjunct professor at the Institute of Telematics of University of Lübeck.

Author's Statement

The authors state no conflict of interest.

5 References

[1] V. Dozein *et al.*, "Determination of benzene, toluene, ethylbenzene, and p-xylene with headspace-hollow fiber solid-phase microextraction-gas chromatography in wastewater and buxus leaves, employing a chemometric approach," *Chemical Papers*, vol. 75, no. 8, pp. 4305–4316, 2021.

[2] J. Hu *et al.*, "Raman spectrum classification based on transfer learning by a convolutional neural network: Application to pesticide detection," *Spectrochimica acta. Part A, Molecular and biomolecular spectroscopy*, vol. 265, p. 120366, 2022.

[3] G. Mercier and M. Lennon, "Support vector machines for hyperspectral image classification with spectral-based kernels," in *IGARSS 2003. 2003 IEEE International Geoscience and Remote Sensing Symposium. Proceedings (IEEE Cat. No.03CH37477)*. IEEE, 2003, pp. 288–290.

[4] M. H. Mozaffari and L.-L. Tay, "Convolutional neural networks for raman spectral analysis of chemical mixtures," in *2021 5th SLAAI International Conference on Artificial Intelligence (SLAAI-ICAI)*, 2021, pp. 1–6.

[5] H. Li *et al.*, "Identification of specific substances in the faims spectra of complex mixtures using deep learning," *Sensors (Basel, Switzerland)*, vol. 21, no. 18, 2021.

[6] OpenCV, "Opencv: Extract horizontal and vertical lines by using morphological operations," 2015. [Online]. Available: https://docs.opencv.org/4.x/dd/dd7/tutorial_morph_lines_detection.html

[7] H. M. Bui *et al.*, "Using grayscale images for object recognition with convolutional-recursive neural network," in *2016 IEEE Sixth International Conference on Communications and Electronics (ICCE)*. IEEE, 2016, pp. 321–325.

[8] C. Goyal, "Multiclass classification using svm," *Analytics Vidhya*, 18.05.2021. [Online]. Available: https://www.analyticsvidhya.com/blog/2021/05/multiclass-classification-using-svm/

[9] Schonlau *et al.*, "The random forest algorithm for statistical learning," *The Stata Journal: Promoting communications on statistics and Stata*, vol. 20, no. 1, pp. 3–29, 2020.

[10] F. Pedregosa *et al.*, "Scikit-learn: Machine learning in Python," *Journal of Machine Learning Research*, vol. 12, pp. 2825–2830, 2011.

Rule-based explanations of CNN classifiers using regional features

William Philipp [1], Raúl Benitez [2]

[1] Medical Informatics, Universität zu Lübeck, william.philipp@student.uni-luebeck.de

[2] Biomedical Engineering Research Center, Universitat Politèctica de Catalunya, raul.benitez@upc.edu

Abstract

What Deep Learning networks gain in performance over traditional machine learning methods, they typically lack in explainability. In order to tackle this issue, several methods have been devised over the years, particularly in the realm of image-related tasks, such as image classification or object segmentation [1–3]. These methods typically yield a visual explanation of a classification problem in form of a heatmap, localising the most relevant regions for the classifier. However, such explanations remain purely visual and unrelated to the features relevant to an expert. We propose a novel Convolutional Neural Network (CNN) explainability method that identifies the most relevant image regions and generates a decision tree based on meaningful regional features to provide a rule-based explanation of the classification model. We first test the method on a synthetic dataset and then apply it to an image classification dataset of cell images.

1 Introduction

1.1 Motivation

The term 'black box' has long been in use to describe the nature of convolutional neural networks. Due to their internal structure, neither the designer, nor the end-user of the network are provided with a human-readable explanation of how the network's output is generated. Still, convolutional neural networks continue to be the architecture of choice for most tasks, mostly attributed to their performance advantage over other architectures. The learned deep features automatically extracted in their convolutional layers are both the reason for their incredible performance and their poor interpretability. It has become clear that ways to explore and explain these networks are needed for various reasons. One clear reason is that in many countries, regulations mandate that machine learning algorithms used in crucial sectors such as healthcare be explainable [4]. As such, the performance advantage of neural networks cannot be fully exploited yet, as many applications still rely on traditional algorithms for their intuitiveness and explainability. Many advances have been made in this research field in recent years, particularly when it comes to visual explanations of image classifications. Some examples include gradient-based methods such as Gradient-weighted Class Activation Mapping (GradCAM) [1], saliency maps [2] and methods based on perturbation of image regions [3].

1.2 Approach

Our approach aims to generate a decision tree based on regional features extracted from segmented regions of the image. We build upon the visual explanations provided by heatmaps which we acquire using GradCAM [1]. GradCAM works by taking the gradients of the output of a CNN with respect to the feature maps of a specific layer and weighting them by the importance of each feature map to the final prediction. The resulting heatmap highlights the regions of the image that the CNN considers most important for making the prediction. This is done by computing a score for each region based on the heatmaps and using this score as the regression target. In the end, the approach yields a decision tree that explains the relevance of each image region to the classification through that region's characteristics. The approach is based on two constraints:

- The algorithm used for generating the heatmaps correctly localises important regions of the image.

- The classification can be explained in terms of interpretable regional features, i.e. the classification is clearly dependent on distinct regions of the image.

The approach can be characterised as post-hoc (i.e. it is applied to the model *after* training) and as a variation of a global surrogate model. Surrogate models, one of the most common being Local interpretable model-agnostic explanations (LIME) [5], work by using a second, explainable model (e.g. a decision tree or a linear model) to explain the 'black box' model. In standard global surrogate approaches, one would train the explainable model by feeding it the original dataset and the predictions acquired through the 'black box' model as the class label. Our approach differs from the standard procedure in the way that we only indirectly use the model's prediction in order to obtain heatmaps, which are then used to assign importance scores to every region of the image. This allows us to exploit features of distinct regions of the image in order to provide an explanation of the classification process based on these features. In contrast, standard global surrogate models only provide explanations based on features extracted on a global scale.

2 Material and Methods

2.1 Dataset

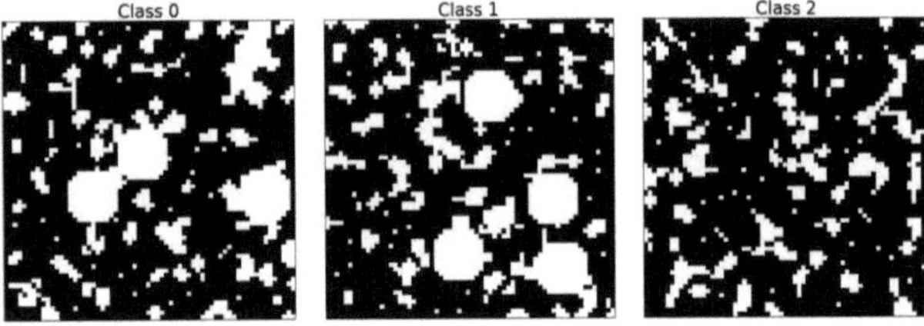

Figure 1: One example of each of the three class labels in the synthetic dataset. The images are binary and of size 64×64.

In order to quantitatively validate our method, we have created a synthetic dataset that automatically generates binary 64×64 images with blob-like structures of different types. It is based on the *binary_blobs* method of the skikit-image Python library [6]. It consists of three classes, as shown in Fig. 1. Class 2 consists of only small blobs, small in this case meaning that the average blob takes up approximately 0.36% of the image, with all blobs in total taking up about 20% of the image. Class 1 adds exactly four large circular blobs with a radius of 5 pixels. Class 0 has exactly three large circular blobs with the same radius as the circular blobs in Class 1 and exactly one large elliptical blob with a major axis length of 13 pixels and a minor axis length of 3 pixels. Additionally, the ellipse is rotated randomly. As both Class 1 and Class 0 use an image of Class 2 as a base and then add the larger blobs on top of that image, the larger blobs overlap and combine with some smaller blobs and thus contain a certain amount of variance. The dataset contains 6000 images balanced among the classes. It is built in this way with three primary goals in mind:

- Clearly distinct classes based on geometrical features, e.g. area, axis length.

- Binary representation to make region segmentation trivial.

- Non-trivial, but sufficiently easy classification problem for quick adaptations and to be able to validate the explainability in terms of relevant regions.

2.2 Methodology

The full pipeline of the method is illustrated in Fig. 2. The key and novel step in the pipeline is the generation of an

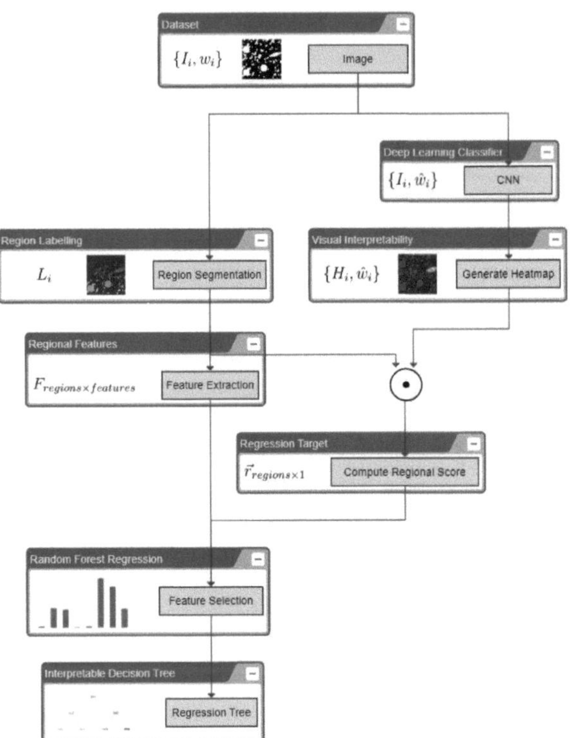

Figure 2: Diagram representing the complete workflow of the approach.

interpretability score for each region and the subsequent regression analysis using regression trees. Let a sample of the dataset be defined as a tuple $\{I_i, w_i\}$ of an image I_i and its corresponding class label w_i. Let f be a classifier, such that $f(I_i) = \hat{w}_i$, where $\hat{w}_i$ is the predicted class label for the image I_i. In our experiments, the CNN model uses three convolutional layers with kernel size 3×3, ReLu as non-linear activation and zero-padding, followed each by a batch normalisation layer and 2×2 max-pooling. The last convolutional block is fed into a fully-connected layer with Softmax activation for classification. After training for 40 epochs, the classifier performs at 99% accuracy on the test set during inference. After the network has been trained, heatmaps H_i are generated for each image of a particular class in the test set. The heatmap is a visual interpretation of what the CNN is using to classify the image. Our implementation uses the GradCAM algorithm [1] for this step. The chosen algorithm needs to be able to localise the important region properly in order for the method to work. As such, other algorithms such as saliency maps [2], GradCAM++ [7] or similar methods might be used as well, as long as they fulfil this criterion. During our testing, we found the chosen padding method to be particularly important for the localisation. Next, the regions of the image are labelled to generate a labelled image L_i. In the case of the synthetic dataset, the segmentation step is straightforward. We then assign a score to each region in L_i by computing the mean heatmap intensity in the region. This is done by taking the Hadamard product $R_i = L_i \odot H_i$. The regional score vector $\vec{r}_{regions \times 1}$

is obtained by pooling every region of R_i. Each entry of the vector contains the mean heatmap intensity of the corresponding region. Features for every region are then extracted from L_i to generate a feature matrix $F_{\text{regions}\times\text{features}}$. In the case of our dataset, those features are geometric features acquired through the *regionsprops_table* method of Scikit-image [6]. We extract area, eccentricity, equivalent diameter area, bounding box area, major axis length, minor axis length, extent and solidity as features. Based on these features and $\vec{r}$ as the regression target, we fit a regression using a Random Forest regressor. The amount of data points in the regression corresponds to the total amount of blobs in all test images, which in our case is approximately 68000. In order to measure the importance of every feature, we use permutation feature importance for model inspection. This technique estimates the importance of each feature by measuring the impact of shuffling a single feature value on the accuracy of the model [8]. Based on the results of the feature selection we train a decision tree regressor using only the most relevant features acquired in the previous step. By constraining the maximum depth of the decision tree, we obtain a condensed representation of the decision process and therefore a simplified explanation of the CNN classifier in terms of regional features.

3 Results and Discussion

3.1 Synthetic dataset

Fig. 3 shows the results of the permutation feature importance for the synthetic dataset. It has identified the major and minor axis length of the blobs as the most relevant distinctive features. Looking at Fig. 4, the regression reaches the highest score by first looking at a major axis length higher than a certain value, and then a minor axis length lower than a certain value. This makes sense as a large major axis length corresponds to a large blob, which distinguishes classes 0 and 1 from class 2. The comparatively small minor axis length leads to elongated blobs, the distinctive feature between classes 0 and 1. In summary, this provides a rule-based explanation of the deep classifier. For quantitative evaluation we compute the coefficient of determination $R^2 = 1 - \frac{u}{v}$, where u is the sum of residual squares and v is the total sum of squares. On the test set, the random forest regressor yields an R^2 of 0.63. This suggests a sufficiently strong correlation between the regression and the CNN classifier.

3.2 Cell images dataset

We applied the same approach to a second, realistic dataset of cell images from the National Library of Medicine of the United States of America [9]. The two datasets are similar in the sense that in both cases, the classes are clearly distinguishable by certain regions of the image present in one class, but not in the other. The cell dataset increases the complexity of the problem formulation by the image being in RGB colour space instead of binary. Fig. 5 shows a

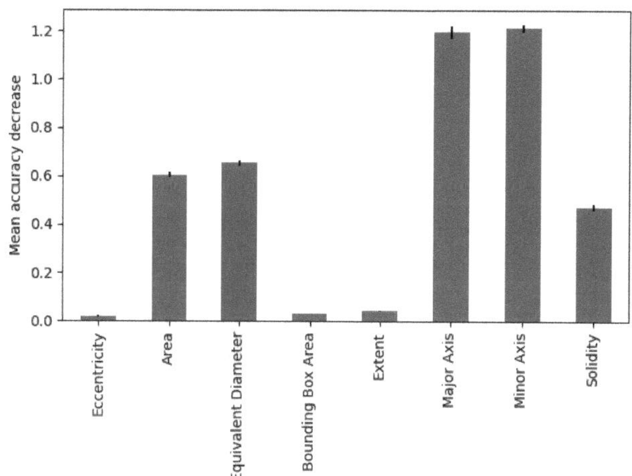

Figure 3: Feature Importance for the synthetic dataset.

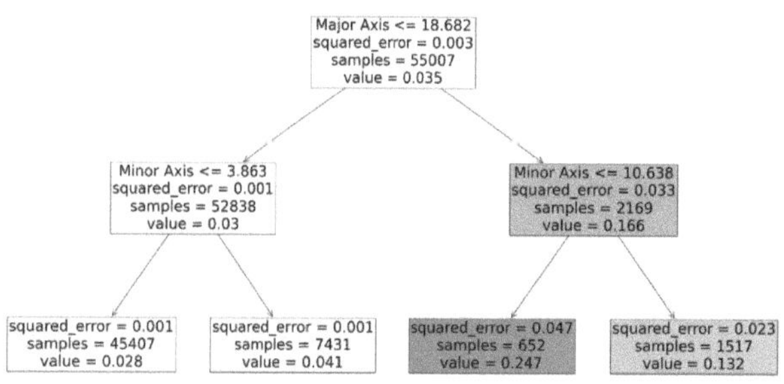

Figure 4: Decision tree for the synthetic dataset using the features determined in Fig. 3.

sample of this dataset. The cells are clearly distinguished by the small, darker spots in the parasitized cells. Inspecting the RGB colour space of the image, the darker shade corresponds to a lower amount of green in the region. The geometrical features used for the Random Forest feature importance model are identical to the ones used for the other dataset. The decision to use exactly the same geometric features has been taken to demonstrate the robustness of the method and to reduce human bias in the pre-selection of features. Additionally, mean values for each of the colour channels are computed for every region, yielding three additional features: Green value, red value and blue value. Gaussian Mixture Models are used to roughly segment the regions in the labelled image. The permutation feature importance identifies major axis length and green value as the most important features. A decision tree based on these features, as shown in Fig. 6 attributes the highest score to regions with a low major axis length, i.e. small regions, and with a small green value in the colour space. It yields an R^2 value of 0.75.

4 Conclusion

The results indicate that for its intended use-case, the method is able to provide a concise and clear explanation

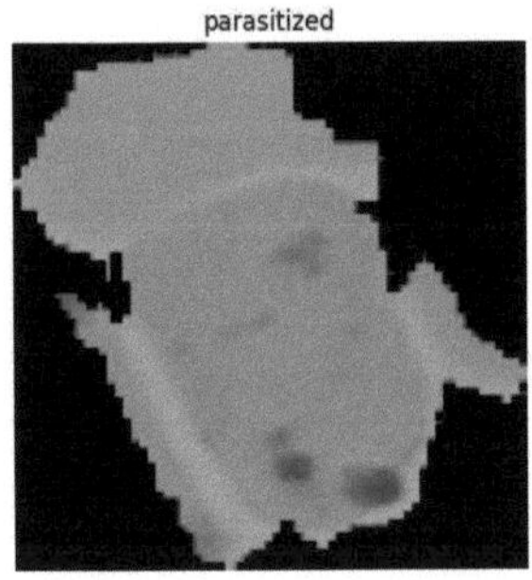
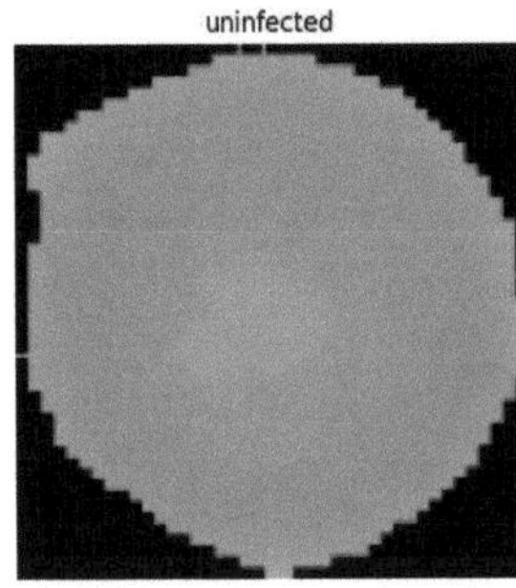

Figure 5: Sample of two cells from the cell dataset, one belonging to each class. The cell on the left has been infected by the parasite *Plasmodium falciparum*, which causes Malaria in humans. The cell on the right is an uninfected, healthy blood cell.

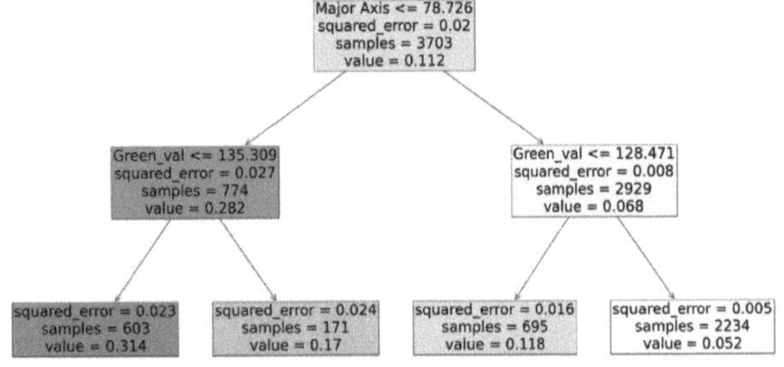

Figure 6: Decision tree for the cell dataset.

of the classification result in terms of regional features. It is important to state that these features likely do not correspond exactly to the ones present in the CNN. However, the fact that the feature importance model identifies features that a human would intuitively use to classify the images suggests a strong correlation between the processes. In conjunction with a visual explainability method, our method is able to obtain two explanations which together make for a simple and intuitive representation. The method's straightforward implementation makes it a useful tool to try on any dataset to identify patterns and regional features. However, the constraints on the problem statement do not make it an all-purpose method and its usefulness has to be evaluated on a case by case basis. The need for a segmentation of the image regions makes it difficult to use for complex problems, although our second example shows that results can be achieved even with a crude segmentation. Future work, focusing on testing the method on more varied and complex datasets in addition to establishing more sophisticated evaluation metrics has to be conducted to further evaluate and ascertain its scope.

Acknowledgement

The work has been carried out at the Biomedical Engineering Research Center, Universitat Politècnica de Catalunya and was supervised by Prof. Dr. Mattias Heinrich, Institute of Medical Informatics, Universität zu Lübeck. It was supported by the research grant from the Spanish Ministry of Science Innovation and Universities 00_PID2020-116927RB–C22.

Author's Statement

Conflict of interest: Authors state no conflict of interest.

5   References

[1] R. R. Selvaraju, M. Cogswell, A. Das, R. Vedantam, D. Parikh, and D. Batra, "Grad-cam: Visual explanations from deep networks via gradient-based localization," in *2017 IEEE International Conference on Computer Vision (ICCV)*, 2017, pp. 618–626.

[2] K. Simonyan, A. Vedaldi, and A. Zisserman, "Deep inside convolutional networks: Visualising image classification models and saliency maps," 2013. [Online]. Available: https://arxiv.org/abs/1312.6034

[3] R. C. Fong and A. Vedaldi, "Interpretable explanations of black boxes by meaningful perturbation," in *2017 IEEE International Conference on Computer Vision (ICCV)*. IEEE, oct 2017. [Online]. Available: https://doi.org/10.1109%2Ficcv.2017.371

[4] D. V. Carvalho, E. M. Pereira, and J. S. Cardoso, "Machine learning interpretability: A survey on methods and metrics," *Electronics*, vol. 8, no. 8, p. 832, jul 2019.

[5] M. T. Ribeiro, S. Singh, and C. Guestrin, ""why should I trust you?": Explaining the predictions of any classifier," *CoRR*, vol. abs/1602.04938, 2016. [Online]. Available: http://arxiv.org/abs/1602.04938

[6] S. Van der Walt, J. L. Schönberger, J. Nunez-Iglesias, F. Boulogne, J. D. Warner, N. Yager, E. Gouillart, and T. Yu, "scikit-image: image processing in python," *PeerJ*, vol. 2, p. e453, 2014.

[7] A. Chattopadhay, A. Sarkar, P. Howlader, and V. N. Balasubramanian, "Grad-cam++: Improved visual explanations for deep convolutional networks," in *2018 IEEE Winter Conference on Applications of Computer Vision (WACV)*. IEEE, mar 2018. [Online]. Available: https://doi.org/10.1109%2Fwacv.2018.00097

[8] L. Breiman, "Random forests," *Machine Learning*, vol. 45, no. 1, pp. 5–32, 2001. [Online]. Available: http://dx.doi.org/10.1023/A%3A1010933404324

[9] S. Rajaraman, S. Jaeger, and S. K. Antani, "Performance evaluation of deep neural ensembles toward malaria parasite detection in thin-blood smear images," *PeerJ*, vol. 7, p. e6977, may 2019.

A Global Regulatory Landscape for AI-based Medical Devices – How to Convey and Address the Emerging Regulatory Landscape for AI Technology in Healthcare –

Merle Streppel [1], Lilly Omland [2], Maria Henke [3]

[1] Medical Engineering Science, Universität zu Lübeck, merle.streppel@student.uni-luebeck.de
[2] Olympus Surgical Technologies Europe, Olympus Winter Ibe GmbH, lilly.omland@olympus.com
[3] Institute of Robotics and Autonomous Systems, Universität zu Lübeck, henke@rob.uni-luebeck.de

Abstract

Medical devices based on artificial intelligence (AI) technology are developed at a rapid pace. AI-based medical devices still present new regulatory territory. This paper presents the realization of a global regulatory landscape for AI-based medical devices. The development of the global regulatory landscape included a literature research and exchange with experts. The focus is laid on the US and EU to address two different types of regulatory approaches, and the aspect of medical device classification. The developed global regulatory landscape addresses and conveys the current developments of regulatory approaches for AI-based medical devices. Further, the results showed the importance of a tailored regulatory approach addressing the specific risks, challenges and opportunities of such devices, while aligning with already existing medical device regulations.

1 Introduction

Artificial intelligence (AI) is a fast-advancing area which poses great possibilities in various medical fields, such as radiology, gastroenterology, and cardiology [1]. Whether in prevention, early diagnosis of disease, supporting treatment, or aftercare, AI-based medical device software has the potential to contribute in establishing better personalized medical care. In the healthcare sector, including medical technology, especially medical device software based on AI technology is developed at a rapid pace across the world. In parallel to the evolving technological advancements of AI-based medical devices, the regulation of such must be developed accordingly.

Medical devices are highly regulated. Depending on a medical device's Intended Use, the medical device class based on risk is determined, and with that, the level of control to ensure reasonable safety and effectiveness of the medical device. Currently, there are no enforced medical device regulations specifically regulating AI-based medical devices. Such medical devices must comply with existing regulatory requirements [2]. However, existing legally enforced medical device regulations are not explicitly designed to address the regulatory challenges of AI technology. Especially continuously learning AI-based medical devices, learning from real-world data, still represent a new regulatory territory. AI algorithms currently are locked to allow the approval and clearance of these type of medical applications.

How regulatory bodies approach the regulation of AI-based medical devices while considering the already existing regulations, standards, and guidance documents, is crucial in shaping the future of AI technology in the healthcare sector including medical technology. The results presented in this paper were obtained as part of a developed extensive global regulatory roundup for AI-based medical devices[1]. The aim is to convey and address regulatory aspects for AI-based medical devices. With focus on the EU and US, the following main aspects are considered: Regulatory approaches for AI-based medical devices, and challenges of AI-based medical device software.

2 Material and Methods

It was decided to create the planned global regulatory landscape in layout of a timeline for January 2019 to July 2022. This regulatory landscape should comprise AI national strategies, available guidance documents, regulations for AI medical devices, and emerging harmonization approaches for regulating AI-based medical devices. The first step in the development of such a landscape included a literature research to determine the applicable resources. The second step comprised the final development and creation of the global regulatory landscape.

---

[1]The research for this paper was conducted during an internship at Olympus Surgical Technologies Europe headquarter in Hamburg. The company specializes in diagnosis, therapy, reprocessing and systems integration, and offers a full range of endoscopic applications.

Table 1: Table presenting a comprehensive overview of the review criteria used during the literature research.

Platform	Review Criteria

Tarius	• **Document type (based on available document types on Tarius) :**
	  - Tarius document type "Guidelines/Guidances", "IMDRF document"
	  (Note: The results were filtered for International Medical Device Regulator Forum (IMDRF) documents to identify harmonization approaches by the IMDRF)
	• **Results regarding either of the following categories:**
	  - AI/ML-based medical devices; AI/ML-based software that is a medical devices; classification of AI/ML-based software that is a medical device
	• **Selected timeframe:** 2019 to July 2022

OECD Website on AI	• **Results regarding either of the following categories:** - Healthcare, Medical Technology • **Selected timeframe:** 2019 to July 2022

OECD.AI Policy Observatory	• **Identification of countries (1ˢᵗ step):**
	  - Countries with a National AI Strategy and/or AI/ML-related regulations and/or guidance documents applicable to the healthcare sector including medical technology
	• **Results in the selected timeframe of 2019 to July 2022 AND under either of the following categories (2ⁿᵈ step):**
	  - Healthcare, medical technology, guidance documents related including medical technology, national strategy

2.1 Determination of Regulations and Approaches for AI-based Medical Devices

The literature research was based on two main parts: Utilizing the web platform Tarius, and a literature research based on resources of the Organisation for Economic Co-operation and Development (OECD), including the OECD website and the OECD.AI Policy Observatory tool. The obtained results were reviewed and filtered based on different aspects, such as document type, relevance to the healthcare sector, including medical technology, and considering a set timeframe (2019 to July 2022). A comprehensive overview of the review criteria can be found in Table 1.

The first part utilized the Tarius platform to which Olympus subscribed. Tarius provides customized web platforms designed to provide access to global regulatory information, such as laws, regulations, standards, and guidance documents, for companies in the healthcare industry that pay a subscription fee for Tarius. Tarius currently monitors more than 250 websites, official journals, and hundreds of governments [3]. Using this web platform ensures access to the most up-to-date reference documents from national authorities and international organizations. The results are reviewed under the criterion of whether it targets especially Artificial Intelligence (AI)/Machine Learning (ML)-based medical devices and AI/ML in the healthcare sector (see Table 1). In addition, those results targeting the classification of AI/ML-based medical devices and global harmonization approaches for regulating AI-based medical devices have been identified.

The OECD addresses policies on the adoption of AI in different fields of applications and discusses recommendations and best practices. The utilized OECD resources included the OECD's website on AI, which provides resources and publications related to AI, and the OECD web tool OECD.AI Policy Observatory. The OECD.AI Policy Observatory provides real-time information on AI policies across the world. In addition, the tool includes a country dashboard providing an interactive map of the world, allowing one to browse through national AI policies and AI strategies in 62 countries and territories.

Additionally, the obtained results were further discussed in an internal and external setting. Internal discussion refers to an exchange with experts in the Regulatory Affairs (RA) department, who know the country-specific regulations and requirements for medical devices. External discussion refers to the exchange with other parties in scope of the presentation "Global Regulatory Roundup Using AI in Medical Devices" as part of the symposium "11th Northern German Dialouge - MedTech for Future (2022)" [5].

2.2 Global Regulatory Landscape

During the global regulatory landscape development, the acquired results were mapped and assessed under several aspects: Vertical and horizontal regulatory approaches, regulatory classification, and approaches for global harmonization.

A horizontal approach means that the regulatory approach applies to several different sectors. In contrast, the vertical approach means that the regulatory approach only applies to the healthcare sector, including medical technology. To the authors' best knowledge, a sufficient global regulatory landscape for AI-based medical devices, especially regarding horizontal and vertical approaches, currently does not exist. Therefore, this paper intends to highlight the aspect and implications of vertical versus horizontal regulatory approaches for regulating AI-based medical devices.

It was decided to develop the final global regulatory landscape in a timeline layout and highlight the regulatory information, such as vertical and horizontal approaches. The presentation of regulatory information and regulatory landscapes of regulations and standards in the layout of a timeline is a widely used practice in RA. Inspiration for the design and presentation of the regulatory landscape was especially drawn from the UK Medicines and Healthcare products Regulatory Agency's (MHRA) "Introductory guide to the MDR and IVDR" [4].

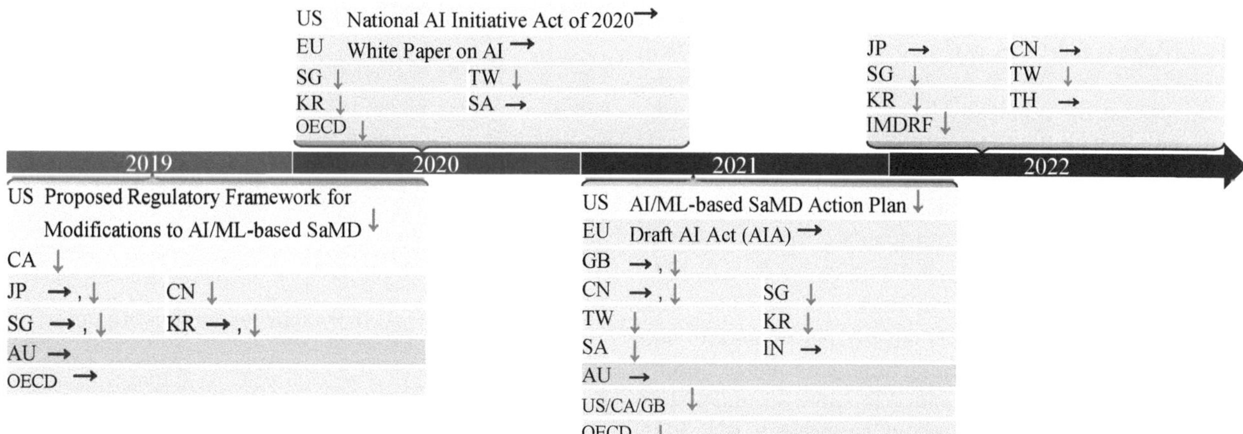

Figure 1: Summary of global regulatory landscape for AI-based medical devices (2019 to 2022). Only the results for the EU and the US are named. Color-coding for continents: Europe, North America, Asia, Australia, others. Arrows indicate whether a results is a horizontal (→) or vertical approach (↓). The number of arrows for a country equals the number of results for that country in that year.

3 Results and Discussion

This section first introduces the developed global regulatory landscape for AI-based medical devices. Then the main focus lays on the regulation of AI-based medical device in the EU and the US. In addition, a brief summary of the results obtained in the assessment of the regulatory landscape from a regulatory classification perspective is also provided.

The results are summarized and mapped in figure 1, presenting a global regulatory landscape for AI-based medical devices in layout of a timeline (2019 and July 2022). In total, the landscape comprises 39 results. Only the results for the EU and the US are explicitly named. The countries of origin are color-coded to highlight the different continents. Results that could not be assigned to a single continent are highlighted by a grey color. These comprise global efforts to harmonize the regulation of AI-based medical devices by the OECD, International Medical Device Regulator Forum (IMDRF), and one publication created within a collaboration of regulatory authorities of the US, Canada, and Great Britain. Besides showing the continent and country of origin, and year of publication, the landscape indicates whether the result is classified as a horizontal/vertical regulatory approach. A horizontal approach or vertical approach is indicated by a horizontal/vertical arrow.

The regulatory landscape does not claim to be exhaustive of global developments. Still, it clearly conveys the rapid ongoing regulatory activity. The regulatory landscape shows that many countries already developed national strategies and action plans in the last four years addressing the new opportunities and specific challenges of AI-based medical devices. Moreover, the landscape indicates the prominent role of the US and ASEAN countries such as China, Singapore, or Korea, in shaping the regulatory landscape for AI medical devices.

Considering the regulatory approach of the EU and the US, the aspect of vertical vs. horizontal approach and the importance of a tailored approach for medical devices is highlighted in the following parts.

The EU Commission published a White Paper on AI, promoting the use of AI while addressing the risks associated with this technology. In April 2021, the EU Commission published a proposal for a risk-based approach with the draft EU Artificial Intelligence Act (AIA), aiming to establish harmonized rules for AI through a legal framework [6]. The draft EU AIA implements horizontal requirements for so-called AI systems. Since the act was not specifically created for medical devices, the scope of the draft act is extremely broad. Pursuant to Article 3 (1) of the current draft EU AIA most AI-based medical devices will fall under the definition of an AI system and therefore under the draft EU AIA. The draft EU AIA is highly discussed and criticized. For instance, most AI-based medical device software would classify as "high-risk" AI systems, pursuant to Article 6 of the draft EU AIA. The proposed risk-based classification system of the draft EU AIA does not allow any further risk stratification for high-risk AI-systems, unlike the EU Medical Device Regulation (MDR). Compared to the EU MDR, the draft EU AIA classification system does not ensure a reasonable risk-benefit ratio for medical devices. Altogether, the current draft EU AIA would cause inconsistent obligations for manufacturers and over-regulation, limiting AI (medical-) technologies to access the EU market. Associations, such as MedTech Europe, explicitly pointed out to the EU Commission that overlaps and duplication of regulatory requirements with the EU MDR should be avoided [7]. During the last year the EU AIA was further amended. In December 2022, a compromised version of the EU AIA was approved, which will next have to be adopted by the EU Parliament [8]. Compared to the EU, the US follows a purely vertical approach. Their proposed framework for AI/ML-based Software as a Medical Device (SaMD) [9] and action plan [10] present the US FDA as a leading regulator. The US FDA addresses new opportunities of AI medical devices, such as adaptive AI algorithms, and their specific challenges, at the regulatory level, in contrast to the EU. In its action plan, the FDA lists specific actions and goals it intends to follow to ensure reasonable safe and effective AI/ML-based SaMD, especially with focus on adaptive technology and increasing transparency for the user of such devices. With the proposed framework the US FDA intends, e.g., to allow SaMD to learn and adapt over time under certain conditions while already placed on the market. One proposed tool is a Pre-determined Change Control (PCC) protocol, which is intended to allow documentation of changes to the SaMD without requiring a new FDA submission as long as those changes remain within the PCC protocol's boundaries. So far, the FDA has not yet established clear guidance on how to submit such a PCC protocol. However, the proposed framework and action plan can be seen as a starting point in efficiently regulating AI-based medical devices and promoting advancements in AI technology.

In the assessment of the regulatory landscape from a regulatory classification perspective, it was found that several countries, including the US [9], currently intend to classify AI-based software that is SaMD under the country's respective principles for the classification of such software. Moreover, it was determined that whether and how the nature of the used AI algorithm might impact the classification has not yet been clearly addressed. Altogether, approaches to appropriately classify such medical devices, seem to be in the early stages of development.

4　Conclusion

The assessment of the EU regulatory approach highlights that over-regulation and duplication of regulatory requirements is an important aspect in regulating AI-based medical devices. The US approach shows the importance of a regulatory approach tailored to the specific opportunities and challenges of AI-based medical devices while also aligning with already existing high-level medical device regulations. In addition, the mitigation of the (AI specific) risks to patients while maintaining a suitable risk-benefit ratio, was identified as a crucial factor for classification of AI-based medical devices. In conclusion, how the regulatory landscape for AI-based medical devices continues to evolve, and how manufacturers manage to adapt to the developments, is important for the future of AI technology in medical devices.
It is planned to update the regulatory landscape on a regular basis to provide a basis for regulatory assessments and development of regulatory strategies of AI-based medical devices. Moreover, the presented regulatory landscape was used for developing a first draft for a tool providing guidance on the classification of AI-based medical device software in the EU and the US, which currently is under further refinement.

Acknowledgement

The work has been carried out at Olympus Surgical Technologies Europe, Hamburg, and was supervised by the Institute for Robotics and Cognitive Systems, Universität zu Lübeck.

Author's Statement

Conflict of interest: Authors state no conflict of interest.

5　References

[1] O. Mehta, et al., *Clinical Applications*. Artificial Intelligence in Medicine, Springer, pp. 84-92, 2022.

[2] Johner Institut, *Regulatory Requirements for Medical Devices with ML*. Available: https://www.johner-institute.com/articles/regulatory-affairs/and-more/regulatory-requirements-for-medical-devices-with-machine-learning/ [last accessed on 2022-12-15].

[3] Tarius, *Countries and Regions covered by Tarius*. Available on: https://http://www.tarius.com [last accessed on 2022-12-18]

[4] MHRA, *Introductory Guide to new medical device regulations launched*. Available on: https://www.gov.uk/government/news/introductory-guide-to-new-medical-device-regulations-launched [last accessed on 2022-12-19].

[5] NSF Prosystem GmbH, *The 11TH Northern German Dialogue – MedTech for Future - Agenda*. Available on: https://www.nsf-prosystem.com/veranstaltungen [last accessed on 2022-12-26].

[6] EU Commission, *Proposal for Regulation of the European Parliament and of the Council Laying Down Harmonised Rules on AI (AIA) and Amending Certain Union Legislative Acts*, Brussels, 2021.

[7] MedTechEurope, *The AIA needs to go hand in hand with sectoral legislations*. Available on: https://www.medtecheurope.org/news-and-events/press-releases/ [last accessed on 2022-10-16]

[8] Holistic AI, *EU AIA: Summary of Updates on Final Compromise Text* Available on: https://www.holisticai.com/blog/eu-ai-act-final-compromise-text [last accessed on 2023-01-02]

[9] U.S. FDA, *Proposed Framework for Modifications of AI/ML-based SaMD*. Available on: https://www.fda.gov/medical-devices/software-medical-device-samd [last accessed on 2022-12-28].

[10] U.S. FDA, *AI/ML-based SaMD Action Plan*. Available on: https://www.fda.gov/medical-devices/software-medical-device-samd [last accessed on 2022-12-28].

Comparative Study Of Different Explainable Artificial Intelligence Algorithms For A Customer Specific Natural Language Processing Model

Julia Richter [1]

[1] Robotics and Autonomous Systems, Universität zu Lübeck, julia.richter@student.uni-luebeck.de

Abstract

It is well-known that artificial intelligence (AI) models are frequently used to solve tasks in natural language processing (NLP). However, improving AI-models is complicated due to the missing insight into the input-output-behavior which limits interpretation of underlying correlations. To solve this problem explainable artificial intelligence (XAI) is frequently used. The goal of this study is to find the best solution for instant user feedback and long-term AI-model improvement. The three XAI algorithms evaluated are SHapley Additive exPlanations (SHAP), Integrated Gradients and local interpretable model-agnostic explanations (LIME). The results showed that SHAP and Integrated Gradients deliver similar quality of explanation, but SHAP was easier to implement. Integrated Gradients was found to be three times faster than SHAP and more suitable for real-time systems, making it a good choice for certain use cases. The computation time of an explanation with LIME was too large to generate meaningful quality statements.

1 Introduction

Artificial intelligence (AI) is a frequently used approach for classification and forecasting of natural language due to the complexity of tasks in natural language processing (NLP) [1]. The advantages of machine learning in NLP are the robustness against unfamiliar input like misspelling or unseen structure, and the scalability of fine-tuning, by just using more data for training. Additionally, during the learning process, AI focuses automatically on the most frequent cases, which represents a significant advantage of this approach.

One of the challenging aspects of AI is that machine learning models remain mostly black boxes [2]. Therefore it is hard to improve those models due to the unknown specific input-output-behavior. Thus the current way to improve existing models is simply to add more training data, which is often inefficient and expensive. Additionally, the trustworthiness of a model can only be evaluated with a lot of test data, and is therefore dependent on the quality of the data set. Biases that exist in both the test and training data sets will not be revealed [3]. Furthermore, unexpected and deviating outputs remain inexplicable [4].

As AI systems increasingly play a role in our daily work, it becomes more important to comprehend the workings of the models in order to verify the trustworthiness, quality, and accountability of outputs, as well as to find more efficient methods for improving AI-models. Explainable artificial intelligence (XAI) is a fast-growing field with various types of approaches and algorithms [3]. All XAI approaches aim to improve the understanding of the rules, impacts and general interpretation of the correlations in the input-output-behavior.

In detail, the explanation's benefits are [5]:

Accountability - XAI helps to make AI systems more accountable by providing a clear understanding of how they arrive at a particular decision or outcome.

Improvement - XAI supports improving the model performance by showing at which point errors occur.

Fairness - XAI helps to ensure that AI systems are fair and unbiased by providing explanations for their decisions, which can help to identify and mitigate any potential biases.

Trust - User of AI systems need to understand how AI systems work in order to trust them. XAI helps to build trust by providing transparent and understandable explanations for AI decisions.

XAI approaches can be categorized in several ways [3]. First there is a difference between model-agnostic and model-specific XAI. Model-agnostic XAI focuses on providing explanations that are independent of the specific machine learning model, while model-specific XAI focuses on model specific explanations. Second there is a difference between post-hoc and intrinsic XAI. Post-hoc XAI provides explanations after a machine learning model has been trained, and intrinsic XAI aims to build explain-ability directly into the model [5].

The objective of this study is to determine the best XAI approach for providing instant user feedback and facilitating long-term improvement of a customer specific AI model. Because this AI model is a NLP model and in the domain of NLP models, mostly model-agnostic post-hoc XAI algorithms are used [5], this study focuses on just these.

2 Material and Methods

In this section the given material and used approaches are discussed to the determine the best XAI approach for the task at hand. First the specific requirements are stated. Second the three XAI algorithms analyzed are introduced and third, the metrics used to compare the algorithms are declared.

2.1 Customer specific requirements

In this study a completely trained NLP model is used. The NLP model is a fine-tuned model of the german-bert-uncased model from the Huggingface-library [6]. The task of the model is to classify, whether a given phrase confirms the customer specific privacy-policy (output-class 'ok') or fails the customer specific requirements (output-class 'not ok'). The model is later used in the relation centers. In these centers agent interact with customers and take notes on their interactions. The model is used to prevent agents from saving notes with sensitive customer information.

There are two use cases the XAI should performe well in. In one use case the agents should get a feedback, why their phrases do not confirm the privacy policy. The requirements for the XAI include a fast computation of an explanation due to the real-time demands of this use case. Additionally, the XAI should have an intuitive and sensible explanation. Moreover, the hardware-requirements contain a setup on a standard computer from the relation center. The other use case is in the development of the model. At the moment, the model has a high false-positive and false-negative-rate. To improve these high rates, it is necessary for the developers to have a precise understanding of where they need to improve the model. For this use case it is important, that the XAI is easy to set up as well as provide a detailed and valid explanation.

2.2 XAI algorithms

The three most common used state-of-the-art algorithms [3] will be evaluated.

One of the most well-known model-agnostic XAI approaches is SHapley Additive exPlanations (SHAP) [4], which aims to explain the output of a machine learning model by identifying the relevance of each input variable to the final prediction. It does this by calculating the Shapley values for each input variable, which represent the contribution of that variable to the model's output.

There is a further development of SHAP, which is called GrammarSHAP [1], which focus on NLP tasks. Due to missing code-examples, GrammarSHAP could not be implemented and therefore not compared to the other algorithms.

Another well-known model-agnostic XAI approach is local interpretable model-agnostic explanations (LIME) [2].

LIME builds for each explanation a local regression model, by varying the input. A regression model is an intrinsic XAI approach by definition. Therefore, using this approach the regression model can easily be explained.

Another approach is Integrated Gradients [7]. It is a mathematical way of understanding the importance of a feature to the result. Integrated gradients are defined as the path integral of the gradients along the straightline path from the given baseline to the input. To understand better, Integrated Gradients calculates the impact of each feature (in NLP tasks, these are tokens) on the model's output by comparing it to a baseline (in NLP tasks, this is often a null-embedding-vector). It does this by creating new inputs that are uniformly spaced apart from the original token and computing the gradients for each step. All these gradients are summed up for each token. In the end these summed up gradients represent the importance of the token for the decision.

2.3 Metrics for Comparison

Due to the requirements, discussed in section 2.1, the runtime, the quality of an explanation and the implementation of the approaches are at most importance.

Runtime

Initial attempts with the XAI have revealed that the time for an explanation is directly related to the length of the input phrase. Therefore, for each explanation, the computation time and the number of tokens from the input phrase are measured.

Quality

All XAI algorithms determine the importance of each token in numerical form. The numerical outputs produced by two different XAI algorithms for explaining the same phrase are too divergent to be compared. In order to make the algorithms comparable, it was necessary to convert the continuous output of the algorithms' importance into a binary output of either "important" or "not important". Therefore, only tokens with an importance greater than 0.1 and all neighbor-tokens with an importance greater than 0.05 where marked as important. For most phrases, 20% of the tokens are marked as important.

The comparison of the algorithms was done in two steps. First, the algorithms were compared in terms of the similarity of the explanations, and second, they were evaluated based on the quality of their intuitive and sensible explanations.

To determine if two algorithms provide a similar explanation for the same input, a threshold of 50% was set. If more than 50% of the same tokens are present in both explanations, the two explanations are considered similar.

Sample sentences that the model should classify as 'not okay', meaning they contain words that need to be modified to comply with the privacy policy, were chosen to evaluate the quality of the explanation. If more than 80% of the words, that have to be modified, are marked, the explanation gives the ability to modify. Therefore, the explanation is marked as 'good'.

2.4 Experiments

Two tests with different phrases where made. All phrases have the true label of 'not ok' and contain tokens that can be identified as important to remove. The first one with 80 phrases, the second one with 20 phrases. The tests differ in terms of the model version. The second test is conducted with a model that is in a later stage of the project. Computation time, number of tokens, similarity to other XAI algorithms' explanations and the ability to modify where tracked for every explanation.

3 Results and Discussion

In this section the results of the experiments are conducted and later discussed. The results are seperated into the runtime analysis, the quality analysis and the implementation analysis.

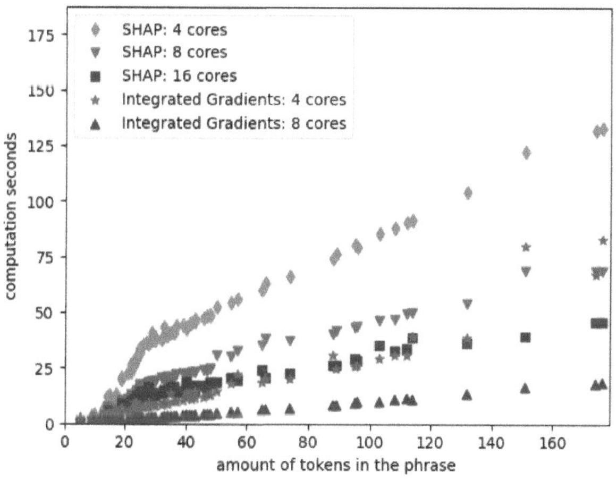

Figure 1: The two model-agnostic post-hoc XAI-algorithms SHAP and Integrated Gradients compared due to the runtime on different virtual machines.

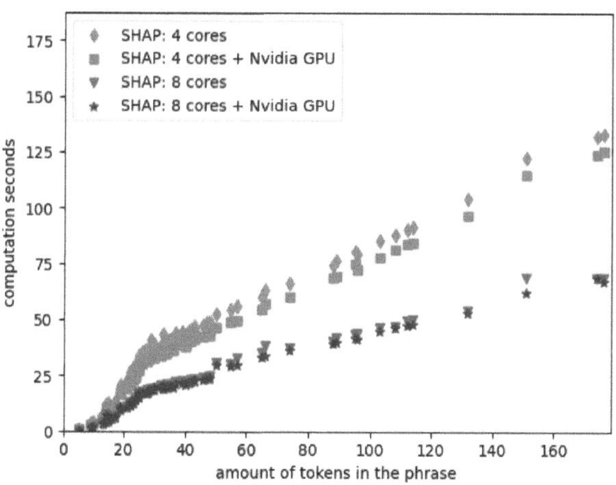

Figure 2: The model-agnostic post-hoc XAI-algorithm SHAP compared due to the runtime on different virtual machines with a GPU (NVIDIA® T4) and without.

3.1 Runtime analysis

Due to the runtime analysis there are three different main results found. The runtime was testet on the google cloud platform (GCP) with different virtual machines. From 15 GB RAM, an Intel® v4 over 30 GB RAM, an Intel® v8 to 60 GB RAM, an Intel® v16. The runtime was also tested with an additional GPU (NVIDIA® T4).

1. *Integrated Gradients is the fastest*: Integrated Gradients computes an explanation faster than SHAP, as can be seen in Fig. 1. SHAP needed even with the best hardware more time, than Integrated Gradients needed with the lowest. LIME takes more than seven minutes to explain one phrase. Further research on this algorithm was not pursued due to resource constraints.

2. *Linearity*: The runtime of both algorithms, SHAP and Integrated Gradients, for one explanation is linear for token-amount greater than 25. For Integrated Gradients it is linear over all number of tokens, for SHAP it is exponential before a length of 25 as is shown in Fig. 2.

3. *Computation with GPU*: There is no significant difference between the computation time with and without an GPU for SHAP as can be seen in Fig. 2.

3.2 Quality analysis

Due to the quality analysis there are two main results found.

1. *Similarity*: SHAP and Integrated Gradients were compared due to the similarity of the explanations. We run two tests, with a different set of phrases. In both tests, almost 60% of the explanations were similar, see table 1. The greatest disparities were observed when the model misclassified the phrase. In contrast, Integrated Gradients often identified tokens that would not have any impact on improving the phrase with regards to the privacy policy, which was determined to happen in 75% of the explanations. On the other hand, SHAP persistently highlighted the important tokens that required modification in order to confirm the privacy policy.

2. *Ability to modify*: In the first test both algorithms had around 80% good explanations, as can be seen in table 1, while Integrated Gradients was better than SHAP. In the second test it was the other way round, with the mean of 70%.

Table 1: Similarity and Ability to modify

compare attribute	Test 1	Test 2
Similar	57,5%	60,0%
Integrated Gradients good	86,8%	63,0%
SHAP good	73,7%	78,9%
not similar, but both good	15,7%	12,5%
not similar, and both bad	17,6%	25,0%

3.3 Implementation analysis

The library for SHAP is easy to understand and the methods can easily be evolved for own use-cases.

For Integrated Gradients it was necessary to write a wrapper-class. With this class it is possible to use every Huggingface-model and explain it.

Both algorithms - SHAP and Integrated Gradients - are able to implement on the customer's agents hardware. Both can be incorporated into the pipeline that the current model is operating within.

3.4 Discussion and Interpretation

Putting all results together, as can be seen in table 2, the XAI-algorithms have different advantages and disadvantages.

Table 2: Summed results of the study

Analysis	Integrated Gradients	SHAP
Runtime	4s	50s
Ability to modify	74,9%	76,3%

The XAI algorithm LIME is unsuitable for use in a work environment because it requires too much time to generate an explanation.

For the ongoing discussion, a closer examination of the pros and cons in the two use cases where the algorithm is intended to be used will be undertaken.

For the first use case, where the agents should receive intuitive explanations to modify their notes properly, it can be stated that there are high real-time requirements. Therefore, even Integrated Gradients almost needs to much time to compute the explanations. The lower quality of Integrated Gradients in the second test can be attributed to the higher rate of missclassification of the model in the second experiment. Because Integrated Gradients is therefore comparable to the explanations of SHAP as long as the model classifies properly, which could be an assumption when the model is used, the XAI-algorithm Integrated Gradients suited well for the requirements in the first use case.

For the second use case, the model improvement, it can be statet, that the runtime is less important than the quality of the explanation. Furthermore, the model missclassifies a lot, due to the need of improvement. In this specific case it is sensible to use SHAP, although it takes more time per explanation. It is advisable to consider both explanations, as this approach provides a comprehensive overview and can increase the accuracy of the modification process.

4 Conclusion

In this study, the XAI algorithms LIME, SHAP and Integrated Gradients are compared regarding runtime and quality of explanations. In general, it is recommended, that regarding the differences of explanations more than one XAI should be used. Especially when the goal is to improve the model properly. XAI improves the understanding of the input-output-behavior and leads to resource-saving trainings.

The XAI-algorithms SHAP and Integrated Gradients are comparable due to the explanation especially as long as the model classifies correctly. So that in real-time systems Integrated Gradients suit better, than SHAP.

Our research is limited to a small number of phrases tested manually in the quality analysis and limited due to the fact, that we only tested one model. In further researches other model should be tested.

Acknowledgement

The work has been carried out at Otto Group Solution Provider (OSP), Dresden and supervised by Prof. Dr.-Ing. Erhardt Barth, Institute for Neuro- and Bioinformatics, Universität zu Lübeck.

Author's Statement

Conflict of interest: Authors state no conflict of interest.

5 References

[1] E. Mosca, D. Defne, L. Mülln, F. Raffagnato, G. Groh, *GrammarSHAP: An Efficient Model-Agnostic and Structure-Aware NLP Explainer*. In: ACL Workshop on Learning with Natural Language Supervision, 2022.

[2] M. T. Ribeiro, S. Singh, and C. Guestrin. *Why should i trust you?" Explaining the predictions of any classifier*. Proceedings of the 22nd ACM SIGKDD international conference on knowledge discovery and data mining, pp. 1135-1144, 2016.

[3] D. Gunning, M. Stefik, J. Choi, T. Miller, S. Stumpf, and G. Z. Yang, *XAI—Explainable artificial intelligence*. Science robotics, vol. 3, no. 37, 2019.

[4] S. M. Lundberg, and S. Lee. *A unified approach to interpreting model predictions*. Advances in neural information processing systems, vol. 30, 2017.

[5] G. Vilone and L. Longo, *Classification of explainable artificial intelligence methods through their output formats*. In: Machine Learning and Knowledge Extraction, MDPI, vol. 3, no. 3, pp. 615-661, 2021.

[6] Hugging Face, *bert-base-german-uncased*. Available: https://huggingface.co/dbmdz/bert-base-german-uncased [last accessed on 2023-02-04]

[7] M. Sundararajan, A. Taly, and Q. Yan. *Axiomatic attribution for deep networks*. International conference on machine learning. PMLR, pp. 3319-3328, 2017.

Machine learning approaches on health insurance data to classify cases related to care grades: first pilot studies

Raphael Berehi Zadeh [1], Xinyu Huang [2], Marcin Grzegorzek [3], and Andreas Witolla [4]

[1] Medical Informatics, Universität zu Lübeck, raphael.berehizadeh@student.uni-luebeck.de
[2] Institute for Medical Informatics, Universität zu Lübeck, x.huang@uni-luebeck.de
[3] Institute for Medical Informatics, Universität zu Lübeck, marcin.grzegorzek@uni-luebeck.de
[4] IKK - Die Innovationskasse, public company, andreas.witolla@die-ik.de

Abstract

Machine learning (ML) techniques have the potential to support the statutory health insurances by their decision taking. This article describes the steps necessary for training and evaluating ML models in the context of a public health insurance. We use a gradient boosted tree as a feature selector and then a random decision forest to classify degrees of care. We show that by applying suitable ML algorithms, we can classify health insurance data even with a sparse data matrix. By applying a suitable feature selection algorithm, we are able to reduce training time and query time. Our results emphasize the potential for using ML techniques to support decision taking of the statutory health insurances.

1 Introduction

Statutory health insurance has been a part of the German social health system since the 19th century, and is the most important pillar of the system. Statutory insurance companies in Germany use a wide range of data to correctly collect health insurance contributions and provide care. As the population ages, health expenditure is expected to increase in the coming years [1]. Preventive measures can help the reduce the chance of acquiring a care grade. [2]. One potential solution is the use of machine learning algorithms to identify potential cases with with the need for long-term care [3]. To achieve this, the existing data must first be examined to detect suitable approaches, and then suitable features must be identified. In this article, we will determine if it is possible to use ML methods to distinguish between insured persons by their grade of care using health insurance data. Following the feature selection process, which identifies the dimensions that most effectively describe the classification problem and eliminates dimensions that are not descriptive, the classifier training evaluation begins. For this we will investigate different machine learning models, including Convolutional Neural Network (CNN), Multi Layer Perceptron (MLP), and Random Decision Forest (RDF) and then compare the feasibility in a health insurance context.

2 Material and Methods

In order to assess the feasibility of applying an ML approach to statutory health insurance data, the aim was to classify the insured into five levels of care [4] on the basis of appropriate characteristics. First, it was necessary to understand how the data is stored in the database and which data can be used for modelling the ML approach. The database consists of demographic data, cost data as well as disease data from the insured persons. It is clear that one approach could be to classify insured persons by their grade of illness. One table in the relational database stores care grades for persons in need of care, ranging from one to five, allowing the care grades to function as different classes. Care grades indicate the level of support a person in need of care requires based on different assessment dimensions. To receive a care grade, the person in need of care must submit an application to the health insurance. The medical service of the health insurance then assesses the person in need of care using the six dimensions mentioned below. The focus was set to model the five care grades with different feature using data from the database. Care grades are described in §14 SGB XI with six criteria dimensions: "mobility", "cognitive and communicative skills", "behavioural and psychological problem", "self-sufficiency", "ability to cope independently with demands caused by illness", and "shaping everyday life and social contacts".

2.1 Data acquisition

In order to define usable features the database was examined by the author and the results were then presented to the team for agreement. The data matrix used for classification consisted of 21,840 rows and 70 columns and included only insured persons who had a care grade and had submitted their application by 01.01.2022. To avoid a matrix with too many zero values, the insured persons had to have used a health care service in the year before the application.

2.1.1 Disease related data

The criterion of *mobility*, which indicates a person's ability to move around the living area independently, is influenced probably by the sum of injuries in the year before submitting the application. In order to realize this, outpatient ICD-10 codes were used. The injuries were mapped to the ICD-10 groups 'S00' to 'S99' to prevent the same injury from being counted more than once per day. It is known, that elderly and severe ill people have a tendency to fall. Another consequence of severely immobile persons is their susceptibility to decubitus ulcers [5], making this diagnosis also suitable for assessing *mobility*. For this purpose, the ICD-10 codes were checked to see whether any decubitus ulcers had been diagnosed until the year before the application. Some diseases can lead to limited self-care, so it was included whether the person in need of care has urinary incontinence. This feature was obtained in the same way as the pressure ulcer. The criteria for *cognitive and communicative abilities*, as well as *behavioural criteria*, were implemented using a variety of disease diagnoses. Thus, if an insured person has been diagnosed with dementia on an outpatient basis until the year before the application, it is assumed that his or her *cognitive and communicative abilities* are declining. The frequency of hospitalizations due to confusion and/or an alcohol-related mental behavioural disorder was also counted, both up to the year before submitting the application. For the criterion of how an insured person can *cope with their illness*, the number of ambulant doctors visited and the number of different outpatient doctors visited in the year before submitting the application were used. The assumption here is that insured persons who see different outpatient doctors more frequently can manage their illness more independently. For the last criterion of *shaping everyday life and social contacts*, no suitable data was found in the database. This is a very broad criterion, but all the other mentioned dimensions can affect this particular criterion. To generate additional features, the twenty most frequent inpatient main diagnoses per care grade were examined. Subsequently, the number of hospitalizations based on the selected diagnoses until one year before submitting the application was modeled as a dimension. The examined diagnoses are overlapping too much between the care grades. Therefore, many of the features generated by the hospitalization diagnosis were discarded throughout the feature selection process. During the feature selection process, features that do not adequately describe the classes are excluded from the classification.

2.1.2 Cost related data

In order to describe the overall physical condition more quantitatively, the monetary expenditure for the insured person in the year prior to the application was modeled as a feature dimension. Total costs were used for this purpose, as well as dividing the costs into additional thirteen dimensions. For example, dental costs to represent self-hygiene, medical product costs to represent *mobility*, or the average hospital- and care- case costs to represent physical state.

2.1.3 Demographic related data

To get more demographic information into the dataset and feature dimensions, data points such as age in the year of application, gender, structural area of residence and marital status were included. Structural areas were included to examine the difference between high density areas and low density areas. As well as the job status of the previous year, the highest reported school-leaving qualification, and the highest vocational qualification of the insured person. In addition, the years of unemployment and occupational activity per year of life were calculated. Another dimension was the number of care applications already made. The "hardship case" feature is a very extensive feature that has been included. Insured persons only get a hardship case as soon as their annual own expenses for the treatment of their illness exceed 2% of the gross annual income. For chronically ill persons it is 1%. This dimension contains information on the gross annual income and the illness. This was taken into consideration if the person in need of care was a hardship case in the year before the application.

2.2 Preprocessing

After data cleansing, the number of rows was reduced to 15,782. With the distribution of the degrees of care shown in Fig. 1. For the objective evaluation, the data were split, with 80% used for training and 20% for testing.

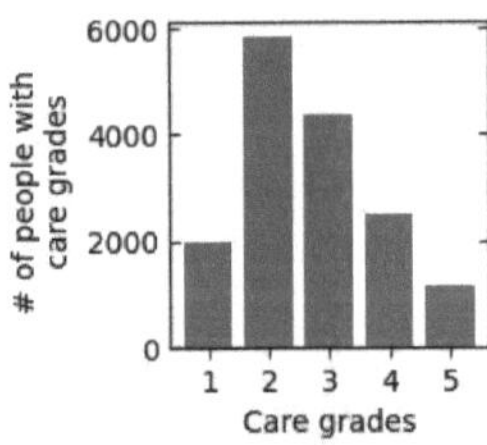

Figure 1: Distribution of care grades in the data

It shows, the distribution of classes is very imbalanced. This leads to the classifier being too oriented towards care grade 2, resulting in poor accuracy. Therefore, the classes represented by the degrees of care have been redistributed. In this way, care grades 1 and 2 form class 0 and care grades 3, 4 and 5 form class 1. This procedure leads to evenly distributed classes.

2.3 Applying ML Models

Following preprocessing, traditional machine learning algorithms and deep learning algorithms were used to find a baseline of the F1-score and accuracy. A CNN was used with two convolutional layers and two fully connected layers, as well as a MLP. The traditional algorithms like RDF and support vector machines with different kernels were also investigated. The neural networks overfitted during the training, an early stopping with a delay of 2 was used to avoid it. During the training of the neural networks, it was not possible for the neural networks to achieve a better validation score than the test score of the traditional machine learning methods. Also in the following evaluation, the neural networks repeatedly performed worse than the other algorithms. The support vector classifier was not able to deliver a result in a reasonable time, therefore no further experiments were conducted with it. Using the existing baseline accuracy and F1-score, filter-based, embedded and wrapper-based feature selection methods were implemented. The chi^2 feature selection, along with a feature selection using a RDF and a recursive feature elimination also based on a RDF, were tested more precisely. Finally, the feature important score of the gradient boosting decision tree with a threshold of 0.1% was used to discard unimportant features. The feature selection did not increase the accuracy significantly, but it did reduce the runtime of the SQL query and the training time of the classifier. In order to avoid the performance variance of the model, we also carried out stratified cross-validation. The data were divided into different groups, maintaining similar proportions for each class, with one group used for testing and the others used for training. After no more changes were noticeable in the evaluation, another approach was tested based on the modeled features. For this purpose, all insured persons with a care grade were considered as one class. Another class was formed with randomly selected persons from the database who do not have care grades. To ensure that the classes are equally weighted, the output was matched to the number of persons in the first class. To avoid the classification being biased by features that only apply to insured persons with a care grade, dimensions such as the number of applications made for a care grade or the care expenditure of the health insurance company for the insured person were removed from the matrix. The result was a data set with 31,740 rows and 52 columns. The feature selection, testing and subsequent training were carried out in the same way as the first approach described above. For the experiments, all data were processed using pseudonyms.

3 Results and Discussion

In order to determine if machine learning methods can be applied in the context of statutory health insurance, one approach was to consider the care grades as a classification problem. Using the gradient boosted trees algorithm, the data matrix could be reduced from 70 dimensions to 32 features when differentiating between the care levels. The feature reduced matrix achieved a relative feature importance of 98.8% compared to all features. The 10 most important features achieve a score of 91.1%, as it can be seen in Fig. 2. For the classification between care grade positive and care grade negative, the matrix could be reduced from 52 to 21 features, which all together give a relative feature importance of 99.5%, while the top 10 features achieving a score of 95.5%. Fig. 3 shows the relative score distribution of the best 10 features. The matrices generated in way were then used to train various classifiers. The best result was obtained using a random forest with 256 trees and a depth of 24. An accuracy of 73.6% was achieved for the clas-

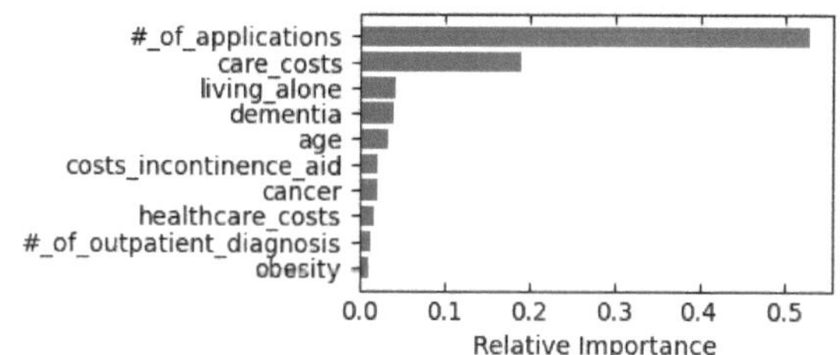

Figure 2: Relative feature importance between care grades

sification of low or high degrees of care. An accuracy of 85.4% was achieved using a random forest with 350 trees and a depth of 12 when classifying care grade positive and care grade negative insured persons.

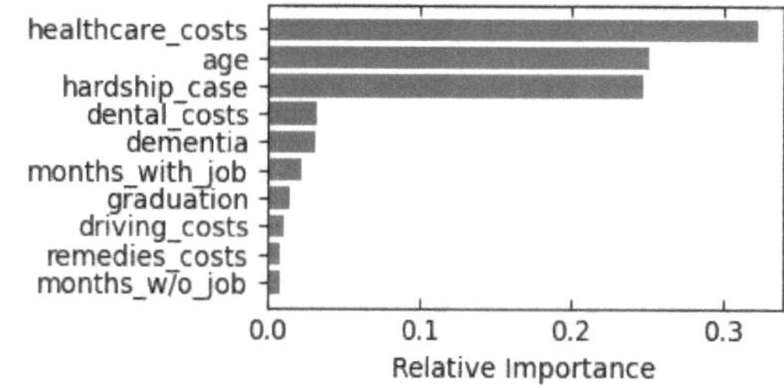

Figure 3: Relative feature importance between care grades and no care grades

Table 1: Accuracy of the classification results given in % / standard deviation in % / duration of a whole training run in sec.

Classifier	Low/High Care grade		Care grade No/Yes	
	All Feature	Limited Features	All Feature	Limited Features
RDF	73.6 / 0.8 / 10.0	**73.6 / 0.8 / 8.8**	85.1 / 0.1 / 16.8	**85.4 / 0.1 / 14.0**
MLP	73.0 / 0.5 / 12.5	73.5 / 0.2 / 13.0	84.4 / 0.2 / 25.0	84.9 / 0.0 / 24.4
CNN	73.0 / 0.1 / 28.5	73.1 / 0.7 / 16.4	83.8 / 0.1 / 73.5	83.5 / 0.4 / 40.2

The results in Table 1 were limited to one decimal place only, as there are statistical deviations when training ML approaches. During the training of the neural networks, it was repeatedly observed that they did not improve their validation score beyond 74% for the classification of low and high care grades and 85% for the binary classification of care grades with the control group. If there is no early stopping, then the deep learning approaches risks overfitting. This is why relatively short training times are realized here. The results show a slight tendency for the classifiers with fewer features to perform better. The traditional machine learning approach with a RDF outperforms the deep learning approaches in terms of accuracy and time. The RDF calculates the importance of the features during its usage, so dimensions that are considered unimportant are given less attention. This means acceptable results can be achieved even without a prior restriction of features.

3.1 Assumptions and Limitations

To model the features for the care grade classification, we made a number of assumptions. Limiting many of the features to the year before the application is one of them. The assumption here is that relevant changes have occurred in the year before the application. Extending the span from one to two years before the application does not result in any significant changes in the evaluation. After the prediction, it is necessary to have enough time for preventive measures. If prevention is started after the prediction, i.e. in the year before the application for a care grade, it is very likely that it will not prevent health problems or the need for long-term care. When modeling the dimensions with different chronic diseases, no attention was paid to the severity of the diseases or the possibility of a cure. For example, the impact of cancer on an individual's life can vary depending on its severity. Similarly, an obese person may lose weight and no longer be considered overweight. The IKK is a health insurance company that developed out of associations of craftsmen. This means that mainly craftsmen are insured in this health insurance fund, even after the opening of the health insurance for everyone. This leads to a disproportionately share of men, which can influence the classification. In 2017, the care grades were introduced, which is why the care data collected before 2017 cannot be used. This limits the number of data sets that can be put to use for training. Data may also be missing if the insured person has recently changed to the health insurance company. Incomplete data may result if an employer reports the activity key, that includes the school-leaving qualification and the highest vocational qualification, incorrectly or not at all. If it's not reported, then the data is not accessible at all. Similarly, diagnoses may be transmitted incorrectly to the health insurance company. As a general rule, health insurance companies in Germany are only allowed to keep data on insured individuals for a maximum of 10 years. This means that in some cases, the data is not available for evaluation. For example, if a former employee has been retired for more than 10 years, data on the former employment relationship is no longer available. All these limitations of possible missing data lead to a sparse data matrix, that makes training difficult and thus restricts the results by limiting the classifiers accuracy.

4 Conclusion

As shown in the results in Table 1, ML methods are feasible for data classification in context of the statutory health insurance. An important factor in this is the selection of suitable dimensions, which requires an understanding of the German healthcare system and background knowledge in medicine. However, proper feature selection not only shortens the training time, it can also bring a significant reduction in query time, which is important for later use in the company. It is always beneficial checking the features used for their importance, as this leads to a better understanding of the data and the problem being modeled. Testing and evaluating different ML approaches is also a good strategy, as the success of an approach depends on the structure of the data set. In this approach, only the classification of care grades was investigated, which is only one possible scenario for a health insurance company; with the available data, multiple scenarios can be modeled. It must also be further examined whether classifying insured individuals makes sense in a business context, as there are strict regulations for statutory health insurance companies that differentiate them from a typical business organisation. As a result, individual insured persons cannot simply be excluded from care, so measures must be taken to implement preventive measures in order to reduce costs. Additionally, having knowledge of potential cost factors can be valuable in strategic planning. For the presented classification problem it is difficult to determine whether early detection and preventive measures of potential person in need of care have an effect on their later obtaining a care grade. Before developing a plan and integrating the trained classifier into the company's daily routine, the implementation must be checked on data security and/or privacy related issues.

Acknowledgement

The work has been carried out at IKK - Die Innovationskasse, public company and supervised by the Institute for Medical Informatics, Universität zu Lübeck.

Author's Statement

Conflict of interest: Authors state no conflict of interest.

5 References

[1] F. Breyer, "Demographischer wandel und gesundheitsausgaben: Theorie, empirie und politikimplikationen," *Perspektiven der Wirtschaftspolitik*, vol. 16, no. 3, pp. 215–230, sep 2015.

[2] D. Koller, G. Schön, I. Schäfer, G. Glaeske, H. van den Bussche, and H. Hansen, "Multimorbidity and long-term care dependency—a five-year follow-up," *BMC Geriatrics*, vol. 14, no. 1, may 2014.

[3] K. Kaushik, A. Bhardwaj, A. D. Dwivedi, and R. Singh, "Machine learning-based regression framework to predict health insurance premiums," *International Journal of Environmental Research and Public Health*, vol. 19, no. 13, p. 7898, jun 2022.

[4] *Long-Term Care Guide - Everything you need to know about long-term care.* Federal Ministry of Health, Feb. 2020, pp. 42–46. [Online]. Available: https://www.bundesgesundheitsministerium.de/fileadmin/Dateien/5_Publikationen/Pflege/Broschueren/200320_BMG_Ratgeber-Pflege_DINA5_ENG_bf.pdf

[5] E. Jaul, J. Barron, J. P. Rosenzweig, and J. Menczel, "An overview of co-morbidities and the development of pressure ulcers among older adults," *BMC Geriatrics*, vol. 18, no. 1, dec 2018.

Benchmarking AI-Accelerators

Frederic Dlugi [1,2]
[1] Robotics and Autonomous Systems, Universität zu Lübeck, frederic.dlugi@student.uni-luebeck.de
[2] New Technologys, Basler AG, frederic.dlugi@baslerweb.com

Abstract

In this work, the focus is on learning about AI accelerators and comparing two solutions from Hailo and NXP, the Hailo-8 and the IMX8m-plus. It involved exploring the various approaches to accelerating artifical intelligence (AI) applications, with a focus on image processing in edge applications and the inference of convolutional neural Networks (CNNs). A significant portion of the work is dedicated to understanding the vendor-specific software development kits (SDK) for using the hardware. The comparison between the solution from Hailo and NXP shows, that the Hailo solution is much faster for supported network architectures, but since the SDK from Hailo is proprietary, some of the tested networks could not be made to run on the solution from Hailo.

1 Introduction

The study begins with the task of researching various AI accelerators available on the market and identifying which ones align with the vision of the company, Basler. The focus then narrowed to two specific accelerators: Hailo-8 and the NPU on the IMX8m-plus system on chip (SoC). These solutions are important to Basler and have unique architectures, so the goal of the work is to compare these two very different hardware solutions. To do this, the focus is on evaluating the software SDK running different network architectures.

1.1 Definition of AI-Accelerator

AI accelerators are specialized chips designed to speed up the process of inferring as well as training convolutional neural networks [1]. To do this, they must be able to accelerate the various mathematical operations used in CNNs, such as matrix multiplications and support for activation functions, pooling and batch normalization. Some AI accelerators may also support preprocessing tasks like color space conversions and postprocessing tasks like non-maximum suppression. AI accelerators can be found in a range of power classes, from below one watt as part of a system on a chip to thousands of watts for training neural networks in data centers. The focus of this paper is on embedded solutions with a power consumption below 20W. These accelerators are typically used only for inference, meaning that the training of the network has already been completed and the finished network is being used. This allows these accelerators to use quantized calculations, rather than the floating-point calculations used in the training phase. Converting a network's calculations from floating point to quantized form typically requires preprocessing outside of the accelerator often on a host computer [2].

1.2 Measuring Performance of AI Accelerators

When looking at the technical specifications for AI accelerators, we will typically see values for tera operations per second (TOPS) and power consumption listed. [1] However, it is important to note that these values represent idealized performance and may not be achievable in most common use cases. To truly evaluate the performance of an AI accelerator, it is worth to consider the supported instructions. For example, does the accelerator support all of the common operators used in neural networks? If not, is it possible to execute those operations on the host processor transparently? These factors can be difficult to evaluate and may require complex software solutions from the chip manufacturer. To measure the real-world performance of AI accelerators, it is helpful to use a benchmarking tool. There are several options available, such as MLPerf by MLCommons, which has a large number of results that can be compared to our benchmarks.

2 Comparison Hailo-8 and IMX8m-plus

The goal of this comparison is to evaluate the performance and ease of use of the Hailo-8 and IMX8m-plus accelerators. To do this, an effort is made to get all of the models in the benchmark suite working on both accelerators. Because of time constraints, if a model could not be made to work through simple debugging steps or by removing preprocessing and post-processing, which where not well supported by Hailo toolchain, further time is not spent on getting a model to run. All networks were only run for throughput, not accuracy. The average number of inferences per second is used as the comparison metric, as there is not a significant difference in inference times between the two accelerators.

All benchmark models, inferred in the comparison, where executed on an IMX8m-plus development board [3], with the Hailo-8 chip being connected to the M.2 2.0x2 slot. A Yocto-Linux with a hardknott kernel is used as operating system.

2.1 MLPerf by MLCommons

Table 1: Sizes of the Inference-Mobile models

Inference-Mobile	Models	Size
Classification	MobileNetEdgeTPU	16.3 MB
Detection	MobileDETs	16.6 MB
Segmentation	DeepLabV3+	9.1 MB
Segmentation	MOSAIC	7.3 MB
Language	Mobile-BERT	100 MB

Table 2: Sizes of the Inference-Edge models

Inference-Edge	Models	Size
Classification	Resnet50-v1.5	102 MB
Detection	Retinanet	148 MB
Segmentation	3D UNET	125 MB
Speech-to-text	RNNT	519 MB
Language	BERT-large	1336 MB

MLPerf is a benchmark for machine learning training and inference[4]. It provides models and target accuracies on datasets for the inference benchmarks, along with a large number of results for different systems. For this paper, the consider all models in the Inference-Edge and Inference-Mobile benchmarks, as most models in these benchmarks are in a size range is feasible for inference on an embedded board and are available in formats that can be used with the hardware being tested (see Table 1 and Table 2).

Using MLPerf with proprietary accelerator SDKs can be challenging due to the open-source nature of MLPerf and the closed-source nature of proprietary accelerator SDKs. To use MLPerf with a proprietary accelerator SDK, it is often necessary to modify the MLPerf code to make it compatible with the proprietary SDK. This process can be time-consuming and technically challenging, especially if the proprietary SDK is not well-documented or if it does not have good support for integration with external tools like MLPerf.

Furthermore, many accelerators do not support all the operators required to run the MLPerf benchmarking suite. This means that even with modifications to the code of the suite, it may not be possible to run all the benchmarks. Since the accelerator can't infer the model. This can limit the usefulness of MLPerf as a benchmarking tool for proprietary accelerators.

2.2 Hailo Toolchain

Hailo has developed its own toolchain, called the Hailo-8 Toolchain, for performing inference on its hardware. The toolchain accepts models in Tensorflow, TFLite and ONNX formats and converts them to a proprietary format for use with the Hailo-8 accelerator. However, not all common operators are supported by the accelerator and may need to be rewritten manually or replaced using configuration files. Hailo provides a model zoo with pre-trained models that have already been converted and compiled for inference. To solve a machine vision problem using Hailo accelerators, it is recommended to select a model from the model zoo and fine-tune it to a task specific dataset. Converting arbitrary models from the internet can be time-consuming and requires a deep understanding of the model and Hailo architecture. At the time of this work, Hailo planned to support the ONNX-Runtime API for their models, but had not yet done so. This development would allow for the inference of arbitrary models from the internet, assuming they can be converted to ONNX. To run a network on the Hailo-8 accelerator, a three-step process using the hailo_sw_suite Docker must be followed.[2]

2.3 IMX8m-plus Toolchain

The NPU (GC9000) in the IMX8m-plus uses an OpenVX interface and can be used as a Tensorflow Lite delegate [5]. Most Tensorflow Lite models found on the internet can be run using the GC9000 as a delegate, which is faster than using the ARM cores or the GPU of the IMX8m-plus, especially for models that are quantized to uint8. However, models that cannot be delegated completely to the NPU must be run on the IMX8m-plus CPU, which is slower. Networks that cannot be converted to Tensorflow Lite models using the default instructions also need to be run on the CPU. The NPU is designed to perform inference on the same network repeatedly, so the first inference caches the weights in dedicated memory. This can result in a significant speedup for small networks. In the future, the IMX8m-plus NPU will support the ONNX-Runtime, which should help to expand the number of networks that can be run on the NPU.[6]

2.4 Yolov5 in GStreamer

This task is chosen to compare the performance of the Hailo-8 and IMX8m-plus in a real-world test. Through comparison of pure inference, see Table 3, we see that a real world example using yolov5s is a network with fitting performance. The task involves using GStreamer to create a stream of images, performing inference with the yolov5s object detection network and drawing bounding boxes around the detected objects. Two GStreamer pipelines were created for this task, which perform object detection on a camera image stream.

NNStreamer is a deep learning plugin for GStreamer that enables us to apply neural network models to multimedia data streams in real time. NNStreamer provides a flexible and efficient way to process multimedia data using neural networks, particularly well-suited for tasks such as image classification, object detection and image segmentation. [7] For the IMX8m-plus pipeline the NNStreamer plugin was used, which integrates with GStreamer and can be used with a wide range of popular deep learning frameworks, such as TensorFlow, PyTorch and Caffe. This makes it easy for us to leverage the power of neural networks in our GStreamer-based applications, opening up a wide range of possibilities for AI-powered multimedia processing.

3 Results

3.1 GStreamer pipeline

Table 3: Isolated benchmark results for yolov5s

Accelerator	Results
IMX8m-plus	6.85 FPS
Hailo-8	**52.92 FPS**

Table 4: Full GStreamer pipeline results for yolov5s

Accelerator	Results
IMX8m-plus	4.62 FPS
Hailo-8	**16.79 FPS**

Comparing the performance isolated to inference shows, that the Hailo-8 is 8 times faster, then the IMX8m-plus (Table 3). Comparing the performance of the IMX8m-plus and Hailo-8 in a GStreamer pipeline doing detection with yolov5s results in the performance shown in Table 4. It is important to ensure proper cooling is applied to the IMX8m-plus and Hailo-8 for this benchmark. No active cooling is needed, but heat sinks are required.

Comparing the performance shows that Hailo-8 is 4 times faster than IMX8m-plus in this full pipeline benchmark. There seem to be bottlenecks in the Hailo pipeline, as the inference of CNN-based networks is much faster on Hailo-8, see Table 3. I suspect that the interface speed of M.2 2.0x2 is a bottleneck when streaming high-resolution video to the chip. Further testing should be done on an x86-based test system to eliminate this bottleneck. It is also suspected that NNStreamer has less programming overhead since it is designed for mobile systems.

3.2 MLPerf Results

Table 5: Inference-Edge Results

Models	IMX8m-plus	Hailo-8
Resnet50-v1.5	1.6 FPS	**67.3 FPS**
Retinanet	**0.01 FPS**	-
3D UNET	-	-
RNNT	-	-
BERT-large	-	-

Table 6: Inference-Mobile Results

Models	IMX8m-plus	Hailo-8
MobileNetEdgeTPU	294.8 FPS	**1615 FPS**
MobileDETs	68.7 FPS	**233 FPS**
DeepLabV3+	**6.3 FPS**	-
MOSAIC	-	-
Mobile-BERT	**0.42 IPS**	-

The results of the Inference-Edge benchmarking are shown in Table 5. The image classification benchmark resnet50-v1.5 performs much faster on the Hailo-8 chip than on the IMX8m-plus, which is expected given the difference in the number of TOPS between the two accelerators [2], [6]. However, the Hailo-8 struggled to run the other benchmark networks. The object detection benchmark ssd-resnet34 is not able to be quantized using Hailo's tools and could only be run on the IMX8m-plus CPU due to the presence of TensorFlow-Lite operations that were not supported on the NPU. The segmentation benchmark 3dunet failed to run on both accelerators and even failed to run on the IMX8m-plus CPU.

The speech-to-text benchmark using dlrm had a model that is too large to load onto the IMX8m-plus and therefore is not run. The language processing benchmark bert-large had a model that is 1 GB in size, which could not be run due to insufficient RAM on the IMX8m-plus. Overall, these results suggest that the Hailo-8 performs well on image classification tasks, but may have difficulty running other types of benchmarks.

The results of the Inference-Mobile benchmark suite are shown in Table 6. The benchmarks were split into those based on CNNs and those using other architectures, as the Hailo-8 currently only supports CNN-based architectures. In the CNN-based benchmarks for image classification and object detection, the Hailo-8 performed significantly faster than the IMX8m-plus NPU. However, the segmentation benchmark could only be run on the IMX8m-plus, as it required an x32 bilinear scaling that is not supported by the Hailo-8. The language processing benchmark also failed on the Hailo-8, as the initialization of parsing to convert the network to Hailo format did not work. The error messages were not conclusive, but I suspect that the transformer attention layer could not be interpreted by the Hailo software. The failure of both the segmentation and language processing benchmarks on the Hailo-8 highlights the potential limitations of proprietary software. In this case the proprietary nature of the software hinders the ability of the user to understand and fix problems, with the software.

3.3 Toolchain Analysis Results

Hailo has a proprietary software stack that accepts Tensorflow, Tensorflow 2, Tensorflow Lite and ONNX models. It converts these models to a proprietary format consisting completely of operations that have been implemented in Hailo's software. If an operator in the model is not supported by Hailo's software, the model cannot be parsed.

The solution offered by Hailo is to cut off the incompatible operators at the beginning and end of the model graph. If an operator in the middle of the model is not compatible, it must be manually replaced by the user. After converting the model to Hailo's format, the proprietary quantization technique optimizes the quantization ranges using a dataset that represents real-world conditions. However, this can sometimes fail without an explanation. Finally, the model is compiled for optimal scheduling on the chip, checking to ensure that chip-specific restrictions, such as a maximum bilinear resizing of 16x, are met.

NXP primarily uses Tensorflow Lite as the inference framework and only supports models that can be fully delegated, which works for most of the tested models. Like Hailo, NXP accelerates quantized operations such as uint8 and int8 using Tensorflow Lite. This works well with Tensorflow-based models, but requires a double conversion for ONNX models that must first be converted to Tensorflow and then to Tensorflow Lite. The Tensorflow Lite framework is not proprietary and many commonly used models in the mobile space are already in this format.

4   Conclusion

Both the Hailo-8 and IMX8m-plus accelerators are able to perform inference on CNNs much faster than CPUs or GPUs with similar power budgets. However, this performance comes with some costs. First, the requirement to only use quantized networks adds an extra step between training and deployment. Efficient quantization also requires knowledge about the input data and the ability of the quantization tool to handle the dynamics of all of the network's operators. Second, to use the full power of hardware acceleration for the inference of arbitrary models, all of the necessary operations must be implemented in hardware or software. This is mainly a software development task, as not all operations are typically implemented in hardware on AI accelerators. The toolchains from Hailo and NXP have different approaches to addressing this issue.

As a workflow, it is recommended to first try using the NXP NPU with Tensorflow Lite. If the performance of a given model does not meet the requirements, it is often possible to convert the Tensorflow Lite model to Hailo because the limited set of operations in Tensorflow Lite is mostly supported by Hailo. However, running ONNX-based models on the IMX8m-plus can be challenging and is often not possible due to the larger set of operations in ONNX compared to Tensorflow Lite. While Hailo does officially support conversion from ONNX, it can also encounter unsupported operators.

Acknowledgement

The internship has been carried out at Basler AG, Ahrensburg and supervised by Matthias Heinrich, Universität zu Lübeck.

Additionally, I would like to express my appreciation to my company supervisor Jens Dekarz for his support and mentorship, as well as for providing access to the necessary resources and equipment.

Author's Statement

Conflict of interest: Authors state no conflict of interest.

References

[1] A. Reuther, P. Michaleas, M. Jones, V. Gadepally, S. Samsi, and J. Kepner, "Ai accelerator survey and trends," in *2021 IEEE High Performance Extreme Computing Conference (HPEC)*, IEEE, 2021, pp. 1–9.

[2] Hailo, *Hailo-8™ ai processor - commercial/industrial datasheet*, version v1.0, 2022.

[3] B. AG, *Basler embedded vision kit for i.mx 8mp*, 2022. [Online]. Available: `https://docs.baslerweb.com/embedded-vision/prb-imx8mp`.

[4] V. J. Reddi, C. Cheng, D. Kanter, *et al.*, *Mlperf inference benchmark*, 2019. arXiv: `1911.02549 [cs.LG]`.

[5] *Tensorflow lite delegates*, TensorFlow, 2022. [Online]. Available: `https://www.tensorflow.org/lite/performance/delegates`.

[6] NXP, *I.mx 8m plus applications processor datasheet for industrial products*, version Rev. 1, 08/2021.

[7] M. Ham, J. J. Moon, G. Lim, *et al.*, "Nnstreamer: Stream processing paradigm for neural networks, toward efficient development and execution of on-device ai applications," *arXiv preprint arXiv:1901.04985*, 2019.

Analysis of Blood Glucose Daily Patterns

Laura Pauline Scherf [1], Oliver Witt [2], Julius Zauleck [3], Lennart Jablonski [4], and Marcin Grzegorzek [5,6]

[1] Medical Informatics, Universität zu Lübeck, laura.scherf@student.uni-luebeck.de

[2] Perfood GmbH, Lübeck, oliver.witt@perfood.de

[3] Perfood GmbH, Lübeck, julius.zauleck@perfood.de

[4] Institute of Medical Informatics, Universität zu Lübeck, l.jablonski@uni-luebeck.de

[5] Institute of Medical Informatics, Universität zu Lübeck, marcin.grzegorzek@uni-luebeck.de

[6] Department of Knowledge Engineering, University of Economics in Katowice, marcin.grzegorzek@uni-luebeck.de

Abstract

Each human has their own unique metabolism and thus blood glucose profiles differ significantly between different individuals. Some humans exhibit many spike-rich blood glucose patterns, whereas others exhibit flat constant patterns. In this paper, two different approaches to analyzing blood glucose daily patterns using continuous glucose monitoring data are proposed. First, a Time Series k-means approach to cluster different patterns is suggested. Second, an approach that identifies the characteristics of blood glucose patterns throughout the day and implements them using rule-based programming is presented. The results show that the first approach is not able to identify desired patterns. The second approach shows first promising results. However, future work is required to improve the results for the proposed characteristics and further evaluation methods are necessary.

1 Introduction

According to estimates, up to 50 percent of all diseases in modern industrialized countries can be attributed to inadequate nutrition and lack of exercise [1]. Hereby, glucose metabolism often plays a key role. The human glucose metabolism is often considered to be the heart of human well-being. For the human body, glucose is the most important source of energy and is among other things, needed for the cardiovascular system, the muscles, and the brain. Having a disturbed glucose metabolism, however, can lead to serious diseases. A low-glycemic diet in which blood glucose levels are kept as constant as possible is intended to help improve or prevent medical conditions. Nevertheless, which foods keep the blood glucose level constant varies from person to person and blanket dietary recommendations can therefore not be standardized. For this purpose, the Perfood GmbH (Lübeck, Germany) has launched a digital nutrition program, which is a digital product for personalized low glycemic nutrition. During a two-week test phase, users wear a glucose sensor on their upper arm, which continuously measures glucose levels. In addition, both diet and other factors that affect glucose metabolism, such as sleep, physical activity, and medication use, are monitored. Furthermore, the participants consume specified test meals. After the test phase, the application evaluates how different foods affect blood glucose levels and issues personalized nutrition recommendations customized to the user to keep blood glucose levels as constant as possible by reducing foods that lead to high-glycemic reactions. Thus, participants in the digital nutrition program receive a personalized low-glycemic nutrition report related to the meals they have tracked [2]. In this paper, blood glucose daily patterns will be analyzed. As each person has their own unique metabolism, the blood glucose profiles differ significantly between individuals. The aim is to identify different patterns in various individuals based on the daily course of blood glucose levels. For example, in some individuals, blood glucose drops sharply at night, in other individuals blood glucose is relatively constant at night. The blood glucose curves of different individuals also differ significantly during the course of the day. For instance, there are groups of people in whom the daily blood glucose pattern shows many high blood glucose peaks. Other groups, on the other hand, show hardly any spikes and have a relatively flat and constant blood glucose curve throughout the day. These different blood glucose patterns throughout the day should be analyzed.

2 Material and Methods

2.1 Medical Background

Blood glucose levels provide information about the amount of glucose in the blood. The blood glucose concentration in the human body is kept up by strict regulation of glucose production and glucose utilization by tissues which can be insulin-dependent or non-insulin-dependent. Blood glucose levels are mainly influenced by individual parameters such as nutrition, activity level, insulin production, and various other factors like stress, for instance. It is not only diabetics who experience fluctuating blood glucose levels during the course of the day. Even the normal blood glucose level of healthy people is not always the same. According to the literature, in the fasting state, the blood glucose level is usually between 70 and 99 mg/dl. In the postprandial state, the blood glucose level can temporarily increase to 140 mg/dl in healthy individuals. A blood glucose level of less than 70 mg/dL is referred to as hypoglycemia [3]. A healthy human body spends a lot of energy to keep blood glucose within a narrow range. Large deviations from this value can be harmful to the body [9].

2.2   Blood Glucose Data

Continuous glucose monitoring (CGM) is an efficient tool for measuring glucose concentration in interstitial fluid at frequent intervals of 5-15 minutes over several days. Minimally invasive CGM technologies are based on a subcutaneously applicable sensor that measures the glucose concentration in the interstitial fluid. Usually, the sensor is placed on the upper arm. Depending on the system used, either a smartphone or measuring device is used to scan or the measured glucose values are transferred directly to the smartphone every minute. The sensors are equipped with data memory to prevent data loss. The intended wear lifetime for the sensors is up to 14 days [4]. Thus, glucose measurements from 14 different days were available from most individuals. The blood glucose data used for the analysis of daily blood glucose patterns are exclusively data from adults. Information on pre-existing conditions, such as diabetes, that may affect blood glucose levels were available. The blood glucose values for the individual persons were available for full minutes in the unit mg/dl with date and time. No predetermined labels or classifications were available for the blood glucose daily patterns to be analyzed. For a few individuals, no readings were available for certain times of the day. This can be attributed to the missing readout of the glucose sensor or an interrupted data transmission. Especially at night, some people are missing data. This can be explained due to the size of the storage space for blood glucose data of 8 hours for certain sensor types, which may undercut sleep time.

Blood glucose data is time series data. The characteristic of time series data, in turn, is that it is a collection of observations that relates to a chronological order [5]. A majority of the recorded CGM data were taken as part of the digital nutrition program of Perfood GmbH (Lübeck, Germany), in which participants undergo a 14-day test phase. As part of this test phase, users are encouraged to track their diet and physical activity using an app. In addition, the participants consume defined test meals. Therefore, further to the available blood glucose data, also other data containing precise information about meal intake, such as carbohydrate amount, nutrient composition, etc., were available, as well as information about sports activities.

2.3   Time Series k-means Clustering

As described in Section 2.2, no predefined labels or classifications were available for the analysis of blood glucose daily patterns. Therefore, an approach involving the use of a clustering procedure was carried out first. For this clustering approach, only the blood glucose data of continuous glucose monitoring (CGM) described in Section 2.2 were used in a retrospective way without any further information on meal intake or sports activities. Clustering analysis is a statistical technique of multivariate unsupervised learning, classifying units of observations into similar groups. Unlike other classification methods, clustering analysis does not determine the groups a priori. Clustering refers to a tool for exploratory data analysis. It intends to group different objects or subjects in such a way that the degree of association between two objects is maximized if they belong to the same group, and minimized otherwise [6]. Accordingly, no labels are required for clustering algorithms. Since blood glucose data is time series data, a clustering method specifically designed for time series data was chosen, aiming to identify the structure of the unlabeled blood glucose data. Contrary to most times series clustering algorithms which calculate the similarity among the whole sequence, the Time Series k-means computes the similarity between two curves with respect to a segment of a time interval rather than the entire sequence. For the blood glucose data, this seems to be a reasonable approach, since it is important for this purpose to identify relevant time spans or subspaces in which similar patterns of blood glucose data occur. The data is then clustered according to the corresponding subspaces [5]. For blood glucose time series data this is corresponding to a part of a longer time span. Dynamic Time Warping (DTW) was used as an algorithm to measure similarity. This is chosen because similarity measures for time series data (in this case blood glucose data) are more difficult to define because the order of elements in the sequences must be taken into account. DTW is able to find the optimal alignment (or coupling) between two sequences of numerical values. In addition, DTW detects flexible similarities by matching the coordinates within the two sequences [7]. DTW allows to detection of similar shapes even if signal changes such as displacements or scalings occur. Thus, similar blood glucose courses of different persons, which may be shifted in time, should nevertheless show a high similarity. The optimal number k of clusters was determined using the Elbow method. By this method, the model is fitted with an increasing value of k, calculating the clusters and the cost that comes with the training. At a certain value for k, the cost decreases drastically and then reaches a plateau if it is further increased. This resembles the optimal number of k [8]. For the analysis of the daily blood glucose patterns, a median pattern was first formed for each person per sensor phase from the available CGM data in a preprocessing step. For this purpose, the median was formed over the sensor days for each time point. Thus, the typical blood glucose daily course for the individuals should be recognizable and outliers can be removed. In addition, only the blood glucose data of the subjects that contained at least the data of 9 sensor days were considered. No other data has been excluded. Time Series k-means clustering using DTW is then performed. For k, the optimal number of 10 was determined. Nevertheless, the approach has been tested with k from 5 to 20.

2.4 Handcrafted Characteristic Approach

For the analysis of blood glucose daily patterns, a further approach was developed and tested, as the results from the Time Series k-means clustering mentioned in Section 3.1 where not sufficient. In this approach, possible characteristics, which are relevant for this and which differ in individual persons, were determined in collaboration with an expert in nutritional medicine and with the help of specialized literature. A special focus was on finding characteristics that could be improved by lifestyle changes, such as changes in diet or more exercise. The goal of this approach design was to automatically detect those previously defined characteristics in order to later make a personalized recommendation to individuals if a certain characteristic is detected. Again, the blood glucose data mentioned in Section 2.2 was used for this purpose. Still, only CGM data of individuals that contained at least 9 sensor days were considered. In addition, the other available data such as information about meal intake and sporting activities have also been considered. The characteristics of the blood glucose patterns of individual sensor days were considered. The most important of the defined characteristics can be taken from Table 1. The implementation of those characteristics was realized by rule-based programming. One of the difficulties in implementing automated detection of the above-mentioned characteristics was the establishment of fixed limits for blood glucose values. First, there is the difficulty that the readings may be inaccurate due to measurement inaccuracies of the blood glucose sensors. For example, a shift in the y-axis intercept is possible. On the other hand, although defined thresholds can be found in the literature as mentioned in Section 2.1, such as which postprandial values are normal for healthy people, these do not necessarily seem to be reliable criteria for values measured with the use of CGM. Due to the availability of continuous measurements, there is a large amount of data, also from healthy individuals, which show that a large proportion of them frequently have postprandial blood glucose values of over 140 mg/dl. To circumvent this, no fixed limits were set for the detection, but only the values of the persons with the highest values in the total cohort are characterized as such. Data from diabetics were excluded. Values above the 90th percentile were set as thresholds.

3 Results and Discussion

3.1 Result of Time Series k-means

To evaluate the results of Time Series k-means clustering explained in Section 2.3, a visual approach was first adopted. For this purpose, the blood glucose median curves

Table 1: Characteristics of Blood Glucose Daily Pattern that are aimed to be detected automatically

Characteristic	Explanation
High Blood Glucose Peak	At certain times of the day, blood glucose levels often rise. Elevated blood glucose levels can damage blood vessels [9].
High Postprandial Blood Glucose Peak	Sharp rise in blood glucose due to the intake of carbohydrates at certain times of the day. Elevated blood glucose levels can damage blood vessels.
Missing Postprandial Normalization	In normal glucose tolerance, glucose levels do rise after a meal is ingested, but usually normalize to pre-meal levels within two to three hours. In case of missing postprandial normalization, the blood glucose level remains elevated for a long time even after this period [10].
Cravings	Meals with lots of carbohydrates are quickly absorbed by the body. The blood glucose level thus rises quickly and the body then secretes a large amount of insulin to bring it back to normal. Excess insulin lowers the blood sugar level to such an extent that slight hypoglycemia occurs. The body in turn reacts with a feeling of cravings [11].
Fast Blood Glucose Rise	Rapid and steep blood glucose rise often occur unnoticed after high-carbohydrate meals. Briefly elevated blood glucose levels are to be considered unhealthy as well. They are suspected of leaving damage to the small blood vessels. In addition, steep blood sugar rises to release large amounts of insulin, which in turn can hinder the weight loss process [9].
Severe Blood Glucose Fluctuations	Large fluctuations in blood sugar are a great challenge for the body. It has to perform a lot of adjustments and in long term, blood glucose levels that are too high or too low weaken the body. It may react with weakness, fatigue, tiredness, lack of concentration, or cravings [9].
No Night Decrease	An occasionally elevated blood glucose level at night is not usually a serious and immediate health problem, but they can affect sleep quality.
Distance Between Meals	Frequent eating alters the intrinsic rhythm of the stomach and intestines. Furthermore, constant snacking leads to increased calorie intake and prevents the insulin level from dropping [12].

were plotted for each cluster. Several observers visually assessed whether similar blood glucose median curves were assigned to the same cluster. Some individuals for whom blood glucose values were available, completed the test phase at least two times, thus at least two blood glucose median curves were available for them. It was assumed that the different curves of these persons are aimed to be assigned to the same cluster. Therefore, a confusion matrix was created using the data of those repeaters. However, since it must be assumed that the data of a person can change due to altered life circumstances, these were additionally displayed visually with the respective cluster membership in order to be able to be evaluated visually. Nevertheless, despite similar patterns, a large number of the repeaters curves were assigned to different clusters. In both assessment approaches, it was found that the clustering approach was not satisfactory because the blood glucose median curves seemed to be assigned to the clusters according to baseline height and not necessarily according to the actual different patterns, such as many spikes or flat trajectories.

3.2 Result of Handcrafted Characteristics

A visual approach was also used to evaluate the results for the approach described in Section 2.4. For this purpose, the blood glucose curves in which the respective characteristics were determined to have been plotted and evaluated. It was found that rule-based programming works well for part characteristics. However, for other characteristics, such as the missing night decrease, the implementation itself should still be improved. In addition, evaluation measures should be further developed and applied. Overall, the handcrafted characteristics seem to be a promising approach to identifying the different properties of blood glucose daily patterns but should be further improved and developed.

4   Conclusion

Two different approaches to analyzing blood glucose daily patterns were presented. For the first method, a Time Series k-means Clustering was used as an unsupervised machine learning method that can handle unlabeled data. However, the clustering did not cluster the data according to different patterns as desired, but rather according to the total height of the blood glucose curves. In a second approach, characteristics were defined with the help of a nutritional physician and then implemented using rule-based programming. This approach seems promising, but needs to be further developed and the implementation should be enhanced to a greater extent. In a further effort, evaluation measures should be further identified and applied to allow objective quality measures.

Acknowledgement

The work has been carried out at Perfood GmbH, Lübeck, and supervised by the Institute of Medical Informatics, Universität zu Lübeck.

Author's Statement

L.S., O.W., and J.Z. have been employed at Perfood GmbH.

5   References

[1] U. Gröber, *Omega 3: Gesünder leben mit den essentiellen Fettsäuren*. Südwest Verlag, 2021.

[2] T. Schröder, G. Kühn, A. Kordowski, S. Jahromi, A. Gendolla, S. Evers, C. Gaul, D. Thaçi, I. König, and C. Sina, *A Digital Health Application Allowing a Personalized Low-Glycemic Nutrition for the Prophylaxis of Migraine: Proof-of-Concept Data from a Retrospective Cohort Study*. Journal Of Clinical Medicine, vol. 11, no. 4, p. 1117, 2022.

[3] A. Carrillo and C. Gomez-Meade, *Blood Glucose*. In: Encyclopedia of Behavioral Medicine, Springer International Publishing, Cham, pp. 265-266, 2020.

[4] C. Fabris and B. Kovatchev, *Glucose Monitoring Devices: Measuring Blood Glucose to Manage and Control Diabetes*, Academic Press, 2020.

[5] X. Huang, Y. Ye, L. Xiong, R. Lau, N. Jiang, and S. Wang, *Time series k-means: A new k-means type smooth subspace clustering for time series data*. Information Sciences, vol. 367, pp. 1-13, 2016.

[6] W. Kirch, *Clustering Algorithms*. In: Encyclopedia of Public Health, Springer, Netherlands, pp. 128-129, 2008.

[7] F. Petitjean, A. Ketterlin and P. Gançarski, *A global averaging method for dynamic time warping, with applications to clustering*. Pattern Recognition, vol.44, pp. 678-693, 2011.

[8] T. Kodinariya and P. Makwana, *Review on determining number of Cluster in K-Means Clustering*. International Journal, vol.1, pp. 90-95, 2013.

[9] M. Kahl-Scholz, *Mensch! Erstaunliches über den Körper*. Springer, 2018.

[10] A. Ceriello, S. Colagiuri, J. Gerich and J. Tuomilehto, *Guideline for management of postmeal glucose*. International Diabetes Federation, 2007.

[11] S. Müller, *Die Müller-Diät*. Schlütersche Verlagsgesellschaft mbH, Hannover, 2009.

[12] B. Kleine-Gunk and A. Wolf, *Präventionsmedizin und Anti-Aging-Medizin*. Springer, 2020.

Comparison of Selected Deep-Learning Approaches for Video-Based Sleep Detection in Neonatal Care

Melina Schönknecht[1] and Fiete Winter[2]
[1] Medical Engineering Science, Universität zu Lübeck, melina.schoenknecht@student.uni-luebeck.de
[2] Drägerwerk AG & Co. KGaA, Lübeck, fiete.winter@draeger.com

Abstract

In this paper, we discuss different deep learning approaches for video-based sleep detection in neonatal care. Our motivation for this is to provide seamless patient care, which can be realized without the need for additional nursing staff. We were able to empirically show that there is no significant effect on model accuracy whether sleep stage classification is performed using 3D CNNs or transformer architectures. Similarly, we found that the length of the input in the form of videos, which were 5, 10, and 15 seconds in length, respectively, had no effect on accuracy. Overall, none of the approaches proved to be suitable for the problem. Consequently, we concluded that there is a need for an architecture that can handle longer video sequences without being too computationally intensive. We assume that a successful sleep-wake classification can be done on the basis of videos whose duration is in the range of minutes.

1 Introduction

If a child is born prematurely or falls ill shortly after birth, it potentially spends some time in a neonatal intensive care unit. In order to create the best possible conditions for the newborns, they are placed in specially designed incubators. However, this measure alone is not sufficient to ensure optimal recovery for children. Rather, it is of great importance that neonates on the ward are monitored continuously to ensure a rapid response to any change in patient behavior. Currently, monitoring is mainly realized by using sensors that are attached to the patient. The recorded data is thereby visualized via monitors. To obtain additional information about the infant, monitoring of patient behavior by staff is also necessary. In practice, nurses can rarely attend to the respective patients all the time. Thus, lag of information consequently leads to gaps in documentation about the condition of the newborn.

Considering the progress made in the past in the field of camera technology, network infrastructure, and machine learning, the idea of using a video-based and automated detection system for the purpose of newborn monitoring in everyday hospital life is reasonable. One aspect of monitoring, which is the focus of this work, is the sleep behavior of newborns. To realize the automated sleep detection, we want to compare three different video classification models for the purpose of sleep-wake classification. We want to investigate which of the three architectures is best suited for our problem and how the length of the processed videos influences the classification result.

In Sec. 2, we will first give a brief overview of the architectures we use as well as their parameterizations. In Sec. 3, we present the dataset and the data preprocessing followed by the hyperparameters and training methods. Finally, an overview of our results is given. Sec. 4 concludes this paper.

2 Video classification models

To realize video-based sleep detection in neonatal care, we consider three different deep learning approaches in this paper: The Video ResNet [7], the S3D [9], and the MViT [3]. All three architectures are easily accessible via pytorch/torchvision allowing for easy implementation and uniform interfacing for training and testing. The following sections provide a brief overview of their main features.

2.1 Video ResNet

In this section, we introduce the so-called Video ResNet [7] for processing spatio-temporal video data. The architectures structure is derived from that of the conventional ResNet [4] for processing 2D data. While the individual subtypes of the Video ResNet differ in how the spatio-temporal convolution operations are implemented within the individual blocks, the basic structure corresponds to that of an exemplary R3D in Tab. 1.

As an input, each Video ResNet receives a tensor of size $C \times T \times H \times W$, where C indicates the number of channels, e.g. RGB channels, while T, H and W refer to the temporal and spatial dimension, respectively, i.e. the length, the height and the width of the tensor.

R3D: 3D convolution. In contrast to the 2D ResNet, the 3-dimensional Video ResNet considers not only the spatial but also the temporal dimension of the input across the en-

layer name	output size	R3D-18	
conv1	$T \times 56 \times 56$	$3 \times 7 \times 7, 64,$ stride $1 \times 2 \times 2$	
conv2_x	$T \times 56 \times 56$	$3 \times 3 \times 3, 64$ $3 \times 3 \times 3, 64$	$\times 2$
conv3_x	$\frac{T}{2} \times 28 \times 28$	$3 \times 3 \times 3, 128$ $3 \times 3 \times 3, 128$	$\times 2$
conv4_x	$\frac{T}{4} \times 14 \times 14$	$3 \times 3 \times 3, 256$ $3 \times 3 \times 3, 256$	$\times 2$
conv5_x	$\frac{T}{8} \times 7 \times 7$	$3 \times 3 \times 3, 512$ $3 \times 3 \times 3, 512$	$\times 2$
	$1 \times 1 \times 1$	spatiotemporal pooling, fc layer with softmax	

Table 1: **R3D-18 architecture**. The convn_x layers denote the different ResNet blocks. Each of them are build out of multiple residual blocks. Their total number is specified by the number behind the parentheses. Each residual block contains, in this case, 2 convolution layers with a kernel size of $3 \times 3 \times 3$. The number after the kernel size represents the number of feature maps. In a residual block, its input is fed into the output of the respective block via skip connections.

tire architecture. For this purpose, 4-dimensional kernels of size $N_{i-1} \times t \times d \times d$ are used in each of the blocks, where N_{i-1} is the number of feature maps, which were generated in the previous block. While d corresponds to the spatial extent of the kernel, t denotes its temporal component. Thus, this kind of kernel is convolved with the tensor not only spatially but also temporally. The schematic structure of a R3D can be seen in Fig. 1a).

R(2+1)D: (2+1)D-convolution. This ResNet variant approximates the actual 3D convolution by a 2D spatial convolution followed by a 1D temporal convolution. Hence, the filter kernel of size $N_{i-1} \times t \times d \times d$, can be separated into two kernels of shape $N_{i-1} \times 1 \times d \times d$, and $M_i \times t \times 1 \times 1$, respectively. Here, M_i determines the dimensionality of the intermediate space into that the activation between spatial and temporal convolution is projected. This hyperparameter is chosen in a way that that the number of parameters in the (2+1)D convolution is equal to the number of parameters in the full 3D convolution [7]. Thereby a major advantage of this decomposition is seen in the doubled number of non-linearities, since another ReLU activation function is added between each of the 2D and 1D convolutional layers [7]. The R(2+1)D is shown in Fig. 1b).

MC3: Mixed 3D-2D convolution. For the architecture with so-called mixed convolution, 3D and 2D kernels are used both. The MCx Video ResNet performs 3D convolutions for the first $x-1$ residual groups switching to 2D spatial convolutions, afterwards. The idea behind this approach is that for the purpose of motion modeling, 3D convolution is mainly useful in the front layers, while in the back layers, i.e., in the 2D convolution layers, such time modeling is no longer necessary, since only semantic abstraction takes place [7]. In this work, we primarily consider the MC3, which is shown in Fig. 1c).

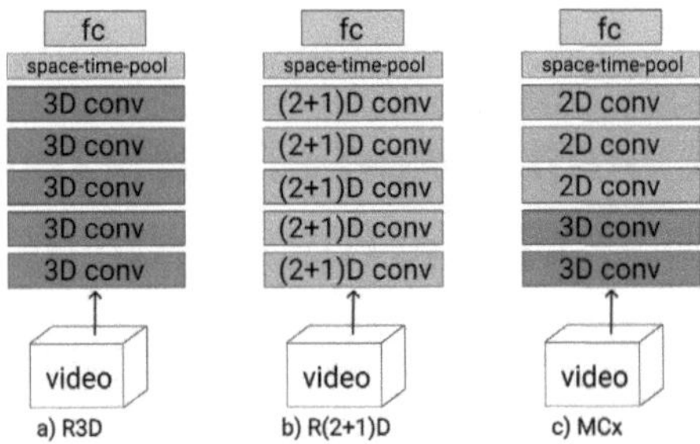

Figure 1: **Subtypes of Video ResNet**. a) R3D, which uses full 3D convolution across all layers; b) R(2+1)D, in which 3D convolution is divided into spatial (2D) and temporal (1D) convolution; c) MC3, where from the third layer and deeper 3D is replaced by 2D convolution.

2.2 Video S3D

The starting point for the S3D architecture is the *I3D* [1]. A (in 2018) state of the art approach where the 2D convolutional layers of a so-called *Inception* network [5], which is a CNN-classifier, have been extended to 3D convolutional layers. Despite the good results that can be achieved with an I3D, it is a very computationally intensive architecture, which caused the authors of S3D to rethink the I3D. In addition to some other architectures, the authors also propose the S3D architecture mentioned at the beginning. In this, the 3D convolutional layers are separated into a spatial and a temporal convolution, as in the R(2+1) Video ResNet. Consequently, the $t \times d \times d$ large kernels are also devided into two consecutive convolution operations with the filter shapes $1 \times d \times d$ and $t \times 1 \times 1$, respectively. This change has allowed the authors to significantly compress the architecture while also increasing speed. The complete S3D architecture can be seen in Fig. 2.

2.3 Video MViT

The structure of a Multiscale Vision Transformer (MViT) is primarily based on that of transformers [8] for Natural Language Processing (NLP): Here, the input is processed

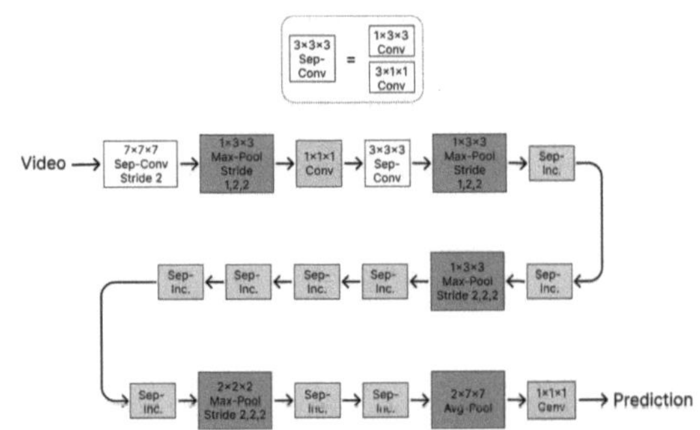

Figure 2: **S3D-Architecture**. The Sep-Conv blocks indicate a 3D convolution separated into spatial and temporal part. The separable inception blocks consist of multiple kernels, where the 3D convolution is also separated, as well as a pooling layer [9].

sequentially by passing it through several encoder/decoder blocks. Each block calculates the so-called self-attention representing the dependencies of the sequence elements on each other. Since this has to be done multiple times, several blocks are combined into Multi Head Attention (MHA). In general, this approach allows to connect information from pixels with larger distances compared to CNNs, where pixels are combined only locally.

Following on from this, the MViT was introduced, a transformer architecture whose core concept is primarily based on the use of stages. Unlike conventional Vision Transformers (ViTs) [2], MViT's can effectively use the temporal information of the input. They utilize the concept of so-called multiscale pyramids: At each stage of the transformer the spatial resolution is successively reduced while the channel capacity is increased. The architecture of the MViT base model is shown in Tab. 2. This processing of the input, which is similar to the concept of convolution, is achieved by using the so-called Multi Head Pooling Attention (MHPA). The concept of pooling attention can be seen in Fig. 3. Contrary to MHA, MHPA reduces the spatial resolution by pooling the sequences of latent vectors. Thus, the MViT architecture is enabled to mainly model simple visual features in its first layers due to the low channel capacity and the high spatial resolution. In contrast, the underlying layers focus mainly on coarse but more complex features [3].

3 Experiments

3.1 Dataset

The dataset consists of 10 videos depicting newborns lying in the incubator. The recording camera was placed outside the incubator in such a way that the patients were filmed either from the head and along their longitudinal axis or from above. The individual recordings had a total length of one to approximately five hours. We visually annotated the videos to determine if the particular incubated infant was either asleep, awake, or if it was unclear which of the above states the baby was in. The videos were subjected to further preprocessing: All passages in which the patient was not in bed, was interacted with, or had an unclear sleep-wake state were excluded from further evaluation.

On this basis, individual snippets of 6, 10, or 15 seconds in length were extracted from the videos. The sleep-wake state of the patient does not change during the duration of each snippet. For the different video lengths, 30 video snippets were created per patient, resulting in a total of 3 data sets with 300 videos each. Whenever possible, the snippets were balanced regarding the two classes (sleeping/not sleeping) for each patient.

3.2 Experimental setup

For our subsequent training and evaluation, we used a 3-fold cross validation. In the validation part of the folds, the not sleeping label was represented with 62.5%, 66.6%

stages	operators		output sizes
data layer	stride $\tau \times 1 \times 1$		$C \times T \times H \times W$
cube_1	$c_T \times c_H \times c_W, C$ stride $s_T \times 4 \times 4$		$C \times \frac{T}{s_T} \times \frac{H}{4} \times \frac{W}{4}$
scale_2	$\begin{matrix} \text{MHPA}(C) \\ \text{MLP}(4C) \end{matrix}$	$\times X_2$	$C \times \frac{T}{s_T} \times \frac{H}{4} \times \frac{W}{4}$
scale_3	$\begin{matrix} \text{MHPA}(2C) \\ \text{MLP}(8C) \end{matrix}$	$\times X_3$	$2C \times \frac{T}{s_T} \times \frac{H}{8} \times \frac{W}{8}$
scale_4	$\begin{matrix} \text{MHPA}(4C) \\ \text{MLP}(16C) \end{matrix}$	$\times X_4$	$4C \times \frac{T}{s_T} \times \frac{H}{16} \times \frac{W}{16}$
scale_5	$\begin{matrix} \text{MHPA}(8C) \\ \text{MLP}(32C) \end{matrix}$	$\times X_5$	$8C \times \frac{T}{s_T} \times \frac{H}{32} \times \frac{W}{32}$

Table 2: **MViT base model.** In layer cube$_1$, the spatial-temporal resolution is reduced from $T \times H \times W$ to $\frac{T}{s_T} \times \frac{H}{4} \times \frac{W}{4}$ by projecting dense cubes of size $c_T \times c_H \times c_W$ onto C channels. Thereby s_T denotes the temporal component of the kernel. In each of the X transformer blocks within a stage, the resolution across the stage is reduced by the MHPA. At the same time, the Multilayer Perceptron (MLP) increases the channel dimension C.

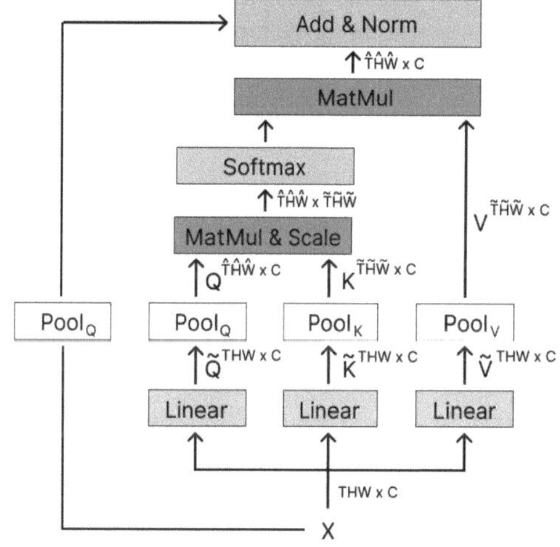

Figure 3: **Pooling Attention.** A form of attention mechanism that uses pooling to successively reduce the temporal-spatial resolution $T \times H \times W$ and thus focus on features of varying complexity. Here, the pooling layers (white blocks) are the extension compared to *traditional* MHA [8].

and 50%, respectively. After rescaling the spatial dimensions of the videos to 256×342, we applied a center crop of size 224×224 and performed normalization of the pixel values. The initial framerate of 30 fps was downsampled to 3 fps. This resulted in a respective video length of 5, 10 and 15 seconds. During training, the whole video snippets were also flipped horizontally with a probability of 0.5. The weights of the models were all pre-trained using the KINETICS dataset [6]. Each model was trained over 10 epochs, with a batch size of 7. We used the Adam optimizer with an initial learning rate of 10^{-3} decreasing by factor 0.4 after each epoch. This setup was used equivalently for all video lengths. The models were compared based on the best classification accuracy that could be accomplished in each of the 3 folds.

video length	5 s				10 s				15 s			
test set	fold 0	fold 1	fold 2	**avg**	fold 0	fold 1	fold 2	**avg**	fold 0	fold 1	fold 2	**avg**
R3D	63.87	69.05	47.62	60.18	65.55	65.48	47.62	59.55	75.63	61.90	63.10	66.88
R(2+1)D	64.71	64.29	47.62	58.87	63.03	77.38	50.00	63.47	62.18	70.24	71.43	67.95
MC3	63.03	64.29	52.38	59.90	63.03	64.29	53.57	60.30	70.59	66.67	47.62	61.63
S3D	63.87	67.86	76.19	69.31	63.03	70.24	66.67	66.65	74.79	64.29	72.62	70.57
MViT	78.99	65.48	51.19	65.22	-	-	-	-	-	-	-	-
avg	66.89	66.19	55.00	62.7	63.66	69.35	54.47	62.49	70.8	65.78	63.69	66.76

Table 3: **Results**. All models were trained with the same videos of different lengths. There was no advantage for any of the models concerning the sleep stage classification. In the case of the MViT, only videos of 5 seconds in length could be considered. This is due to the fact that the MViT could only process an input shape of 16 frames.

3.3 Results

Our results are shown in Tab. 3. We were not able to consider the MViT for all experiments, since only an input of 16 frames could be used for it. The question which model seems to be the most suitable for our problem cannot be answered by the results, because in no case a model accuracy could be produced which was constantly above the percentage of the stronger class. Likewise, the results do not allow us to draw any conclusions about the influence of the length of the snippets on the accuracy. While in some cases the accuracy increased successively with increasing snippet length, we also observed the opposite case. It also happened that the accuracy first increased and then decreased again for the next longer snippets, vice versa.

4 Conclusion

In this work, selected deep learning approaches for video-based sleep stage classification in neonatal care were compared. We observed that the models used produced results that were better than chance in only a few cases.

For better classification results it would be beneficial to use an architecture that can handle longer snippets without making the processing too computationally intensive. We assume, that the movements relevant for classification often span a period of several minutes. Moreover, all models were pre-trained with the KINETICS dataset, whose classes are more distinct from the ones we used. Since the sleeping and awake states are very similar, it might be more challenging for the models to make a distinction here. Thus, accuracy could also be inmproved by using more than two classes where the various sleep phases are further differentiated.

Acknowledgement

The work has been carried out at Drägerwerk AG & Co. KGaA, Lübeck and supervised by Prof. Dr. Barth, Institute of Neuro- and Bioinformatics, Universität zu Lübeck.

Author's Statement

Conflict of interest: Authors state no conflict of interest. At the time of writing, the authors are employed by Drägerwerk AG Co. KGaA. Informed consent: Informed consent has been obtained from all individuals included in this study.

5 References

[1] J. Carreira and A. Zisserman, *Quo vadis, action recognition? a new model and the kinetics dataset*. CVPR, 2017.

[2] A. Dosovitskiy, L Beyer, A. Kolesnikov, D. Weissenborn, X. Zhai, T. Unterthiner, M. Dehghani, M. Minderer, G. Heigold, S. Gelly, J. Uszkoreit, N. Houlsby . *An image is worth 16x16 words: Transformers for image recognition at scale*. ICLR, 2021.

[3] H. Fan, B. Xiong, K. Mangalam, Y. Li, Z. Yan, J. Malik and C. Feichtenhofer, *Multiscale Vision Transformers*. ICCV, 2021.

[4] K. He, X. Zhang, S. Ren and J. Sun, *Deep Residual Learning for Image Recognition*. CVPR, 2016.

[5] S. Ioffe and C. Szegedy. *Batch normalization: Accelerating deep network training by reducing internal covariate shift*. arXiv:1502.03167v3, 2015.

[6] W. Kay, J. Carreira, K. Simonyan, B. Zhang, C. Hillier, S. Vijayanarasimhan, F. Viola, T. Green, T. Back, P. Natsev, M. Suleyman, and A. Zisserman. The kinetics human action video dataset. CoRR, abs/1705.06950, 2017.

[7] D. Tran, H. Wang, L. Torresani, J. Ray, Y. LeCun and M. Paluri, *A Closer Look at Spatiotemporal Convolutions for Action Recognition*. arXiv:1711.11248v3, 2018.

[8] A. Vaswani, N. Shazeer, N. Parmar, J. Uszkoreit, L. Jones, A. N. Gomez, L. Kaiser, and I. Polosukhin. *Attention is all you need*. arXiv:1706.03762v5, 2017.

[9] S. Xie, C. Sun, J. Huang, Z. Tu and K. Murphy, *Rethinking Spatiotemporal Feature Learning: Speed-Accuracy Trade-offs in Video Classification*. arXiv:1712.04851v2, 2018.

Clinical evaluation of a Deep Learning approach for glenohumeral joint segmentation in CT images

Bjørn Keohane [1], Liliana Duarte [2], Bartosz Silski [3], Sven Goebel [4],

[1] Biomedical Engineering, Luebeck University of Applied Sciences, bjoern.keohane@stud.th-luebeck.de

[2] ApoQlar GmbH, Hamburg, liliana.duarte@apoqlar.com

[3] TheBlue.ai, Hamburg, bartosz.silski@theblue.ai

[4] Perth Shoulder Clinic, Perth AUS, sven@me.com

Abstract

In recent years, the number of shoulder replacements performed worldwide has increased and the requirements for improving clinical decision making have become more challenging. Techniques for successful planning and execution of implantation in surgery are becoming increasingly important, and recently the use of Deep Learning has become a highly regarded and researched topic in surgery. We present an algorithm that enables segmentation of the scapula and glenoid. This algorithm preserves the anatomical structures to be assessed when a surgeon wants to plan the course of his surgery. The algorithm achieved an accuracy of 87%, the glenoid version angle, a key factor in preoperative planning, could be reproduced and showed a competitive mean value of -8.23° with respect to -8.07° in the original CT images. Therefore, to some extent, this approach paved the way for an automated clinical workflow for shoulder prostheses, maintaining the precision required for a successful outcome.

1 Introduction

Shoulder replacement is a widely used method for the treatment of various shoulder pathologies. Despite advances in shoulder replacement, loosening and failure of the glenoid component remain the main reasons for medium- and long-term complications and revisions. An improperly positioned glenoid component is potentially at risk for numerous biomechanical complications and component wear. Therefore, accurate positioning is critical for the longevity of the glenoid component [1].

Computed tomography (CT) provides detailed two-dimensional (2D) or three-dimensional (3D) imaging of the glenohumeral joint. Advances in computations have allowed preoperative planning to be performed using CT. Hence, questions about differences in planning between 2D and 3D representations were raised [1].

In recent years, convolutional neural networks (CNNs) have been successfully applied in various industries and have achieved many research results in automated image segmentation. CNNs are based on the traditional neural network and *convolutional filter kernels*, whose main function is to learn and extract the features necessary for efficient medical image understanding [2], [3].

Our work aimed towards the development of a segmentation algorithm using the U-Net, a famous CNN for image segmentation, to segment the glenoid fossa adequately. The measurements of the glenoid version angle are usually made on a 2D image plane prior to surgery, to select the optimal component. Glenoid version is thus a key factor in surgical interventions on the glenoid, especially for shoulder replacement [4]. Therefore, our segmentation algorithm serves as a preliminary tool for surgeons later on to perform planning and image-guided surgery in 3D mixed reality (MR).

2 Material and Methods

2.1 Data Acquisition

Prior to this work, a set of 35 CT scans of 36 shoulder joints was obtained. The images were reviewed for patient positioning, slice thickness and reconstruction interval (distance between slices). The CT shoulder protocol according to [5] was used to assess the quality of the collected images. Here, a supine position of the patient, a slice thickness of ≤ 1.25 mm and a reconstruction interval of ≤ 0.625 mm are recommended. Our dataset showed slice thicknesses ranging from 0.8 mm to 1.5 mm (mean = 0.99 ± 0.24). The reconstruction intervals ranged from 0.31 mm to 1.5 mm (mean = 0.57 ± 0.37). All patients were in the supine position. All images had a resolution of 512x512 pixels. Images showing artefacts such as an implant or missing bone structures were excluded. This protocol is intended to provide a general concept of a CT protocol for shoulder assessment. The details of the protocol will depend on the type of CT scanner, the specific hardware and software, and the preferences of the radiologist. Therefore, we have included scans that deviate from the recommended values in order to achieve better generalisability of the algorithm. The dataset included six left-sided joints and 30 right-sided joints. Patient demographics included an age range of 21 to 88 years (mean = 65.21 ± 15.29) and a distribution of approximately 50% male and female. The images were labelled by the author using image processing software (3D Slicer, v3.0.5) and active learning (MONAI Label, v0.6.0rc6). In this way, the pixels were assigned to either the humerus, the scapula or the adjacent bones, which was verified and confirmed by an orthopaedic surgeon.

2.2 Image Preprocessing

All images of the dataset were normalized per subject. The mean μ and the standard deviation σ of the pixel intensity values X were calculated, and a z-normalization was performed according to (1).

$$X_n = \frac{X - \mu}{\sigma} \tag{1}$$

Therefore, all pixels in the images had values $\mu = 0$ and $\sigma = 1$. The intensity distributions of CT images are expressed in Hounsfield units (HU) and range from -1024 HU to 3071 HU, corresponding to 4096 gray level values. These values were normalized according to (2) so that they range from 0 to 1, which makes the calculations in the algorithm faster. Furthermore, CNNs must be trained with a large dataset to achieve the best performance. Data augmentation increases the size of the existing set of images through random flips and croppings [3]. The preprocessed, augmented image data were then fed into the CNN.

$$X_s = \frac{X_n - min(X_n)}{max(X_n) - min(X_n)} \tag{2}$$

2.3 Algorithm Design

A dynamic U-Net architecture was implemented with a pre-trained ResNet-34 encoder, which is pre-coded and available in the FastAI library (v2.7.10). This library works with the Python language (v3.8.3) and the PyTorch library (v1.10.0) as a backend. At the point of maximum compression (lowest part of the architecture, see Fig. 1), the decoder is connected following the principle of the classical U-Net architecture to finally obtain an output equal to the size of the input image.

The dataset was divided into 21 training, two validation and 12 test datasets. The algorithm took the training dataset to adjust the filter kernels to extract characteristic features in the images. The validation dataset is considered a subset of the training dataset and serves as an unbiased early assessment of the algorithm performance. Finally, the test dataset consists of a sample of data used for an unbiased evaluation of the final filter kernels fitted to the training dataset.

The algorithm was trained on the training datasets and corresponding labels in 20 epochs. The training and validation processes were evaluated using binary cross entropy (BCE), according to (3).

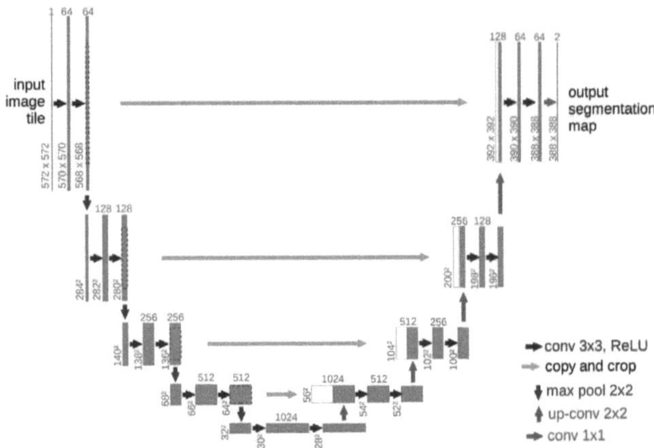

Figure 1: The U-Net is a popular segmentation architecture tailored for pixel-wise prediction. It consists of two paths, namely, the encoder path and the decoder path. The deep features are learned in the encoder path, and the segmentation is performed based on the learned features in the decoder path. Spatial information is transferred to the deeper layers, resulting in a much more accurate segmentation map. The arrows indicate the different operations [6].

$$H(y,p) = -(ylog(p) + (1 - y)log(1 - p)) \tag{3}$$

The BCE measures the efficiency in classifying pixels whose output corresponds to a probability between 0 and 1, smoothed by the log component. The BCE increases when the predicted probability p differs from the actual label y. Since the log is negative in the range between 0 and 1, the BCE equation has a sign. BCE aims to converge to a minimum and thus represents the smallest error between true-positive (TP)/true-negative (TN) and false-positive (FP)/false-negative (FN) pixel classifications [7].

The Dice-Sörensen Coefficient (DSC) was used to numerically evaluate the segmentation or prediction compared to the original labels or ground truth. The DSC measures the similarity between the two images (prediction and ground truth) by comparing the pixels in the images to determine the ratio of TP pixels, FP pixels, and FN pixels, as shown in (4) [8].

$$DSC = \frac{2TP}{2TP + FP + FN} \tag{4}$$

The procedures of training, validation and testing of the algorithm was carried out using Microsoft's InnerEye toolbox. The InnerEye toolbox is capable of training any PyTorch-based algorithm inside of Microsoft AzureML, making use of logging the algorithm's training progress and distributed training on a dedicated GPU (NVIDIA Tesla K80, 6 cores, 56 GB RAM) without code changes. Therefore, the data used for training and validation, the code for image preprocessing and the pre-coded dynamic U-Net were encapsulated into a special container, from which a class was derived that carried all the necessary information needed for training. By passing the container class to the toolbox via terminal commands, training, validation and testing were executed automatically on the AzureML cloud.

2.4   Clinical Evaluation

To evaluate the performance of the algorithm, the angle of glenoid version was measured in 12 CT scans used in the test dataset and corresponding output segmentation map. For this purpose, the measuring tools of an image processing software (3D Slicer, v3.0.5) were used. The evaluation was done by the author and reviewed by an orthopaedic surgeon. That is, the glenoid version values were examined for equality and whether retroversion or anteversion could be reproduced by the segmentations. In Fig. 2 the Friedman method is shown, a common measurement method for glenoid version. It should be noted that the variance in the dataset, and thus in the glenoid version, is prone to error because patient positioning in the various scanning sessions affected the projection of the anatomical structures onto the detector, and the patient population within the dataset was of advanced age and thus showed various signs of arthritic disease such as osteoarthritis.

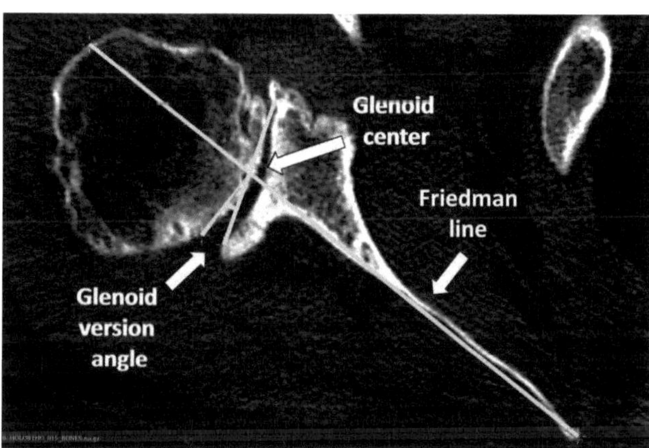

Figure 2: Measurement of glenoid version in the axial view according to the Friedman method. The scapular axis (Friedman line) is perpendicular to the line across the glenoid fossa (intermedial joint line) and passes through the center of the glenoid. The line connecting the edges of the glenoid and the intermedial joint line form the angle of the glenoid version [4].

3   Results and Discussion

3.1   Algorithm Evaluation

The binary cross-entropy loss converged after 15 training epochs, so a successful fit of the filter kernels to the training data was observed, as shown in Fig. 3. In terms of accuracy, the DSC reached a value of about 0.92 after 20 epochs while algorithm training. In the validation dataset, the algorithm stabilized its accuracy at about 0.75 after 16 epochs, indicating that training on 21 training datasets resulted in an early performance on the two validation datasets of 75%.

Our U-Net algorithm achieved a mean DSC value of 0.87 ± 0.08 on the 12 test datasets, ranging from 0.63 to 0.94. This means that the algorithm predicts a segmentation map that overlaps with the label map by 87% on average. Compared

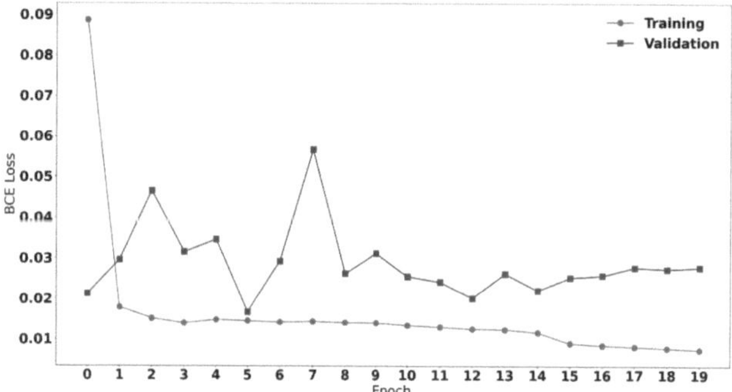

Figure 3: The binary cross-entropy loss as a function of training epochs. The loss decreased over time and converged to an asymptotic value in both the training and validation datasets. This indicates successful learning of image features by the algorithm.

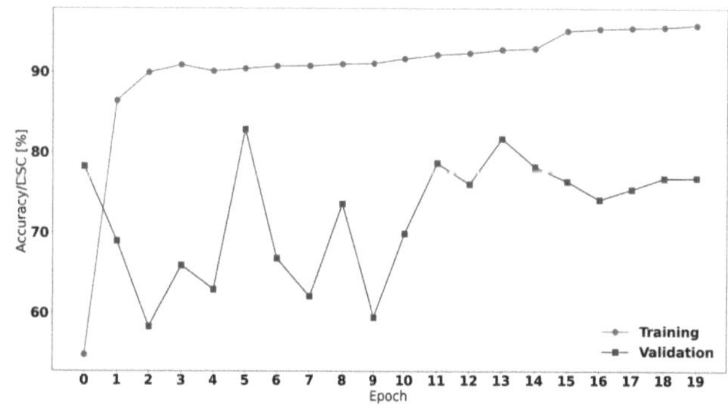

Figure 4: The DSC, or accuracy, as a function of training epochs. The DSC value increased continuously in both the training and validation datasets.

to the DSC values reached by literature references (Table 1), our approach is still below the target limit values.

Table 1: The mean DSC of scapula segmentation algorithms with U-Net, by comparison with the literature.

Experiment	Modality	Training data	Mean DSC
Our approach	Helical CT	21 scans	0.87
Reference [2]	MRI	500 scans	0.91
Reference [8]	2D to 3D reconstruction	1200 biplanar images	0.96

3.2   Clinical Evaluation

Measurements of the glenoid version in the segmentations yielded the results shown in Fig. 5. The negative values of glenoid version apply to retroversion, while the positive values apply to anteversion [4]. The mean values of the results show that most glenoids were in retroversion. The glenoids of the 12 segmentations of the test datasets showed a version from $-20.9°$ to $+5.6°$ (mean= $-8.07° \pm 8.43°$). The glenoids of the 12 corresponding CT images from the test dataset showed a version of -19.3° to +5.5° (mean= -8.23° ± 8.4°).

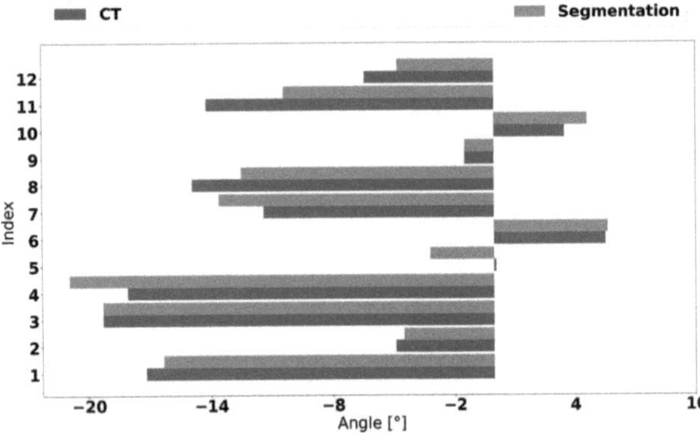

Figure 5: Comparison between glenoid version angle on CT and segmentation map predicted by the U-Net algorithm.

According to [4], the average results of glenoid version measurement show that most glenoids were also in retroversion. Here, the glenoids achieved retroversion in the center of the glenoid in a range from -16.7° to +11.6° (mean= -2.09° ± 6.67°). Thus, because the dataset used in our work was much smaller, the variation is present, but the values are within a plausible range. Fig. 5 shows that the glenoid version in the segmentation maps differed from that in the CT in most cases. In a single case, a change from retroversion to anteversion was observed.

The measurements resulted in a standard error of 2.43° for the segmentations and 2.42° for the test datasets. Looking at the whole dataset of 35 CT scans of 36 shoulder joints, the standard error of the glenoid version was 1.44°. In [4], 104 CT scans were evaluated and the standard error was reported as 0.65°. Since the dataset used in our study was smaller than the dataset evaluated in [4], the accuracy of comparing the glenoid version on CT data with the glenoid version on segmentations should be improved by expanding the dataset and retraining the algorithm with more data.

4 Conclusion

The algorithm achieved an accuracy (DSC) of 87%. However, it still leaves room for improvement. Due to the relatively small dataset used to train the algorithm, compared to [2] (500 scans; DSC = 91%) and [8] (1200 biplanay images; DSC = 96%), the DSC of 87% can be considered reasonable. However, the accuracy of the segmentations was sufficient to determine glenoid version angles that were close to the angles in the CT datasets, comparing a mean version of -8.23° with -8.07°. To achieve better accuracy in both segmentation and glenoid version measurement, more CT scans need to be collected and labelled, thus increasing the training dataset on which to retrain the algorithm.

Therefore, the next steps include the assembly of a larger training dataset to achieve higher DSC values. In addition, automation of the determination of the glenoid version angles on the segmentations should be integrated. Furthermore, by adding post-processing steps to enable the algorithm to output the segmentation as an STL object, a planning tool for implant positioning can be developed using 3D mixed reality devices such as Microsoft HoloLens.

Acknowledgement

The work has been carried out at apoQlar GmbH, Hamburg and was supervised by Dr.-Ing. Erhardt Barth, Institute of Neuro- and Bioinformatics, Universität zu Lübeck.

Author's Statement

Conflict of interest: Authors state no conflict of interest.

References

[1] Oluwatobi Olaiya et al. "Templating in shoulder arthroplasty – A comparison of 2D CT to 3D CT planning software: A systematic review". In: *Shoulder Elbow* 12 (5 Oct. 2020), pp. 303–314.

[2] Xinhong Mu et al. "In-depth learning of automatic segmentation of shoulder joint magnetic resonance images based on convolutional neural networks". In: *Computer Methods and Programs in Biomedicine* 211 (Nov. 2021), p. 106325.

[3] D. R. Sarvamangala and Raghavendra V. Kulkarni. "Convolutional neural networks in medical image understanding: a survey". In: *Evolutionary Intelligence* 15 (1 Mar. 2022), pp. 1–22.

[4] Petr Fulin et al. "Study of the variability of scapular inclination and the glenoid version - considerations for preoperative planning: clinical-radiological study". In: *BMC Musculoskeletal Disorders* 18 (Dec. 2017), p. 16.

[5] Joachim Feger. "Shoulder protocol (CT)". In: https://radiopaedia.org/articles/ct-shoulder-protocol-1 [last accessed on 2023-02-03].

[6] Olaf Ronneberger, Philipp Fischer, and Thomas Brox. "U-Net: Convolutional Networks for Biomedical Image Segmentation". In: *arXiv - Computer Vision and Pattern Recognition* (May 2015).

[7] Floris van Beers et al. "Deep Neural Networks with Intersection over Union Loss for Binary Image Segmentation". In: *Proceedings of the 8th International Conference on Pattern Recognition Applications and Methods* (2019), pp. 438 445.

[8] Catherine Namayega et al. "Contour detection in synthetic bi-planar X-ray images of the scapula: Towards improved 3D reconstruction using deep learning". In: *Proceedings - IEEE 20th International Conference on Bioinformatics and Bioengineering, BIBE 2020* (Oct. 2020), pp. 303–307.

Adaptive Contrast Enhancement with Image-to-Image Translation for Digital X-Ray Images

Ann-Kathrin Popp [1], Mona Schumacher [2], and Marian Himstedt [3]

[1] Medical Informatics, Universität zu Lübeck, annkathrin.popp@student.uni-luebeck.de
[2] MeVis Medical Solutions AG, mona.schumacher@mevis.de
[3] Institute of Medical Informatics, Universität zu Lübeck, marian.himstedt@uni-luebeck.de

Abstract

Digital radiography in medicine is a widely used imaging method for obtaining visual information about the inside of a body. To prepare the acquired raw image for diagnostic evaluation, the contrast must be adjusted depending on the examined part of the body. The contrast enhancement of an image can be considered as a style transfer or an image-to-image translation which is an important field in deep learning. Based on common methods like the pix2pix network that only translate from one domain into one other, we propose a method for translating into multiple domains in one training. We provide additional information about the examination to the network for a specific adjustment of the contrast. Compared to the pix2pix network, our method reduces the mean squared error by a factor of six and achieves an improvement of approximately seven percentage points for the histogram intersection with the histogram of the target image.

1   Introduction

Medical radiographic imaging is a widely used procedure for visual representations of different body structures such as bones, soft tissue, organs or vessels. The acquired raw image needs to be processed to enhance the contrast and thus receive an evaluable image for the radiologist. Depending on the body part and examination (exam), some structures shall be enhanced while others shall be suppressed. For instance, hand examinations mainly aim to visualise bones to diagnose typical injuries like fractures. Images of the abdomen are intented to especially highlight internal organs. There are also cases in which the same body part is scanned but different anatomical structures are of interest. For thoracic images, the focus can either lie on the lung which requires the suppression of rib bones (chest exam), or on ribs, disregarding lung structures (rib exam). In order to meet these various requirements, the exposure voltage and duration can be modulated or image processing techniques can be utilised. Classical image processing algorithms often require a number of various parameters or settings that need to be adjusted for each body region or exam. But the processing can also be considered as a style transfer. This is realised by image-to-image translation which has become a major research field in deep learning in recent years.

Isola *et al.* [1] proposed a conditional generative adversarial network (cGAN) called *pix2pix* which translates images from one domain into a target domain. In [2], Denck *et al.* extended this approach by additionally providing acquisition parameters to the pix2pix network to adjust the contrast in magnetic resonance images after their acquisition. To in-

sert these conditions, they add an auxiliary classifier (AC) to the discriminator and conditional instance normalisation layers to the generator.

The original pix2pix network is able to apply one style transfer to one image and thus, for thoracic images, can either show ribs or lung structures enhanced. To address this limitation, we propose a method that allows the application of two distinct style transfers to the same image and therefore is able to show different body regions enhanced for the same raw image. For this purpose, we derive from [2] and insert a class condition (type of exam) into the pix2pix network. Contrary to [2], we concatenate an additional channel to the input containing the class information. We compare our method with the original pix2pix network and evaluate it visually and quantitatively.

2   Material and Methods

2.1   Network Architecture

Our approach is adopted from the original pix2pix network described in [1] which is based on a GAN architecture. It consists of a U-Net generator, G, and a PatchGAN [1] discriminator, D. The discriminator classifies the images in patches of 70×70 pixels by using the least squares error from the Least Squares GAN (LSGAN) [3] which helps to prevent gradient vanishing. In addition to the L1 loss [1], the LSGAN loss is included in the generator objective function, L_G, as well. We extended L_G by a structual similarity index measure (SSIM) [4] loss $L_{\mathrm{SSIM}}(x, y) = 1 - \mathrm{SSIM}(x, y)$. The resulting objective function for the

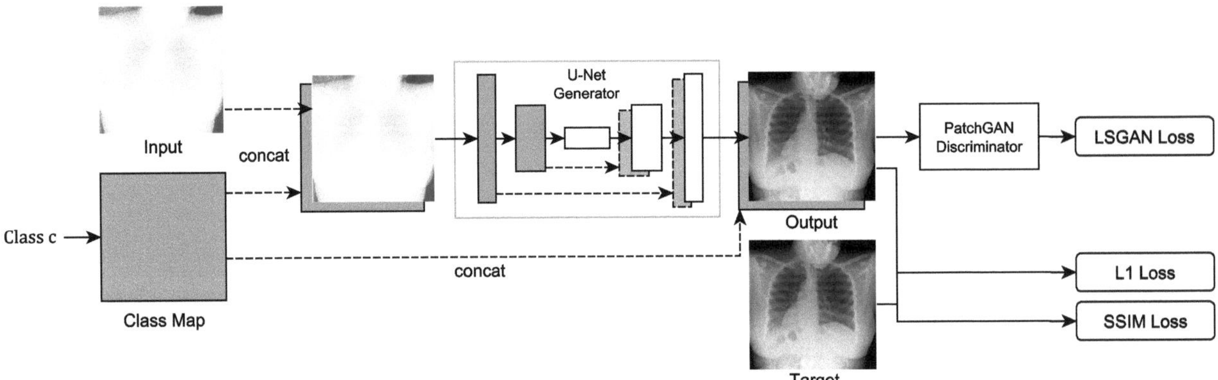

Figure 1: Network architecture of our approach. The input is expanded by concatenating a map containing the class c (type of examination). The unprocessed input image is given to the U-Net generator which aims to mimic processed images. The PatchGAN discriminator then decides whether the generated image is real or generated. The network is trained by a combination of L1 loss and SSIM loss between the generator output and the target image, as well as the adversarial loss of the discriminator. The generator and discriminator architectures are adopted from the original pix2pix network [1] and were adjusted by an additional input channel and an additional block in both paths of the U-Net.

generator is

$$L_G(x, y) = L_{\text{LSGAN}}(D(G(x), x), 1) + \lambda_1 L_{\text{L1}}(G(x), y) \\ + \lambda_2 L_{\text{SSIM}}(G(x), y) \tag{1}$$

with x as the input image, y as the target and $G(x)$ as the generated image. As in [5], $\lambda_1 = 100$, $\lambda_2 = 5$ are used for weighting the individual functions. Moreover, we extend the U-Net generator by one layer in depth to enable training on images of 1024×1024 pixels. An overview of the network is depicted in Fig. 1.

For providing class information to the network, in our case the type of exam, we generate class maps of the same size as the input image which represents its corresponding label y. The encoding of y is inspired by the CMP Facade Database [6] which was also used in [1]. In this dataset, each label is assigned to an integer class value $c \in [0, C - 1]$ for C different classes. As we have image-wise labels, all values in one class map correspond to the same c.

2.2 Data

The dataset used for this work contains 164 unprocessed 16-bit X-ray DICOM images acquired using Nexus DR (Varex Imaging, USA) software. The ground truth was obtained by Nexus DR as well by performing classical image processing on the raw images. All images have a pixel size of either 0.100 or 0.139 mm and a total size between 2421×2107 and 3483×4247 pixels. Included body exams are Chest in posteroanterior (PA) view and Ribs in PA and anteroposterior (AP) view with 82 images each. Each exam is assigned a class label $c \in [0, 1]$ for $C = 2$ classes. Raw and processed images are subsequently resized to 1024×1024 pixels via bilinear interpolation to obtain an equal resolution and normalised to intensity values within [-1, 1]. The dataset is then split into three sets for training (60%), validation (20%) and testing (20%).

2.3 Experiments

To show the ability of our approach to learn to perform different contrast adjustments on images depending on (class) information provided to the network, we trained and evaluated our method on the described chest and rib dataset depicting the same body region and image details.

To determine the impact of adding class information to the task of image-to-image translation and different contrast adjustments, we first trained a standard pix2pix with only X-ray image data as input. Afterwards, we extend that with our approach and add class labels to the network input to learn various contrast styles independently.

For both trainings, the generator and discriminator are respectively trained by using Adam optimisers with initial learning rates of 2×10^{-4} adapted by a LambdaLR scheduler starting after 50 epochs. Our method is trained for 1,200 epochs while the pix2pix network is stopped after 800 epochs as its GAN loss is starting to diverge. Moreover, on-the-fly data augmentation is applied incorporating random flips and rotations. For evaluation, the mean squared error (MSE) is used for pixel-wise intensity comparison of output images with their target. Furthermore, we compare the similarity between the generated and target images by analysing their histograms and intersection as the network is meant to learn a transfer in style and therefore a distribution of intensities. However, background pixels (intensity < 5000) are not taken into account here.

3 Results and Discussion

We compare the results from pix2pix with those from our approach and qualitatively evaluate the effect of processing the same images with different label inputs in our proposed work. Quantitative results are listed in Table 1. In comparison to pix2pix, our method results in a reduction of

Table 1: Quantitative results for experiments with common pix2pix and additional class condition between generated and target images. The MSE of image intensities was computed on normalised images with intensities in [0, 1] while the histogram intersection is obtained on 16-bit images. The intersection is a measure of the similarity of the histograms for the generated and target image. The values are given as average $\pm$ standard deviation.

	Examination	Class / Label	MSE	Histogram Intersection [%]
pix2pix	Ribs	-	0.012 ± 0.009	75.7 ± 5.3
pix2pix	Chest	-	0.007 ± 0.008	78.6 ± 7.1
proposed method	Ribs	0 / "Ribs"	0.002 ± 0.002	83.8 ± 2.0
proposed method	Chest	1 / "Chest"	0.001 ± 0.002	84.1 ± 2.5

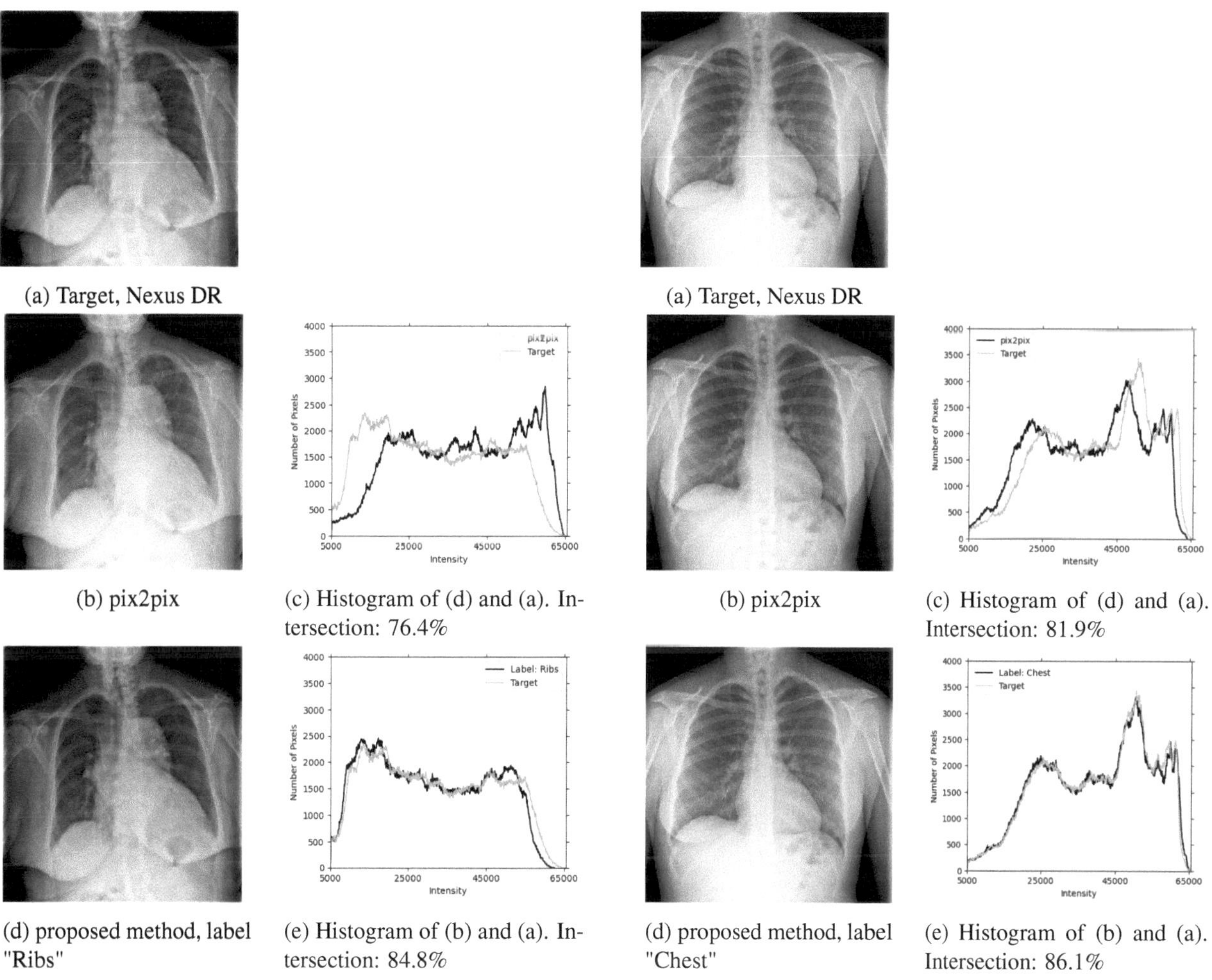

(a) Target, Nexus DR

(b) pix2pix

(c) Histogram of (d) and (a). Intersection: 76.4%

(d) proposed method, label "Ribs"

(e) Histogram of (b) and (a). Intersection: 84.8%

(a) Target, Nexus DR

(b) pix2pix

(c) Histogram of (d) and (a). Intersection: 81.9%

(d) proposed method, label "Chest"

(e) Histogram of (b) and (a). Intersection: 86.1%

Figure 2: Example of processed X-ray images of a rib exam in PA view. Target images are obtained with Nexus DR (a). Generated, processed images are obtained through our method (d) which gets the label "Ribs" as additional input and by the pix2pix network (b). The histograms of the images and their targets are depicted next to them (e), (c).

Figure 3: Example of processed X-ray images of a chest exam in PA view. Target images are obtained with Nexus DR (a). Generated, processed images are obtained through our method (d) which gets the label "Chest" as additional input and by the pix2pix network (b). The histograms of the images and their targets are depicted next to them (e), (c).

the MSE by a factor of six for both rib and chest examinations. Moreover, the histogram intersection of rib images can be improved by approximately eight percentage points (p.p.) while that of chest images is improved by 5.5 p.p. These results match the impression gained from the visual inspection of the generated images. Fig. 2 and Fig. 3 show target images and generated ones of pix2pix and our approach for ribs and chest images along with corresponding

histograms. In these examples, the intensity distribution of generated images by pix2pix deviates more from the target than those generated by our method. Furthermore, by utilising our method with differing input labels on the same image, it is possible to generate images with characteristics of the respective class. An image fed into our network with the label "Ribs" will produce a darker image in the lung re-

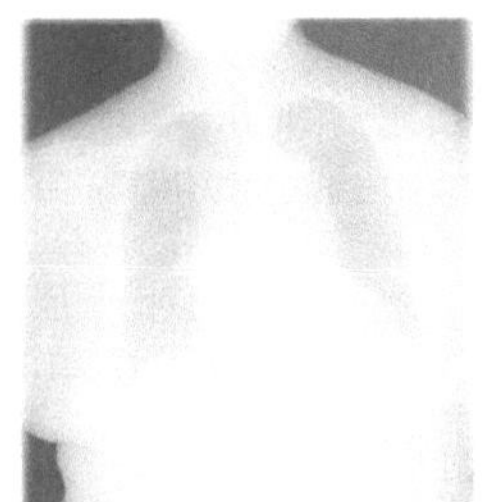

(a) Raw image (ribs)

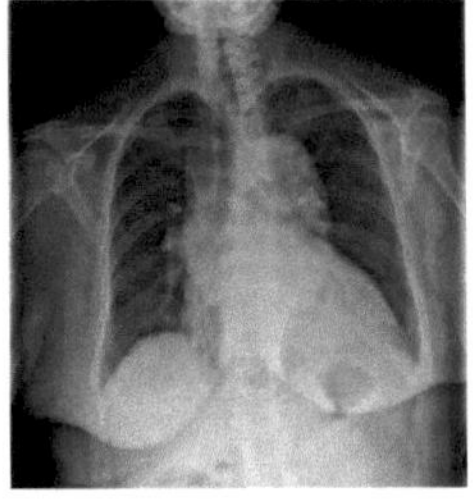

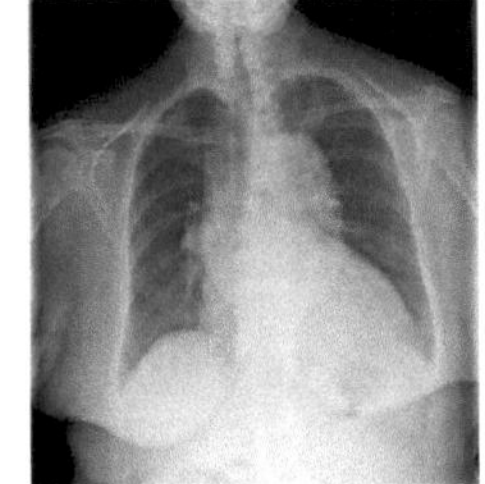

(b) Generated image by our method, label "Ribs"

(c) Generated image by our method, label "Chest"

Figure 4: Different processings of a rib exam raw image (a) by our method. Depending on the input label ("Ribs"/"Chest"), our method generates either a rib enhancing image (b) or a lung enhancing one (c).

gion compared to the same image with the label "Chest", which is more likely to reveal structures in the lung area. This can be seen in Fig. 4.

Regarding to the histograms of generated rib images, the traditional pix2pix method frequently produces images with an intensity distribution that is more consistent with chest images than its actual target rib image. This phenomenon is observed in 56% of rib images, which all have a larger histogram intersection (approximately 10 p.p. on average) with images generated by our method with "Chest" as the incorrect input label. An example of this is shown in Fig. 5. For chest images, only approximately 13% of cases show a similar pixel value distribution as rib exams.

4   Conclusion

We presented a method to adaptively enhance image contrasts using a conditioned image-to-image translation. In comparison with the original pix2pix network, we could improve the histogram intersection by eight percentage points for rib and by 5.5 points for chest images, using images obtained from a commercial X-ray imaging software as target. The MSE could be decreased by a factor of six compared to pix2pix generated images. Furthermore, we have shown that it is possible to create two different images from the same input image highlighting different structures with a single network, depending on a label input.

In future work, we will include more body regions and more class labels into the training to expand the network to more different contrast adjustments. However, since the training is supervised, it is not to be expected that the quality of generated images exceeds the quality of the target images.

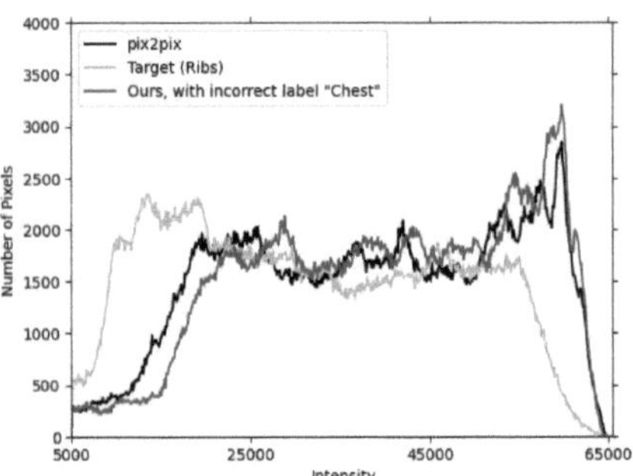

Figure 5: Histogram of a rib examination image processed by pix2pix (Fig. 2b), our approach with "Chest" as the incorrect label (Fig. 4c) and Nexus DR as target (Fig. 2a).

Acknowledgement

The work has been carried out at MeVis Medical Solutions AG, Bremen and supervised by the Institute of Medical Informatics, Universität zu Lübeck. Special thanks to Dr. Hauke Haehne and Moritz Wernke-Schmiesing (MeVis Medical Solutions AG) for valuable discussions. All images are used with courtesy of Varex Imaging, USA.

Author's Statement

Conflict of interest: Authors state no conflict of interest.

5   References

[1] P. Isola, J.-Y. Zhu, T. Zhou, and A. A. Efros, "Image-to-image translation with conditional adversarial networks," in *Computer Vision and Pattern Recognition (CVPR), 2017 IEEE Conference on*, 2017.

[2] J. Denck, J. Guehring, A. Maier, and E. Rothgang, "MR-contrast-aware image-to-image translations with generative adversarial networks," *International Journal of Computer Assisted Radiology and Surgery*, vol. 16, no. 12, pp. 2069–2078, 2021.

[3] X. Mao, Q. Li, H. Xie, R. Y. Lau, Z. Wang, and S. P. Smolley, "Least squares generative adversarial networks," in *2017 IEEE International Conference on Computer Vision (ICCV)*, 2017, pp. 2813–2821.

[4] Z. Wang, A. Bovik, H. Sheikh, and E. Simoncelli, "Image quality assessment: from error visibility to structural similarity," *IEEE Transactions on Image Processing*, vol. 13, no. 4, pp. 600–612, 2004.

[5] Z. Hua, L. Qi, Z. Yang, and Y. Sun, "The improved pix2pix generative adversarial networks for sand-dust image enhancement," 2022. [Online]. Available: https://doi.org/10.21203/rs.3.rs-2191083/v1

[6] R. Tylecek and R. Sára, "Spatial pattern templates for recognition of objects with regular structure," in *Pattern Recognition*, 2013, pp. 364–374.

Bodypart segmentation in radiography using Time-of-Flight Cameras

Ferdinand Petrat [1],

[1] Medical Engineering Science, Universität zu Lübeck, ferdinand.petrat@student.uni-luebeck.de

Abstract

When performing X-ray examinations the patients and radiographers safety is always of upmost importance. To make sure that the exposure to X-rays is kept to a minimum a neural network is trained to segment body parts hoping to increase safety by recognizing those body parts positioned falsely. Utilizing Time-of-Flight cameras 3D data in the form of point clouds are captured, containing the X-ray room and the people therein. The neural network chosen is PointNet as it is simple to use and can be trained on point clouds directly. An average accuracy of 86.6% is achieved indicating the applicability of PointNet for the presented task.

1 Introduction

3D geometric data such as point clouds and meshes are becoming more and more prevalent in everyday tasks. Cars, self-driving or not, and autonomous robots need to be able to recognize people and objects [1]. In clinical settings the ability to track doctors, nurses and patients can improve efficiency of the surgical workflow and increase the patients safety [2].

Especially X-ray imaging poses a safety risk to the people involved, ionizing radiation can damage cells leading to cancer [3]. Only those parts of the patients body that need to be examined should be exposed. A weary inexperienced radiographer who is pressed for time can make mistakes causing additional costs due to the need of a repeated examination and future health problems for the patient. Therefore a system that can automatically detect people and body parts in an X-ray room and in this way help by decreasing risks is explored in this paper. To detect body parts a neural network first needs to be trained to perform semantic segmentations on 3D data. One common approach is the voxelization of captured 3D point clouds [4]. Voxelization is the process of plotting a point cloud onto a grid of equally spaced 3D voxels, which then can be processed by established convolutional neural networks. This process however makes the data much more voluminous, resulting in more inefficient training whilst also introducing quantization artifacts. PointNet on the other hand can be trained on point clouds directly, bypassing the problems of voxelization and allowing for efficient learning [5]. Figure 1 shows the main process from input data to predictions of body parts.

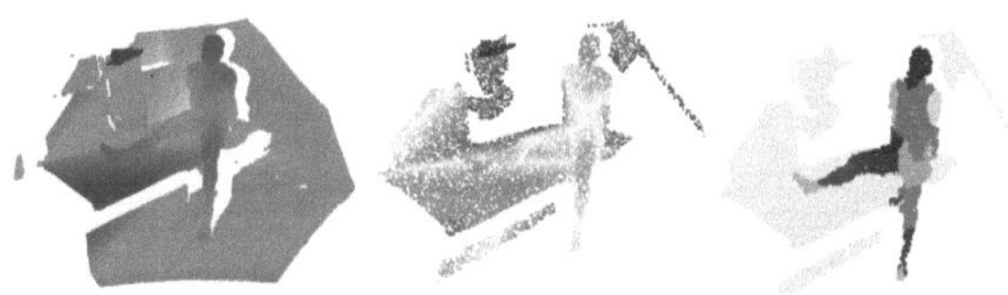

Figure 1: Main process: input point cloud (left), preprocessing, sampling and augmentations (middle), output point cloud with labeled body parts (right)

2 Dataset

The dataset consists of 498 point clouds and depicts clinically relevant scenes in an X-ray room. Three Time-of-Flight (ToF) cameras (Microsoft Azure Kinect DK [6]) were used. Alongside RGB-data ToF cameras can also detect depth information by measuring the round-trip time of reflected light. One camera was placed on a tripod, the other two were mounted on the X-ray unit. Figure 2 shows labeling data from two points of view. On the left the point of view of an X-ray unit mounted camera is shown, depicting an X-ray examination of a patients right leg. On the right the whole patients body can be seen.

Four different people were captured in poses imitating common examinations in radiography such as for ankle injuries or abdominal pain. Most data captured by the X-ray unit mounted cameras show the abdomen, the knee joints and the upper ankle joints. Additionally the X-ray room was captured by itself, primarily showing the X-ray unit and the examination table alongside parts of walls and floor.

Each of the 498 point clouds contains 368.640 points in 3D-

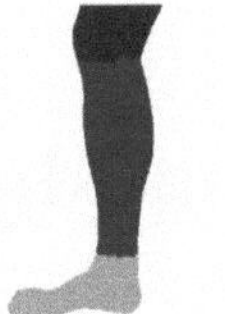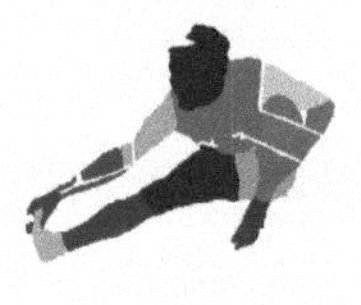

Figure 2: Label data showcasing the ToF cameras points of view: cameras 2 and 3 mounted on the X-ray unit (left), camera 1 on tripod (right).

space. Every point cloud was labeled manually corresponding to the following classes: background, head, torso, left upper arm, right upper arm, left lower arm, right lower arm, left hand, right hand, left thigh, right thigh, left lower leg, right lower leg, left foot and right foot. The distribution of classes is shown in Fig 3.

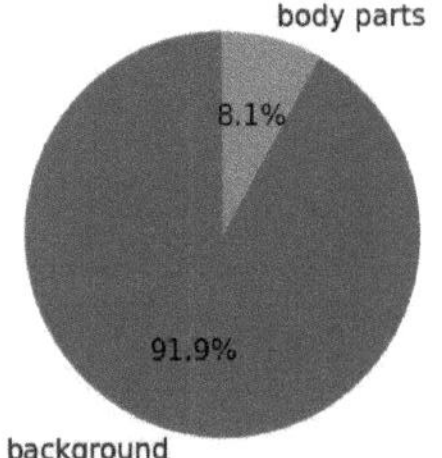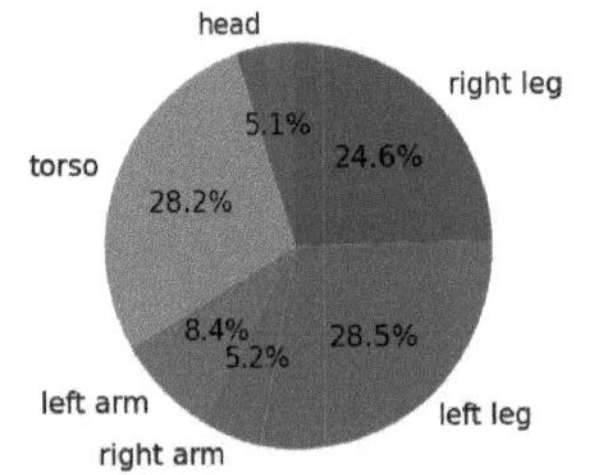

Figure 3: Class distribution: share of all points labeled as a body part compared to the background, indicating a vast majority of background points (left). Distribution of classes without background, for comprehensibility combined into head, torso, left arm, right arm, left leg and right leg (right).

Class imbalance is a problem that is prevalent in many datasets [7]. A common way to deal with this problem is called undersampling. By removing a portion of samples of the majority class, in this case background points, the dataset is more balanced. Before training begins the following steps are taken to reduce the amount of background points. First, points that are part of the floor and points that are far away from the point clouds center are erased. Second, invalid points are erased. Invalid points occur when the depth camera cannot return correct values, for instance due to saturation of the infrared signal [6]. These points are labeled as background. Those two steps reduce the share of background labels to about 80%. Another way of dealing with imbalanced classes is the use of class-specific weightings. By calculating the percentage of each label a weight is determined that influences the loss function during training. Less represented classes will have a higher impact on the learning process. To help the network generalize and make it more robust the following augmentations are applied: rotations, scaling, jitter, and shuffling of the points order. These augmentations provide a natural variation to the input data.

3 Training and Testing

3.1 PointNet

The PointNet [5], developed by Charles R. Qi, Hao Su, Kaichun Mo and Leonidas J. Guibas, is a neural network that specializes in object classification and semantic segmentation of shapes in unordered 3D point clouds. The basic network architecture is shown in Fig. 4. First the input which is comprised of points in x-, y- and z-coordinates is transformed to provide invariance to permutations and geometric transformations such as rotation and translation. This alignment into a canonical space is done in two steps by the so called T-Net and a multi-layer perceptron which increases the amount of features. A vector containing global features is then created by aggregation of found features using max-pooling. For semantic segmentation, the assignment of a label to each point, these global and features are concatenated with local features, which in turn is used to output point specific scores for every label.

3.2 Training process

Before training the dataset is split into two parts. The training dataset contains about 90% of the data. For evaluation of the training the remaining 10% are used. To improve efficiency of the training 10.000 points are sampled randomly from each point cloud. For training the negative log likelihood is applied to calculate the loss, utilizing the aforementioned weightings for each label. To track the training progress and evaluate the networks performance the accuracy is measured. The accuracy is defined as the amount of points whose labels are predicted correct when compared to the ground truth. The Adam optimizer [8], a learning rate of 0.001 and a batch size of 16 are used to train PointNet for 40.000 epochs. In addition an experiment is performed to determine the impact of class imbalance: classes are combined in three ways as seen in Table 1 and each combination is trained for 10.000 epochs. Especially the third combination, training on just the two labels background and body, is expected to achieve a much higher accuracy compared to the original training.

Table 1: Combinations of classes

#	Combined class	Labels
1	upper body	thorax, head
	left arm	left upper and lower arm, left hand
	right arm	right upper and lower arm, right hand
	left leg	left thigh, left lower leg, left foot
	right leg	right thigh, right lower leg, right foot
2	upper body	head, thorax, both arms
	lower body	both legs and feet
3	whole body	all non-background labels

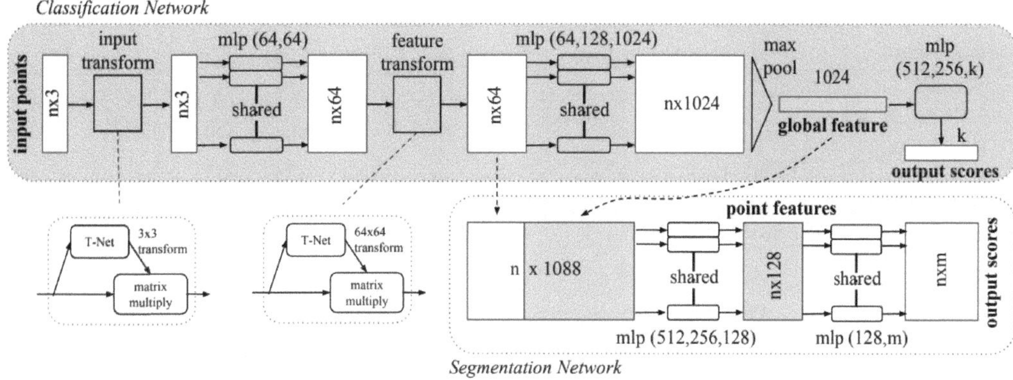

Figure 4: Illustration of the PointNet architecture [5]: a vector of n points is used as input, a matrix of size n x m is the output, with m containing class-specific scores for each point.

3.3 Post-processing

One possible post-processing step is a cluster analysis, utilizing the *fcluster*-module from *scipy* [9]. Points featuring the same label that are in close proximity are considered to be of the same body part. This enables the algorithm to make more precise assumptions about the quantity of present body parts and their locations. An example of this post-processing step is shown in Fig. 5.

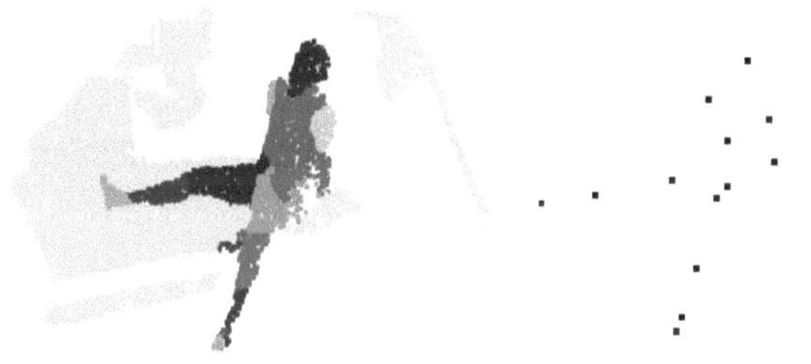

Figure 5: Post-processing: cluster analysis on segmentation results (left) to find each body parts central point (right)

4 Results and Discussion

An example of a labeled point cloud is shown in Fig. 6. While there are some mislabeled points, mainly parts of the examination table in contact with the body, most points are labeled correctly. The average accuracy for predicted labels is 86.6%. But whereas the background is labeled with an accuracy of more than 95%, for some body parts an accuracy of just 10% is achieved. Table 2 lists accuracies for selected body parts.

The low accuracy for the right hand is caused by class underrepresentation. It can also be seen that for the body's right side (right arm/leg) a higher accuracy was achieved compared to the body's left side (left arm/leg). This is due to the way the point clouds are captured, the left side being occluded more often than the right. Another problem is a *near-miss* case. For example a point located at the ankle, that is part of the foot but is mislabeled as part of the lower

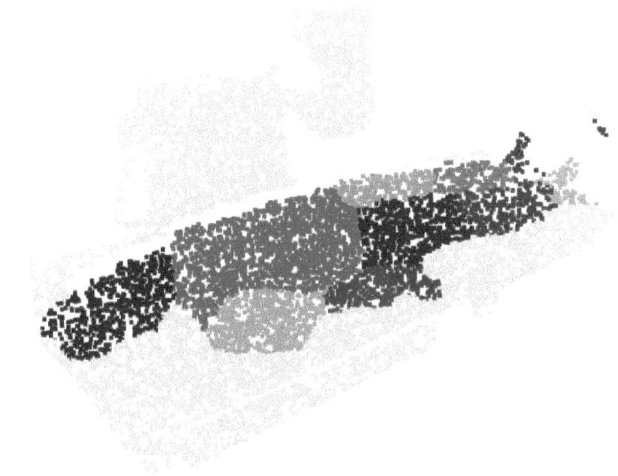

Figure 6: Segmentation results: A human laying on an examination table can be seen.

leg is considered wrong and has a negative effect on the accuracy. Depending on the task at hand it can be debated if the networks performance is sufficient. A task that does not need accurate segmentations of every body part might be satisfied with these results. This aspect becomes more evident when looking at the results of the training on the combined classes. Reducing the classes to upper body, left arm, right arm left leg, right leg and background results in an accuracy of 89%, reducing the classes to background, upper and lower body results in an accuracy of 93%, while training on just background and body achieves an accuracy of 96%. Figure 7 illustrates these results: Most points are labeled correctly, with just a few points misclassified located at the right hand and hip.

5 Conclusion

This paper presents an application of PointNet for a simple way to efficiently perform semantic segmentation of body parts in 3D data. Given the rather small dataset and the issues discussed the resulting performance of the trained model can be considered sufficient. A task such as recognizing certain body parts to assure safety during an X-

Table 2: Accuracies

Body part	Accuracy
Thorax	80.6%
Left thigh	56.7%
Right hand	10.5%
Background	95.4%
Whole point cloud	86.6%
Left arm	37.1%
Right arm	44.7%
Left leg	66.1%
Right leg	74.6%

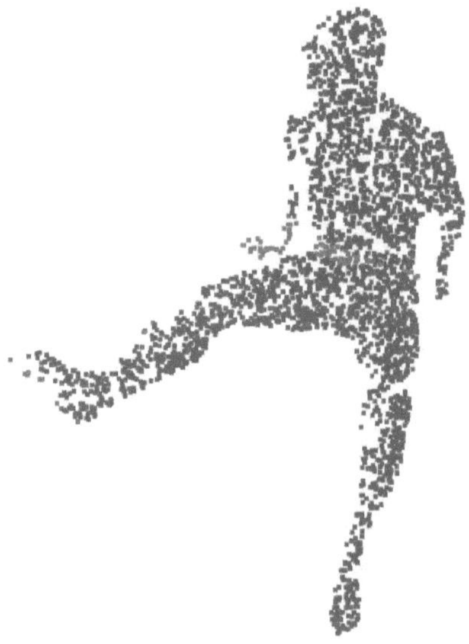

Figure 7: Comparison with ground truth: most labels correct, few points at the hip and right hand wrong.

ray examination could be accomplished. Increasing the datasets size especially in regards to the underrepresented classes can lead to even more accurate predictions. Also, there are newer more proficient models such as PointNet++, which exploits the points distances in metric space allowing the network to learn the local features contexts [10], or the PVCNN which combines the advantages of both voxel- and point-based neural network models [11]. For the task of segmenting body parts both of these models need to be explored.

Acknowledgement

The work has been carried out at the Institute of Neuro- and Bioinformatics, Universität zu Lübeck.
Many thanks to Celina-Christin Schubbe for providing the dataset, including the labeled data.

Author's Statement

Conflict of interest: Authors state no conflict of interest.

6   References

[1] K. Zheng, W. and C. Xiaoping, *Laser-Based People Detection and Obstacle Avoidance for a Hospital Transport Robot.* Sensors, vol. 21, 2021.

[2] D.C. Birkhoff, A. v. Dalen and M.P. Schijven *A Review on the Current Applications of Artificial Intelligence in the Operating Room.* Surgical Innovation, vol. 28, pp. 611-619, 2021.

[3] E.C. Lin. *Radiation risk from medical imaging.* Mayo Clinic Proceedings, vol. 85, pp. 1142-1146, 2010.

[4] Y. Zhou and O. Tuzel. *VoxelNet: End-to-End Learning for Point Cloud Based 3D Object Detection.* arXiv e-prints, 2017.

[5] C. R. Qi, H. Su, K. Mo, and L. J. Guibas, *PointNet: Deep Learning on Point Sets for 3D Classification and Segmentation.* Proceedings of the IEEE Conference on Computer Vision and Pattern Recognition, 2017.

[6] *Azure Kinect DK documentation,*
URL: https://learn.microsoft.com/en-us/azure/kinect-dk/depth-camera [last visited 2023-01-18].

[7] M. Buda, A. Maki and M.A. Mazurowski, *A Systematic Study of the Class Imbalance Problem in Convolutional Neural Networks.* Neural Networks, vol. 106, pp. 249-259, 2018.

[8] P. Diederik, J. B. Kingma. *Adam: A Method for Stochastic Optimization.* 3rd International Conference on Learning Representations, 2015.

[9] *SciPy documentation.* URL: https://docs.scipy.org/doc/scipy/reference/generated/scipy.cluster.hierarchy.fcluster.html [last accessed on 2023-01-18].

[10] C. R. Qi, L. Yi, H. Su, and L.J. Guibas. *PointNet++: Deep Hierarchical Feature Learning on Point Sets in a Metric Space.* Proceedings of the 31st International Conference on Neural Information Processing Systems, pp. 5105–5114, 2017.

[11] Z. Liu, H. Tang, Y. Lin and S. Han. *Point-Voxel CNN for Efficient 3D Deep Learning.* Proceedings of the 33rd International Conference on Neural Information Processing Systems, vol. 2, pp. 965-975, 2019.

Segmentation of medium-sized Pulmonary Vessels based on a 3D U-Net Approach

Karoline Heber [1]

[1] Medical Engineering Science, Universität zu Lübeck, karoline.heber@student.uni-luebeck.de

Abstract

Automated pulmonary vessel segmentation supports radiologists and is a challenging task to accomplish. In this paper, a 3D U-Net to predict medium-sized vessel masks in the lung lobes is presented. For data preparation, reference masks based on a heuristic method called vesselness have been generated and the cases were chosen which fulfill predefined visual criteria. As a result, the network is able to mimic the reference masks over the test dataset with a mean Dice score of 93.62%. The other topological and volumetric metrics reach mean values beyond 90% as well. The visual evaluation shows incomplete segmentation results in the transition area from the mediastinum to the lung lobes and also reveals difficulties with the connection of smaller vessel structures which need further research.

1 Introduction

A challenging structure to observe for a radiologist is the pulmonary vessel tree which is complex, highly inter-twined, and consists of a huge number of branches. Its assessment is relevant in the diagnosis of serious lung diseases like pulmonary emboli and pulmonary hypertension [1], but also for planning, investigating and follow-up of lung surgeries [2]. Moreover, its results can for instance improve the detection of the airway tree [2]. In order to support clinicians in providing an accurate diagnosis or treatment, an effective automatic vessel segmentation can be useful. One example of a heuristic method is the vesselness approach which identifies the vessels by their tubularity under consideration of the vessel brightness and curvature in terms of the Hessian matrix. As a benefit, this technique can distinguish well between lung tissue and vessel structures, but in combination with a region growing technique, it suffers in the evaluation of tissue with similar grey value intensities, measured in Hounsfield Units (HU), like tumor nodules or dense lesions [2].

In 2015, a deep learning architecture called U-Net was proposed which revolutionized the voxelwise detection of target structures. It has become one of the most important semantic segmentation frameworks for supervised learning and many attempts for extended techniques have been made [3]. One of its strengths is the capability to learn contextual information by aggregating global context and observing relevant spatial details. But a supervised approach for an U-Net requires a lot of data with associated annotation masks. This requirement is hard to fulfill because the manual voxelwise extraction of 3D data like Computed Tomography (CT) is a tedious and time-consuming task for experts.

In this paper, a 3D U-Net with an adapted deep learning training is used in order to predict the pulmonary vessels. To that end, pulmonary vessel masks in the lung lobes were generated as references with a vesselness method. Besides a visual evaluation of the results, the performance of the U-Net is assessed using volumetric and topological metrics. This semantic segmentation approach concentrates mainly on medium-sized vessels without distinguishing between veins and arteries. It should be pointed out that the generated annotations of the dataset have not been observed and evaluated by an expert yet. Therefore, no statement can be made as to whether the outputs of the U-Net are suitable for radiological reporting, hence further clinical validation is required.

2 Material and Methods

2.1 Dataset

The contrasted 3D chest CT scans used in this work were compiled from both public and internal datasets. 85 cases stem from the public dataset by The Lung Image Database Consortium and Image Database Consortium [4] and 15 cases from the public Extraction of Airways from CT 2009 challenge [5] were used. Additionally, an internal dataset from the Ruhrlandklinik Essen and Missions-ärztliche Klinik Würzburg consisting of 18 cases as well as a dataset with 327 cases supplied by the Diagnostik Image Analysis Group (DIAG) at Radboud University Medical Center were included. The patients show a broad range of health statuses from healthy to illnesses with abnormalities in the airway and lung parenchyma e.g. tumor nodules. For the compilation of the dataset, annotations were created for all images and evaluated individually by visual constraints which will be described in the next subsection.

The best 50 annotations with associated CT scans, with a best possible balancing of manufacturers of CT devices, sex and ages of the patients were used as test set. The rest were split randomly into 338 training and 57 validation images.

2.2 Generation of Reference Segmentations

As a preprocessing step, the original CT image voxels are resampled to isotropic size with a length of 0.7mm which lead to annotations with smooth vessel branches in general. CT scans with a large slice thickness over 1.5mm often result in coarse, pixelated vessels despite resampling so they must be sorted out. As a further step towards the unification of the dataset, the minimum grey value is set to -1000 HU. This value corresponds to air, which makes up the majority of the lung volume, and provides a clear contrast to the vessels. Smaller values are cut off.

An already implemented method to create vessel references has been introduced in the VESSEL12-Challenge [1] and works as follows: at first, a lung mask consisting of lung lobes is generated with a classical image processing approach. For further usage, the volume 15mm away from the outer lung boundary is excluded which results in a smaller mask. Other anatomical structures to ignore are the airways, which can be detected by a simple coarse bronchi segmentation. Afterwards, the actual vessel segmentation based on the multi-scale vesselness method [6] begins within the lung masks. This approach is used as a filtering process that computes the likelihood of a voxel to belong to a tubular geometrical structure. To that end, the orthogonal principal components can be determined by the eigenvalue analysis with the second-order derivatives, obtained by the Hessian matrix. The vesselness results were set at any voxel above the 97% of intensity values afterwards to define seed points. To define which seed points should be used in the further steps, the vesselness threshold needs to be set. This value depends on the grey-scale range of the image and excludes seed points below a response strength. The default of 30 leads to a dense vessel tree which includes also really fine vessels. To facilitate the assessment of the vessel trees, a larger threshold of 70 is defined in order to exclude the finest vessels but obtain a lung-filling vessel tree. The resulting seed points will be connected by a region growing method in the direction of descending vessel branches.

The sorting part of the references should assure good and usable vessel masks for training and evaluation. To that end, a few visual criteria need to be defined. Only coherent and smooth branches are included. With increasing distance to the mediastinum, the vessel diameter should get smaller. Encapsulated spherical tumors which are easy to locate are removed from the mask by hand. Tumors or any kind of mass in connection with vessels could not be evaluated by a non-clinician such that these images had to be sorted out. Artifacts like incomplete plate-like vessel segmentations repeatedly catch the eye. They belong to the large vessels in the mediastinum and were not cohesive to the branches, so had to be removed as well.

2.3 Training Procedure

For the semantic segmentation task, a four-level 3D U-Net has been chosen. A 2D approach with less computational effort would not take into account the dimensional information of adjacent slices which would result in low efficiency and the loss of context [3]. To distinguish between vessels and other structures and obtain coherent branches, the field of view should be as large as possible. Therefore, patches with a fixed size of $92 \times 92 \times 92$ voxels were extracted. Due to the variation of image sizes, an overlapping tile strategy [7] is used. Padding with image information or otherwise with voxel values of -1000 HU with a dimension of $44 \times 44 \times 44$ is added to the patches. Due to the shrinking effect of convolutions, the output size ends up as the same extracted patch size. As loss metric, the combined soft Dice and categorical cross-entropy like in [8] is chosen. In order to prevent the network bottleneck [8], batch normalization follows every convolutional layer. To enhance the performance of the network, data augmentation techniques are applied to mimic realistic CT scans. The first method simulates the different positioning of the patient and triples the original dataset by rotating around the z-axis at angles of $-10°$, $0°$, and $10°$. For an increased diversity of the data, an additive Gaussian noise is applied to the extracted patches. Sigma, the standard deviation of the normal distribution, is randomly selected between 0 and 7 for every patch which leads to a maximum change of 20 HU. During training, the validation is performed every 1000 iterations. The training lasts 250,000 iterations with 2 training patches per batch. To specialize the network on evaluating only lung tissue, only the patches with vessel annotations enter the training loop as input. They consist of 71,832 training and 12,578 validation patches. The Adaptive Moment Estimation (Adam) is used as optimizer. The linearly decaying learning rate initialized at 0.001 and ending at 0.00001 simplifies the fine-tuning in the end. The trained model with the best Jaccard index as a similarity metric on the validation set is kept. The model should optimize its performance within the lung, hence loss weights were set in the lung to the value 1 with a lung mask.

2.4 Evaluation

The performance of the U-Net on unseen test data will be evaluated with volumetric and topological metrics, and also with visual criteria. As volumetric metrics, the Dice score, sensitivity, and precision are used to evaluate the similarity of the masks and how well the deep learning method is able to mimic the annotations. In addition, these metrics are suitable for an imbalanced class problem with vessels as a minority in the volume. As a further volumetric measurement, the volumes of the predicted and reference masks are observed. Because the coherent branches were used as one criterion for well-looking tubular and curvilinear vessel structures, the topological measurement plays an important role. It measures the connectivity by generating a skeleton of the vessel tree and evaluating the intersection with the mask to be compared. As topological similarity metrics, the centerline (cl)Dice [9], clprecision and clsensitivity are applied. The criteria to assess the visual impression are in correspondence with the decision rules for sorting the dataset such as connectivity, artifacts, smoothness, and descending vessel diameter with increasing distance to the mediastinum. Another focus will be put on vessel masks with smaller and larger diameters separately. The smaller vessels in the CT images exhibit lower and less bright HU values than larger ones and may have a width of only a few voxel. Therefore, it is interesting to observe how well the deep learning model will perform on such a multi-scale problem. Being performed by a non-clinician, only similarities, recurring patterns, and abnormalities that catch the eye over a major part of the test data were considered and mentioned. Probably more information about the performance of the U-Net and how accurate the masks are will be obtained by an expert.

3 Results and Discussion

3.1 Numerical Evaluation

The topological and volumetric results from the numerical evaluation are shown in Table 1. Because the results should be as close to 100% as possible, all mean values over 90% of the test dataset seem to indicate the capability of the U-Net to mimic the vesselness annotations mostly reliably. The same applies to all individual test images which can be interpreted with standard deviation less than 2%. At the review of single test image values, no outliers could be detected. To sum up the first impression of this Table, good connectivity of the branches and the high similarity of the masks appear to be essentially achieved. The compiled test dataset should be mentioned for interpretation of the numerical evaluation as well. Only the generated references which fulfill the criteria best were chosen for evaluation of the training performance. Therefore, anomalies and pathological manifestations might be poorly represented in this dataset, so the U-Net has to observe cases which are easier to cope with. In comparison of my numerical results to other publications, the common basis for discussion is missing. In literature, topological evaluation metrics are rather rarely used, the target references can be defined as seed points or volume and mostly, also the finest vessels are included which represents a challenging task in general.

The volumes of the vessel masks are shown in Table 2. The predicted mask volume is on average slightly larger than the mean of the reference data, in 47 cases out of 50. That means, that the deep learning method defines more voxels as the actual vessel structure. If the U-Net either achieves a high false-positive rate or can locate vessels that could not be captured by the vesselness method is hard to determine. The high variance between the volumes can be explained by the different age and sex of the patients.

Table 1: Volumetric and topological evaluation results of the test dataset

metric	mean / %	std / %
clDice	93.23	0.90
clprecision	91.98	1.29
clsensitivity	94.52	1.00
Dice	93.62	0.71
precision	92.51	0.76
sensitivity	94.76	1.03

Table 2: Evaluation of the mask volumes of the U-Net outputs and the vesselness annotations

metric	mean / ml	std / ml
U-Net	131.02	29.78
Reference	127.93	29.05

3.2 Visual Evaluation

The connection of the vessel branches works quite well over the test dataset. The medium-sized vessels are overall cohesive. Only a few single thin long vessels are not connected with the vessel tree in contrast to the vesselness results. Unexpectedly, the network captures a few more small tubular structures with a diameter of a few voxels that are mostly connected with the tree and fulfill the visual criteria. That suggests, it possibly predicts vessels correctly, that could be missed through the high vesselness threshold in the annotation data. The finest vessels of the vesselness method were interpreted differently by the deep learning method. Sometimes, they are not perfectly connected, in some cases, voxels are missing or added. The described phenomena of the small vessels are shown in Fig. 1. The finest, connected vessels in the lung are hard to capture in general. There are much more voxels in the large branches than in smaller ones, so the latter ones have no big impact on the training procedure. In order to improve this, a weighting strategy for increasing the focus on smaller vessels might be helpful. The criterion of descending branches has been met in general. Another striking recurring pattern are small little chunks within the outer boundary of the lung lobes. The preprocessing of the vesselness method includes an eroded lung mask that excludes the outer volume. The precision might be better if only the model output in this area will be evaluated. Some plate-like artifacts at the boundary to the mediastinum, introduced in Section 2.2, are usually ignored correctly. Another area to focus on is the transition from the mediastinum to the lung lobes. The lung mask sets the boundary between these two areas where the division into many vascular branches takes place. For the vesselness method and the U-Net these vessels seem to be hard to capture. The former one could have problems with the junctions not to be clearly tubular and the latter one might be limited by the available annotations. Therefore, holey or incomplete segmentations can be the consequence and require further research.

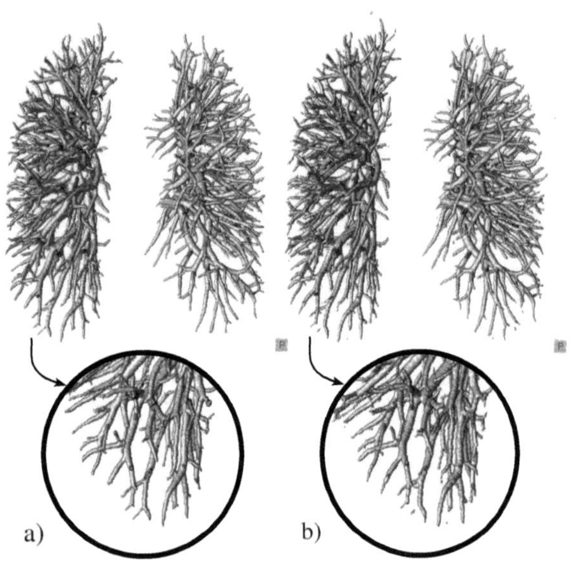

Figure 1: a) an example of a reference mask with vessel branches of the test set, b) the matching, predicted mask of the U-Net which shows different vessel results like elongated or missing small vessels.

4   Conclusion

In conclusion, the U-Net is able to mimic the medium-sized vessel annotations generated by the vesselness method quite well. Moreover, it fulfills the predefined visual criteria well in general. Only an expert may evaluate, how well the annotations and the output of the U-Net correspond to the real vessels. Weaknesses of the deep learning approach seem to be for this specific segmentation task probably the connection and prediction of smaller vessel structures which should be observed by further research. In addition, the transition area also needs more attention. Another interesting approach might be the usage of different deep learning networks like for example nnU-Net [8] for better performance. Moreover, the evaluation of the performance of data with specific pathologies or abnormalities might be interesting as well. To ensure a robust training convergence and similar parametrization of the weights in the network, the training session needs to be repeated.

Acknowledgement

The work has been carried out at Fraunhofer Institute for Digital Medicine MEVIS, Bremen and supervised by Prof. Dr. Mattias Heinrich, Institute of Medical Informatics, Universität zu Lübeck. This work was funded by the project NFDI4Health Covid-19. Furthermore, I would like to thank Felix Thielke and Dr. Bianca Lassen-Schmidt for their support.

Author's Statement

Conflict of interest: Authors state no conflict of interest.

5   References

[1] R. D. Rudyanto, S. Kerkstra, E. M. v. Rikxoort, C. Fetita, P.-Y. Brillet, C. Lefevre, *et al.*, "Comparing algorithms for automated vessel segmentation in computed tomography scans of the lung: the VESSEL12 study," *Medical Image Analysis*, vol. 18, no. 7, pp. 1217–1232, 2014.

[2] W. Tan, Y. Yuan, A. Chen, L. Mao, Y. Ke, and X. Lv, "An Approach for Pulmonary Vascular Extraction from Chest CT Images," *Journal of Healthcare Engineering*, vol. 2019, pp. 1–11, Jan. 2019.

[3] G. Du, X. Cao, J. Liang, X. Chen, and Y. Zhan, "Medical Image Segmentation based on U-Net: A Review," *Journal of Imaging Science and Technology*, vol. 64, Mar. 2020.

[4] S. G. Armato, G. McLennan, L. Bidaut, M. F. McNitt-Gray, C. R. Meyer, A. P. Reeves, *et al.*, "The Lung Image Database Consortium (LIDC) and Image Database Resource Initiative (IDRI): A Completed Reference Database of Lung Nodules on CT Scans," *Medical Physics*, vol. 38, pp. 915–931, Feb. 2011.

[5] P. Lo, B. van Ginneken, J. M. Reinhardt, T. Yavarna, P. A. de Jong, B. Irving, *et al.*, "Extraction of Airways From CT (EXACT'09)," *IEEE Transactions on Medical Imaging*, vol. 31, pp. 2093–2107, Nov. 2012.

[6] A. F. Frangi, W. J. Niessen, K. L. Vincken, and M. A. Viergever, "Multiscale vessel enhancement filtering," in *Medical Image Computing and Computer-Assisted Intervention — MICCAI'98* (W. M. Wells, A. Colchester, and S. Delp, eds.), Lecture Notes in Computer Science, (Berlin, Heidelberg), pp. 130–137, Springer, 1998.

[7] O. Ronneberger, P. Fischer, and T. Brox, "U-net: Convolutional networks for biomedical image segmentation," in *International Conference on Medical image computing and computer-assisted intervention*, pp. 234–241, Springer, 2015.

[8] F. Isensee, P. F. Jaeger, S. A. A. Kohl, J. Petersen, and K. H. Maier-Hein, "nnU-Net: a self-configuring method for deep learning-based biomedical image segmentation," *Nature Methods*, vol. 18, pp. 203–211, Feb. 2021. Number: 2 Publisher: Nature Publishing Group.

[9] S. Shit, J. C. Paetzold, A. Sekuboyina, I. Ezhov, A. Unger, A. Zhylka, *et al.*, "cldice-a novel topology-preserving loss function for tubular structure segmentation," in *Proceedings of the IEEE/CVF Conference on Computer Vision and Pattern Recognition*, pp. 16560–16569, 2021.

4

Signal Processing

Electrical Bioimpedance Spectroscopy for the characterization of the tissular properties of the myocardium using a transcatheter method

Kimberley Lühring [1], Gerard Amorós-Figueras [2] and Javier Rosell-Ferrer [3]

[1] Biomedical Engineering, Luebeck University of Applied Sciences, kimberley.luehring@stud.th-luebeck.de

[2] Department of Cardiology, Hospital de la Santa Creu i Sant Pau, IIB-Sant Pau, Universitat Autònoma de Barcelona, Barcelona, Spain, gamorosf@santpau.cat

[3] Electronic and Biomedical Instrumentation Group, Department of Electronic Engineering, Universitat Politècnica de Catalunya, Barcelona, Spain, javier.rosell@upc.edu

Abstract

When treating cardiac arrhythmias by radiofrequency ablation, it is important to know whether the tissue causing the interfering stimuli has been inactivated. Fast broadband electrical impedance spectroscopy, EIS for short, can be used for this purpose. To determine the suitability of this method for tissue characterization, data from human clinical trials were evaluated using MATLAB algorithms. The effects of cardiac condition, catheter orientation and applied force on the impedance curve were examined. It was found that arrhythmic phases and the state of tissue are reflected in the impedance measurement. However, force and orientation angle must be recorded within a certain range to obtain comparable recordings. By analyzing the data, it became apparent that especially the catheter position has a strong influence on the measurements, which must be taken into account in future experiments. In general, EIS is shown to be a useful method for assessing the condition of the tissue.

1 Introduction

The treatment of cardiac arrhythmias, e.g. atrial fibrillation, due to pathological changes of the tissue as a result of a myocardial infarction has remained a challenge in today's clinical practise [1]. Here, the conduction of impulses in the heart tissue is disturbed leading to reentry and arrhythmias. To prevent this, radiofrequency ablation can be performed, in which the affected tissue is treated with high-frequency currents. This destroys the cells that are responsible for the formation or transmission of the impulses. To further improve this process, it is important to know where the affected regions are and if they were inactivated by ablation. Currently, approaches for identifying arrhythmogenic regions rely on electrogram-based features. However, these depend on the cardiac activation sequence, which changes during arrhythmic phases. The new method of fast broadband electrical impedance spectroscopy (EIS) will be applied, which provides information about tissue properties by measuring the local impedances using a transcatheter method, independent of the activation sequence [2]. This makes use of the fact that biological tissue conducts electricity differently depending on the frequency [3]. That can be explained by the cell membrane behaving like a capacitor with parallel resistance due to its ion channels [4]. At DC and low frequencies, the so-called membrane effect occurs, i.e. the channels of the cell membrane prevent the passage of current and it is conducted around the cell [5]. At higher frequencies, however, the current can pass through the cell. EIS is done by measuring the electrical impedance at 26 frequencies from 1 to 1000 kHz between the ablation catheter and an electrode placed on the patient's skin [6]. Therefore, data from 14 human patients were used, in which the impedances in the left atrium were measured before and after ablation. Position and orientation of the catheter were determined using the Carto3 system, which generates magnetic fields and calculates their influence on the catheter. The purpose of this work is to develop algorithms for the processing of impedance data and investigate the effects of catheter position, orientation and force on the tissue on the measurements.

2 Material and Methods

2.1 Experimental data

In this work, data from 14 human patients recorded in the left atrium before and after ablation were used for analysis. The impedance was measured for 26 frequencies between 1 and 1000 kHz using the ablation catheter. Each recording was taken in about five seconds before the measurement was initiated. In addition to impedance, a local electrocardiogram (ECG) was recorded, reflecting the condition of the heart. For each measurement, Biosense Webster's Carto3 system was used to determine the position and orientation of the catheter in the heart.

2.2 Impedance during cardiac cycle

To analyze the behavior of impedance during the cardiac cycle, local ECG data and the impedance curve of two selected frequencies, 15 and 95 kHz, were compared by overlaying the curves. Systole and diastole were located in the local ECGs and then assigned to the closest extreme points in the impedance curve. In order to calculate the systolic and diastolic impedance values, the magnitude of the impedance at the respective points were averaged for each frequency. For comparison of values, systolic and diastolic impedances were plotted along with their standard deviation and the mean value of the entire recording.

2.3 Classification of contact force

The force vector of the catheter on the tissue could be calculated using a spring in the catheter tip and is given in three axes, but here only the magnitude of the force is needed to indicate the stability of the contact to the tissue. A stable contact is important to be able to reproduce and compare the measurement results. Therefore, each recording was assigned to three possible categories: floating, stable or unstable. A low variation in amplitude indicates a stable contact, whereas a high variation indicates a rather unstable contact. Recordings taken in the blood pool of the atrium were considered as floating and used as a reference measurement.

Force vectors with a magnitude of less than 1 g and a variation of less than 0.5 g were considered as floating since almost no pressure was exerted on the catheter tip in this case. Stable recordings are characterized by an approximately constant pressure of the catheter on the tissue. A maximum variation of 1.6 g during an acquisition was selected for this purpose. If the cases just mentioned have not occurred, the recordings are termed unstable.

Classification of the contact force indicates the quality of the recordings and enables pre-selection of the recordings suitable for analysis.

2.4 Determination of orientation angle

In addition to the contact force, information about the direction of the catheter was also obtained during the measurements. The orientation angle is defined as the angle between force vector and catheter direction and gives further information about the contact of the catheter on the tissue.

Due to the large amount of data, only the average values of a record are considered for both the force and the orientation angle to compare the data. Records with different force magnitudes and orientation angles will be compared to show the effect of the catheter positioning on the measurement.

3 Results and Discussion

3.1 Impedance curves during cardiac cycle

When examining the ECGs, it has been noticed that the P-wave, which is the beginning of diastole, usually appears at a local minimum and the R-peak, which denotes the beginning of systole, is at a maximum. Therefore, for all recordings, it was determined that the mean of the local maxima corresponded to the systolic impedance value and the mean of the minima corresponded to the diastolic impedance value.

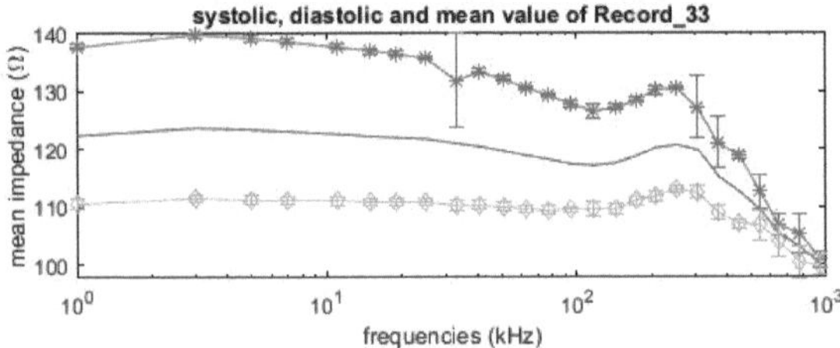

Figure 1: Systolic, diastolic and mean impedance values for each frequency for record 33. The maximum difference between systolic and diastolic impedances is 30 Ω.

As an example this is shown in Fig. 1 for record 33. At low frequencies the systolic and diastolic impedance values differ by about 30 Ω at a mean impedance of 120 Ω, whereas at higher frequencies the difference is decreasing. This shows that above 100 kHz the membrane effect disappears so that the shape of the cell has no influence on the impedance and systolic and diastolic values converge.

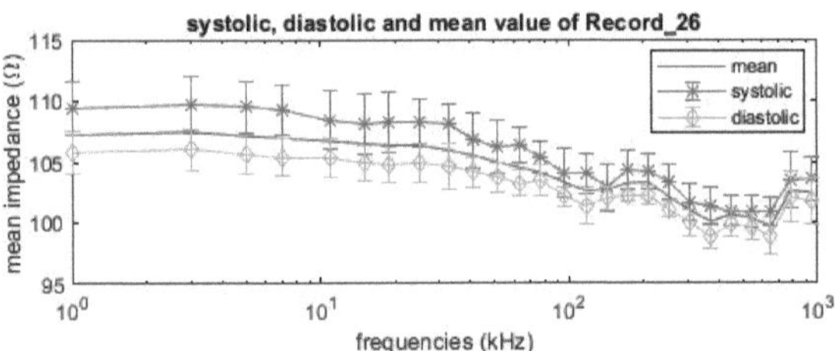

Figure 2: Systolic, diastolic and mean impedance values for each frequency for record 26. The maximum difference between systolic and diastolic impedances is only a fifth of that from record 33.

When comparing phasic changes of different recordings it has been noticed that systolic and diastolic magnitudes varied, e.g. in record 33 the maximum difference between systolic and diastolic values was about 30 Ω, whereas in record 26 (Fig. 2) the difference was 6 Ω at most with a lower mean value. This indicates that either in some places of the heart the impedance is more affected by the movement or that the contact of the catheter with the tissue might have changed between the recordings.

To further examine the reason for the change in systolic and diastolic values the effect of the applied force is analyzed.

3.2 Effect of force and orientation angle on the impedance

Impedance may change if the force of the catheter on the tissue is too high or too low. For example, if the catheter-tissue contact is low, the impedance amplitude decreases as the proportion of blood impedance in the total impedance increases. This is shown in Fig. 3, in which towards the end of the recording the contact decreases and the impedance drops below 100 Ω, which corresponds to the impedance of blood.

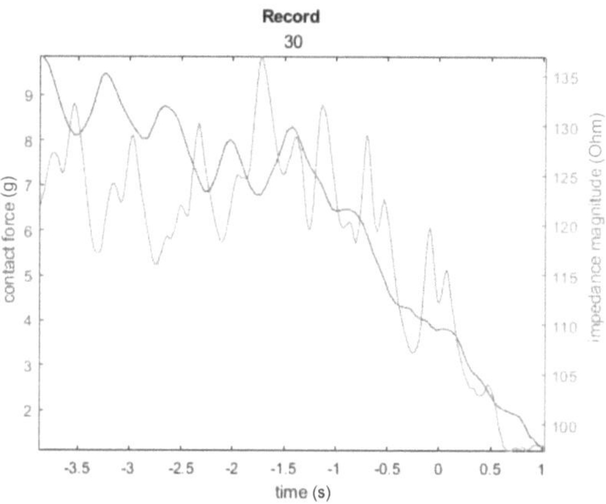

Figure 3: Contact force and impedance magnitude for 11 kHz of record 30. During recording the contact to the tissue is lost which is also reflected in the decreasing impedance magnitude that drops to blood level.

Some changes in impedance can be explained by a varying contact force, as can be seen in Fig. 4. The contact force varies over the recording from a minimum of 7 g to a maximum of 17 g. The local minima of the impedance coincide with the decreasing force, while the maxima are hardly affected by the changing contact. Since not both maxima and minima change, it can be assumed that the varying amplitudes are not due to the subject's breathing, but are

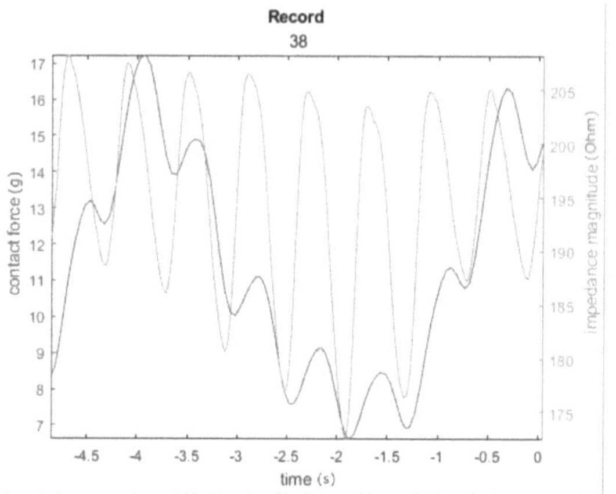

Figure 4: Impedance magnitude for 11 kHz and contact force of record 38. During recording, the catheter-tissue contact varies, which is manifested in the impedance curve as a change in magnitude of the local minima.

clearly caused by the contact force. The altering minima also change the average diastolic impedance, which could be a possible reason for the difference in Figs. 1 and 2.

A comparison of recordings with the same mean contact force and different orientation angles is shown in Fig. 5. Recording 94 has a mean orientation angle of 9 degrees, while recording 50 has an angle of 48 degrees. Apparently, the orientation of the catheter affects the systolic and diastolic values, but also the mean impedance values. The recording with a lower orientation angle has a mean impedance magnitude of about 100 Ω and a difference between systolic and diastolic impedance of 20 Ω, whereas for a larger angle the mean amplitude is increased. Here, the impedance level is about 40 Ω higher than at an angle of 9 degrees.

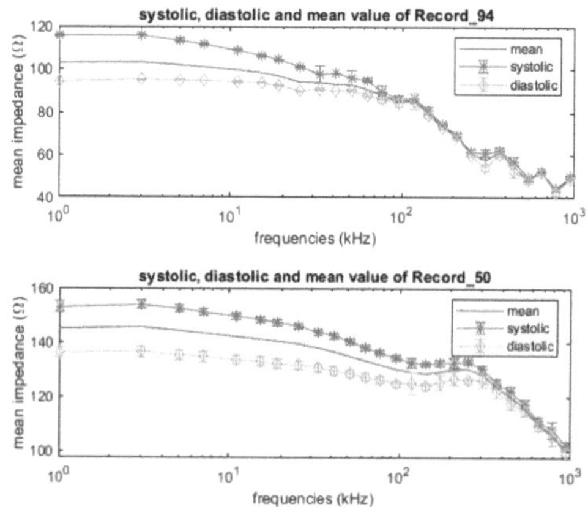

Figure 5: Comparison of records with similar mean force of 11 g and mean orientation angles of 9 degrees (above) and 48 degrees (below).

It can be assumed that the different impedance behaviors in Figs. 1 and 2 are due to a combination of different force magnitudes and orientation angles.

In addition, recordings 33 and 26 were recorded at different locations in the heart, so it also cannot be ruled out that different impedances are due to different tissue characteristics.

3.3 Suitability for tissue characterization

From the previous sections, it is clear that impedance measurement can be affected by various factors in the measurement. However, it is also important to know how the impedance curve is altered by physiological factors. In Fig. 6 an ECG with arrhythmias is shown and also the impedance curves for 15 and 95 kHz. It can be seen that the impedance curve behaves differently from recordings with normal sinus rhythm.

The impedance curve has a waveform with approximately constant amplitude during regular heartbeat. With abnormal ECG, it can now be seen that the impedance becomes irregular and the amplitude of the main peaks decreases. This suggests that changes in the state of the heart are reflected in the impedance and thus the impedance can also give information about the tissue in arrhythmic phases.

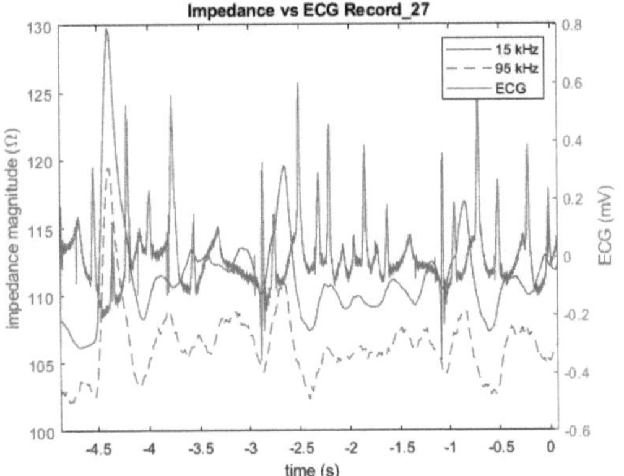

Figure 6: Impedance at 15 and 95 kHz together with local ECG. The arrhythmia can be seen in the ECG as well as in the impedance curve.

To determine the suitability of impedance measurement for evaluating the success of radiofrequency ablation, postablation recordings must be considered. In Fig. 7 systolic, diastolic and mean impedance values are shown for a record that was taken after ablation. It is noticeable that systolic and diastolic values hardly differ and are only just above 100 Ω, i.e. significantly below the impedance values of the previous examples. The recording was taken with a mean contact force of 11 g in the left atrium, but the values are typical for the measurements in the blood pool. This shows that the cells no longer have any influence on the measurement, which means that they must have been destroyed during ablation.

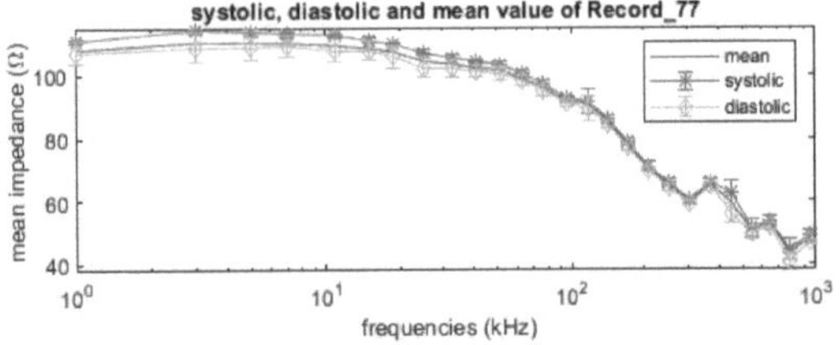

Figure 7: Systolic, diastolic and mean impedance values of each frequency recorded after radiofrequency ablation. The values are much closer together, indicating the inactivity of the tissue.

Thus, the EIS method is shown to be a useful technique to demonstrate the effects of ablation on tissue. However, to assess the success of ablation, measurements must be taken at the same point before and after ablation. Evaluation of this requires more data than accessible in the scope of this work.

4   Conclusion

In this work, impedance data from 14 subjects were studied, which additionally included local ECGs and catheter positioning. It was found that impedance is a good indicator for tissue characterization and thus can distinguish healthy from inactive cells. Moreover, electrical impedance is influenced by the state of the heart, which was shown by its change during an arrhythmic phase. However, it was observed that impedance also depends on the positioning of the catheter, so that its influence must be taken into account in future experiments. It seems that the contact force influences the systolic and diastolic impedance values and orientation angles affect the mean impedance level significantly. To obtain results that are as reliable as possible, the contact force and the orientation angle must be similar for the recordings that are to be compared.

Acknowledgement

The work has been carried out at Universitat Politècnica de Catalunya, Barcelona, Spain and supervised by A. Mertins, Institute for Signal Processing, Universität zu Lübeck.

Author's Statement

Conflict of interest: Authors state no conflict of interest. Ethical approval: The research related to human use complies with all the relevant national regulations, institutional policies and was performed in accordance with the tenets of the Helsinki Declaration, and has been approved by the authors' institutional review board or equivalent committee.

5   References

[1] L. A. Unger et al., *Local Electrical Impedance Mapping of the Atria: Conclusions on Substrate Properties and Confounding Factors*. Frontiers in Physiology, vol. 12, 2022.

[2] G. Amorós-Figueras et al., *Endocardial infarct scar recognition by myocardial electrical impedance is not influenced by changes in cardiac activation sequence*. Heart rhythm: the official journal of the Heart Rhythm Society, vol. 15, no. 4, 2017.

[3] Y. Salazar Muñoz, *Caracterización de tejidos cardíacos mediante métodos mínimamente invasivos y no invasivos basados en espectroscopia de impedancia eléctrica*. doctoral thesis, UPC, Departament d'Enginyeria de Sistemes, Automàtica i Informàtica Industrial, 2004.

[4] S. Grimnes and O. G. Martinsen, *Chapter 4 - Passive Tissue Electrical Properties*. In: Bioimpedance and Bioelectricity Basics (Third Edition), Academic Press, Oxford, pp. 77–118, 2015.

[5] J. Malmivuo and R. Plonsey, *Bioelectromagnetism: Principles and Applications of Bioelectric and Biomagnetic Fields*. Oxford University Press, New York, 1995.

[6] G. Amorós-Figueras et al., *Recognition of Fibrotic Infarct Density by the Pattern of Local Systolic-Diastolic Myocardial Electrical Impedance*. Frontiers in Physiology, vol. 7, 2016.

Speech Emotion Recognition Using wav2vec 2.0 Embeddings

Felix Jorczik [1], Mathias Eulers [2], Alfred Mertins[3]
[1] Medical Engineering Science, Universität zu Lübeck, felix.jorczik@student.uni-luebeck.de
[2] Institute for Signal Processing, Universität zu Lübeck, m.eulers@.uni-luebeck.de
[3] Institute for Signal Processing, Universität zu Lübeck, alfred.mertins@uni-luebeck.de

Abstract

In recent years, state-of-the-art machine learning techniques have increasingly relied on transformer networks. In the field of Speech Emotion Recognition (SER), self-supervised architectures such as wav2vec 2.0 and HuBERT have been successfully applied, leading to the current state-of-the-art in SER. To evaluate the performance of these architectures, in this study we utilize a previous solution using wav2vec 2.0 with a classification head and fine-tune it on the MSP-Podcast dataset. Subsequently, we test the downstream model on a German audio dataset for emotion classification and evaluate its performance in terms of arousal, dominance, and valence.

1 Introduction

Speech emotion recognition (SER) is an important area of research in affective computing that aims to recognize, understand and respond to human emotions through the analysis of speech signals. It has a wide range of applications, particularly in human-computer interaction and in healthcare [1]. Previous SER models have primarily relied on hand-engineered feature extraction and traditional machine learning techniques [2]. These methods have limited success in achieving high levels of accuracy in recognizing emotions from speech and do not generalize well across different datasets and languages. In recent years, however, the advent of transformer-based models has led to a significant improvement in the performance of SER. Transformer models such as wav2vec 2.0 have been shown to be highly effective in capturing the complex patterns of emotional speech [3].

These architectures are self-supervised and pre-trained on large amounts of speech data, allowing them to learn rich representations of speech that can be fine-tuned for various tasks such as emotion recognition. Unlike traditional models, transformer models are able to handle large input sequences and have the ability to model long-term dependencies in speech signals.

In the field of SER, there are two distinct ways of labeling emotions: discrete labels and dimensional labels [4]. The former refer to a categorical system in which each label belongs to a specific emotional category, such as happy, surprised, fearful, or angry. The latter, on the other hand, refer to a continuous scale where emotions are represented as points in a multidimensional space, such as valence, arousal, and dominance. The relation between the two approaches is depicted in Fig. 1. Valence represents the degree of positivity or negativity of emotion, arousal is the level of physiological or psychological activation, and dom-

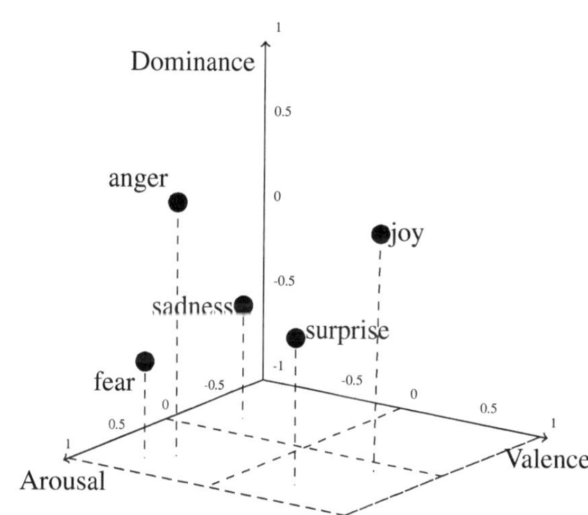

Figure 1: 3D representation of VAD model showing distribution of discrete emotion labels across valence, arousal and dominance dimensions.

inance stands for the degree of control or influence emotion has over the individual experiencing it. Dimensional labels provide a more nuanced understanding of the emotion conveyed in a speech sample, while discrete labels provide a broader categorization of the speech. The approach described below uses dimensional labels.

In this paper, we utilize wav2vec 2.0 with a classification head and fine-tune it on a specific dataset for emotion classification [9]. We will evaluate the performance of the model in terms of arousal, dominance, and valence. Our goal is to evaluate the effectiveness of transformer-based models on recognizing emotions from speech of the German language and to contribute to the advancement of SER in the field of affective computing. Initially, we provide an overview of the datasets and their properties. Subsequently, we explain the selected loss function, followed by a detailed examination of the architecture. Finally, we present the obtained results and provide a conclusion.

2 Material and Methods

2.1 Datasets

The limited availability of authentic audio datasets for speech emotion recognition poses a significant challenge for the advancement of SER, as datasets consisting of acted speech may not accurately reflect spontaneous spoken language.

2.1.1 MSP-Podcast

The MSP-Podcast corpus is a large dataset that contains speech segments from podcast recordings that have been labeled with discrete and dimensional emotional information [5]. The labels are within the range of 1 to 7. The current version of the dataset includes 73000 samples (114 hours), and it is an ongoing effort, intending to reach 400 hours. This dataset is unique as it is a naturalistic speech dataset collected from real-life conversations, which makes it more relatable and realistic. The emotional content is balanced, providing enough samples across the valence-arousal-dominance space. The dataset is divided into four partitions: Test set 1 (15000 samples), Test set 2 (5000 samples), Validation set (8000 samples) and Train set (45000 samples). The samples range from 1 second to 29 seconds with an average of 6 seconds.

2.1.2 Vera am Mittag German audio-visual emotional speech database

The Vera Am Mittag Database (VAM) is a German audio-visual emotional speech database, containing audio and video recordings from guests on the German talk show "Vera am Mittag" recorded in 2005 [6]. This corpus includes unscripted and genuine conversations from talk show guests, featuring spontaneous and highly emotional speech. The emotion labels are in the form of valence, activation, and dominance. The labels are within a range of -1 to 1. The data includes 947 sentences spoken by 47 different speakers and has a total length of 47 minutes. The minimum length of a sample is 1 second, while the maximum reaches 17 seconds. VAM was collected and segmented by researchers at the University of Karlsruhe in Germany.

2.2 Loss Function

A loss function is a mathematical function that quantifies the difference between the predicted output of a model and the ground truth. Its purpose is to guide the optimization process during training by providing a measure of model performance, allowing the model to learn from its mistakes and adjust its parameters to improve its predictions. In our work, we use the Concordance Correlation Coefficient (CCC) [7]. The CCC is defined as

$$CCC = \frac{2\rho_{xy}\sigma_x\sigma_y}{\sigma_x^2 + \sigma_y^2 + (\mu_x - \mu_y)^2},\tag{1}$$

where x and y are the vectors of labels from prediction and ground truth. The values of μ and σ represent the mean and standard deviation, respectively. The correlation between x and y is the Pearson coefficient correlation

$$\rho_{xy} = \frac{\sum (x - \mu_x)(y - \mu_y)}{\sqrt{\sum (x - \mu_x)^2 \sum (y - \mu_y)^2}}.\tag{2}$$

The CCC takes into account not only the linear correlation but also the agreement between the two variables, building upon the Pearson coefficient. The CCC ranges from -1, indicating perfect disagreement, to 1, indicating perfect agreement. The CCC loss function (CCCL) is used for optimization, which is defined as

$$CCCL = 1 - CCC,\tag{3}$$

where the range of values lies between 0 to 2. It is calculated separately for arousal ($CCCL_V$), valence ($CCCL_A$), and dominance ($CCCL_D$). The $CCCL_T$ is a composite of these three individual loss functions.

$$CCCL_T = \\ \alpha CCCL_V + \beta CCCL_A + (1 - \alpha - \beta)CCCL_D\tag{4}$$

Parameters α and β add up to 1. However, it is important to individually determine these parameters for each dataset as evaluated in [8].

2.3 Architecture

Wav2vec 2.0 is a neural network (NN) architecture for unsupervised learning of speech representations from audio data [3]. It is based on the transformer architecture, which is a type of NN that is well-suited to processing sequential data [10]. The architecture consists of a Convolutional NN (CNN) and a transformer, which consists of several transformer layers. The model is depicted in Fig. 2.

The key innovation of wav2vec 2.0 is the use of a masked autoregressive model to predict the next sample in the audio signal, given the preceding samples. The model is trained using contrastive learning, which involves learning to distinguish between positive examples (pairs of similar audio samples) and negative examples (pairs of dissimilar audio samples). This helps the model to learn a representation of the audio data that captures the most important features.

Several variations of wav2vec 2.0 exist. The wav2vec 2.0 base model (12 transformer layers and 768 feature dimensions) and wav2vec 2.0 large (24 transformer blocks and 1024 feature dimensions) are pre-trained on a length of 960 hours of English speech audio data. The model wav2vec2-xlsr-53 is trained on 56000 hours of speech in 53 languages.

After training, it can be used to extract high-dimensional

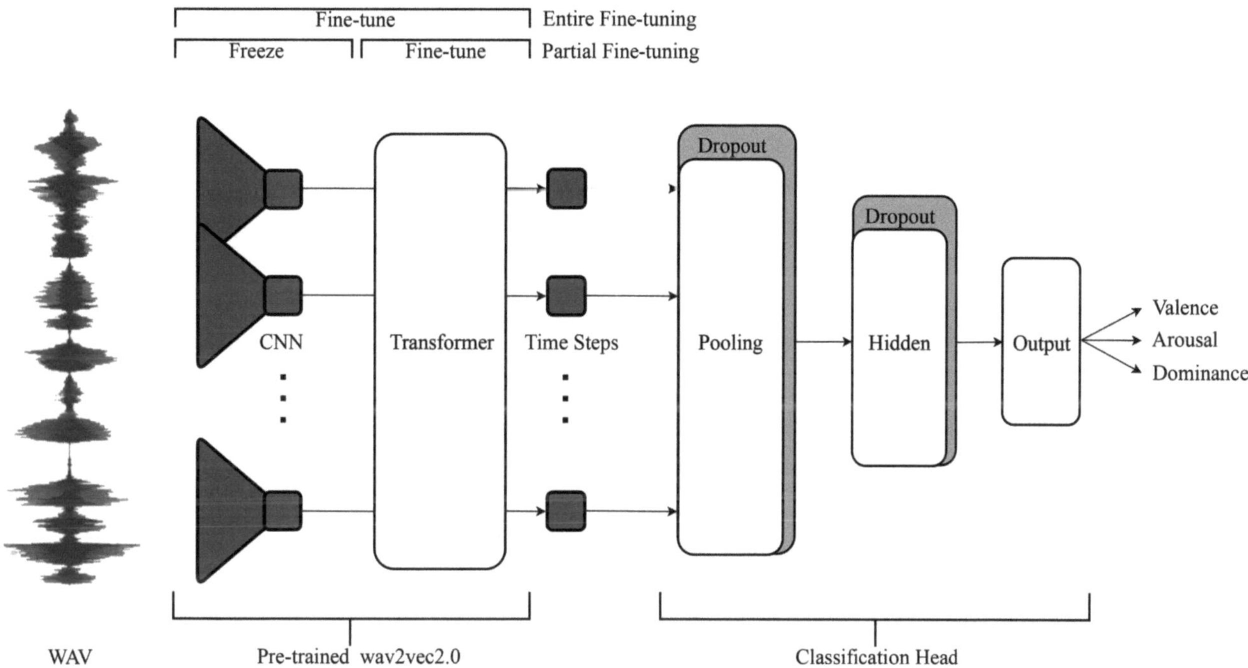

Figure 2: Classification head constructed on top of the pre-trained wav2vec 2.0 architecture with different training procedures. While partial fine-tuning only adjusts the transformer, entire fine-tuning optimizes the gradients of all layers. The classification head is trained by the conventional method.

representations of audio data, which can be useful in a wide range of speech-related applications, such as speech recognition, speaker identification or in our case SER.

As proposed in [9], it is possible to extend these architectures by adding a classification head. This is shown in Fig. 2. The classifcation head is a NN of relatively limited complexity. The complete model consists, besides the pre-trained wav2vec 2.0, of a 1-D average pooling layer, a fully connected linear hidden layer and fully connected linear output layer. The pooling layer and hidden layer are followed by a dropout. Not updating the CNN component of the pre-trained model during training is referred to as partial fine-tuning (PF). The reason for this approach is that the pre-trained CNN already possesses the ability to effectively extract features from the audio input. Fine-tuning that includes the CNN is specified as entire fine-tuning, which is typically implemented at later stages of training when the model has already achieved a satisfactory level of performance on its assigned task. It is typically performed with more subtle changes to the model's parameters to make slight adjustments to the model's performance. We will use partial fine-tuning. Due to computational limitations, we will only train the model on 20% of the training data.

3   Results and Discussion

Firstly, we address the parameters from (4). Linear search between 0 and 1 with 0.1 increments dependent on each other yields the optimum of training. As a full training is very time consuming, we compared the loss after several training iterations and chose the setting with the smallest CCC loss magnitude. Thus, we determined for MSP-Podcast values of $\alpha = 0.4$ and $\beta = 0.5$.

Table 1: Results of different wav2vec 2.0 models on MSP-Podcast and VAM. The Concordance Correlation Coefficient (CCC) is displayed for valence (V), arousal (A), and dominance (D). In addition, accuracy is included.

Dataset: MSP-Podcast (English)

Model	V	A	D	Accuracy
wav2vec 2.0 base	0.191	0.478	0.319	0.552%
wav2vec 2.0 base (Wagner)	0.363	0.728	0.636	-

Dataset: VAM (German)

Model	V	A	D	Accuracy
wav2vec 2.0 base	0.09	0.351	0.312	0.457%

The results on MSP-Podcast and VAM are shown above in Table 1. To make these results more comprehensible we calculated an average accuracy. An output was defined as accurate if the absolute difference to the label was smaller than 0.1, where the labels have a range between 0 and 1. We did this along each dimension and divided the total value of accurate labels by the number of labels. As demonstrated in the table, Wagner's results were significantly better, however, it should be noted that their model was trained on the full training dataset compared to ours. The CCC values of arousal and dominance are close to each other, while valence is comparably low in both cases. In addition, the results of our model evaluated on the German speech dataset are worse in comparison to the English dataset, but the accuracy was still acceptable.

4 Conclusion

In this work, we explored the performance of the wav2vec 2.0 base model on the German language. There are a variety of approaches that can be taken to refine the model and produce outcomes akin to those achieved by Wagner. There is a larger model wav2vec 2.0 large we will implement in the future. Additionally, there is the model wav2vec 2.0 xlsr-53, which is trained on 56000 hours of speech in 53 languages, which might show better results on VAM. An alternate approach could be to start with partial fine-tuning, then gradually move on to full fine-tuning as the training progresses. During this process, small modifications can be made to the model's parameters to refine its performance gradually. Lastly, it is worth examining if a different model such as HuBERT[12], which shares a similar architecture to wav2vec 2.0, would perform better for the German language.

Acknowledgement

The work was supervised by Prof. Dr.-Ing. Alfred Mertins and conducted with support of Mathias Eulers at the Institute for Signal Processing, Universität zu Lübeck.

Author's Statement

Conflict of interest: Authors state no conflict of interest.

5 References

[1] Lugovic, S., Dunđer, I. & Horvat, M. Techniques and Applications of Emotion Recognition in Speech. (2016,5)

[2] Schuller, B. Speech Emotion Recognition: Two Decades in a Nutshell, Benchmarks, and Ongoing Trends. *Commun. ACM.* **61**, 90-99 (2018,4), https://doi.org/10.1145/3129340

[3] Baevski, A., Zhou, H., Mohamed, A. & Auli, M. wav2vec 2.0: A Framework for Self-Supervised Learning of Speech Representations. (arXiv,2020), https://arxiv.org/abs/2006.11477

[4] Gunes, H. & Schuller, B. Categorical and Dimensional Affect Analysis in Continuous Input: Current Trends and Future Directions. *Image Vision Comput..* **31**, 120-136 (2013,2), https://doi.org/10.1016/j.imavis.2012.06.016

[5] Martinez-Lucas, L., Abdelwahab, M. & Busso, C. The MSP-Conversation Corpus. *Interspeech 2020.* pp. 1823-1827 (2020,10)

[6] Grimm, M., Kroschel, K. & Narayanan, S. The Vera am Mittag German audio-visual emotional speech database. *2008 IEEE International Conference On Multimedia And Expo.* pp. 865-868 (2008)

[7] Lin, L. A concordance correlation coefficient to evaluate reproducibility. *Biometrics.* **45**, pp. 255–68 ISSN0006-341X, 1989.

[8] Atmaja, B. & Akagi, M. Evaluation of error- and correlation-based loss functions for multitask learning dimensional speech emotion recognition. *Journal Of Physics: Conference Series.* **1896**, 012004 (2021,4), https://doi.org/10.48550/arXiv.2003.10724

[9] Wagner, J., Triantafyllopoulos, A., Wierstorf, H., Schmitt, M., Burkhardt, F., Eyben, F. & Schuller, B. Dawn of the transformer era in speech emotion recognition: closing the valence gap. (arXiv,2022), https://arxiv.org/abs/2203.07378

[10] Vaswani, A., Shazeer, N., Parmar, N., Uszkoreit, J., Jones, L., Gomez, A., Kaiser, L. & Polosukhin, I. Attention Is All You Need. (arXiv,2017), https://arxiv.org/abs/1706.03762

[11] Conneau, A., Baevski, A., Collobert, R., Mohamed, A. & Auli, M. Unsupervised Cross-lingual Representation Learning for Speech Recognition. (arXiv,2020), https://arxiv.org/abs/2006.13979

[12] Hsu, W., Bolte, B., Tsai, Y., Lakhotia, K., Salakhutdinov, R. & Mohamed, A. HuBERT: Self-Supervised Speech Representation Learning by Masked Prediction of Hidden Units. (arXiv,2021), https://arxiv.org/abs/2106.07447

Fast and High-Resolution Synthetic Aperture Radar Mapping with a Multi-Radar System

Mohamed Aboeljereed

Robotics and Autonomous System, Universität zu Lübeck, mohamed.aboeljereed@student.uni-luebeck.de

Abstract

Computing Synthetic Aperture Radar (SAR) images involves processing a large amount of radar data and can be time-consuming when done on a computer's Central Processing Unit (CPU) or utilizing a Graphics Processing Unit (GPU) improperly. However, some SAR algorithms allow for efficient parallelization on modern GPUs, which can dramatically reduce the computation time and make an algorithm a good candidate for real-time applications. In this work, we implement SAR backprojection algorithm in C++ and utilize an NVIDIA GPU to process simulated and real radar datasets. We show that high-resolution (1 cm) SAR images of a 40 x 40 m scene can be computed at a frame rate of 5 fps on an NVIDIA GeForce GTX 1070 Ti device by using special GPU features. Initial results show that our implemented C++ CUDA kernel using the GPU computes same SAR image 78 times faster than a MATLAB implementation using a CPU.

1 Introduction

Synthetic Aperture Radar (SAR) technology utilizes motion of a platform carrying one or multiple radars to construct a large virtual antenna aperture, which, in turn, enables producing a high-resolution image of a scene traversed. The concept was first introduced in 1951 by Carl A. Wiley [1] and then took many years of development until it reached its current shape and renamed as SAR. Initially being used for military reconnaissance, it has then been used by airborne or spaceborne radars to produce high-resolution images of the earth's surface and in other applications. Recently, more research was done to explore SAR applicability to solving the automated driving tasks. Indeed, SAR allowing for a centimeter-level image accuracy can achieve more accurate environment perception in typical driving scenarios as compared to a conventional radar detection pipeline [2]. Though, proper SAR imaging requires accurate localization of a moving ego-vehicle which can be achieved, for example, by fusing the data of such vehicle sensors as a GNSS (Global Navigation Satellite System) sensor, IMU (Inertial Measurement Unit), and odometers [2].

Yet, there exist other mapping methods, for example, Occupancy Grid Mapping (OGM). Its comparison to SAR in [3] revealed better level of SAR map details, though. These advantages of SAR can make it a good candidate for automotive applications, because mapping accuracy is essential for completing the autonomous driving tasks, including trajectory planning and localization. However, processing time of SAR algorithms (in particular, backprojection [4]) is still considered a challenge, because big amount of data has to be processed for a map update at a single radar frame.

Many imaging modes have been developed for SAR, with the stripmap being the most commonly used one. Variants of the image formation algorithm also exist, such as backprojection, polar format, range migration, and matched filter, with the last being the most accurate but the slowest ($O(N^4)$) [4], and the first being a good trade-off between speed ($O(N^3)$) and accuracy.

SAR working principle is the coherent accumulation of radar echo signals reflected by the objects while the ego vehicle traverses a scene. A longer virtual antenna aperture is created over the vehicle trajectory, where same parts of the scene are repeatedly captured by consecutive small real apertures. Subsequent constructive accumulation of the received signals improves the overall angular resolution.

Various methods were designed to accelerate SAR backprojection algorithm using Field Programmable Gate Arrays (FPGA) [5] and Graphics Processing Units (GPU) [6]. This paper uses the CUDA toolkit, a closed-source project by NVIDIA. As compared to [6] pursuing a similar approach, our implementation features some aspects that speed up the processing. In particular, we only use the GPU texture memory for the purpose of interpolation, otherwise using the default memory that has similar cache size and speed as the texture one, but no input data size limit. Thanks to this, we eliminate the problem of fitting a large-size high-resolution SAR image into a limited-size texture memory.

2 Material and Methods

2.1 Dataset

To asses if our GPU implementation of SAR backprojection algorithm computes a plausible map of a scene, a simulated dataset was initially used, where full ground truth was available. An ego-vehicle with two identical side-looking radars

Table 1: Radar parameters.

Parameter	Value	Unit
Transmit center frequency	~79	GHz
Bandwidth	~3	GHz
Number of chirps	384	-
Baseband sampling frequency	10	MHz
Chirp length	51.2	μs
Number of receiver antennas	4	-
Angle of view	80	degree

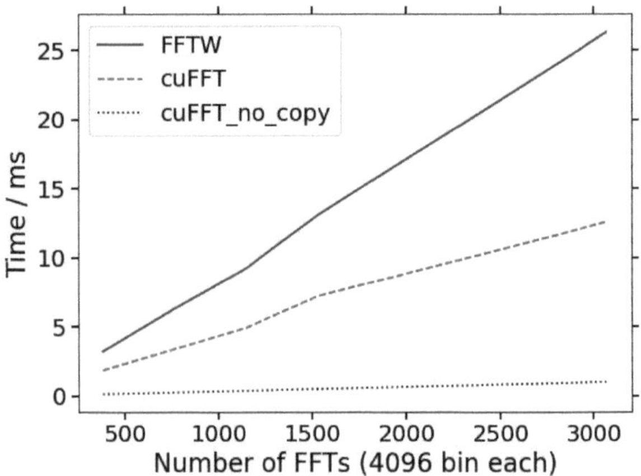

Figure 2: FFT compute time comparison.

was simulated. Some relevant radar parameters are shown in Table 1. Same parameters were used later for algorithm evaluation on real data (Section 3.4).

The simulated scene contained several parked cars, fences, trees, and curbstones, all represented as collections of discrete points as shown in Fig. 3. The ego-vehicle was traversing the scene in a straight-line trajectory.

2.2 SAR Algorithm and Signal Model

We implement the well-known SAR backprojection algorithm and its derivation is similar to the one in [7]. The steps of the algorithm are shown in Fig. 1.

Since we consider only a single transmit antenna, the algorithm input data (Section 2.1) can be thought of as a three-dimensional array with fast-time, slow-time, and the antenna dimensions. The Fast Fourier Transform (FFT) is applied only on the fast-time dimension with oversampling factor of 8. A long virtual aperture is created by sampling at discrete locations along the ego-vehicle trajectory, while the map is updated as the vehicle is traversing the scene.

2.3 Pre-implementation: Benchmarks

For each frame of radar data, updating the SAR map takes multiple matrix operations such as computation of a differential range from radar to every map pixel, linear interpolation of the FFT results at each pixel range, complex-valued matrix addition, multiplication and exponential. These steps are repeated for each chirp and each radar antenna used. Our resulting SAR map is a 4000 x 6000 matrix representing a 40 m x 60 m grid with a resolution of 1 cm.

We have tested various GPU linear algebra libraries for operations on similar-size data as described above. It was

found out that superior performance of the NVIDIA GPU devices can be achieved by implementing the operations using customized low-level CUDA kernels. Those are compiled for a GPU, where many operations can be combined in a single line which will be ran by many threads, each for a matrix element. The kernels also make use of the cache which results in less memory fetches (requiring 600 clock cycle each) compared to the other libraries. Moreover, CUDA supports linear algebra operation on complex data which makes it suitable for algorithm calculations.

Although the FFT requires less time than the other repeated operations of the algorithm, the frame rate per second can be slightly improved by choosing whether the FFT should be implemented on CPU or GPU. In particular, the time for transferring the data to GPU can increase total processing time if the number of FFT bins is not large enough, which makes it a memory-bounded operation. Fig. 2 shows the time taken by the FFTW and cuFFT libraries to compute different number of repeated 4096-point FFTs on CPU and GPU of a used device, respectively. It also shows the time taken by the cuFFT library excluding the time to copy the data from host to device, as it can depend on a GPU type. For example, on devices with unified memory, copying data can take less time compared to other GPU architectures.

2.4 Implementation

One possible reason to do the FFT on the CPU is to utilize it while the GPU is computing differential ranges, phase corrections, and map updates. However, in our case, the data must be present in the GPU for subsequent steps after the FFT. Also a planned target device uses a unified memory. This makes the cuFFT overall a better choice for our task.

The interpolation operation is necessary because the FFT bins are spaced equally, which corresponds to circular ranges from the radar while the pixels of the grid map might not hit them exactly. Linear interpolation can be time-consuming, when done on a CPU or on a GPU using software libraries. In this work, however, we use a special type of memory available in NVIDIA GPUs, called texture memory. It can implement linear interpolation and other

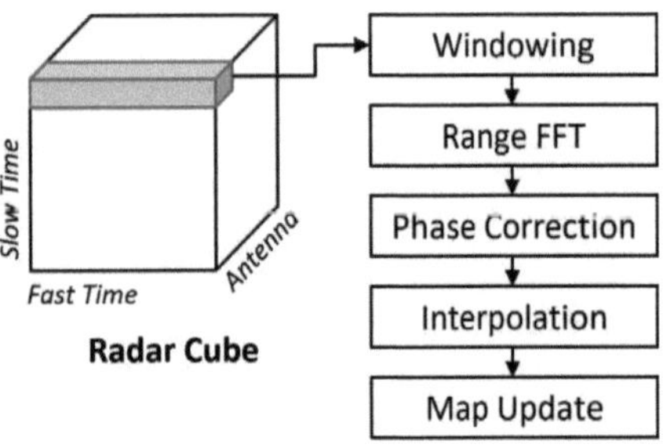

Figure 1: Algorithm flowchart.

types of filters when fetching FFT data at almost no extra time thanks to caching and hardware filtering.

Our implementation assumes that the vehicle is not moving during the fast-time sampling. The errors associated with this approximation are neglected, because the radio signal propagates faster than the vehicle's movement. All operations were done in single precision except for linear interpolation on texture which can only fetch values at 8 bit fixed-point precision allowing for only 265 possible values between two integer indices. The used CPU is an Intel Xeon E3-1240 v6 @ 3.70GHz and the GPU is NVIDIA GeForce GTX 1070 Ti. The frame rate can be further improved by using half precision supported by the CUDA toolkit.

Since similar operations are done on every pixel, parallel CUDA threads are spawned through the kernel, one for each pixel. Threads are organized into thread blocks and every block is processed by one of the 19 Streaming Multiprocessors (SMs) of the device. It has not been studied whether parallel threads working on the same pixel would be faster. Only the accumulated SAR image, current inter-frame radar position information, and the FFT output are kept in the GPU memory during calculation, which makes it more suitable for low-memory GPUs.

3 Results and Discussion

3.1 Results on Simulated Data

Fig. 3 shows a bird's-eye view of the simulated scene described in Section 2.1. For this scene, we compare the SAR maps computed with our GPU implementation (Fig. 4) and a reference MATLAB implementation using the CPU. The map in Fig. 4 involves processing a total of 592 radar frames collected while the ego-vehicle (depicted as a blue box) was driving a straight line along the X-axis of the image.

3.2 Pixel Comparison

Fig. 5 compares the distributions of SAR map values computed by the reference MATLAB implementation and the CUDA version. A good match between the two confirms the consistency of our CUDA implementation.

3.3 Performance Results

For the part of the SAR algorithm implemented on the GPU, the CUDA version provides a 18 to 22 times speed-up as compared to the MATLAB GPU implementation, depending on the number of receive antennas processed. It also provides a 78 times speed-up compared to the MATLAB CPU case as shown in Table 2. Benchmarking was done in the settings of Section 3.1 with 4 receivers processed.

3.4 Results on Real Data

Section 3.1 presented a proof of concept that the GPU SAR implementation can produce same maps on simulated data as the reference MATLAB implementation, but faster.

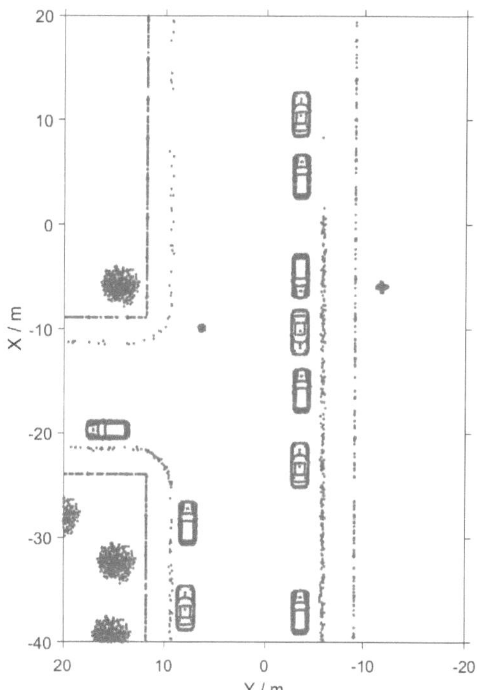

Figure 3: Simulated scene: Bird's-eye view.

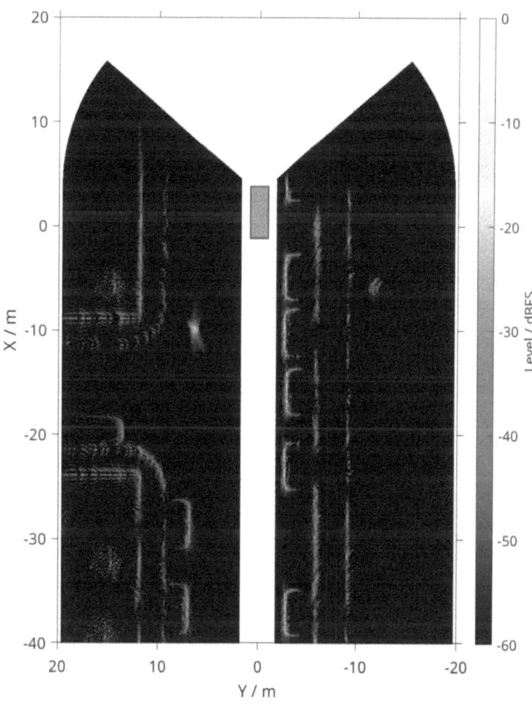

Figure 4: CUDA SAR map of a simulated scene.

Table 2: Algorithm run-time evaluated for a 4000 x 6000 pixel grid, 592 radar frames, 2 radars.

Method	Time / s	Speedup
MATLAB (CPU)	59142	1
MATLAB (GPU)	15560	3.8
CUDA	755	~78

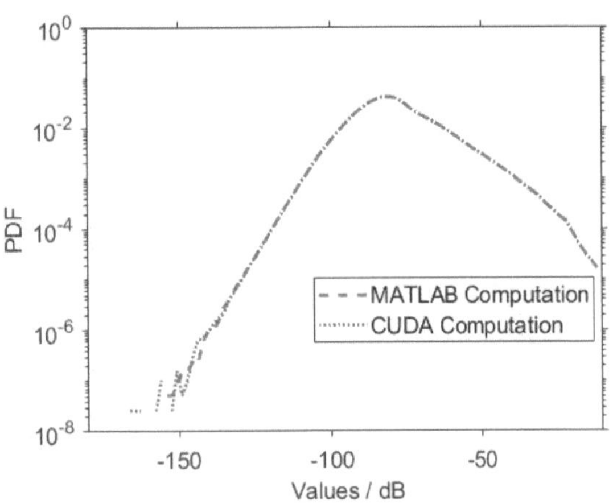

Figure 5: Comparison of probability distribution functions (PDF) of CUDA and MATLAB SAR map pixel values.

Next, our GPU SAR algorithm was applied to a real-world data recorded with the same radar parameters as in Table 1, again showing a good qualitative and quantitative match of GPU-computed results to the reference MATLAB implementation. Fig. 6 shows the output of the GPU-accelerated version of the SAR backprojection algorithm executed on the real-world data sequence.

4   Conclusion

We showed that using the CUDA toolkit and some special GPU features enables dramatic speed-up of the otherwise time-consuming SAR backprojection algorithm. Qualitative and numeric results computed on real and simulated data showed correctness of our CUDA SAR processing.

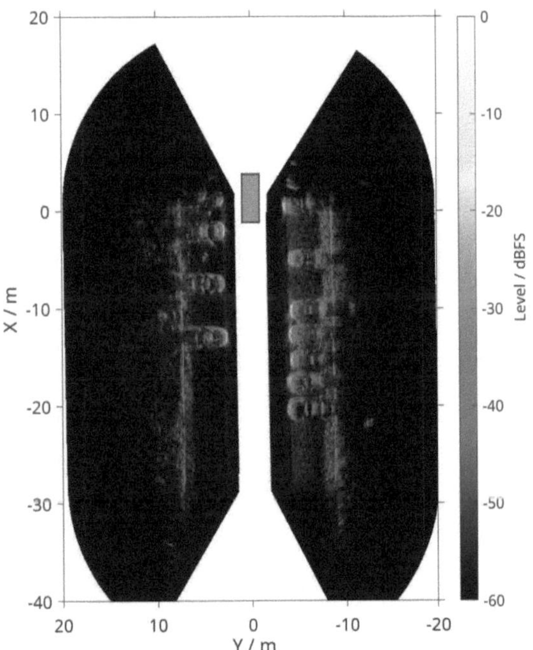

Figure 6: CUDA SAR map of a real-world scene.

Acknowledgement

The work has been done at Sony Europe B.V., Zweigniederlassung Deutschland, R&D Center Europe Stuttgart Laboratory 1 and co-supervised by Dmytro Rachkov of Sony Europe B.V., Stuttgart Laboratory 1 and Georg Schildbach of Institute of Electrical Engineering in Medicine, Universität zu Lübeck. The author thanks the engineers of Stuttgart Laboratory 1 for providing the radar simulator and reference MATLAB implementation of the SAR algorithm and fruitful discussions throughout the work.

Author's Statement

Conflict of interest: Authors state no conflict of interest.

5   References

[1] A. Love, "In memory of Carl A. Wiley," *IEEE Antennas and Propagation Society Newsletter*, vol. 27, no. 3, pp. 17–18, 1985.

[2] D. Tagliaferri, M. Rizzi, M. Nicoli, S. Tebaldini, I. Russo, A. V. Monti-Guarnieri, C. M. Prati, and U. Spagnolini, "Navigation-aided automotive SAR for high-resolution imaging of driving environments," *IEEE Access*, vol. 9, pp. 35 599–35 615, 2021.

[3] T. Grebner, P. Schoeder, V. Janoudi, and C. Waldschmidt, "Radar-based mapping of the environment: Occupancy grid-map versus SAR," *IEEE Microwave and Wireless Components Letters*, vol. 32, no. 3, pp. 253–256, 2022.

[4] L. A. Gorham and L. J. Moore, "SAR image formation toolbox for MATLAB," in *Algorithms for Synthetic Aperture Radar Imagery XVII*, E. G. Zelnio and F. D. Garber, Eds., vol. 7699, International Society for Optics and Photonics.   SPIE, 2010, p. 769906. [Online]. Available: https://doi.org/10.1117/12.855375

[5] D. L. N. Hettiarachchi and E. J. Balster, "Fixed-point processing of the SAR back-projection algorithm on FPGA," *IEEE Journal of Selected Topics in Applied Earth Observations and Remote Sensing*, vol. 14, pp. 10 889–10 902, 2021.

[6] A. Fasih and T. Hartley, "GPU-accelerated synthetic aperture radar backprojection in CUDA," in *2010 IEEE Radar Conference*, 2010, pp. 1408–1413.

[7] A. Haderer, P. Scherz, J. Schrattenecker, and A. Stelzer, "Real-time implementation of an FMCW backprojection algorithm for 1D and 2D apertures," in *2011 8th European Radar Conference*, 2011, pp. 53–56.

Development of a Sensor Prototype for Monitoring Wireless Communication

Pascal Petri [1], Abdullah Yaqout [1], Horst Hellbrück [1]

[1] Department of Electrical Engineering and Computer Sciences, Luebeck University of Applied Science
{pascal.petri@stud., abdullah.yaqout@, horst.hellbrueck@}th-luebeck.de

Abstract

Wireless communication continues to be a growing technology. Communication between machines and devices in industry is becoming increasingly important. As more signals are transmitted, the number of interferences grows. These interferences degrade reliability and increase latency. Measures need to be implemented to counteract these effects. In this paper, using a Software Defined Radio (SDR) and the open-source software GNU Radio, a prototype sensor is developed to receive specific signals. Based on the knowledge that data is being sent or that communication is taking place between one or more devices, other devices can react and send their signals at a certain time. This time can be determined, for example, by the priority of the devices. The three standards, IEEE 802.15.1, known as Bluetooth, IEEE 802.11, known as WLAN, and 802.11.4, known as ZigBee are described in this paper. These three standards were chosen because they all operate on the same frequency band.

1 Introduction

Wireless communication continues to be a growing field. Both at home (lamps, dishwashers, etc.) and in industry, more and more devices are communicating with each other, with the Internet of Things also playing a major role [1]. This means that more and more signals are being sent and received, which can lead to more interference in communication[2]. To reduce or minimize this interference, signals can be divided into categories and prioritized. However, in order to first detect which signals have been sent, there must be one or more sensors that monitor signal transmission on specific frequencies. Furthermore, it has to be decided which communication has to take place next. In this paper, we will look at three different standards that are among the most widely used wireless communication standards. All three have different tasks, requirements, and protocols. However, they all operate in the same frequency range and can also interfere with each other. The three standards are presented and compared in section 2.1. Subsequently, in section 2.2, the possibilities are presented, including how the communication can be supervised and which prerequisites have different methods. Afterwards, in section 2.3, the software GNU radio is introduced. In section 3, the implemented program is described, which is currently only capable of detecting WLAN signals.

In section 4, a summary is drawn and possible continuations and extensions of the sensor are listed.

2 Material and Methods

This section explains the standards studied, the different methods used for signal detection, and the software and hardware used to implement the sensor.

2.1 Communication Standards

Three of the most widely used wireless communication standards published by the IEEE are IEEE 802.11, IEEE 802.15, and IEEE 802.15.4, all of which use the unlicensed 2.4 GHz frequency band. Other frequency bands are also used by these standards, but we will limit ourselves here to the 2.4 GHz band as well. Table 1 lists the most important characteristic values of the three standards.

Table 1: Comparison of Wifi[4], Bluetooth [6] and Zigbee [5]

Data	WiFi	Bluetooth	Zigbee
Frequency	2.4GHz	2.4GHz	2.4GHz
Data rate	up to10Gbit/s	1Mbit/s to 2Mbit/s	250kbit/s
Power consumption	medium to high	low	low
Range	100m	10m	100m
Topology	infrastructure, ad-hoc	point-to-point,point-to-multipoint	mesh
Security	WPA, WPA2, WPA3	AES-128	AES-128

2.1.1 IEEE 802.11 WLAN

IEEE 802.11 describes a radio standard commonly known as WLAN or Wifi. It uses frequencies in the range of 2.4 GHz to 2.4835 GHz. This range is divided into 13 channels, each with a bandwidth of 20–22 MHz and a channel spacing of 5 MHz. It employs, among others, direct sequence spread spectrum and complementary code modulation techniques. The range is highly dependent on the transmission rate, but it can reach up to 100 m. 802.11 describes a protocol that requires the receiver to confirm the reception of a data packet. The sender waits for a certain time. If the transmission of the data is not confirmed, the data is sent again. The area of application of WLAN is very large. The IEEE 802.11n and 802.11ac WLAN standards achieve transmission rates of more than 100 Mbps. The devices are usually permanently connected to the power grid due to their relatively high power requirements[3] [4].

2.1.2   IEEE 802.15.4 and ZigBee

IEEE 802.15.4 describes a transmission protocol for wireless personal area networks. This standard is used by several other standards. In this paper, the ZigBee standard is described. Zigbee also uses the frequency band from //2.4 GHz to 2.4835 GHz. This band is divided into 16 channels with a channel width of 5 MHz each. The maximum transmission rate is 250 kb/s. ZigBee devices communicate in a mesh network. There are two types of devices that use Zigbee. There are full-function devices (FFD) and reduced-function devices (RFD). FFDs can use any type of topology, but RFDs can only use a star topology. Every network needs at least one FFD, which coordinates the signals. RFDs are usually battery-powered devices, such as light switches or sensors, with very low power consumption. FFDs act as coordinators, have much higher energy consumption, and are usually connected directly to the power grid. The Coordinator stores data and can, for example, be connected to a WLAN network to forward the data from the RFDs to computers or smartphones. The range of ZigBee is up to 100 m[5].

2.1.3   IEEE 802.15 Bluetooth

IEEE 802.15 describes a set of standards for wireless personal area networks. The most used standard is Bluetooth. It also uses the frequency band of 2.4 GHz to 2.48 GHz. In general, Bluetooth uses up to 79 different channels with a bandwidth of 1 MHz. The number of channels and bandwidth available in different Bluetooth versions can vary. It uses a frequency-hopping spread spectrum (FHSS) to communicate. It uses the FHSS to hop between different channels, i.e., frequencies, in a pseudo-random pattern to minimize interference and maintain a stable connection. The highest data rate of Bluetooth is 24 Mb/s, but this also depends on the used version of Bluetooth, the used devices, and the distance between these devices. The typical range of Bluetooth is around 10 m. Bluetooth is commonly used in devices like smartphones and laptops. It uses a low amount of power, even less when using Bluetooth Low Energy[6].

2.2   Spectrum Sensing

This section shows the basics of signal sensing, compares different options, and explains which type was used. There are many types of spectrum sensing. Three of them are energy detection, matched filter detection, and feature detection. The main topic of this paper will be energy detection.

All three types are based on the detection of signals from a sensor through local observation. Matched-filter detection is based on the design of a matched or optimal filter. A matched filter is a filter that is designed to maximize the signal-to-noise ratio of a known signal that has been corrupted with white Gaussian noise. To design a matched filter, we need prior knowledge of the signal. Because of that, matched filter detection is not suitable here.

The second option to sense the signals is Feature detection. Feature detection captures specific features of a signal. Such as the matched filter detection Feature detection needs prior knowledge of every signal we want to detect. Therefore, feature detection is also not suitable.

2.2.1   Energy Detection

The third option for signal sensing is energy detection. The main advantages of energy detection are that no prior knowledge of the signal to be captured is necessary and that its low complexity does not require complex algorithms. That makes it a good method to be implemented into a SDR. Energy detection detects the signals by measuring the energy in a specific frequency band. The energy of a received signal can be defined by the integral of its squared magnitude over a certain time period, as seen in equation 1, where s(t) is the received signal.

$$E = \int |s(t)^2|dt \qquad (1)$$

If the signal to be detected is unknown, this is the best option. [8] The biggest problem with energy detection is noise. In order to distinguish whether a signal has been picked up or whether only noise has been picked up, a threshold is set. This limit value is compared with the energy of the captured signal. If the received energy is greater than the threshold, a signal has been captured. To clearly detect a signal, accurate knowledge of the noise level is necessary. If the threshold is not set correctly to distinguish a signal from noise, the detector will not work properly.

Since we have no knowledge of the signals we want to sense, energy detection is the method we use in our SDR. Fig. 1 shows the energy detection as a block diagram. First, the signal is received. It is then filtered with the aid of a bandpass filter in order to further process a signal that is as clean as possible. Then an FFT is performed. Equation 1 is now applied. The signal is squared and then summed with an integral. Now this calculated energy is compared with the threshold.

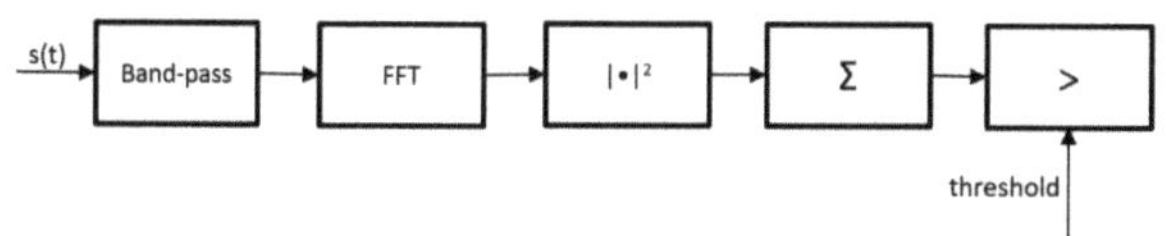

Figure 1: Block diagram for energy detection

2.3 GNU Radio

GNU Radio is a free and open-source software development toolkit for building SDRs. It provides a wide range of tools and libraries for signal detection, filtering, modulation, demodulation, and processing. GNU Radio uses signal processing blocks that can be arranged into a flow chart. GNU Radio also supports a wide range of hardware platforms, particularly Universal Software Radio Peripheral Devices (USRP), which are frequently used for SDR applications. It is also possible to write your own blocks in C++ or Python and use them in a GNU Radio flowchart. The main advantage of GNU Radio, and the reason we used it for the sensor, is that it allows rapid prototyping without specialized hardware and equipment.

2.4 Hardware

For this project, we used the *Ettus Research USRP B205mini-i*. It is a small SDR with a frequency range of 70 MHZ to 6 GHz and a bandwidth of 56 MHz. It allows full duplex operation and is fully supported and maintained for GNU Radio by Ettus Research[9].

3 Implementation and Results

In this section, the implemented GNU Radio flowchart and its features will be explained. In addition, the measurements performed are explained, and the results are presented.

3.1 Experimental setup

In this section, the flowchart for energy detection, shown in fig. 2, is explained. The flowchart starts with a UHD: USRP Source. This block is the interface to the SDR. Bandwidth and sample rate are set to a fixed value, while the frequency is a variable and can be changed by hand during the measurement to turn on different channels. After this block, the flowchart splits into two directions. One direction connects a frequency sink, which performs a FFT and shows the unfiltered frequency spectrum of the received signal. The other path leads to a Band Pass filter. This filter is supposed to filter out some noise. After that, the signal will be increased, and the format will be changed to perform an FFT. After that, the complex number is transformed into a magnitude and gets squared and integrated. At this point in the flowchart, we have a number that can be compared to a threshold. This threshold is variable because it has to be adjusted to the environmental conditions. If the input value of the block is lower than the threshold, the block returns zero

as an output. If it is higher, the block returns one. When a zero is returned, no signal is detected. If one is returned, a signal is detected.

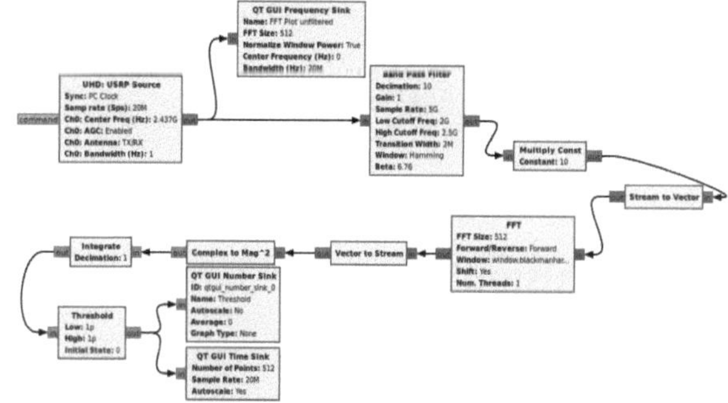

Figure 2: GNU Radio flowchart of the sensor

3.2 Measurements

Fig. 3 and 4 show the output of the flowcharts. Fig. 3 shows a signal recorded at 2.4187 GHz, i.e., channel 6 of IEEE 802.11, in the frequency spectrum. Due to the performance of the used hardware, especially the used laptop, not the full bandwidth of 20 MHz is covered.

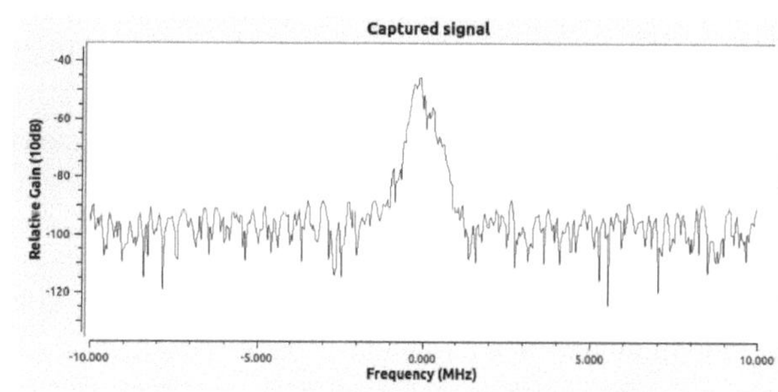

Figure 3: Captured signal in frequency band

Fig. 4 shows the corresponding threshold over a period of $25\mu s$. This is at one over the entire period. At the time of the measurement, several WLAN routers were transmitting on this channel.

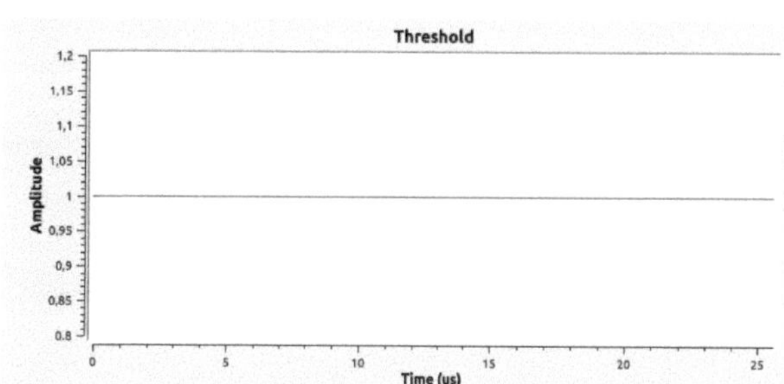

Figure 4: Threshold over time

The controls shown in fig. 5 can be used to change the frequency and height of the threshold during the measurement.

This makes it possible to switch between different frequencies in real time.

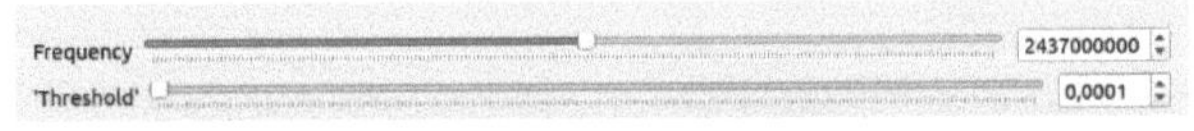

Figure 5: Control elements

4 Conclusion and future work

We have developed a prototype sensor using an SDR to measure whether signals are being transmitted. This is possible with the preset values in the frequency range of 2.4 GHz–2.4835 GHz. It was only tested with the IEEE 802.11 standard. The threshold must be manually adjusted for each environment since the signal-to-noise ratio is different for each environment. To be able to use this sensor, an implementation as an integrated circuit is necessary. Furthermore, an interface is needed to decide which signals are transmitted when the frequency band is free. To cover large areas, several sensors are necessary, which also communicate with each other. It is important to consider how the sensors communicate with each other so that they do not interfere with each other. This would be a spectrum-sensing network. The frequencies on which the sensor operates can be adjusted very easily, so other frequency ranges that may be required can also be monitored easily. For example, WLAN also works on the 5 GHz frequency band. Cognitive radios (CR) are similar to a network of sensors that monitor specific areas. CRs adapt to the environment by monitoring communication and adjusting their parameters accordingly. Among other things, they use machine learning to evaluate their environment. They can adjust their frequency, power level, and other parameters in real time. In contrast to the spectrum-sensing network, no extra sensors are needed, but the transmitters take over this task[7] [10].

Acknowledgement

This publication is a result of the research of the Center of Excellence CoSA at the Technische Hochschule Lübeck.

5 Author's Statement

Conflict of interest: Authors state no conflict of interest.

6 References

[1] Jan Phillip Behrens, *Wireless Communication: WLAN and WPA2* Available: https://www.cs.uni-potsdam.de/bs/teaching/docs/courses/ss2020/scn/material/Behrens-WLAN.pdf Universität Potsdam, 2020.

[2] Nasser, Abbass; Al Haj Hssan, Hussein; Chaaya, Jad Abou; Mansour, Ali and Yao, Koffi-Clément *Spectrum Sensing for Cognitive Radio: Recent Advances and Future Challenge*, MDPI, 2021

[3] *IEEE Standard for Information Technology–Telecommunications and Information Exchange between Systems - Local and Metropolitan Area Networks–Specific Requirements - Part 11: Wireless LAN Medium Access Control (MAC) and Physical Layer (PHY) Specifications*, in IEEE Std 802.11-2020 (Revision of IEEE Std 802.11-2016) , vol., no., pp.1-4379, 26 Feb. 2021, doi: 10.1109/IEEESTD.2021.9363693.

[4] S. Kapp, *802.11: leaving the wire behind*, in IEEE Internet Computing, vol. 6, no. 1, pp. 82-85, Jan.-Feb. 2002, doi: 10.1109/4236.989005.

[5] S. Safaric and K. Malaric, *ZigBee wireless standard*, Proceedings ELMAR 2006, Zadar, Croatia, 2006, pp. 259-262, doi: 10.1109/ELMAR.2006.329562.

[6] *IEEE Standard for Low-Rate Wireless Networks*, in IEEE Std 802.15.4-2020 (Revision of IEEE Std 802.15.4-2015) , vol., no., pp.1-800, 23 July 2020, doi: 10.1109/IEEESTD.2020.9144691.

[7] Mitola, J.; Maguire, G.Q, *Cognitive radio: Making software radios more personal.* IEEE Pers. Commun. 1999, 6, 13–18.

[8] W. Wang, *Spectrum Sensing for Cognitive Radio*, 2009 Third International Symposium on Intelligent Information Technology Application Workshops, Nanchang, China, 2009, pp. 410-412, doi: 10.1109/IITAW.2009.49.

[9] *Comparative features list - B200/B210/B200mini*,Ettus Research, URL https://files.ettus.com/manual/page_usrp_b200.html

[10] S. Haykin, *Cognitive radio: brain-empowered wireless communications*, in IEEE Journal on Selected Areas in Communications, vol. 23, no. 2, pp. 201-220, Feb. 2005, doi: 10.1109/JSAC.2004.839380.

5

Radio Technology and Locating

Mavlink Based Communication Protocol Implementation

Fazli Faruk Okumus

Robotics and Autonomous Systems, Universität zu Lübeck
fazli.okumus@student.uni-luebeck.de

Abstract

Nowadays, most autonomous systems, including aircrafts, require communication with the control centers or other vehicles in the network to share information and enable remote control. The communication protocol allows the autonomous aircraft to be observed, controlled, and tested remotely without risking human life. A well-known MAVLink messaging protocol is used to implement communication protocol, which is helpful for systems targeting less latency. This work includes embedded software implementation details of MAVLink based protocol in the flight control unit, which has resource constraints. As a result, this communication protocol handles different messages necessary for the autonomous navigation of aircraft in the case of different communication hardware mediums. This system works optimally if range and bandwidth constraints are satisfied; otherwise introduces latency into the system, which can lead to undesired results.

1 Introduction

Autonomous aircrafts are popular because they have remote operation, safe testing, and interoperability capabilities. One of the cornerstones of the operability of the aircraft is the communication between the aircraft, ground control station(GCS), and other components. Through this communication, the state of the aircraft can be observed and logged in real time. Aircraft can be remotely controlled by a human pilot, can be interrupted, and can be planned for its autonomous navigation. This communication protocol also needs to enable control of many mission-critical tasks like surveillance and reconnaissance. Therefore, the GCS software and communication protocol backbone must prove themselves in industry-standard applications. Communication protocol also needs to be secure and should consist of necessary handshakes to ensure correct messages are sent and taken.

1.1 Background

This section is designed to introduce common tools, and software chosen and used throughout the project.

1.1.1 QGroundControl

In this project, as a GCS, QGroundControl (QGC) software is chosen [1]. Because of its good user interface (UI) and very good user experience (UX). Other good properties of QGC are 1. QGC is open-source software, which enables the developer can reach its components easily and can change the UI and functionality. 2. QGC is still developing. There are active and reliable developers behind it. Its community could be beneficial in case of any issue during software development. 3. QGC's UI is practical and easy to understand. Because of that, pilot training time could be

dramatically reduced. 4. QGC is based on native C++. For that reason, QGC can be used cross-platform(e.g. Android, Linux, Windows, etc.). 5. It satisfies industry-standard applications. 6. It is based on the Mavlink protocol. 7. It can work with all types of vehicles, like fixed-wind,multicopter, VTOL [1].

1.1.2 Pixhawk, PX4

In this application, it is intended not only to communicate with the aircraft and ground control station but also with other components like Pixhawk and PX4 firmware.
Pixhawk is hardware designed to use with open-source autopilot software like PX4 and Ardupliot. It includes many peripherals and is based on an STM32 chip [2]. This hardware includes redundant inertial sensors like a gyroscope, accelerometer, magnetometer, barometer, and so on. However, also it is possible to connect many more external sensors to it. These specifications allow hobbyists to use prepared autopilot hardware [3].
PX4 is Professional Autopilot software. Developed by world-class developers from industry and academia, and supported by an active worldwide community, it powers all kinds of vehicles from racing and cargo drones through to ground vehicles and submersibles [4]. This open-source software allows using plug-play autonomous mini-micro vehicles. It can be directly used with Pixhawk and QGC software. PX4 supports different types of frames and vehicles, and all these functionalities are open-source, which means developers can change the vehicle's behavior for their use case. In this project, the communication protocol was also designed to connect with Pixhawk, in which PX4 firmware was installed to use its capabilities during the test and quick prototyping [5].

1.1.3 MAVLink

MAVLink is a messaging protocol backbone for communicating with remote vehicles. MAVLink is designed as a publisher-subscriber and point-to-point pattern [6]. All messages and commands are defined via XML file. Users can create their XML file to specify their set of MAVLink messages [7]. It is also possible to create a unique MAVLink message using the MAVLink generator if the already-defined messages are unsuitable for the application. In this application, the C library of MAVLink is used [8].

2 Material and Methods

The general scheme of the overall communication can be seen in Fig. 1. The communication protocol is implemented in the onboard flight computer that is located inside the aircraft.

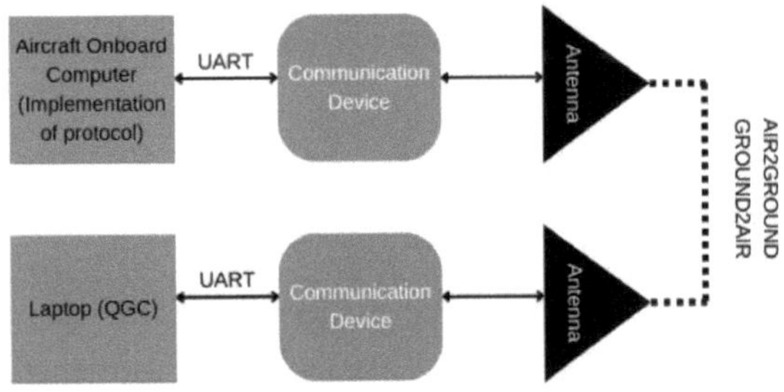

Figure 1: General Scheme of the communication of air vehicle and GCS. Aircraft and GCS send the messages to the communication device over the universal asynchronous receiver-transmitter (UART). Communication devices deliver messages by using antennas.

In this section, the implemented protocol is to be explained. Communication between aircraft and ground consists of microservices (individual protocols), and common messages received periodically from aircraft. This protocol also includes a connection with PX4.

2.1 Microservices

2.1.1 HeartBeat-Connection Protocol

To create a connection, firstly existence of the components in the MAVLink network has to be advertised. A Heartbeat message is used for this functionality. Like getting a post request in the traditional world wide web, in the MAVLink network heartbeat message needs to be advertised to connect to other components in the MAVLink network. Heartbeat message includes the identification of the component.

2.1.2 Parameter Protocol

After the connection is set, the ground control station will request the aircraft's configuration. Each parameter in the configuration is represented as pair of keys/values. The key is the human-readable description of the configuration element, and the value is the corresponding number of the key. Therefore, getting the parameters of the component needs some message exchange between the GCS. Fig. 2 shows the parameter protocol details and necessary message exchange between the air vehicle and GCS.

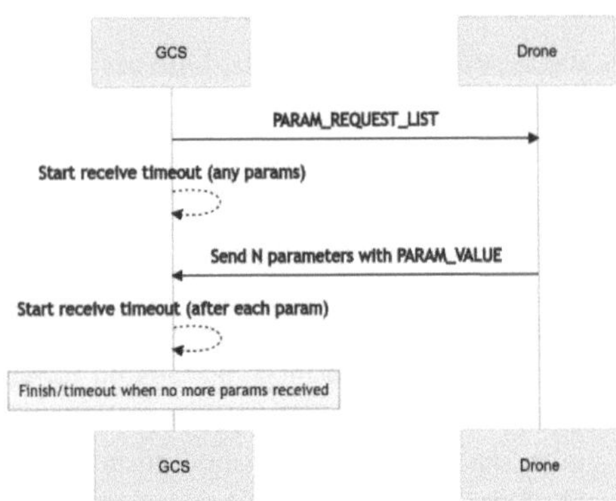

Figure 2: Parameter Protocol [7] of the communication. GCS needs to send *PARAM REUQEST LIST* message to the aircraft. Then, the aircraft side will respond with the *PARAM VALUE* messages for each parameter.

On the other hand, parameters need to be saved in memory in a non-volatile way inside the onboard flight computer. There are many ways to do it. YAML, JSON, and XML formats can be used to store and parse the parameters.

2.1.3 Mission Protocol

This protocol exchanges autonomous mission waypoints, geofence, and safe points with the aircraft. This subprotocol is more complex than others because it needs to make sure that guidance information in aircraft is exactly as intended. Otherwise can cause failures and crashes.
The first part of this protocol is *Upload Mission* to the aircraft. Fig. 3 shows the communication sequence between the GCS and the aircraft. Implemented as described below in Fig. 3. The second part is *Download Mission* from the aircraft. This subprotocol is the same but the reverse of the *Upload Mission* to the vehicle. This subprotocol is important because it is the only way to validate mission items saved on the onboard computer. The third part is the *Clear Mission* subprotocol, which deletes all the waypoints inside the aircraft. These waypoints also need to be saved in the onboard computer's memory in a non-volatile way.

2.1.4 ARM Authorization

ARM and DISARM are essential functionalities in aviation. When the aircraft is armed, that means its motors are activated, and the aircraft is ready for flight. This functionality is also vital for the safety of both vehicles and ground support people. It is a state machine that checks the internal parameters and states of the vehicle to decide whether the aircraft is suitable to be armed.

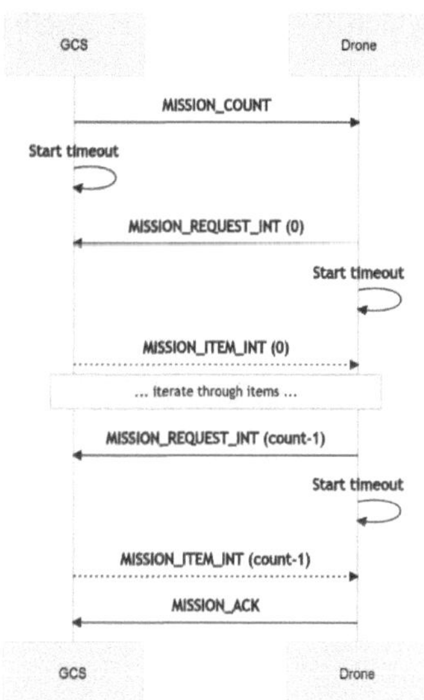

Figure 3: *Upload Mission* subprotocol to the Vehicle [7]. GCS has to send the number of waypoint information with *MISSION COUNT* message to the aircraft. Then for each waypoint, the aircraft sends a request with *MISSION RE-QUEST INT* message and GCS responds with *MISSION ITEM INT* message.

2.1.5 Flight Mode

One of the central core functionality of this communication protocol is the implementation of flight mode management. Autonomous vehicles have different flight modes. The purpose is that the operator may want different flight behavior during the flight envelope, and if an emergency occurs, the operator may want to get full control of the vehicle itself. Flight mode changes can be implemented using the *MAV CMD DO SET MODE* command, which can be seen in Table 1.

Param	Description	Values
1: Mode	Flight Mode	0-10
2: Custom Mode		
3: Custom Submode		

Table 1: *MAV CMD DO SET MODE* command [7]. *Custom Mode* and *Custom Submode* are system specific areas in the message. But in this case, these are not used.

Depending on the application and regulation, a state machine can be established to check whether the allowance of the intended mode changes is valid. This state machine needs to take the flight mode of the system and the custom mode request coming from the GCS into consideration.

2.2 Periodic Messages

Some messages are sent periodically by aircraft, like its orientation, global location, and position. Therefore, handling and extracting the information embedded inside the message is important.

2.2.1 Handle Messages

Another part of the implementation is parsing, reading, and categorizing the incoming message. After this implementation, information coming with the messages can be extracted. These messages also include mission items, commands, and flight modes. After categorization, the associated part of the code is fired up and responds accordingly. For example, if the incoming message is *MISSION COUNT*, GCS requires sending the mission items to the vehicle, so the vehicle has to respond to this with *MISSION REQUEST INT* and expects a mission-related message back. Because of that, after getting some specific messages, the communication protocol automatically closes some periodic messages and opens some microservices to respond back.

2.3 Connection with PX4

For this use case, the onboard computer has low-level controllers and controls the aircraft's attitude, altitude, and position. By communicating with Pixhawk, the onboard computer can enhance its features thanks to PX4's commander, navigator, path planner, and tracker modules. The user can have fully autonomous aircraft by setting the communication between the Pixhawk and the onboard low-level controller. Pixhawk uses its onboard sensors, external sensors, the commander, and the path planner, to calculate the position, velocity, and acceleration setpoints to send a low-level controller according to commands from the GCS.

This implementation is essential in terms of quick prototyping and flight safety. If the aircraft needs to be tested repeatedly, that would give the pace to the overall testing procedure, and the human pilot is not needed every time. In Fig. 4, a diagram of the hardware setup of the overall communication system can be seen.

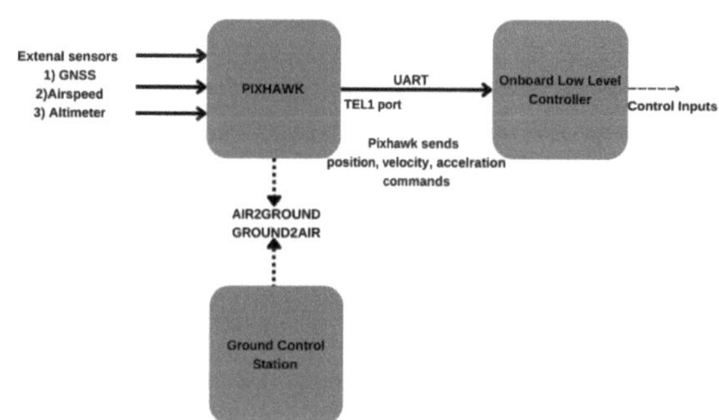

Figure 4: Pixhawk and low-level controller communication. Pixhawk calculates all setpoints by using external sensors and sends them over its *TEL1* port by using UART. GCS communicates with Pixhawk.

3 Results and Discussion

This communication protocol implementation is intended to communicate with the QGC and Pixhawk, in which PX4 firmware was uploaded. This implementation was tested in Software in the loop simulation, which uses UDP protocol to communicate with QGC. Afterward, the protocol was tested on real hardware. This way of development is to decouple hardware and software issues. For the part of the GCS connection, as a communication device, RFD900 telemetry, can be seen in Fig. 5, was used for communication. RFD900 is working on a 900 Mhz band. With this hardware, every protocol described and implemented was working except the mission subprotocol, which is more complex than the other subprotocols. To debug this issue, RFD900 was removed. Then, air and ground are connected with FTDI cable. In this case, every subprotocol worked flawlessly, meaning RFD900+ caused the problem. The problem is that mission protocol requires lots of message exchange, which RFD900+ could not handle. Afterward, RFD900+ was changed to a different company-specific communication device that works on a 5GHz band. In this way, this issue was fixed.

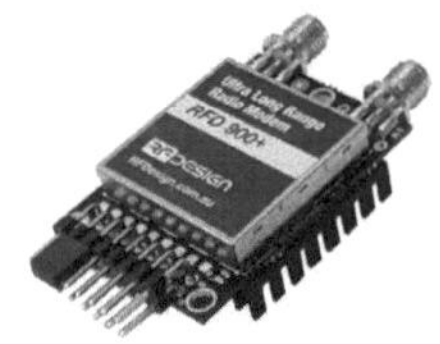

Figure 5: RFD900+ Telemetry Device

For the part of communication with Pixhawk, the implementation is tested on the actual hardware. After solid communication, a flight test was conducted. The mission is designed with QGC and uploaded to Pixhawk, and the onboard controller gets the position, velocity, and acceleration setpoints from Pixhawk. But, both devices estimated different altitudes, positions, and horizontal velocities during the flight test. This can be a massive problem because it causes flight termination, wrong setpoint calculation, or an autonomous mission to get stuck. The real reasons behind these problems are 1. Both devices use different sensors. 2. Both devices have different fusion and estimator algorithms. These problems can be reduced by doing the following 1. Make sure that both devices use the same set of sensors. 2. Close the internal sensor usage, especially the barometer, of Pixhawk by changing its configuration. After these steps, the Pixhawk and onboard controller pair worked in hold mode and maintained their position against external disturbances given.

Overall, during the six months internship exact measurements of latency and the number of message drops during communication could not be performed. Conducted tests depended on the safety pilot perspective and comparison of logged data by both aircraft and GCS.

4　Conclusion

In this project, the communication protocol is implemented based on MAVLink. This protocol implementation is targeted to communicate with the ground control station and Pixhawk, in which PX4 software is installed. Pixhawk, PX4, and QGroundControl were chosen according to their capabilities and the communities behind them. Necessary ground and flight tests were conducted, and issues were detected and fixed. The proposed code was working perfectly with both Pixhawk and QGC. However, there is still room for improvement. By conducting latency measurement tests on communication protocol, code quality can be improved.

Acknowledgement

The work has been carried out at Volocopter GmbH, Munich. Supervised by Dr. Ing. Burak Yueksel, Volocopter GmbH, and Prof. Dr. Georg Schildbach, Universität zu Lübeck.

Author's Statement

Conflict of interest: The author state no conflict of interest.

5　References

[1] QGC-Community, "Qgroundcontrol developer guide, and documentation." available https://docs.qgroundcontrol.com/ [last accessed on 2023-01-18], 2022.

[2] L. Meier, P. Tanskanen, F. Fraundorfer, and M. Pollefeys, "Pixhawk: A system for autonomous flight using onboard computer vision," in *2011 IEEE International Conference on Robotics and Automation*, pp. 2992–2997, 2011.

[3] D. Foundation, "Pixhawk." available https://pixhawk.org/ [last accessed on 2023-01-18], 2022.

[4] L. Meier, "Px4 autopilot user guide (main)." available https://docs.px4.io/main/en/ [last accessed on 2023-01-18], 2022.

[5] L. Meier, D. Honegger, and M. Pollefeys, "Px4: A node-based multithreaded open source robotics framework for deeply embedded platforms," in *2015 IEEE International Conference on Robotics and Automation (ICRA)*, pp. 6235–6240, 2015.

[6] A. Koubâa, A. Allouch, M. Alajlan, Y. Javed, A. Belghith, and M. Khalgui, "Micro air vehicle link (mavlink) in a nutshell: A survey," *IEEE Access*, vol. 7, pp. 87658–87680, 2019.

[7] P. Community, "Mavlink developer guide." available https://mavlink.io/en/ [last accessed on 2023-01-18], 2022.

[8] P. Community, "Mavlink c library." available https://github.com/mavlink/c_library_v2 [last accessed on 2022-09-12], 2022.

Development and evaluation of a localization system based on magnetic field measurements for identification of current carrying conductors

Niklas Thom [1], Sven Ole Schmidt [2], and Prof. Dr. Horst Hellbrück [3],

[1] Department of Electrical Engineering and Computer Science, Technische Hochschule Lübeck - University of Applied Sciences, Germany, niklas.thom@th-luebeck.de

[2] CoSA, Center of Excellence, Technische Hochschule Lübeck - University of Applied Sciences, Germany, sven.ole.schmidt@th-luebeck.de

[3] CoSA, Center of Excellence, Technische Hochschule Lübeck - University of Applied Sciences, Germany, horst.hellbrueck@th-luebeck.de

Abstract

By german law, high-voltage DC cables are required to not exceed the minimum bury depth of 1 m under the sediment. The current in these cables result in a magnetic field. At the moment, no device found in the literature can determine the buried depth of a current carrying conductor under the sediment. In this paper, a new approach for localization by magnetic fields will be developed. Based on a model simulated in Matlab, the consequent magnetic field of a current carrying conductor is estimated by the Biot-Savart theorem and will be evaluated with measurements from a fixed setup of a developed system of multiple magnetometers. The results show that with the approach used an estimate of the location of the cable is made, but more complex mathematical approaches are required to calculate the distance accurately.

1 Introduction

The topic of locating high-voltage submarine cables has received little focus to date. However, with the increasing construction of offshore wind parks in the North and Baltic Seas, this topic is gaining importance. Due to the current flow, the cables emit electromagnetic fields as well as heat. The resulting consequences for wildlife and sediment are still unknown, but initial observations have shown that the hunting behavior of bottom-dwelling sharks and rays is affected by these fields [1]. According to current research, a temperature increase of less than 2 Kelvin at 20 cm below the sediment is still tolerable [2]. This is only to be complied with if the laying depth is more than one meter. If a cable is to be laid crosses another cable or pipeline, additional safety measures in the form of riprap are necessary. For the safety and maintenance of power transmission systems and in order to ensure that the previously named requirements are met despite deep sea current and sediment shifts, developing a reliable method for localization of submarine cables is a crucial task.

This paper focuses on the development of a system that allows the localization of these high-voltage submarine cables by means of magnetic field measurements.

This paper is structured as follows. Section II provides an overview about related work on the field of magnetic field localization. Section III starts with an introduction of the theory, the methods as well as the hardware and software used. Section IV provides an overview of the implementation of the hardware and the structure of the measurement system. Section V discusses the evaluation of the measurement results. Section VI summarizes the conclusion and provides an outlook on future work on this topic.

2 Related Work

Previous studies have investigated the use of magnetic field measurements for the detection and localization of high-voltage submarine cables.

One example of the use of magnetic field sensors for underwater localization in combination with numerical algorithms is given by Vibhav Bharti, David Lane and Sen Wang [3] who filtered out the earth's magnetic field by the geo-coordinates and data from the world magnetic model (WMM). However, the provided method only takes into account a 2D plane (x,y plane) of the magnetic field. Another example is given by Xianbo Xiang, Caoyang Yu, Zermin Niu and Qin Zhang [4] in which the authors present a system of two magnetometers and an evaluation algorithm to locate and follow submarine cables for a fixed depth plane. These studies demonstrate the potential of magnetic field measurements for the detection and localization of high voltage submarine cables,

3   Material and Methods

Following Ampere's circuit law and neglecting the displacement current, the flow of electric current results in a magnetic field:

$$\nabla \times \vec{B} = curl(\vec{B}) = \mu_0 \cdot \vec{J} \qquad (1)$$

where $curl$ is a vector operator describing the infinitesimal circulation of a vector field in three-dimensional space, $\vec{B}$ is the vector of the magnetic flux density, μ_0 the permeability of free space and $\vec{J}$ the vector of the current density. Solving this equation for a circular conductor in 3-dimensional space leads to the Biot-Savart theorem:

$$\vec{B} = \frac{\mu_0 \cdot I}{4 \cdot \pi \cdot r^3} \qquad (2)$$

with which the strength of the magnetic field for of a specific point can be calculated in relation to the distance r.

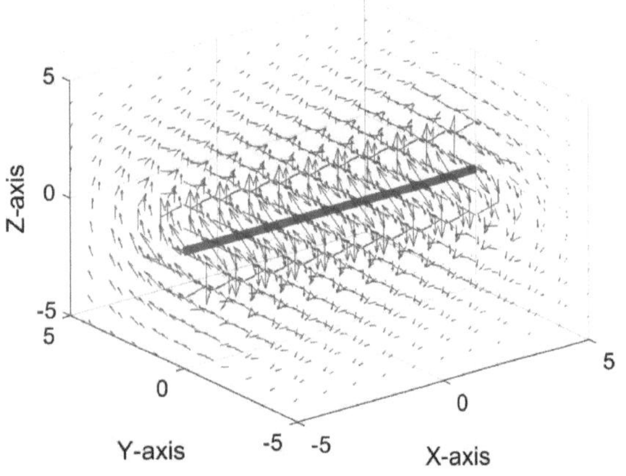

Figure 1: B-field of a current carrying conductor along the X-axis

Fig. 1 shows a current carrying conductor along the X-axis and the resulting magnetic field vectors, depending on the distance to the conductor. At every point of the conductor's surface, the magnetic field has the tangential direction. The magnetic vector field created by the current flow has an x, y and z-orientated component with the magnitude of the magnetic field:

$$B_{Mag} = \sqrt{B_X{}^2 + B_Y{}^2 + B_Z{}^2}. \qquad (3)$$

With the ratio of the B_X, B_Y and B_Z component of the magnetic field, the direction in which the current carrying conductor lies, can be estimated. Furthermore, with the difference in magnitude of the magnetic field measured by the different magnetometers of the system, the orientation of the conductor can be estimated.

4   Implementation of a measurement system

For creating the measurement system, the *SENSYS MX3D UW* data acquisition unit with four freely arrangeable *FGM3D/100 UW II* 3-axis fluxgate sensors are used. The sensors have a measurement range of $\pm$ 100,000 nT and a depth rating of up to 300 m [5]. Each magnetometer is sampling three spatial components x, y and z of the magnetic field caused by the current carrying conductor iteratively with a sampling rate of 2 kHz, taking into account the polarity [6].

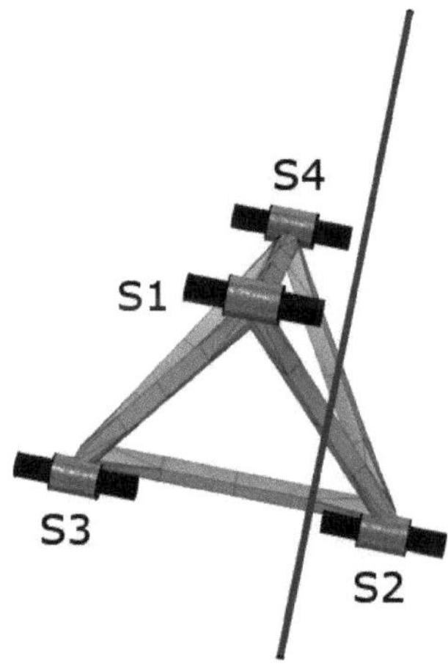

Figure 2: Three-dimensional arrangement of the measuring system in relation to the conductor

Fig. 2 shows the setup used to perform the measurements. The four sensors S1 - S4 are represented by black cylinders insider their mounting. The tetrahedron shaped arrangement of the four magnetometers has a height of 74 cm from the floor to Sensor S1. The upper Sensor S1 is placed in a Distance of 13.5 cm from the middle of the Sensor to the cable, which is shown in red. This equals a distance of 8.4 cm from the Sensors point of reference. Due to this tetrahedron shaped arrangement, the individual sensors measure different magnitudes, spatial components and polarities of the magnetic field vectors from the same conductor.

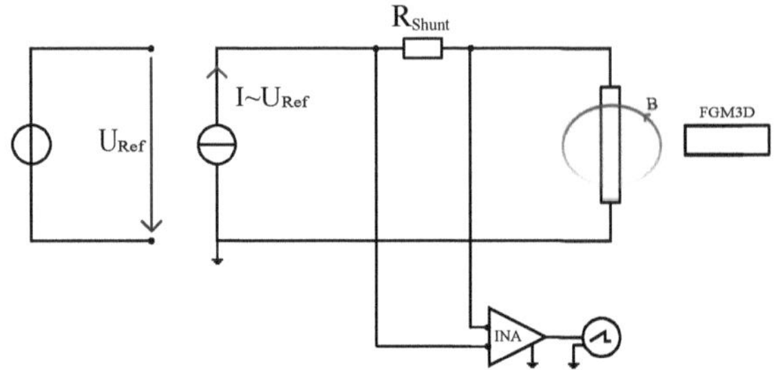

Figure 3: Magnetic field measurement setup including a sinusoidal current of 0.45 A

Fig. 3 shows the setup used to send a defined sinusoidal current of 0.45 A and 20 Hz through the cable whereby the red circle indicates the expected magnetic field.

It consists of a linearly regulated, voltage-controlled current source with an output current in the range of 0-1 A at a control voltage of $\pm$ 15 V. The voltage is measured via a shunt of $R_{Shunt} = 10 \ m\Omega$ and displayed on an oscilloscope via an instrumentation amplifier (INA) with a gain of $A = 100$. The magnetic field resulting from the current flow is then measured with the FGM3D UW II magnetic field sensors at a fixed distance.

A comparison measurement without a current flow is performed as well in order to determine external influences on the measurement. Furthermore, a measurement input of the data acquisition unit is not used to ascertain influences of the measurement noise and to take them into account during the evaluation.

5   Evaluation

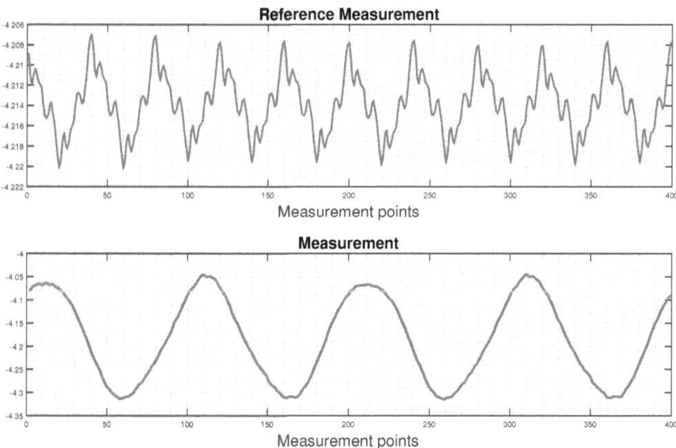

Figure 4: Measurement results of the magnetic field without and with current flow in the conductor

Fig. 4 shows the comparison of the measured magnetic field resulting from the defined current flow of 0.45 A and the reference measurement. The graph clearly shows the offset, a 50 Hz ambient signal and the resulting deformation of the 20 Hz measurement signal. Both graphs fit the expectation, that the 50 Hz signal from the power grid and other influences, such as the earth's magnetic field, affect the measurement signal.

A Fast Fourier Transformation (FFT) is performed to convert the data from the time domain into the frequency domain to determine the spectral components of the magnetic field. Thereafter, a bandpass filter is used to filter out all components of a deviating frequency as well as the offset caused by external influences such as the earth's magnetic field from the measured signal of 20 Hz. With an inverse FFT, the spectrum is transformed back into the time domain.

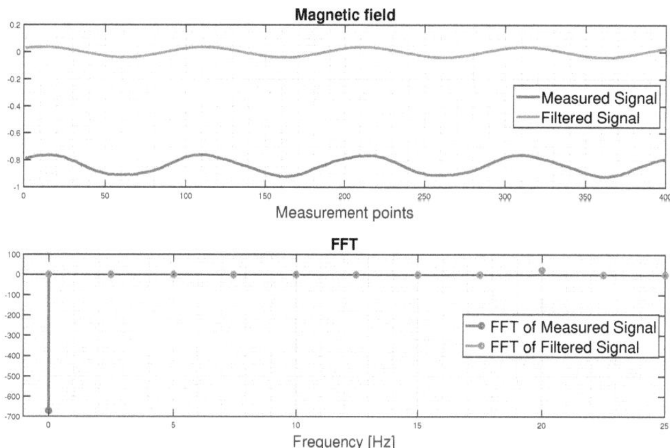

Figure 5: Signal curve and FFT of measured Signal before and after filtering

Fig. 5 shows the signal curve and the spectrum before and after the bandpass filter. As the graph clearly shows, a sinusoidal signal around the zero axis is obtained from the deformed signal with offset. This fulfills the expectation, since the measurement signal is sinusoidal without an offset. By determining the difference between the filtered measurement data and the filtered reference measurement data, further interferences caused by various electronic devices and external factors on the same frequency of 20 Hz are cut out.

Table 1: Approximated and expected vertical angles between Sensor and Conductor

Device	Angle [Deg]	Approximated Angle [Deg]	Deviation [Deg]
Sensor 1	10	19	9
Sensor 2	109	108	1
Sensor 3	54	44	10
Sensor 4	79	74	5
Average			6.25

By the ratio of the filtered magnetic field components, the angle can be determined mathematically. The results of this calculation as well as the angles of the measurement setup are shown in Table 1.

Table 2: Approximated and expected distance between Sensor and Conductor

Device	Distance [cm]	Approximated Distance r [cm]	Euclidean norm
Sensor 1	8.52	39.36	30.84
Sensor 2	78	93.53	15.53
Sensor 3	89	120.1	31.1
Sensor 4	74	95.2	21.3
Average			24.69

With the measured values for the magnitude of the magnetic field, the distance can be determined mathematically by rearranging the previously approximated formula to

$$r = \sqrt[3]{\frac{\mu_0 \cdot I}{4 \cdot \pi \cdot B}}. \tag{4}$$

Table 2 shows the distance of the setup and the distance approximated as well as the euclidean norm.

Despite the less than ideal conditions of the measurement setup, the angles are determined relatively reliable with a maximum deviation of 10 Degree and an average deviation of 6.25 Degree. However, with an euclidean norm between 15.53 and 30.84 there are larger deviations when determining the distance. Taking into account the fact that German law requires cables to be buried at least one meter deep, this estimation of the distance is not sufficient to ensure that compliance with this law is given at any time this approach is used.

By evaluating the polarity of the spatial components of the measurement data with logic operations, it is possible to determine whether the current carrying conductor is located behind, below or ahead of the measurement setup or between two sensors at the same height of the mounting which poses the risk of a collision. In combination with the determined angle, the localization of the cable is estimated.

6   Conclusion and future work

Comparison of expected and calculated values show, that this method provides an approximation to in which direction and angle the conductor is located. As shown in Table 1, the estimated angles fit the angles of the used setup with an average error of 6.25 Degree. However, the determination of the distance under the assumption that the measured magnetic field is caused by the closest point of a straight conductor is not sufficient to locate current carrying conductors with accuracy. One assumption for this deviation is, that the formula doesn't take into account, that the magnetic field at a specific point is not caused by the closest point of a straight conductor, but by the entire length of the current carrying conductor [7].

For further improvement of this method, the fraction contributing to the measured magnetic field over the entire length of the experimental setup has to be considered. Another point that needs to be revised is the setting of a fixed reference point for the contemplation of the angle. Due to the trigonometric calculation of the angle from the spatial components, the hypotenuse is always a positive value, which leads to a rotation of the reference point depending on the polarity of the catheti. Furthermore, the skewed position of the sensors due to the mountings and the associated differences in the vectorial quantities of the magnetic field cannot be easily normalized by a calibration factor. For further improvement, a new mounting of the sensors must be made to meet the new requirements.

Nevertheless, it was shown that the measurement setup can identify the individual magnetic field components independently of environmental disturbances even under less than ideal conditions. Furthermore, it is possible to determine

the position of the cable in the premises with the help of the determined angle and direction. These conclusions can now be used to further refine the setup and evaluation, taking into account the newly identified problematic factors.

Acknowledgement

This publication abstract results from the research of the Center of Excellence CoSA at the Technische Hochschule Lübeck and is funded by the Federal Ministry of Economic Affairs and Energy of the Federal Republic of Germany (Id 03SX467B, Project EXTENSE, Project Management Agency: Jülich PTJ). Horst Hellbrück is an adjunct professor at the Institute of Telematics of University of Lübeck.

Author's Statement

Conflict of interest: Authors state no conflict of interest.

7   References

[1] Bundesamt für Strahlenschutz, Blanka Pophof, Dirk Geschwentner, "Umweltauswirkungen der Kabelanbindung von OffshoreWindenergieparks an das Verbundstromnetz"

[2] Bundesamt für Naturschutz, Available: https://www.bfn.de/seekabel#anchor-4035 [last accessed on: 2023-01-21]

[3] Vibhav Bharti, David Lane and Sen Wang, "A Semi-Heuristic Approach for Tracking Buried Subsea Pipelines using Fluxgate Magnetometers" *2020 16th IEEE International Conference on Automation Science and Engineering (CASE) August 20-21, 2020, Online Zoom Meeting*

[4] Xianbo Xiang, Caoyang Yu , Zemin Niu and Qin Zhang , "Subsea Cable Tracking by Autonomous Underwater Vehicle with Magnetic Sensing Guidance"

[5] SENSYS Magnetometers & Survey Solutions, "Multi-Channel Survey System for Underwater Applications MAGNETO MX3D UW", Datasheet.

[6] SENSYS Magnetometers & Survey Solutions, "Multi-Channel Survey System for Underwater Applications MAGNETO MX3D UW", Matrix of Housing types and Pin Layout.

[7] Heine Henke, "Elektromagnetische Felder - Theorie und Anwendung", *Springer Verlag, 2011, ISBN: 978-3-642-19745-1 pp. 45.*

Evaluation of Position Estimations for a Bluetooth Low Energy Angle-of-Arrival Localization System

Ben Kampen [1], Sven Ole Schmidt [1] and Horst Hellbrück [1]

[1] Department of Electrical Engineering and Computer Science, Technische Hochschule Lübeck - University of Applied Sciences, ben.kampen@stud.th-luebeck.de, {sven.ole.schmidt, horst.hellbrueck}@th-luebeck.de

Abstract

Bluetooth Low Energy has become an established technology for indoor localization. With the introduction of Bluetooth 5.1, it is possible to determine the direction from which the Bluetooth signal is coming. This property enables the Angle of Arrival method to determine the position of the Bluetooth transmitter with respect to the fixed installed receivers. In this paper, we have built a Bluetooth 5.1 system based on the Angle of Arrival localization system and evaluated its accuracy of it. For this purpose we established the mathematical model developed the system architecture and implemented the position algorithm. The evaluation showed that in 80 % of the measurements, the position error is less than 1.5 m and in 60 % less than 1 m.

1 Introduction

The use of indoor position determination has a wide range of applications. One example is the use in hospitals for the localization of medical equipment as well as the medical staff. Another large application area is Industry 4.0. As processes become more and more transparent and every step is to be mapped in the system, the application of localization systems is an essential part of digitalization.

The Internet of Things describes devices equipped with sensors and software networked via the internet to exchange data. To collect data the devices should be mobile, portable or stationary. An important factor is the interpretation of the data which is made possible by the position [1].

There is a number of localization solutions that need to be weighed for each application. Decisive parameters for the selection of the localization system are the accuracy and the environment in which the system is to be used. For example, the Global Positioning System (GPS) is not suitable for indoor localization because of the walls and ceilings which leads to a weakness of the GPS signal [2]. There are a variety of technologies that can be used in the field of indoor localization. One possible technology for indoor localization is Bluetooth Low Energy [3]. The approach in this context is to measure the signal strength of the Bluetooth signal from a beacon. With this technology accuracies in the range of 3-4 meters can be achieved. With the introduction of Bluetooth 5.1 in the year 2019, the so-called radio direction finding is possible [4]. Methods for determining position with this technology are Angle of Arrival (AOA) and Angle of Departure (AOD). For this purpose locators and beacons are used to determine the angle, which allows the position to be determined using geometric tri-/multilateration.

A great advantage of this system is the low power consumption, which is ideal for the use of beacons with batteries. In addition, procurement and maintenance costs are low [5].

In this paper, a mathematical model based on geometric multilateration is developed for an AOA Bluetooth 5.1 system with 4 locators. In this model, the Received Signal Strength Indication (RSSI) values are not used for position determination. Following this approach, to the best of our knowledge only systems including artificial intelligence exists [6]. Furthermore, a suitable system architecture is designed. Finally, the position measurements are evaluated and a conclusion is drawn.

The paper is organized as follows. Section 2 presents the Bluetooth 5.1 technology features required for direction finding and the AOA method. Section 3 describes the measurement setup as well as the system architecture and evaluation. Finally, in section 4 the conclusions are drawn.

2 Methods

2.1 Bluetooth 5.1 Direction Finding

Before the introduction of Bluetooth 5.1, the signal strength was used to determine the position. The direction finding feature makes it possible to determine the direction from which a Bluetooth signal is coming.

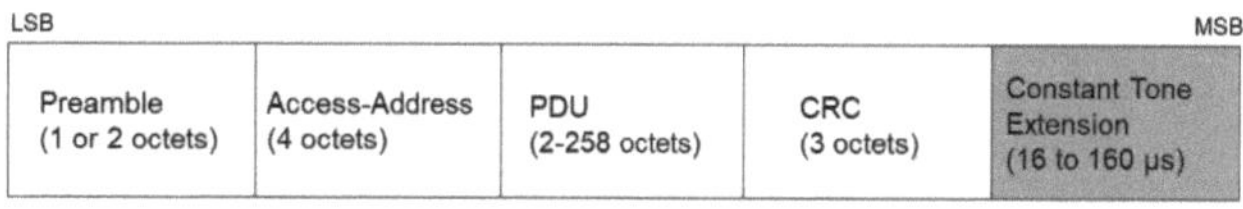

Figure 1: Bluetooth 5.1 link layer packet

Fig. 1 shows the extension by Constant Tone Extension (CTE). To perform direction finding the Bluetooth link layer adds a CTE to each Bluetooth packet. The CTE is an unmodulated sine, sent on the Bluetooth carrier frequency (plus 250 kHz) between 16 and 160 μs. The sine comprises a 1 s noise-free sequence that is transmitted long enough for the receiver to extract the data without modulation interference. Since the CTE signal is transmitted last, the cyclic redundancy check (CRC) of the packet is not affected [7].

2.2 Direction Finding using Angle of Arrival

In the AOA method, a signal is transmitted by a beacon and received by an antenna array. The signal reaches the individual antennas at different times due to the respective path that the signal travels. This results in a phase difference. The angle θ from which the signal was transmitted can be determined. For this the distance d between two antennas, the wavelength λ and the phase difference γ of the incident signal is needed [7]. In the μ-blox XPLR-AOA-2 kit, 5 dual-polarized antennas are used, which increases the accuracy of angle determination. The relationship from the previously explained shows (1) :

$$\theta = \arccos\left(\frac{\gamma \cdot \lambda}{2 \cdot \pi \cdot d}\right) \tag{1}$$

To estimate the position of a beacon within a given area, geometric multilateration can be used.

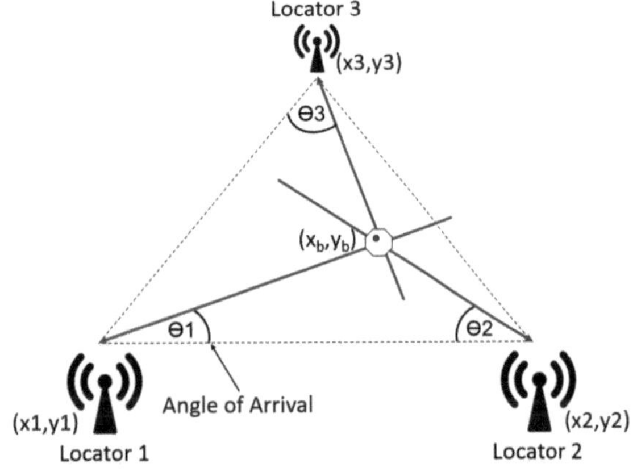

Figure 2: Principle of Angle of Arrival estimation in 2 dimensions

Fig. 2 shows the position estimation with the AOA method. Therefore the previously calculated angles are required. To estimate the position of a beacon at least two AOA measurements from two different references are necessary. In practical applications, more than two references are often used to improve accuracy due to limited angular resolution, multipath effects and noise. An advantage of AOA-based methods are that they do not require clock synchronization. But for accurate angular determination, directional antennas, multiple-element antenna arrays and computationally intensive algorithms are needed [8].

For the position determination in 3 dimensions the azimuth angle θ (horizontal) and the elevation angle ψ (vertical) are needed. Both angles can be calculated with 1. The position of the beacon in 3 dimensions can be determined by rearranging and substituting (2) and (3) for each of the locators:

$$\tan(\theta_i) = \frac{x_b - x_i}{y_b - y_i} \tag{2}$$

$$\tan(\psi_i) = \frac{z_b - z_i}{x_b - x_i} \tag{3}$$

2.3 Position Estimation Algorithm

Algorithm 1 Position Estimation

---

i_{th} $Locator$ is at $L_i = [x_i, y_i, z_i]$ $\quad i = 1, 2, 3, 4$

$\theta_i, \ \psi_i \quad i = 1, 2, 3, 4$

$$x_1 = \frac{\frac{-L_1(1)}{\tan(\theta_1)} + L_1(2) + \frac{L_3(1)}{\tan(\theta_3)} - L_3(2)}{\frac{1}{\tan(\theta_3)} - \frac{1}{\tan(\theta_1)}}$$

$$x_2 = \frac{\frac{-L_2(1)}{\tan(\theta_2)} + L_2(2) + \frac{L_4(1)}{\tan(\theta_4)} - L_4(2)}{\frac{1}{\tan(\theta_4)} - \frac{1}{\tan(\theta_2)}}$$

$$y_1 = \frac{-L_1(2) \times \tan(\theta_1) + L_1(1) + L_3(2) \times \tan(\theta_3) - L_3(1)}{\frac{1}{\tan(\theta_3)} - \frac{1}{\tan(\theta_1)}}$$

$$y_2 = \frac{-L_2(2) \times \tan(\theta_2) + L_2(1) + L_4(2) \times \tan(\theta_4) - L_4(1)}{\frac{1}{\tan(\theta_4)} - \frac{1}{\tan(\theta_2)}}$$

$$z_1 = \frac{\frac{-L_1(3)}{\tan(\psi_1)} + L_1(1) + \frac{L_3(3)}{\tan(\psi_3)} - L_3(1)}{\frac{1}{\tan(\psi_3)} - \frac{1}{\tan(\psi_1)}}$$

$$z_2 = \frac{\frac{-L_2(3)}{\tan(\psi_2)} + L_2(1) + \frac{L_4(3)}{\tan(\psi_4)} - L_4(1)}{\frac{1}{\tan(\psi_4)} - \frac{1}{\tan(\psi_2)}}$$

$$x_B = \frac{x_1 + x_2}{2} \quad y_B = \frac{y_1 + y_2}{2} \quad z_B = \frac{z_1 + z_2}{2}$$

Algorithm 1 represents the position estimation. First, the locator positions L_i and the azimuth and elevation angle θ_i and ψ_i are determined. The following equations x_1 to z_2 are used for the final position estimation of the beacon at position (x_B, y_B, z_B). This is achieved by averaging the previously mentioned equations.

3 Results and Discussion

This chapter begins with a presentation of the materials used for the subsequent measurement setup and the system architecture. This is followed by an evaluation of the measurement results.

3.1 Material

The system used is the μ-blox XPLR-AOA-2 kit. This is an indoor positioning system which allows to use Bluetooth 5.1 technology. It contains 4 locators (C211) and 4 beacons (C209). The system has a mean angle accuracy of 5 degrees. It is possible to use up to 50 beacons within the locating range. Through a USB interface, the locator data can be transferred by connecting to a PC or other host system [4].

3.2 Measurement setup

The measurement setup consists of 4 locators, a beacon and a measurement grid. To position the beacon accurately a measurement grid was used. The measurement grid was fixed on the ground and has a dimension of 3x3 meters with a spacing of 0.5 m. The locators have a distance to the measurement grid of 2 m and were fixed at a height of 1.6 m.

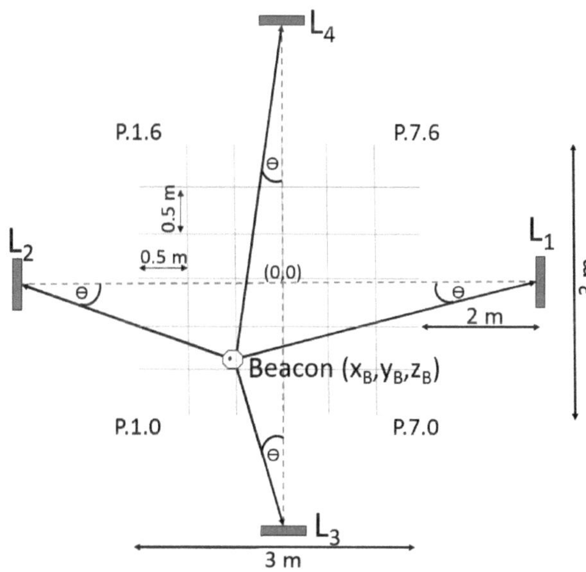

Figure 3: Top view of the measurement setup

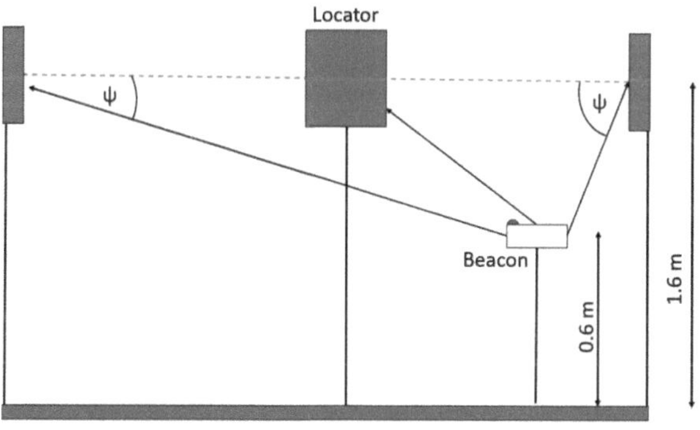

Figure 4: Side view of the measurement setup

Fig. 3 and Fig. 4 show the top and side views of the system. The distance between the locators and the grid points must be at least 2 m according to the data sheet [4]. Otherwise significant measurement errors will occur. The beacon which is placed on the grid has a height of 0.6 m. A total of 49 measuring points with 250 measured values are recorded.

3.3 System architecture

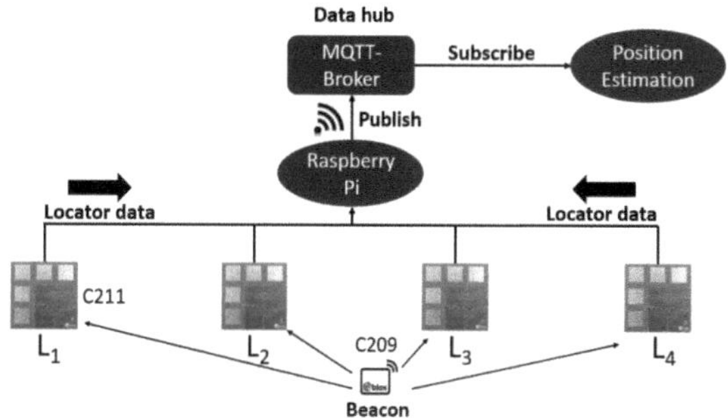

Figure 5: System architecture

The system architecture is represented in Fig. 5. The beacon (C209) sends out a Bluetooth signal that the locators (C211) receive and process. The data of the locators are read in through the serial interfaces of a Raspberry Pi and published wireless to a Message Queuing Telemetry Transport (MQTT) broker that serves as a data hub. The azimuth and elevation angle are transmitted as locator data. By subscribing to the respective topics, it is possible to receive the data and perform position determination as shown in Algorithm 1.

3.4 Evaluation

In this chapter the measurement results are evaluated with the previously explained measurement setup.

The position errors were determined by the euclidean distance. The estimated positions are an average of the 250 recorded measurements per measuring point. The Euclidean distance was calculated by (4):

$$d\left(p_j, \hat{p}_j\right) = \sqrt{\left(p_{xj} - \hat{p}_{xj}\right)^2 + \left(p_{yj} - \hat{p}_{yj}\right)^2 + \left(p_{zj} - \hat{p}_{zj}\right)^2}$$
(4)

where:
$p_j = (p_{xj}, p_{yj}, p_{zj})$ Expected position at measuring point j
$\hat{p}_j = (\hat{p}_{xj}, \hat{p}_{yj}, \hat{p}_{zj})$ Estimated position at measuring point j

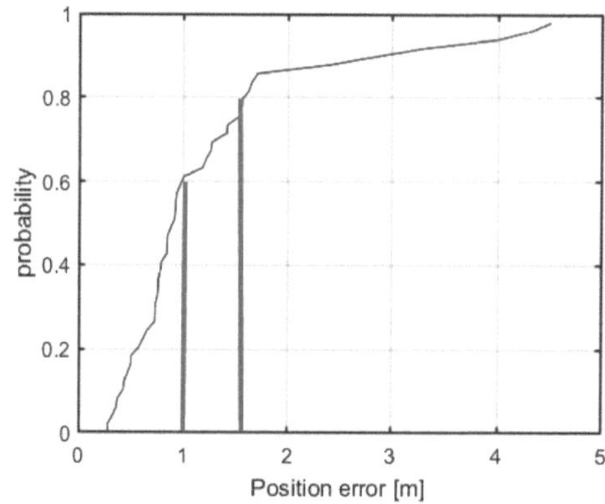

Figure 6: eCDF of position error $d\left(p_j, \hat{p}_j\right)$

Fig. 6 shows the empirical Cumulative Distribution Function (eCDF) for the position errors. The eCDF shows that the estimated positions have a position error of less than 1 meter in 60 % and less than 1.5 meters in 80 % of the cases.

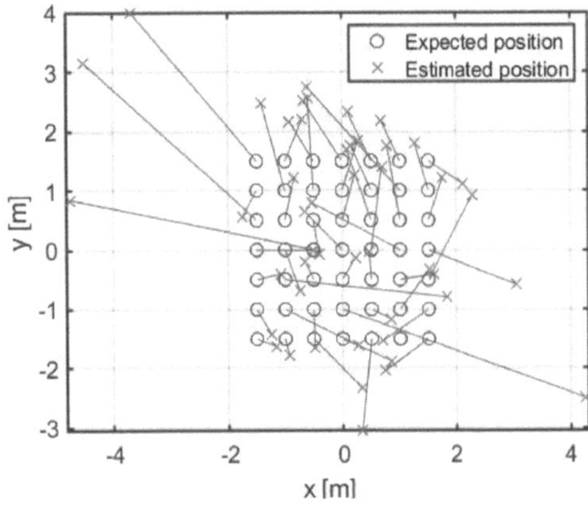

Figure 7: Expected and estimated positions

Fig. 7 shows the expected and estimated positions. There are three main characters:

Significant errors in position estimations
Particularly conspicuous are the position estimations which in some cases vary strongly from the expected positions. Especially the measurement points P1.4, P1.6, P3.3, P4.1 result in a large error of up to 4 meters. It is assumed that the large errors in the areas of the grid points are due to obstacles and multipath propagation. A subsequent investigation of this problem will be conducted in the future. However, the points with large errors represent only a small fraction.

y-axis offset
In the lower and upper range of the measurement series, a y-axis offset can be seen. In the lower area, the offset of the estimated position is in the negative y-direction. This can be seen in the following positions P1.0 to P7.0 and P1.1 to P7.1. On the other hand, a positive y-axis offset in the estimation of the positions can be seen in P1.5 to P7.5 and P1.6 to P7.6. The exact cause is still unknown.

Position estimation with smaller errors
There are smaller errors between expected and estimated position in the centre area of the measurement grid, which is in the range between $x \pm 0.5$ and $y \pm 0.5$. One assumption is that the distance to the locators is greatest in the centre area and the errors become smaller for this reason. In this case, the error is on average about 0.6 meters.

4 Conclusion

In this paper, a model for Bluetooth Low Energy position estimation was evaluated. The model uses the AOA method together with Bluetooth 5.1 technology. We have found that the accuracy of the position determination is in the meter range and partly depends on the position of the beacon. In 60 % of cases, there is a deviation of less than 1 meter and in 80 % of cases less than 1.5 meters. The accuracy of the technology is in accordance with the literature. In the future, the large deviations between expected and estimated positions will be investigated and analyzed. Due to the smaller deviations in the centre area of the measurement grid, an upscaling of the measurement setup is a possibility to increase the distance to the locators. For a more accurate analysis of large deviations, it is recommended to set up the system in an outdoor environment, which minimizes influences such as multipath propagation and interference.

Acknowledgement

The work has been carried out at the CoSA Center of Excellence at the Technische Hochschule Lübeck - University of Applied Sciences. I would like to thank to Sven Ole Schmidt and Prof. Dr. Hellbrück for supervising the work.

Author's Statement

Conflict of interest: Authors state no conflict of interest.

5 References

[1] S. O. Schmidt and H. Hellbrück, "Detection and identification of multipath interference with adaption of transmission band for UWB transceiver systems," 2021, (2022, December 8). [Online]. Available: http://ceur-ws.org/Vol-3097/paper4.pdf

[2] A. Lindemann, B. Schnor, J. Sohre, and P. Vogel, "Indoor positioning: A comparison of wifi and bluetooth low energy for region monitoring," in *International Conference on Health Informatics*, 2016, (2022, December 8).

[3] Bluetooth special interest group. (2022, December 15). [Online]. Available: https://www.bluetooth.com/

[4] Xplr-aoa-2 kit user guide. (2022, December 23). [Online]. Available: https://content.u-blox.com/sites/default/files/XPLR-AOA-Explorer-kits_UserGuide_UBX-21004616.pdf

[5] Bluetooth. (2022, December 17). [Online]. Available: https://www.u-blox.com/en/technologies/bluetooth

[6] Z. HajiAkhondi-Meybodi, M. Salimibeni, A. Mohammadi, and K. N. Plataniotis, "Bluetooth low energy and cnn-based angle of arrival localization in presence of rayleigh fading," 2021, (2023, January 29).

[7] G. Pau, F. Arena, Y. E. Gebremariam, and I. You, "Bluetooth 5.1: An analysis of direction finding capability for high-precision location services," (2022, December 15). [Online]. Available: https://www.mdpi.com/1424-8220/21/11/3589

[8] D. Munoz, F. Bouchereau, C. Vargas, and R. Enriquez, "Chapter 3 - location information processing," in *Position Location Techniques and Applications*, 2009, (2022, December 10). [Online]. Available: https://www.sciencedirect.com/science/article/pii/B9780123743534000090

Adaptable, LIDAR based, mobile platform for performing localized indoor measurements

Carl Revander [1], Björn Sievers [2] and Horst Hellbrück [3]

[1] Applied Information Technology, TH Lübeck - University of Applied Sciences, Germany, carl.revander@stud.th-luebeck.de

[2,3] Department of Electrical Engineering and Computer Science, TH Lübeck - University of Applied Sciences, Germany, {bjoern.sievers, horst.hellbrueck}@th-luebeck.de

Abstract

In this paper, we develop a mobile platform for performing localized indoor measurements. Whereas in outdoor environments GPS would likely be used for localized measurements, this is not viable within buildings. Alternative indoor positioning systems, meanwhile, often rely on infrastructure to certain degree, which is not guaranteed to exist in every environment. We therefore implement a versatile mobile measurement platform in this paper, which does not depend on the availability of such infrastructure, by utilizing simultaneous localization and mapping. After first mapping a previously unknown environment, our mobile platform subsequently calculates locations which to autonomously navigate to and perform measurements at.

Navigating to these points, however, proved difficult to implement and currently stands in the way of a full implementation of the system. While the hardware modalities we use in this paper certainly are a promising approach for the task at hand, our results are characterized by obstacles still standing in the way of a complete implementation of our platform.

1 Introduction

Currently, there is no real standard approach for indoor environments, for performing localized measurements in order to map them and gain insights about the measured quantities.

One scenario that could benefit from a system that delivers this kind of capability is the placement of 5G access points. Compared to previous standards, traits, such as higher data rates, lower latencies or an increased reliability have made it an interesting technology, not just for providing better mobile networks for cellphones, but also for industrial automation contexts among many other applications [1].

The resulting and increasing usage of 5G in indoor settings presents unique challenges regarding the planning and placement of access points. Measurements to evaluate current signal strengths in different locations, for example, would typically rely on GPS for localization. In indoor scenarios, however, GPS signals are weaker, making acquiring and tracking them a challenging task [2].

For this reason, many different alternative approaches for indoor localization have already been devised in the past [3]. This paper explores the use of Simultaneous localization and mapping (SLAM), based on a Light detection and ranging (LIDAR) sensor, as one of them. Utilizing the distance measurements of a LIDAR sensor, a SLAM algorithm can generate maps of local environments as it moves through them. Since a global context, like the one provided by GPS, is likely not necessary for most indoor measurement tasks, SLAM and LIDAR can often provide a suitable and simpler solution in such cases. In addition, higher precision in localization and mapping forms an important basis for the subsequent equipment of measurement systems with autonomous behavior. This would be especially valuable in use cases, such as mapping the distribution of gases indoors, as performing remote controlled or autonomous measurements would help risks to humans.

To provide a basis for performing indoor measurements using LIDAR and SLAM for localization, we implement a platform that is designed to be flexible regarding measurement devices and measurement tasks. For this, we equipped a mobile robot with a 5G modem and a LIDAR sensor, for which we implement a semi-autonomous measurement procedure in a Python script.

This paper is structured as follows. Section 2 gives an overview of the methods and materials we used. In Section 3, we describe the implementation of our platform. We discuss the results of this in Section 4 and conclude the paper in Section 5.

2 Methods and Materials

2.1 LIDAR

LIDAR, is an optical measurement method for determining the distance to objects. It is similar to RADAR, with the main difference being, that instead of radio waves, light from or near the visible spectrum is used for LIDAR. Measuring the Time of Flight t, i.e. the time it takes for emitted light pulses to be reflected back to the sensor, a LIDAR sensor is used to calculate a distance d with the speed of light c [4]:

$$d = ct/2 \qquad (1)$$

By rotating a LIDAR sensor and continuously taking measurements, horizontal scans of the entire environment are performed.

2.2 SLAM

Simultaneous localization and mapping is a term referring to algorithms, that address the problem of robots having to navigate in unknown environments, by providing accurate approximations of its location, as well as detailed models of an environment [5].

2.3 Hardware

2.3.1 LIDAR sensor

An M2M2 two-dimension LIDAR sensor by Slamtec [6] constitutes one of the main hardware components of the overall setup for performing the necessary laser scans in the horizontal plane. A SLAM algorithm is already integrated on a computing unit in the sensor and with the corresponding SDK provided by Slamware as an interface, the generated maps are directly accessible. It has a measuring range of 0.1m to 40m, a mapping resolution of 0.05m and a maximum inclination angle of up to $3°$.

With the intention of reducing tilt compared to a handheld application and providing a basis for a more autonomous measurement process, the LIDAR sensor is mounted on a robotic platform, which we describe next.

2.3.2 Mobile robotic platform

The quadruped A1 robot by Unitree [7] serves as a mobile platform for the LIDAR sensor. It is controlled via an accompanying remote control, a phone with the UnitreeRobotics app or commands within the Robot Operating System (ROS) framework.

2.3.3 Miscellaneous

We use a SIM8200EA-M2 5G modem by Simcom to provide external connectivity for sending and visualizing measurements and SLAM maps or for receiving commands. Furthermore we mounted a Jetson Nano embedded computing board by Nvidia [8] to the robot as well, in order to ensure sufficient computing power. In the current implementation, however, it is not utilized and computations are handled by the robot itself and on a laptop, connected to the robot via 5G.

Two power banks are also mounted to the robot to provide power for the LIDAR sensor, the 5G modem and the Jetson Nano. This saves energy from the robots own battery pack

and increases operating time. The described overall setup can be seen in Fig. 1.

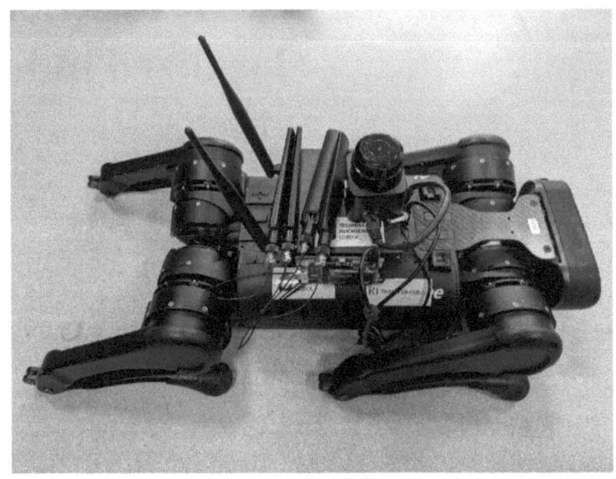

Figure 1: Overall setup with the robot, Jetson Nano, LIDAR sensor and 5G modem visible

2.4 Software

Ubuntu serves as the operating system for the Jetson Nano, laptop, as well as the robot.

Additionally, ROS , an open-source framework for communication with robots, is installed on all of these. By subscribing or publishing to so called ROS topics, where information is exchanged in the form of messages, another device can send or receive data (e.g. instructions or measurements) to or from a robot, respectively. ROS also offers a tool for visualization, called RVIZ, which is used in this paper for displaying the current SLAM map during mapping.

The Slamware ROS SDK supplied with the LIDAR sensor provides the interface to ROS by means of various ROS topics that can be used to address the sensor, for example to change settings or retrieve information. Particularly important for this work is the */map* topic, which can be subscribed to in order to receive the SLAM maps that the sensor automatically generates and publishes in this topic.

The A1 also offers the possibility of being used in conjunction with ROS. For example, it automatically subscribes to the standard ROS topic */move_base/goal*, which can then be used to send it a message with a destination to which it should navigate.

The overall measurement procedure is handled by a custom python script, using the rospy library for interfacing ROS topics.

The next section goes into detail about this and the results of it.

3 Implementation

We implemented a Python script to handle the mapping and measurement process, with the goal of automating as much of the whole procedure as possible in the long term. In its current state this script is divided into a mapping and a measurement phase, as illustrated in Fig. 2

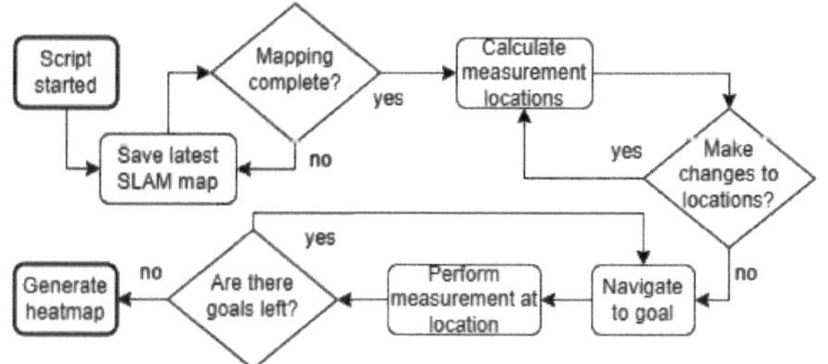

Figure 2: Schematic sequence of the Python script

First, the former is performed manually, by the user, via the remote control of the robot. For this the robot is maneuvered around for as long as the user wishes and builds up a SLAM map along the way. Meanwhile the script receives map updates, by being subscribed to the ROS topic */map*, to which the LIDAR sensor publishes those updates. In those messages obstacles, unmapped and accessible areas are each represented by a corresponding numeric value within a grid. Once the map, displayed in RVIZ during this process, has reached a sufficient state, the script can be advanced to the next phase by the press of a button in the script terminal window. At this point the script ceases listening to newer messages published to the */map* topic.

The measurement process begins with the script using the latest received state of the map to calculate and suggest positions at which measurements shall be performed. Here, the idea was to arrange those uniformly in a grid, rather than having them at arbitrary locations, which, depending on the user and the implementation, would likely be the case if they were performed during the mapping phase. Thus, such predefined measurement points provide a more even distribution of data that is not dependent on specific durations needed for certain measurements. Furthermore, potential problems of measurements that take a long time to perform and a robot that is moving simultaneously can be circumvented by remaining stationary for as long as a measurement takes.

By default those measurement points are spaced 20cm apart and at least 20cm away from obstacles or unmapped areas. Both those values can be changed by the user in the next step, after a map with preliminary measurement locations is displayed (see Fig. 3).

Increasing the distance to obstacles is helpful in ensuring, that areas that are more difficult or impossible for the robot to traverse are avoided. If fewer waypoints and measurements are needed than originally proposed, their number can be reduced by increasing the distances between points. This is demonstrated in Fig. 4, where both distances were doubled, thereby eliminating points in harder to reach areas. However, the downside is, that some areas remain without any measurements.

Once the user has confirmed a certain configuration of measurement points, the script sends them to the robot via the */move_base/goal* topic one after the other, whenever the robot has finished measuring at its current position. At this

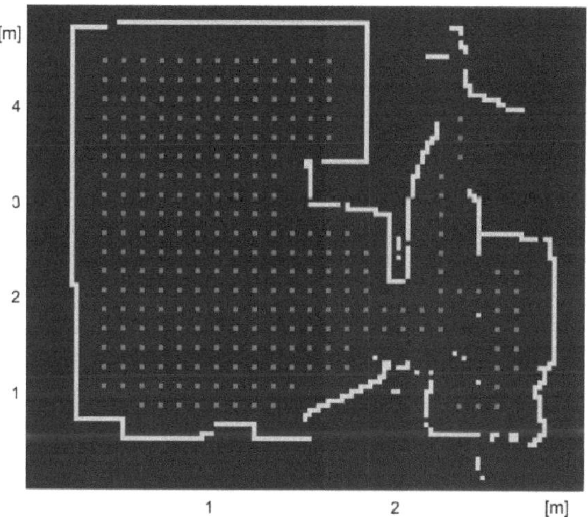

Figure 3: Waypoint locations displayed in the mapped environment

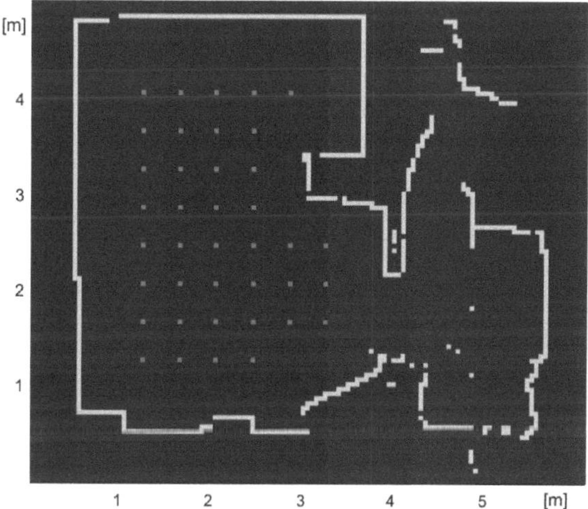

Figure 4: Waypoint locations with adapted distance setting.

point a custom ROS topic can be integrated for the measurements, by subscribing to it from the script to receive the measured values.

4 Results and Discussion

Using the information on obstacles and accessible spaces present in the */map* topic, we were able to calculate a modifiable grid of measurement points, which we then send the measurement platform to, in order gather its readings.

However, since the robot does not respond to the navigation targets sent to it by the script via */move_base/goal* or the alternative */move_base_simple/goal* topic, these steps could not be implemented. Unfortunately, this problem persisted despite us testing many different combinations of available navigation ROS topics with the various approaches for publishing to ROS topics from within a Python script. The issue does not seem to be necessarily in the interface between ROS and Python, since subscribing, e.g. in the case of */map*, does work and we also managed to successfully publish navigation goals at some point, yet with the robot still not moving.

In contrast to this, sending goals to the robot works fine, if done via a corresponding button in RVIZ. However, this is not a suitable solution for our platform, since defining measurement points in this way would require user input throughout the measurement process, and it would also not be possible to obtain uniform point grids like the ones shown previously. Of course, not performing grid-based measurements at all is an alternative, but dependence on user input would still increase, at least if goals have to be given via RVIZ, and measurements of areas would often be less consistent.

Fig. 5 shows how the results of measurements are meant to be presented after interpolating their values. In this case random values were used for demonstrative purposes, as we did not yet perform real measurements, due to the problems described above.

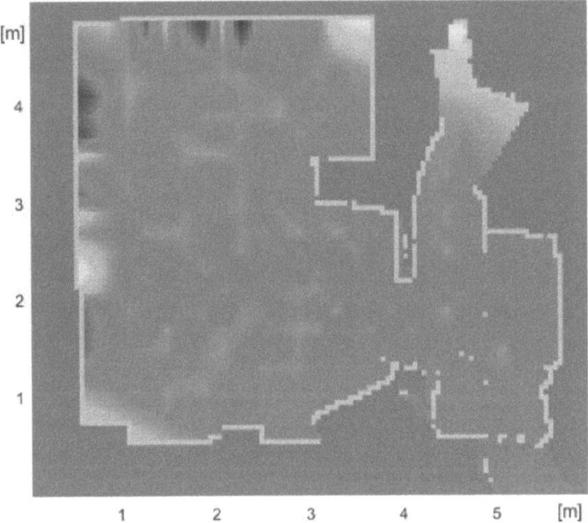

Figure 5: Map with interpolated random values at measurement locations

5   Conclusion

In this paper, we devise a method for gathering localized indoor measurements. Among other devices, we use a quadruped robot and a LIDAR sensor mounted on top of it as a hardware platform for this task. With a SLAM algorithm we were able to map unknown environments, meanwhile using ROS for the communication between the different components. Once finished with the mapping process, our script then calculates grids of measurement locations, which are then sent to the robot.

Unfortunately however, we were not successful at implementing the next steps of navigating to those location and gathering readings there.

Besides those remaining steps, future work could also address the mapping phase, by automating it to a point, where only user supervision, instead of user control, is required. In addition to this, it might be worthwhile investigating how measurements could be integrated into such an autonomous

mapping phase, rather than keeping mapping and measuring separate. One benefit of this might be, that the overall distance traveled by the robot would be far shorter, thus also reducing power consumption and extending the availability of the robot for the overall procedure. Another helpful addition would be an option to individually add, remove or change measurement locations, rather than just controlling their spacing, as is the case in the current implementation.

Acknowledgment

This work has been carried out at the Center of Excellence CoSA of the TH Lübeck - University of Applied Sciences.

Author's Statement

Conflict of interest: Authors state no conflict of interest.

6   References

[1] S. Gangakhedkar, H. Cao, A. R. Ali, K. Ganesan, M. Gharba, and J. Eichinger, "Use cases, requirements and challenges of 5g communication for industrial automation," in *2018 IEEE International Conference on Communications Workshops (ICC Workshops)*, 2018, pp. 1–6.

[2] G. Dedes and A. Dempster, "Indoor gps positioning - challenges and opportunities," in *VTC-2005-Fall. 2005 IEEE 62nd Vehicular Technology Conference, 2005.*, vol. 1, 2005, pp. 412–415.

[3] A. Yassin, Y. Nasser, M. Awad, A. Al-Dubai, R. Liu, C. Yuen, R. Raulefs, and E. Aboutanios, "Recent advances in indoor localization: A survey on theoretical approaches and applications," *IEEE Communications Surveys Tutorials*, vol. 19, no. 2, pp. 1327–1346, 2017.

[4] H. Gotzig and G. O. Geduld, *LIDAR-Sensorik.* Wiesbaden: Springer Fachmedien Wiesbaden, 2015, pp. 317–334. [Online]. Available: https://doi.org/10.1007/978-3-658-05734-3_18

[5] S. Thrun, *Simultaneous Localization and Mapping.* Berlin, Heidelberg: Springer Berlin Heidelberg, 2008, pp. 13–41. [Online]. Available: https://doi.org/10.1007/978-3-540-75388-9_3

[6] *SLAMTEC Mapper Laser Mapping Sensor*, Slamtec, 2019. [Online]. Available: https://cdn.robotshop.com/media/r/rpk/rb-rpk-15/pdf/slamtec_mapper_datasheet_m2m2_v1.0_en.pdf

[7] *Unitree A1*, Unitree, 2018. [Online]. Available: https://www.mybotshop.de/Datasheet/Unitree_A1_User_Manual_v1.0.pdf

[8] *NVIDIA Jetson Nano System-on-Module*, Nvidia, 2019. [Online]. Available: https://tinyurl.com/33fy5p3u

Demonstrating Side Effects of Digital Modulation and Demodulation in Educational Laboratories

Mattes Köppe [1] and Peter Bartmann [2]

[1] Applied Information Technology, TH Lübeck - University of Applied Sciences, mattes.koeppe@stud.th-luebeck.de
[2] Department of Electrical Engineering and Computer Science, TH Lübeck - University of Applied Sciences, peter.bartmann@th-luebeck.de

Abstract

The paper proposes experiments teaching students fundamentals in digital modulation. The contribution focuses on modulation and demodulation signal processing paths, which are not covered in related work. A simple mathematical model is introduced supporting students in their understanding. Different equipment is used and reviewed, as well as their limitations and possible problems are examined. The proposed experiments then allow a more hands-on way of experiencing the concepts of digital modulation. The different experiments are evaluated and compared regarding complexity and possible educational usage.

1 Introduction

In an ever-growing digital and interconnected world, the understanding of communication technologies is becoming more critical for students in this field. The concept of digital modulation is one of the fundamental concepts enabling interference-resistant and spectral-efficient data transmissions [1]. Modulation generally describes the process of shifting information on a carrier signal, i.e. on a sine and cosine waveform, thus transmitting complex data symbols. Despite the transmitter and receiver being asynchronous, carrier frequency and phase alignment is essential for digital modulation to work. In many off-the-shelf components and implemented technologies, many aspects of this processing chain are hidden, e.g. in fully integrated radio frequency transceivers like the AD9363 by Analog Devices. Translating theoretical knowledge to practical implementation becomes an unnecessary challenge for students.

To overcome this problem, this paper shows how some aspects of digital modulation and demodulation can be visualized and demonstrated in educational laboratories for students. The work focuses on modulation and demodulation rather than digital modulation schemes. Hardware with dedicated measurable processing paths and fully integrated Software Defined Radios (SDR) are used.

The paper is structured as follows: First, we look at similar works in Sec. 2. We then introduce the used materials in Sec. 3. A mathematical model is presented in Sec. 4, which is essential for understanding the focus of the following experiments in Sec. 5, demonstrating side effects in modulation and demodulation processing paths. Finally, we briefly summarize the experiments in their capabilities and conclude the paper in Sec. 6.

2 Related Work

Prust provides course materials in [2], teaching communications systems with the use of SDR hardware in an educational environment. The course is designed for undergraduate electrical and computer engineering students. It presents various laboratory exercises with hardware like the ADALM-PLUTO in combination with software simulations using Simulink models and Matlab scripts. The material is divided into six topics. For each topic, a description and examples are prepared. For example, the script for lab 4 in [2] covers the effect of frequency offset between transmitter and receiver. However, students were provided with ready-to-use blocks to cope with it.

Boulmalf et al. follow a similar approach in [3]. Here, methods using Matlab and Simulink are proposed for teaching undergraduate Information Technology students in digital and analog modulation. This is done by simulating different modulation techniques. A survey of students indicated a good understanding of the modulation techniques as well as a high level of satisfaction with this approach. However, the approach simplifies the theoretical background, e.g. the derivation of a mathematical model for modulation and demodulation is neglected. By doing so, students do not have to come up with a strong foundation in mathematics.

In contrast, this work aims to demonstrate the need for bandpass filters in modulation. Furthermore, simple methods were introduced making the result of frequency inaccuracy visible in educational laboratories using a signal generator and oscilloscope in the demodulation path. Experiments are supported by the popular ADALM-PLUTO SDR [4] and the R&S FPC-Z10 teaching kit [5].

3   Materials

This section provides a brief overview of the equipment and material used. Important technical capabilities are outlined.

3.1   Signal Generator and Oscilloscope

As a signal generator, the SDG6022X of Siglent is used. It is a function or arbitrary waveform generator with two channels and a maximum bandwidth of 200 MHz. One used feature is the output of custom, arbitrary waveforms, which can be generated with Matlab for example. The optional I/Q signal generator function makes it easy to output I/Q signals up to 37.5 MSymb/s of different modulation techniques.

As exemplary oscilloscopes, the RTO2004 and RTO6 by Rohde & Schwarz are used. The RTO2004 has a rather limited maximum bandwidth of 600 MHz in its smallest configuration. This makes it incapable of capturing radio band signals in typical and free of use Industrial, Scientific and Medical (ISM) bands starting at around 800 MHz. Hence, supportive devices shifting or removing the carrier are needed. In contrast, the RTO6 has a maximum bandwidth of 6 GHz. This allows for direct capture of radio signals if properly attenuated. Both have four channels and math functions, with filter and multiplication possibilities for signals. Utilizing those capabilities, a complete demodulation path is implementable.

3.2   R&S FPC-Z10

The FPC-Z10 of Rohde & Schwarz is a teaching kit for showcasing different RF measurements. It consists of two signal paths for modulation and demodulation also called upconverter and downconverter, respectively. Both signal paths feature a variety of signal processing sections, e.g., attenuator, amplifier and bandpass filter. Each section can be used or bypassed.

The I/Q modulator AD8345 and demodulator ADL5387 on the teaching kit work at an intermediate carrier frequency of 200 MHz. This frequency places lightweight requirements on measurement equipment. This allows the FPC-Z10 to become a core element in student laboratories.

3.3   ADALM-PLUTO SDR

The ADALM-PLUTO Active Learning Module or PlutoSDR is an SDR developed by Analog Devices, based on their RF agile transceiver AD9363. In a learning environment, it is particularly useful in teaching the fundamentals of SDRs, radio frequencies, or wireless communications. It features one receive and one transmit channel in full-duplex mode, supporting carrier frequencies between 325 and 3800 MHz with a 20 MHz bandwidth. The PlutoSDR offers a flexible programming interface using Matlab, Matlab Simulink, GNU Radio, or any custom code. This makes it very versatile as well as easy to use with an environment like Matlab and therefore a good candidate to teach the fundamentals of digital modulation to students. Together with the well-documented Wiki [4], the ADALM-PLUTO became a standard in communication laboratories at universities.

4   Mathematical Background

In digital modulation, binary data is mapped onto complex-valued symbols $d[k] = d'[k] + jd''[k]$ at the discrete time k. The finite set of possible symbols $d[k]$ is described by the modulation scheme, whereas the real part is denoted as the in-phase component I and the imaginary part as the quadrature component Q. After passing the values through a transmit filter $g_{tx}(t)$ the complex envelope $s(t)$ is generated.

$$s(t) = \sum_k d[k] g_{tx}(t) \tag{1}$$

Eq. (1) also has the form $s(t) = a \cdot e^{j2\pi ft + \varphi}$. Digital modulation schemes change one of the attributes amplitude a, frequency f, or phase φ of the signal [6]. The modulation schemes are named amplitude shift keying (ASK), frequency shift keying (FSK), or phase shift keying (PSK), accordingly. Another form is quadrature amplitude modulation (QAM), which can be viewed as a combination of two independent ASK symbols or the combination of ASK and PSK.

In digital modulation the I-component is modulated with a $\cos(2\pi f_c t)$ and the Q-component with $-\sin(2\pi f_c t)$.

$$s_{tb}(t) = \sqrt{2}\, \Re\{s(t)\} \cdot \cos(2\pi f_{c,tx} t + \varphi_0) -$$
$$\sqrt{2}\, \Im\{s(t)\} \cdot \sin(2\pi f_{c,tx} t + \varphi_0), \tag{2}$$

where $s_{tb}(t)$ is the equivalent transmission band signal of $s(t)$ on the carrier $f_{c,tx}$.

The R&S FPC-Z10 has an intermediate frequency (IF) f_i due to its low-frequency modulator and demodulator. A local oscillator (LO) frequency f_{lo} with $f_{c,tx} = f_{lo} + f_i$ is used to shift the final signal to the transmission band. This is modelled for the real part of $s(t)$, i.e. $s'(t)$, neglecting φ_0 as:

$$s'_{tb}(t) = \sqrt{2}\, s'(t) \cdot \cos(2\pi f_i t) \cdot \sqrt{2}\, \cos(2\pi f_{lo} t) \tag{3}$$
$$= s'(t) \cdot (\cos(2\pi(f_{lo} - f_i)t) -$$
$$\cos(2\pi(f_{lo} + f_i)t)) \tag{4}$$

This shows that a bandpass filter is needed to filter out the unwanted frequency at $f_{lo} - f_i$.

In the receiving path, the same principles hold. Even if an IF is not used, demodulation creates additional frequency components. In contrast to (4), higher frequencies are unwanted and thus low pass filtered. The received baseband signal is then

$$r'(t) = s'(t) \cdot \cos(2\pi(f_{c,rx} - f_{c,tx})t) \tag{5}$$

As the transmitter and receiver are usually not sharing the same clock, a frequency offset remains if $f_{c,tx} \approx f_{c,rx}$ and $f_{c,tx} \neq f_{c,rx}$ holds. This results in a rotation of the constellation diagram of the actual digital modulation scheme. A frequency compensation can be used to prevent this effect [7].

5 Experiments

5.1 Modulation

Using the introduced materials, there are two ways to apply digital modulation schemes to a signal. The first one utilizes the modulation signal path of the FPC-Z10. The signal generator feeds the I/Q-input of this board with either random symbols or an actual message which needs to be decoded at the receiver. Depending on the actual target, it is possible to export the modulated baseband signal either with an intermediate frequency of $f_i = 200\,\text{MHz}$ or a higher modulated signal further shifted by a configurable local oscillator with $f_{lo} = 233.5\,\text{MHz}$ or $f_{lo} = 636.5\,\text{MHz}$.

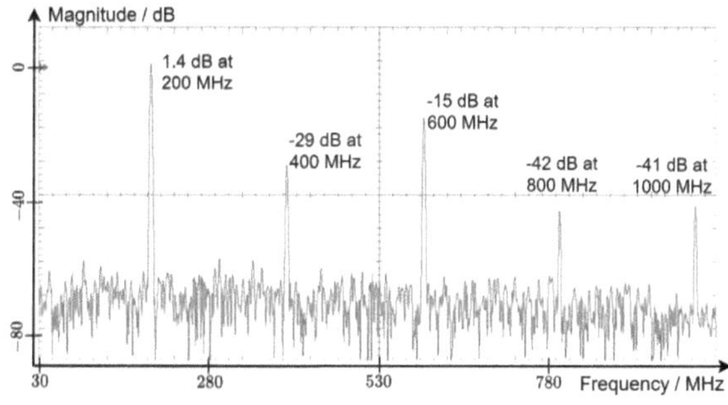

(a) After the IQ-Modulator of the FPC-Z10

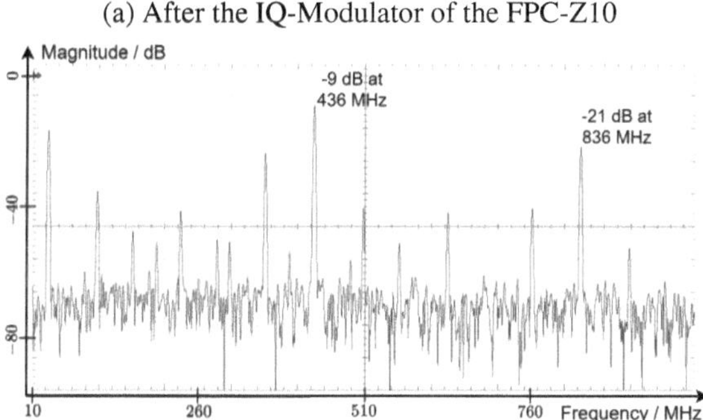

(b) After additional upshift with local oscillator frequency $f_{lo} = 636.5\,\text{MHz}$

Figure 1: Power density spectrum at different processing stages of the FPC-Z10

Fig. 1 shows the frequencies appearing at each processing stage. In Fig. 1a the spectrum of the carrier outputted by the AD8345 modulation chip is shown. It is obvious that even at this point multiple frequencies appear whereas not visible in (2). This possibly results from a weak interpolation filter. The situation becomes even worse after the signal shift by $f_{lo} = 636.5\,\text{MHz}$. Instead of having just one unwanted frequency at $f_{c,tx} = f_i - f_{lo}$ as by (4), a peak in the spectrum appears at about every $100\,\text{MHz}$, which Fig. 1b illustrates. Hence, removing these components is mandatory in a communication system. The FPC-Z10 implements a non-configurable bandpass filter at $f_{pass} = 836.5\,\text{MHz}$ for this purpose.

A second approach solely uses the ADALM-PLUTO and its incorporated features. Using the ADALM-PLUTO is a lot simpler e.g. by using the Transmitter example from Matlab [8]. The digital modulation scheme as well as the carrier frequency $f_{c,tx}$ can be chosen and many more options can be modified. In contrast to the approach using the FPC-Z10, the modulation and mixing of the signal are hidden in the used AD9363 chip. This chip utilizes a bandpass filter removing unwanted frequencies.

5.2 Demodulation

For the demodulation part, two options are evaluated. Both of them utilize the ADALM-PLUTO to generate a modulated signal of random data.

The first approach is the most basic one, but also the most complex. It uses a signal generator as well as an oscilloscope to show the constellation diagram of the transmitted signal. To achieve this, the signal generator is used to generate phase-aligned sine and cosine waves with the wanted carrier frequency $f_{c,tx}$. An oscilloscope captures the transmitted signal of the ADALM-PLUTO at one channel and the sine and cosine wave on two other channels. The task of the oscilloscope is then to apply demodulation processing, which requires a powerful processing unit inside the oscilloscope.

To display the constellation diagram the transmitted signal needs to be multiplied by the sine and cosine waves. After low-pass filtering, the result - a rotating constellation diagram - appears on the oscilloscope. Fig. 2 shows the result for a 16-QAM transmitted by the ADALM-PLUTO on a carrier with $f_{c,tx} = 100\,\text{MHz}$. The constellation diagram rotates as (5) explains. Fine-tuning $f_{c,tx}$ determines the rotation speed of the constellation diagram.

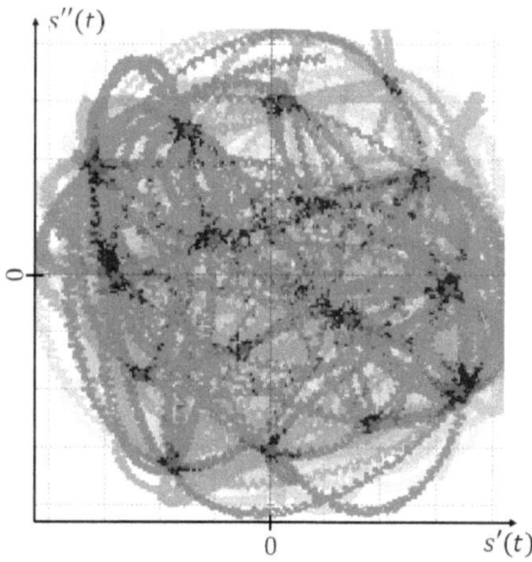

Figure 2: Demodulated 16-QAM signal with constellation points

A nearly identical approach uses the FPC-Z10 to demodulate the signal, instead of the manual demodulation done in the oscilloscope. However, the carrier frequency of the ADALM-PLUTO is not very precise and can only be tuned coarsely. Also, the carrier frequencies of the FPC-Z10 are not tune-able. Therefore, it is virtually impossible to generate a visible, rotating constellation diagram. A difference of some tenth of a Hertz between carriers $f_{c,rx} - f_{c,tx}$ is sufficient to rotate the constellation diagram with such a speed that it isn't recognizable anymore for a human eye.

5.3 Carrier Synchronization

By using the signal generator and FPC-Z10, as mentioned in Sec. 5.1, a text message on a certain carrier is transmitted. In contrast to Sec. 5.2, where the effect of carrier offset is being demonstrated, the demodulation is implemented using the ADALM-PLUTO. The Matlab receiver example [8] configures the SDR to receive the message and to estimate a bit error rate (BER). The example code incorporates also a carrier offset compensation for QPSK symbols. Depending on the deviation between the transmitter and receiver carrier frequency the BER changes.

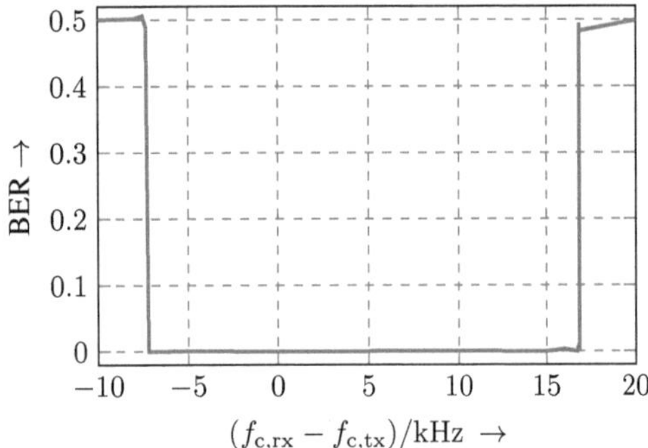

Figure 3: Bit error rate for different center frequencies of the receiver $f_{c,rx}$ shifted around $f_{c,tx} = 836.5\,\mathrm{MHz}$

Fig. 3 shows the actual response of the BER vs. the offset. On one hand, the width of the trough represents the efficiency of the frequency correction. The compensation works in a range of $25\,\mathrm{kHz}$. On the other hand, there is a slight offset compared to $f_{c,rx} - f_{c,tx} = 0$. This demonstrates again that a target frequency of $f_c = 836.5\,\mathrm{MHz}$ differs between receiver and transmitter.

6 Summary and Conclusion

This work examined the usage of the FPC-Z10 in an educational lab environment in detail and is the first to do so in the public domain to the best of our knowledge. It was found that the board has many useful and beneficial components for experimenting with the fundamentals of digital modulation and demodulation.

For the modulation part, it was shown that many unwanted frequencies occur which results in the need for a bandpass filter. From a didactic point of view, using the FPC-Z10 demonstrates effects better since all intermediate steps can be examined, whereas the ADALM-PLUTO hides this process.

In the demodulation part, a constellation diagram was generated only using a signal generator and oscilloscope. This is especially useful as only basic laboratory equipment is needed. Although this approach is more complex than just using the ADALM-PLUTO, it demonstrates the rotation effect of not matching carrier frequencies in a better way. However, the example code provided with the ADALM-PLUTO demonstrates that simple carrier synchronization

is sufficient to achieve zero BERs if the offset is within a certain margin.

Overall it was shown that is possible to demonstrate and explain the fundamentals of digital modulation and demodulation to students in laboratory environments. The work fills the gap where other public student laboratories just introduce mathematical formulas without demonstrating them. The proposed methods are implementable without the need of investing in expensive hardware.

Acknowledgement

The work has been carried out at Technische Hochschule Lübeck, Department of Electrical Engineering and Computer Science.

Author's Statement

Conflict of interest: Authors state no conflict of interest.

7 References

[1] M. Werner, *Nachrichtentechnik - Eine Einführung für alle Studiengänge*. Vieweg+Teubner, 2009, vol. 6.

[2] C. Prust, "Introductory Communication Systems Course Using SDR," Available at https://www.mathworks.com/matlabcentral/fileexchange/69417-introductory-communication-systems-course-using-sdr (2023/01/11).

[3] M. Boulmalf, Y. Semmar, A. Lakas, and K. Shuaib, "Teaching digital and analog modulation to undergradute Information Technology students using Matlab and Simulink," in *IEEE EDUCON 2010 Conference*, 2010, pp. 685–691.

[4] Analog Devices, "ADALM-PLUTO Overview," Available at https://wiki.analog.com/university/tools/pluto (2023/01/11).

[5] Rohde & Schwarz, "Teaching Kit R&S®FPC-Z10 User Guide," 2020.

[6] J. Schiller, *Mobile Communications*, 2nd ed. Addison-Wesley Educational, 2003.

[7] K.-D. Kammeyer and A. Dekorsy, *Nachrichtenübertragung*, 6th ed. Springer Vieweg, 2018.

[8] The MathWorks, Inc., "Digital Modulation," Available at https://de.mathworks.com/help/supportpkg/plutoradio/digital-modulation.html (2023/01/11).

6

Sensor Data Analysis

Dynamic Time Warping to investigate the difference between two paths

Christopher Schmale [1]

[1] Robotics and Autonomous Systems, Universität zu Lübeck, christopher.schmale@student.uni-luebeck.de

Abstract

An important area of autonomous driving is the path planning and path following of a vehicle. However, it is hard to tell if the vehicle follows the path well in different situations. This project investigates dynamic time warping as a measurement metric to determine the distance between paths. Therefore, the concept of dynamic time (DTW) warping is investigated as well as the performance of two different implementations (Python and C++) is measured. A C++ implementation is set up for usage in the robot application construction kit(RACK). Afterwards the parameters are tuned, and their influence on the distance and the run time is determined. The distances and run times are measured and evaluated in an experiment. Closing this article, a conclusion is drawn on how to DTW can be used for comparing path data.

1 Introduction

Autonomous driving is currently one of the most revolutionary technologies in society and promises key advances. Next to the optimisation of traffic management, the reduction of traffic jams and traveling time, the vehicle usage time via car sharing can be increased and the CO2 emissions can be decreased.

To be able to reach a destination the vehicles must calculate a path. After planning the path, the vehicle tries to follow the path until it has reached the target.

In this topic lies a lot of potential to create efficient trips. With a vehicle, which drives a well-planned path, the destination can be reached quickly. However, the vehicle needs feedback, how well it drove the planed path in order to optimize the next trip or to report back that something is wrong on the way. Maybe some obstacles block the street, so the time, the street takes to be driven, increases.

2 Material and Methods

To be able to understand the metric mechanics and to integrate DTW into the RACK, the data set and the robotic framework is explained. Moreover, it is important to understand the general concept of DTW to evaluate the results and determine the quality. Of cause, there are alternatives to DTW, which are stated in [1]. However, the project focus was on the investigation of DTW, so only this metric is discussed.

2.1 Dataset

In this project, the focus lied on three datasets, which are described below. Fig. 1 shows the plot of the three paths.

These three different paths were used for testing the DTW metric and benchmark the performance of the different DTW implementations (Python and C++).

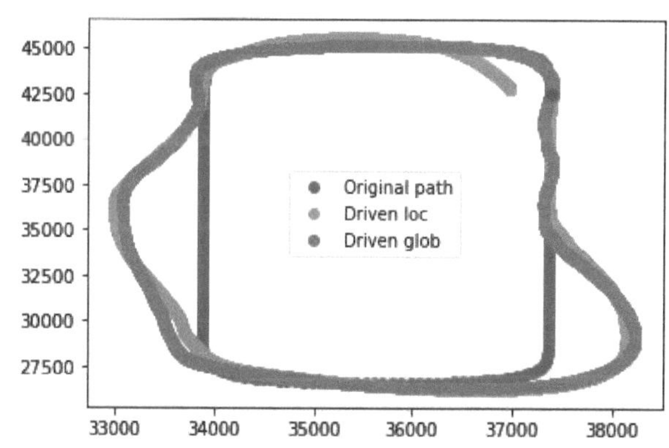

Figure 1: Visualised path data: Original path, driven path using local optimisation, driven path using global localisation, Difference in the driven paths and planned path can be observed.

The blue path is the path planned by the path planner of the vehicle. The orange and the green paths are two tracked vehicle positions, which the vehicle came across following the path by using either only a local localisation system or by using a local and a global localisation system. The tracked position is the vehicle position delivered by the simulation.

2.2 Robotic application construction kit

The RACK[2] is a robotic middle ware framework like Robotic Operating System (ROS)[7]. It was developed at the University of Hanover for Systems Engineering by the

"Real-Time Systems Group". The idea compared to ROS is basically the same.

A module structure of different abstraction layers communicates with a messaging system. This messaging system works as interface between the modules. However, the RACK has one big difference, which is real-time capability. This allows the RACK to be used in real-time critical application. Moreover, the RACK is mainly programmed in C++ and can import libraries written in C++. The "dtadistance" library[3] offers a C version of DTW. With some adaptions, this creates the C++ library.

2.3 Dynamic time warping

In general time series analysis, DTW measures the similarity between two datasets, without taking time into account. In the project case, two of the three datasets are compared to each other, and the similarities could be detected[4].

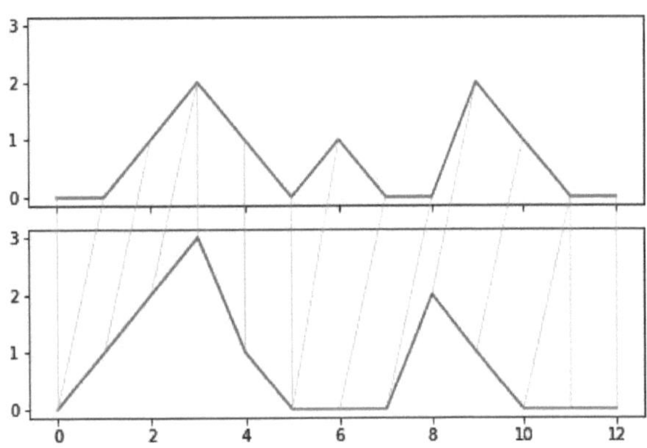

Figure 2: DTW example, how two different series are matched to each other[3]

As Fig. 2 shows, the type of sequence is irrelevant. Not only path data can be compared, video, audio or other sequences like movement can be evaluated as well.

The general DTW algorithm sets up a distance matrix. Therefore, it iterates over the two datasets and checks the state distance of every state of the two datasets. In the end, a matrix with the state distances of the two datasets is given, which can be used for the analysis of distance[5].

For the distance analysis the last value of the matrix can be used. The best path to the start of the matrix can be generated by using the Needleman–Wunsch algorithm [6].

2.4 Test concept of DTW

The carried out tests have been divided in two groups: Conceptional/functional tests and parameter/performance tests. Only the DTW function was tested with input data.

The conceptional/functional tests were done to understand the different possible outcomes of DTW. Therefore different simple data sequences were compared and analysed by creating the corresponding heat map by using DTW.

For the parameter/performance tests, the different changable parameters of DTW were changed using

the idea of grid search.After the parameter change, the distance between the paths was calculated using DTW and the time was measured. To create more reliable results, the python tests were done five and the C++ tests were done ten times, which generated 525 python results and 1050 C++ results.

3 Results and Discussion

A lot of time was spend on testing the created C++ library. The python results look the same as the C++ results, therefore, only in the performance part, the two implementations are looked at separately.

3.1 Outcomes of conceptional/functional tests

The results of the simple datasets are the distance matrices shown in Fig. 3. In general, the darker areas of the heat map, which represents the single values of the matrix, are smaller distances between the states than the lighter ones. The colours of the heat map are normalized over the minimum and maximum distance value.

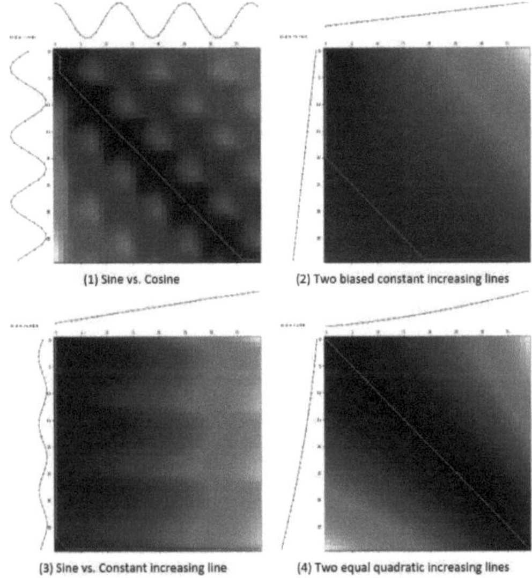

Figure 3: DTW results of comparing simple datasets with each other to understand the heat map and the best path. The best path is plotted in red.

On the top and the left of the heat map the two compared datasets are given. If they are a one-dimensional array. The general shape of the datasets can be taken from Fig. 1 as well. The DTW distance calculation of the heat map is stated in the top left corner.

The red line through the heat map is the best path. This path shows the optimal match of the two datasets, in other words it shows the steps it takes to go from the end to the start with minimal cost. The cost in this case is the distance in the cells of the matrix. For visualisation the visualisation tool of the "dtaidistance" library[3] is used.

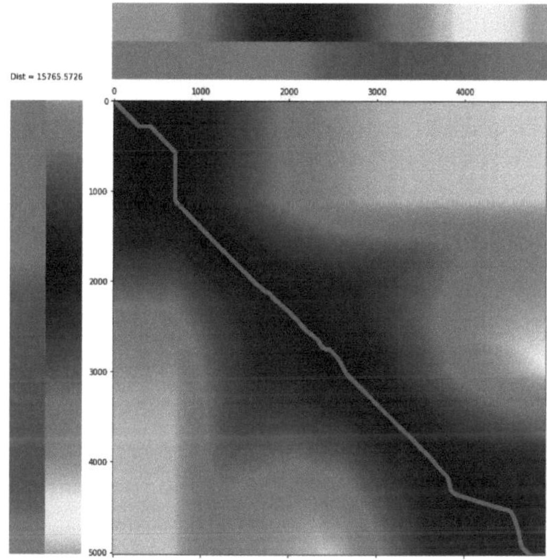

Figure 4: Driven path with global localisation compared to planned path. Observable dips in the best path, which means, that the driven path is not completely equal to the planned path.

Using actual path data with two input dimensions, the heat map becomes more complex and the best path changes from a straight line with some corners to a more complex shape. As Fig. 4 shows, the two paths have some areas, where the single sequences of the paths match better than other sequences.

3.2 Discussion of the conceptional/functional outcomes

As the heatmap of sinus and cosine (Fig. 3) shows, there is a curve in the best path until the sequence of sinus and cosine match. When the first matching point is found the distance does not increase until the end of the dataset. The best path shows where the sequences are equal. If the last point of the best path is diagonal to the current point, the sequences match in this part.

Going to the top right and bottom left corner of the heat map, it shows sine wave shaped difference in distance. If one point of the sinus dataset is matched to the cosine dataset, its distance is always sine wave shaped.

Like the sine and cosine comparison, the heat map of the two straight lines with an offset looks like. In the beginning, the distance slides parallel to one axis of the heat map until a match is found. Then the distance stays the same until the end of one sequence and the distance is increased again.

However, the distance going towards the bottom left corner does not increase in the shape of a sine wave, in this case, it increases linearly. Two linear datasets produce a linear increasing distance by matching a single point to the other dataset.

This is different in the third comparison. It can be seen, that the distance increases in sine wave shape away from the best path. The amplitude of the waves is not as strong as in the as in the sine-cosine comparison, due to the linear increasing dataset. Therefore, the waves are smoother, and no reputation of a wave can be observed, because the linear function only has one match with the sine function.

When two equal functions are compared, the DTW distance is zero. By going away form the best path, the distance increases like the shape of the function arc. In this case, the functions are quadratic, therefore the distance increases quadratic moving away from the best path.

In the comparison of the paths in Fig. 4, it can be seen that the best path is in large parts of the heat map on the main diagonal. This is the case, because the vehicle drove with almost the same speed the almost same path, which is shown in Fig. 1. There are also curves in the best path, which could be a sign of different speeds at that measurement time or a difference in path, by driving for example a corner with different speeds and different steering angles. Those differences can be seen in Fig. 1 as well. The path is mainly followed, however, looking closer to some parts of the datasets, the driven path sometimes does not match the planned path.

3.3 Performance

The variety of carried out tests is to big to state in this article. Therefore, the performance and parameter results are summarised. The most important parameters are mentioned.

Starting with the distance results, it can be seen, that the distances calculated in python and in C++ stay the same over tests in the single test cases. The distance changes accordingly by using different datasets. In some last digits, the C++ and the Python distance is not equal. A reason for this could be different rounding mechanics in the programming languages.

By using pruning (setting the maximum distance to the Euclidean distance) the distances differ as well. This can be explained by the way the Euclidean distance is calculated. In python the Euclidean distance in both dimensions is calculated at the same time (like the dependent DTW distance). In the C++ version, the Euclidean distance is calculated dimension after dimension (like the independent DTW distance). Therefore, a different upper bounds exist and the distance matrix differs.

In the run time analysis it can be seen that the change of parameters has an influence on the run time. They have a similar impact on every distance calculation and programming language. According to the tests, it can be stated, that the python calculation takes around 10^{15} times longer than the C++ one, due to the fact, that C++ is a compiler language and therefore more efficient than python as interpreting programming language.

The fastest run time was achieved by setting the window parameter to one. In this case, just the main diagonal of the distance matrix is calculated, and the rest of the matrix is not specified. Therefore, the calculations are highly reduced and the run time decreases. Moreover, by using higher window parameters, the general run time can be reduced compared to not setting the parameter.

For other parameters, this is the reason as well. The maximum distance parameter stops calculation when the limit is exceeded as well as the maximum step size parameter. It works more dynamically, depending on the distance value than the window parameter. The window parameter always calculates the tube around the main diagonal independent from the single distances while the maximum distance and maximum step size parameter stop the calculation depending on the value and not on the distance to the main diagonal.

3.4   Real-time capability

Using the runtime test, a guaranteed time can be stated in which the DTW distance can be calculated for the datasets. The datasets can be adjusted to a defined length before using the algorithm. However, by looking into the DTW function, there is memory allocated dynamically. Therefore, no workaround has been found yet. In conclusion, the real-time capability is not reached yet.

4   Conclusion

The tests show, that DTW can be used as a metric, which states, how equal two datasets are. Since the distance is a unit free value, it just can be said, that dataset one matches dataset two better compared to dataset three. In the case of the original path and the two tracked path it can be said that the path is better followed by the vehicle with global than by the one without global localisation.

Using this information, systems, algorithms or control parameters can be evaluated and changed. With the achievable goal of a minimal distance, parameters of a controller can be tuned automatically. This approach is thinkable for a path following controller.

Furthermore, if a special sequence in a live system has a high DTW distance something is wrong in that area. There may be an obstacle in the way which needs to be removed. Moreover, the parameter have no influence on the distance. Since the distance is relative, there is no "correct" distance between to datasets. Therefore, the parameters can be optimized due to run time with the condition, that different datasets have different distances to each other.

With DTW as metric to measure the distance between paths, it can be used for collective robotics. In a group of robots following each other, DTW can be determine, how good the path or the motion of the robot ahead is reproduced. When the DTW distance increases, the controller must change the policy of the of the robot.

By looking at the whole swarm movement, DTW can be used to determine how good the swarm with current parameters performs. A task for the swarm is defined. After a test run, the parameters of the swarm mechanics are changed and DTW measures the performance.

To be able to run the C++ library in a live system in the RACK more functionality is needed. The file wrapper must be replaced with a data wrapper which is fed with live data.

For this purpose, a ring buffer can be used to store the current data to do the DTW calculation on. Every time new data is available, old data is deleted from the buffer and the DTW calculation is started on a constant amount of data. Moreover, the dynamic memory allocation must be changed into static memory allocation. With a constant sized ring buffer this is implementable. All needed memory is allocated in the start-up process of the module and freed by termination.

Acknowledgement

The work has been carried out at the company STILL and has been supervised by Prof. Dr. Heiko Hamann, Institute of Computer Engineering, University of Lübeck and Tino Krueger-Basjmeleh, Software Engineer, KION Mobile Automation.

Author's Statement

Conflict of interest: Authors state no conflict of interest.

5   References

[1] Bagnall, A. *The Great Time Series Classification Bake Off: An Experimental Evaluation of Recently Proposed Algorithms. Extended Version.* Available: https://arxiv.org/abs/1602.01711 [last accessed on 02-08-2022].

[2] University Hanover *Real Time Systems Group.* Available: https://www.rts.uni-hannover.de/125.html [last accessed on 01-08-2022].

[3] wannesm *wannesm/dtaidistance.* Available: https://github.com/wannesm/dtaidistance/tree/v2.3.5 [last accessed on 10-08-2022].

[4] Zhang, J. *Dynamic Time Warping.* Available: https://towardsdatascience.com/dynamic-time-warping-3933f25fcdd [last accessed on 14-06-2022].

[5] Ricardo Portilla, B. H. *Understanding Dynamic Time Warping.* Available: https://www.databricks.com/blog/2019/04/30/understanding-dynamic-time-warping.html [last accessed on 14-06-2022].

[6] Lang, H. W. *Needleman-Wunsch-Algorithmus.* Available: https://www.inf.hs-flensburg.de/lang/algorithmen/bio/needleman-wunsch.htm [last accessed on 10-08-2022].

[7] Open Robotics *Robot operating system.* Available: https://www.ros.org/ [last accessed on 13-08-2022].

Method to evaluate the accuracy of external and on-board weather information

Helen Lokowandt [1], Julian Knödler [2], and Georg Schildbach [3]

[1] Robotics and Autonomous Systems, Universität zu Lübeck, helen.lokowandt@student.uni-luebeck.de
[2] Dr. Ing h.c. F. Porsche AG, Stuttgart, julian.knoedler2@porsche.de
[3] Institute for Electrical Engineering in Medicine, Universität zu Lübeck, georg.schildbach@uni-luebeck.de

Abstract

In order to use forecast weather information for an advanced range calculation for battery electric vehicles (BEVs), the quality of weather service information must be evaluated. This evaluation is executed in two separate steps. Firstly, historical records of selected weather services are matched to historical on-vehicle records. Secondly, weather forecasts are downloaded before test drives and compared with vehicle sensor data. The quality of different historic parameters varies. Temperature records can be better generalized with the introduced modelling and in first tests even seem to be transferable to forecast.

1 Introduction

Range calculation is an important feature for electric cars. Several factors can be considered when creating a car-, world-, and driver model as a base for the range calculation. For the world model, an essential factor is weather. Weather, especially temperature, has a significant effect on range and charging [1]. Additionally, the driver's reaction to weather conditions could increase travel time and hence range needs. Analysis of long distance test drives shows that temperature can change over 10 K on a drive. This leads to increased energy demands with regard to battery and interior air conditioning. Air conditioning can reduce range up to 54 % [2]. Therefore, precise knowledge about weather condition is desirable for range calculation.

2 Material and Methods

2.1 Data sources

2.1.1 Vehicle Sensor Data

Measurements of weather conditions from the vehicle's perspective are the ground truth for all evaluation. These measurements are taken from recorded test drives within Germany. Ambient temperature, ambient relative humidity, rainfall and sun intensity are measured by vehicle sensors. The different sensors in the vehicle have different sampling rates. For analysis, all sensor information is generalized to 10Hz. The test routes are already sectioned in segments, so called links. A link is a uniform segment of road. Crossroads, speed limits, or changes of the road class require a new link. For all generalized sensor data points, the number of the link is recorded. All samples from one link are combined, hence the weather service data is compared to a mean within the link. The length of links is neither fixed in length nor in time but is small enough to be combined into

one geographic coordinate. For each link, the maximum and minimum value of the considered recordings as well as the mean value are saved and used for later evaluation.

2.1.2 Historical Weather Records

The vehicle sensor data is compared with weather service data. Historical records are analysed. Three weather services are compared with different mappings of geographical position to weather station information. Deutscher Wetterdienst (DWD) returns only the measurement of the closest weather station. Meteostat returns measurements of the closest stations combined with model data, this process is called reanalysis and is used to achieve a higher local resolution [3]. Openweathermap (OWM) as a commercial weather service does not share its mapping of weather station to geographical position. The recorded variables and their units can be taken from table 1.

Table 1: Units of historical variables

Variable	Vehicle	DWD	Meteostat	OWM
Mean Temp.	[°C]	[K] 2 m / 5 cm	[°C]	[K]
Max. Temp.	[°C]	-	-	[K]
Min. Temp.	[°C]	-	-	[K]
Humidity	[%]	[%]	[%]	[%]
Precipitation	[%]	-	[mm]	-
Pressure	-	[kPa]	[hPa]	[hPa]
Update rate	100 ms	10 min	1 h	1 h

2.1.3 Weather Forecast

Forecast information is taken from Openweathermap and DWD's Model Output Statistics MIX (DWD MOSMIX). Openweathermap accepts geographic coordinates as forecast input. DWD only accepts station numbers as input for the position. The variables of interest from the forecasts are shown in table 2.

Table 2: Units of forcast variables

Variable	Vehicle	DWD	OWM
Mean Temp.	[°C]	[K] 2 m / 5 cm	[K]
Max. Temp.	[°C]	[K] 2 m	[K]
Min. Temp.	[°C]	[K] 2 m	[K]
Humidity	[%]	-	[%]
Pressure	-	[kPa]	[hPa]
Update rate	100 ms	1 h	1 h

2.2 Experimental Procedure of Forecast Test Drives

As there exists no long-term archive for historical weather forecasts, none of the existing records of historical test drives could be used to evaluate the forecast quality. This means that the historical drives can only be evaluated in relation to weather station data and not forecast information. New test drives had to be arranged to test forecast quality. As these test drives should challenge the weather forecast services, the route was planned to cover different conditions. Open fields, motorways, altitudes, different velocities were taken into account. On October 18, 2022, a first test drive was conducted. Whenever possible, the driver used adaptive cruise control for reproducibility. From the first test drive, the time deltas between passing two links and the geographical coordinates of the links were saved. On November 17, 2022, a nightly test drive was conducted. On November 18,2022, a test drive in the rain was conducted. Half an hour before the test drives, the forecasts were downloaded from DWD and OWM with the geographical coordinates from the first test drives and the times resulting from the scheduled start time plus the time deltas. The reason for this procedure was to have a time point for each link of the route. If the route and the resulting time points were planned with an external navigation, this would not be easily possible. The major limitation of this approach is the susceptibility to traffic delays.

2.3 Regression and Quality Evaluation of Recorded Weather

The weather service recordings are modelled via Multiple Linear Regression (MLR) to fit the vehicle ground truth. Only external sources should be used to model a vehicle internal variable. For the three weather services a model including the variables of the corresponding service and the altitude is generated. The hypothesis is that the temperature and humidity measured by the vehicle is a linear combination of the corresponding variables from the weather services, the altitude, an offset between measured vehicle variable and weather service variable and potentially other weather service variables. The population model for the vehicle variable y_i with k external variables x_i as regressors and n data points can be written as

$$y_i = \beta_0 + \beta_1 \cdot x_{i,1} + \beta_2 \cdot x_{i,2} + ... + \beta_k \cdot x_{i,k} + \epsilon_i \quad (1)$$

where the model is linear in the coefficients $\beta_1, ... \beta_k$ [4]. MLR estimates the β coefficients as b coefficients at fitting the predicted value $y_{fitted,i}$ to the actual value y_i. In matrix notation, (1) can be written as

$$\mathbf{y} = \mathbf{X}\boldsymbol{\beta} + \boldsymbol{\epsilon} \quad (2)$$

with $\mathbf{y} = [y_1, y_2, .., y_n]^T$, $\mathbf{X} = [\mathbf{x_1}, \mathbf{x_2}, .., \mathbf{x_n}]^{\mathbf{T}}$ where $x_i = [1, x_{i,1}, x_{i,2}, ..., x_{i,k}]$ and $\boldsymbol{\beta} = [\beta_1, \beta_2, .., \beta_k]^T$ and $\boldsymbol{\epsilon} = [\epsilon_1, \epsilon_2, .., \epsilon_n]^T$. The fitted value y_{fitted} is calculated as

$$y_{fitted,i} = b_0 + b_1 \cdot x_{i,1} + b_2 \cdot x_{i,2} + ... + b_k \cdot x_{i,k} \quad (3)$$

where the b-values estimates the linear coefficients. $\mathbf{b} = [b_0, ..., b_k]$ is calculated with the MATLAB *regress* method. The quality of a regression model can be described with the R^2 statistic. R^2 can be calculated as

$$R^2 = 1 - \frac{\sum_{i=1}^{n} {y_i - y_{fitted,i}}^2}{\sum_{i=1}^{n} {y_i - y_{mean}}^2} \quad (4)$$

where $y_{mean} = \frac{1}{n} \sum_{i=1}^{n} y_i$. R^2 represents the percentage of variability in $\mathbf{Y}$ attributed to the linear combination of regressors $\mathbf{X}$ [5]. For this research, an R^2 greater 0.75 is accepted as sufficiently explaining the vehicle measurements with weather service and altitude information.

Additionally, as more intuitive quality measurement, the mean absolute error for the MLR modelled variables is used as:

$$e_{fitted} = \frac{|\mathbf{y_{fitted}} - \mathbf{y}|}{n} \quad (5)$$

This error is compared to the weather service error calculated with the unaltered weather service variable:

$$e_{weatherservice} = \frac{|\mathbf{y_{weatherservice}} - \mathbf{y}|}{n} \quad (6)$$

2.4 Implementation

For DWD, Meteostat and OWM, the data quality is evaluated separately. 23 test drives with historical weather data are available. The test drives are varying in duration, distance, times and location. For the 23 trips, the historical records from DWD, Meteostat, and OWM are retrieved. Only for the last two test drives, forecast information is existing as explained in 2.1.3. In the first step, for each weather service a cross validation is implemented. The sample pool of 23 test drives is, in a random order, divided into 5 parts. In 5 iterations, 19 test drives are used as training data for the MLR and the remaining, in each iteration changing, 4 test drives are the validation data testing the coefficients $\mathbf{b}$ calculated in the training. In each iteration, the training data is joined into one vector and the coefficients $\mathbf{b}$ are calculated on this joined vector to weigh the length of the drives. As validation, the calculated $\mathbf{b}$ is tested on the individual validation drives. If the mean absolute error of the regression (5) and the weather service (6) in both training and validation is comparable in all 5 iterations, the MLR is seen as generalizable. If the MLR is both generalizable and has an R^2 greater 0.75 in all iterations of the cross validation, the weather service is classified as eligible otherwise it is discarded in the examined variable. For DWD, the regressor variables are $x_{i,DWD} = [1, H_{i,HERE}, T_{i,DWD,2m}, \phi_{i,DWD}, T_{i,DWD,5cm}]$, where

$H_{i,HERE}$ is the altitude given by the HERE location platform, $T_{i,DWD,2m}$ and $T_{i,DWD,5cm}$ are the temperatures recorded by DWD in 2 m and 5 cm height respectively and $\phi_{i,DWD}$ is the relative humidity by DWD. For DWD, a second regression without humidity is realised for temperature modelling as MOSMIX forecasts do not contain predictions of humidity. Accordingly, the regressor variables are reduced to $x_{i,DWD2} = [1, H_{i,HERE}, T_{i,DWD,2m}, T_{i,DWD,5cm}]$. For Meteostat, the regressor variables are $x_{i,Meteo} = [1, H_{i,HERE}, T_{i,Meteo}, \phi_{i,Meteo}, P_{i,Meteo}, S_{i,Meteo}]$ with $T_{i,Meteo}$ being the Temperature returned by Meteostat, $\phi_{i,Meteo}$ the relative humidity as given by Meteostat, $P_{i,Meteo}$ is the volume of precipitation in mm as given by Meteostat and $S_{i,Meteo}$ is the sunshine duration from Meteostat. The OWM regressor variables are $x_{i,OWM} = [1, H_{i,HERE}, T_{i,OWM}, \phi_{i,OWM}, T_{i,OWM,min}, T_{i,OWM,max}]$ with $T_{i,OWM}$, $T_{i,OWM,min}$ and $T_{i,OWM,max}$ being the mean, minimal and maximal temperature as given by OWM. $\phi_{i,OWM}$ is the relative humidity from OWM. The vehicle variables modelled with MLR are in the first step temperature $T_{vehicle}$ and secondly humidity $\phi_{vehicle}$. Other variables are not examined as they do not exist in both vehicle and all weather service records.

3 Results and Discussion
3.1 Historical Weather Databases
3.1.1 Temperature

Over the five training iterations of the cross validation, the mean of $e_{weatherservice}$ as calculated in (6) is 3.0 K for DWD. After MLR, the training mean of e_{fitted} as calculated in (5) is 2.0 K. The validation mean of $e_{weatherservice}$ is 3.4 K and the validation mean of e_{fitted} is 2.8 K. This means only an improvement of 0.6 K on the validation set can be achieved while training has an improvement of 1 K. The R^2 statistic for this case falls below 0.75 in the last iteration as can be seen in table 3. Hence, DWD does not fulfil the quality criteria required by the MLR. A second MLR on the DWD data but without humidity leads to the same mean error values over the five iterations with minimal differences in some iterations. The R^2 values can be taken from table 3. As with the MLR on DWD data with humidity, the MLR on DWD data without the DWD value for humidity is not sufficient in either the R^2 statistic nor the transferability of the mean errors between training and validation phase. For Meteostat, the mean of $e_{weatherservice}$ (6) on the training data over the five iterations is 2.2 K. After MLR, the mean e_{fitted} (5) is 0.9 K in training. On the validation data over the five iterations, the corresponding errors are 2.3 K and 0.8 K. This indicates that the MLR is generalizable. The R^2 as shown in the fourth row of table 3 shows that the variability in the vehicle temperature can be very well attributed to a combination of the variables $x_{i,Meteo}$. Lastly, OWM has a mean of $e_{weatherservice}$ (6) over the five iterations on the training data of 2.9 K. After MLR, the mean of e_{fitted} (5) on the training data is 1.4 K. For the validation data, the corresponding errors are 3.0 K and 1.4 K. This indicates that the MLR is generalizable. R^2 never falls below 0.857

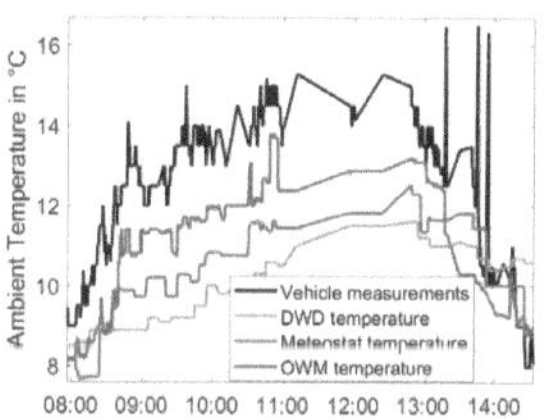
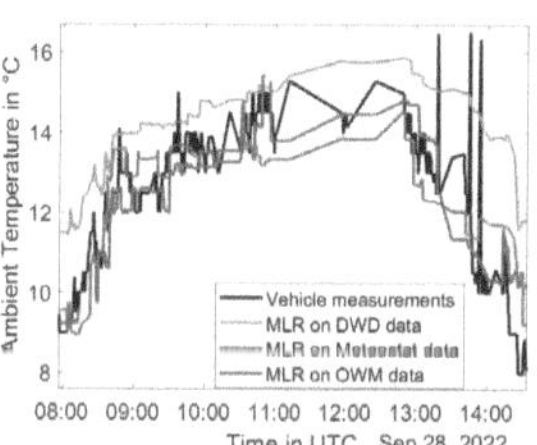

Figure 1: Ambient temperature, recorded by weather services

Figure 2: Ambient temperature as modelled by MLR

in table 3, and hence is of acceptable quality. The improvement can be seen exemplary for the test drive September 28, 2022, from the third validation iteration in the change from fig. 1 to 2.

Table 3: R^2 statistic for historical temperature MLR

Iteration	1	2	3	4	5
DWD	0.754	0.782	0.792	0.773	0.736
DWD without humidity	0.754	0.779	0.791	0.773	0.736
Meteostat	0.958	0.962	0.953	0.958	0.949
OWM	0.875	0.868	0.857	0.865	0.896

3.1.2 Humidity

As humidity can vary between surroundings, an 10 %-window additional to the minimum and maximum vehicle humidity is considered as acceptable. DWD has a mean of $e_{weatherservice}$ (6) on the training data over the five iterations of 30.1 %. After MLR, the mean of e_{fitted} (5) on the training data over the five iterations is 7.7 %. The corresponding errors on the validation data are 30.8 % and 8.2 %. Hence, the improvement on training and validation data is transferable. R^2 is never more than 0.53 as shown in table 3. This means that DWD and HERE data combined can not sufficiently explain the variability in vehicle measured humidity. For Meteostat, the mean of $e_{weatherservice}$ (6) on the training data over the five iterations is 26.0 %. After MLR, the mean of e_{fitted} (5) on the training data over five iterations is 4.2 %. The corresponding errors on the validation data are 25.2 % and 6.2 %. In combination with no R^2 value under 0.76, this means that Meteostat can be used to model vehicle humidity with external weather service data. For OWM, the mean of $e_{weatherservice}$ (6) on the training data over the five iterations is 34.0 % and after MLR, the mean of e_{fitted} (5) decreases to 5.4 %. On the validation data over the five iterations the corresponding errors are 33.1 % and 7.1 %. As R^2 never passes 0.69, OWM and HERE data combined can not sufficiently explain the variability in vehicle measured humidity. The change can be seen exemplary for the test drive April 22, 2022, from the fourth validation iteration in the fig. 3 and fig. 4.

Table 4: R^2 statistic for historical humidity MLR

Iteration	1	2	3	4	5
DWD	0.310	0.418	0.529	0.340	0.298
Meteostat	0.827	0.794	0.784	0.766	0.784
OWM	0.681	0.657	0.639	0.609	0.659

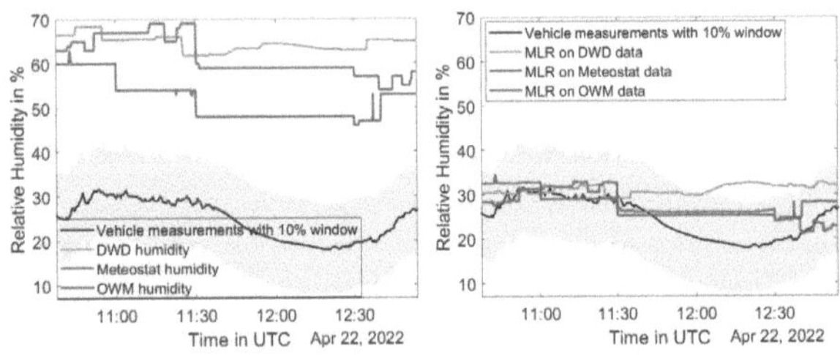

Figure 3: Ambient humidity, recorded by weather services

Figure 4: Ambient humidity as modelled by MLR

3.2 Weather Forecasts

3.2.1 Temperature

As explained in section 3.1.1, MLR on DWD data does not fulfil the demands introduced in section 2.3. Hence, MLR is not transferred from historical records to forecast. The error $e_{weatherservice}$ (6) from the DWD predicted temperature to the measured temperature over the geographical coordinates is 1.1 K for the first and 0.7 K for the second test drive. It is remarkable, that the predicted temperature is much closer to the vehicle temperature than the mean of DWD historical data. For the OWM forecast, the error $e_{weatherservice}$ (6) for the predicted temperature is 1.0 K for the first and 2.0 K for the second test drive. Using the coefficients b resulting from the MLR in section 3.1.1 and transferring it to the OWM forecast results in mean errors e_{fitted} of 0.9 K for the first and 0.5 K for the second test drive. As it was not possible in the time frame to conduct more test drives, this is only an indication that OWM characteristics gained from historical records can be transferred to future forecasts. The same can not be said about DWD which shows poor performance on historical data and much higher performance on the two forecast test drives.

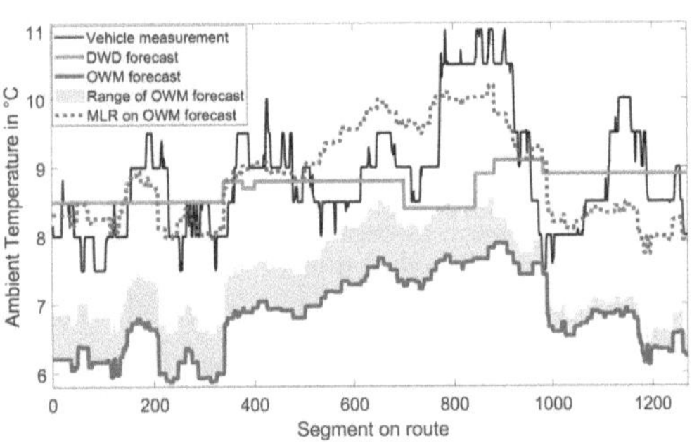

Figure 5: Measured ambient temperature of the vehicle and original DWD and OWM forecast of temperature and modelled OWM forecast with historical MLR on OWM forecast temperature, test drive of November 18, 2022.

3.2.2 Humidity

Only OWM forecast contains humidity, DWD MOSMIX forecast does not predict humidity. OWM does not fulfil the demands introduced in section 2.3. Hence, MLR is not transferred from historical records to forecast. The error $e_{weatherservice}$ (6) from OWM predicted humidity to vehicle measured humidity over geographical position is 28.7 %

for the first and 29.7 % for the second test drive. While this is comparable to the mean errors in section 3.1.2, this is a highly insufficient result.

4 Conclusion

External weather services can offer important information for BEV world models. The first step, to use historical weather records to evaluate the quality of temperature and humidity, results in a good and generalizable model with MLR for temperature for OWM and especially Meteostat. Meteostat data can even be used to model humidity via MLR. On two exemplary test drives, transferability between historical records and forecast was tested. Transferring the MLR results from OWM temperature records to forecast indicates that the resulting fitted temperature only deviates in acceptable range from the measured temperature and is closer to the measured vehicle temperature than the forecast temperature. This research can be expanded to model forecasts and analyse driver responses.

Acknowledgement

The work has been carried out at Dr. Ing h.c. F. Porsche AG, Stuttgart and supervised by the Institute for Electrical Engineering in Medicine.

Author's Statement

Authors state no conflict of interest.

5 References

[1] J. R. M. Delos Reyes, R. V. Parsons and R. Hoemsen, *Winter Happens: The Effect of Ambient Temperature on the Travel Range of Electric Vehicles.* In: IEEE Transactions on Vehicular Technology, vol. 65, no. 6, pp. 4016-4022, 2016.

[2] Z. Zhang, W. Li, C. Zhang and J. Chen, *Climate control loads prediction of electric vehicles.* In: Applied Thermal Engineering, vol. 110, pp. 1183-1188, 2017.

[3] F. Kaspar et al., *Regional atmospheric reanalysis activities at Deutscher Wetterdienst: review of evaluation results and application examples with a focus on renewable energy.* Advances in Science and Research, vol. 17, pp.115-128, 2020

[4] PennState Eberly College of Science, STAT 462 Applied Regression Analysis. *5.4 - A Matrix Formulation of the Multiple Regression Model.* Available: https://online.stat.psu.edu/stat462/node/132/ [last accessed on 2022-12-10].

[5] K. Backhaus, B. Erichson, W. Plinke and R. Weiber, *Multivariante Analysemethoden: eine anwendungsorientierte Einführung.* pp.16-26, Springer, Berlin Heidelberg, 1990.

Implementation of Hovering and Obstacle Avoidance of MONSUN Autonomous Underwater Vehicle

Neelam Sattur [1],
[1] Robotics and Autonomous Systems, Universität zu Lübeck, n.sattur@student.uni-luebeck.de

Abstract

The project aims to implement an underwater robot swarm's hovering behaviour and obstacle avoidance. Autonomous underwater vehicles (AUV) shall be used in the MOVE project to monitor macrophytes in lakes, which play an essential role in assessing water quality. A small and compact AUV known as MONSUN microAUVs are used for monitoring, which has to move constantly over the lake bed at a certain distance to take close-up pictures of the macrophytes with a camera for monitoring purposes using a SONAR altimeter. This behaviour is called *hovering*. The obstacle avoidance was implemented using a front-facing SONAR altimeter. Both principles were implemented as a new behaviour using MONSUN microAUVs, Robot Operating System (ROS) and Python.

1 Introduction

Monitoring the water quality of lakes and ponds is important in protecting the environment. Due to human influence, namely agriculture, there is an oversupply of nutrients which leads to the turbidity of the water. This water causes changes in the living conditions of aquatic plants and animals. There is a lot of interest in developing small Autonomous Underwater Vehicles (AUV) called microAUVs to monitor and explore lakes and ponds since microAUVs can reduce the cost and increase the efficiency of the monitoring process. MicroAUVs are also preferred due to their small size and robust structure. Sensors can be attached to microAUVs to measure underwater pressure, depth, and imaging. MicroAUVs can perform several tasks with the help of different sensors. Due to their small size, microAUVs can reach spaces on the lake bed better than humans. This research paper demonstrates AUVs' hovering and obstacle avoidance, particularly the MONSUN microAUVs.

The MONSUN microAUVs shall be used in the MOVE project to monitor the presence of a large class of aquatic plants known as macrophytes in lakes, which play an essential role in assessing water quality. MONSUN microAUV has to move constantly over the lake bed at a certain distance to take close-up pictures of the macrophytes with a camera. This behaviour is called *hovering*.

One of the goals presented here is to install an altimeter for measuring the distance to the lake ground and its integration into the ROS software of MONSUN. This new implementation includes the investigation of a sensor fusion with the pressure sensor for depth measurements. The other goal is to implement *obstacle avoidance* using a front-facing single-beam pinger SONAR altimeter. The MONSUN uses this function to navigate around any potential obstacles present near the lake bed.

The implemented behaviours can be scaled to be used in a swarm of MONSUN microAUVs. The paper follows the general structure: The materials and methods used are discussed in the first section. The results obtained are briefly explained.

2 Material and Methods

This section presents an overview of the MOVE project and a closer look into the working of the MONSUN AUV and pinger SONAR altimeter.

2.1 The MOVE project

Monitoring vegetation and water quality in lakes with underwater robot swarms or the MOVE project aims to automate the tracking of small water bodies such as lakes and ponds. The MOVE project's primary motivation is to monitor the ecosystem of aquatic plants and animals due to climate change, pollution or over-exploitation and to convert the water bodies back to their optimal ecological status. This goal is achieved by individually analysing the existing environmental conditions of the water bodies. In addition to recording the parameters such as temperature, pH value and oxygen content, the water quality is determined by the presence of aquatic plants known as macrophytes. These macrophytes represent an important sub-criterion for assessing the condition of the water.

The automation of the recording and analysing of the water body is done by using the MONSUN AUV deployed as underwater robot swarms, as shown in Fig. 1.

The MONSUN is used for area-wide investigation and mapping of lakes. The robots are equipped with measuring

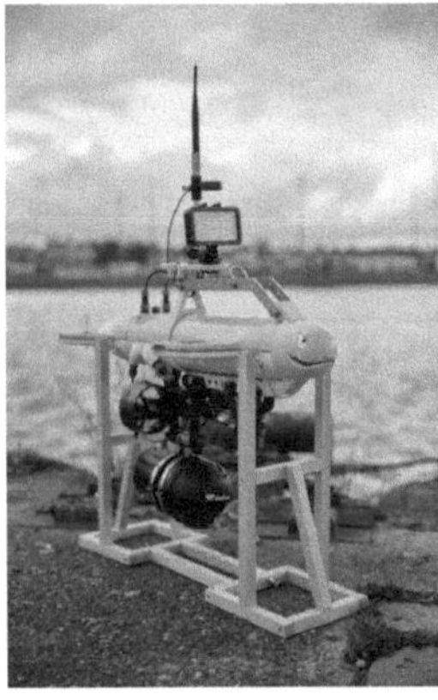

Figure 1: MONSUN AUV mounted with cameras, antennas and sonars.

probes, cameras and sonars, which give a direct view of the water so that the aquatic plants and the parameters for optimal macrophyte growth can be identified and recorded. MONSUN intends to collect the characteristics of macrophytes and other related data, which will be processed in further steps based on the assessment guidelines provided by the EU- Water Framework Directive and Fauna-Flora-Habitat Directive [1].

2.2 Autonomous Underwater Vehicles

An Autonomous Underwater Vehicle (AUV) is a submersible robot that can travel underwater autonomously, i.e., not requiring input from the operator. AUVs are preferred over manned vehicles for underwater research and exploration due to their versatility and autonomous operation. Various sensors can be attached to AUVs to measure the concentration of elements and compounds, the depth, pressure, or the presence of microscopic life. Some sensors are conductivity-temperature-depth (CTDs) and cameras.
The size of AUVs ranges from man-portable, lightweight vehicles to large-diameter vehicles of over 10 metres in length. AUVs with a cylindrical or torpedo shape and a powered propeller is considered optimal designs for size, hydrodynamic efficiency, and handling. When the AUV dives underwater, it will lose its GPS signal since radio waves cannot penetrate water for a larger depth range. The most common way for AUVs to navigate is through an underwater acoustic positioning system and dead reckoning, a process used in navigation that calculates the current position of a moving object using a previously determined position along with the estimates of speed, direction and the elapsed time.
The propulsion techniques for AUVs use brushed, or brushless electric motors, a gearbox, a propeller and a thruster unit [2].
Since most AUVs are bulky and torpedo-shaped, they are often too big to manoeuvre in tight spaces or require structures like ships to be deployed in the water. This makes them expensive and complex. Smaller and more inexpensive AUVs, called microAUVs, are built. Since there is no

clear definition for the term micro AUV currently, there is an assumption that microAUVs are small, easy to develop, usually less than 1 m in length and low in weight. Due to their small size and low cost, microAUVs can be deployed in a swarm. MicroAUVs are better suited for shallow waters or near the coastline [3].

2.3 MONSUN AUV

The MONSUN is an AUV developed at the Institute of Computer Engineering, Universität zu Lübeck, and is used in robot swarms. Due to its small size, it is known as a microAUV [4]. The MONSUN's design is robust and modular, allowing for various tasks such as monitoring and inspection to be carried out. The design concept is scalable to be used in a swarm consisting of several AUVs which cooperate independently. The AUV is designed to be highly robust to external influences such as water pressure at depths of 100 m and mechanical stress during boarding off/on a ship. The AUVs can measure at the surface and multiple depths with environmental sensors equipped on the robot and use a combination of Wi-Fi communication at the surface and while diving acoustic modems with a data rate of 13.9 kbit/s and operating frequency range of 18 to 34 kHz is used.
This enables underwater communication to coordinate and navigate the swarm of robots and transmit data to the surface simultaneously. The swarm robots communicate with each other via acoustic modems. The localisation and communication concept of the robot assumes that some of the robots stay at the surface and others dive to the given depth. The surface robots obtain their position by GPS coordinates and communicate with each other and a control station through Wi-Fi. The dived robots measure the depth by pressure sensors and keep it stable using a depth control and pose control algorithm [5].

The main control unit of the MONSUN robot is a Raspberry Pi 3 with a quad-core 1.2 GHz Broadcom BCM 2837 64-bit ARM CPU with 1 GB RAM. It has a Linux operating system capable of implementing the ROS framework. The I2C bus with the Raspberry Pi as the master node is provided for communication with sensors, actuators and other devices. The propulsion system consists of six independent brushless Motors, each driven by a separate motor controller. The MONSUN is equipped with the temperature-compensated MS5803-14BA pressure sensor, which measures the depth with an accuracy of 2 cm to a maximum depth of 100 m.

The MONSUN software is divided into three levels sense/act level, behaviour level and task level; as shown in Fig. 2, the uppermost level is the task level, where the missions are defined and organised at the highest abstraction level. These levels are realized using ROS and Python.

The basic principle of ROS is to run a great number of ex-

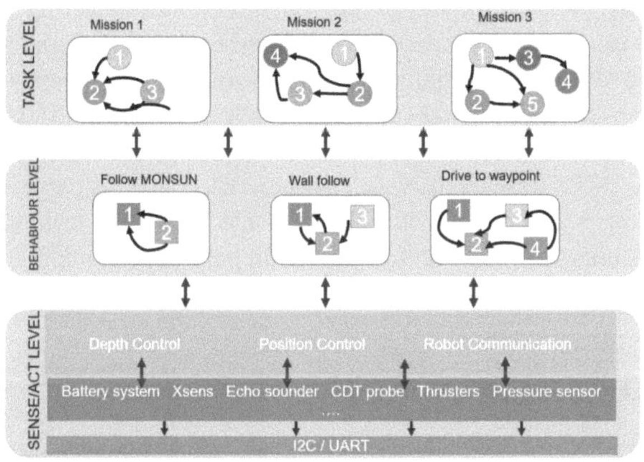

Figure 2: ROS-based software architecture of the MON-SUN AUV is divided into three hierarchical levels: a Sense/Act Level, a Behaviour Level and a Task Level.

ecutables in parallel that need to be able to exchange data synchronously or asynchronously.

The ROS Master is a declaration and registration service (network server), which makes it possible for these executables (nodes) to find each other and exchange data. Every node registers with the ROS Master at startup. The nodes interested in data subscribe to the relevant topic, and nodes that generate data publish to the relevant topic. There can be multiple publishers and subscribers to the same topic. Each topic has a message type given by the ROS message used to publish; the node can only receive messages of the same type [6]. There is no consistency for the publishers, but subscribers will only establish message transport if the type matches.

2.4 Pinger Sonar Altimeter

The single beam echo sounder (SBES), or a depth sounder, determines water depth by measuring the travel time of a short acoustic pulse or a *ping*. The *ping* is emitted from a transducer positioned below the water surface, and the SBES listens for the return echo from the bottom of the lake bed. Accurate depths are obtained by filtering out spurious signals in the reflected echo.

The Blue Robotics Ping Echosounder and Altimeter is a low-cost underwater single-beam sonar module that measures the distance to underwater objects. The ping sonar has a range of 50 m, a beam width of 30 deg and a depth rating of 300 m. The module can be used as an altimeter and for obstacle avoidance sonar.

The ping device works on the principle of echo sounding. It emits a short 115 kHz acoustic pulse from the transducer and then measures the strength of the returned acoustic pulse. The acoustic pulse reflects or echoes off solid objects and travels back to the device while travelling through water. The device calculates the distance to the object using the following equation:

$$D = v(t/2) \tag{1}$$

where D is the distance, v is the velocity of sound in water, and t is the acoustic signal travel time.

The device runs a tracking algorithm that locks on to the most significant target in the range of the device. It is designed to track a flat surface but can also be used as a proximity sensor. The algorithm considers the strongest return signal, which is most likely the object and prior measurements to determine the object. The tracking algorithm produces the confidence measurement corresponding to the probability that the object is identified correctly. The device's output is the distance, and the corresponding confidence level [7].

3 Results and Discussion

The following algorithms were implemented and tested using dummy messages in ROS.

3.1 Hovering Node

Hovering is implemented as a new behaviour of the AUV. The hovering behaviour is realised using ROS nodes and written in Python.

Fig. 3 shows the behaviour level missions and the sense/act level for the hovering task. Hovering is enabled from the task level using ROS services. The hovering node subscribes to the pinger node, which publishes the topic distance and confidence, and the ms5803 pressure sensor node, which publishes the depth.

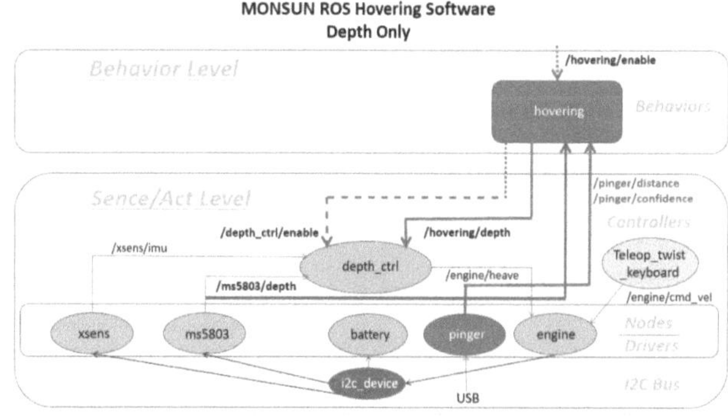

Figure 3: Software architecture of the hovering operation

The hovering node takes the data from the pinger node and filters the noisy data using the in-built lambda filter from the Python Library, where all the sonar readings above the confidence level are extracted. This filtered distance value is then published to the depth control node (already present as a node in the MONSUN software).

The AUV is made to hover at a constant distance of, e.g. 80 cm above the lake bed. The hovering distance is kept constant, independent of the depth. The hovering distance is calculated using the following equation:

$$H = S + F_d - H_d \qquad (2)$$

where H is the set depth value at which the AUV should move to start hovering, which is sent to the depth control node (depth_ctrl), S is the current depth of the AUV. It is obtained from the pressure sensor node (ms5803), F_d is the distance obtained from the pinger node after filtering, H_d is a constant depth at which the AUV should hover (e.g. 80 cm).

3.2 Obstacle Avoidance Node

The obstacle avoidance node is implemented for MONSUN to detect and avoid obstacles while performing tasks for the MOVE project. This behaviour is known as escape behaviour.

The node is written in Python and ROS. The Blue Robotics Ping Echo sounder is used here as a forward-looking sonar mounted at the front of MONSUN. If the distance gets lower than a set threshold (distance taken from the sonar readings), MONSUN shall drive backwards for a short time; then, the robot will turn right for another given time and continue moving forward.

This node subscribes to the pinger node to obtain the distance values and then publishes to the engine node (engine), which is already integrated into the MONSUN software. The engine node controls the brushless motors; 4 vertical and two horizontal thrusters. It subscribes to linear and angular velocities with values ranging from $(-1.0, \cdots, 0, \cdots, +1.0)$ for drive(x), dive(z) and roll(x), pitch(y) and yaw(z), respectively.

The obstacle avoidance node publishes Twist messages containing the two sub-messages, the linear and angular velocity, defined by the variables x, y and z, to the engine node. Fig. 4 shows the obstacle avoidance node's behaviour and sense levels. If the distance readings from the sonar are less

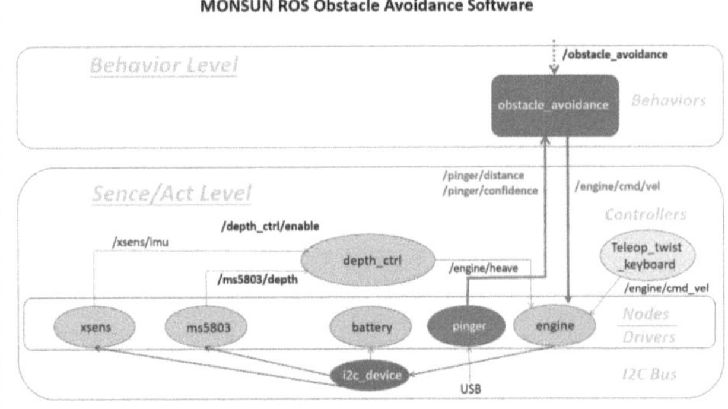

Figure 4: Software architecture of obstacle avoidance behaviour

than the given distance threshold, it implies that there is an object in front of the AUV. The obstacle avoidance node has to publish to the engine after every change in the linear and angular velocities so that the AUV can manoeuvre around the obstacle.

4 Conclusion

This paper presents an implementation of hovering behaviour and an obstacle avoidance technique for microAUVs using a single-beam echo sounder, the ping sonar. The implementation of hovering allows the MONSUN to hover at a constant distance over the lake ground, enabling the AUV to perform various other tasks, such as capturing images at the lake bed. The obstacle avoidance technique ensures that the MONSUN does not get trapped or damaged during navigation.

Acknowledgement

The work has been carried out at the Institute of Computer Engineering, Universität zu Lübeck and supervised by Prof. Dr.-Ing. Erik Maehle.

Author's Statement

Conflict of interest: Author(s) state no conflict of interest.

5 References

[1] ITI Lübeck, *The MOVE Project.* Available: https://www.iti.uni-luebeck.de/en/research-areas/mobile-robotics/move.html [last accessed on 2023-01-07].

[2] M. Saghafi, R. Lavimi *Optimal design of nose and tail of an autonomous underwater vehicle hull to reduce drag force using numerical simulation.* In: Part M: Journal of Engineering for the Maritime Environment, 2019 [last accessed on 2023-01-10].

[3] E. Maehle, B. Meyer, C. Isokeit and U. Behrje *MONSUN: a swarm AUV for environmental monitoring and inspection.* In: Ehlers, Frank (editor): Autonomous Underwater Vehicles - Design and Practice. IET - The Institution of Engineering and Technology, pp. 329–355, 2020.

[4] ITI Lübeck, *MONSUN.* Available: https://www.iti.uni-luebeck.de/en/research-areas/mobile-robotics/monsun.html [last accessed on 2023-01-07].

[5] B. Meyer, C. Isokeit, U. Behrje and E. Maehle *A Robust Acoustic-Based Communication Principle for the Navigation of an Underwater Robot Swarm.* In OCEANS'18 MTS/IEEE, Kobe, Japan 2018.

[6] Robot Operating Software, *ROS Documentation.* Available: http://wiki.ros.org/ROS/Tutorials/WritingPublisherSubscriber [last accessed on 2023-01-10].

[7] Blue robotics, *Ping Echosounder Sonar User Manual.* Available: https://bluerobotics.com/learn/ping-sonar-technical-guide [last accessed on 2023-01-10].

Designing a Study to observe the Incidence of Falls by means of a Sensory Floor System

Solveig Kathleen Najork [1], Axel Steinhage [2], Christl Lauterbach [3], Laura Liebenow [4], and Marcin Grzegorzek [5] [6]

[1] Medical Informatics, Universität zu Lübeck, solveig.najork@student.uni-luebeck.de
[2] SensProtect GmbH, axel.steinhage@sensprotect.com
[3] SensProtect GmbH, christl.lauterbach@future-shape.com
[4] Institute of Medical Informatics, Universität zu Lübeck, laura.liebenow@student.uni-luebeck.de
[5] Institute of Medical Informatics, Universität zu Lübeck, marcin.grzegorzek@uni-luebeck.de
[6] Department of Knowledge Engineering, University of Economics in Katowice, marcin.grzegorzek@uni-luebeck.de

Abstract

This paper describes the designing of a study, which observes the effects of the capacitive sensor floor system. The SensFloor® can recognise falls and, depending on the type of resolution, also offers the possibility of gait analysis. For the study described in this paper, the effects of this system now are investigated. Thereby, the study design process is discussed in detail and preliminaries of the study planning are explained. In particular, the given preconditions and questions about the practical implementation are also discussed. This paper only describes the planning of the study but not the execution or the results of the study, as this is only planned for the future.

1 Introduction

This paper presents the process and the final result of planning a study. Nevertheless, the study itself has not yet been carried out, which is why this paper only describes the structure of the planned study. The SensFloor® is a capacitive floor sensor system that examines the living and working conditions of residents as well as caregivers in healthcare. Thereby, this study is urgently needed to have an objective evaluation of the SensFloor® and its functions, since so far only reports from different facilities regarding implementation and usage are available. These reports are quite beneficial and suggest that there is a positive impact of the SensFloor® on the nursing operation and the reduction of falls. However, these do not represent an objective observation, which may be achieved by a study. This study will examine the effects on the different participants, looking at both physical and psychological effects. The focus, however, is on the frequency of falls.

Falls are a major hazard in old age. Due to the naturally occurring frailty of old age, many elderly people can no longer get up independently after a fall In these cases, rapid recognition of such a fall is essential. Otherwise, downtimes of several hours may occur, leading to serious consequences for the health of the person who has fallen. This detection task can be solved by the SensFloor®. In the planned study discussed here, the most important aspects are now considered and, above all, viewed objectively [1].

2 Material and Methods

In the following the large application field of ambient assisted Living of the SensFloor, as well as the considered methods of study planning are explained.

2.1 Ambient Assisted Living

As a result of demographic change and the ever-increasing shortage of care workers, care assistance systems are urgently needed. The fact that more and more people want to remain autonomous in their own flat or house for as long as possible also contributes to this phenomenon. One possible solution to the problems mentioned above is Ambient Assisted Living, which is intended to support people in need of help in their everyday lives [2]. The aim is to support a self-determined life into advanced age. An additional goal is to improve the quality of services and to increase the quality of life for the respective persons. Hereby, it is important to focus on the users and their ability to use the technology independently in their everyday life.

2.2 SensFloor®

The study aims to examine the effects of the SensFloor® on the frequency of collapses, as well as the sense of security of the residents and their relatives. Furthermore, the impact on the carers requires consideration.

In this examination, a capacitive floor sensor system is used. The considered system is the SensFloor® by FutureShape GmbH. This technology allows measuring the activity of a person by electrical capacitances. Capacitance is defined as the ability of a capacitor to absorb and store electrical charge. In this application, a plate capacitor is comparable, whereby the upper plate is represented by the foot of the subject that steps on the floor. Thus, an increase in capacitance follows as soon as one or more people step on the floor [3].

The SensFloor® consists of three distinct layers. Here the lowest layer is aluminium foil. Attached to this sheet there is a three-millimeter-thick layer of polyester. On the top, there is a thin layer of polyester which is coated with metal closing the base. The upper layer is interleaved by gaps so that measurements can be made for the individual sensory fields. These gaps build a triangle shape of sensor fields. In comparison to alternative field shapes, this solution offers the advantage that more sensor areas can be reached, and thus, higher resolutions become achievable. Eight of these triangles are building one module where each module contains one sensor. This sensor measures the capacitance for each of the sensory fields. The floor consists of an individual number of rectangular modules, which can be chosen freely according to the room's architecture. These modules are independent of each other such that only one of them is connected directly to the power supply. The remaining modules are connected by stripes of the upper layer among each other. The SensFloor® may be installed under the usual floor structure so that neither heavy objects nor water are a problem [3].

2.3 Study design fundamentals

The study design is defined as the use of "evidence-based procedures, protocols, and guidelines that provide the tools and frameworks for conducting a research study" [4]. The choice of the study design is a consequence of the circumstances of the study such as the research question or the objective, phenomena. Also, the sampling strategies and the population of interest have a great impact on this choice [5]. The concrete planning of the study should be preceded by the development of its hypotheses. For this purpose, it is important to first formulate the respective points of consideration and examine their testability. In the further course, the null and alternative hypotheses should then be developed. Hereby the null hypothesis is considered and tested in the course of the study. If this hypothesis is rejected, the alternative hypothesis can be considered proven.

The study design can be divided into observational and experimental designs. The *observational design* does not alter variables or the environment itself during the study. Here, only a consideration of the circumstances takes place. The *experimental design* requires a change in variables or manipulation of the given circumstances. Whenever it is possible to choose the study design, the experimental design should be preferred, as it can show much stronger evidence of an association than the observational design [4].

In this paper, two different study designs are considered in more detail. These are the cross-over and parallel group design presented in Fig. 1, Fig. 2. The *cross over design*, as shown in Fig. 1, divides the participants of the study into two groups. For this study design, it is indispensable that effects are visible immediately with the chosen treatment method, which, however, also disappear again after a certain period and a state similar to the starting state is reached. Both study groups then alternate between the two different treatments, with a break between the two phases. The motivation for such a strategy is that the effects of the first treatment phase should fade away and only the effects of the second treatment phase are measured in the following. In the evaluation of the study, the results achieved by the two treatment methods are now considered against each other. The advantage of this procedure is, that the participants are observed for both treatments and thus selection bias can be avoided [4]. The *parallel group design*, shown in Fig. 2, also divides the participants into two different groups. Here each group receives an individual treatment and the results of the two groups are compared.

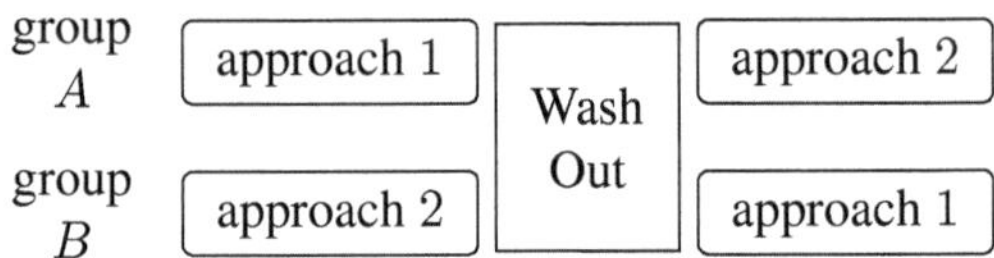

Figure 1: Cross-over design schematic

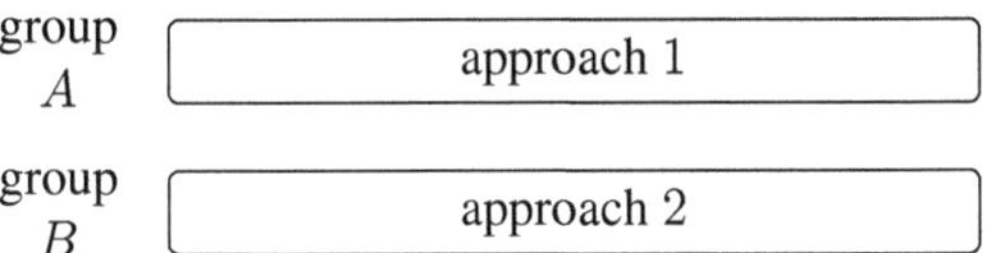

Figure 2: Parallel group design schematic

Another important instrument of the study design is *randomisation*. This is the process in which the participants are randomly assigned to the different treatments. The idea behind this process is to avoid errors, such as an uneven distribution of influencing factors, which are called *confounding factors* [6], [7]. A further tool to avoid errors is *blinding*. The aim here is to avoid errors due to pre-study assumptions by participants or implementers. The group to which the participant is assigned is kept secret and, depending on the type of blinding is not disclosed to either the participants or the treatment providers. There are different variants, whether the participants themselves do not know which group they belong to, or the study investigators do not know this information. In another variant, neither party knows the assignment of the groups. This is to prevent unconscious unequal treatment and the placebo effect. The use of these instruments should be well discussed and the reasons for not using these techniques should be given in the study design, as these are established methods that fundamentally increase the quality and validity of the study.

Another major decision is the choice of study participants. Here it is important to think about the *population of interest*. The population of interest represents the group, that is affected by the treatment under consideration. As in most cases, a study with the complete population of interest is not possible, due to the limitation of the treatment or the capacities, a representative group for this population of interest must be found. For this process, it is important to think about possible confoundings and formulate certain limitations. These are called *eligibility criteria* and can be subdivided into the *inclusion* and *exclusion criteria* [4]. Inclusion criteria are a formulation of the objectives that must be indispensably achieved to participate in the study and represent the main characteristics of the population of interest [4]. Exclusion criteria make participation impossible, as they are intended to avoid confounders. The idea behind the criteria is to strengthen the knowledge gained in the study and to protect against possible biases. After the selection has been made by applying the criteria, there is usually still a larger number of people left than those who can participate in the study. Now, the tool of *sampling* can be applied, whereby with different strategies, which depend on the characteristic of the population, a selection of the participants of the study is made [4], [8].

2.4 Planning of the study

In planning the study, the hypotheses were first worked out. After this was done, different possibilities for the study concept were discussed with the involved parties and a joint decision was made for a study design. Subsequently, the concrete planning was continued with the support of the biometric counseling of the University of Lübeck and an ethics application was prepared.

As preliminaries, the following circumstances for the planning of the study were given. A study planning for a study on the frequency of falls and the consequences of falls with installed SensFloor® was to be carried out. The effects of the SensFloor® on the mentioned aspects as well as the effects on the daily care routine and especially the well-being of the carers, relatives, and residents are considered. There is already an institution for which the study is intended, that will be completely equipped with the SensFloor®.

Adapted to the given framework conditions, the planning of the study started with an elaboration of the hypotheses. For the choice of study design, serval of options were considered. Due to the practical and ethical circumstances, an observational design was chosen. In detail, a cross-over and parallel study design were discussed and the parallel study design was chosen. In the course of planning, further opportunities arose in such a way that with this design another facility can be considered in the study. This further facility has no SensFloor® installed and builds the second group for the parallel design. Due to the average time, residents usually live in such an institution, the choice of study duration is limited. Therefore, the length of the study was planned to be three months to set a reasonable period and to have sufficient time to compare the results on the one hand. In this study, the population of interest is people living in a care facility. Thus, the inclusion criteria are living in one of the two study facilities. Exclusion criteria were deliberately not set here, as the SensFloor® is expected affect on residents who are at high risk of falling. This concerns, among others, people with dementia or other illnesses that lead to susceptibility to falls. The aim is to have an average resident population of the facilities as the study population and thus also to be able to conclude about other facilities.

Due to the circumstances, the study population is formed from the existing residents. Thus, the possibility of randomising the study participants is not given, since the residents are only considered for the facility in which they currently live. An important detail is that the two facilities are run by the same care provider and are also very similar in terms of the structure of the home. Consequently, it is assumed that the circumstances for the residents and the nursing staff are as similar as possible, apart from the crucial difference that the SensFloor® is only installed in one facility. To create the greatest possible structural similarity between the study participants, pairwise matching is carried out. For this process, criteria such as age, gender, any medical conditions that may be present, and the need for care are considered.

3 Results and Discussion

The outcome is the planning of the study with the formulation of the hypotheses, as well as the writing of the necessary applications and the statistical planning associated with the study. Biometric counselling at the Institute for Medical Biometry and Statistics has been in the amount of approx. 10 hours. As explained in more detail above in 2.3, this is an *observational study* with a *parallel group design*.

The course of the study can be divided into five sections. First, the study starts with the preparatory organisation, which is taking place in parts. These are, on the one hand, the preparatory organisation, such as the presentation of the study in the two institutions. This is followed by the introduction of the study, this work package consists to a large extent of the recruitment of the study participants. The third package is the enrolment period, during which the data is collected, followed by the final phase of the study, during which interviews will be conducted. Concluding the study, results are evaluated and findings are formulated.

During the study the following hypotheses are investigated, the first and main hypothesis is that a reduction in the number of falls is possible, if the SensFloor® is installed. The other secondary hypotheses to be investigated are listed below.

- There is no change in the stress of the caregivers.

- The activity does not change after the control visits.

- There is no change in the length of time caregivers spend with residents in need of assistance.

- There is no change in the unnecessary distances travelled by the nursing staff.

- The SensFloor® does not have a positive influence on the feeling of safety of the relatives.

- The feeling of safety of the residents is not positively influenced by the SensFloor®.

- An improvement in the attractiveness of the workplace cannot be observed.

For all hypotheses except the consideration of nocturnal activity, the measurements and observations from the two different facilities are compared against each other and will provide a statement about the effects of the SensFloor®.
One issue that has already been addressed is the question of study design. In an optimal case, a different study design would have been chosen for the study, since in the parallel group design there is a risk of errors due to an unequal distribution of persons with confounders. This is intensified by missing blinding, which is not possible due to the mode of operation of the SensFloor®. This is further exacerbated by the lack of randomisation. However, it is also important to question whether this optimal solution is feasible in practice and ethically justifiable. It is important to consider that randomization would require the willingness to recruit a study group and randomly assign them a place of residence and living, which seems very questionable both practically and ethically. Another alternative in the study design would have been a cross-over design. In this case, the study would have taken place in one institution only and there would have been two study groups and two study phases that both groups would have gone through. However, the question arises of how the two treatment phases should be structured. Of course, it would be optimal for the study if the SensFloor® functioned normally in one study phase, while recordings were made in the other study phase, but these were not forwarded to the nurses. However, this would also mean that in the event of a fall being detected by the SensFloor®, no notification would be made. In the worst case, such a procedure could lead to residents lying helplessly on the floor and possibly suffering further physical harm, which is why it is not ethically justifiable, even if this would provide the clearest proof of the functions. An alternative would be to simply display the information on whether there is an activity in a room. In this case, the fall alarm would work regularly in both study phases and only the information about activity would not be displayed on the ward overview. However, since there is already a presumption in the planning of the study that falls can be prevented by this information, this is also ethically difficult to justify since it is questionable whether the residents themselves and their relatives would agree to participate in the study under these conditions. The chosen solution avoids these problems by choosing an ethically justifiable option. Thus, the second device without SensFloor® installed corresponds to a common device and the number of falls between the devices can be compared. It is important to note that while no randomisation was included, the matching of subjects will occur to create as similar a study group as possible for the two facilities.

4 Conclusion

In this paper, the planning of a study to investigate the effects of a capacitive sensor floor was presented. In particular, the possible study designs and the question of choosing a study design were discussed. Further, an ethics proposal was prepared. An important continuation is the implementation of the study discussed here and the consideration of the results achieved.

Acknowledgement

The work has been carried out at Sensprotect GmbH, Höhenkirchen-Siegertsbrunn and supervised by the Institute of Medical Informatics, Universität zu Lübeck.

Author's Statement

Conflict of interest: Authors state no conflict of interest.

5 References

[1] M. Terroso, N. Rosa, A. Torres Marques, and R. Simoes, "Physical consequences of falls in the elderly: a literature review from 1995 to 2010," *European Review of Aging and Physical Activity*, vol. 11, no. 1, pp. 51–59, 2014.

[2] A. Braun, F. Kirchbuchner, and R. Wichert, "Ambient assisted living," in *eHealth in Deutschland*, pp. 203–222, Springer, 2016.

[3] R. Hoffmann, H. Brodowski, A. Steinhage, and M. Grzegorzek, "Detecting walking challenges in gait patterns using a capacitive sensor floor and recurrent neural networks," *Sensors*, vol. 21, no. 4, p. 1086, 2021.

[4] U. Majid, "Research fundamentals: Study design, population, and sample size," *Undergraduate research in natural and clinical science and technology journal*, vol. 2, pp. 1–7, 2018.

[5] U. Majid, "Research fundamentals: The research question, outcomes, and background," *Undergraduate Research in Natural and Clinical Science and Technology Journal*, vol. 1, pp. 1–7, 2017.

[6] S. R. Cummings, D. Grady, and S. B. Hulley, "Designing a randomized blinded trial," *Designing clinical research*, vol. 3, no. 1, pp. 147–61, 2007.

[7] D. A. Grimes and K. F. Schulz, "Bias and causal associations in observational research," *The lancet*, vol. 359, no. 9302, pp. 248–252, 2002.

[8] F. Kamangar and F. Islami, "Sample size calculation for epidemiologic studies: principles and methods," *Archives of Iranian medicine*, vol. 16, no. 5, pp. 0–0, 2013.

Providing medical data from an external database for reports and statistics to create a visualization dashboard for a maternal-child monitoring ward

Svea Störmer [1], Nils Hombeuel [2]

[1] Medical Engineering Science, Universität zu Lübeck, svea.stoermer@student.uni-luebeck.de
[2] Philips Medical Systems Böblingen, nils.hombeuel@philips.com

Abstract

Considering the increasing shortage of nurses, midwives and gynecologists in hospitals, more efficient monitoring of pregnant patients and the unborn child, such as by providing a statistical overview of the current situation on the various wards, would reduce the workload. To achieve this, the medical patient data collected by a mother-child monitoring software is processed in an external database for statistical analysis and provided to the open-source software Grafana for visualization. The considered open-source software does not have a direct plugin for capturing the data from the external database, so the two time series databases InfluxDB and Prometheus for capturing the data are identified, analyzed and compared based on requirements. Depending on the analysis, the more suitable time series database InfluxDB with its agent Telegraf is implemented and a representation of the statistical data in the form of individually configurable charts is enabled in a Grafana dashboard for visualization.

1 Introduction

A mother-child monitoring software collects medical patient data and prepares them in an external database for statistical analysis. These data are used for medical reports and provide hospital staff with a statistical overview of the current situation on the various wards. An example is the number of high-risk patients currently under care or the average length of stay of patients, which can be informative for the nurses. For a maternity ward, the average age of expectant mothers or an overview of the genders of newborns and the number of births, among other data, may also be of interest. A clear, individually configurable dashboard that visualizes the statistics of the external database would make the work of midwives and physicians significantly easier and more efficient.

1.1 Maternal and fetal monitoring systems

Delivery room data management systems are used in perinatal medicine for the documentation of pregnancy, gynecological examinations, labor, birth, and the unborn child. In the data management system, antepartum and intrapartum alarm and monitoring functions are combined with detailed documentation and storage of patient data in patient reports. The data management system can be used for documentation of an entire pregnancy or as a pure monitoring system in an emergency, as well as for fetal monitoring. Monitoring parameters include oxygenation, fetal and maternal heart rate, and fetal movements [1].

Furthermore, a delivery room data management system can be used as a pure cardiotocogram system focusing on the single cardiotocogram. Cardiotocography is a method of monitoring labor activity and fetal heart rates during labor and delivery. The monitoring is done with transducers. The transducers can be used to measure the parameters using the Toco measurement method. The Toco measuring method is used to record labor activity via pressure-sensitive measuring sensors that measure the hardening and tension of the uterine muscle [1].
If the delivery room data management system receives abnormal curves based on the analysis of the cardiotocogram, a warning signal is emitted [1].

1.2 External database for statistical analysis

A mother-child monitoring software has an internal and an external database. The external database is a replication of the internal database where statistical analysis can be run without interfering with ongoing clinical operations [2].
Generally, the developer can access the external database through a SQL client application. This application provides a tabular overview of all data as well as the possibility to view all attributes of the data records. For example, the attributes of a patient record stored in the external database can be listed, which include the patient ID, the first and last name, and the date of birth of the respective patient [2].
However, medical personnel (hereinafter referred to as user) can only query and visualize the statistics from the external database via a Microsoft Excel spreadsheet, as program-

ming skills are required for the developer tool. The Excel spreadsheet is generated directly from the delivery room data management system by the nurse or physician after manually selecting the desired statistics in a toolbox [2]. To improve this process to be made more user-friendly, a visualization tool like Grafana for statistics is required.

1.3 Visualization Tool Grafana

The open source software Grafana is a platform that can be used to visualize data in dynamic, interactive dashboards. Grafana is often used for monitoring tasks, such as the visualization of metrics or for alerting. The software provides the ability to create, analyze and also share dashboards independently and easily, regardless of the location of the data used. This makes it possible to display data from different databases on one screen in parallel [3]. The elementary component of Grafana is a HTTP(S) server that serves as a graphical web interface for the user. The web interface is used to configure the connections of the data sources using a plug-in system and the visualization of the metrics. Grafana works with two types of databases. On the one hand, it supports time series databases such as InfluxDB or Prometheus. On the other hand, Grafana also supports relational databases, such as MySQL or PostgreSQL [3].

The principle on which Grafana was developed is based on granting access to data to all employees, not just to individuals. This additionally enables the joint analysis of data in the team and thus promotes cooperation [4]. Since Grafana does not provide a plug-in to collect the data directly from the external database, the two time series databases InfluxDB and Prometheus were analyzed to store data outside the database and then visualize it with Grafana. Both Prometheus and InfluxDB are enterprise database management systems used to collect, store, process and visualize metrics. Preferably InfluxDB and Prometheus are used as a time series database that stores time series. This means that the data is time-stamped and stored [5],[6].

2 Material and Methods

2.1 Requirements for time series databases

To achieve the desired visualization result, requirements for the two time series databases have been defined. The time series databases needs to have a Plug-in for querying the data from the external database. Additionally a compatibility to Grafana is needed. The mother-child monitoring software is a medical device and as a result the statistics are patient data, a high level of data security and a storage period of at least 25 years must be ensured [2]. Since the software captures patient data at seconds resolution, InfluxDB and Prometheus should also provide this resolution.

2.2 Comparison of the suitability of the use of Prometheus and InfluxDB

Since Grafana does not provide a direct plug-in to capture data from the external database, InfluxDB and Prometheus are compared against the requirements to evaluate whether the respective time series databases are suitable for capturing and storing the metrics.

The visualization tool Grafana offers a direct plug-in for InfluxDB as well as for Prometheus. Thus a compatibility for Grafana is given for both databases. Also the necessary data security is fulfilled by both applications by means of API keys for authentication [7],[8]. Despite the fact that the resolution of the time stamp of InfluxDB in the nanosecond range is better than the resolution in the millisecond range of Prometheus, both fulfill the requirement, since for the mother-child monitoring software only a resolution in the second range is necessary [6].

InfluxDB and Prometheus differ significantly in the storage time of the data and in the provision of a plug-in for retrieving the data from the external database. Both InfluxDB and Prometheus do not provide a direct plug-in that allows data retrieval from the database. However, the InfluxDB agent Telegraf offers a so-called exec input plug-in [9]. This exec plug-in can be configured to query user-defined metrics from any source. Prometheus does not have such a plug-in. Furthermore, the local memory of Prometheus is not intended as a long-term memory and thus data is deleted after only 15 days instead of the required 25 years required by legal retention requirements [10]. Therefore, the time series database Prometheus is not suitable for retrieving data from the external database.

Based on the result of the analysis, the time-series database InfluxDB is used for the implementation. For the realization of the connection of the external database with Grafana via InfluxDB, a linkage of the external database with the data collection agent Telegraf of InfluxDB has to be realized first, as shown graphically in the Fig. 1, before the connection from InfluxDB to Grafana can be established.

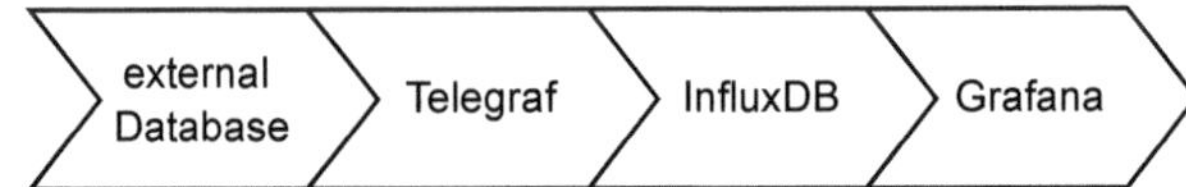

Figure 1: Schematic flow of the data export from the external database to Grafana

2.3 Implementation of data delivery from an external database to InfluxDB

To connect the external database and InfluxDB, the locally installed InfluxDB application is started on the server using PowerShell. The start of the application also causes the output of the default listening port 8086. If the localhost:8086 is then opened in the browser, the InfluxDB user interface can be started. After a successful log-in the user gets to the homepage of the InfluxDB User Interface. By connecting to the localhost, a so-called bucket is automatically created, which is a database and is used to store the data.

Subsequently, the InfluxDB agent Telegraf is configured and started. By installing Telegraf, a configuration file is automatically generated. This configuration file can be customized depending on the application. For example, the output plug-in is configured first. Since the data is to be exported to the InfluxDB application, InfluxDB must be activated and configured as an output plug-in. This includes specifying the appropriate URLs, token, organization name and bucket name. Since only one bucket can be accessed per configuration file, one configuration file is created per bucket.

For the access to the external database the individual and freely configurable exec input plug-in is used. Thus, the exec plug-in must be activated and configured in the configuration file. The exec plug-in is configured to execute a PowerShell script, which then establishes the link to the external database and executes the database query requested by the user. To comply with the InfluxDB line protocol shown in Fig. 2, the database query first captures the desired metric and then the associated timestamp. After the data is captured, the format of the data is modified to match InfluxDB's line protocol so that Telegraf can read the data.

```
• Measurement name  ············
• Tags  - - - - ·
• Fields  ·········
• Timestamp  ———

measurement,<tag_key>=<tag_value> <field_key>=<field_value> timestamp
············ - - - - - - - - - - - :::::::::::::::::::::: ———

weather,city=london temperature=32.2,wind_speed=6i 1465839830100400200
············ - - - - - - - - - - - - - - - :::::::::::: ———
```

Figure 2: Line protocol of Telegraf consisting of measurement name, tags, fields and the timestamp [11]

After successful configuration, the Telegraf service is started. However, before the captured data can be displayed in InfluxDB, the individual command and authentication token generated by InfluxDB specifically for each bucket must be specified. Afterwards, the desired bucket can be selected in the data explorer of the InfluxDB user interface and the desired metrics can be displayed graphically by filtering.

Furthermore, the manual selection of the bucket and filters automatically generates a source code from InfluxDB that describes the graph. The source code is important for linking InfluxDB with Grafana.

2.4 Implementation of data delivery from InfluxDB to Grafana

After successfully collecting the metrics from the external database with InfluxDB and its agent Telegraf, the metrics can be displayed in a Grafana dashboard. For this purpose, the Grafana Service is started as a first step by executing the

Grafana.exe application. If the application startup process is successful, Grafana can be accessed in the browser by using the localhost:3000. The localhost:3000 is the default TCP for Grafana unless the configuration file has been changed. After successful entry of the login data, the user is taken to the Grafana homepage.

Subsequently, a data source can be added to Grafana. Grafana offers a number of compatible data sources which can be selected in the configuration. In this use case, the open source time series database InfluxDB is selected as the data source, since Grafana should display the metrics that have already been collected by InfluxDB.

The next step is to configure the details to connect to InfluxDB. Grafana has two options for query languages with InfluxDB, Flux and InfluxQL. In this case, Flux is used because Flux is less error prone. Additionally, the default URL for InfluxDB is defined in the configuration, which is the localhost:8086. Lastly, the correct InfluxDB organization name and token are captured to ensure a successful link to the existing InfluxDB database. If the entries are error-free, the number of buckets already created in InfluxDB is displayed.

A Grafana dashboard can then be created containing panels that interface to query the data from InfluxDB. Once the user creates a new dashboard, a page appears with the option to add a new panel. When a new panel is added, a configuration page opens in Grafana's user interface. In this page, the user has the option to select the InfluxDB data source and copy in the source code that was automatically generated by InfluxDB. After copying in the code, the metrics can be displayed in a freely configurable dashboard as in Fig. 3 visualized.

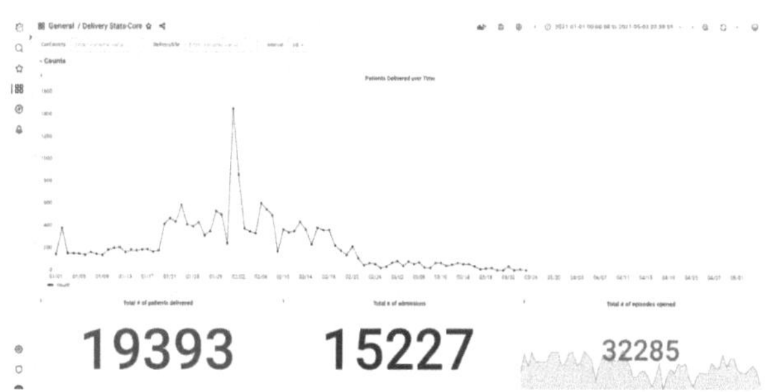

Figure 3: Individual display of the panels in a Grafana dashboard (top: Number of births over time, bottom left: Total number of births, bottom middle: number of admissions, bottom right: number of opened episodes)

3 Results and Discussion

Grafana offers a variety of display and configuration options. For example, the user can choose between different display formats, create titles, determine query periods and insert descriptions for the panel. In addition, a library of different panels can be created so that the user can select from the library which metrics they would like to have displayed.

However, the implementation shows a drawback in the Telegraf configuration, as a PowerShell script can only make one explicit data request to the external database, otherwise the line protocol for Telegraf is no longer satisfied. This results in the need to write a separate PowerShell script for each metric to be captured from the external database. Additionally, since the exec plug-in can only run one PowerShell script at a time and and each PowerShell script stores its data in a different bucket to still be able to distinguish the data, an individual bucket must still be created for each metric. Also, Telegraf can only run one configuration file at a time and therefore can only pass data from one configuration file to InfluxDB.

Since the external database has over 1000 metrics, all of which may be of interest to the attending physician, over 1000 buckets and configuration files would need to be created and run sequentially to provide all metrics to the Grafana dashboard. On the one hand, this results in a very large amount of data having to be read into InfluxDB and a time delay in capturing the data. On the other hand, due to the high number of buckets that have to be created in InfluxDB, just as many panels would have to be preconfigured in Grafana. As a result, data entry becomes very time-consuming and complicated for the user.

Due to the fact that InfluxDB and its agent Telegraf is interposed between Grafana and the external database, no direct query from Grafana to the data from the external database is possible, so all metrics have to be stored in InfluxDB. This is accompanied by a very high memory requirement and a very high workload.

4   Conclusion

During the analysis and comparison of InfluxDB and Prometheus, it was found that InfluxDB meets all requirements, while Prometheus does not. As a result, the time series data bank InfluxDB and its agent Telegraf were used for the implementation of the data export. The implementation has shown that data delivery from the external database to Grafana via InfluxDB is feasible. However, the amount of PowerShell scripts, buckets, and Grafana panels that need to be created, as well as the resulting time lag in data collection and high memory requirements, represent a high workload and complexity for the user.

Using a Docker container that contains InfluxDB, its agent Telegraf with the input-exec plug-in, and the PowerShell script would minimize the user's workload by enabling automated management. However, a Docker container would not reduce the number of buckets in InfluxDB, Telegraf configuration files, and PowerShell scripts that need to be created to query the database. Therefore, the next step is to find and analyze another method that simplifies the implementation of the data export. One possibility is the analysis of the novel, paid and commercial Sqlyze data source plug-in from Grafana.

Acknowledgement

The work has been carried out at Philips Medical Systems Böblingen and supervised by H. Paulsen of the Institute of Physics, Universität zu Lübeck.

Author's Statement

Conflict of interest: Authors state no conflict of interest.

5   References

[1] R. Kramme, *Medizintechnik - Verfahren - Systeme - Informationsverarbeitung*. Springer Medizin Verlag, Heidelberg, 2007.

[2] Philips Medizin Systeme Böblingen GmbH, *Gebrauchsanweisung IntelliSpace Perinatal Software-Rev. K.002x*. Böblingen, 2020.

[3] S. Luber and N. Litzel, *Definition - Was ist Grafana?*. Available: https://www.bigdata-insider.de/was-ist-grafana-a-1016619/ [last accessed on 2022-09-21].

[4] Grafana Labs, *Your Stack*. Available: https://grafana.com/?plcmt=nav-solutions-cta1 [last accessed on 2022-08-24].

[5] InfluxData, *Introduction to InfluxDB*. Available: https://awesome.influxdata.com/docs/part-1/introduction-to-influxdb/ [last accessed on 2022-09-21].

[6] The Linux Foundation, *Prometheus - COMPARISON TO ALTERNATIVES*. Available: https://prometheus.io/docs/introduction/comparison/#prometheus-vs-influxdb [last accessed on 2022-09-22].

[7] InfluxData, *Documentaion - Manage InfluxDB security*. Available: https://docs.influxdata.com/influxdb/v1.8/administration/security/ [last accessed on 2022-09-22].

[8] The Linux Foundation, *Security Model*. Available: https://prometheus.io/docs/operating/security/ [last accessed on 2022-09-22].

[9] InfluxData, *Documentaion - Plugin directory*. Available: https://docs.influxdata.com/telegraf/v1.23/plugins/ [last accessed on 2022-09-22].

[10] The Linux Foundation, *Prometheus - Storage*. Available: https://prometheus.io/docs/prometheus/latest/storage/ [last accessed on 2022-09-22].

[11] InfluxData, *Data Collection with Telegraf*. Available: https://university.influxdata.com/courses/data-collection-with-telegraf-tutorial/course/ [last accessed on 2022-09-21]

7

Medical Electronics

Development of a Digital Continuous Wave NMR for Search for Hemoglobin Patterns

Christian Grundman [1], Max Urban [2]

[1] Biomedical Engineering, Lübeck University of Applied Sciences, christian.grundman@stud.th-luebeck.de

[2] Biomedical Engineering, Lübeck University of Applied Sciences, max.urban@th-luebeck.de

Abstract

This paper outlines the early-stage development of an NMR device, capable of low-field, Continuous-Wave Nuclear Magnetic Resonance (CW-NMR). It was found that detection of Hemoglobin-Oxygen pairings through NMR Spectroscopy is possible for more sophisticated machines. While the electronics available today make a benchtop NMR machine feasible, there are still bottlenecks to the creation of such a device. The requirement for high frequency signal generation and amplification forces the use of greater equipment than can be expected in a standard electronics laboratory. Further, use of Fourier-Transform NMR (FT-NMR) provides better analysis resolution. This requires a higher B0 field and thus significantly higher hardware costs. It is however still relevant to create a CW-NMR machine that can be adapted for FT-NMR analysis in future research trials.

1 Introduction

This paper will outline the feasibility of constructing a benchtop Continuous Wave (CW) Nuclear Magnetic Resonance (NMR) machine for mobile spectroscopy. Compact, low-field instruments are allowing for mobile testing and faster analysis times [1]. Benchtop NMR machines are being used in the field for identifying metabolic diseases [2], suggesting a potential for disease outbreaks and access to advanced testing equipment for more

This paper will serve as an initial study and feasibility report. This paper will not deliver a full outline for the technological solutions for all requirements. As a first project of its kind for this lab, the requirements are not formed from a perspective of expertise but rather a position of exploration. With initial assumption, the following architecture is proposed, as shown in Fig. 1:

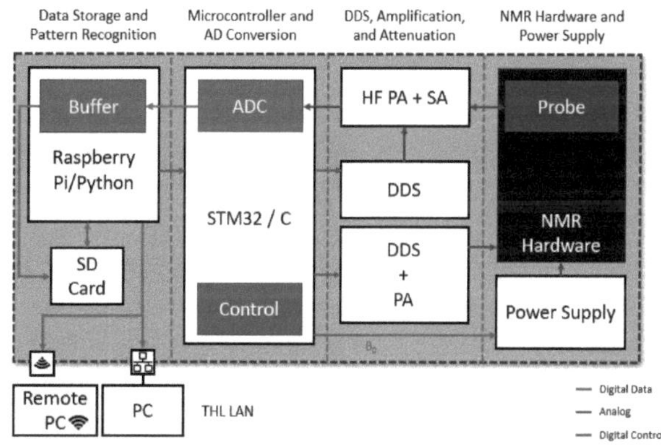

Figure 1: The goal of the project is to outline a System Architecture of the Device. After conducting numerous tests and concepts, this best represents the architecture for an initial device.

1.1 Chemistry of Hemoglobin

Human blood is consists of red blood cells containing oxygen-carrying hemoglobin. Chemical changes, such as anemia, to hemoglobin affect the amount of oxygen it can carry. Studies have confirmed the link of Anemia to Covid-19 [3] and [4]. These changes can be detected by NMR spectroscopy.

1.2 NMR Spectroscopy

In order to judge the efficacy of any NMR device developed, the field as a whole must be examined. The timeline as described by Louis-Joseph [5], serves as sufficient description. This description is enumerated in Table 1.

Table 1: NMR Advances

NMR Method.	Larmor Frequency	Introduction
CW-NMR		
	30-90 (MHz)	1950's
FT-NMR		
1D	180-400 (MHz)	1960's
2D homonuclear	500-750 (MHz)	1970's
2D heteronuclear grad.	750-850 (MHz)	1990's
3D, 4D, TROSY	850-950 (MHz)	late 1990's
FAST NMR	950-1000 (MHz)	2000's

Table 1 shows the continual development of the NMR field since the first device made in the 1950's. For even more detail about the measurement subgroups, Emwas [6] describes the introduction of Principle Component Analysis (PCA) and analysis along multiple chemical bond types for proton spin.

The device that this paper outlines is a benchtop CW-NMR machine. CW-NMR is the oldest technology of NMR, allowing it to be the least expensive and an appropriate development baseline. Advances in all aspects of the technology (magnetic induction, Microcontrollers, HF-signal generators) greatly shrink these devices in size (benchtop) and cost.

1.3   NMR Metabolomics

The final consideration into the efficacy of benchtop CW-NMR is its potential for application in Metabolomics. Metabolomics is the. The general baseline for NMR-based metabolomics is a 600MHz system [7], because spectral dispersion is sufficient above 600MHz. Benchtop CW-NMR falls well short of this, and most systems no longer use CW technology.

2   Material and Methods

To better understand the technical requirements for an NMR device, real components must be tested for their function. This report will detail the capability of various items for this task.

2.1   Digital CW-NMR Requirements

This lab aims to improve the state-of-the-art of NMR devices by building an inexpensive benchtop NMR device operating at 20-80MHz to identify Hemoglobin-O2 ratios with a pattern search. In order to achieve this goal, the following is a list of initial requirements int Table 2:

Table 2: Requirements of the NMR System

Requirements
Benchtop NMR capable of detection within blood
Generate analog signals need for resonance
Operate current coils, probe, and setup and produce:
Up to 500 mT for the B0 field
A 20-30 MHz sinusoidal signal
A variable circuit
Amplify and attenuate signals appropriately
Function automatically without manual adjustment
Convert analog output (16kHz) into digital output
Store digital data
Perform a pattern search to analyze data patterns

2.2   Components Discussed

There are several development components used for this project. These are electronic systems designed for a wide range of applications that were adapted to satisfy system requirements.

The Microcontroller is the most important consideration for the project. For timing and data conversion requirements, most available inexpensive Microcontrollers are inadequate.

The main component used are listed below in Fig. 2:

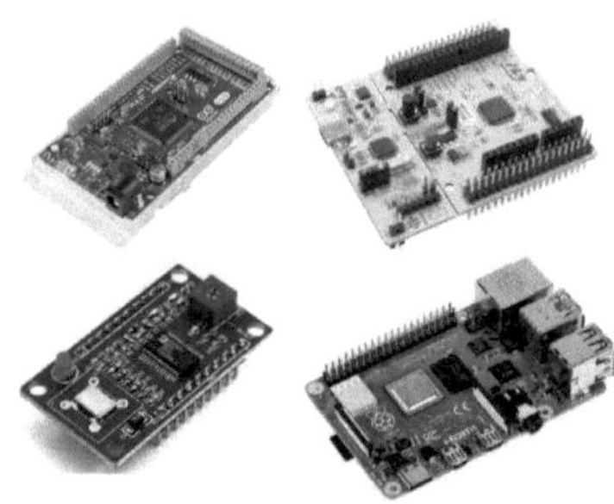

Figure 2: Components (upper left) Arduino DUE (upper right) STM32 (lower left) AD9850 Direct Digital Synthesizer (lower right) Raspberry Pi 4 Model B

The Arduino DUE has a faster clock speed (84MHz) and thus the most promise of the Arduino offering line. The simplified language of the Arduino makes troubleshooting and problem solving easier.

The STM32 has an even faster clockspeed (100MHz). The STM32 is however more difficult to program, as the board runs on C or C++ languages. This may be much faster, but would make development time longer and require stronger programming skills.

Another challenge in creating an NMR system are the high frequency generation. This can be done through Direct Digital Synthesis (DDS) devices. The output signal of the AD9850 is up to 30MHz.

The final selected component is the Raspberry Pi. This Microprocessor can theoretically run all applications and programs any computer can run, albeit slower than professional workstations.

3   Results and Discussion

Full results and discussion must take place at the subsystem level. These subsystems include: Microcontroller and ADC; DDS, Amplification, and Filtering; NMR Hardware and Power Supply; Data Storage and Pattern Recognition.

3.1   Microcontroller and ADC

This subsystem includes the microcontroller and the analog-to-digital converter (ADC). This is all included on the Arduino DUE and the STM32. This subsystem is outlined below in Figure 3:

3.1.1   Microcontroller

The main component used automate the NMR setup is the microcontroller. The microcontroller controls the settings

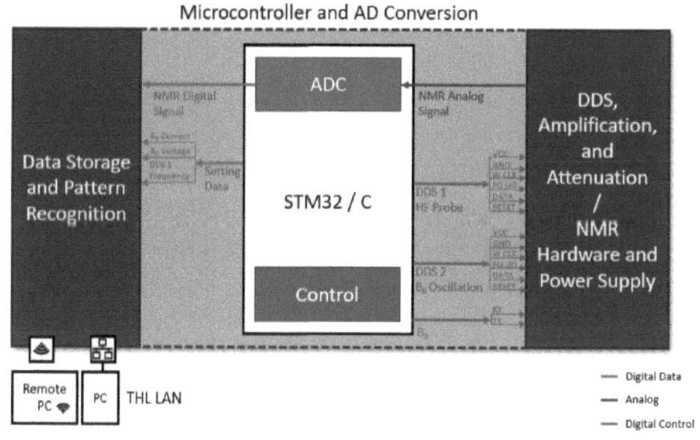

Figure 3: Microcontroller and ADC Schematic

and the inputs/outputs to the system.

3.1.2 Analog-to-Digital Conversion

The signal returned from the NMR device but then be converted to digital data. The analog-to-digital converter (ADC) must do this at the signal speed (16kHz). This must also take in the B0 oscillation field in order to place the relative location of the resonance in the oscillation.

The analog to digital conversion proved to be integral in micro-controller selection. On paper, the Arduino DUE promised to be capable of this task with an internal clock peed of 84MHz. However the Arduino programming language was too slow for this application. The clock speed of the STM32 is higher (100 MHz) and it is programmable through the C Programming language. ADC conversion requires 12.5 clock cycles, which is roughly 8 MHz sampling frequency.

3.2 DDS, Amplification, and Filtering

From the microcontroller, the digital control signals must be transferred to analog signals used for the NMR Probe and the oscillation field. Figure 4 contains the schematic for this system:

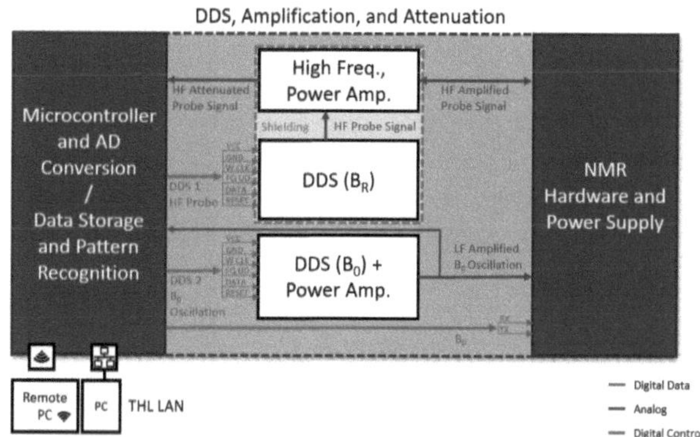

Figure 4: DDS and Amplifier Schematic

3.2.1 Direct Digital Synthesis

The DDS module outputs a clean signal up to 30MHz, with noise being introduced at the 20-30MHz range.

In this case, two DDS modules are required. One for the high frequency signal to later generate the BR field (referred to as DDS 1) and another to generate the signal for the B0 oscillation field (referred to as DDS 2). Shielding is required for the high frequency signal. The DDS signals need to be amplified appropriately for their functions.

3.3 NMR Hardware and Power Supply

The NMR signal creation occurs within the NMR Hardware and Power Supply seen in Figure 5. As you can see in the above image, the connection points are weighted according to their relative power usage and their resultant magnetic field.

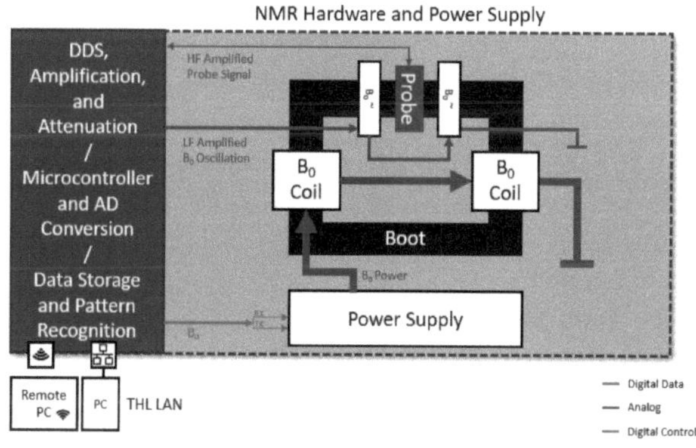

Figure 5: This figure outlines the main hardware components for the NMR function. This contains power supply, magnetic coils, and boot for the device.

Figure 6 shows how these fields are added together to produce a constant 28Hz magnetic field:

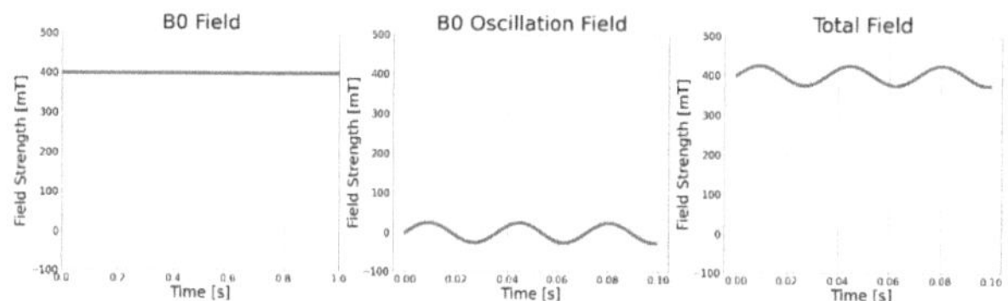

Figure 6: Components of the induced magnetic field, B0.

3.3.1 NMR Hardware

The hardware consists of a magnetic boot to carry the magnetic field, a set of large coils for the B0 field, a set of smaller coils for the B0 oscillation circuit, and a probe.

3.3.2 Power Supply

The power supply supplies the high current to the coils to produce the B0 field. The power supply can be successfully communicated with (via SPCI) to sweep through the range of currents to find resonance.

3.4 Data Storage and Pattern Recognition

Data Storage and Pattern Recognition can be handled by a Raspberry Pi. This board can control the microcontroller, store all data to an onboard SD card, handle interfacing (wired, wireless, and via onboard display), and run machine learning models for pattern recognition. This schematic can be seen below in Figure 7:

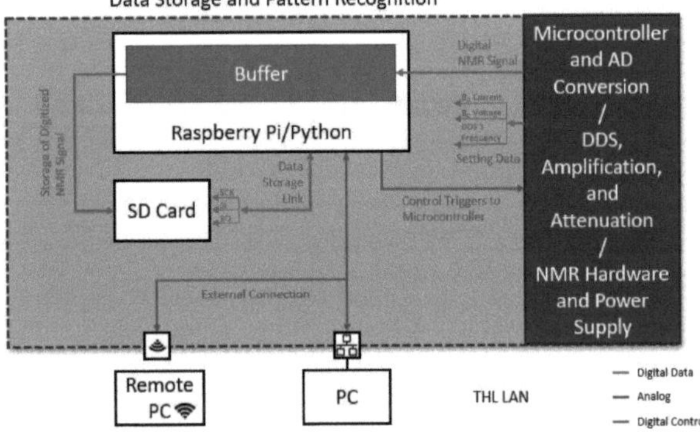

Figure 7: This figure outlines the connections for the Raspberry Pi and SD storage device, interface with the other devices, and connection with the Micro-controller.

3.4.1 Data Storage

The signal from the NMR setups has to be stored and processed. The data packages for each sample are less than 1kB. For 100 repeats per sample and 100 sequences per repeat, the data package for any material sample is around 10GB. SD card capacity has greatly surpassed this.

3.4.2 Pattern Sequencing

The data must be sequenced and turned into a spectrum after storage. Each repeat of the samples stacks and creates the same amount of data as one sample. This reduces the total data size from the above estimate to 10MB, easily fit on 1GB of RAM on the Raspberry Pi tested.

3.4.3 Pattern Recognition

The roughly 10MB sequence can then be fed into a machine learning model for evaluation. Many of these AI models can be implemented easily on the Raspberry Pi.

4 Conclusion

After the completion of this project, several paths can be followed for a successful outcome. Incites about the future opportunities and challenges were obtained from the technical accomplishments limitations.

4.1 Recommendations

The main limitation found was with the high frequency NMR signal. Appropriate prototyping HF signals requires advanced equipment. Traditionally, PCB's are used are for high frequency signal handling. It is thus recommended to create a partnership with an institution or research group with these capacities.

On the task of Hemoglobin-Oxygen pairing analysis, CW-NMR machines are not capable. It is thus the recommendation of this paper to include FT-NMR in future iterations of this system development.

Acknowledgment

The work has been carried out and supervised at the Labor für Medizinische Sensor- und Gerätetechnik, Technische Hochschule Lübeck.

In addition, this work owes much to Agastya Heryudhanto and Ahmed Abdo, without whom these results would not be possible.

Author's Statement

Conflict of interest: Authors state no conflict of interest.

5 References

[1] B. Blümich *Introduction to compact NMR: A review of methods*. Elsevier, 2016.

[2] B.C. Percival, M. Grootveld, M. Gibson, Y. Osman, M. Molinari, F. Jafari, T. Sahota, M. Martin, F. Casanova, M.L. Mather, M. Edgar, J. Masina, and P.B. Wilson *Low-Field, Benchtop NMR Spectroscopy as a Potential Tool for Point-of-Care Diagnostics of Metabolic Conditions: Validation, Protocols and Computational Models*. MDPI, 2019.

[3] Fetler BK, Simplaceanu V, Ho C. 1H-NMR investigation of the oxygenation of hemoglobin in intact human red blood cells. Biophys J. 1995.

[4] Tao Z, Xu J, Chen W, Yang Z, Xu X, Liu L, Chen R, Xie J, Liu M, Wu J, Wang H, Liu J. Anemia is associated with severe illness in COVID-19: A retrospective cohort study. J Med Virol. 2021.

[5] A. Louis-Joseph, P. Lesot *Designing and building a low-cost portable FT-NMR spectrometer in 2019: A modern challenge*. Elsevier, 2019.

[6] A.H. Emwas, R. Roy, R.T. McKay, L. Tenori, E. Saccenti, G.A.N. Gowda, D. Raftery, F. Alahmari, L. Jaremko, M. Jaremko, D.S. Wishart *NMR Spectroscopy for Metabolomics Research*. metobolites, MDPI, 2019.

[7] D.S. Wishart, *NMR metabolomics: A look ahead*. Elsevier, 2019.

Performance Evaluation of Lithium-ion Batteries for Application in a Mobile Medical Device

Shehabeldin Ahmed [1], Reza Behroozian [2], Benjamin Kern [2], and Stefan Müller [2]

[1] Biomedical Engineering, Luebeck University of Applied Sciences, shehabeldin.ahmed@stud.th-luebeck.de

[2] Medical Sensors and Devices Laboratory, Luebeck University of Applied Sciences, reza.behroozian@th-luebeck.de benjamin.kern@th-luebeck.de stefan.mueller@th-luebeck.de

Abstract

The purpose of this experiment was to assess the performance of lithium-ion batteries as a power source for mobile blood gas analyzers under various temperature and load conditions. This experiment used Panasonic NCR18650B, LG MJ1, and LG M36 lithium-ion batteries. The batteries' voltage and current were measured and recorded after they were subjected to a variety of load conditions and temperatures. The results of the study indicate that the LG M36 battery performed particularly well, displaying the highest power output and energy capacity among the three batteries tested. The Panasonic NCR18650B performed second best, followed by the LG MJ1. These results suggest that the LG M36 battery may be the most suitable choice for use in the mobile blood gas analyzer, ensuring its dependability and performance under different conditions. Further research is necessary to fully assess the performance of lithium-ion batteries in this application and identify any potential limitations or issues.

1 Introduction

The purpose of this research is to assess the voltage, current, and performance of three different lithium-ion batteries as the power source for mobile blood gas analyzers under a variety of temperature and load conditions. Portable medical devices, such as mobile blood gas analyzers, rely heavily on the performance of their power source [1]. Because of their high energy density, long lifespan, and low self-discharge rate, lithium-ion batteries are commonly used in mobile blood gas analyzers[2]. Furthermore, these batteries are free of the memory effect, which can shorten the overall lifespan and performance of some batteries[3]. The primary goal of this research is to evaluate the suitability of lithium-ion batteries for this application; however, factors influencing the selection of lithium-ion batteries for mobile blood gas analyzers will also be discussed. The temperature has a significant impact on the performance and lifespan of lithium-ion batteries[4]. Low temperatures can slow down chemical reactions and charge transfer, leading to decreased energy and power capabilities and potential performance failure[5], and high temperatures can lead to internal damage, loss of capacity and power, and even thermal runaway and explosion if not properly managed[6]. The effect of temperature and current on the performance of batteries was the main focus of this study. By tracking the discharge time, capacity retention, and energy efficiency under various current and temperature conditions, the battery's performance was evaluated. A constant current was applied to the batteries during the testing process, which also included monitoring the voltage and discharge time. Throughout the testing, the temperature was regulated and kept constant. These findings contribute to a better understanding of how temperature and current affect battery performance and can help guide future battery research.

2 Material and Methods

The characterization test required a set of specialized equipment and software to accurately record the performance of lithium-ion batteries under various load and temperature conditions. XTAR-X4 battery charger was used to fully charge the batteries, the climate chamber WEISS SB22/160/40 was used to simulate different environmental temperatures, a battery holder was used to securely hold the batteries, and a custom-made variable load circuit was used to apply different loads to the batteries during the experiments as shown in the block diagram Fig.1. The circuit tests and samples Li-ion batteries' voltage and current under various load currents. a PWM signal controls the current load driver, which applies the load current to the batteries. A low-pass filter filters out noise in the signal, and the µC board samples voltage and load for analysis. The test setup was controlled by a Teensy 3.2 µC board running Arduino software, which was programmed to measure the voltage and current of the batteries over time as well as adjust and regulate the load. The code was written for monitoring the voltage and current of three batteries using a Teensy µC board. Additionally, the method can be adapted to monitor batteries in various applications. The

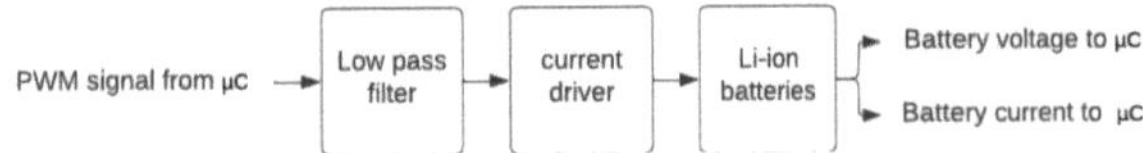

Figure 1: block diagram for the custom-made load circuit.

shown flowchart in Fig.2 depicts the process for one channel, but it could be replicated for the other channels as well. The Panasonic NCR18650B, LG MJ1, and LG M36 batteries were used in the tests. To begin, the circuit was customized, designed, and configured with the teensy board and the desired load range Fig.3, and the computer was linked to the teensy board via a USB cable Fig.4. The code was then uploaded to the teensy board using the Arduino software, and the circuit was tested by observing the circuit's behavior and measuring voltage, current, and time. The code was set up to achieve the intended load. During the test, time, batteries voltages, as well as currents, were collected, recorded, and analyzed. The climate chamber

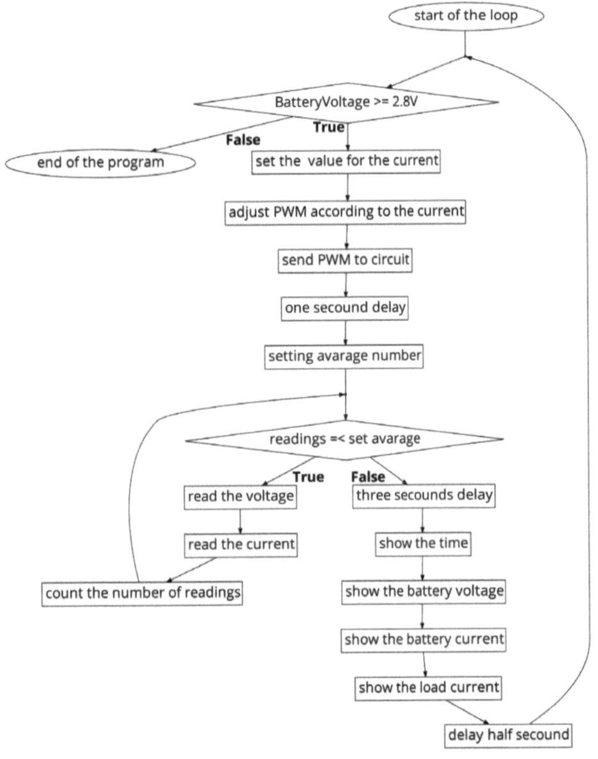

Figure 2: flowchart for the code written on Arduino.

was used to adjust the ambient temperature of the batteries. Tests were carried out at five different temperatures of -20, -10, 0, 20, and 50°C, each using four different load levels of 1A, 2A, 3A, and 3.8A. The batteries were placed in the climate chamber before the tests began as in Fig.5, and the required temperature was set. After reaching the desired temperature, the batteries were given an hour so that they were properly tempered to the new temperature. To begin the tests, all three batteries were fully charged. They were planned then to be discharged until their voltage dropped to 2.8V to protect them. According to the specification sheet for each battery, this limit voltage represented the point at

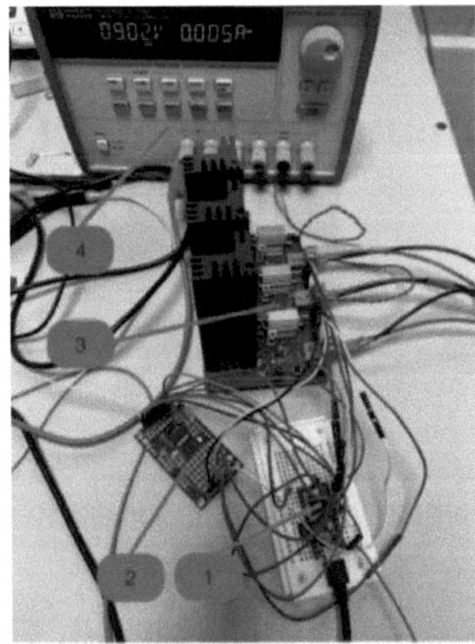

Figure 3: 1: μC board. 2: an analog-to-digital converter 3: custom made variable load circuit. 4: power supply

which the batteries were considered fully discharged and should no longer be used without being charged again. To prevent damage to the batteries during the charging process, they were recharged after the tests when their temperatures had reached at least +10°C. The batteries were discharged continuously until they reached the voltage of 2.8V. A total of 20 tests were conducted to ensure that all the batteries had been thoroughly evaluated.

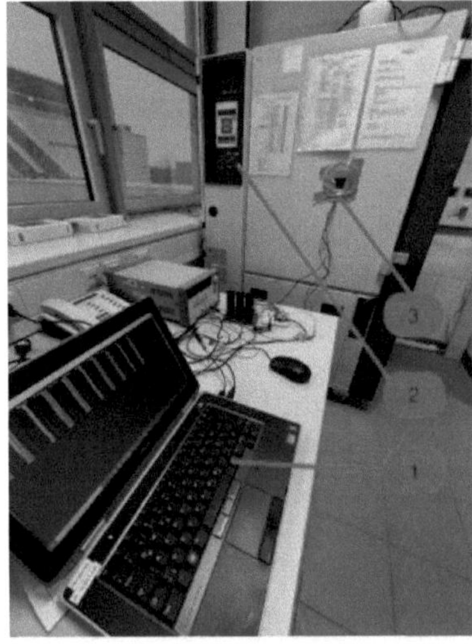

Figure 4: 1: PC to collect the results 2: climate chamber. 3: connection from the batteries to the circuit

3   Results and Discussion

This study examined the discharge characteristics of Panasonic NCR18650B, LG MJ1, and LG M36 lithium-ion batteries. Under varying load and temperature conditions. The data was collected at a range of load conditions, including 1A, 2A, 3A, and 3.8A, and plotted on a graph with time on the x-axis and voltage on the y-axis. The results of the

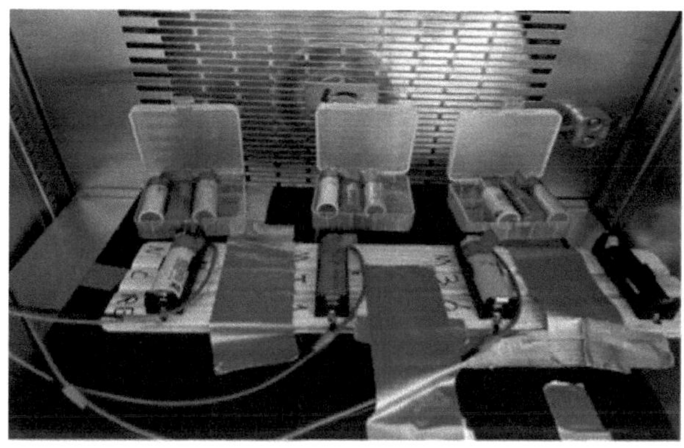

Figure 5: Lithium-Ion batteries placed in the holder in the climate chamber.

discharge curve analysis for three batteries at a load current of 1A and a temperature of -20°C, as shown in Fig.6, indicate that the NCR18650B battery had a starting voltage of 3.28V and was fully discharged after approximately 55 minutes. The MJ1 battery had a starting voltage of 3.55V and was fully discharged after 97 minutes. The M36 battery

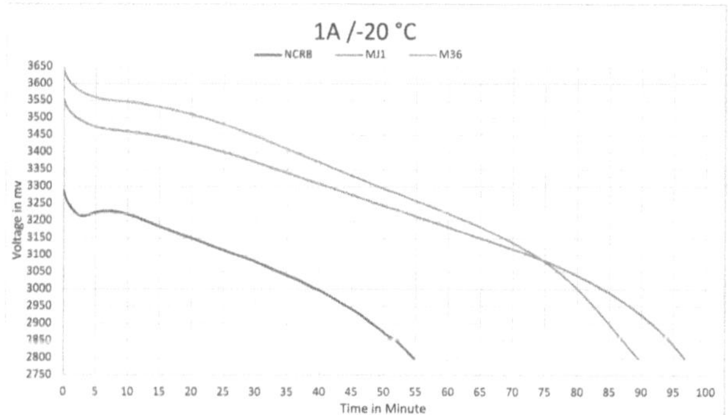

Figure 6: discharge curve for the three batteries at -20°C while supplying 1A loads.

had a starting voltage of 3.64V and was fully discharged after 89 minutes. While the MJ1 battery lasted longer than the M36 battery, the M36 battery provided more power and energy as it maintained a higher voltage throughout the majority of the discharge period, reaching a voltage of 3V after 75 minutes before starting to discharge at a higher rate than the MJ1 battery. In contrast, the results of the discharge curve analysis for the same three batteries at a current of 3.8A and a temperature of -20°C, as shown in Fig.7, reveal that all three batteries were fully discharged within a relatively short period. While the M36 battery was fully discharged after 23 minutes, the M36 battery provided more power and energy due to its higher starting voltage and its ability to maintain a higher voltage until reaching the cut-off load point. At 1A and 50°C, as shown in Fig.8, all three batteries had a starting voltage of approximately 4.1V. The batteries NCR18650B and M36 were both fully discharged after approximately 195 minutes, while the MJ1 battery was after 200 minutes. These results suggest that the batteries behaved similarly in terms of discharge time when loaded with a current of 1A and a temperature of 50°C. On the

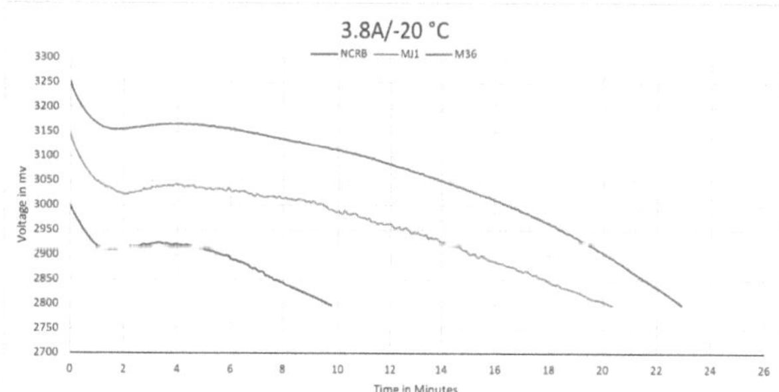

Figure 7: discharge curve for the three batteries at -20°C while supplying 3.8A loads.

other hand, the results of the discharge curve analysis for the same three batteries at the current of 3.8A and the temperature of 50°C, as shown in Fig.9, indicates that all three batteries were fully discharged within a relatively short period of time. All three batteries had a starting voltage of approximately 3.8V and were fully discharged within 50 minutes. However, the M36 battery provided more power and energy due to its ability to maintain a higher voltage for a longer period until reaching the cut-off load point. The results of

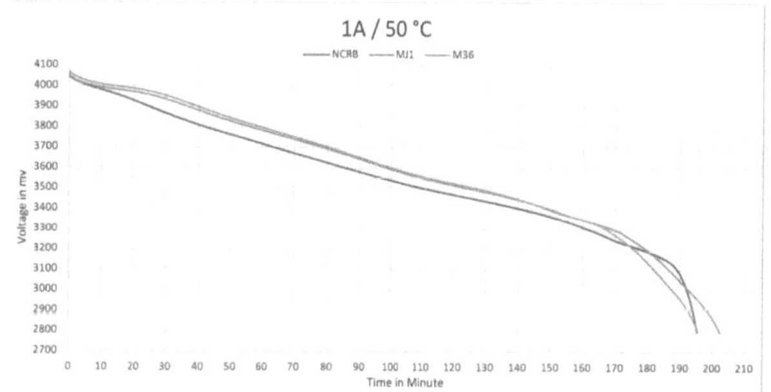

Figure 8: discharge curve for the three batteries at 50°C while supplying 1A loads.

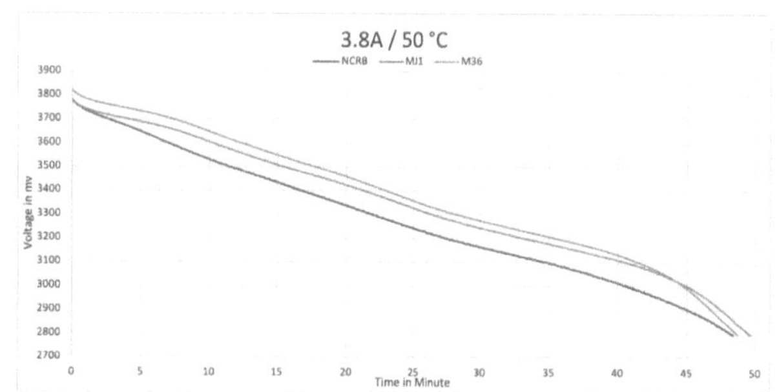

Figure 9: discharge curve for the three batteries at 50°C while supplying 3.8A loads

the discharge curve analysis indicate that both temperature and load current have a significant impact on battery performance. At higher temperatures and lower load currents, the batteries had longer discharge times and higher power output and energy capacity as shown in Fig10. As temperature decreased and the load current increased, the discharge times shortened, and the power output and energy capacity

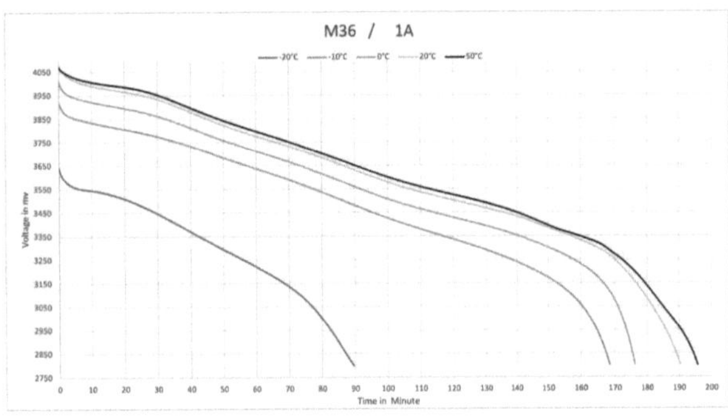

Figure 10: discharge curve curves for the battery M36 when loaded with 1 A at different temperatures.

decreased as in Fig.11. The M36 battery performed particularly well at all temperatures and all loads compared to the other two batteries, providing higher power output and energy capacity. Findings were consistent across various loads 1A, and 3A and temperatures condition -10°C, 0°C, and 20°C, these findings provide important insights into the factors that influence the battery performance.

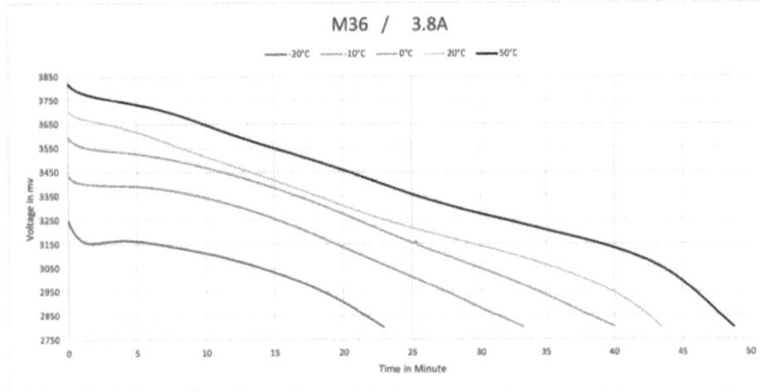

Figure 11: discharge curves for M36 loaded with 3.8A at different temperatures.

4   Conclusion

Finally, this research has shed light on the discharge characteristics of lithium-ion batteries under varying load and temperature conditions. The results of tests conducted at load conditions of 1A, 2A, 3A 3.8A, and temperatures of -20°C, -10°C, 0°C, 20°C, and 50°C show that temperature and load current have a significant impact on battery performance. According to the data collected, the batteries had longer discharge times and higher power output and energy capacity at high temperatures and low load currents. On the other hand, the discharge times were shorter at lower temperatures and higher load currents, which leads to lower power output and energy capacity. Furthermore, compared to the other two batteries tested, the M36 battery performed exceptionally well, with higher power output and energy capacity at a load current of 3.8A and temperatures of -20°C and 50°C. The results of this study provide insight into the selection and use of batteries in various applications. The findings, in particular, contribute to a better understanding of the discharge characteristics of lithium-ion batteries and can serve as a foundation for future research in this field. Because of their ability to provide more power, batteries with higher starting voltage and superior discharge rate, such as the M36 battery in this study, may be more suitable for high-current draw applications. Furthermore, the study suggests that temperature has a significant impact on battery performance, and battery selection may be critical in applications where the high current draw is expected as it can significantly impact the performance and efficiency of the device[7]. Further research and testing are required to confirm and extend these findings, as well as to determine the best battery for specific high-current draw applications.

Acknowledgement

The work has been carried out in the Medical Sensors and Devices Laboratory at the Lübeck university of applied sciences.

Author's Statement

Conflict of interest: Authors state no conflict of interest.

5   References

[1] Rand, D. A. J. *Lithium-ion batteries for portable electronic devices.*. In: Journal of Power Sources, 61(1-2), 37-47, 1996.

[2] Dahn, J. R. *Lithium-ion batteries for portable electronic devices.*In: Materials Today, 5(3), 46-53, 2002

[3] Ma, C., Du, J, *A review of the memory effect in lithium-ion batteries.* 117,160–169. . 2003.

[4] G. Ning, B. Haran, B.N. Popov, J *Power Sources* In: Renewable and Sustainable Energy Reviews, 82, 2198-2212, 2018

[5] R. Spotnitz, J. Franklin, J, *Power Sources* . 113 81–100. 2003.

[6] J.R. Belt, C.D. Ho, C.G. Motloch, T.J. Miller, T.Q. Duong, J. *Power Sources.* 123,241–246 2003.

[7] Shoaib, M., Tariq, M., Imran, M. A. *Battery Selection for High-Power Applications* In: A Review. Renewable and Sustainable Energy Reviews, 67, 1338-1347, 2017.

Development of an MRI receive-only coil-array prototype with adjusted geometrical overlap to improve the sensitivity profile and the signal to noise ratio in the area of the overlap

Henrik Volkens[1], Luca Belloi[2]

[1] Medical Engineering Science, Universität zu Lübeck, henrik.volkens@student.uni-luebeck.de
[2] LMT Medical Systems, Lübeck, belloi@lmt-medicalsystems.com

Abstract

To decouple adjacent channels, MRI surface receive-only coil-arrays use the geometrical overlap. To achieve decoupling of the next nearest channels it is common to use preamplifier decoupling. For two adjacent channels the geometrical decoupling leads to a drop in the shared sensitivity profile and hence in the signal to noise ratio (SNR) in the area of the overlap. A two-channel prototype of an MRI receive-only coil-array was built with an improved matching network to increase the preamplifier decoupling and the possibility to change the overlap of the two channels. As a proof of concept of the prototype, tests in a 1.5 T MRI system were performed. Both the sensitivity profile as well as the SNR in the area of the overlap were shown to be improved. This leads to images with higher quality, since the channels are stronger decoupled, and the sensitivity profile is more homogeneous.

1 Introduction

MRI is a noninvasive imaging modality that generates a signal from the human body through the sum of magnetic moments of the nuclei of interest. Thus high resolution anatomical 3D data as well as functional imaging is possible. The density of magnetic moments in the body, the magnetization, aligns with an external, static magnetic field B_0. If a second oscillating magnetic field B_1 of appropriate frequency is applied, this magnetization can be flipped. For every nucleus of interest there is a specific frequency to flip the magnetization, which is called the Larmor frequency,

$$\omega_0 = \gamma B_0, \tag{1}$$

where γ is the gyromagnetic ratio of the nucleus and B_0 the static magnetic field strength. The flipped magnetization precesses about B_0, which can be picked up by a receive coil. A radiofrequency (RF) receive coil can be understood as a LC-circuit. To pick up the signal from the body, the coils resonance frequency must be as close to the Larmor frequency of interest as possible. Parameters influencing this frequency are the inductivity and the capacitance of the circuit:

$$f = \frac{1}{2\pi\sqrt{LC}}. \tag{2}$$

Accordingly, the equivalent circuit of the receive coil consists of an inductivity, resistor and capacitors connected in series. The frequency response to an alternating magnetic field is a voltage induced in this coil. With a known inductivity, resistance and capacitance, the coil can also be

described with its respective quality-factor (Q-factor):

$$Q = \frac{1}{R}\sqrt{\frac{L}{C}}. \tag{3}$$

The higher the Q-factor of the coil, the smaller is the bandwidth and more electromagnetic energy can be stored in the LC-circuit. Accordingly, is the current induced in the coil of higher amplitude, which leads to a higher signal due to a higher Q-factor of the LC-circuit [1]. It is common to use receive surface coil-arrays instead of single receive volume coils in MRI. Volume coils have a higher penetration depth and larger field-of-view (FOV), but surface coils achieve a higher SNR. The coil-arrays consist of multiple receive surface coils that are overlapped, and all have independent processing chains containing at least one preamplifier [2]. Such preamplifiers are of utter importance for the signal processing, as the voltage induced in the receive coils is in the range of microvolts and has to be amplified to be thoroughly processed. A low noise figure of the first preamplifier mainly determines the overall noise gained in the amplification of the signal [3]. The signal gained from those single coils is then combined at the end of the processing chain and an image from the sum of all receive coil inputs is formed. Thus a larger FOV can be achieved while the high SNR associated with surface coils can be preserved [2]-[4]. But RF coils that are brought close to each other will interact through their mutual inductance. As soon as an alternating magnetic field is applied the induced voltage will create a current in the coil. Following the principle of reciprocity, this current will generate an alternating magnetic field, which can induce a voltage in nearby coils and hence interfere with the signal from the patient. So, the mutual inductance leads to a split in the resonance frequency of the receive coil. This means a significant decrease of the SNR. The overlap of adjacent coils is used to prevent this resonance split, as at a certain degree of overlap the mutual inductance becomes zero. Hence, the adjacent coils can be considered decoupled. For two adjacent coils the geometrical decoupling leads to a drop in the shared sensitivity profile and thereby as well in the SNR in the area of the overlap in a certain depth. In [5] it was shown that the SNR in this overlap region can be improved if sufficient preamplifier decoupling (PreAmp Decoupling) is achieved, and the coils overlap more than required for geometrical decoupling. With a low input impedance, a preamplifier can activate a parallel LC-trap. In this an inductivity and a capacitor are connected in parallel and electromagnetic energy can be stored as it is exchanged between the two components of the circuit and can't progress any further. This induces a high impedance on the respective coil channel. This prevents current flow on the channel and finally, significantly lowers the effect of the mutual inductance and interaction with other coils [1],[2].

2 Material and Methods

The basis of this work is the matching network that is highlighted in the bottom right of Fig. 1. It is the interface between the coil channel and the preamplifier, hence responsible for the noise matching. The goal of such noise matching is to minimize the noise figure of the preamplifier as well as reducing the impedance seen from the coil to the preamplifier. To achieve improved PreAmp decoupling the impedance should be as low as possible. The network is part of a preexisting spine coil-array. This coil-array consists of 8 receiver channels and their respective preamplifiers connected through the above-mentioned matching network.

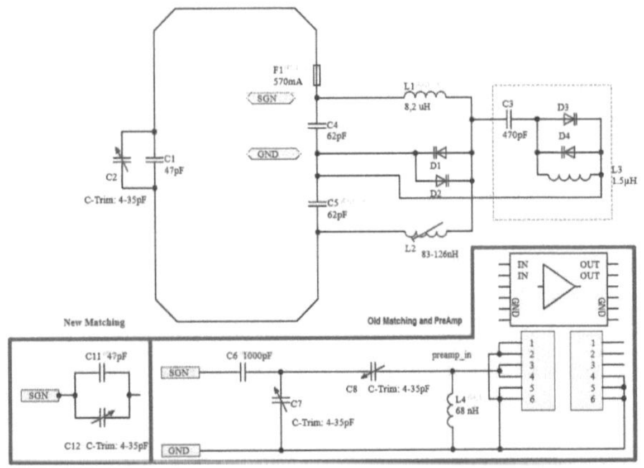

Figure 1: On the top the new circuit of one coil-channel can be seen. On the bottom left the new matching network and on the bottom right the old matching network as well as the connection to the preamplifier can be seen.

2.1 Prototyping

As a proof of concept, a 2-channel prototype of the spine coil-array was built. Two versions of prototypes were built: One with the old matching network referred to as prototype A in the following and the second one with the new matching network, referred to as prototype B. Both prototypes consisted of two electrically nearly identical channels realized as a printable circuit board. One of the channels has been fixed on an MRI-safe plastic board, while the other was positioned slightly higher on the board such that it could be slid across the fixed channel. It featured a printed ruler to measure the offset to the geometrical decoupling position.

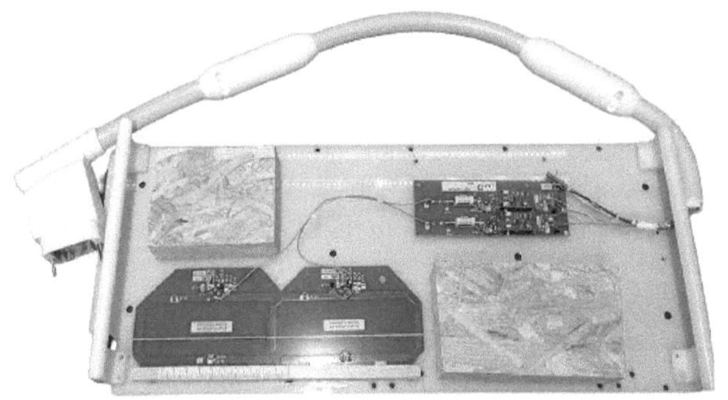

Figure 2: Two-channel MRI receive coil prototype featuring the two coil-channels on the bottom left, the preamplifier board on the top right and the cable to connect to the MRI system on the top.

Coaxial cables connected the channels to the preamplifier board which was also fixed to the plastic board. The coil plug to connect to the MRI system was attached to the preamplifier board. To make the construction more stable when loaded with a phantom, two wooden blocks, tested to not interfere with the MRI signal, were also placed on the board. Fig. 2 shows the above-described construction. The design of the new matching network in prototype B was carried out using LT Spice XVII (Analog Devices, MA, USA, 2021) for modeling the behavior of the matching network and experimental tests on a test bench with a network analyzer (E5061A, ENA Series Network Analyzer, Agilent Technologies) before the experiments in the MRI system have been done.

2.2 Experiments

As mentioned above, experiments on the network analyzer were conducted to prove the functionality of the prototypes before testing them in the MRI system. The scattering parameters of the network analyzer describe the electrical behavior of the coil as a response to a broadband transmission signal. The S21 parameter transmits from port 1 of the network analyzer and receives from port 2. Measurements that were carried out were the tuning and PreAmp decoupling of the prototypes. Those have been done with the scattering parameter S21 using a decoupled double-pick probe. Additionally, the S21 response from the coil output port has been measured to get the coil sensitivity to external alternating magnetic fields. The frequency response of the network analyzer describes the ratio of electromagnetic energy stored in the coil to the energy sent by the network analyzer. At 0 dB, 100% of the energy would be stored in the coil. Respectively, in linear values this would mean that 1 "unit" of current would flow in the coil. Accordingly, for tuning the frequency response at the Larmor frequency should be as close to 0 dB as possible, while for the PreAmp decoupling it should be as low possible.

Following the tests on the network analyzer, the experiments in the MRI system were conducted. They were performed on a 1.5 T whole-body MRI system (Magnetom Espree, Siemens Healthineers, Erlangen). On top of the board, connected to the MRI-scanner, a standard phantom provided by the manufacturer (Siemens) was placed. The phantom was positioned at the system's isocenter. Before the experiments were performed, the "RF-noise" and "RF-spectrum" sequences were done. Those are official Siemens sequences to test that no oscillations occur in the coil. For the experiments a gradient echo sequence with a TR of 150 ms, TE of 10 ms and a flip angle of 90° was performed. The slice thickness was set to 2.5 mm, the resolution to 320 x 320 while the size of the FOV was 30 cm x 30 cm. Those parameters were used as a trade-off between resolution and imaging time. For both prototypes 10 measurements were performed. The overlap of the two coil-channels was increased by 2.5 mm for every measurement, starting at the position of geometrical decoupling. Measuring the signal in the area of the overlap as well as the overall noise was directly possible through the computer-interface of the MRI system. To get the SNR the ratio of signal and noise was calculated. The signal was measured in the overlap of the coils in a depth of approximately 3.25 mm for all measurements at the position of the pixel with the lowest signal in this depth. For the noise in three regions of the same size located at the bottom, middle and top of the left side containing only air the standard deviation of the signal was taken.

3   Results and Discussion

A new matching network as an interface between a receive coil and its respective preamplifier has been developed. This interface is not directly connected to the coil: Between the preamplifier board and the coil there is a 23 cm coaxial cable as well as a common-mode current trap, introducing another 16 cm of cable. Additionally, it is important to notice that the matching capacitor on the coil loop has also been changed to 62 pF which before was 120 pF. Both this connection and the matching capacitor are part of the matching network. As it can be seen in the bottom left of Fig. 1, the new matching network on the preamplifier board consists of a 47 pF capacitor in parallel to a 4-35 pF trimmer capacitor. Through the trimmer capacitor the frequency of the PreAmp decoupling can be adjusted. Other than the old one, the new matching network is floating. The control over tuning the coil from the preamplifier board is thereby

lost. However, with the lower capacitance, according to (3), the Q-factor determining the PreAmp decoupling is higher. Consequently, the current attenuation curve gets narrower and deeper. Overall, the new matching network achieves improved PreAmp decoupling. This has been shown both in network analyzer measurements as well as tests in an MRI system, as detailed below.

3.1   Network analyzer tests

To verify that the prototypes are working before conducting measurements in the MRI system, the parameters that had to be checked at the network analyzer were the tuning, sensitivity and the PreAmp decoupling. Table 1 shows the measured values for prototype B (B) and prototype A (A). Directly for the tuning a significant difference can be seen with prototype B having a higher frequency response at the Larmor frequency. Which is due to the lower capacitance of the matching capacitor and adjusted matching network and therefore higher Q-factor. For the sensitivity measurement prototype B shows with 3.45 dB a smaller value than prototype A with 4.69 dB. Since the PreAmp decoupling is stronger for prototype B, the coil is made insensitive to alternating magnetic fields more effectively [1]. The PreAmp decoupling for Prototype B reaches under -70 dB, while prototype A only reaches about -60 dB. In linear values, the current induced in the coil by an alternating magnetic field with approximately 300 micro units is about three times lower for prototype B. This already suggests a better performance regarding SNR for prototype B.

Table 1: Network analyzer measurement values

	Tuning	PreAmp decoupling (linear)	Sensitivity
A	-25.28 dB	-59.24 dB (975.15 µU)	4.69 dB
B	-14.56 dB	-70.83 dB (311.37 µU)	3.45 dB

3.2   MRI system tests

The tests in the MRI-scanner also proved the improved PreAmp decoupling. In Fig. 3 the SNR in the area of the overlap between the two coil channels depending on the overlap of the two channels in mm can be seen. For both prototypes a higher SNR can be observed for an overlap of 2.5 mm more than the geometrical decoupling. In this position the geometrical decoupling still has an influence and suppresses noise, while the signal rises due to the overlapped channels. The drop after this first rise, which is also present in both lines, shows that the effect of geometrical decoupling vanishes at this point. After this comparable behavior of the two prototypes the SNR of prototype A decreases significantly, while the opposite happens to the SNR of prototype B. The highest SNR can be seen for an overlap of 12.5 mm more than the geometrical decoupling. At this point the SNR has increased by nearly 7% for prototype B and dropped by 5% for prototype A. Afterwards the SNR is dropping for both prototypes. Still, the level of SNR is higher for prototype B compared to prototype A. Here the effect of the increased PreAmp decoupling can be observed. The induced current in the coils by the mutual inductance of stronger overlapped channels is suppressed by the high impedance introduced by the PreAmp decoupling. Hence, the increase in noise is limited and the rise in signal dominates the overall behavior, leading to a peak in SNR. At a higher overlap and therefore stronger coupling the PreAmp decoupling is not strong enough and the SNR is dropping.

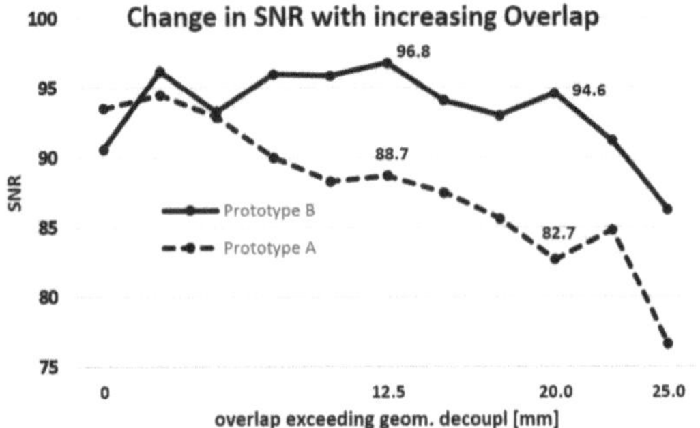

Figure 3: Relation between the SNR in the overlap between the two coil-channels and the overlap in mm. The solid line shows the new matching network. The dashed line shows the old matching network.

In Fig. 4 MR images of a Siemens water phantom with prototype B can be seen. In the images the position of geometrical decoupling and 12.5 mm additional overlap, where the highest SNR was measured, can be seen for comparison. It is evident for the position of geometrical decoupling that above each the two coil-channels the signal forms a semicircle. This is due to the sensitivity profile of a single coil. In the area of the overlap this leads to drop in signal in a certain depth. In the image for the 12.5 mm additional overlap, the two semicircles are overlapping stronger. The rise in signal in the area of the overlap is most significant near the surface of the coils. But at the same depth the achieved signal is also higher than for the two geometrical decoupled coil-channels.

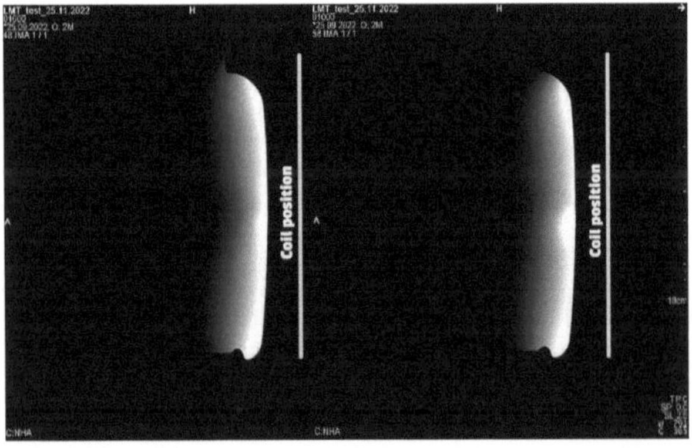

Figure 4: Sagittal MR images of a Siemens water phantom from prototype B. On the left, the two coil-channels are geometrically decoupled. On the right, the two channels are 12.5 mm further overlapped than the geometrical decoupling. B_0 is parallel to the vertical axis.

4 Conclusion

A two-channel MRI receive-only coil-array prototype was built with a new matching between coil and preamplifier. The PreAmp decoupling between the two channels has been improved. This allows for a stronger overlap associated with a more homogeneous sensitivity profile of adjacent coil-channels. Hence, the sensitivity profile has been made more homogeneous and the SNR in the area of the overlap has been improved. The two-channel prototype can be scaled up to a coil-array with more channels, this would lead to receive-only coil-arrays with higher image quality and more homogeneous sensitivity profile.

Acknowledgement

The work has been carried out at LMT Medical Systems in Lübeck and was supervised by Prof. M. Koch, Institute of Medical Engineering, Universität zu Lübeck.

Author's Statement

Conflict of interest: Authors state no conflict of interest.

5 References

[1] H. Kopka, T. Zheng, X. Yang, M. J. Finnerty and S. Handa, *RF Surface Receive Array Coils: The Art of an LC Circuit.*Journal of Magnetic Resonance Imaging, vol. 38, pp. 12–25, 2013.

[2] P. B. Roemer, W. A. Edelstein, C. E. Hayes, S. P. Souza and O. M. Mueller, *The NMR Phased Array.* Magnetic Resonance in Medicine, vol. 16, pp. 192-225, 1990.

[3] X. M. Cao, D. L. Zu, X. N. Zhao, Y. Fan and J. H. Gao, *The design of a low-noise preamplifier for MRI.* Science China Technological Sciences, vol. 54, no. 7, pp. 1766-1770, 2011.

[4] B. Gruber, M. Froeling, T. Leiner and D. W. J. Klomp, *RF Coils: A Practical Guide for Nonphysicists.*Journal of Magnetic Resonance Imaging, vol. 48, pp. 590-604, 2018.

[5] S. B. King, S. Varosi, D. A. Molyneaux and G. R. Duensing, *The Effects of Ultra Low Input Impedance Preamplifiers on Phased Array Coil Design.* Proceedings of the International Society for Magnetic Resonance in Medicine, vol. 10, 2002.

Explorative analysis of microRNA expression in liquid biopsy DNA sequencing data

Luisa Lekat [1], Martin Kircher [2,3]

[1] Medical Informatics, Universität zu Lübeck, luisa.lekat@student.uni-luebeck.de

[2] Institute of Human Genetics, Universität zu Lübeck, martin.kircher@uni-luebeck.de

[3] Computational Genome Biology, Berlin Institute of Health at Charité - Universitätsmedizin Berlin, martin.kircher@bih-charite.de

Abstract

MicroRNAs (miRNA) have emerged as interesting biomarkers in various diseases. They are interesting marker genes because of their high specificity and the small number of highly expressed miRNAs per tissue. Liquid biopsies, a term used for sequencing data derived from cell-free DNA (cfDNA), carries signals of DNA regulation in its tissue of origin. Here, we explored whether miRNA promoter regions might show a signal informative of their expression. The expression data of miRNAs from Ludwig et al. [8] were considered and processed using a Snakemake workflow to calculate the Windowed-Protection-Score (WPS). The results could be compared with graphics of protein-coding genes, so that a statement about the nucleosome positioning could be made. The investigations showed that there are two miRNAs that cause a strong signal in the data. After these outliers were removed, it was found that no consistent pattern correlating with miRNA expression could be identified in the cfDNA data.

1 Introduction

CfDNA is DNA that is not located in cells but is found freely in body fluids such as blood plasma. It was first discovered in human plasma in 1948 [1] and is believed to be a product of apoptosis, the cell death. CfDNA is described as short and double-stranded DNA fragments with a length distribution that suggests association with nucleosome-bound DNA (between 120-180 base pairs (bp)). Nucleosomes are protein complexes that are used in the eukaryotic cell nucleus for DNA packaging and gene regulation. Approximately 147 bp of DNA is wrapped around a nucleosome, and an approximately 20 bp-long linker-fragment can also be bound [2]. MiRNAs are small, non-coding RNAs that play a significant role in the post-transcriptional regulation of gene expression. They are about 22 nucleotides long [3] and bind to complementary sequences in mRNA molecules, which usually leads to a reduction in protein production or the available RNA copies [4]. Regulation by miRNAs can affect, among other things, the development and progression of diseases [3].

It is known that open chromatin regions of protein-coding genes are present in the promoters and have regular nucleosome positioning [2]. The aim of this research is to show whether the miRNA promoters in cfDNA also have regular nucleosome positioning and whether this correlates with gene expression.

2 Material and Methods

2.1 Snakemake

Snakemake is a Python-based workflow management system that allows to build and run complex analysis pipelines. As a data analysis tool, Snakemake offers readability, portability, modularization, transparency, and scalability. Through integration with the Conda package manager and container virtualization, all software dependencies of each workflow step are automatically provided upon execution. With Snakemake, data analysis can be broken down into well-separated modules and reusable tool wrappers can be created [5].

2.2 WPS and coverage

The WPS is a measure of the number of DNA fragments spanning a 120 bp window with a given genomic coordinate minus the number of fragments with an endpoint within that window. High WPS values indicate increased protection of the DNA from cleavage by DNase enzymes [10], while low values indicate that the DNA is unprotected.

The coverage of a fragment is defined by all positions between the two ends of the fragment, including the endpoints [2]. Coverage describes the number of reads that align with or cover known reference bases. The higher the coverage, the more sequence reads will cover each base, allowing base calls to be made with a higher degree of certainty. Coverage is a key factor in determining the quality of a sequencing project [6].

2.3   Sequencing data

For the analysis in this paper, the cfDNA sample "BH01" by Snyder et al. [2] was used. The sample consists of the combination of the blood plasma of different people, which gives the sample high coverage and representativeness.

2.4   WPS implementation

The Windowed-Protection-Score (WPS) script resides in the lab's cfDNA GitHub (https://github.com/kircherlab/cfDNA) [7] and runs via a Snakemake pipeline. As described in section 2.2, the WPS is a measure of cfDNA protection. The plots are generated by averaging the values across multiple aligned genomic regions and then normalized by subtracting the trimmed mean across the overlay region.

2.5   WPS script by Snyder et al. 2014

Various scripts were used while working on this topic. The script by Snyder et al. [2] for analyzing epigenetic signals detected by fragmentation patterns of cfDNA was the basis for the Snakemake workflow described in section 2.3 and was also considered in this research work.

2.6   Correlation of DNA fragmentation at miRNA transcriptional start sites (TSS) with their expression

MiRNAs cell-type expression data was obtained from Ludwig et al. [8] and were divided into five expression bins based on the monocyte cell-type, the 20th, 20th-40th, 40th-60th, 60th-80th and 80th-100th percentiles, resulting in five lists containing the same number of miRNAs. Genomic windows centered at the TSS of these miRNAs could then be processed with the WPS script, resulting in tables of regions and associated WPS values. By modifying a plotting routine script, the various percentiles were then combined in one figure.

2.7   Nucleosome protection at TSSs of protein-coding genes

The TSS and the expression data of protein-coding genes were also considered as a point of comparison. Data and figures from previous analyses were already available for this purpose, so that it was possible to compare whether the results obtained were correct. We used this information to validate that the two scripts (the WPS Snakemake workflow [7] and the Snyder et al. scripts [2]) produce equivalent results. Here, updated expression data from the protein expression atlas (proteinatlas.org) was used. Using the statistical software R, the expression percentiles of the protein-coding genes in monocytes were determined and lists of

the respective Ensembl gene IDs were generated whose expression values were within the specified percentiles (below 20, 20-40, 40-60, 60-80 and 80-100). Corresponding TSS positions were obtained with the web-based extraction tool BioMart of the Ensembl genome browser. This resulted in 5 lists. The individual lists were processed using the WPS scripts and the resulting data used for the graphical representation in R.

3   Results

3.1   WPS signal around the TSS of protein-coding genes

Fig. 1 shows nucleosome protection around protein-coding TSSs from the paper by Snyder et al. that should be recreated [2]. There is a clear pattern for the positioning of nucleosomes, relative to the start of transcription (zero position of the plot). Peaks show the position of a nucleosome.

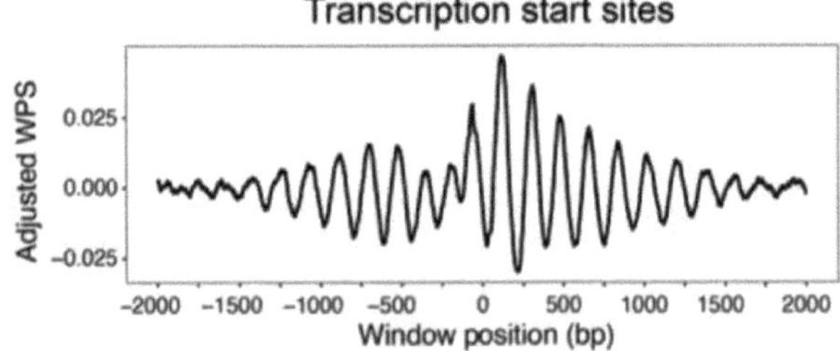

Figure 1: Expected WPS signal around the TSS of protein-coding genes from Snyder et al. [2].

An attempt was made to recreate this graph using two different methods. First, the curve in Fig. 2 was created with the WPS Snakemake workflow. Note that it looks at a smaller window than the original plot.

The range between -600 and -300 is striking. The zero values were not as expected. If one compares with Snyder et al. and the results in Fig. 2, it becomes clear that they do not match and that they deviate significantly, especially at the beginning. The WPS Snakemake workflow uses various corrections and filters that can be switched on and off individually. We speculate, that this is the source of the difference. Fig. 3 shows the data without normalization and filters (plotted in R).

This method shows agreement with the graph from the paper by Snyder et al.[2]. Therefore, we were able to identify an error in one of the normalization steps of the WPS plotting routine of the Snakemake workflow.

3.2   WPS signal around the TSS of the miRNAs

Fig. 4 shows the adjusted WPS around the TSS of miRNAs. The lines for the five expression bins appear to be quite different, with strong deflections being evident in the under-20-line and the 80-100-line in particular.

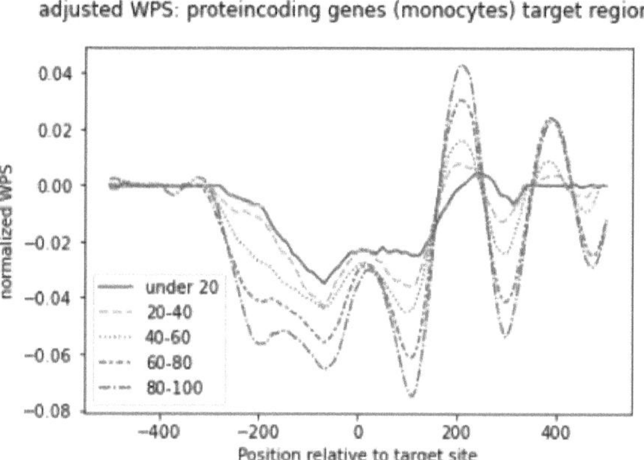

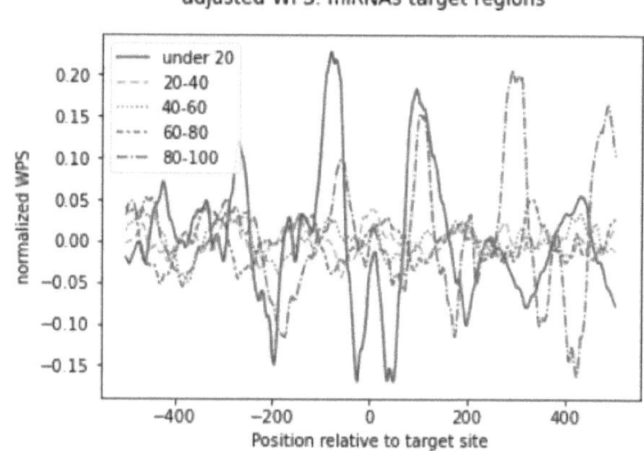

Figure 2: Nucleosome protection around protein-coding TSSs plotted for the Snakemake WPS script. The graph shows the low expressed genes in a solid line. Dashed line shows expressed genes between the 20th and 40th percentiles. The genes with expression values between 40th-60th percentiles are shown in a dotted line, the line with a short and a long dash covers the 60th-80th percentiles and the highly expressed genes are shown in the dotdash line.

Figure 4: Adjusted WPS of expression data classification of miRNAs. The graph shows the low expressed genes in a solid line. The dashed line shows values between the 20th and 40th percentiles. The expression values of 40th-60th percentiles are shown in a dotted line, the line with a short and a long dash covers the 60th-80th percentiles and the highly expressed genes are shown in the dotdash line.

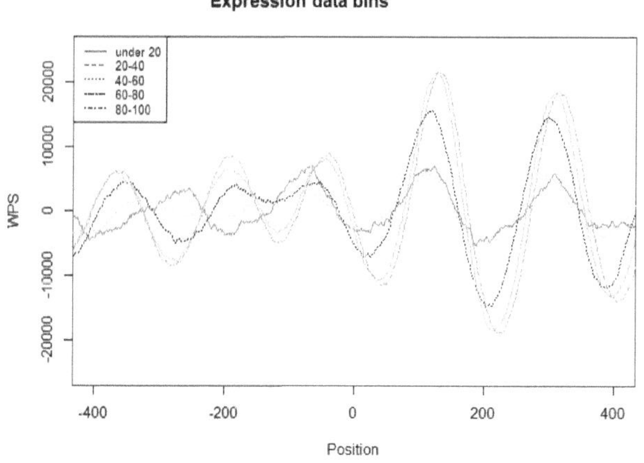

"hsa-miR-3648". Other row sum values from each range are close together, making it clear that these two miRNAs are outliers that strongly affect the signal.

After the two miRNAs are removed from the expression bins, Fig. 5 emerges. There is no apparent expression effect with nucleosome positioning as with the protein-coding genes. However, miRNAs do not seem to exhibit any pattern in the positioning of the nucleosomes.

Figure 3: Nucleosome protection around the TSS of protein-coding genes from the paper by Snyder et al. (Source: own illustration). The solid line shows the low expressed genes, the dashed line genes between the 20th and 40th percentile, the dotted line the moderately expressed genes, the line with a short and a long dash genes with expression values between the 60th and 80th, percentile and the dotdash line the highly expressed genes.

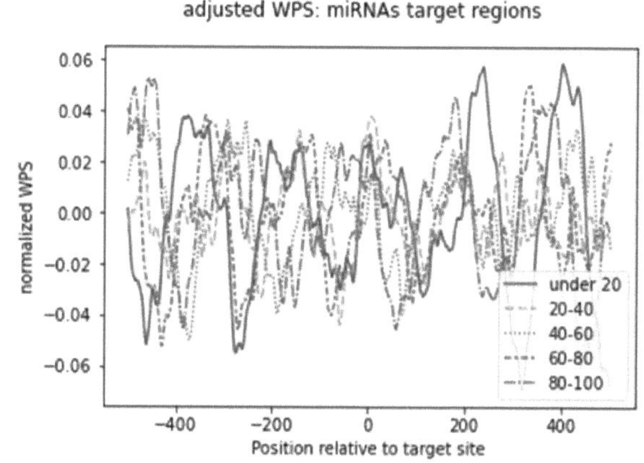

Figure 5: Adjusted WPS around the TSS of miRNAs without the outliers. Lines as in Figure 4.

The further division of the bins into three random gene lists should clarify whether these peaks exist across many regions or whether the mean value is shifted due to an extraordinarily strong signal from individual regions, i.e., a few miRNAs with a high signal dominate the result. Apparently, a few high values in individual regions pull the mean (data not shown). The Two lines show remarkably high values. MiRNAs from the respective expression bins, which had the highest WPS series sum, are in the first bin (seen in Fig. 4 in the solid line) the microRNA "hsa-miR-3687" and in the fifth area (the dotdash line in fig. 4) the miRNA

4   Discussion

When comparing the WPS Snakemake workflow and the original scripts by Snyder et al., it could be noticed that the intermediate results of the WPS calculation do not differ. It became clear that plotting makes the difference. Plotting in the WPS script has a few options that can be turned on or off. It turned out that unexpected effects occured due to the different programming languages used for plotting. The running mean definition in Python versus the earlier R implementation resulted in the null values in Fig. 2.

The results of this work have shown that there is no consistent pattern in the WPS around the TSS of miRNAs. The TSS of miRNA genes were chosen because TSS of protein-coding genes showed regular nucleosome positioning in previous analyses. In these genes, the TSSs are well annotated and this is where the real start of a biological process, the transcription, is found. Two miRNAs were identified that dominate the signal in the respective expression bin. These two genes have a high coverage or a strong WPS signal, which means that the course is clearly deflected. The exceptionally high coverage (and resulting WPS signal) might be due to misalignment or errors in the reference assembly. After removing the two miRNAs, it becomes clear that no consistent pattern can be seen in the data. This is possibly due to the annotation and sequencing of miRNAs. In the work by Wang et al. from 2020 it could be shown that the processing of the pri-miRNA takes place too fast for it to be detected with conventional mRNA sequencing approaches [9], which means that the transcription starts of the miRNAs cannot be detected directly. Genome-wide TSS sequencing (CAGE, SAGE and PET) was able to significantly influence and facilitate the annotation of miRNA [9]. In these considerations, it is also important to note that miRNAs are not always transcripts from their own promoter. MiRNAs belong to larger transcripts.

5 Conclusion

The results show that there is a difference in plotting when comparing the two methods of calculating and displaying the WPS. In addition, it was shown that when displaying the WPS signal around the TSS of miRNAs, two miRNAs strongly influence the signal. After removing the two outliers, no consistent pattern can be seen in the data. With these results, further research can now be carried out. For example, one could look at the distribution of cfDNA fragments around experimentally identified miRNA promoters.

Acknowledgement

The work has been carried out at the Berlin Institute of Health together with the Regulatory Genomics group, Institute of Human Genetics, Universität zu Lübeck and supervised by the Institute of Human Genetics, Universität zu Lübeck. Special thanks to the lab members Sebastian Röner, Kristin Köhler and Lea Burkard, for their support while working on the project.

Author's Statement

Conflict of interest: Authors state no conflict of interest.

6 References

[1] P. Mandel and P. Metais, *Nuclear Acids In Human Blood Plasma [Les acides nucléiques du plasma sanguin chez l'homme]*. In: Comptes rendus des seances de la Societe de biologie et de ses filiales, no. 142 (3-4), pp. 1241–243, 1948.

[2] M. Snyder, M. Kircher, A. Hill, R. Daza and J. Shendure, *Cell-free DNA Comprises an In Vivo Nucleosome Footprint that Informs Its Tissues-Of-Origin*. In: Cell, no. 164(1-2), pp. 57–68, 2016.

[3] D. Bartel, *Metazoan MicroRNAs*. In: Cell, no. 173(1), pp. 20–51, 2018.

[4] M. Ha and V. Kim, *Regulation of microRNA biogenesis*. In: Nature Reviews Molecular Cell Biology, no. 15, pp. 509–524, 2014.

[5] F. Mölder, K. Jablonski, B. Letcher and M. Hall, *Sustainable data analysis with Snakemake*. F1000Research, vol. 10, no. 33, 2021.

[6] Illumina, *Coverage depth recommendations*. Available: https://www.illumina.com/science/technology/next-generation-sequencing/plan-experiments/coverage.html [last accessed on 2023-01-09].

[7] S. Röner, *Snakemake workflow: Analysis of epigenetic signals captured by fragmentation patterns of cell-free DNA*. Available: https://github.com/kircherlab/cfDNA#readme [last accessed on 2023-01-10].

[8] N. Ludwig, P. Leidinger, K. Becker and C. Backes, *Distribution of miRNA expression across human tissues*. Nucleic Acids Research, no. 44(8), pp. 3865–3877, 2016.

[9] S. Wang, A. Talukder, M. Cha and X. Li, *Computational annotation of miRNA transcription start sites*. In: Briefings in Bioinformatics, vol. 22, pp. 380–392, 2021.

[10] D. Han, M. Ni, R. Chan, V. Chan, K. Lui, R. Chiu, Y. Lo, *The Biology of Cell-free DNA Fragmentation and the Roles of DNASE1, DNASE1L3, and DFFB*. In: Am J Hum Genet, no. 106(2), pp. 202–214, 2020.

Evaluation and characterization of a galvanometer scanner

Thies Hörcher [1] and Matthias Neef [2]
[1] Medical Engineering Science, Universität zu Lübeck, thies.hoercher@student.uni-luebeck.de
[2] Thorlabs GmbH, Tech Center OCT, mneef@thorlabs.com

Abstract

To map any scan pattern in optical coherence tomography (OCT), it is necessary to have an adequate, fast and vibration-free control of the laser beam. To achieve this, a galvanometer scanner is used. To analyse the controlled system the response is recorded the proportional-, integral-, differential- (PID) control signal and the galvanometer feedback are measured. For analysing the frequency response of a galvanometer scanner, the international laser display association (ILDA) has developed a pattern that visualizes information like the cut off frequency. In this work, two galvanometer scanners are compared. One already and a second scanner never used in OCT systems before. The results of the comparison reveal that the second scanner has slower response but can reduce the damping of the system. Comparing the advantages and disadvantages of both scanners regarding the application in OCT, the new system is not recommended due to the lower performance at high-speed.

1 Introduction

Tomographic imaging methods have become indispensable in research, development, and medical diagnostics [1]. Optical coherence tomography (OCT) is one of the few methods that can be used to reproduce pictures in real time. A field of application is ophthalmology, where OCT is used to precisely image the front and the background of the eye with an accuracy of only a few micrometer (μm).

Thies section gives an overview of how OCT works and what control engineering is.

1.1 Optical coherence tomography

Unlike conventional microscopy, it is possible to create a depth profile with an OCT system. In Fig. 1 the generation of an OCT signal is shown schematically. An OCT system consists of a coherent light source, an interferometer, and a detector. The light is divided into the reference arm and sample arm by a beamsplitter. By including a so-called galvo-scanner in the sample arm path, a pattern on the sample can be applied. The reflected light from the sample interferes with the reflected light from the reference arm and the resulted light is detected by the detector. For different wavelengths, the detector detects different intensities, so that a depth profile can be constructed [1]. The depth profile at a point is named A-scan [1]. It is generated by the measured reflection of the light with different wavelengths on a sample. For a diagnostic image, a series of A-scans is recorded and is called a B-scan. To obtain a 3D-image, a series of B-scans is considered, than the so-called C-scan is obtained. To generate B- and C-scans, the OCT system must contain a light guiding system that can scan the desired patterns. Most commonly, galvanometers (galvos) are used

for that. A galvo converts electrical current into mechanical movement. In combination with a mirror, a galvo can move a light beam in one axis. For a 2D pattern, two mirror galvos are used, than every point of the sample can be mapped with small rotation angels of the galvos [2]. The rotation is called "mechanical angle ($\theta_{mech.}$)" and the exit angle is called "optical angle ($\theta_{opt.}$)", where $\theta_{mech.} = 2 \cdot \theta_{opt.}$. Further parts of a galvo-scanner are a voltage source and a driver. The latter acts as an amplifier and controller.

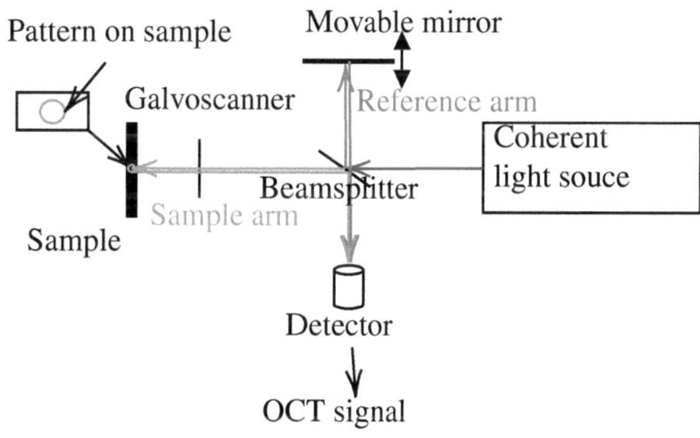

Figure 1: Schematic representation of an OCT system.

1.2 Fundamentals of control engineering

Control engineering is used to regulate a system's output to a desired value. In a closed-loop system this happens over a feedback path, that compares the output (y(t)) and input (r(t)) until no error (e(t)) remains [5]. A distinction is made between three components: The control system, the control unit, and the controller.

A control system consists of actuators (galvanometers,

valves, etc.) and the measuring device, with the input *u(t)* and the output *y(t)*.

The control unit generates a time process $u_s(t)$ (feedforward) independent from the current process $y(t)$. The set point $r(t) \approx y(t)$. The main difference to the controller is the feedforward process.

The controller generates the signal $u_r(t)$ based on feedback of the actual value of $y(t)$ and compares it with the set point $r(t)$. If the two signals are not equal, the error $e(t) = r(t) - y(t)$ remains. The task of the controller is to eliminate this error.

The most common controller is the proportional-, integral-, differential- (PID) controller. Mathematically, the controller can be described by

$$y(t) = K_p \cdot e(t) + K_i \cdot \int_0^t e(\tau)d\tau + K_d \cdot \frac{de(t)}{dt}, \quad (1)$$

where K_p, K_i, and K_d stands for the PID-components.

The p-component sets the output to a specific value that is as close as possible to the target value. That means the p-component is basically the gain factor K_p of the controller. As shown in Eq. 1 with only the p-component ($K_p \neq 0$ and $K_i, K_d = 0$), the error cannot be eliminated [5].

Using the i-component, the control error can be eliminated completely [5]. Unlike the p-component, the i-component can take past values into account since all control errors are summed up in this. The i-component can be described by the second part of Eq. 1. K_i is the integral gain and it depends on the reset time (T_n) of the closed-loop system ($K_i = \frac{K_p}{T_n}$). Thus, due to the i-component, there is a slow approach to the set point until it is exactly reached [5].

The d-component takes into account the change of the control error by differentiating it. The d-part is defined with the last part of Eq. 1. Where K_d is the derivative gain and depends on the derivative action time (T_v) of the system ($K_d = K_p \cdot T_v$) [5]. This allows the controller to respond considerably faster, but the error remains [5].

To check the control behaviour, the step response of the system is often analysed. Where the set point is changed from zero to a specific value. The output of the system due to the step is then the step response.

The Thorlabs GmbH develops and distributes systems for OCT. The objective of this work is the evaluation and characterization a galvanometer scanner for use in OCT.

2 Material and methods

There are three important parameters for imaging with OCT. The three most important parameters of an OCT system are the usable depth range, the sensitivity (the size of the smallest detectable signal), and the speed given in the number of depth slices per second [1]. However, the galvo scanner only has a decisive influence on the speed, therefore, the following methods for evaluation refer to the speed of the controller. The speed of the controller is its response to input changes as well as its frequency behaviour of the controller.

To do so, the controller must be tuned. To tune a PID-controller there are several ways. A common way is the Ziegler-Nichols (Z&N) method. This method assigns a value to each component of the controller depending on the rise time and the time delay (time until the controller reacts). For analog controllers, where it is not possible to put certain values, the adjustments are done by hand with the help of the step response [4].

Therefore it is necessary to know the function of each component. The gain has the hardest impact on the control loop and is responsible to move the system response as quickly as possible towards the desired output value. Unfortunately, when the p-component is set too strongly the system starts to oscillate. The i- and d-components are used to reduce the control error. These two components are also known as high and low frequency damping (HFD, LFD). Large values of K_p and T_v lead to a large manipulated variable, whereas a large T_n slows down the control behaviour [5].

2.1 Step response

A step response is basically the system's response to a high amount of frequencies with a defined amplitude. To improve the controllers speed, the settling time, i.e. the time the controller takes to reach the input value and stays there, is taken into account. The settling time must be as short as possible. For OCT imaging, the controller of the galvo scanner must be able to deliver both high amplitudes and high frequencies at the input signal. This means, the control must be optimally adjusted for both small and large steps.

2.2 Frequency behaviour

For lasers emitting in the visible spectrum, the international laser display association (ILDA) provides technical standards for sufficient control [7]. Therefore, the ILDA developed the ILDA test pattern [6]. The pattern is used to visualize values such as scanner speed, correct output amplitude as well as overshoots in the control [7, 6]. The structure of the pattern is displayed in Fig. 2. In OCT, xy-scanners are used. Therefore, the marked sections $A1 - A6$ are of particular importance. Most information of the pattern is also seen in the step response. For a fast evaluation of the frequency behaviour the ILDA test pattern is a useful tool. The circle (sine as input signal) A1 of the pattern shows the damping at various frequencies. An attenuation of -3dB, i.e., a reduction of the input signal to the output of 70% is considered as good [7]. This corresponds to the reduction of a circle previously touching all corners of a square and then touching all edges of the same square.

3 Results

Two scanner systems are compared for use in OCT. A completely new one (scanner A) and one already used in OCT (scanner B). The system parameters of the two scanners are recorded and compared. It must be ensured that the actual mirror movement and not the input voltage are the same.

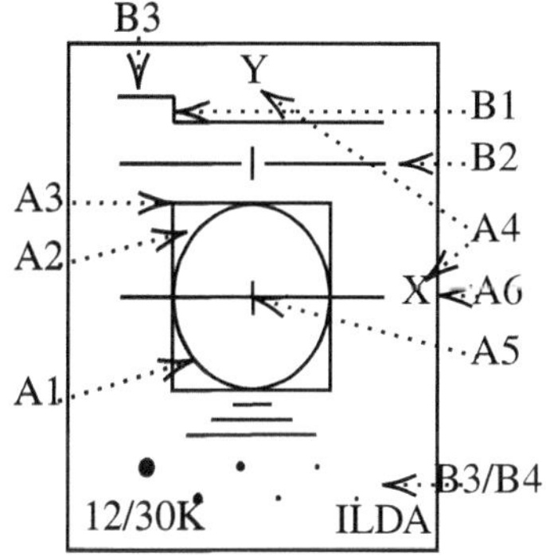

Figure 2: ILDA test pattern.
This type of pattern can be used to determine the correct scanner speed, amplitude, attenuation, and centering. For two-dimensional scanners (A1-A6) and for blanking scanners (B1-B4) are the relevant parts. The 12/30K indicates the output speed for this test pattern in points per second. Taken from [6] according to the standards from the ILDA.

In order to characterize scanner A, the comparison to the data sheet was made first. In Tab. 1, a discrepancy between the data sheet and the real data is shown. However, it can be assured that scanner A has a so-called Slew Rate Limit (SRL). The SRL ensures that no real stepping is specified at all for large amplitudes of the stepping function. Instead, for large steps at the input, only a ramp is given to the galvo. With the SRL, it is possible to regulate the power of the driver and optimize the controller for small or large steps. Further step responses are shown in Fig. 3 under the spec-

Table 1: Comparison with data sheet of the galvo A

Galvo: A	Settling time	Step
Step response 0,40°	in ms	in V
Measured with mirror	0,35	0,09
Measured without SRL	0,75	0,09
Data sheet	0,25	0,18

ification as scanner A, where the influence of the SRL can be seen clearly.
Scanner B is a system already used for the OCT imaging. However, even this setup cannot reach the declarations of its data sheet as shown in Tab. 2. For the comparison of

Table 2: Comparison with data sheet of the galvo B

Galvo: B	Settling time	Step
Step response at 10°	in ms	in V
Measured with mirror	0,52	5
Measured without mirror	0,45	5
Data sheet	0,30	10

the two scanners, first the step responses were compared. All subsequent values were thereby recorded with the mirror, since the mirror is an essential component in the overall setup. Thus, the times are only relevant with the mirror. For the evaluation of the scanners for arbitrary patterns, step

responses for different steps of scanner A and scanner B are shown in Fig. 3. However, the comparison parameter is not the specified step, but the actual deflection of the scanners. In this way, the speed can be evaluated for the same movements.

As Fig. 3 shows, the SRL has a huge impact on the step

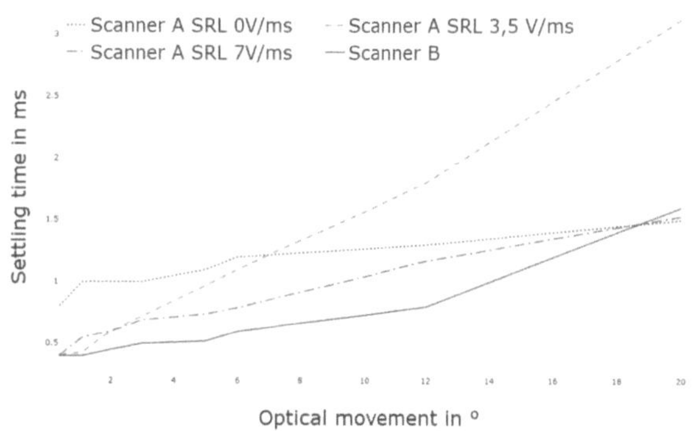

Figure 3: Comparison of the two scanners for a rectangular drive signal (different SRLs also have different controls).

response. For small optical movement, corresponding to a small step response, a rather small SRL is requested, so that scanner A catches up with scanner B. However, for large steps, a high SRL is needed for scanner A. due to Fig. 3 the most consistence response of scanner A can be fond without the SRL. Here, all settling times are in the range of $1,5$ ms.

To analyse the frequency response behaviour from the

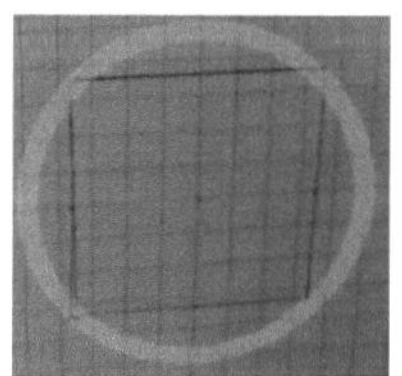 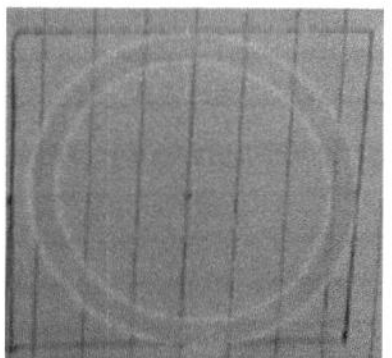

Scanner A at 150 Hz   Scanner A at 750 Hz
Deflection angle 8°   Deflection angle 5,5°

Figure 4: Characterization of scanner A with parts $A1 - A3$ from Fig. 2. Left the behaviour for low frequencies (circle outside the square), right the cut-off frequency at -3dB (circle touches all the sides of the square).

scanners, a commonly used tool is the Bode-plot, but the ILDA pattern can visualise the frequency response as well. Since we are working with an xy-scanner, only the corresponding part of the ILDA pattern must be generated.
In Fig. 4 the parts of the ILDA pattern for scanner speed, a damping with scanner A is shown. To see if the galvos interact well with each other, the circle should optimally only reduce its radius with increasing frequency, but not change in its shape. The scanner shows this behaviour up to the cut-off frequency of 750 Hz.
For scanner B the same experiment shows the cut-off frequency at 1,1 kHz.

4 Discussion

The main issue is the speed of the scanner. The results show, that neither scanner A, nor scanner B can catch up with the settling times specified in the data sheets. This discrepancy can have several reasons. Since the mirrors play an important role, there is the first approach to the measured data. In addition, the information was given with different drivers. The other driver can thereby provide an input voltage twice as high. A higher voltage of the signal also results in a slightly less noisy signal and thus better measurement [8]. Another adaptation for the scanner A is the SRL. There is no information about the setting in the data sheet. However, in Fig. 3, depending on the change of the SRL, there is also a strong change of the settling times for different step sizes. Despite the SRL, scanner A is clearly slower than scanner B. However, it is also clear from Fig. 3 that the settling times converge for smaller and smaller steps and can even reach the times from scanner B. Since scanner B meets the requirements for OCT, this means that scanner A can also fulfil them for small steps.

With the ILDA pattern it as possible to determine the frequency behaviour easily. As expected, the size of the circle changes over the frequency and shows the damping of the system. In Fig. 4 is shown that the scanners have a perfect response at low frequencies, but at higher frequencies scanner A gets faster to the borderline of -3dB. Despite this, the ILDA pattern shows an acceptable behaviour from scanner A up to 750 Hz.

Additionally, scanner A has some technical improvements. The scanner has a notch filter. That filter prevents the scanner from oscillation with the natural frequency [9]. Another advantage of scanner A is that a saturation state is almost prevented by more setting options on the driver. For example, power can be reduced for large steps via a SRL.

However, to be able to use the scanner, it must be clarified whether the scanner meets all the requirements for use in OCT systems.

5 Conclusion

This work gives an overview over the handling and characterization of galvo scanners for step and frequency response. For the characterization of the scanners, methods from other areas, such as show laser technology, were also used. The experiments show that scanner A cannot completely keep up with the speed of scanner B. All though Fig. 3 shows differences in the speed depending on the setting of the SRL. Thereby, an improvement can be achieved for large or small steps compared to scanner B. Admittedly, it is neither possible to create a faster scanner in the step response nor in frequency behaviour.

Summarizing, the results show that scanner A is slower than scanner B, but their speed is in a similar range. Thus, scanner A could be used for OCT systems. If a more stable scanner is required, scanner A could be preferred as it is more stable than scanner B due to a better regulation via SRL.

To upgrade scanner A, smaller mirrors could be used to increase the scanner speed. Another interesting aspect would be the merging of both scanner systems, to test every part of each system. This could be used to find out which part of scanner A is the slowest. This would then be exchanged with the corresponding part of scanner B. So the more stable sides of scanner A could come together with the speed of scanner B.

Acknowledgement

The work has been carried out at Thorlabs GmbH OCT, and supervised by the Institute for Electrical Engineering in Medicine, Universität zu Lübeck.

Author's statement

Conflict of interest: Authors state no conflict of interest.

6 References

[1] W. Wieser *Optische Kohärenztomographie mit Millionen Tiefenschnitten pro Sekunde und hoher Bildqualität.* Ludwig-Maximilians-Universität München, 2015.

[2] T. T. Nguyen *Entwicklung eines optischen Multi-Lasertracker-Systems zur berührungslosen Positionsbestimmung in kinematischen Systemen.* Technischen Universität Ilmenau, 2014.

[3] K. Kniel and others *Ein Beitrag zur Entwicklung eines laserinterferometrischen Trackingsystems für die Genauigkeitssteigerung in der Koordinatenmesstechnik.* Bremerhaven: Wirtschaftsverl. NW, Verl. für neue Wiss., 2007.

[4] M. Gärber *PID Regler einstellen in der Praxis.* TLK energy Blog, 2021. Available: https://tlk-energy.de/blog/pid-regler-einstellen [last accessed on 2022-07-05].

[5] G. Franklin and others *Feedback Control of Dynamic Systems.* Pearson Higher Education, 2015.

[6] C. Stach and B. Müller and S. Huggins *ILDA Test Pattern.* ILDA Tecnical Cemmittee, 1995.

[7] ILDA Tecnical Cemmittee *ILDA Technical Standards.* ILDA Tecnical Cemmittee, 2021. Available: https://www.ilda.com/technical.htm [last accessed on 2022-05-05].

[8] MediaLas Laserproducts GmbH *HighSpeed-Treiberkarte MicroAmp Tuning und Einstellung.* MediaLas Laserproducts GmbH, 2016.

[9] C. Winter *Optimierungdes Scans.* Memo von Thorlabs, 2018.

8

E-Health

Definitions and applications of digital biomarkers: a systematic mapping of the biomedical literature

Ana Karen Macias Alonso [1], Julian Hirt [2,3], Perrine Janiaud [2,3], and Lars G. Hemkens [2,3]

[1] Biomedical Engineering, Luebeck University of Applied Sciences, ana.karen.alonso@stud.th-luebeck.de
[2] University Hospital Basel and University of Basel, Department of Clinical Research, Basel, Switzerland
[3] University Hospital Basel and University of Basel, Research Center for Clinical Neuroimmunology and Neuroscience Basel (RC2NB), Basel, Switzerland

Abstract

This article presents how digital biomarkers are being defined and applied in biomedical research. Biomarkers are objective measures used to predict or correlate with feelings, functions, and survival of patients. These measurements contribute as indicators for assessing the existence and progression of illnesses and health outcomes. Technological daily devices such as wearables, sensors, and virtual assistants deliver an opportunity to gather data that may be used as so-called "digital biomarkers", expanding the spectrum of biomarkers or even providing a viable and quickly evolving alternative to conventional biomarkers. We identified 86 PubMed-indexed articles in which definitions, features, and applications of digital biomarkers were analysed by performing a systematic mapping. The results show that there is no clear consensus on definitions and standards for the use of digital biomarkers leading to confusion about terminology, which demonstrates that exists a demand to create official concepts and regulations regarding this contemporary type of biomarkers.

1 Introduction

Biomarkers are defined as a set of characteristics that are objectively measured and used as an indicator of normal biological processes, pathogenic processes, or biological responses that appear due to exposure or therapeutic interventions [1]. This set of characteristics comprises physiologic, molecular, histologic and radiographic measurements [2]. The Food and Drug Administration (FDA) defines the next categories of biomarkers as: susceptible/risk, diagnostic, monitoring, prognostic, predictive, response and safety [1]. One of their guidelines is that a full biomarker description must include the source or matrix, the measurable characteristic(s), the methods used to measure the biomarker, among others. [1].

The digital transformation is influencing healthcare and medicine steadily enabling practical daily used devices, such as wearables, sensors, and virtual home assistants, to provide a new category of biomarkers, the digital biomarkers.

The definitions of conventional biomarkers and digital health technologies provided by the FDA [1] led several sources to define digital biomarker(s) as "objective, quantifiable, quantitative, physiological and behavioural data that are collected and measured by means of digital devices such as portables, wearables, implantables, or digestible. The data collected are used to explain, influence, and/or predict health-related outcomes" [2], [3], [4]. Many of the everyday digital tools, traditional medical devices and equipment used mainly for entertainment purposes can be considered as a source of helpful information that can transform into these biomarkers, bringing another perspective about their health status.

In recent years, digital biomarkers increasingly started to be present in everyday clinical practice and research. Numerous examples of digital biomarkers have been developed in many areas of medicine, such as cardiology, oncology, in the most recent event of COVID-19, among others. For instance, the results of a clinical trial show how smartphone-recorded cough sounds can be used to detect asthma and respiratory infections [5], [6]. However, predominantly this type of biomarkers had spread in the neurology field, which has a large unfulfilled need mostly for non-invasive and objective biomarkers [4]. Another example is the attempt to provide a digital biomarker-based individualized prognosis for people at risk of dementia where data were collected from their smartphones and tablets within 3 years. [7].

Due to its novelty and recent development, there is a current absence of established regulations and standards provided by organizations and regulatory bodies. This provokes the creation of several definitions of the term digital biomarker(s) outlined in the academic literature, however, some of them are presenting difficulties and confusion when attempting to describe and classify these data.

We aimed to describe the definitions and applications of digital biomarkers in biomedical research by performing a systematic mapping. The specific goals were: i) to identify the most important and cited definitions; ii) to characterise which authors and institutions are discussing them; iii) to discuss the features and areas of application.

2 Material and Methods

A literature search was carried out using PubMed-indexed publications that refer to the term "digital biomarker(s)" in the title or abstract on May 19, 2022. All types of articles were included, regardless of the publication year.

The eligible publications were obtained from their sources and stored using the software Citavi for data management (Swiss Academic Software GmbH 2022, version 6.14).

2.1 Study selection and data extraction

A Microsoft Excel (Microsoft 365 MSO, version 2211) sheet was elaborated containing a table with the desired information to extract. The screening process started and animal-related research was excluded to reduce the sample for human-related studies only. Additionally, repeated articles (corrigendum or erratum) were also removed. Once the list of publications to analyse was narrowed down, the data extraction began.

2.1.1 Publications characteristics

The following categories regarding the attributes from every article were extracted: authors, year of publication, title, journal, Digital Object Identifier (DOI), volume, issue, page, correspondence author and country, and publication type. The last mentioned group was divided into three main classes: primary research, reviews (any type), and others (opinions, perspectives and editorials).

2.1.2 Definitions of digital biomarker(s)

Every publication was examined in search of definitions of "digital biomarker(s)" created by the authors. In this step, articles with an absence of any type of definition were excluded to fulfil the primary goal of this research of analysing the existing definitions.

To have a more comprehensive outlook of the definitions, each one was divided into sections that were identified during the extraction and to follow the guideline provided by the FDA [1]: type of data, acquisition mode and applications.

For instance, the definition of digital biomarkers specified above can be segmented into:

- Type of data which corresponds to what is measured and its characteristics: "objective, quantifiable, quantitative, physiological and behavioural data..."

- Acquisition method or source, corresponding to how is measured: "... collected and measured by means of digital devices such as portables, wearables, implantables, or digestibles..."

- Applications, for what are digital biomarkers useful: "...used to explain, influence, and/or predict health-related outcomes."

2.1.3 Description of digital biomarker(s) in primary studies

For the description of the digital biomarker(s), only original research was included. In this part, the primary studies were categorised depending on their type.

Then, a profound examination was performed on the content of the studies by scanning and using the text search tool to identify the medical field in which digital biomarker(s) were applied, as well as considering if digital biomarker(s) were developed and/or went under a validation process by the authors or were taken from other research.

2.2 Data analysis

Finally, an analysis of the extracted data was conducted focusing on the articles that provided a definition. For the first group, publications characteristics, the number of publications per category was counted with the intention of having an overall knowledge of the most prominent authors, institutions and journals involved, the countries with the major impact in the digital biomarkers scene, from which year the digital biomarker development started to increase in the scientific community, and so forth.

For the group regarding the definitions and their categories, a word cloud was created to see the importance and frequency of the most used words in the given definitions. This helped to visualize the concepts and used terms and get insights on trends and patterns. Concerning the identified sections that compose the interpretations, a deductive approach was done to answer a question: to what degree do definitions fulfil the criteria of being formed by the three fundamental components (type of data, acquisition, and applications)?

In the third group, the description of digital biomarker(s) discussed in primary studies, and the number of publications per category were also reviewed to understand which type of primary studies are notable, which medical field has seen more growth with respect to the use of digital biomarkers, and how many authors are developing and validating their own biomarkers.

3 Results and Discussion

A total of 333 articles were identified in PubMed, from which 14 were excluded (animal related-research and repeated publications).

319 articles published between 2014 and 2022 were the eligible ones, of which:

- 213 are primary research

- 69 are reviews (any type)

- 37 are others (e.g. opinions, perspectives, and editorials)

86 provided a definition:

- 39 are primary research

- 34 are reviews

- 13 are others

For the characteristics of the publication, the year category (Table 1) showed that from 2019, there was increasing attention to exploring more about digital biomarkers and 2021 was the most prolific one with 32 articles. The low number of 9 articles found in 2022 can be explained with the fact that the search for publications had been finished in May 2022.

The analysis of the journals exhibited that Digital Biomarkers (Karger, USA) journal is the main source with 12 publications (14%), followed by Frontiers in digital health (Frontiers, Switzerland) with 6 publications (7%).

The countries that produced the majority of the research were Canada (10 publications; 12%), the United Kingdom (12 publications; 14%), Germany (12 publications; 14%), Switzerland (17 publications; 20%), and the United States (47 publications; 55%).

Table 1: Year of publication (n=86)

Year	Total n (%)
2015	1 (1.2)
2017	4 (4.7)
2018	5 (5.8)
2019	14 (24.4)
2020	21 (24.4)
2021	32 (37.2)
2022	9 (10.5)

The results observed in the exploration of the definitions extraction were:

The word cloud (Fig. 1) showed that the following terms are the most used and relevant when creating the definitions: "digital", "data", "devices", "biomarkers", "health", "activity", "clinical", "wearables", "sensors", "behavioural", "technologies", among many others.

The deductive approach applied to the main components of the definitions (type, acquisition, and applications) revealed that from the 86 provided only:

- 36 (42%) definitions contain the type component.

- 52 (60%) definitions possess the acquisition component.

- 27 (31%) definitions explain the application component.

- 12 (14%) definitions have all three components.

The considerable variation in the definition segments and the fact that only just 12 of them provide a full description containing the components, shows how broad is the current understanding of a fundamental concept that needs to be regulated and standardized as the conventional biomarkers which are actively controlled by certified organizations.

Finally, for the description of digital biomarker(s) in primary studies only, the type of primary studies and the medical field/topic results were analysed.

For the type of primary studies, validation studies, technical studies, preclinical, and clinical studies were among the identified ones. Preclinical and validation studies are the most influential types with 12 and 17 publications respectively. This shows the quite advanced progress in the pipeline of research where most of the created digital biomarkers are currently, either in the stage prior to clinical trials in humans or already in the validation processes.

The medical topics where digital biomarkers are being developed showed areas such as cardiology and oncology, and also disease specific in particular Parkinson's disease with 5 publications, dementia, cognitive impairment (CI) and mild cognitive impairment (MCI) with 8 publications, and the general discussion about digital biomarkers with 9 publications. The most prominent area where this type of biomarker is currently focusing is Neurological diseases. Nevertheless, this outcome opens a discussion about all the opportunity areas in which digital biomarkers can be beneficial for patients, clinicians and researchers.

For the development and validation of digital biomarker(s) in the articles with original research (39 publications), 30 articles developed one or more digital biomarkers and 21 articles conducted a validation process on those digital biomarkers. Such results mean that exists a great number of scientists creating and analysing constantly how such information generated by everyday digital tools could turn into a relevant aid in the prevention, diagnosis or treatment of several diseases.

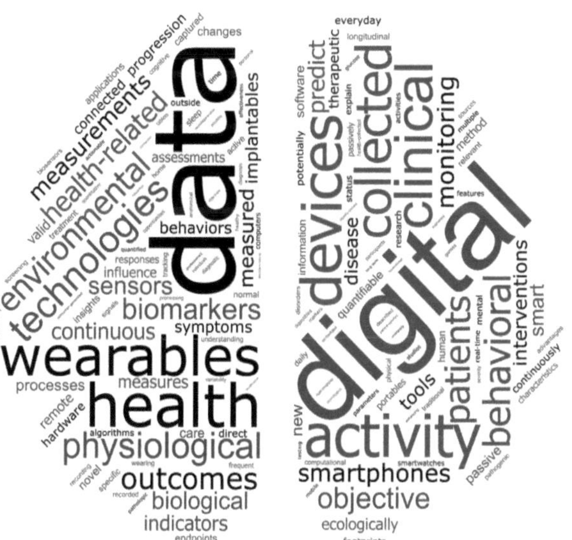

Figure 1: Word cloud with the most important terms in the analysed digital biomarker(s) definitions

4   Conclusion

Digital biomarkers offer an opportunity to collect objective, clinical and significant data in a cost-efficient way. The expected value of this work is to show the available definitions, features, and applications of digital biomarkers. The results point to a variability of definitions for digital biomarkers indicating that authors have attempted to create their own concept and give an identity to this type of biomarker. There is an increasing need for a more harmonized concept and guidelines which can unify, regulate, and prevent any confusion with the terms.

Given the deficiency of standards and regulations, an outlook for future work is to analyse the current challenges regarding the privacy risk that the collected data can be exposed to and concerns about patient data protection. Additionally, raising awareness towards the scientific community and regulatory organizations to consider the importance of creating an established benchmark which could lead to having a fundamental base from which further research innovations could be developed for the health of humans.

Acknowledgement

This work has been carried out at the Pragmatic Evidence Lab part of the Research Center for Clinical Neuroimmunology and Neuroscience Basel (RC2NB) by the University Hospital Basel and the University of Basel led by PD Dr. med. Lars G. Hemkens, MPH; and supervised by Dr. med. Dagmar Lühmann, Universitätsklinikum Hamburg-Eppendorf (UKE), Zentrum für Psychosoziale Medizin Institut und Poliklinik Allgemeinmedizin, and Technische Hochschule Lübeck.

Author's Statement

RC2NB (Research Center for Clinical Neuroimmunology and Neuroscience Basel) is supported by Foundation Clinical Neuroimmunology and Neuroscience Basel.

Conflict of interest: Authors state no conflict of interest.

5   References

[1] FDA-NIH Biomarker Working Group, *BEST (Biomarkers, EndpointS, and other Tools)*. Silver Spring (MD): Food and Drug Administration, National Institutes of Health and Bethesda, 2016. Available: https://www.ncbi.nlm.nih.gov/books/NBK326791/pdf/Bookshelf_NBK326791.pdf [last accessed on 2022-12-10]

[2] H. Motahari-Nezhad, M. Péntek, L. Gulácsi, Z. Zrubka, *Outcomes of Digital Biomarker-Based Interventions: Protocol for a Systematic Review of Systematic Reviews*. JMIR Res Protoc, vol 10(11):e28204, 24 Nov. 2021. DOI: 10.2196/28204

[3] S. Vasudevan, A. Saha, M. E. Tarver, B. Patel, *Digital biomarkers: Convergence of digital health technologies and biomarkers*. NPJ Digit Med., vol 5(1):36, 25 March 2022. DOI: 10.1038/s41746-022-00583-z

[4] L. M. Babrak, J. Menetski, M. Rebhan, G. Nisato, M. Zinggeler, N. Brasier, et al., *Traditional and Digital Biomarkers: Two Worlds Apart?*. Digit Biomark 2019, vol. 3, no. 2, pp.92-102, 2019. DOI: 10.1159/000502000

[5] RespApp, *Diagnosing respiratory disease in children using cough sounds 2 (SMARTCOUGH-C-2)*. 2018, Available: https://www.clinicaltrials.gov/ct2/show/NCT03392363 [last accessed on 2022-10-30]

[6] A. Coravos, s. Khozin, K. D. Mandl, *Developing and adopting safe and effective digital biomarkers to improve patient outcomes*. npj Digital Medicine, article 2, vol. 14, 2019. DOI:10.1038/s41746-019-0090-4

[7] M. Buegler, R. Harms, M. Balasa, I. B. Meier, T. Exarchos, et al., *Digital biomarker-based individualized prognosis for people at risk of dementia*. Alzheimer's & dementia, vol. 12(1):e12073, 2020. DOI:10.1002/dad2.12073

Experiences of adding FHIR support to a legacy system

Jesse Kruse [1], Jonas Böttcher [2], Joshua Wiedekopf [3] and Josef Ingenerf [3]

[1] Medical Informatics, Universität zu Lübeck, jesse.kruse@student.uni-luebeck.de
[2] ISG INTERMED Service GmbH & Co. KG, Geesthacht, j.boettcher@intermed.de
[3] Institute of Medical Informatics, Universität zu Lübeck, j.wiedekopf, josef.ingenerf@uni-luebeck.de

Abstract

Over the past few years *Fast Healthcare Interoperability Resources* (FHIR) gains increasing traction, but the ongoing use of old standards never fostered the incorporation of modern Internet technologies in current systems. Over their live span sometimes thousands of interfaces to other software were implemented, what makes it nearly impossible to replace them within reasonable cost. This leads to a necessity to incorporate support for new technologies. The goal of this work was to enable such a system to process real world FHIR resources in a robust and flexible way. A FHIR interface and an example web application to request and process FHIR resources was implemented. To accomplish this a *parser* and a *serializer* were written in the proprietary programming language of the example system. These were then tested to ensure data integrity after processing. To evaluate the practical use of the system's ability to generate resources from its existing data, FHIR resources were produced that conform to drafts of profiles from the *Kassenärztliche Bundesvereinigung (KBV)*. The generation mechanisms turned out to be versatile and robust (> 98.37% valid resources against the profiles).

1 Introduction

The use of the latest *HL7* standard *Fast Healthcare Interoperability Resources (FHIR)* increased significantly over the past few years [1]. German legislation fosters the use by establishing it for a variety of use cases. For example, the *Medizinische Informationsobjekte (MIOs)*, that are planned to become central parts of the German electronic patient record (ePA), are based on FHIR [2]. This raises the necessity for health care providers to support it. Often that is not an easy task, because the systems lack modern capabilities used by FHIR like *Representational State Transfer* (REST) and support for formats like JSON and XML. Also, until recently there were no strong incentives to implement them because the over 30 years old *HL7 v.2* is still the most common exchange standard in the medical domain worldwide [3]. Therefore, some software modules from products maintained by major players in the field of medical information systems are in part about the same age and have no, or just very rudimentary support for the mentioned technologies.

Additionally, these systems can feature thousands of interfaces to providers like hospitals and medical practices that are to a high degree customized. The day-to-day work of these providers is based on data that is provided via these interfaces and a longer shut down of these services is not feasible. This makes it nearly impossible to replace the system within reasonable time and cost.

Systems like that are often referred to as legacy systems. The term means a software that has been in production and was extended over a long period of time. This leads to problems in maintaining and updating it to meet upcoming requirements. To reduce some effects of the described problems the goal was to add support for FHIR to such a system. Since the internship was done at *INTERMED Service GmbH*, a company that provides IT-services for the *LADR Laboratory Group*, the system in question was a large laboratory information system (LIS).

Besides robustness and flexibility, there was an additional focus on practical use by developing a web application that communicates with the interface, as well as interoperability by ensuring conformance to profiles published by the KBV.

2 Material and Methods

2.1 Fast Healthcare Interoperability Resources (FHIR)

FHIR is an interoperability standard developed and published by the *HL7* organization with a strong focus on implementation. It is structured around resources. These are the smallest information units that provide meaning on their own. For example, blood pressure needs to have additional context information, like the time of measurement, to be interpretable. On the other hand, a whole patient record has far too much information to be a basic building block. Examples for resources are *Patient* and *Observation* as well as *MedicationRequest*. But there are also more technical resources like the *Bundle*, which bundles resources or the *StructureDefinition* that is itself a resource but is also used to describe the structure of all resources in FHIR.

To foster interoperability, FHIR uses terminologies like *SNOMED-CT* or *LOINC* [4]. Most fields should be filled with codes instead of free text. This leads to an increase of machine readability as well as a better understanding across different systems and institutions because of shared concept definitions through common terminologies.

The FHIR standard is very flexible and does not make many strong requirements about which fields in a resource have to be filled and how. To tailor a resource to a specific use case *Profiles* are used. These can then be published, for example by the KBV, and developers can automatically check their own resources against these *Profiles* to see if they match the given requirements. While FHIR provides other communication paradigms like messaging, the focus clearly lies on *Application Programming Interface (API)* and more specifically on REST. An advantage of REST is, that it is build on HTTP, and familiar to many developers.

2.2   Laboratory Information System (LIS)

While the code of the LIS, that should acquire the FHIR support, is not open for changes, there exists a build in script language. Many functionalities and customizations can be implemented with the help of this tool, but it has certain drawbacks. For example, there are no real collection structures or functions, and most things are achieved by string processing.

Besides strings and numbers, a heavily used data structure within the LIS is called *EI-Structure*. This is in some ways similar to a *HashMap* in other common languages. It can be nested leading to a tree structure. Fig. 1 shows an example of how the *EI-Structure* is used. The expression with the $-sign marks a variable and is like a root node. From there, data fields can be nested by adding them with a dot. To retrieve a value they can be addressed the same way. The *EI-Structure* is internally represented as a string. Therefore, by building a string that conforms to this structure an *EI-Structure* can be generated programmatically.

```
$var.Patient.name.family = "Mustermann"
$var.Patient.name.given = "Max"
$var.Patient.name.given2 = "Fred"

$xml = z_EI2FHIR($var)
```

```
<Patient>
  <name>
     <family value="Mustermann"/>
     <given value="Max"/>
     <given value=„Fred"/>
  </name>
</Patient>
```

Figure 1: Example of how the *EI-Structure* is used. `z_EI2FHIR()` calls the serializer. The variable `$xml` holds the XML-string depicted in the lower box.

2.3   Communication Server

Mirth-Connect (Mirth), is a communication server for the health care domain [5]. These servers are used as a middleware to route and transform messages between systems. The core constructs in *Mirth* are called *channels*. These are objects that provide one-to-many connections with one *source connector* that takes an incoming input message, which is then distributed to *n destination connectors*. The source, as well as the destination connector can have multiple *transformers* which transforms a message based on given rules [6]. Besides other options these transformers can be scripts in *JavaScript*. This gives the implementer great flexibility. Additionally, the *JavaScript* interpreter *Rhino* is employed and by that native *Java* classes can be used within the *JavaScript* code [7]. This way external *Java* libraries like *HAPI-FHIR* [8] can be utilized to enable the processing of FHIR resources.

Sources and destinations can have different types of connections. The two important protocols in the project are HTTP, that is used by FHIR and the Minimal Lower Level protocol (MLLP), that is based on TCP and is often used in conjunction with *HL7 v.2* and therefore supported by the LIS. MLLP defines an optional mechanism to send responses (ACK/NAK) depending on whether a message is successfully persisted in the receiving system [10].

2.4   Web server and client

To test the interface in a practical use case, a web application was implemented. For serving a dynamic website to users, an application server is needed. As a basis the *jetty* application server was used, mainly for two reasons [9]. First, *jetty* is implemented in *Java* and therefore, the integration with the FHIR library *HAPI-FHIR*, that is also written in *Java*, is simple. The second reason is that there is an embedded version of the *jetty* server, so it can be integrated within the custom web application code. The resulting artifact is one *jar* file what makes it easy to deploy as a *docker* container. Deployment as a *docker* container on the other hand results in fast and flexible deployment across different systems.

Additionally, an *SQLite* database was used to enable some desired features explained below. *SQLite* is a relational database system that stores all the data in one single file, so it can also be embedded into the container and a separate database deployment is not needed.

3   Results and Discussion

3.1   System architecture

Fig. 2 shows an overview of the systems architecture. Users interact with the application via a web interface. Information can be retrieved from the LIS, displayed, manipulated and stored in the LIS database. The communication is based on HTTP and REST. Since the LIS does not support HTTP, *Mirth* is used as a facade for the LIS, so that the web appli-

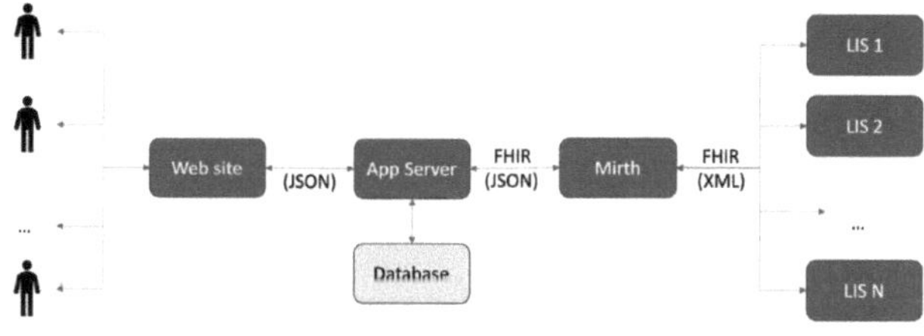

Figure 2: Overview of the involved systems. N is the number of attached LIS instances.

cation sends its requests to the communication server. From there they are passed to the LIS via MLLP. The use of the communication server has additional advantages: First, the laboratory has different locations and each one has its own LIS instance with its own database. The user can choose the location with which he or she would like to interact with. The location is then inserted into the URL of the request. The Mirth-Channel has one *destination-connector* per location and the request is routed within *Mirth* to the right destination based on the URL. Since the *destination-connector* and the LIS-side logic are the same across all locations apart from the IP-address in the *destination-connector*, adding new locations to the system is simple and fast.

Another advantage of *Mirth* is the capability to include external libraries like *HAPI-FHIR*. This is handy, because communication with the frontend using JSON is convenient, since modern web browsers support it natively. The LIS does not support JSON but has a very rudimentary support for XML. FHIR resources coming from the web application in JSON are parsed by *HAPI-FHIR* and then encoded again as XML before they get send to the LIS. Responses from the LIS are treated the other way around. Additionally, this way a basic check is done if the sent resources stick to the FHIR standard.

The LIS supports interface definitions to connect external systems. In these definitions custom scripts can be selected to get executed whenever a new message arrives. As stated before, the LIS has build in support for the MLLP. This is used as the basis for the communication. Since HTTP-methods like GET or POST do not exist in MLLP, they have to be extracted from the incoming request. This is done by an implementation in the LIS's own scripting language. Based on the HTTP-verb different functionalities are invoked like storing data or returning a requested resource. As mentioned, the MLLP provides a mechanism to send ACKs. Since there is no check that prevents sending something else, these ACK-messages are instead used to send back responses that hold the requested resources.

3.2 Resource generation within the LIS

It is possible to extract a specified XML-tag and its content within the LIS, but no attributes. FHIR stores its values in most cases as an attribute. Also, it is not convenient nor flexible, if one has to know exactly how a message is structured up front. This led to the implementation of an XML parser that converts a FHIR resource from XML into an *EI-*

Structure. The *EI-Structure* follows the naming scheme that is used by FHIR with one exception. Since *EI-Structures* do not support indexing multiple fields with the same name, collections in FHIR resources are converted by enumerating consecutive items that occur more than once. In the resulting *EI-Structure* fields can thereby be addressed conveniently for data extraction.

If a resource is requested, data is queried from the database and stored in an *EI-Structure* that has the same structure as the FHIR resource. To convert it into an XML representation, a serializer was implemented. One problem was that the addressing of the *EI-Structure* is not case-sensitive, while FHIR is. So, for every tag the correct notation in *CamelCase*, has to be provided and looked up during encoding. The parser and serializer were tested in an end to end setup. First, a FHIR resource in XML format was generated from values in a *HashMap*. The XML was then given as input to the parser resulting in an *EI-Structure* as output. This *EI-Structure* was then used as an input for the serializer. In the last step, the resulting XML was parsed with *HAPI-FHIR* and the extracted values were compared to the corresponding values in the initial *HashMap*. It was tested with six different resources (*Practitioner*, *Organization*, *Appointment*, *Observation*, *Composition* and *Bundle* filled with before generated resources). In all cases no data was lost or altered during these tests. Note that the use with other resources may require adding the spelling of tags used.

3.3 Limitations and Discussion

When fitting data from an already existing system to another one, in many cases there are discrepancies in the data models. For example, the LIS has a database table named "Einsender". Here are all entities stored that can send in requests for laboratory tests. These can be doctors but also practices, stations or whole hospitals. FHIR, having a much broader scope, does differentiate between *Practitioners* (doctors) and *Organization* like stations or hospitals. To transform the data it was not always clear to decide automatically whether a data entry is a person, hence a *Practitioners* or an *Organization*. To differentiate between them, the "Lebenslange Arzt Nummer" (LANR) was used to identify doctors and hospital codes to identify hospitals [11]. This leads to 62% of data entries that are identifiable as one or the other. The other part are in many cases practices or doctors without LANR but in rare cases also companies. Since in the test app all "Einsender" need to be queried, the unidentifiable portion is in doubt assumed to be practices named after the doctors and are modeled accordingly as organizations. Since the test application required names, addresses and IDs, that are provided by both, *Practitioners* and *Organization*, this was not a problem in practice. But in other scenarios this might be different and could potentially be fixed by providing a database entry that holds the FHIR resource type that should be generated from a record if it is not unambiguous.

From the identifiable portions, *Practitioners* and *Organiza-*

tion are generated that match the profiles included in the KBV *MIO Laborbefund*. One entry returned an error during generation, because of corrupt data. From the generated *Practitioners* 99.82% were valid against the KBV profile. The generation of the *Organization* resulted in 98.37% valid resources.

While the scripting language gives users great flexibility and extensibility, during the project some limitations were encountered. One might assume that the language was first and foremost designed to enable string processing of individual messages. This assumption is supported by the fact that querying capabilities are very limited, what might also be due to security concerns. As a workaround the *SQLite* database was used. When users logged into the web app all *Compositions* created by the user previously should be displayed. Since there is no way to search the database for all *Compositions* created by one user, the ID of every *Composition* has to be stored with the user ID who created it. If the user logs into the app, all IDs of that particular user can be queried from the web apps database and with this IDs query all of his or her *Compositions* one at a time from the LIS database. This adds additional overhead due to many individual requests. It also involves a deviation from the RESTful-paradigm of statelessness and inhibits requests users would expect from an FHIR-API. This aspect could potentially be reduced if a database is not connected to the client but to Mirth, to store data necessary for search operations, what would mimic a more organic FHIR-API. Another problem encountered is an error that occurs if messages are too long. The LIS starts to send the message but never sends the terminal symbols needed by MLLP. The communication server waits for that particular symbol that never arrives and runs into a timeout. To resolve this, *paging* was implemented for *Bundles*. They can contain a link that returns the next n resources if the number of items would otherwise be too big.

4   Conclusion

It was possible to implement in a relatively short amount of time a versatile interface to add FHIR support to a legacy system that had little prerequisites for supporting modern technologies. The implemented parts were tested to show their capabilities of robustly producing a variety of resources that could potentially be utilized in upcoming communication with major players of the German health care sector. The implementation for the test use case can be easily expanded to support more FHIR resources like *Observation* or *DiagnostikReport*, for other uses in the laboratory context. Nevertheless, limitations occurred that demanded for solutions that sometimes introduce a fair amount of new complexity to the system and stretches the capabilities of the underling software. While some provided solutions may be also applicable to other scenarios, the prerequisite of extensibility, like the scripting language in this case, must be given to allow such system extensions in the first place.

Acknowledgement

The work has been carried out at the ISG INTERMED Service GmbH & Co. KG, Geesthacht and supervised by the Institute of Medical Informatics, Universität zu Lübeck. Furthermore, a special thanks to the whole team at the INTERMED and the LADR Laboratory Group for their great impetus, support and supervision during the project.

Author's Statement

Conflict of interest: Authors state no conflict of interest.

5   References

[1] HL7 FHIR Foundation, *HL7 FHIR*. Available: http://hl7.org/fhir// [last accessed on 2022-11-21].

[2] Kassenärztliche Bundesvereinigung, *MIOs, Erklärung FHIR*. Available: https://mio.kbv.de/pages/viewpage.action?pageId=30146985 [last accessed on 2022-11-11].

[3] T. Benson, G. Grieve, *Chapter 12 HL7 Version 2*. In: Principles of Health Interoperability, Springer-Verlag London, p. 223, 2016.

[4] HL7 FHIR Foundation, *Terminologies - FHIR v4.3.0*. Available: https://hl7.org/fhir/terminologies.html [last accessed on 2023-02-03].

[5] NextGen Healthcare, *Healthcare Integration Engine | Mirth® Connect by NextGen Healthcare*. Available: https://www.nextgen.com/solutions/interoperability/mirth-integration-engine [last accessed on 2023-02-03].

[6] P. Köppen, S. Langenberg, *Erfahrungsbericht über den Einsatz des open source Kommunikationsservers Mirth Connect am Universitätsklinikum Bonn*. In: Informatik 2014, Bonn, pp. 1465–1474, 2014.

[7] S. Nizamov, *Unofficial Mirth Connect v3.6 Developer's Guide*. Shamil Publishing, p. 21, 2016.

[8] HAPI Community, *HAPI FHIR*. Available: https://hapifhir.io/hapi-fhir/ [last accessed on 2022-11-12].

[9] J. McConnell, *Eclipse Jetty | The Eclipse Foundation*. Available: https://www.eclipse.org/jetty/ [last accessed on 2023-02-03].

[10] Oracle Corporation and/or its affiliates, *MLLP V2*. Available: https://docs.oracle.com/cd/E19509-01/820-5508/ghadt/index.html [last accessed on 2022-11-12].

[11] S. Rass, *Richtlinie der Kassenärztlichen Bundesvereinigung nach § 75 Absatz 7 SGB V zur Vergabe der Arzt-, Betriebsstätten-, Praxisnetz- sowie der Netzverbundnummern*. Available: https://www.kbv.de/media/sp/Arztnummern_Richtlinie.pdf [last accessed on 2023-02-03].

Developing a validation tool to evaluate data quality and improve data uniformity for a federated feasibility query platform

Paul Behrend [1], Joshua Wiedekopf [2], Josef Ingenerf [2], and Lorenz Rosenau [2]

[1] Medical Informatics, Universität zu Lübeck, paul.behrend@student.uni-luebeck.de
[2] IT Center for Clinical Research (ITCR-L), Universitat zu Lubeck, Lubeck, j.wiedekopf, josef.ingenerf, lorenz.rosenau@uni-luebeck.de

Abstract

Although data generation is ever-increasing, the great potential of medical data outside of routine care applications is largely untapped. One such project addressing this issue is the development of the *German Portal for Medical Research Data*. However, sufficient data quality and uniformity are necessary prerequisites to the reuse of clinical data for research purposes, especially when data is integrated from disparate systems as it is in this case. To better gauge the extent of data quality issues and inconsistencies in the existing data pool, we developed specialized FHIR profiles and validated local FHIR instance data at participating sites against them using a dedicated validation tool we developed for this purpose. With the analysis of the resulting reports, data quality issues and discrepancies could indeed be identified, thus validating initial concerns and providing a foundation for improving data harmonization.

1   Introduction

While far from fully digitalized, data generation, transfer, and storage in the health sector are increasingly automated through integration into the digital space. The primary purpose of these processes is to improve immediate patient care and serve administrative requirements stipulated by local and national legislation. However, such data presents an enormous potential for areas not connected to direct support of the healthcare system. Indeed it is key to furthering advances in many fields of study, such as healthcare process optimization or genomics [1, 2]. Thus, increasing the accessibility of medical data for research applications is crucial. One such endeavor is the establishment of the *German Research Data Portal for Health* (FDPG) under the ABIDE project. It aims to develop and implement a platform for federated feasibility queries to quantify and identify suitable patient cohorts for a given study [3]. Due to the contribution of 28 different german hospitals, there is no guarantee of interoperability regarding the data provided by each site. Despite the employment of previously established data integration centers (DIZ) to serve as data warehouses for secure access to clinical data and agreement upon a standardized data model using HL7 FHIR and the core data set (KDS) profiles of the Medical Informatics Initiative (MII) [3], a lack of specificity of the profiles introduced doubts on whether the data produced by the DIZs exhibited the required uniformity for the application. Consequently, the data present at each site has to be analyzed with respect to its conformity to the agreed-upon data model with the goal of improving data quality.

2   Material and Methods

2.1   Fast Healthcare Interoperability Resources (FHIR)

The data model used as a template for data standardization inside the DIZs is the HL7 FHIR standard. It is an exchange standard for medical data focussing on ease of implementation and interoperability[4]. FHIR uses already established standards such as XML, JSON, and RDF to lower implementation barriers to improve acceptance. Additionally, FHIR employs among other things a RESTful architecture approach [8] to manage clinical data transfer and interfacing of modern distributed systems. In this standard, the communication of data is abstracted to resources, each representing a foundational entity involved in clinical data exchange. They are regarded as distinct logical entities serving one or more unique purposes while being flexible enough to support a large variety of transactions. Each resource contains elements holding information specific to the clinical object or event it represents, i. e. the Patient resource contains the patients' gender. In this regard, FHIR incorporates only data points necessary in 80 percent of use cases [4]. Through extensions, the standard allows for the integration of additional information if desired. For adapting the base resources to more specific use cases or requirements, in FHIR the user can constrain their content via the definition of profiles. Through this process, the cardinality of elements can be changed, and their content is confined to application-specific value ranges. One such example is the Core Data Set (KDS) used in the MII to harmonize german health data. To provide semantic interoperability, FHIR encourages using standardized code systems for defining allowable values through dedicated resources for code systems and derived value sets. The creation, modification, and interaction with FHIR instance data are facilitated by RESTful web services using the standard HTTP operations GET, POST, PUT and DELETE. Such interfaces, as well as interfaces for the terminology data and message transfer, are also part of the FHIR standard.

2.2 Research Data Portal for Health

Being envisioned as a nationwide research data and feasibility portal, the *German Portal for Medical Research Data* (Forschungsdatenportal für Gesundheit [FDPG]) of the MII aims to provide centralized access to distributed clinical data present at university hospitals across Germany. In this regard, this project is a first attempt to establish a central data access point for the entire MII. Using this tool, researchers are able to get information on available clinical data and patient cohort sizes fitting custom criteria. Once feasibility is established, they are able to apply for using the data in subsequent research endeavors on the same portal [3]. Thus, access to nationwide routine care data and biosamples is streamlined. The structure devised and implemented to handle the distributed feasibility queries consists of four major components. Firstly, the user interacts with the feasibility UI, which enables the creation and management of user-defined queries. Here, the specific inclusion and exclusion criteria identifying the desired patient cohort are chosen. Upon submission, a backend service transforms them into the implementation-agnostic *Structured Query* format. This process involves a custom ontology developed for the project enriching the original criteria e.g. via code system concept expansion using an ontology tree [3][5]. Afterward, the query is securely distributed to each participating sites' DIZ through a middleware broker. After arrival, the query is translated into an FHIR-specific target format. Following query execution, the number of matching patients is returned to the central feasibility platform and the aggregated result is provided to the requester. As the combined queryable pool of data currently covers over 20 different hospitals, medical information originating from many disparate source systems have to be integrated. While fractional efforts towards standardization have been undertaken, an MII-wide approach to data harmonization is essential. For this purpose, the participating members chose the FHIR standard to ensure interoperability. More specifically, they mandated the processed routine care data in each DIZ to conform to the KDS profiles of the MII [3].

3 Results and Discussion

3.1 Aspects of Data Quality

Before discussing the proposed solution, identifying relevant aspects of data quality and conformance concerning this use case is paramount to retaining an appropriate scope on the subject matter. As defined by Kahn et al. [6],

our efforts cover two out of three central data quality categories: conformance (syntactical and structural correctness) and completeness (coverage of and extent to which data elements contain data). Both are essential to allow querying of the data inside the combined data pool as they ensure the presents of necessary data elements where expected.

3.2 Feasibility Query Data Validation

Following the above considerations, we identified three conformance levels covering both data quality categories that are necessary for the execution of distributed feasibility queries on the present data. Firstly, the data must be valid FHIR instance data, meaning conformance to the FHIR base resource definitions is required. At this lowermost level of conformance, the data would exhibit syntactical and structural correctness. Secondly, it has to conform to the KDS profiles as stipulated via the joint decision of all participating members. While adherence to the KDS provides sufficient data harmonization during routine care and administrative scenarios at each site, this is not the case for distributed feasibility queries. Even though it restricts possible values of critical elements inside the instance data to standardized code systems like ICD10-GM, SNOMED CT, or LOINC, the optionality introduces deviations between the sites. Mapping between code systems is not only very time intensive but also often ambiguous and sometimes impossible. Another issue arises for laboratory values. Irrespective of the fact that UCUM units are mandatory if a quantity is recorded in observational data and LOINC codes have to be used to specify its type, the profiles stipulate no fixed combinations of LOINC codes and UCUM units, i.e., the body height shall be indicated in cm. Although unit conversion during query answering might seem like a valid solution, it introduces performance issues and does not work for all unit combinations. Furthermore, the querying process uses the patient resource as context. Therefore, all instance data must refer to patients to be findable. Consequently, the constraints introduced by the KDS profiles aren't strict enough for the FDPG use case. Based on the identified limitations and using the KDS Profiles as base definition, we created profiles for all FHIR resource types relevant for query answering and that required adjustments: Condition, Observation, Procedure, Medication, MedicationStatement, MedicationAdministration, Specimen. For Condition, Procedure, and Medication, we require the use of one specific code system to encode the relevant information, demanding the presence of an ICD-10 GM, OPS, and ATC code, respectively. While both MedicationStatement and MedicationStatement can contain the information on the prescribed medication directly, we allowed only references to a dedicated Medication instance data to ensure consistency. For Specimen, a custom extension was added, containing a reference to the associated diagnosis represented by a Condition resource instance. For the Observation resource, multiple profiles were used to cover all necessary constraints. Since we needed to define sensible combinations of LOINC codes and UCUM units, each was represented by a single profile. Using previous standardization efforts in the MII, we specified over 800 valid code unit and code answer list pairs, which are present if the identifying LOINC code describes a qualitative assessment instead of a quantitative measurement. In addition, fallback profiles were defined to capture Observation instance data with LOINC codes not covered by any profile. Through these measures, we can assess and address local differences sensibly while later having the means to centrally provide conformance templates with the knowledge collected in the previous step and ensure data quality. Data not adhering to any of the conformance levels cannot be found. Currently, not all sites validate the FHIR instance data generated by ETL-Jobs. Consequently, we cannot make any assumptions about the conformance. Furthermore, we decided to provide the necessary tooling to use the defined profiles for the validation process. This serves two purposes: On the one hand, this allows fixing present issues at the relevant DIZ and improving conformance. On the other hand, the insights gained by analyzing how each hospital encodes specific clinical events can help make decisions on how to represent such information consistently across all sites. This is necessary, as in the current state, the profiles only represent assumptions made by the FDPG search ontology, which are not mandatory. Our goal is an iterative process in which our initial top-down profile definition is adapted based on a bottom-up approach as depicted by Figure 1.

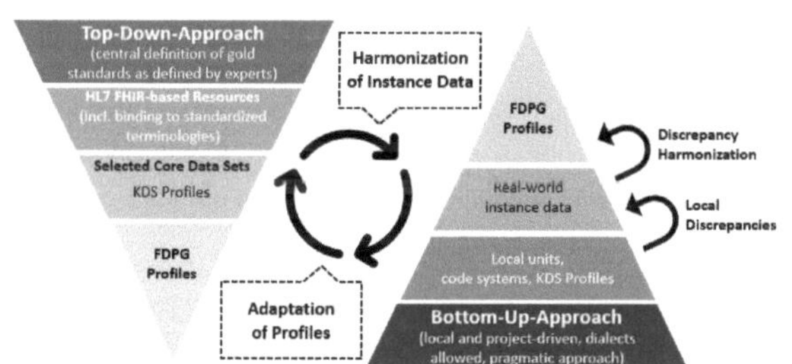

Figure 1: Description of both approaches as described in [7] and adapted to the FDPG use case

3.3   Validation Tool

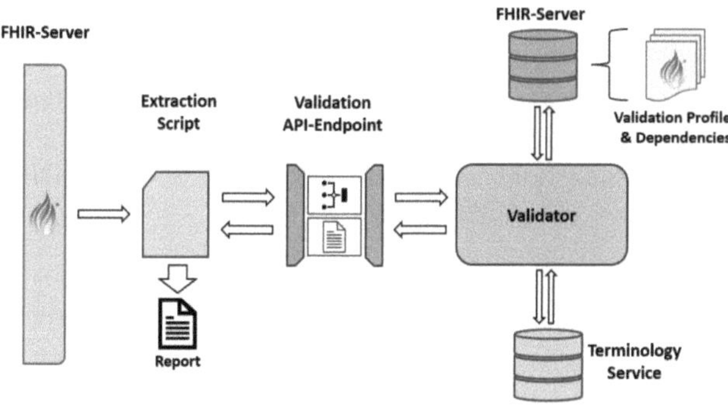

Figure 2: Schematic display of involved components

Employing these profiles to validate the data of the DIZs however, required additional tooling and infrastructure.

Thus, we developed a custom validation tool to validate the local data at each site against our profiles and those of the KDS, aggregate the results and generate a report, which can be analyzed regarding data quality and conformance. A schematic display of the tools' components and their interactions is depicted in Fig. 2. FHIR instance data is requested from the local FHIR server by the extraction script. It manages the entire validation process and distills the final report from the validation results. In addition to requesting data to validate, it performs distribution analyses to ascertain what code systems are most prevalent to encode condition, procedure, and medication data. The script passes the requested data to the validation endpoint, where instances are assigned suitable profiles based on their content. For example, depending on the LOINC code used in observational data, a fitting profile containing the expected Code-Unit combination is chosen to validate against. Once this is done, the augmented data gets transferred to a validator, which generates the validation results. To enable easy deployment on-site, we provide our validation profiles via a local FHIR server to which they are uploaded. It also automatically pulls necessary dependencies from a remote repository. Since code systems and value sets play a central part during the validation of FHIR instance data, a terminology service providing related operations and terminology data is a requirement. Due to the fact that most hospitals do not have the infrastructure available, we provide our own built-in terminology service covering the required operations on terminology resources during validation and based on the FHIR Terminology Service specification. To circumvent needing to make assumptions on the local execution environment, all components can be deployed with Docker. We refrained from including patient references in the generated report to protect patient privacy and promote acceptance of the tool.

3.4   Validation Results

In order to verify the correctness and usefulness of the validation tool, a first run in collaboration with three member university hospitals was conducted. Before discussing the results, it is important to mention that while some of the issues exhibited by the data might be critical to query execution, this is not the case for all categories. At the current state, it is more appropriate to regard many occurring issues as deviations from the baseline we provided. Consequently, our profiles do not represent an authoritative source of truth but rather identifiers of potential inconsistencies. To solve such disparities between sites, an overview of the entire data pool has to be established and a concerted decision has to be made. However, such an undertaking is outside of the scope of the first run. The analysis of the resulting reports showed KDS conformance for most resource types, except for Medication and Observation, which also contained discrepancies regarding our profiles. Of particular relevance to us was that diverging Code-Unit combinations were identified. One such example can be seen in Figure 3. This was not limited to unit mismatches, however. We also discerned

```
{
    "severity": "error",
    "code": "processing",
    "diagnostics": "Value is 'ng/ml' but must be 'pg/ml'",
    "location": [ ... ]
}
```

Figure 3: Diverging unit code combination

```
{
    "severity": "error",
    "code": "processing",
    "diagnostics": "The Profile ... definition allows for the
                    type Quantity but found type CodeableConcept",
    "location": [ ... ]
}
```

Figure 4: Qualitative/quantitative value mismatch

inconsistencies regarding quantitative and qualitative observational values as depicted by Figure 4. The report itself contains much more detailed information on the types of issues occurring and their distribution. To present our findings in a compact fashion, an extensive analysis was performed and its results were forwarded to the corresponding DIZ support team. This included recommendations on how to address issues if they could be solved locally and without correspondence with other members of the FDPG project. Due to the large size of the available data inside the DIZs FHIR servers, we sampled the data and did not analyze it in its entirety. While this might seem like a limitation, due to the nature of the ETL jobs used for data transformation, most issues can be identified using a small sample size with relative certainty. However, creating a complete picture of data quality across the entire data pool by analyzing all data is desirable.

4   Conclusion

When integrating data from many disparate source systems, ensuring data quality is a difficult and complex process. Prior to our efforts, no overarching efforts were made to systematically assess the validity of the harmonization process thus far. Even if through concerted decision compliance to a baseline data model is demanded, sufficient data quality cannot be assumed without proper data auditing and enforcement. While mandating compliance with the KDS is a good first step, it does not provide sufficient constraints for distributed feasibility query execution. Through the definition of a stricter compliance baseline and subsequent data analysis, we were able to highlight remaining quality issues and disparities between sites. To paint a full picture of this matter, the entire distributed data pool should be analyzed. Since not all issues can be addressed by each DIZ independently, this is especially important. Only if these efforts and possibly periodic quality examinations in the future are considered can data quality be maintained.

Acknowledgement

This research was carried out as part of an internship at the ITCR-L, Universität zu Lübeck.
We want to express our gratitude to the participating sites in the first validation run.

Author's Statement

Conflict of interest: none declared.

5   References

[1] T. Hulsen et al., *From Big Data to Precision Medicine.* Frontiers in Medicine, 2019, DOI: 10.3389/fmed.2019.00034.

[2] K. Feldman, R. A. Johnson and N. V. Chawla, *The state of data in healthcare: Path towards standardization.* Nature, 2018, DIO: 10.1007/s41666-018-0019.

[3] J. Gruender et al., *The Architecture of a Feasibility Query Portal for Distributed COVID-19 Fast Healthcare Interoperability Resources (FHIR) Patient Data Repositories: Design and Implementation Study.* JMIR MEDICAL INFORMATICS, 2022 vol. 10 iss. 5, DIO: 10.2196/36709.

[4] D. Bender, K. Sartipi, *HL7 FHIR: An Agile and RESTful Approach to Healthcare Information Exchange.* Proceedings of the 26th IEEE International Symposium on Computer-Based Medical Systems, 2013-6, DIO: 10.1109/CBMS.2013.6627810.

[5] L. Rosenau et al., *Generation of a Fast Healthcare Interoperability Resources (FHIR)-based Ontology for Federated Feasibility Queries in the Context of COVID-19: Feasibility Study.* JMIR MEDICAL INFORMATICS, 2022 vol. 10 iss. 4, DIO: 10.2196/35789.

[6] M. G. Kahn, T. J. Callahan, J. Banard and A. E. Bauck, A Harmonized Data Quality Assessment Terminology and Framework for the Secondary Use of Electronic Health Record Data. eGEMs, 2016 vol. 4 iss. 1, DIO: 10.13063/2327-9214.1244.

[7] A.-K. Schoppenhauer et al., Medical Data Engineering – Theory and Practice. Communications in Computer and Information Science, 2021 vol. 1481, DIO: 10.1007/978-3-030-87657-9_21.

[8] R. T. Fielding, Architectural styles and the design of network -based software architectures. 2000, University of California, Irvine.

An app for documenting the progress of therapy in movement disorders

Rica Schulze [1], Roland Stenger [2], and Sebastian Fudickar [2]

[1] Medical Informatics, Universität zu Lübeck, rica.schulze@student.uni-luebeck.de

[2] MOVE Group, Institute of Medical Informatics, Universität zu Lübeck, {roland.stenger,sebastian.fudickar}@uni-luebeck.de@uni-luebeck.de

Abstract

Movement disorders are characterized by a paucity or an excess of movement. Access to specialists is difficult due to underserved areas and long distances, making regular visits impractical. Some studies have discussed telemedicine options for therapy monitoring, such as videoconferencing, which have been accepted by physicians and patients. Asynchronous methods such as video recording allow more temporal freedom but have the disadvantage that physicians and patients cannot interact with each other, which can lead to a decrease in quality. This article presents a prototype of an app that aims to enable asynchronous therapy monitoring that still offers the same quality as videoconferencing or face-to-face meetings. The app can be used to record guided videos from home. In the future, it will be possible to upload the data, providing direct access. There are also plans to test the usefulness and acceptance of the app and the videos in a study.

1   Introduction

Movement disorders are neurological diseases. A distinction is made between hypokinetic and hyperkinetic movement disorders. Hypokinetic movement disorders such as Parkinson's disease are associated with a paucity of movement, whereas hyperkinetic movement disorders such as dystonia are marked by an excess of movement. In addition, movement disorders are divided into idiopathic movement disorders, which are caused by the disease itself, and symptomatic movement disorders, which occur due to other neurological diseases. Symptomatic movement disorders manifest differently in each person and may change over time [1]. The diagnosis and therapy of movement disorders are usually carried out by specialists. However, access to them is increasingly difficult, due to the limited number of specialists, movement restrictions, underserved areas, and long travel time [2]. It is important, though, to monitor the therapy on a regular basis. For symptomatic movement disorders, continuous therapy monitoring can be a great achievement because movement disorders can change over time or as a result of therapy. The physician should be able to react to changes immediately. Another example is cervical dystonia, where the patients show an abnormal head posture. It is treated with botulinum toxin injections, which are repeated every 3 months. Continuous monitoring would be a great achievement as the injections' effect varies from patient to patient. In addition, side effects, which can be caused by high doses, can be detected and corrected [1]. Telemedicine interventions such as video conferencing are increasingly used to address the problem of limited access

to specialists, underserved areas, and long distances [2]. It was found by [3] that 50% of Movement Disorder Society members, mostly physicians, from 83 countries around the world already use and plan to continue using telemedicine interventions such as videoconferencing and video education in the context of movement disorders. In addition, [2] showed that Parkinson's patients are satisfied with a video consultation or even prefer it to an on-site consultation. A study on telemedicine visits in the treatment of dystonia came to the same conclusions [4]. Whereas [2] considers synchronous videoconferencing an improvement, [5] points out that asynchronous video can overcome the problem of poor internet connections and low resolutions. In addition, asynchronous methods are suitable for exchanges over a longer period of time, so that the patient and doctor do not have to agree on an appointment each time and are freer in their time management. However, there are problems with asynchronous videos too. [2] noted that the information gain is not as good with asynchronous video because clinicians and patients can interact better in video conferences, and [5] sees the problem that, for example, some features in dystonic disorders can only be detected through task-specific and site-specific situations.

In this article, an app prototype is presented, with which a patient can record guided videos from home, where defined movements should be performed suited to the given movement disorder. In addition, a questionnaire on well-being can be filled out. The goal of the app is to provide an asynchronous telemedicine method for therapy progress monitoring in movement disorders. The instructions in the videos should provide a high usefulness of the videos and should have an equivalent quality as video conferences or face-to-face meetings.

2   Methods and Material

To monitor the progress of therapy in patients with movement disorders, an app has been developed to record guided videos. The developed prototype of the app provides a framework, which can be adapted to a required movement disorder. However, it is planned to test the app on a group of patients with cervical dystonia, which is characterized by an abnormal posture of the head [1]. Therefore, the implemented version of the app is suited to this disorder and allows the recording of a typical video protocol to assess the severity of cervical dystonia.

2.1   Requirements of the App

As the app provides a framework, which should be able to use for several movement disorders, the requirement must be general. On the basis of the user base, there are a couple of requirements that need to be considered in particular. Smartphone use is increasing in all age groups. However, a statistic shows that people older than 65 are still overwhelmed with smartphones as they have difficulty using it. The majority of them use their smartphones only in a very limited way because they are afraid of making a mistake and accidentally deleting programs or losing important stored information [6]. However, movement disorders can occur at different ages. For example, dystonia may manifest in childhood, adolescence, or in adulthood [1]. Cervical dystonia often starts between 30 and 50 years of age, whereas dystonia in cranial regions first appears in the fifth or sixth decade of life [7]. Especially for this reason, it is important to make the app as simple and intuitive as possible, so that even users who have little knowledge of smartphones can utilize the app without any problems. In addition, the app is developed for patients with movement disorders. Therefore, they may have limited movement, which could make it difficult to control an app. For example, tremors can occur in the case of Parkinson's or dystonia, which makes operation challenging [1]. It is therefore particularly important - especially for important functions such as deleting or transferring data - to consider and catch user errors.

2.2   The Framework of the App

In the following, the features of the current version of the app are introduced. As the framework is developed with *Android Studio* [8], it uses standardized functional graphical units and therefore, will be familiar to android users, which may increase intuitive usage. The therapy monitoring was realized in two different ways: by a guided video recording and by a questionnaire about general well-being. Recording videos is the more important feature of the app. It has already been shown that the therapy of movement disorders in the form of video conferencing is accepted by physicians and patients [2], [4]. The advantage of video

conferencing over video is that the doctor and patient can interact more effectively [2]. In order for doctors and patients to act independently of appointments, video recordings provide an asynchronous alternative to video conferencing. To increase the quality and usefulness of the videos, patients are guided by instructions before and during the recording. This is to ensure that patients perform appropriate movements so that clinicians can better identify and assess disease-specific symptoms. Since the app has been adapted for the case of cervical dystonia, the instructions are also matched to it. However, these instructions can be quickly modified to suit other movement disorders with just a few changes.

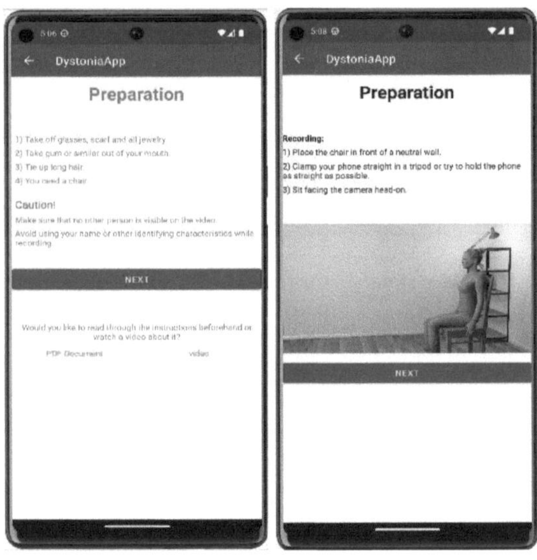

(a) First page of the preparation for the recording

(b) Second page of the preparation for the recording

Figure 1: This figure shows the preparation pages for the recording, which contain some pre-information.

The video recording contains some preparation on two pages, which can be seen in Fig. 1. This includes information about positioning, setting, and ensuring privacy. On the first page, the user can also view a log of the instructions given in the video or watch a sample video directly. As the instructions are adapted to typical movements for assessment of the specified disease, the patient might be familiar with them. Nevertheless, the user has the option to see these commands before recording the video to feel confident and better prepared. The second page explains to the user the environment in which the video should be recorded and the position of the camera in relation to the user. For example, in the case of cervical dystonia, the user is instructed to position the camera so that the head and shoulders are clearly visible, as cervical dystonia affects the muscles in the head and neck. Also, this page allows checking the volume of the spoken commands so that it can be adjusted and the instructions are easily understood during the recording. Once the preparation is complete, the camera can be opened, as seen in Fig. 2. The modified camera contains a text field for the written instructions, an image for illustra-

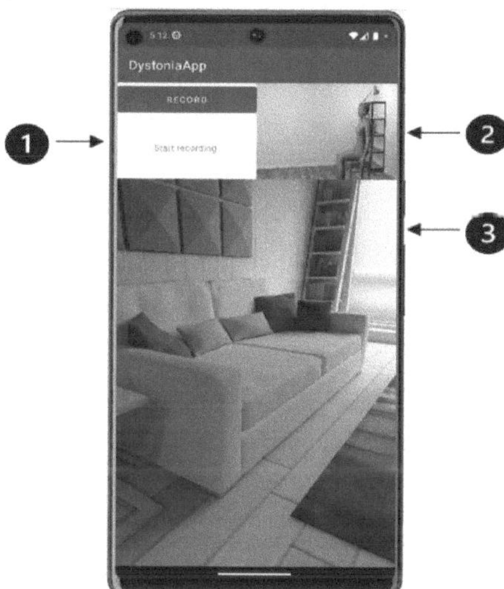

Figure 2: This graphic shows the camera. It is divided into three sections: the written instructions (1), the animated images (2), the camera view (3).

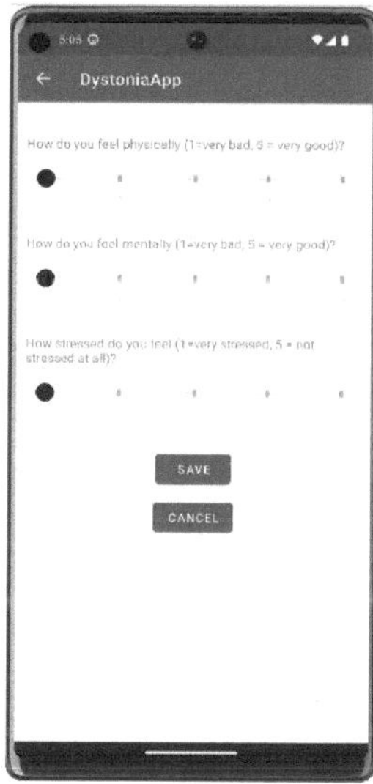

Figure 3: A questionnaire is displayed where the user can evaluate his physical and mental condition as well as his stress level with the slide bars.

tion, and a camera view. In addition, the commands are also spoken aloud. This is to ensure that everything is explained to the user in a clear manner. The instructions are given at short intervals and after the last one, the video ends automatically. The recorded videos are listed on the main page of the app. They are named by the date and time they are recorded. The videos can be viewed or deleted. To avoid accidental deletion, the user must confirm again that the video should actually be deleted. In addition, it should be possible to upload the videos to a secure server here. This functionality is not implemented yet. For this, it is planned as well that confirmation is requested from the user when the video is to be uploaded so that only data is shared where the user wants this. Currently, the videos and questionnaires are stored locally on the cell phone.

Since it may not be necessary to record a video every day, there is also the option to fill out a questionnaire that assesses the patient's overall well-being, as seen in Fig. 3. From the home page, the user can navigate to an overview page where both the completed questionnaires can be seen, and new questionnaires can be completed. In this, the user evaluates his physical and mental condition, as well as his stress level. Since movement disorders are physical limitations, the question of physical condition arises. The question about the mental condition comes from the fact that movement disorders can be accompanied by depression or other mental illnesses. [7] showed that about one-third of all patients with cervical dystonia suffer from depression. Triggers for this may be social embarrassment or a decrease in self-esteem due to their disorder. Therefore, it can be assumed that mental health also decreases with decreasing effect of therapy. In addition, one study investigated the effect of botulinum toxin on depression and showed a positive correlation. This could be another reason that as botulinum injections wear off, mental health declines [9]. The last question about stress level is asked because stress can

be a cause of diseases. For example, [10] shows in an experiment on mice that an increased stress level over six weeks can lead to movement restrictions. In order to minimize the sources of error and to create comparability, the patients can only rate their well-being by moving a slider. When saving a questionnaire, it will be closed directly. If the page is left without saving, the user is asked whether the questionnaire should be saved or discarded. The questionnaire is completed within a few seconds and should provide the doctor with information about the therapy. It can be filled out instead of or in addition to a video recording.

In addition to the video recording and the questionnaire, there are some auxiliary features to simplify the usage. Before using the app for the first time, the user is asked to confirm the privacy policy, which he can view at the same time. Only then the app can be used. To make it easier to get started with the app, the user is also asked if he would like to watch an explanatory video about the app. The privacy policy and the explanatory video can be viewed again at any time via a menu on the home page. Another feature is that the app reminds the user to record videos or fill out questionnaires every day. The user can set any time for the reminders or disable the notifications.

3 Future Work

As mentioned in chapter 2.2 the videos and questionnaires are currently saved locally on the smartphone. The app will be expanded in a further step by uploading the videos and questionnaires to a secure server that the physician can access at any time. This will ensure that clinicians have direct access to the data and can control and adjust the therapy immediately. The biggest challenge here is the encoding and security of the videos, as they contain sensitive patient data. So that only patients that are known to the clinicians have access to the secure server and in order that the patient's data can be clearly assigned, the users of the app will need to log in via a QR-Code, given to them by the doctor.

Since the app has not yet been tested, it is not known whether it actually provides support and improvement in the therapy progress monitoring of movement disorders. Therefore, a survey is planned which has the aim to positively fulfill the following research questions:

- Is the app accepted by patients and therefore suitable for regular use?

- Do the videos have a high quality and bring an advantage for the physician in the monitoring of therapy progress?

- Are the assessments of well-being from the questionnaire related to the progress of therapy and can therefore support progress monitoring?

The survey consists of two parts. First, the participants should use the app on-site and give their feedback via a questionnaire. This is intended to test the understandability, user-friendliness, and attractiveness of the app. In addition, any handling and coding errors can be discovered and adjusted. In the second step, the test participants should use the revised app from home over a longer period of time. For the reason of data privacy, the recorded videos and questionnaires will be stored on the smartphone and the data will receive during a face-to-face meeting at the end. The purpose is to clarify the acceptance of the app. It can be checked whether and how often the app is actually used by the participants by counting the number of saved data. In addition, doctors will provide feedback on the quality of the videos and if they see an advantage in recording them. Hopefully, the doctors can evaluate the therapy progress through the videos, so that the assessments of the well-being from the questionnaire can compare to it and the relation can be analyzed.

4 Conclusion

An app was developed with the aim to improve therapy progress monitoring of movement disorders from home. Monitoring is done on the one hand through guided videos and on the other hand by questionnaires in which patients can assess their general well-being. However, there is still some future work to make. Currently, the data is stored locally on the mobile phone. Instead, the videos and questionnaires should be uploaded to a secure server where the doctors can view them immediately. The challenge here will be data privacy. In addition, a study is planned to test the acceptance and usefulness of the app and the recorded data.

Acknowledgement

The work has been carried out and supervised by the MOVE Group of the Institute of Medical Informatics, Universität zu Lübeck.

Author's Statement

Conflict of interest: Authors state no conflict of interest.

5 References

[1] I. Donaldson, C. D. Marsden and S. Schneider, *Marsden's book of movement disorders*. Oxford University Press, Harlow, 2012.

[2] H. Ben-Pazi, P. Browne, P. Chan, E. Cubo, M. Guttman, A. Hassan, and others, *The promise of telemedicine for movement disorders: an interdisciplinary approach.* Current Neurology and Neuroscience Reports, vol. 18, no. 5, pp. 1–10, 2018.

[3] A. Hassan, E. R. Dorsey, C. G. Goetz, B. R. Bloem, M. Guttman, C. M. Tanner, and others, *Telemedicine use for movement disorders: a global survey.* Telemedicine and e-Health, vol. 24, no. 12, pp. 979–992,2018.

[4] A. Fraint, G. T. Stebbins, G. Pal, and C. L. Comella, *Reliability, feasibility and satisfaction of telemedicine evaluations for cervical dystonia.* Journal of Telemedicine and Telecare, vol. 26, no. 9, pp. 560–567, 2020.

[5] R. Srinivasan, Ragini, H. Ben-Pazi, M. Dekker, E. Cubo, B. Bloem, E. Moukheiber, an others *Telemedicine for hyperkinetic movement disorders.* Tremor and Other Hyperkinetic Movements, vol. 10, 2020.

[6] Emporia, *Smartphone-Studie: Senoiren fühlen sich technisch überfordert.* Presseportal,2018. Available: https://www.presseportal.de/pm/106450/4133442 [last accessed on 2023-02-01].

[7] A. M. Escobar, T. Pringsheim, Z. Goodarzi, and D. Martino, *The prevalence of depression in adult onset idiopathic dystonia: Systematic review and metaanalysis.* Neuroscience & Biobehavioral Reviews, vol. 125, pp. 221–230, 2021.

[8] *Android Studio Dolphin,* 2021.3.1, Google, 2022, https://developer.android.com/studio.

[9] E. Finzi, and E. Wasserman.*Treatment of depression with botulinum toxin A: a case series.* Dermatologic Surgery, vol. 32, no. 5, pp. 645–650, 2006.

[10] A. Hosseini-Sharifabad, S. Naghibzadeh, and V. Hajhashemi, *The effect of lead, restraint stress or their coexposure on the movement disorders incidence in male mice.* Research in pharmaceutical sciences, vol. 14, no. 4, p. 343, 2019.

WASP - Web application supporting SNOMED CT-based postcoordination

Tessa Ohlsen [1], Cora Drenkhahn [2], and Josef Ingenerf [3]

[1] Medical Informatic, University of Lübeck, tessa.ohlsen@student.uni-luebeck.de
[2] IT Center for Clinical Research, University of Lübeck, c.drenkhahn@uni-luebeck.de
[3] Institute for Medical Informatics, University of Lübeck, josef.ingenerf@uni-luebeck.de

Abstract

SNOMED CT with its approximately 350,000 precoordinated expressions, is regarded as an expressive interlingua for computerized medical data. This statement can only considered to be truly valid if SNOMED CT's potential for postcoordination is utilized. There is some hesitation to use postcoordination, partly due to the lack of IT support for creating and processing postcoordinated expressions (PCEs). This research paper aims to show the development of a web application to support the user in the generation of PCEs. A user-friendly interface was designed so that the user is not confronted with the complexity of SNOMED CT Concept Model or the SNOMED CT Compositional Grammar. The implementation was realized by using advanced services of the terminology server Ontoserver based on the Fast Healthcare Interoperability Ressources (FHIR)-standard. A validation with practically used PCEs has shown that it is reliably possible to form both syntactically and semantically correct PCEs using the web application.

1 Introduction

SNOMED CT (SNOMED Clinical Terms) is considered the most expressive terminology in medicine with over 350,000 SNOMED CT concepts. The goal is to provide a machine-usable interlingua to minimize country- and specialty-specific coding problems [1]. Despite the large number of precoordinated and predefined SNOMED CT concepts, not all medical expressions of interest can be accurately coded. An example is "Fracture of left humerus due to an accident" and can not be represented by a precoordinated SNOMED CT concept, because only the SNOMED CT concept *"32121000119107 |Fracture of bone due to accidental fall|"* exists. The information that the fracture is located at the left humerus is missing. One way to avoid inaccurate coding is to use postcoordinated expressions (PCE). Here, multiple precoordinated SNOMED CT concepts are combined into new expressions by using SNOMED CT Compositional Grammar, removing the necessity to provide a precoordinated SNOMED CT expression for each combination of SNOMED CT concepts. This prevents an explosive increase of further new concepts [2, 3]. Instead of just one precoordinated concept the following expression allows to represent the meaning of the mentioned example:

64572001 |Disease| :
{ 363698007 |Finding site| =
719460003 |Bone structure of left humerus|,
116676008 |Associated morphology| =
72704001 |Fracture| },
{ 42752001 |Due to| = 217082002 |Accidental fall| }

The generation of precise PCEs allows to record medical data in a detailed and targeted way. This could lead to an improvement of the quality of data in patient records and databases and given the potential of their computerized processing. The generation of PCEs is quite complex because the rules of the SNOMED CT Compositional Grammar and the SNOMED CT Concept Model have to be considered. For example, some PCEs exist in the Medizinischen Informationsobjekten of the Kassenärztlichen Bundesvereinigung [8]. The majority of these have syntactical issues. This shows support for the generation of PCEs is needed. This research paper aims to show the development of a web application for the generation of syntactically and semantically correct postcoordinated expressions based on SNOMED CT Expression Templates. By using the web application WASP (Web application supporting SNOMED CT-based postcoordination), users avoid being confronted with the complexity of the SNOMED CT Compositional Grammar and SNOMED CT Concept Model.

2 Material and Methods

2.1 SNOMED CT

2.1.1 SNOMED CT Compositional Grammar

The SNOMED CT Compositional Grammar specifies the correct syntax for PCEs. It contains a set of rules that allow the representation of SNOMED CT expressions as strings. The SNOMED CT Compositional Grammar is human-readable as well as machine processable. A PCE can be classified into two components - one or more focus concepts and a refinement (see Fig. 1). A SNOMED CT identifier is required for a focus concept, as well as an optional description. The refinement consists of one or more attribute relationships, which can be ungrouped or grouped (RoleGroup) depending on the definition in the SNOMED CT Concept Model [2, 3].

Therefore contributing in the generation of PCEs, making it an essential component in reaching this paper's main objectives.

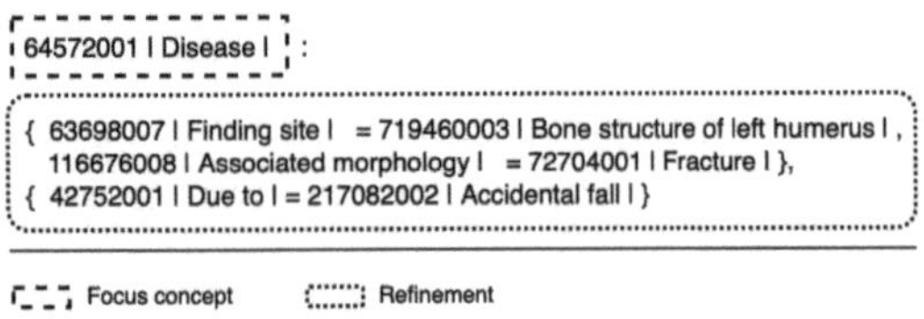

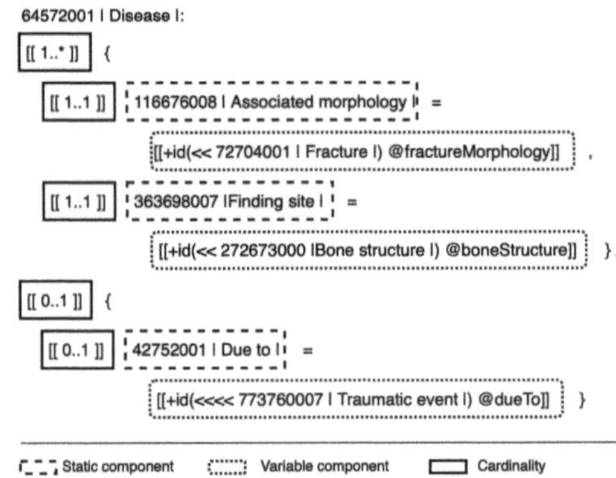

Figure 1: PCEs based on SNOMED CT Compositional Grammar and classified into the two components.

2.1.2 SNOMED CT Concept Model

The SNOMED CT Concept Model contains a set of rules specifying "the types of relationships that are permitted between concepts in particular branches of the hierarchy." [1]. For each SNOMED CT attribute, a domain (subset of source concepts for attribute relationship, mostly SNOMED CT hierarchy) and a range (subset of attribute values for the relationship) is defined. The use of Expression Constraint Language (ECL, a language developed by SNOMED International) expressions specifies which SNOMED CT concepts can be associated with which attributes. This restricts the set of all possible SNOMED CT expressions. The SNOMED CT Concept Model is used to specify an attribute's cardinality and if RoleGroups are required [1, 2]. The Machine Readable Concept Model (MRCM) contains the rules of the SNOMED CT Concept Model in machine-readable form. The MRCM Domain ReferenceSet is one of the four ReferenceSets and contains a template for the generation of SNOMED CT expressions for each domain (predominantly subhierarchies). Figure 2 shows an extract of the domain "Clinical finding". Here, "id" is replaced by a SNOMED CT identifier [2, 4].

The SNOMED CT Concept Model or the MRCM Domain ReferenceSet are mainly used in this research to obtain the allowed attributes and the associated cardinalities and value ranges of a corresponding focus concept.

```
[[+id(<< 404684003 I Clinical finding I)]]:
  [[0..*]] {
    [[0..1]] 363698007 I Finding site I =
      [[+id(<< 442083009 I Anatomical or acquired body structure I)]]
    [[0..1]] 116676008 I Associated morphology I =
      [[+id(<< 49755003 I Morphologically abnormal structure I)]]
    ...
  }
```

Figure 2: Extract of the domain "Clinical finding".

2.1.3 SNOMED CT Expression Templates

The SNOMED CT Expression Templates serve as reusable templates for the definition of similar concepts as well as the creation of PCEs. This allows semantically correct and precise concepts or PCEs used in a particular use case, where SNOMED International provides templates for some use cases. The SNOMED CT Expression Templates are based on the rules of the SNOMED CT Compositional Grammar and the SNOMED CT Concept Model. They contain attributes that are relevant for a specific use case and permitted according to the SNOMED CT Concept Model, as well as an associated value range. The SNOMED CT Expression Templates are structured like fill-in-the-blank texts. They consist of three components - the static components (SNOMED CT attributes), the variable fields (attribute value range or concrete attribute values), and the cardinalities [5]. Fig. 3 shows an extract of a SNOMED CT Expression Template for fractures.

In this research, the SNOMED CT Expression Templates provide a basis for the generation of PCEs on one side, and on the other side they serve as a syntactic template when creating a new template.

Figure 3: SNOMED CT Expression Templates structured like fill-in-the-blank texts.

2.2 HL7 FHIR Standard

FHIR (Fast Healthcare Interoperability Resources) is an international standard in healthcare for medical data exchange between different information systems. FHIR provides, amongst other services, terminology services with corresponding predefined resource types and operations. With the use of these and a terminology server, access to various terminologies, such as SNOMED CT, is enabled.

Table 1 presents the operations that are relevant for this research [6]. The FHIR operations "$expand" and "$lookup" are needed during PCE and template generation. The FHIR operation "$expand" is needed for an ECL request to Ontoserver to get a set of SNOMED CT concepts. Using the FHIR operation "$lookup" the Fully Specified Name of a SNOMED CT concept can be determined. The FHIR operation "$subsumes" is used for the template creation to find relevant SNOMED CT Concept Model constraints for a focus concept.

Table 1: Summary of relevant FHIR operations.

Operation	Definition
$expand	Expanding an implicitly defined ValueSet
$lookup	Look up details about a code
$subsumes	Checking the subsumption relationship between two codes

2.3 Ontoserver

Ontoserver is a terminology server for clinical coding systems, which was developed and provided by the Australian company CSIRO, based on the HL7 FHIR standard. Ontoserver supports and facilitates the work with important coding systems, such as SNOMED CT. A complete implementation of the Expression Constraint Language and Postcoordinated Expressions of SNOMED CT exists for the Ontoserver [7].

3 Results and Discussion

3.1 Web application WASP

WASP is realized based on two interrelated subtasks - the generation of PCEs and the creation of new templates (see Fig. 4). The pipeline for generating a PCE is also shown in Fig. 4 and here the SNOMED CT Compositional Grammar is of particular importance. In addition, Fig. 4 shows the pipeline for the creation of a template. The SNOMED CT Concept Model, the three named FHIR operations and Ontoserver are important components (see section 2). Based on the previously explained components and considerations, WASP was developed with the web development framework Angular and with Spring Boot.

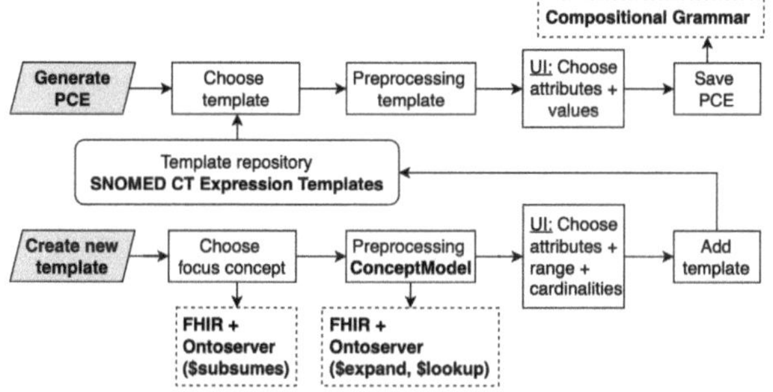

Figure 4: Pipeline of two main functions of WASP.

3.1.1 Generation of a PCE based on a template

Fig. 5 shows a screenshot of WASP to create a PCE based on a template. Initially, a SNOMED CT Expression Template must be selected. This is processed and the user interface is generated. The desired SNOMED CT concepts for the individual attributes can be selected. For each attribute, additional information such as a definition, the value range or possible SNOMED CT concepts are displayed to the user. After checking the entries and cardinalities, the PCE is generated based on the SNOMED CT Composi-

tional Grammar and can be stored in a CodeSystem Supplement.

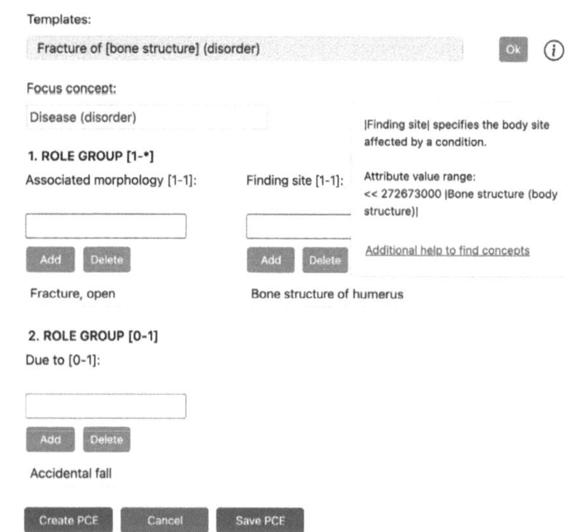

Figure 5: Screenshot of WASP to generate a PCE based on a template.

3.1.2 Template creation

Fig. 6 shows a screenshot of WASP to create a template. To enable flexible coding of arbitrary medical facts, the creation of custom templates is of importance. In the first step, the focus concept for the postcoordinated SNOMED CT expression must be entered into a displayed input field. The correct domain of the SNOMED CT Concept Model is automatically determined by checking the subsumption between the respective SNOMED CT Concept Model domains and the focus concept. Then, the SNOMED CT attributes based on the SNOMED CT Concept Model domain that are relevant for a use case can be selected and the cardinalities can be specified (see "Attribute summary"). The value range of the attribute can be specified (see "Attribute value range"). Furthermore, the user is provided with further information about the attribute, such as definition, cardinalities or value range, in an information window. Further RoleGroups can be created, if they are allowed by the SNOMED CT Concept Model. After checking the inputs and cardinalities, the template is generated and saved.

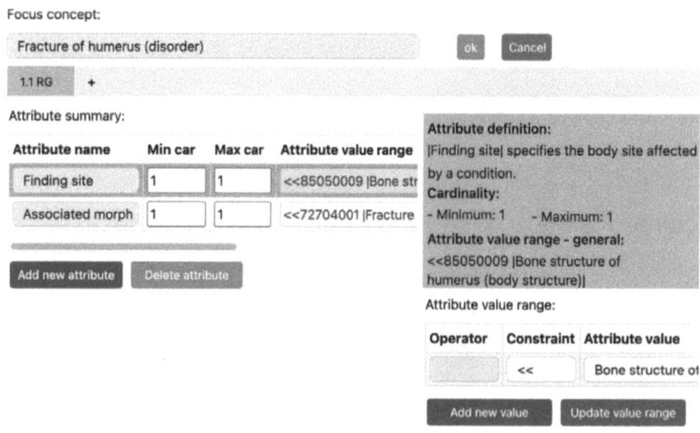

Figure 6: Screenshot of WASP to create a new template.

3.2 Validation using already existing PCEs

To validate the process for generating of PCEs, already existing PCEs are considered. For this purpose 41 PCEs are used, which were defined in the Medizinische Informationsobjekte (MIOs) of the Kassenärztliche Bundesvereinigung (KBV) [8]. First, the 41 PCEs of the MIOs were validated based on the domains of the SNOMED CT Concept Model using FHIR operation "$validate-code" and Ontoserver. The validation revealed that the majority of the PCEs violated SNOMED CT Concept Model rules, such as missing attributes with a minimum cardinality of 1 or incorrect grouping attributes. These peculiarities will be discussed with the KBV in the future and shows the necessity of an application guiding users through the creation of PCEs. For each remaining PCE an appropriate template was constructed in WASP, which were successfully used to recreate the original expressions. All PCEs could be built without rule violations, showing that the developed process can successfully and reliably create templates and PCEs based on templates. Thus, it would be possible to form the syntactically incorrect post-coordinated SNOMED CT expressions from the MIOs without errors using the developed web application WASP.

3.3 Validation of the SNOMED CT Expression Templates

SNOMED International provides over 70 templates. These were evaluated based on the SNOMED CT Concept Model constraints. The evaluation identified that 19 templates violated at least one rule of the SNOMED CT Concept Model. Table 2 lists the various rule violations and their frequencies. SNOMED International was contacted and has confirmed the rule violations and and will fix them.

Table 2: Violations of SNOMED CT Concept Model in SNOMED CT Expression Templates.

Rule violation	Freq.
Specified value range versus SNOMED CT Concept Model value range	11
Missing constraints	6
Incorrect groupings of attributes	6
No longer existing SNOMED CT concepts	4
RoleGroup- versus attribute cardinality	2

4 Conclusion

This paper focused on the development of a web application for the generation of syntactically and semantically correct PCEs, which is based on SNOMED CT Expression Templates. To ensure syntactically and semantically correct PCEs the rules of the SNOMED CT Compositional Grammar as well as the SNOMED CT Concept Model have been considered. Using the MRCM, the FHIR operations as well as the terminology server Ontoserver were essential for a straightforward implementation. It was possible to develop a user interface, which supports the user to generate templates and PCEs. Furthermore, the validation performed with the PCEs of the MIOs showed that it is possible to create arbitrary PCEs syntactically and semantically correct as well as reliable. In the future the web application will be extended to create MRCM-compliant PCEs without templates.

5 Acknowledgement

The work was supervised at the Institute for Medical Informatics Lübeck under the direction of Prof. Dr. Josef Ingenerf. I would like to thank Cora Drenkhahn for providing her expertise on SNOMED CT.

Author's Statement

Conflict of interest: Authors state no conflict of interest.

6 References

[1] SNOMED International. *SNOMED CT Starter Guide. International Health Terminology Standard Development Organisation.* In: International Health Terminology Standard Development Organisation (2019).

[2] J. Ingenerf, C. Drenkhahn. *Referenzterminologie SNOMED CT; Interlingua zur Gewährleistung semantischer Interoperabilität in der Medizin.* Springer Fachmedien Wiesbaden, 2023.

[3] SNOMED International. *SNOMED CT Compositional Grammar Specification and Guide.* In: International Health Terminology Standard Development Organisation (2020).

[4] SNOMED International. *SNOMED CT Machine Readable Concept Model Specification.* In: International Health Terminology Standard Development Organisation (2017).

[5] SNOMED International. *Template Syntax DRAFT Specification.* In: International Health Terminology Standard Development Organisation (2017).

[6] CSIRO. *FHIR API - Ontoserver.* Available: https://ontoserver.csiro.au/docs/5.0/api-fhir.html [last accessed on 2022-12-18].

[7] A. Metke-Jimenez, J. Steel, D. Hansen, M. Lawley. *Ontoserver: a syndicated terminology server.* In: Journal of Biomedical Semantics 15, pp.9—24, 2018.

[8] KBV. *KBV-BASIS-PROFILE.* Available: https://mio.kbv.de/display/BASE1X0/KBV-Basis-Profile [last accessed on 2022-12-18].

9

Medical Imaging

Experimental Validation of a software Tool used for determining the Pulse Wave speed in blood Vessels from 2D MRI data

Tessema Tameru Dominikos[1], Annika Sommer[2], Constantin Schareck[4], Michael Scharfschwerdt[3], Maren Balks[4], Christian Damiani[5]

[1] Biomedical Engineering, Luebeck University of Applied Sciences, tessema.tameru.dominikos@stud.th-luebeck.de
[2] MSGT Lab, Luebeck University of Applied Sciences
[3] Klinik für Radiologie und Nuklearmedizin, UKSH, Lübeck
[4] Klinik für Herz- und thorakale Gefäßchirurgie, UKSH, Lübeck
[5] MSGT Lab, Luebeck University of Applied Sciences, christian.damiani@th-luebeck.de (corresponding author)

Abstract

Arteriosclerosis is a symptomless disorder that is primarily responsible for cardiovascular diseases. There is currently no standardized, clinically used way to identify it. The condition of an artery may be determined by measuring the pulse wave velocity (PWV), a biomarker that is closely related to arterial stiffness. A software was developed at the University Hospital of Luebeck to calculate the PWV using MRI data. Its accuracy needs to be verified using more direct methods. In this work, the accuracy of this software was verified using an in-vitro model. An experimental set-up was built using a pulse-generating pump and a simplified arterial model. The PWV was determined using two different kinds of pressure sensors and then compared to the one obtained from 2D flow-MRI data. This led to an average PWV of 23,62 m/s with the pressure sensors and 16,00 m/s from the MRI data. The discrepancy of results suggests that the data acquisition for the MRI should be improved in order to get reliable PWV values.

1 Introduction

Cardiovascular diseases are the leading cause of mortality globally. Arteriosclerosis is a symptomless disorder and one of the major risk factors responsible for the disease [1]. It is a degenerative disease with hardening or thickening of arterial walls. Early identification of atherosclerosis is crucial to minimize long-term effects and start early treatment. Since the pulse wave from the heartbeat travels through the arteries in accordance with the elasticity of the wall, the Pulse Wave Velocity (PWV) is used as a biomarker in clinical settings to identify the disease [2]. The clinical gold standard for PWV determination in the aorta is invasive pressure catheter measurement. This method offers high temporal resolution, but it is invasive. Magnetic resonance imaging (MRI) can also be used to obtain the PWV non-invasively. Software to calculate PWV using 2D and 4D MRI was developed in 2018 at Lübeck University Hospital. Previous tests have demonstrated that the accuracy of the data and software needs further verification given the complicated measurement setup and the chosen measurement technique. This study attempts to improve knowledge of the physical processes in wave propagation and fluid flow by simulating a worst-case situation regarding PWV level while preventing artifacts and reflections that could affect the software or the sensors.

A previous work in the literature [3] gives an insight into the methods to determine arterial stiffness and the PWV. The relation between the PWV and arterial compliance is defined by the Bramwell-Hill equation [3]:

$$PWV = \sqrt{\frac{A}{\rho} \cdot \frac{\partial P}{\partial A}} = \sqrt{\frac{1}{\rho D}} \qquad (1)$$

$$where,\ D = \frac{\partial A}{A \partial P} \qquad (2)$$

where A represents the lumen area, ρ the fluid density, ∂A the lumen area change, and ∂P the pressure change, and D is arterial compliance. In the resting state, the blood pressure lies between 80 and 120 mmHg. A decrease in arterial compliance results in an increase in peak pressure values and the PWV. For the arteries, a nonlinear relation between pressure and area is observed, so that PWV is dependent on the operating pressure [3]. Furthermore, measuring the PWV instead of the compliance over a segment gives the average stiffness and does not require a simultaneous pressure and area measurement. As an approximation, the PWV for the physiological range is calculated by

$$PWV = \frac{\Delta L}{\Delta t} \qquad (3)$$

where ΔL is the distance between the pressure sensors and Δt the transit time of the arterial pulse. The range of PWV for healthy patients lies between 6 and 12 m/s [3]. The governing equations of fluid mechanics are the Navier-Stokes equations in their differential form. This research is interested in the pressure curve profile, which is represented by the control volume approach.

2 Material and Methods

2.1 Experimental setup

The experimental setup was realized with a simplified, straight, uniform silicone tube representing the aortic arc (see Table 1) and a pump system. A model closer to the physiological conditions was not used for this first set of measurements. The aim was to increase understanding of physical processes in wave propagation and fluid flow by modeling a worst-case scenario for PWV level while avoiding artifacts and reflections that might influence the software or sensors. The modulus of elasticity shown in Table 1 was obtained by performing tensile tests on the material of the silicone hose.

Table 1: Specifications of the silicone hose for length, inner diameter, outer diameter, shore strength and elastic modulus

Length	Inner	Outer	Shore strength	E
997 cm	2 cm	2.4 cm	A60°+/-5°	$2.7*10^7 \frac{dyn}{cm^2}$

The setup is shown in Fig.1. The custom-made pump was built by the heart surgery department at the University Hospital Lübeck. The pulses are generated by a piston pump with cam drive (1) where the movement of the piston is transferred to a latex membrane (4). The flow volume can be adjusted via the lever ratio between the cam disk and the piston (2). During the measurements, a stroke volume of 80 ml with a frequency of 60 bpm was used. The atrial pressure load is modeled by an atrial reservoir (5). A chamber filled with air at the outlet of the pump represents the ventricular resistance. The generated pulse is transmitted via a 4 m long rigid tube (6) connected to the aortic model to maintain sufficient distance between the MRI device and the pump metallic objects. The model, including the connection between the model and the rigid tube, was inside a Plexiglas box to prevent possible water leakage from reaching the MRI device. The model was connected to a water column (9), with a height of 80 cm to model a constant diastolic pressure of 59 mmHg. In addition, the outlet system is represented by a non-linear resistance element and an adjustable air compliance chamber.

2.2 Experimental Pressure Measurements

WIKA Pressure Transducer Type S-11, WIKA Alexander Wiegand SE & Co. KG, Germany, and Millar Microtip Catheter Pressure Transducer, Millar Instruments, Inc., USA, are used individually to take pressure measurements at the locations denoted as A and B in Fig. 1. The Wika S-11 sensors are pressure transducers that determine pressure as a voltage-dependent variable with the help of a flush

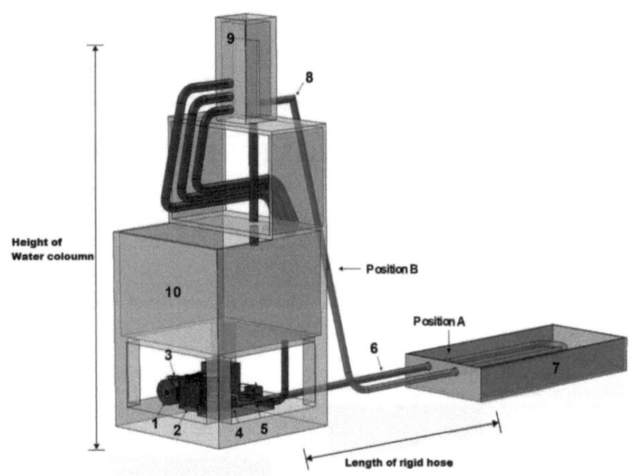

Figure 1: The set-up for Experimental and MRI measurement. Labels indicating 1 cam, 2 device for adjusting the lever ratio, 3 lever, 4 latex membrane, 5 atrial reservoir, 6 rigid tube (green) with length 4m, 7 Plexiglas box with aortic model (shown in light blue), 8 connecting tube to pump (green), 9 water column, 10 water reservoir.

diaphragm. These sensors were inserted into the setup via a 3D-printed hard connector, and recorded data was analyzed with Cassy Lab 2 software. On the other hand, the ultra-miniature sensors located at the distal end of Millar pressure catheters generate an electrical signal proportional to the magnitude of the perceived pressure. The signals from the sensors were fed into a National Instruments USB-6259 via a Transducer Control Unit Model TC-510, and the pressure values were recorded using Leonard MX software, University of Lübeck, Germany. The measurements were evaluated with a self-written Julia notebook. The pressure measurement was repeated five times with a temporal resolution of 10 kHz for both sensor types, and the mean values were calculated.

2.3 MRI Measurements

The MRI measurements were carried out on the 3T Siemens MRI device at UKSH. After attaching the model to the pump, 18 l of 20°C water was poured into the reservoir, and 50 ml of Gadovist® contrast medium was injected. Two coils mounted on top of the Plexiglas box defined the recording region. At the start of each flow pulse, the light barrier recorded the movement of the cam in the pump and sent a pulse (equivalent to a QRS complex). The trigger signal was then read into the MRI machine's software as an external signal, setting the start for the acquisition time of the MRI. The sagittal, transversal, and coronal layers were acquired, and parameters were selected separately for each slice. The 2D flow MRI data was then analyzed using a Matlab-based PWV MRI software tool. Four distinct algorithms were used to calculate the temporal change: peak-to-peak (P2P), upstroke-to-upstroke (U2U), foot-to-foot (F2F), and cross-correlation (CC).

3 Results and Discussion

3.1 PWV from Pressure Measurements

The pressure curves obtained from the Wika sensors are shown in Fig. 2. The maximum pressure values were 189 mmHg and 116 mmHg at sensors 1 and 2, respectively. The maximum deviation at sensors 1 and 2 was 8.2 mmHg and 3.4 mmHg respectively. The P2P and CC methods resulted in a PWV of 2555 cm/s and 2337 cm/s, respectively. The values differ by 218 cm/s, or 8.53 %, from one another.

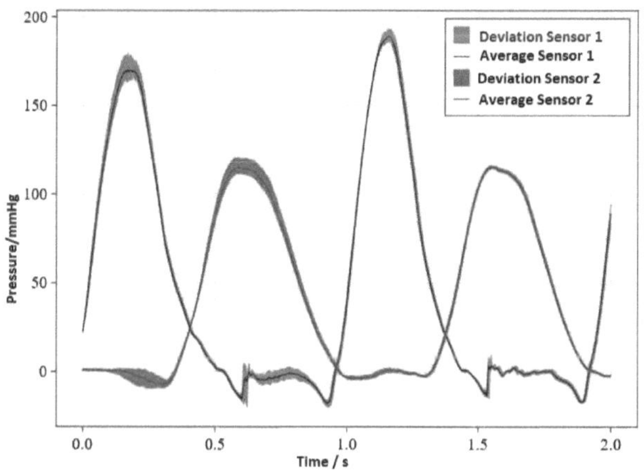

Figure 2: Pressure curves measured with WIKA sensors, displaying pressure in mmHg plotted against time in seconds.

The resulting pressure curves for the experiment carried out with Millar sensors are presented in Fig. 3. The pressure

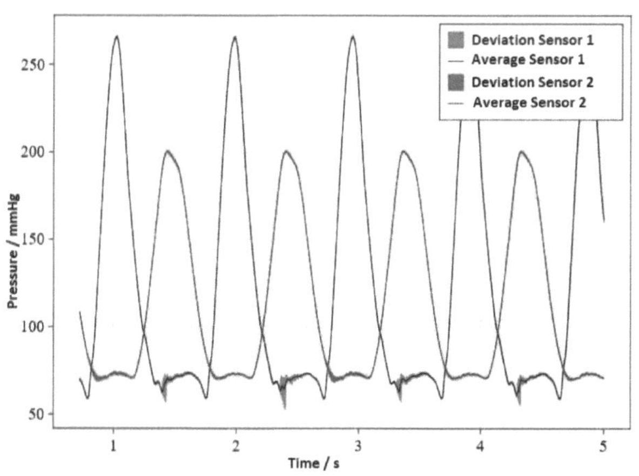

Figure 3: Pressure curves measured with Millar sensors, showing pressure in mmHg plotted against time in seconds.

values recorded at their maximums were 266 mmHg and 201 mmHg at sensors 1 and 2, respectively. The maximum deviation of the pressure values at sensors 1 and 2 were 13.9 mmHg and 2.7 mmHg, respectively. The mean PWV from the P2P and CC methods resulted in 2360 cm/s and 2362 cm/s, respectively.

The choice of evaluation method for the transit time should be made individually for each pressure curve according to

the spatial distance, broadening of the peak, and identifiable local minima. The measurement accuracy of the WIKA sensors is ±0.5 % (22.5 mmHg) in the range of 0 mmHg to 4500 mmHg. For the millar sensor, it is reduced to 1.75 mmHg, with an accuracy of ±0.5 % for a range of -50 to +300 mmHg. As a result, the Millar sensors provide more accurate measurements. As described in [4], CC method is better when there is a large spatial distance between the inlet and outlet sensors. Therefore, the CC method should be considered to determine the PWV. WIKA sensors measured pressure relative to hydrostatic pressure. The maximum deviation between the WIKA and Millar sensors was 2.29% after subtracting the offset of 70.9 mmHg from the Millar sensor. All measurements at the inlet sensors show a sudden increase in pressure with a steeper curve at the start of the pulse cycle, possibly due to the pump's mechanical flap suddenly closing. This could cause reflections, which would explain the high pressure deviations from the mean value in the inlet sensors.

3.2 MRI Measurement Results

Fig. 4 and 5 show examples of the 2D flow MRI measurements evaluated with the PWV MRI software. First, the ROI was determined at two separate points on the vessel, and based on that, the distance could be determined.

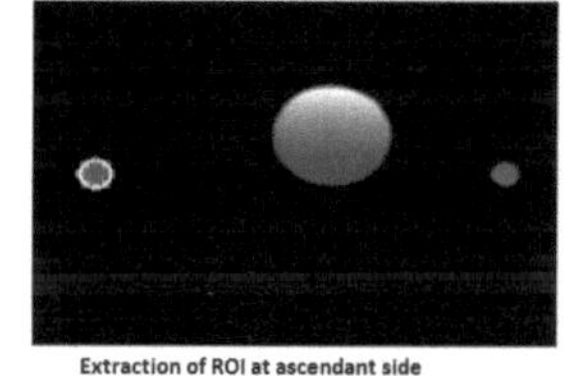

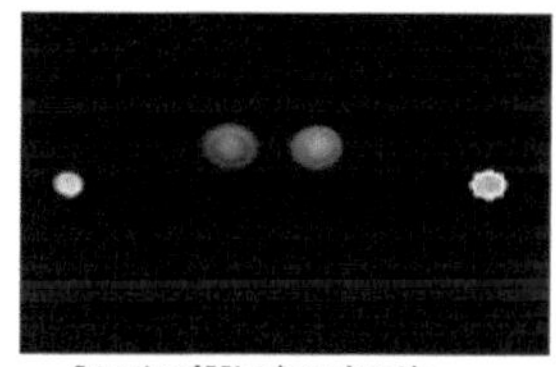

Figure 4: Representation of the ROI, on the left the inlet side and on the right the outlet side.

In Fig. 5, the nodal points represent the starting point for spline interpolation. The folding artifacts due to the edge of the coil have no effect on the accuracy of the results since only the flow in the center of the recording area is needed for the PWV MRI software, and only the arch section is used to determine the path length. Fig. 6 shows the graphical results of the four methods used for determining the temporal shift of the flow rate curve. The mean PWVs for the evaluation methods P2P, F2F, U2U, and CC were 1850 cm/s, 1600 cm/s, 2510 cm/s, and 1912 cm/s, respectively. A comparison of the results for the four evaluation methods shows a maximum deviation of 910 cm/s from each other. The U2U approach showed a considerable variance when compared to the other methods; nonetheless, it is the only value that is closer to the sensor measurements. As a result, this value may be the most accurate. Nevertheless, this requires more validation. The results of the other methods are comparable to the findings in Gaddum, et al. [4], in terms of the influence of noise, temporal resolution, and waveform similarity. In all of their evaluations, the transit time was overestimated with the F2F method. The CC method

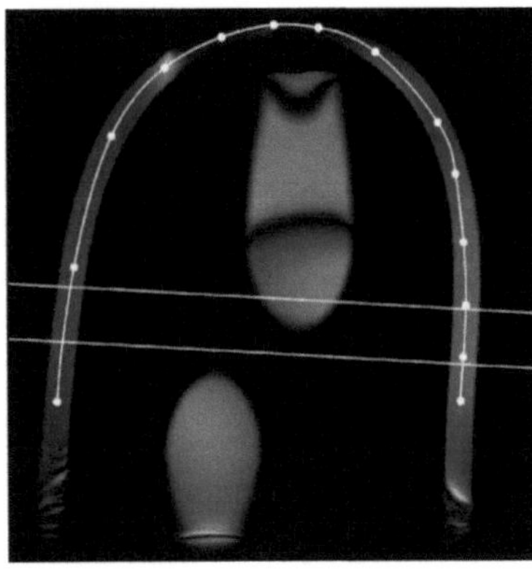

Figure 5: Representation of the extracted path length from evaluation.

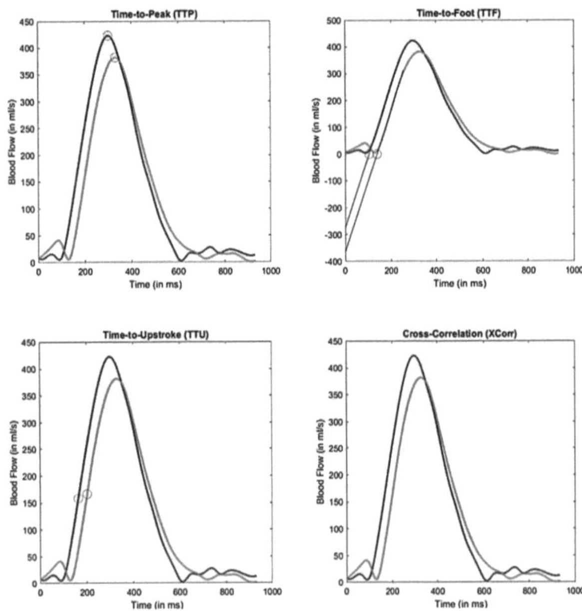

Figure 6: Results of the time shift of evaluation 1, showing the P2P (top left), F2F (top right), U2U (bottom left) and CC (bottom right) methods.

showed the lowest sensitivity in terms of noise and temporal resolution. However, the transit time in the CC method was always underestimated when the spacing of the waveforms increased or the similarity of the waveforms decreased [4]. These findings are also reflected in our results. As it can be seen in Fig. 6, there is a broadening of the peak at the outlet, which would account for the 332 cm/s difference between the P2P evaluations. In the F2F method, the lowest PWV is present due to the overestimated running time. The PWV with the CC method is larger compared to the P2P and F2F methods, which may be due to an underestimation of the transit time caused by broadening of the peaks.

One reason for the high deviations in the PWV-MRI software in comparison to the pressure measurements shown in Fig. 2 and 3 could be that the PWV was calculated for a distance of 56.5 cm on average, whereas 997 cm was used for the setup with pressure sensors. The large difference in PWV between the tested setups and a non-pathological

healthy person (6–12 m/s) can be explained by the fact that there is a big elasticity difference between the actual aorta and the simplified model, as we only used a straight silicon tube to model a worst-case scenario for PWV level while avoiding artifacts and reflections that might influence the software or sensors. In general, the PWV values determined in both cases lie within the range indicated as pathological [5].

4 Conclusion

Future measurements should focus on further verifying why the software cannot render the right PWV values. The data acquisition with the MRI and evaluation methods need further validation, as only the U2U approach showed value that was closer to the sensor measurements while having a considerable variance when compared to the other evaluation methods. This way further measurements need to performed to confirm the software can distinguish between a pathological and a non-pathological aorta. Since the patient's heart rate is not constant over the duration of the measurement period, the relationship between variable heart rate and possible errors due to imprecise recording times should also be investigated.

Acknowledgement

The work has been carried out at MSGT Lab, Luebeck University of Applied Sciences and supervised by Dr. Christian Damiani. Special thanks to UKSH for their collaboration.

Author's Statement

Conflict of interest: The authors state there is no conflict of interest.

5 References

[1] Cardiovascular diseases. Available: https://www.who.int/health-topics/cardiovascular-diseases [Last accessed on 2022-11-05].

[2] P. Salvi and et al., *Comparative study of methodologies for pulse wave velocity estimation*. J Hum Hypertens, vol. 22, no. 10, pp. 669–677, Oct. 2008.

[3] P. Segers, E. R. Rietzschel and J. A. Chirinos, *How to Measure Arterial Stiffness in Humans*. ATVB, vol. 40, no. 5, pp. 1034–1043, May 2020.

[4] N. R. Gaddum and et al., *A technical assessment of pulse wave velocity algorithms applied to non-invasive arterial waveforms*. Annals of biomedical engineering, vol. 41, pp. 2617-2629, 2013.

[5] T. Mengden, M. Hausberg and C. Heiss, *Arterial stiffness - causes and consequences*. Cardiologist, vol. 10, pp. 38-46, 2016.

Colon Segmentation and Centerline Estimation in Abdominal CT Scans

Harish Kurla Shankarareddy [1], Marian Himstedt [2]

[1] Robotics and Autonomous Systems, Universität zu Lübeck, harish.kurlashankarareddy@student.uni-luebeck.de
[2] Medical Informatics, Universität zu Lübeck, marian.himstedt@student.uni-luebeck.de

Abstract

In this paper, we present a pipeline for segmenting the colon and determining its centerline from abdominal CT scans. Firstly, segmentation is performed using the 3D-slicer application using the Grow from Seeds algorithm. For centerline extraction, initially, Thinning-based skeletonization is applied to get an approximated centerline with branches. The colon is a tube-like structure, and a single centerline without branches is expected for safe navigation; hence, a graph-based approach is used to discard undesirable branches to obtain a single centerline. Further, a B-spline based smoothing algorithm is implemented to obtain a smooth, continuous centerline. The proposed method was validated using several segments of colon data and different levels of segmentation.

1   Introduction

The centerline must be situated in the center of the colon. This is particularly beneficial during medical procedures such as biopsy or endoscopic interventions, where precision is of the utmost importance. Colon segmentation allows for the detection of specific areas of the colon that may be infected with disease, such as polyps or tumors. This information can be used by the surgeon to plan any necessary treatments and to guide themselves throughout the procedure. The colonoscope's centerline, which is the path taken by the scope's tip during the examination, is used as a reference to create synthetic views of the colon while navigating. This centerline can be estimated from real colonoscopy movies and used to simulate the movement of a virtual colonoscope through a 3D model of the colon using image processing techniques. In addition, centerline estimation enables the construction of realistic and anatomically accurate virtual environments for training and assessing endoscopic navigation systems, making it a crucial step in the automatic generation of synthetic colonoscopy videos for domain randomization [1].

Endoscopic navigation systems can be trained and tested in a controlled and realistic environment by using synthetic colonoscopy movies with a known centerline. When applied to real-world scenarios, this can lead to improved system performance and safety [2]. Furthermore, randomizing the textures of the virtual environment can help to improve the generalization of the taught system. As a result, we can use centerline estimation to create a variety of synthetic films that mimic real-world situations. Virtual colonoscopy (VC) is a diagnostic technique that allows for the creation of three-dimensional images of the colon and rectum using information obtained from appropriate imaging modalities, most commonly spiral computed tomography (CT). The procedure is also known as a CT colonoscopy or CT colonography when a CT scanner is used. The VC's minimal invasiveness, increased patient compliance, and value for colorectal cancer screening are among the primary advantages that justify its wider use in medical practice [3].

Thinning based method convert an image into a thin, skeletal representation of an object and the centerline is determined from this representation. Active contour based techniques utilize a flexible model, such as a snake or level set to evolve and fit the object's contours in the image with the centerline estimated as the center of the contour. Methods utilizing distance transforms which gives each voxel a distance value depending on how close it is to the nearest background voxel. The centerline is determined by finding the shortest route between its start and end points. Deep neural networks are used in machine learning to estimate the centerline from an image. For training this approach requires a lot of labeled data. Centerline estimation is required during a colonoscopy in order to precisely maneuver the colonoscope and comprehend the shape and structure of the colon. The path taken by the tip of the colonoscope during the examination or the centerline of the colonoscope, provides important details about the structure of the colon and can aid in directing the surgeon's movements throughout the surgery.

In the case of a colon image centerline estimation is critical for evaluating colonic haustra, measuring the colonic lumen and detecting any abnormalities.

The CT image colon segmentation process is carried out in a 3D slicer and centerline estimation is then performed on the segmented colon image. The extracted centerline can be used for virtual colonoscopy and domain randomization (Figure. 1).

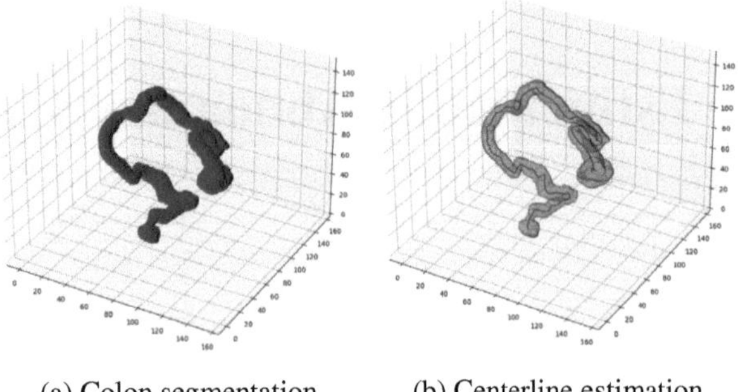

(a) Colon segmentation   (b) Centerline estimation

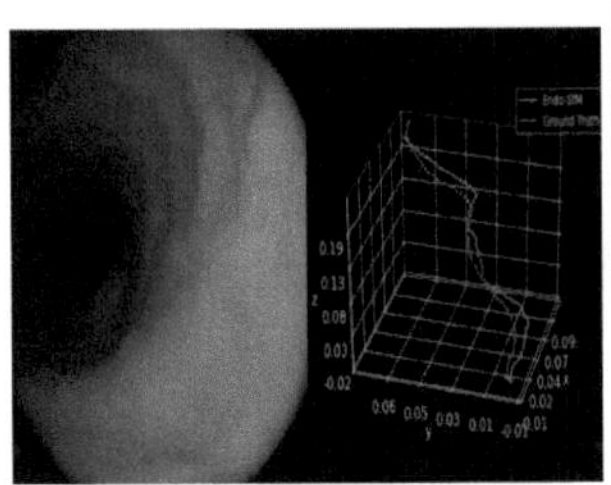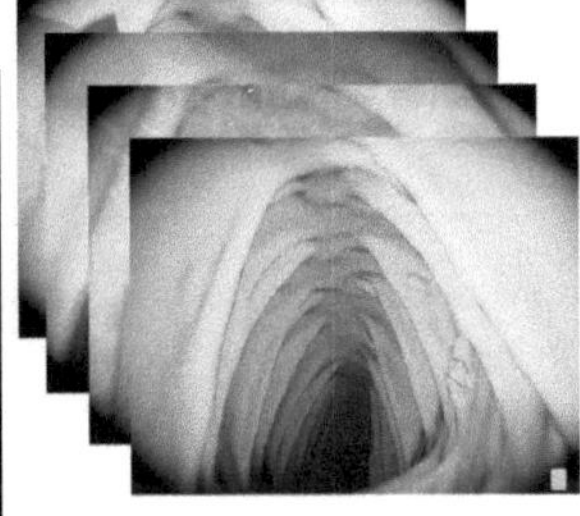

(c) Robotic capsule endoscopy (d) VC, domain randomization

Figure 1: Illustrating a) colon segmentation is visualized in matplotlib, b) centerline estimation for the segmented colon, c) centerline application for robotic capsule endoscopy [4] and other centerline application d) virtual colonoscopy and domain randomization [1].

2 Material and Methods

In this section the whole pipeline of our approach is introduced as follows:

1. Segmentation

2. Centerline Esitimation

2.1 Segmentation

The CT colonography is retrieved from The Cancer Imaging Archive (TCIA) and imported in 3D slicer for segmentation. The segment editor in 3D slicer software offers quick, thorough, and simple manual and semi-automated segmentation procedures [5]. For this work we use semi-automated procedures such as threshold and Grow from Seeds. The Threshold option allows the user to specify a threshold range and Grow from Seeds is a technique for segmenting medical images that makes use of a modified Grow Cut algorithm. The original Grow Cut algorithm is a pixel-based interactive image segmentation technique that divides an image into foreground and background regions using a graph-cut method. By adopting a quick and effective implementation of graph cuts, the Fast Grow Cut approach outperforms the original algorithm and enables real-time segmentation of big medical images [6]. The method's main idea is to represent the image as a graph, with each voxel (3D pixel) acting as a node and the edges between the voxels weighted by the similarity of their intensities. The algorithm begins by populating the graph with a set of labeled

voxels that correspond to the user's seed points. These seed points can be chosen by hand or obtained during a pre-processing step. The algorithm then propagates the labels from the seed points to the neighboring voxels iteratively. The algorithm examines the neighboring voxels of the current set of labeled voxels in each iteration and assigns the label with the highest probability to each of the voxels. When the voxel labels no longer change or when the maximum number of iterations is reached, the algorithm terminates. It also has a user-interaction capability that enables the user to manually modify the segmentation results. In the end smoothing process can be performed to achieve a smooth segment, with one method being the Gaussian technique which eliminates all fine details. Although excessive smoothing is possible it results in a reduction of the segment size and therefore should only be applied to specific segments.

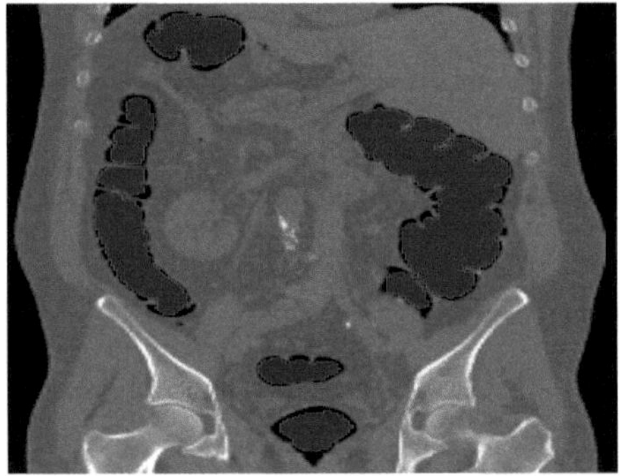

Figure 2: Colon segmentation in 3D slicer.

2.2 Centerline Estimation

Once volumetric segmented data is obtained from 3D slicer as mentioned in Section 2.1, the idea is to estimate centerline in segmented colon. As discussed in Section 1 there are several approaches implemented so far over the years, we use Thinning-based technique to estimate centerline. The function *skimage.morphology.skeletonize3d()* [1] is used for skeletonization, which is a simplified version of the data that preserves its topology. The thinning algorithm is used based on the Zhang-Suen thinning technique [7], which involves iteratively eliminating pixels from the image based on the values of their neighbors. The method returns the skeletonized version of the 3D binary data. That skeletonized image is then transformed into a graph. From the graph shortest path obtained between the start and end point by using shortest path technique . This path represents the centerline of the object. Finally, by using cubic B-splines to approximate the skeleton, we construct a smooth approximation of the centerline. The process is carried out as follows.

1) First, a colon segment image that has been skeletonized by using *skimage.morphology.skeletonize3d()*.

2) consequently the skeletonized image is converted into a

---

[1] https://scikit-image.org/

graph using *sknw* [2] [8]. $G = (V, E)$ is the image's mathematical representation as a graph (G), with each voxel acting as a node (V) and edges (E) connecting neighboring voxels.

3) To make our centerline estimation process automatic, while finding shortest path [3] for G start point and end point is needed, in this approach we assumed start point as first point in the G and last point as end point.

4) The centerline obtained through graph search is a piece wise path consisting of multiple voxels, which is not ideal for navigation purposes. To make it suitable, smoothing techniques are applied to make the path smoother. In this work we use cubic B-splines to achieve smooth centerline [9].

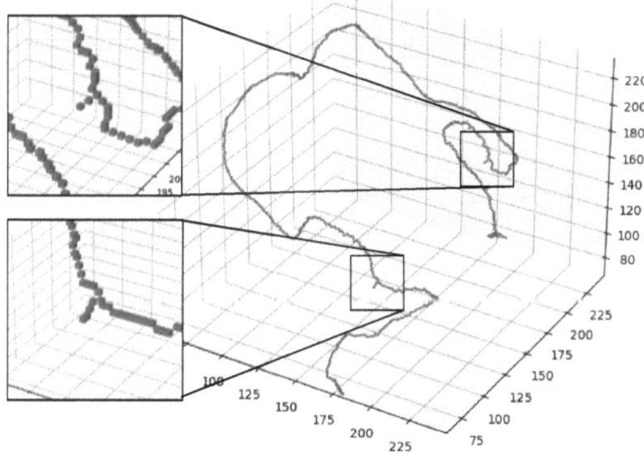

Figure 3: Centerline with branches is the result of skeletonized method alone.

When the skeletonization is alone performed on colon segment, a centerline with small branches is produced(Figure. 3).

When three processes i.e, skeletonization, graph search algorithm and cubic B-splines approximation are together performed on colon segmented image resulting centerline is free from branches [10] (Figure. 4).

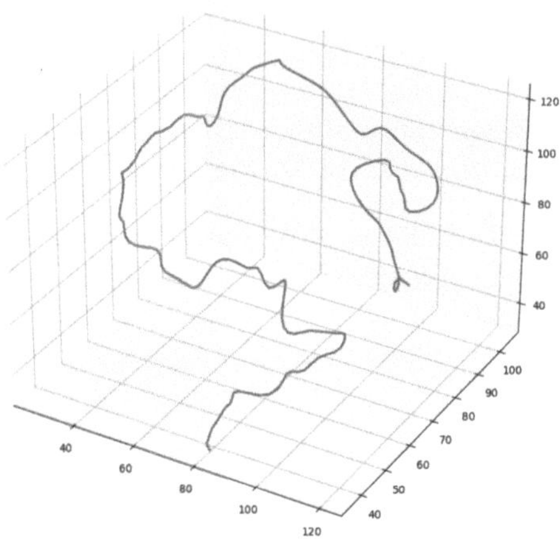

Figure 4: Centerline without branches.

---

[2] https://github.com/Image-Py/sknw
[3] https://github.com/networkx/networkx

3   Results and Discussion

The centerline without branches offers a reliable and effective means of navigation through the colon, making it an essential tool for safe and precise medical procedures. With our centerline estimation method undesired branches can be removed, this enables medical practitioners to precisely guide instruments or devices reducing the risk of damage to surrounding tissue and improving overall procedure accuracy. The method qualitatively evaluated using various image scales and different levels of segmentation smoothness. The method works well with providing start and end points as well as without start and end points.

We compared the runtimes of segmented colon image (307, 307, 301) and segmented colon image after downscaling (154, 154, 150) in spyder. The former had a runtime of 4819.80 ms and the latter had a runtime of 423.58 ms.

Our proposed method was found to produce better results when applied to well-segmented and smooth colon images (Figure.5a and Figure.5b). However, when tested on images with poor segmentation and roughness, the results were less accurate (Figure.5c and Figure.5d).

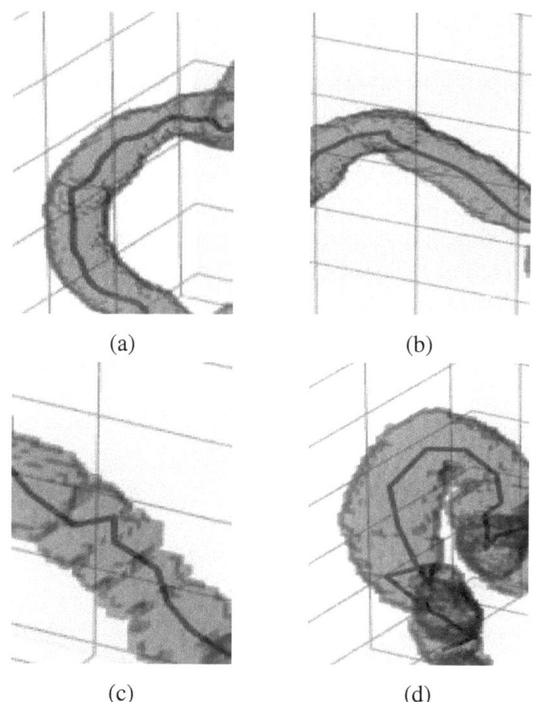

Figure 5: a) and b) Centerline estimation in segmented image section after performing smoothing process, c) and d) Centerline estimation in segmented image section before performing smoothing process and in one more case.

We have tried another approach, first an image of a colon segment that has been skeletonized using the *skimage.morphology.skeletonize3d()* function. After that shortest path estimated by using *dijkstra3d* [4] for this we have provided start and end points. Cubic B-splines are used for that path in order to obtain a smooth centerline. The resulted centerline is smooth as shown in (Figure. 6).

---

[4] https://pypi.org/project/dijkstra3d/

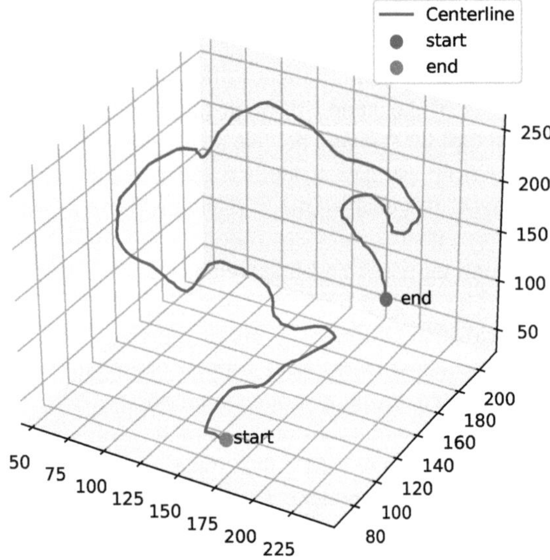

Figure 6: Centerline with source and target using proposed method.

4   Conclusion and Future Works

This paper presents a pipeline for segmenting the colon and finding its centerline from abdominal CT scans. The process involves using the 3D-slicer application and the Grow from Seeds algorithm for segmentation, followed by Thinning-based skeletonization and a graph-based approach to extract a centerline. For a smooth and continuous centerline we used a B-spline based algorithm. In Virtual colonoscopy and Domain Randomization centerline is hugely significant. In the future, we plan to build a learning-based pipeline that will automatically segment and estimate centerlines from abdominal CT scans.

Acknowledgement

The work has been carried out at Institute of Medical Informatics, Universität zu Lübeck.

Author's Statement

Conflict of interest: Authors state no conflict of interest.

5   References

[1] A. D. Jagtap, M. Heinrich, and M. Himstedt, "Automatic generation of synthetic colonoscopy videos for domain randomization," 2022. [Online]. Available: https://arxiv.org/abs/2205.10368

[2] A. Pore, M. Finocchiaro, D. Dall'Alba, A. Hernansanz, G. Ciuti, A. Arezzo, A. Menciassi, A. Casals, and P. Fiorini, "Colonoscopy navigation using end-to-end deep visuomotor control: A user study," in *2022 IEEE/RSJ International Conference on Intelligent Robots and Systems (IROS)*, 2022, pp. 9582–9588.

[3] A. Skalski, M. Socha, T. Zielinski, and M. Duplaga, "Virtual colonoscopy - technical aspects," in *Colonoscopy*, P. Miskovitz, Ed. Rijeka: IntechOpen, 2011, ch. 17. [Online]. Available: https://doi.org/10.5772/19329

[4] K. B. Ozyoruk, G. I. Gokceler, G. Coskun, K. Incetan, Y. Almalioglu, F. Mahmood, E. Curto, L. Perdigoto, M. Oliveira, H. Sahin, H. Araujo, H. Alexandrino, N. J. Durr, H. B. Gilbert, and M. Turan, "Endoslam dataset and an unsupervised monocular visual odometry and depth estimation approach for endoscopic videos: Endo-sfmlearner," 2020. [Online]. Available: https://arxiv.org/abs/2006.16670

[5] C. Pinter, A. Lasso, and G. Fichtinger, "Polymorph segmentation representation for medical image computing," *Computer Methods and Programs in Biomedicine*, vol. 171, pp. 19–26, 2019. [Online]. Available: https://www.sciencedirect.com/science/article/pii/S0169260718313038

[6] L. Zhu, I. Kolesov, Y. Gao, R. Kikinis, and A. R. Tannenbaum, "An effective interactive medical image segmentation method using fast growcut," 2014.

[7] T. Y. Zhang and C. Y. Suen, "A fast parallel algorithm for thinning digital patterns," *Communications of the ACM*, vol. 27, no. 3, pp. 236–239, 1984.

[8] A. Wang, X. Yan, and Z. Wei, "ImagePy: an open-source, Python-based and platform-independent software package for bioimage analysis," *Bioinformatics*, vol. 34, no. 18, pp. 3238–3240, 04 2018. [Online]. Available: https://doi.org/10.1093/bioinformatics/bty313

[9] A. Ravankar, A. Ravankar, Y. Kobayashi, Y. Hoshino, and C.-C. Peng, "Path smoothing techniques in robot navigation: State-of-the-art, current and future challenges," *Sensors*, vol. 18, p. 3170, 09 2018.

[10] Y. Ge, D. R. Stelts, J. Wang, and D. J. Vining, "Computing the centerline of a colon: a robust and efficient method based on 3D skeletons," *J Comput Assist Tomogr*, vol. 23, no. 5, pp. 786–794, Sep. 1999.

Classification of Prostate Cancer in 3D Magnetic Resonance Imaging Data based on Convolutional Neural Networks

Malte Rippa [1], Ruben Schulze [2], and Marian Himstedt [3]

[1] Medical Informatics, Universität zu Lübeck, malte.rippa@student.uni-luebeck.de
[2] FUSE-AI GmbH, ruben.schulze@fuse-ai.de
[3] Institute of Medical Informatics, Universität zu Lübeck, marian.himstedt@imi.uni-luebeck.de

Abstract

Prostate cancer is a commonly diagnosed cancerous disease among men world-wide. Even with modern technology such as multi-parametric magnetic resonance tomography and guided biopsies, the process for diagnosing prostate cancer remains time consuming and requires highly trained professionals. In this paper, different convolutional neural networks (CNN) are evaluated on their ability to reliably classify whether an MRI sequence contains malignant lesions. Implementations of a ResNet, a ConvNet and a ConvNeXt for 3D image data are trained and evaluated. The best result was achieved by a ResNet3D with an initial learning rate of $8e{-}6$, trained over 14 epochs. It yields an average precision score of 0.4583 and AUC ROC score of 0.6214. This implies that it is a non-trivial task to obtain a reliable classifier with a CNN backbone in this setting. Further experiments are necessary to find a classifier with satisfactory performance.

1 Introduction

With 1,276,106 newly diagnosed cases world-wide in 2018, prostate carcinomas (PCa) are the second most frequently diagnosed cancer disease and account for 3.8% of all deaths related to cancerous diseases among men [1]. The methods for PCa diagnosis are constantly improving and have reached a new pinnacle with the introduction of multi-parametric magnetic resonance imaging (mpMRI). mpMRI describes the usage of multiple imaging sequences such as T2-weighted (T2W), diffusion weighted image (DWI), dynamic contrast enhanced (DCE) and apparent diffusion coefficient (ADC) sequences. Every sequence reveals different characteristics of the abdominal tissue, which allows a broad assessment of the prostate [4]. However, the analysis of mpMRI sequences for PCa diagnosis remains a time consuming task and requires further assessment of the severity and clinical significance of the identified lesion(s) e.g. by conducting biopsies. In the current state of the art in medical image processing, neural networks have been shown to provide reliable predictions about the clinical significance of lesions on different types of images [2]. It was shown that a convolutional neural network (CNN) can predict the Gleason grade (see Sec. 2.2) of a histological slice of a prostate biopsy [6]. Recently, it was proven that CNNs can reliably detect carcinomas in liver images, when trained with MRI sequences and histopathological ground truth [3].

The scope of this paper is to compare the performance of different CNN architectures, that predict whether a prostate contains malignant lesions, based on mpMRI sequences and information gathered from histopathological tissue assessment as image level ground truth label during training. All experiments and implementations were carried out within the framework of the existing product *Prostate.Carcinoma.ai*, which is a software product to detect and segment malignant lesions in the prostate, developed by *FUSE-AI*.

2 Material and Methods

2.1 Image Data

The data for the experiments was taken from a non-public dataset exclusively provided to *FUSE-AI* by *Kantonspital Aarau*, Switzerland. Data in the dataset is structured in cases, studies and sequences, where a case contains one or more studies and a study contains one or more mpMRI sequences. Studies that contain a T2W image of insufficient quality because of artifacts that hide the prostate in the image e.g. due to endorectal coils, hip implants or anatomical phenomena (bladder protruding into the prostate or similiar) were excluded from the dataset. After refinement a dataset consisting of 453 studies and 2173 image sequences has been obtained. Each image has a size of $149 \times 149 \times 32$. The dataset was assessed manually *FUSE-AI*.

2.2 Labels

For every study that contains image data, a histopathological report was provided, from which the labels for the images could be extracted. The reports contain region level information such as the Gleason score per sextant. The Gleason grading system is considered one of the most powerful grading systems in prostate cancer analysis. It provides information about the condition of the tissue as described in [5]. The information from the reports are refined to image level binary labels, by condensing the Gleason scores into one score (either 0 or 1). A Gleason score of 3+3 and higher is considered as malignant/clinically significant, therefore, if one sextant contains a lesion with a Gleason score that indicates clinical significance, the entire image is labeled with 1, else 0 for indicating benign/clinically insignificant lesions or no lesions at all. Inconsistencies, errors and incompleteness in human annotation make the ground truth unreliable or incomplete for some cases. The entire study including the image data was excluded from the dataset, if the ground truth is found to be of insufficient quality. In total 246 benign labels and 119 malignant labels were generated.

2.3 Models

Generally, CNNs are considered appropriate for fast image processing and are widely used in computer vision tasks. References [2][3] suggest using CNNs for the classification of prostate cancer in mpMRI data by delivering strong results when applying CNNs for similar problems. For this paper ConvNet3D, ResNet3D and ConvNeXt3D are chosen. All these models rely on a CNN backbone and use fully connected layers for the final classification. Depending on the model, the order, amount, and parameters of the layers change. Also, residual and skip connections are handled differently. The ResNet3D is a standard residual network for three dimensional data. It consists of eight convolutional blocks containing convolution operations, batch normalization and ReLU. The residual connections are realized by using "bottleneck blocks", which are convolutional blocks that add the output after the convolution block to the input before the convolution block. Six bottelneck blocks are used. In total 4,527,906 parameters have to be learned. The ConvNet3D is a vanilla CNN that uses two convolutional blocks to increase the channel/feature dimension while decreasing the spatial resolution. It has 168,705 trainable parameters. ConvNeXt3D is a modified mixture of ConvNet and ResNet. It uses features such as grouped convolutions, inverted bottlenecks with modified normalizations, and activation functions, as can be seen in [7]. The combination of three convolution blocks, three inverted bottleneck blocks containing three convolutional layers each and a fully connected layer results in 31,321,561 trainable parameters.

All models output a single class activated using sigmoid, indicating the confidence of containing a malignant lesion. As baseline, the inhouse lesion segmentation model that is currently deployed in *Prostate.Carcinoma.ai* was run on the same dataset. The model, an anisotropic U-Net, is supposed to create a segmentation for benign and malignant lesions. It therefore must be able to classify the clinical significance of detected lesions. For comparability to the other models mentioned earlier, the model output is aggregated using global max pooling to generate a classification score. The

baseline model was trained on a different dataset.

2.4 Training

Selecting only data with sufficient image and ground truth quality leaves merely 365 cases with a total of 1095 sequences for training. Three MRI sequences (T2W, ADC and DWI) are stacked in the channel dimension to compose a three channel 3D image as input for the model. It was shown that incorporating DWI and ADC sequences leads to increased performance when aiming to recognize anomalies in the prostate [8].

The data is then split into a training, test, and validation partition by 70, 15, and 15 percent, respectively. Due to the small amount of data, data augmentation in form of mirror transforms, changes in contrast and resolution, addition of noise, and spatial transforms is applied to the images.

To enhance the focus on the important regions of the image, an existing model from *FUSE-AI* is utilized to generate a segmentation of the prostate, that is then passed to the classification network for further processing. See Fig 1.

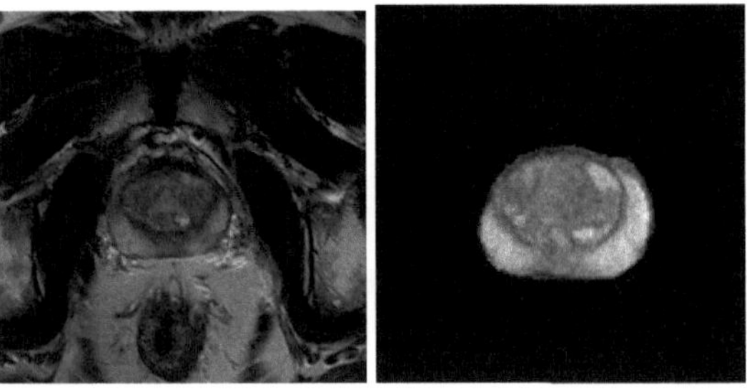

Figure 1: Left: The raw input image (here T2W), Right: The cropped prostate as image input for the model

The models were trained multiple times with different hyperparameters and loss calculations, to encounter a training setup that delivers reasonable results. Once the results showed that the performance of the networks was stable, the setup was considered successful and fine tuning of the hyperparameters could commence. To counter the imbalances in class distribution, the binary cross entropy (BCE) loss was weighted with inverse class frequencies. Additionally, the networks were trained on different partitions of the entire dataset and smaller subsamples of the entire dataset (40 to 50 samples), to determine if the composition of data impacts the outcome of the model training.

3 Results and Discussion

After running multiple different trainings for each network, a valid training setup could be found. The performance of the different network implementations was measured by calculating the area under the curve of the receiver operating characteristic (AUC ROC) and the average precision (AP). Table 1 shows the best score for each model in its best epoch measured on the test partition.

The ResNet3D was trained for 300 epochs with an initial learning rate of $8e-6$ and exponential and weight decay by

Table 1: Performance of the different networks (all entries for the respective best test epoch)

Model	AUC ROC	AP
Baseline model	0.6343	0.6967
ResNet3D	0.6214	0.4583
ConvNet3D	0.5964	0.3743
ConvNeXt3D	0.5732	0.4801

$1e-4$ every 100 steps, with a batch size of 2, a dropout rate of 70% and an AdamW optimizer. It was observed that the network started to overfit the training data after approximately 19 epochs. Decreasing the initial learning rate prevented overfitting but led to worse results for the validation and test partition.

In the next step, the ConvNet3D was trained in the same setup as the ResNet3D. After fine tuning the learning rate to $1e-6$, the AUC ROC score and AP did increase slightly to 0.6214 and 0.4583 respectively in the best epoch for the test partition.

The last step was the training of the ConvNeXt3D within the same setup. The ConvNeXt3D overfitted the training data in the first epochs on an initial learning rate of $8e-6$, as well, however further fine tuning did not improve the results.

It is to mention, that the training with smaller learning rates did not lead to any learning at all. The loss of the classification of the training data is oscillating throughout the entire training of 300 epochs and thus the scores for AUC ROC and AP are not improving over time. The evolution of loss and AUC ROC over the first 120 epochs are displayed in Fig. 2 for the training of the ConvNeXt3D as an example. The best performance of this network was achieved in the earlier epochs of the training and the score decreases over time, while the loss remains constant.

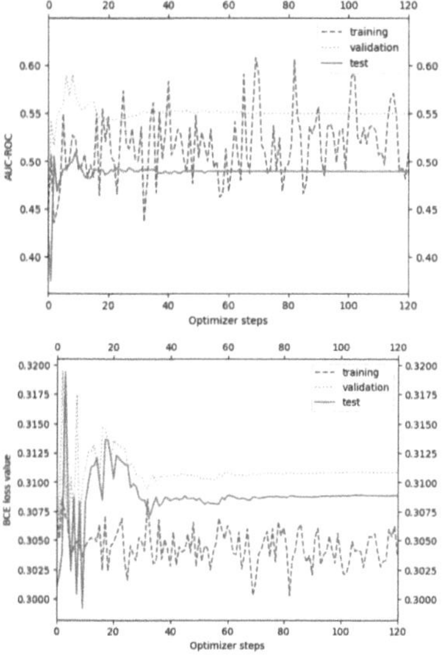

Figure 2: Evolution of the scores for training, test and validation during the training of the ConvNext3D, Top: loss Bottom: AUC ROC

Training the models on small subsets of the dataset, delivers strong models with AUC ROC and AP at 1 for training and over 0.8 for validation and test. The results are not reliable, however, as discussed later in this section.

It can be seen that the models perform similarly with AUC ROC slightly better than chance, but still below comparable results [8]. The ResNet3D performed best. It yielded an AUC ROC of 0.6214 and AP of 0.4583. In terms of AUC ROC the performance is similar to the inhouse solution, but the AP is far lower than the baseline.

Comparing the results of the different trainings, it can be observed that the models do not generalize well on small learning rates. The best epochs often are in the earlier epochs of the entire training. Increasing the learning rate leads to overfitting, which delivers a model that learned the distribution of the training data instead of learning to find a generalized representation of the input. Furthermore, the good performance of the models on smaller subsamples of the dataset, support the observation of the networks learning distributions instead of representation. Especially on the smaller sets, it is more likely to randomly select a set for which the distribution of training data matches the distribution of validation and test data, which results in perfect but unreliable results. The subsamples are very small considering that a median dataset size of 127 patients/studies is reported when comparing other approaches on PCa classification on MRI data [2].

Fig. 3 shows the confusion matrices for training and test after 300 epochs of training. Analyzing the confusion matrices, the majority of correctly classified samples are benign (clinically insignificant) cases. This adheres directly to the distribution of the class labels. Also the high rate of false positives and false negatives leads to decreasing scores considering AUC ROC and AP. There is no significant difference in applying weighted BCE or regular BCE loss.

The generally mediocre performance of the models could be due to many factors including the dataset, the network architecture, the preprocessing including the augmentation or the fine tuning of hyperparameters. In future work, more than one data source should be considered, which would help concluding if the data quality is insufficient or if the hyperparameters are wrongly chosen. Additionally, it would be useful to assess other machine learning algorithms such as logistic regression, SVMs or visual transformers, instead of using merely different CNN architectures. Also, it may be helpful to have more than two classes for the network to choose from. Adding a class for uncertain samples, expanding the network with out of distribution detection or having one output class for every Gleason score could increase the accuracy of the classifier. It would also be helpful to use the entirety of information from the histopathological report instead of the aggregated label. Moreover, the implementation of cross validation could help to measure the performance more accurately. The results in this paper are based on only one run with static partitioning, thus the results can be impacted by the random initialization of the weights of the layers. Additionally, further quality assurance regarding the ground truth of the dataset might be necessary.

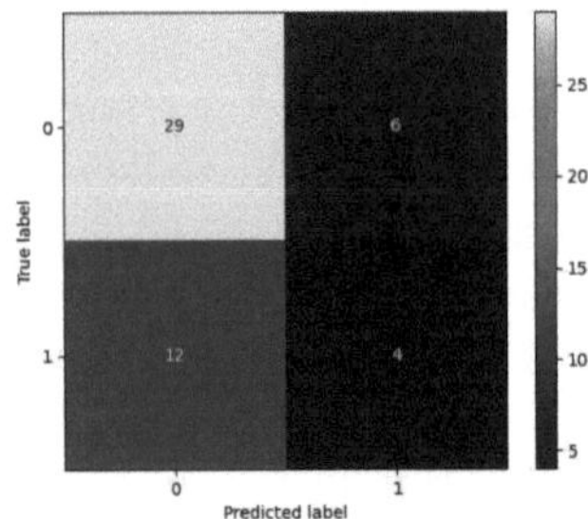

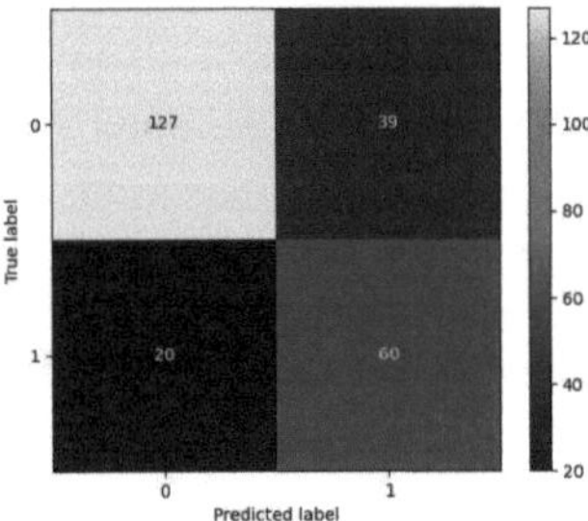

Figure 3: Confusion matrices for the ResNet3D after 300 epochs, Top: test partition, Bottom: training partition

4   Conclusion

Several different convolutional neural networks were tested in different training configurations to obtain the best performance for each network. The performance was measured by calculating AUC ROC and AP for training, test and validation. The test scores were used for comparison of the models. Still, the scores were comparably low, with an AUC ROC of 0.6214 and AP of 0.4583 at best. In terms of AUC ROC the ResNet3D performed similar to the in-house solution on this dataset, but the low AP shows that predictions are not precise.

Generally, the results show that the chosen networks are not able to provide reliable predictions of the clinical significance of lesions in the prostate by processing only MRI sequences of the prostate without additional information or improvements in the training process. In literature an AUC ROC of 0.8 or higher is reached for lesion classification [8], which sets the minimum score to be reached to certainly contribute to the PCa diagnosis workflow. It is not trivial to find factors to improve, since it can not be concluded clearly why the models fail to return a solid prediction of the clinical significance. It should also be considered to train other models than merely CNN-like architectures, to check if CNNs in general are suitable in this setup. Still, it can be seen that the networks that were trained are able to perform better than chance leaving room for future improvement on the basis of the trained models.

Acknowledgement

The work has been carried out at FUSE-AI GmbH in Hamburg and supervised by the Institute of Medical Informatics, Universität zu Lübeck. Furthermore we would like to thank Quang Thong Nguyen for the extensive help on the preparation of the dataset and the implementation of ResNet3D, ConvNet3D and ConvNeXt3D.

Author's Statement

Conflict of interest: Authors state no conflict of interest.

5   References

[1] P. Rawla. *Epidemiology of Prostate Cancer.* In: World journal of oncology vol. 10, no.2, pp. 63-89, 2019, Available: https://doi.org/10.14740/wjon1191

[2] J. M. Castillo T., M. Arif, W. J. Niessen, I. G. Schoots, and J. F. Veenland, *Automated Classification of Significant Prostate Cancer on MRI: A Systematic Review on the Performance of Machine Learning Applications.* In: Cancers, vol. 12, no. 6, p. 1606, Jun. 2020. Available: http://dx.doi.org/10.3390/cancers12061606

[3] P. M. Oestmann, C. J. Wang, L. J. Savic, C. A. Hamm, S. Stark, I. Schobert, et. al. *Deep learning-assisted differentiation of pathologically proven atypical and typical hepatocellular carcinoma (HCC) versus non-HCC on contrast-enhanced MRI of the liver.* In: European radiology, vol. 31, no. 7, pp. 4981–4990, 2021. Available: https://doi.org/10.1007/s00330-020-07559-1

[4] O. Rouviere and P. C. Moldovan. *The current role of prostate multiparametric magnetic resonance imaging.* In: Asian Journal of Urology, vol. 6, no. 2, pp. 137-146, 2019. Available: https://doi.org/10.1016/j.ajur.2018.12.001.

[5] J. Gordetsky, J. Epstein. *Grading of prostatic adenocarcinoma: current state and prognostic implications.* In: Diagn Pathol vol. 11, no. 25, 2016. Available: https://doi.org/10.1186/s13000-016-0478-2

[6] D. Karimi, G. Nir, L. Fazli, P. C. Black, L. Goldenberg and S. E. Salcudean. *Deep Learning-Based Gleason Grading of Prostate Cancer From Histopathology Images - Role of Multiscale Decision Aggregation and Data Augmentation.* In: IEEE journal of biomedical and health informatics, vol. 24, no. 5, pp. 1413–1426, 2020. Available: https://doi.org/10.1109/JBHI.2019.2944643

[7] Z. Liu, H. Mao, C. Wu, C. Feichtenhofer, T. Darrell and S. Xie. *A ConvNet for the 2020s.* 2022. Available: https://arxiv.org/abs/2201.03545

[8] H. Li, C. H. Lee, D. Chia, Z. Lin, W. Huang and C. H. Tan. *Machine Learning in Prostate MRI for Prostate Cancer: Current Status and Future Opportunities.* In: Diagnostics (Basel, Switzerland) vol. 12, no. 2, 2022, Available: https://doi.org/10.3390/diagnostics12020289

Analysis and Correction of Thermally Induced Errors of Time-of-Flight Cameras

Hanna Stolle [1,2], Iris Ellerkamp [2]
[1] Medical Engineering Science, Universität zu Lübeck, h.stolle@student.uni-luebeck.de
[2] R&D Innovation – Research, Basler AG Ahrensburg, [hanna.stolle]/[iris.ellerkamp]@baslerweb.com

Abstract

A significant problem in Time-of-Flight imaging are thermally induced measurement errors. They are caused by different surrounding temperatures and changing internal parameters like the exposure time and framerate, resulting in errors of multiple centimetres. In this work we investigated these error dependencies with experiments at constant room temperature and at varying temperatures from 0 °C to 45 °C. Further, we tested two correction methods: M1 is based on the temperature T_S at the camera's sensor board, the exposure time and framerate. M2 is based on T_S and the temperature T_I at the camera's illumination board. The results suggest that influences by camera parameters and surrounding temperatures all can be incorporated in one combined dependency of T_S and T_I. Thus, M2 yields better results than M1 when both internal and external influences take effect. With M2, temperature dependent errors could be reduced from about 12 cm to < 7 mm.

1   Introduction

1.1   Time-of-Flight Imaging

Time-of-Flight (ToF) imaging is a method for generating depth measurements of a scene. In addition to the brightness it measures a depth value – the distance to an object – for each pixel. It is applied in logistics, medical technology or robotics [1][2]. The imaging process is based on the time light needs for traveling to an object and back to the camera sensor. Therefore, ToF cameras use an active illumination of the scene. The emitted light is modulated in intensity in form of rectangular or sinusoidal pulses with MHz frequency. The reflected light is detected in four time intervals A_1, A_2, A_3 and A_4 at each sensor pixel, shown in Fig. 1. With the four samples the phase shift φ between the emitted and detected signal is determined, see (1). The depth D is then calculated with the phase, the modulation frequency f_{mod} and the speed of light c, see (2). [3]

$$\varphi = arctan\left(\frac{A_1 - A_3}{A_2 - A_4}\right) \tag{1}$$

$$D = \frac{1}{2} \cdot \frac{c}{f_{mod}} \cdot \frac{\varphi}{2\pi} \tag{2}$$

To guarantee high measurement accuracy it is important that the shape of the emitted light pulses constantly stays the same. Also, the signal propagation times of the emitted light and the detection intervals must be very precisely matched to each other. One major limiting factor here are temperature changes at the sensor and at the light sources [4]. Temperature differences are caused by different

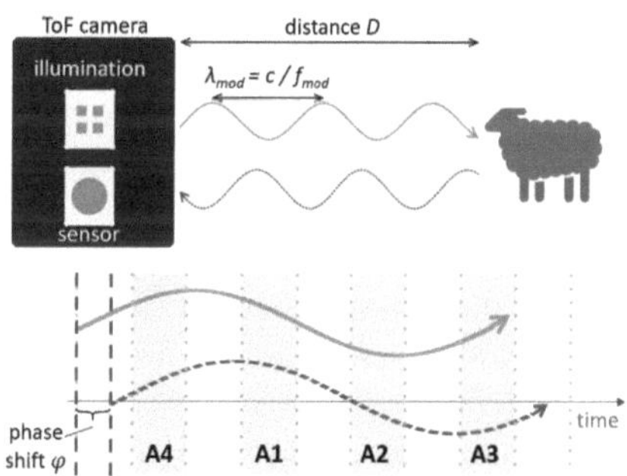

Figure 1: A ToF camera emits modulated light at frequency f_{mod} which is reflected at an object and detected at the camera sensor in four intervals A_1, A_2, A_3 and A_4 to determine the phase shift φ and the distance D.

surrounding temperatures and by internal factors such as the exposure time and framerate [4]. They influence the shape of the emitting pulses and the time shift between emitting pulses and detecting intervals, leading to errors in the range of centimetres [5]. This paper investigates these error dependencies and proposes two possible correction methods based on the empirically acquired model.

1.2   Related Work

Several attempts have been made to deal with the temperature issue. One possibility is to combine each measurement with a reference measurement of known distance and adapt the result according to the error of the reference measurement. This reference can be obtained with an optical fibre which guides a small amount of the emitted light directly to the sensor [5], or with the emitted light that is reflected from the cover glass to the sensor [6].

Other attempts use empirically developed models for the correction like it is done in this paper. One example detects temperatures and errors during some heating processes of the camera to identify a system constant K and a time constant τ [7]. These are then used for estimating a phase offset P_0 according to (3) with the measured temperature T, the derivative $d(T)/dt$ and the calibration temperature T_{ref} during operation [7]. Similarly, the coefficients d_i can be obtained for (4) which is another example using the two temperatures T_S at the sensor and T_L at the light source to calculate correction terms for the measured phase [8].

$$P_0 \approx K \cdot (T - T_{ref} + \tau \cdot d(T)/dt) \tag{3}$$

$$f(T_L, T_S) = d_0 + d_1 \cdot T_S + d_2 \cdot T_L + d_3 \cdot T_L^2 + d_4 \cdot T_L^3 \tag{4}$$

2   Material and Methods

2.1   *blaze* – the Basler ToF Camera

This work has been carried out with Baslers ToF camera, the *blaze*. The camera works with rectangular pulses as described above, having built in the Sony DepthSense^{TM} IMX556 sensor and four VCSEL diodes (940 nm) for the illumination. To guarantee high depth resolution for far distances it combines two images with different modulation frequencies: one with 15 MHz pulses (range up to 10 m) and one with 100 MHz pulses (up to 1.5 m, with a better depth resolution compared to 15 MHz). The sensor and VCSELs are installed on two separate boards, each board being equipped with a temperature sensor. So, the temperatures T_S and T_I can be measured at the sensor board and the illumination board. Currently the *blaze* has implemented a correction method **M0** according to (5) based on the assumption of linear error dependencies of T_I and the exposure time exp with slopes c_I and c_{exp}. All terms Δx refer to the difference of a calibration value and a measured value of x with the error D_{ref1} resulting during calibration.

$$D_{M0} = D + c_I \cdot \Delta T_I + c_{exp} \cdot \Delta exp - D_{ref1} \tag{5}$$

2.2   Hypotheses

Considering temperature dependencies, we formulate four hypotheses: **H1:** Longer exposure times and higher framerates each lead to higher temperatures and therefore to larger errors. **H2:** After starting the camera or changing a parameter, the camera temperatures rise or fall exponentially over time until reaching the temperature determined by the current parameters. During that time the error is linearly dependent on the camera temperature. **H3:** Changes in the surrounding temperature influence the camera temperature resulting in larger absolute errors for higher temperature differences. **H4:** The errors listed in H1, H2 and H3 can be modelled by linear functions which can be used for the error correction.

2.3   Experimental Design

To test the hypotheses the following experiments had been set up. For investigating H1 and H2 a *blaze* camera had been mounted to a motorised axis in a laboratory at constant room temperature. It was directed towards a plane white target. Each measurement included two parts: first a 45 min warm-up with constantly taking images at a fixed distance from the target and second, moving the camera on the axis from 0.25 to 6 m distance whilst taking images at 5 cm steps. Several data sets have been created: **E1:** two sets with a fixed framerate (E1.1: 10 fps, E1.2: 20 fps) and exposure times varying from 100 µs to 1000 µs; **E2:** two sets with fixed exposure time (E2.1: 550 µs, E2.2: 1000 µs) and framerates varying from 2 fps to 20 fps; **E3:** two sets with ten different combinations of exposure time and framerate, one with warm-up measurements as described above and one with only the second part of the measurement. For investigating H3 a set of measurements **E4** has been created in a climate cabinet with the camera at a fixed distance of about 60 cm. Four measurements with different combinations of exposure time and framerate have been done. For each one, temperatures from 0 °C to 45 °C have been generated in 5 K steps in the cabinet, each lasting for 30 min. All experiments have also been considered for proving H4. For the error correction, two methods have been developed: **M1** is designed like M0 but includes the framerate as a third variable to incorporate a possible temperature dependency of the framerate as well, see (6). Similarly to the method in [8], **M2** works with the two temperatures T_S and T_I to include several temperature dependencies, but here with a linear function, see (7). In contrast to [8], it operates on the depth value and not on the detected phase. Furthermore, it does not apply the correction separately for the two modulation frequencies. Instead, it takes the merged result as input for the correction. The methods M0, M1, M2 have been tested on the data E1-E4 and compared to each other. For the comparison the mean error range r for an experiment E_i was determined with the ranges at all n positions k on the axis, calculated with the maximum and minimum errors of all measurements j included in E_i, see (8) and (9).

$$D_{M1} = D + c_I \cdot \Delta T_I + c_{exp} \cdot \Delta exp + c_{fr} \cdot \Delta fr - D_{ref1} \tag{6}$$

$$D_{M2} = D + c_I \cdot \Delta T_I + c_S \cdot \Delta T_S - D_{ref2} \tag{7}$$

$$error = D_{measured} - D_{real} \tag{8}$$

$$r(E_i) = \frac{1}{n} \cdot \sum_{k=1}^{n} \left(\max_{j \in E_i} (error_{j,k}) - \min_{j \in E_i} (error_{j,k}) \right) \tag{9}$$

3   Results and Discussion

3.1   Results from the Experiments

Fig. 2 shows the uncorrected data of five warm-up measurments of E2.2. The plot over time (b) shows an exponential growth as proposed in H2. The error, plotted over temperature in (a), can be approximated by a linear function for

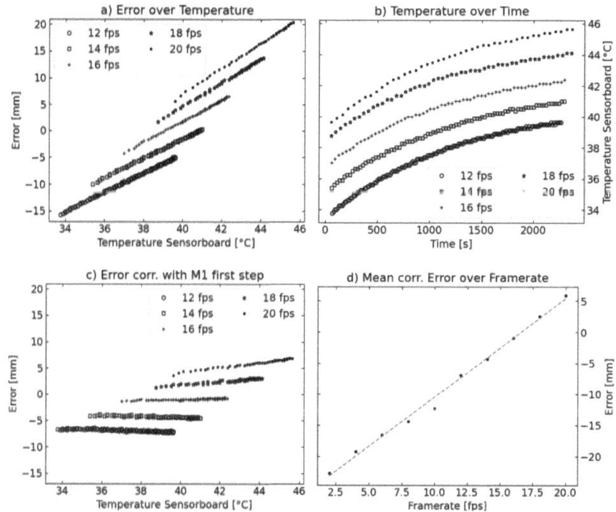

Figure 2: E2.2 warm-ups with five framerates: The uncorrected error is plotted over the temperature T_S (a) and over time (b). An exponential growth over time and linear dependencies of T_S can be seen. After a correction with the mean slope of the lines in (a), the error over T_S now shows nearly horizontal lines (c) and a linear dependency of the framerate becomes visible (d).

each measurement. All the lines have similar slopes. Analogously, the other E1 and E2 sets yield linear functions as well. As the relations are more linear for the temperature T_S compared to T_I, T_S is used in the following for M0 and M1 instead of T_I. The results of E4 are similar: Like for the warm-up data, there is a linear dependency between the error and the camera temperature during an exponential growth of the temperatures. These findings from E1, E2 and E4 support the validity of H2 and H3.

To examine H1 and M1, c_S was calculated as the mean slope of all linear fits from the E1 and E2 data and applied as a first correction step using 37.5 °C as reference temperature, resulting in Fig. 2c. After this correction, linear dependencies of the exposure time and framerate become visible as shown in Fig. 2d. This strengthens H1. But looking at it in detail, the relations seem to be more complex: Fig. 3 showing the temperature corrected data from E1 and E2 indicates that the exposure time–error dependency is additionally dependent on the framerate as the slope of the lines from E1.1 and E1.2 are different. Analogously, this is also true for the framerate-error dependency. Therefore, it seems to be necessary to adapt (6) and add the term $c_{exp,fr} \cdot \Delta exp \cdot \Delta fr$ to include the combined error-dependency of exposure time *and* framerate, resulting in (10). The coefficients c_{exp}, c_{fr}, $c_{exp,fr}$ and D_{ref1} for the updated M1 were determined by the fitted surface in Fig. 3 and are listed in Table 1.

$$D_{M1} = D + c_S \cdot \Delta T_S + c_{exp} \cdot \Delta exp + c_{fr} \cdot \Delta fr +$$
$$c_{exp,fr} \cdot \Delta exp \cdot \Delta fr - D_{ref1} \tag{10}$$

To determine c_S and c_I for M2 the uncorrected E1 and E2 data are plotted over the temperatures T_S and T_I in Fig. 4.

All data – including different exposure times, framerates *and* different warm-up temperatures – lie on one plane. So one can assume that the dependency of the exposure time and framerate in fact is only a dependency of T_S and T_I. Therefore, there should be no need in correcting the temperature separately from the exposure time and framerate (like M1), but a correction only based on T_S and T_I (like M2) should work. The fitted plane provides the coefficients c_S, c_I and D_{ref2} which are listed in Table 1.

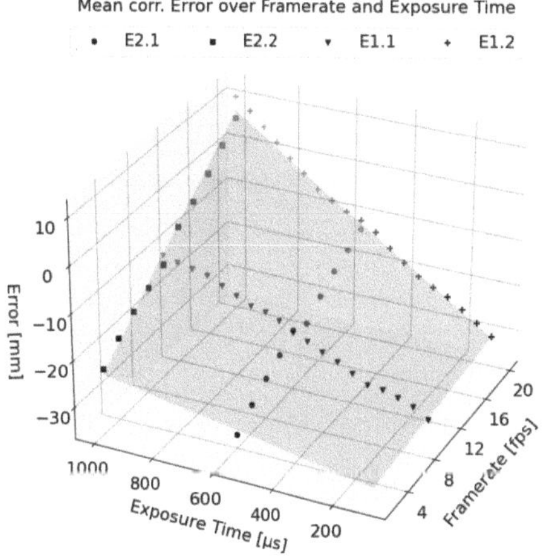

Figure 3: E1, E2 warm-up data: Temperature corrected errors plotted over exp and fr with fitted surface according to (10) reveal a combined error-dependency of exp and fr.

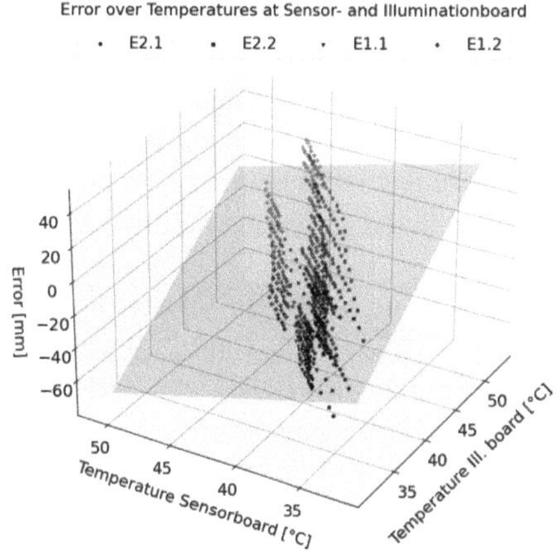

Figure 4: E1, E2 warm-up data: uncorrected errors plotted over T_S and T_I. All data points lie on a plane with linear dependency of T_S and T_I according to (7).

3.2 Test and Comparison of M0, M1 and M2

For testing the correction methods, (5), (10) and (7) were applied to all data with the coefficients determined by E1 and E2. A special interest lies on the results from E3 and E4 as these data were not used for determining the coefficients. The resulting mean ranges are listed in Table 2. Fig. 5 shows the mean errors with the mean error ranges for the E3 data.

Table 1: Coefficients for M0, M1 and M2

M0, M1	c_S	1.90 mm/K
	c_{exp}	0,0042 mm/µs
	c_{fr}	1.75 mm/fps
	$c_{exp,fr}$	-0.0018 mm/(µs·fps)
	D_{ref1}	7.5 mm
M2	c_S	-1.92 mm/K
	c_I	4.00 mm/K
	D_{ref2}	-7.9 mm

Table 2: Mean error range [mm] for E1-E4 data

	uncorr.	M0	M1	M2
E1, E2	41.8	10.1	3.6	3.8
E3	52.5	27.4	4.1	5.6
E4	122.5	27.1	10.0	6.7

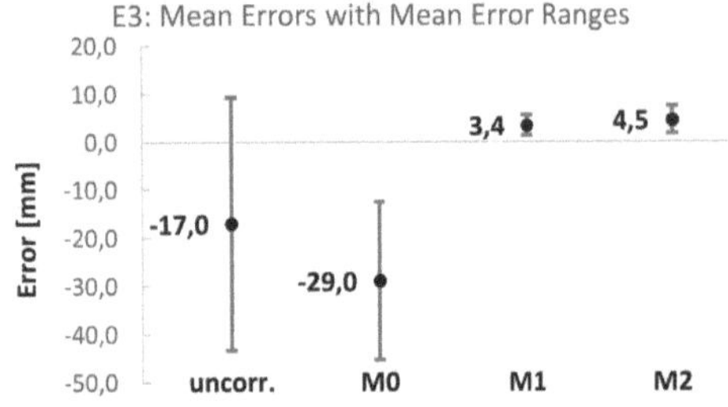

Figure 5: Results for E3 with M0, M1 and M2. M1 and M2 both clearly reduce the error range and the abs. mean error.

All three methods clearly improve the results. The data corrected with M0 still show a big mean range, especially compared to M1 and M2. This supports the finding that exposure time and framerate both should be considered – and in fact in combination, if only one of the temperatures T_S or T_I is included in the correction. M1 and M2 yield pretty similar results for E1, E2 and E3. The resulting error ranges are smaller than 6 mm and slightly better for M1. For E4, the error range of M2 is still similar, but the one of M1 is about twice the ones for E1-E3. So, M1 only compensates for external temperature changes to some extent, even though it is the more complex method that tries to consider influences by camera parameters and different temperatures separately. The simpler method M2 ignores the origin of temperature changes and directly considers T_S and T_I. For the correction it seems to be better suited than M1. The success of the test of M1 and especially M2 gives evidence for H4. So together, all hypotheses could be confirmed.

4 Conclusion

This paper investigated the relations between the measurement error of a ToF camera and the camera's temperatures. The results indicate linear relations between the error and the camera's temperatures induced by different surrounding temperatures, by different exposure times and framerates and by the camera warm-up. Further, two methods for correcting these errors have been designed and tested.

The correction with one temperature T_S, exposure time and framerate (M1) works fine on the data acquired at constant room temperature, but insufficiently on those acquired in the climate cabinet. The correction based on T_S and T_I (M2) yields good results for the data collected at constant as well as at varying room temperatures. Therefore, M2 better incorporates all three temperature-error relations and in total is superior to M1. The next steps will be to implement the methods in the calibration process of the camera and test them on several cameras in real applications.

Acknowledgement

The work has been carried out at Basler AG, Ahrensburg and supervised by Erhardt Barth, Institute of Neuro- and Bioinformatics, Universität zu Lübeck.

Author's Statement

Conflict of interest: Authors state no conflict of interest.

5 References

[1] T. Ringbeck and B. Hagebeuker, *A 3d time of flight camera for object detection*. Proceedings of Optical 3D Measurement Techniques, 2007.

[2] C. Schaller, *Time-of-flight – a new modality for radiotherapy*. Doctoral thesis, University of Erlangen and Nürnberg, Erlangen, 2011.

[3] T. Möller, H. Kraft, J. Frey, M. Albrecht and R. Lange, *Robust 3D measurement with PMD sensors*. Range Imaging Day, Zürich, vol. 7, no. 8, 2005.

[4] T. Kahlmann, F. Remondino and H. Ingensand, *Calibration for increased accuracy of the range imaging camera SwissRanger*. Proceedings of the ISPRS Commission V Symposium 'Image Engineering and Vision Metrology', vol. 36, pp. 136–141, 2006.

[5] J. Seiter, M. Hofbauer, M. Davidovic, S. Schidl and H. Zimmermann, *Correction of the temperature induced error of the illumination source in a time-of-flight distance measurement setup*. 2013 IEEE Sensors Applications Symposium Proceedings, pp. 84–87, 2013.

[6] M. Dielacher, M. Flatscher, H. Plank and A. J. Schoenlieb, *Method and apparatus for characterizing a time-of-flight sensor and/or a cover covering the time-of-flight sensor*. United States Patent 20210382153A1, Dec. 9, 2021.

[7] B. Patil, A. Sharma, S. C. V. Sadhu and R. Ayyagari, *Phase compensation in a time of flight system*. United States Patent 10663566B2, May 26, 2020.

[8] J. P. Godbaz, *Time-of-flight measurements using linear inverse function*. United States Patent 20200326426A1, Oct. 15, 2020.

Proof of Concept of a Vital Sign Control System for in Vivo Measurements of Adult Zebrafish for a PET Prototype

Maja Frerkes [1], Steven Seeger [2], Magdalena Rafecas [2]

[1] Medical Engineering Science, Universität zu Lübeck, maja.frerkes@student.uni-luebeck.de

[2] Institute of Medical Engineering, Universität zu Lübeck, {seeger, rafecas}@imt.uni-luebeck.de

Abstract

The MERMAID project aims to develop a bimodal in-vivo imaging system for adult zebrafish, a species increasingly used as an animal model for human disease. To allow for dynamic studies and long in-vivo scans, as well as to ensure the welfare of the zebrafish, an aquatic environment needs to be integrated into the imaging chamber, together with a vital signs monitoring system. As a first approach for monitoring the vital signs, a pulse sensor is used. For its development, two options are investigated: transmission and reflection. Since the reflection-based sensor produces a stronger signal, the integration of this sensor system has been pursued to support upcoming in-vivo measurements.

1   Introduction

Animal models are of great importance in medical research to support the understanding of several diseases and the subsequent development of therapies. In addition to laboratory animals such as mice and rats, the use of zebrafish has grown steadily. This is mainly due to their transparent embryos and development outside the uterus, which makes them particularly suitable for microscopic methods [1]. Zebrafish are interesting for genetic and biochemical research since a large part of genes present in humans (about 70 %) are also present in zebrafish. These genes can have similar or identical functions as in humans. In addition, the entire zebrafish genome, consisting of 26 000 protein-coding genes, has been decoded [2]. Compared to other laboratory animals such as rats and mice, zebrafish have a high reproduction rate and a short reproduction time. Due to the high number of direct offspring, comparative studies can be made with high statistical significance in relation to the number of test animals.

Especially the range of in-vivo research methods for adult zebrafish is limited. Yet, they are important to study for example tissues that do not exist during earlier developmental stages, like the intracranial lymphatic vascular system [3]. One particularly challenging aspect for in vivo scans is the need to integrate the aqueous environment of the fish into the measurement setup.

From this need, first measuring chambers were developed [4], [5]. Such a fish chamber was presented as part of the MERMAID project [6]. MERMAID is an acronym for "Multi Emission Radioisotopes - Marine Animal Imaging Device". The MERMAID project aims to implement functional imaging for adult zebrafish with high spatial resolution. To this aim, a first Positron Emission Tomography (PET) prototype has been developed. PET can be used to visualize biochemical and physiological functions of living organisms. It is based on the tracer principle, where radioactive substances are used to label the desired molecule. Since PET is based on the administration of radioactive substances, it is essential that the handling is quick and clean to protect the personnel and ensure the well-being of the fish. PET is commonly combined with Computer Tomography (CT) to obtain anatomical information [5].

Within the scope of this work, the existing PET prototype is to be expanded to include a vital sign system, based on [7]. Monitoring well-being is complicated by the fact that fish do not express facial expressions compared to mammals. However, one possibility that exists, is to use a heartbeat sensor.

The expected range for the zebrafish heart rate is 88-127 bpm at level IV anesthesia [7]. Level IV anesthesia is characterized by a loss of mild external stimuli and a normal respiration rate [8]. This level is planned to be used for the in-vivo measurements within the MERMAID project since it reduces the stress caused by the handling of the fish.

Two pulse sensor systems are presented in [7] to detect the heartbeat of a zebrafish. One system is based on infrared transmission (IR). The IR transmitter and receiver are placed on opposite sides of the zebrafish. By changing the volume of the blood during a heartbeat, the number of transmitted photons changes and a signal correlating to a heartbeat is generated. This system, based on IR transmission, has been validated using a camera system that uses Computer Vision algorithms and a commercial heart rate meter (Oximeter MD300C29, ChoiceMMed) [7].

2   Material and Methods

The material and methods for integrating a pulse sensor system into the existing chamber, used within the MERMAID project, are presented in this section.

Particularly challenging in the implementation is the small amount of blood of the zebrafish (total blood volume 20-25 µL, based on the maximum obtainable blood sampling volume) and the resulting required sensitivity of the sensors [9]. Moreover, as little metal as possible should be used in the field-of-view to not decrease the imaging quality by scattering and absorption.

2.1   Setup

In order to integrate the fish into the aqueous environment, an imaging chamber was designed within the MERMAID project. This imaging chamber currently consists of a tube made of polymethylmethacrylate with a diameter of 38 mm and a length of 144 mm. The tube contains a 3D printed holder made of flexible material. It is designed to fix fishes of different sizes and thus prevent them from moving due to water flow. The flexible material of the internal holder ensures that the skin of the zebrafish is not damaged. No metal parts were used in the field-of-view to ensure the image quality [6].

To perform a measurement, the zebrafish must first be placed in the holder, which is inserted into the chamber. The chamber is then closed by screwing on the lid. Afterwards, a pump system is connected. The chamber and its components as well as the used fish dummy are shown in Fig.1.

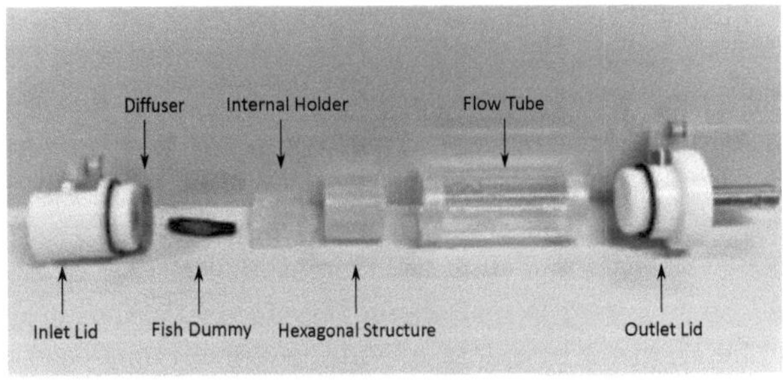

Figure 1: The disassembled flow chamber shown consists of several components. On the left edge is the inlet cover, which has a hose connection and is connected to the diffuser via adhesive. To the right is the fish dummy. This can be positioned in the inner holders further to the right, which can then be integrated into the hexagonal structure that follows. This assembly can then be inserted into the flow tube and finished with the outlet cover.

In order to perform long in-vivo PET measurements, a heart beat sensor is added to the chamber. It is based on the change of absorbed/reflected photons as a function of the blood volume. The data is then converted from an analog signal to a digital signal via an Arduino®. The digital data can be either directly monitored live using the serial plotter/ monitor function or sent to a Python® program for later analysis.

For first trials to test the methodology we used a sample vessel produced by Sarstedt®. With a diameter of 25.5 mm and a length of 116 mm, this vessel has dimensions comparable to the fish chamber. A necessary modification to transfer this approach to the imaging chamber shown in Fig. 1, is to add a passage for the cables of the sensor. Furthermore, for space reasons, we chose an external thread instead of an internal one in the flow tube. The lids are attached to the fish holder and extended by cables to integrate the sensors. The joints between the cables and the cover are sealed with Elastosil® E43-transparent.

Transmission-based sensor system

For this approach we used a high-power IR emitter at 850 nm (IRL 81A) and a silicon PIN photodiode (BPW82).

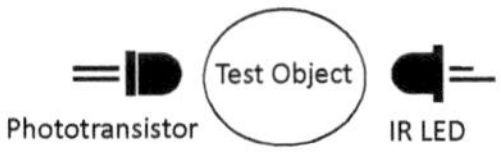

Figure 2: Transmission based pulse sensor approach.

The IR source and the diode are positioned on opposite sides with respect to the test object, so that the diode collects the light passing through the animal as shown in Fig.2. Since the number of absorbed photons is related to the blood volume, the pulse can be detected by this methodology.

Reflection-based sensor system

We used two different sensor combinations for the reflection approach. First, the IRL 81A IR emitter and the BPW82 photodiode were used in reflection from a human finger. Alternatively, we used the pulse sensor module (SE050) especially designed for Arduino®.

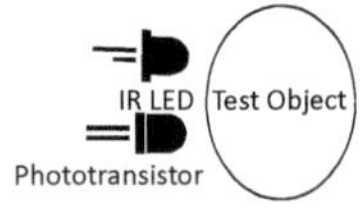

Figure 3: Reflection based pulse sensor approach.

The pulse sensor module (SE050) combines a simple optical heart rate sensor based on reflection with amplification and noise reduction circuitry. It has a current consumption of 4 mA at 5 V.

2.2   Integration of the sensors into an aqueous environment

We carried out measurements with water between the sensors and with air between the IR emitter (IRL 81A) and the photodiode (BPW82).Measurements were taken three times for one minute per measurement at a distance of 7 mm from emitter to receiver. The mean values were then compared after substracting the dark noise. Furthermore, attention was paid to the watertightness of the system. In addition, the intensity values of the receiver were compared to a setup with static water and a setup where the water was put into motion.

2.3 Validation

To gain an initial impression of the reliability of the pulse sensor, a human fingertip, that has a size comparable to the zebrafish, was first used as the source of the heartbeat. The data was evaluated using the Arduino® pulse sensor playground, an Arduino® library, and compared with a manual heart rate check and a Smartwatch (Fossil Collider HR®).

3 Results and Discussion

3.1 Setup

A first setup was realized as shown in Fig. 4. We used a sample vessel from Sarstedt®. After filling the vessel with water, a fish is placed into the fish holder between an IR emitter and detector. The sensors connect the lid of the sample vessel to the fish holder. The handling process was not slowed down or complicated by the integration of the sensors, compared to the existing chamber shown in Fig. 1. By directly connecting the lid and fish chamber, no additional handling step is required.

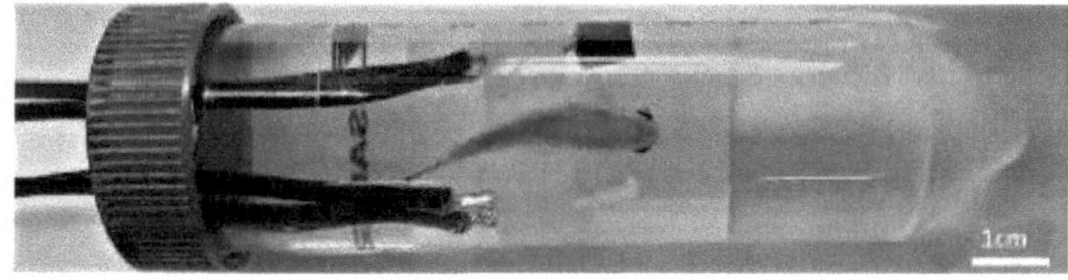

Figure 4: First approach of the integration of the sensors into the fish chamber in a transmission setup with a vessel from Sarstedt®.

3.2 Integration of the sensors into an aqueous environment

No leaks were detected in the assembly during the tests carried out. Therefore, the approach of sealing with Elastosil® is maintained for further experiments.

The mean intensity value of the transmission-based sensor system is 10 ± 1 % lower than without water at a transmitter/receiver distance of 7 mm. The water flow did not affect the mean value but increased the fluctuations by 3 %. The system is therefore also suitable to be used in an aqueous environment. Since the singal-to-noise ratio decreases as the thickness of the water layer increases. The latter should be kept as thin as possible. This is ensured within the reflection-based approach

3.3 Validation

Transmission-based sensor system

The transmission-based sensor system was not able to produce a signal strong enough to extract the heartbeat from it. This could be due to the attenuation and scattering by the tissue. The dependence of the signal on the thickness of the transmitted tissue also is a possible source of error. Since no signal correlating with the heartbeat can be recognized in figure 5 this approach is not being pursued further.

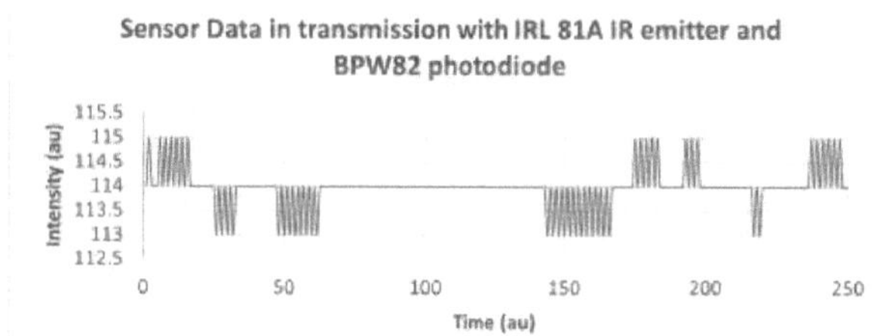

Figure 5: Signal from the IRL 81A IR emitter and the BPW82 photodiode when transmitted through a human finger. The x-axis corresponds to time units and the y-axis to intensity units.

Reflection-based sensor system

The arrangement in reflection of the IRL 81A IR emitter as well as the BPW82 photodiode resulted in a stronger signal than in transmission. The graph shown in Fig. 6 shows visualizes a pulse. Further amplification and noise reduction would be desirable.

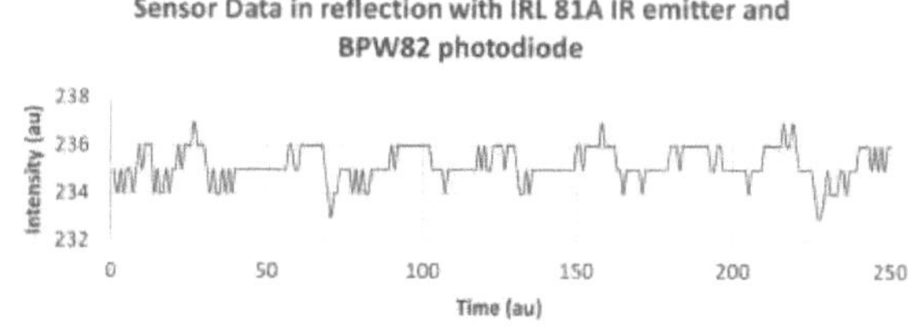

Figure 6: Signal from the IRL 81A IR emitter and the BPW82 photodiode when reflected by a human finger. The x-axis corresponds to time units and the y-axis to intensity units.

A clearer signal has been obtained with the reflection-based sensor module (SE050) with built-in amplification and noise reduction. The sensor module (SE050) produces a stable signal and is not susceptible to ambient light. The system was able to generate a signal that correlates with the subject's heartbeat.

The data has been visualized by an Arduino® program. The intensity curve is shown in Fig. 7 directly. Alternatively, the heartbeats are determined by setting a threshold. The number of peaks per minute is determined and then given through an output. Both the graph and the beats per minute output are displayed in real-time.

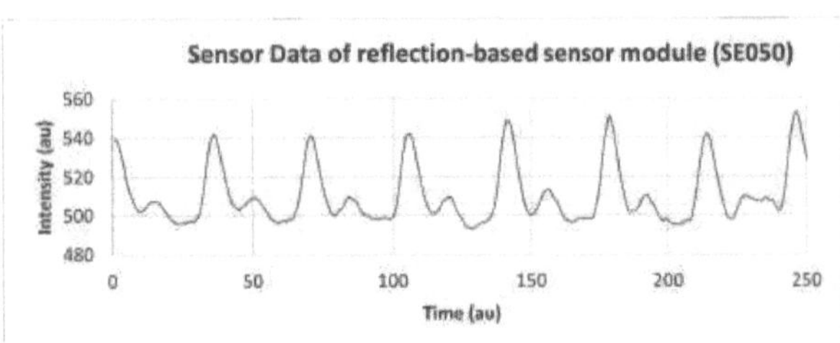

Figure 7: Visualization of the heartbeat of a human test subject with the serial Arduino® plotter. The x-axis corresponds to time units and the y-axis to intensity units.

4 Conclusion

The integration of the sensors in an aqueous environment was implemented using the infrared emitter IRL 81A and the diode BPW82. Emphasis was placed on making the handling quick and uncomplicated to ensure the well-being of the fish as well as the safety of the test personnel. However, no heartbeat could be detected with this system in transmission due to insufficient sensitivity. The quantity of tissue through which one measures is relevant here, since this increases both scattering and absorption and thus reduces the signal-to-noise ratio. When using the sensors in reflection a stronger signal was detected. An even stronger and less noisy signal was detected using the pulse sensor module (SE050). For this reason, the pulse sensor module (SE050) was considered suitable for the further development of the pulse sensor. With this sensor, two types of visualizations of the heartbeat have been implemented.

To place as little metal as possible in the field-of-view, it would be desirable to implement the sensor unit spatially separated from the amplification and noise reduction circuitry, so that the image quality is affected as little as possible by the components and the design is as space efficient as possible. Subsequently, the influence of the sensors on the perfomance of the imaging system should be checked. On the one hand, this includes the influence of metal artifacts. On the other Hand, the development of static pressure in the chamber as well as on the influence of flow dynamics, such as turbulence could be investigated. As a further step, the lids of the chamber shown in Fig. 1 can be adapted so that the sensor is permanently integrated into the current setup. The next important step is to test the sensor on living zebrafish, taking into account animal welfare guidelines. In the process, the signal-to-noise ratio is expected to increase because of motion artifacts and the low blood volume of the fish. Therefore it might be necessary to implement further filter and amplification conditioning circuits. The data sent to the computer could then be further processed with a bandpass Butterworth filter.

Acknowledgement

This work has been carried out at the Institute of Medical Engineering. Special thanks to Dirk Steinhagen, for technical support, as well as Christian Schmidt and Leoni De Graaf for suggestions and advice.

Author's Statement

The authors state no conflict of interest.

5 References

[1] T. Choi, T. Choi, Y. Lee, S. Choe, and C. Kim, *Zebrafish as an animal model for biomedical research*. In: Experimental & Molecular Medicine, vol. 53, no. 3, pp. 310–317, 2021. doi: https://doi.org/10.1038/s12276-021-00571-5.

[2] K. Howe et al., *The zebrafish reference genome sequence and its relationship to the human genome*. In: Nature, vol. 496, no. 7446, pp. 498–503, 2013. doi: https://doi.org/10.1038/nature12111.

[3] D. Castranova, B. Samasa, M. Venero Galanternik, H. M. Jung, V. N. Pham, and B. M. Weinstein, *Live imaging of intracranial lymphatics in the zebrafish*. In: Circulation research, vol. 128, no. 1, pp. 42–58, 2021. doi: https://doi.org/10.1161/CIRCRESAHA.120.317372.

[4] J. Koth, M. L. Maguire, D. McClymont, L. Diffley, V. L. Thornton, J. Beech, et al. (2017). *High-Resolution Magnetic Resonance Imaging of the Regenerating Adult Zebrafish Heart*. In: Sci. Rep. 7 (1), 1–12. doi:10.1038/s41598-017-03050-y.

[5] M. Zvolský, S. Seeger, M. Schaar, C. Schmidt, and M. Rafecas, *Mermaid - a pet prototype for small aquatic animal imaging*. In: 2019 IEEE Nuclear Science Symposium and Medical Imaging Conference (NSS/MIC), 2019, pp. 1–2.

[6] S. Seeger, M. Zvolský, M. Frerkes and M. Rafecas, *Dedicated Chamber for Multimodal In Vivo Imaging of Adult Zebrafish*. In: ZEBRAFISH, vol. 19.2, 2022, doi: 10.1089/zeb.2021.0066.

[7] A.C.M. Magalhães et al., *New Enclosure for in vivo Medical Imaging of Zebrafish With Vital Signs Monitoring*. In: Frontiers in Physiology, vol. 13, 2022, doi: 10.3389/fphys.2022.906110.

[8] T. Martins, A. M. Valentim, N. Pereira and L. Antunes, *Anaesthesia and analgesia in laboratory adult zebrafish: a question of refinement*. In: Laboratory Animals2016, Vol. 50(6) 476–488. doi: 10.1177/0023677216670686.

[9] Humane Endpoints, *Zebrafish: Physiological parameters* Available: https://www.humane-endpoints.info/en/zebravis/fysiologische-parameters. [last accessed on 2023-01-03].

10

Biochemical Physics

Reaction coordinates of protein folding: Comparison between the number of native hydrogen bonds and the RMSD of the crystal structure

Jessica Rückert [1], Niclas Ludolph [2] and Hauke Paulsen [3]

[1] Biophysics, Universität zu Lübeck, jessica.rueckert@student.uni-luebeck.de
[2] Institute of Physics, Universität zu Lübeck, n.ludolph@student.uni-luebeck.de
[3] Institute of Physics, Universität zu Lübeck, hauke.paulsen@uni-luebeck.de

Abstract

The denaturant-independent protein unfolding often occurs at high temperatures or pressures over long time periods. Given this, it is harder to perform in lab experiments. Molecular dynamic simulations bridge this gap and provide information about the unfolding. The process of unfolding can be described by reaction coordinates such the RMSD or native contacts, which were compared in this paper. Using the software GROMACS, the native contacts were defined as hydrogen bonds from 100 simulations of Ubiquitin, which was unfolded at 1 kbar and 600 K. A correlation between the two parameters was observed. Further, both coordinates show a maximum in Gibbs free energy at about 3 ns in average, suggesting the formation of a transition state. Overall both parameters appear as suitable reaction coordinates for the unfolding. However, since the calculated energy differences deviate between the coordinates, they do not yield identical results and are not interchangeable.

1 Introduction

Due to the continuous improvement of computer systems over the last decades, computer simulations have become an important tool in research. One of the newest tools, alpha fold, allows a rather accurate predicament of the folded three dimensional protein structure [1]. The three dimensional structure of a protein is defined and important for its function [2]. It describes the protein's native structure and consists of a primary, secondary, tertiary and sometimes a quaternary structure [2]. The primary structure describes the amino acid sequence of the protein [2]. A secondary structure arises from the interaction of individual amino acids through hydrogen bonds, which leads to the local formation of a three-dimensional structure such as alpha helices or beta sheets [2]. Through further aggregation of the secondary structures, using hydrogen bonds and disulfide, the tertiary structure is formed [2]. A quaternary structure is formed when the tertiary structures of separate amino acid chains interact [2]. Using molecular dynamic simulations (MD simulations), computers can also simulate the reversed process, the unfolding of a protein. The unfolding occurs when every native structural level except for the primary structure is destroyed [2]. It can be induced by temperature, pressure or addition of denaturants [2]. While denaturant-independent unfolding simulations at room temperatures provide information under biological conditions, a major obstacle at such temperatures is that they are time consuming. They are therefore accelerated by performing them at higher temperatures. Since proteins are simulated in an aqueous environment, which represents biological conditions, the high temperatures lead to a phase transition of the simulated water into the gas phase. In order to keep the water in a liquid state, the pressure is increased simultaneously. This leads to a slight decrease in the density of the water, which does not affect the simulations. From such simulations, unfolding rates and times can be calculated and later on extrapolated to lower temperatures and pressures.

The transition from a folded, native state of a protein to an unfolded state can be described by so-called reaction coordinates. In general, reaction coordinates describe the progress of a reaction as a trajectory from an initial state over an energetically higher transition state into its final state [3]. Two such reaction coordinates are (a) the root of the mean square distance (RMSD) between the same atoms in two aligned structures and (b) the number of close contacts between different residuals [4]. Regarding the protein unfolding, the RMSD compares the similarity of the native, folded structure with the simulated structure by aligning identical atoms (1). For each atom i the distance d_i is calculated between the equivalent atoms and evaluated for all N atoms. A higher RMSD value indicates less similarity between the aligned structures.

$$RMSD = \sqrt{\frac{1}{N}\sum_{1}^{N} d_i^2} \qquad (1)$$

The "number of native close contacts" or "native contacts" only consider the contacts, which are present in the native state of the protein [4]. In order to determine the degree of unfolding, all native contacts are defined. With these defined contacts, the relative number of native contacts Q can be calculated (2). It describes the ratio of the number of defined native contacts N_{native} in the native state to the number of native contacts, which are still present in a MD simulated structure N_{MD} and thereby indicating their similarity [4]. A Q value close to 1 indicates that a lot of the defined native hydrogen bonds are still present in the MD simulated structure N_{MD}. The "non-native" contacts which form during unfolding are not considered [5].

$$Q = \frac{N_{\text{MD}}}{N_{\text{native}}} \tag{2}$$

2   Material and Methods

Using already calculated trajectories, the native contacts were determined by hand with the help of GROMACS (Version 2019.4). GROMACS is a software, which enables the simulation and evaluation of MD processes for different biomolecules [6]. The native contacts were then compared with previously generated RMSD data of the same simulation. The comparison of these reaction coordinates could provide information which one is more suitable for molecular dynamics simulation of the protein unfolding. The analyzed data was taken from 100 trajectories of the human protein variant Ubiquitin [7], which was unfolded at 600 K and 1 kbar over 10 ns. Ubiquitin is a small protein, which consists of 76 amino acids [7]. The trajectories contain the simulated structure of the protein, sampled every 20 ps. For the visualization of the protein the graphic software PyMOL (Version 1.7.2.1) was utilized.

3   Results and Discussion

3.1   Defining native contacts

GROMACS does not have a command to report native contacts, therefore the native contacts were defined by hand. In the following only the hydrogen bonds, which can be determined in GROMACS, were considered as native contacts. Hydrogen bonds play a crucial role in the folding and unfolding of the tertiary structure, therefore the restriction to the hydrogen bonds seems sufficient for investigating the reaction coordinates.

Since the structure always differs slightly for each simulation, the most frequent hydrogen bonds in all 100 trajectories were calculated between 20 ps to 200 ps. This time frame was chosen, because previous RMSD calculations of Ubiquitin showed strong change in the RMSD from 0 ps to 20 ps. This change is attributed to the crystal structure loaded into GROMACS at 0 ps, which does not correspond to the most favorable structure according to GROMACS and is therefore corrected accordingly in the first picoseconds by the program. After 200 ps the structure could be

influenced by the high temperature or pressure and thereby altered. For the length of the hydrogen bond GROMACS default settings with a cut-off at 3.5 Å were used. The 50 most frequent hydrogen bonds are visualized in Fig. 1 using PyMOL.

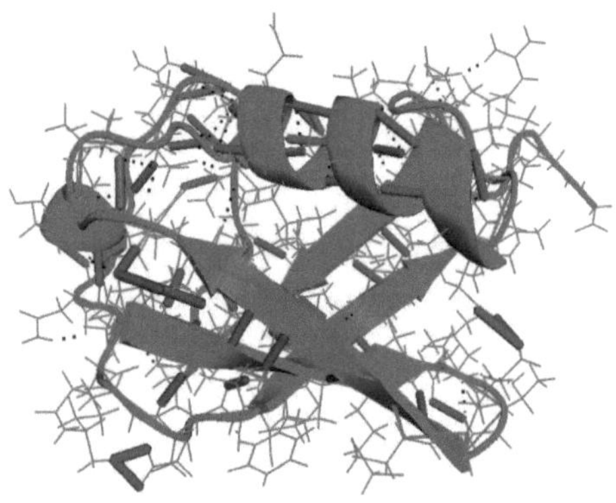

Figure 1: Spatial distribution of the 50 most frequent hydrogen bonds between 20 ps to 200 ps according to GROMACS (thick red lines) and all hydrogen bonds calculated by PyMOL (dotted lines).

Three different thresholds of 30 %, 50 % and 70 % for the native hydrogen bonds were defined, describing the existence of the hydrogen bonds in the 1000 time points between 20 ps to 200 ps in all trajectories to a certain percentage. The threshold and their number of hydrogen bonds can be found in Table 1. While a threshold of 30 % might seem too low, the simulations take place at 600 K. The protein and its bonds vibrate more strongly at such high temperatures, leading to faster unfolding. Further, these movements could lead to the cut-offs being exceeded more easily. Because of this, hydrogen bonds with a low relative frequency could occur with a greater cut-off distance and therefore be neglected by GROMACS. Regarding the number of the residues between the amino acids forming the hydrogen bonds, no additional restrictions as mentioned in [4] were introduced, since the position and importance of the hydrogen bonds in regard of the tertiary structure was checked in PyMOL.

Table 1: Hydrogen bond number for different thresholds

Threshold	number of hydrogen bonds
30 %	45
50 %	30
70 %	14

3.2   Correlation of the native contacts and RMSD

In Fig. 2 the number of native hydrogen bonds were averaged over all trajectories for the different thresholds and correlated against the averaged RMSD. Each dot represents a time point of the averaged data starting with 0 ps (top left) and ending with 10 ns (bottom right). The RMSD data comes from previous calculations performed by this research group. The native hydrogen bonds were normalized with (2). With increasing RMSD the relative hydrogen bonds number drops, leading to a negative correlation. All three curves display a decrease in their number of hydrogen bonds for later time points, indicating that the defined native hydrogen bonds are lost. While the hydrogen bonds decrease, the RMSD value increases over time, implying that the distance between the identical atoms grows. In both coordinates a strong change in value is observed between the time points 0 ps and 20 ps, which is attributed to the crystal structure loaded into GROMACS (Fig. 2). For the curves of the threshold 50 % and 70 % the offset is at a higher relative hydrogen bond count, showing that the selected hydrogen bonds occur in more trajectories. Around an RMSD of approx. 0.2 nm the curves for the 30 % and 50 % threshold have a slight bend. However, the bend occurs early on and can therefore be neglected in consideration of the unfolding.

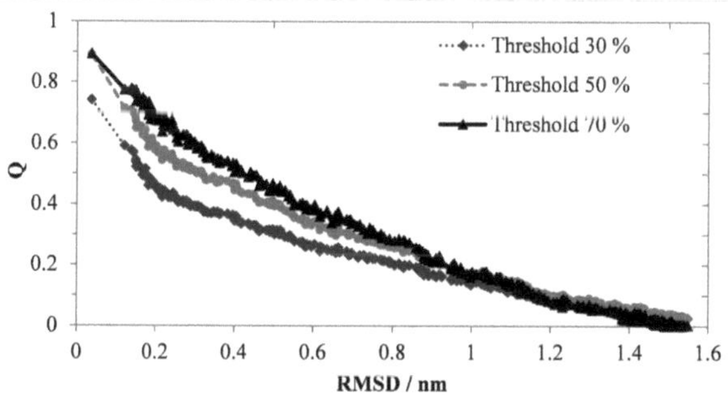

Figure 2: Correlation between the RMSD and relative number of hydrogen bonds for the thresholds of 30 %, 50 % and 70 %.

3.3 Comparison of the Gibbs free energy

In order to obtain the Gibbs free energy of the two reactions coordinates, the probability for native hydrogen bond number and RMSD values was determined and summed up for different intervals. The Gibbs free energy G is calculated with (3) [8].

$$G = -kT \ln \left(w_n \right) \qquad (3)$$

The Gibbs free energy depends on the Boltzmann constant k, the temperature T and the probability w_n of conformation n and differed depending on the chosen probability intervals. In Fig. 3 the Gibbs free energy of the native hydrogen bonds is illustrated for a threshold of 30 %. Independent of the probability intervals, the native hydrogen bonds had a maximum in energy around a number of 10 to 12 hydrogen bonds, representing a possible, energetically unfavorable transition state (Fig. 3). The minimum in the Gibbs free energy at 0 hydrogen bonds suggests the energetically favorable unfolded state, while the small minimum at 16 to 20 hydrogen bond may represent the folded state (Fig. 3). It appears, that the folded state is formed by less hydrogen bonds than defined for the thresholds of 30 % and 50 %. However this native conformation at 20 hydrogen bonds

could be formed by different combinations of those defined hydrogen bonds and thereby occur more frequently.

In Fig. 3 the energy maximum of the possible transition state is at 18 kJ/mol with an energy difference between the folded and transition state of 1.52 kJ/mol. Depending on the chosen probability interval, this energy difference ranged between 0.62 to 2.34 kJ/mol.

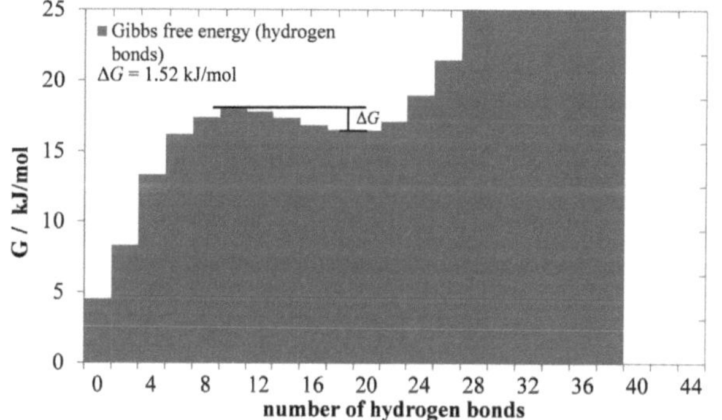

Figure 3: Gibbs free energy of the 45 different numbers of hydrogen bonds (threshold 30 %) for intervals of 2 hydrogen bonds.

As seen in Fig. 4, the RMSD has a maximum at 0.8 nm in the Gibbs free energy with 19.9 kJ/mol. This maximum at 0.8 nm suggests a transition state. Further the energy minimum at 0.2 nm may be equivalent to the folded state, while the minimum at 1.4 nm can be interpreted as the unfolded state. In Fig. 4, the energy difference between the folded and transition state is 8.17 kJ/mol. For other intervals it ranged between 4.48 to 9.65 kJ/mol. In comparison to the native hydrogen bonds, the RMSD has higher values in the energy difference.

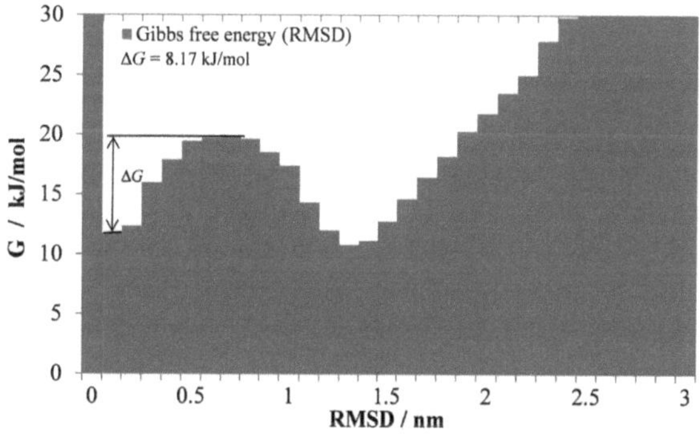

Figure 4: Gibbs free energy of RMSD for intervals of 0.2 nm.

Since the native hydrogen bonds are discrete and limited, only certain interval sizes were possible until the maximum and minimum in Gibbs free energy started to overlap. Further, the energy difference between the folded state and transition state for the native hydrogen bonds and RMSD depend on the chosen intervals.

A possible explanation for discrepancy between the reaction coordinates regarding the energy differences could be, that due to the environmental conditions some hydrogen bonds exceed the cut-off and are thereby neglected in the conformations. This would result in a shift to lower hydrogen bond numbers. For the folded conformation at 16 to 20 hydrogen bonds this possible shift could create the impression that the folded state occurs less frequently and therefore higher in the Gibbs free energy of the native hydrogen bonds.

After assigning energies to the native hydrogen bonds numbers and RMSD values, the change of the energy over time was considered using the data of the RMSD and native hydrogen bonds averaged over all trajectories. Additionally, the averaged trajectory of the native hydrogen bonds was also rounded. As seen in Fig. 5 both reaction coordinates display a maximum in the Gibbs free energy at approx. 3 ns, indicating the time after which the transition state is formed. While Gibbs free energy at maximum differs between parameters, this possible transition time of 3 ns appears to be identical for both coordinates.

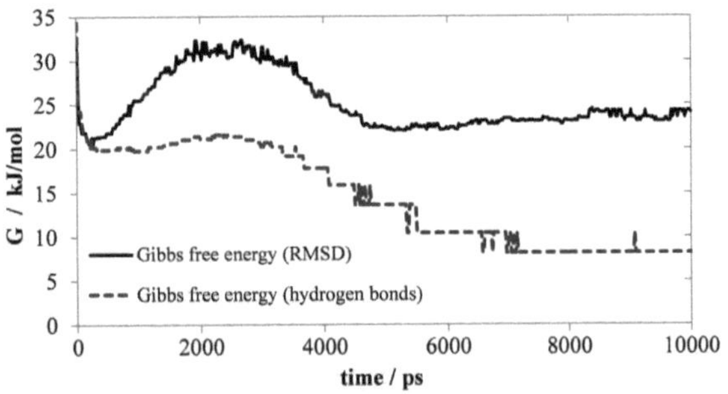

Figure 5: Change of the Gibbs free energy for the averaged RMSD and number of hydrogen bonds (threshold 30 %) over time.

4   Conclusion

It can be concluded that the native contacts defined as hydrogen bonds correlate with the RMSD. Since both parameters show three possible states in their Gibbs free energy, each one appears as suitable reaction coordinate for the unfolding. Both reaction coordinates display a maximum and two minima in the Gibbs free energy, proposing a transition state as the maximum and the folded and unfolded state as the two minima. For the native hydrogen bonds the transition state appears at a number of 10 to 12 hydrogen bonds, while in the RMSD it is positioned at 0.8 nm. Furthermore, both parameters yield an identical transition time of 3 ns. While the Gibbs free energy and energy difference between the folded and transition state depend on the chosen summation intervals for the probabilities, the range of these values is not identical for the coordinates, therefore they are not interchangeable.

For future projects, further reaction coordinates, describing the unfolding process, can be considered. An example for another possible reaction coordinate is the change of the native angles of a protein. By evaluating and comparing other parameters with the RMSD and native hydrogen bonds, the unfolding process could be described in further dependence of the Gibbs energy for different reaction coordinates.

Acknowledgement

The work has been carried out at the Institute of Physics, Universität zu Lübeck.

Author's Statement

Conflict of interest: Authors state no conflict of interest

5   References

[1] AlphaFold Protein Structure Database. *AlphaFold.* Available: https://alphafold.com [last accessed on 2022-12-12].

[2] J. M. Berg, J. L. Tymoczko and L. Stryer. *Biochemie.* Springer Spektrum, 2013.

[3] P. Atkins and J. de Paula. *Physical chemistry Vol. 8.* Oxford University Press, 2006.

[4] B. Fernández Del Río and A. Rey. *Behavior of proteins under pressure from experimental pressure-dependent structures.* Journal of Physical Chemistry B 125(23), pp. 6179-6191, 2021.

[5] R B. Best, G. Hummer and W. A. Eaton. *Native contacts determine protein folding mechanisms in atomistic simulations.* Proceedings of the National Academy of Sciences of the United States of America 110(44), pp. 17874-17879, 2013.

[6] B. Hess, D. van der Spoel and E. Lindahl. *GROMACS user manual version 4.6.* Available: https://www.gromacs.org [last accessed on 2022-11-13].

[7] RCSB Protein Data Bank. *1UBQ.* Available: https://www.rcsb.org/structure/1UBQ [last accessed on 2022-10-09].

[8] M. B. Jackson. *Molecular and cellular biophysics.* Cambridge University Press, 2006.

Atomic Force Microscope analysis of binding forces of *E. coli* bacteria to Sahara mineral dust particles collected on the Cape Verde Islands

Mareen Mey [1], Thomas Gutsmann [2], and Christian Nehls [2]

[1] Biophysics, Universität zu Lübeck, mareen.mey@student.uni-luebeck.de
[2] Research Center Borstel, Division of Biophysics, Borstel, Germany, (tgutsmann; cnehls)@fz-borstel.de

Abstract

Dust storms can pick up dust in the Sahara desert and carry it for hundreds of kilometres. These storms are linked to severe health issues for humans, which may be caused by minerals or bio-aerosols. Unfortunately, there are still major knowledge gaps when it comes to dust storms and their biochemical composition, making it difficult to properly understand their impact on human health. In this paper dust from Sahara storms collected on the Cape Verde Islands was analysed under the Atomic Force Microscope to better understand its structural composition as well as adhesion forces between bacteria and dust particles. It was found that *E. coli* bacteria were attached with forces around 0.06 nN or 0.19 nN. The sum of these individual forces could lead to an agglomeration of bacteria and mineral dust which could explain how transport of bacteria within dust storms is facilitated.

1 Introduction

Every year 2000 Mt of dust are emitted into the atmosphere of the earth. The Sahara desert in Africa is the largest dust source worldwide [1]. During a dust storm not only dust particles but also bio-aerosols and minerals are carried over many miles [2], both of which can cause severe health issues for humans [3], such as diseases of the respiratory tract and cardiovascular diseases as well as allergic skin reactions [4], [5]. Bio-aerosols can contain bacteria, fungi, viruses and other biological possibly infectious particles [6].

In the past, research on dust storms didn't attract much attention from scientists. In Africa, for example, there weren't any studies conducted on the storms and their health effects on humans in the last years [5]. This results in a huge knowledge gap which researchers have started to work on recently.

On the Cape Verde Islands the storms carrying dust from the Sahara have a seasonal pattern and are thus suitable to further research the characteristics of the storms [7]. The international DUSTRISK project of the Leibniz Institute for Tropospheric Research in Leipzig aims to fill the knowledge gap regarding dust storms as well as to develop a risk index for the associated health risks to be implemented in local weather news. This risk index takes the biochemical composition of the dust as well as included bio-aerosols and minerals into account [8].

In tie with this project the division of Biophysics at the Research Center Borstel analyzes the dust collected on the Cape Verde Islands with an Atomic Force Microscope (AFM) to determine the binding strength of *E. coli* bacte-

ria to the dust particles. Additionally, some insight into the structural composition and surface topography of the collected particles is gained.

2 Material and Methods

The dust samples for this project were collected on the Cape Verde Islands with air filters allowing a particle size of 10 μm or smaller to pass. To elude the dust from the filters, they were sonicated in distilled water for 15 min and the solution was filtered using a cell strainer (Corning, Corning, USA) with a pore size of 40 μm in order to remove fibres from the filter material. Four samples were examined in this paper, namely DR2, DR8, DR11 and DR17, the names refer to the dust collection site (station in Praia, Cape Verde) and the collection date (four different days).

To determine the concentration of the resulting samples, a concentration curve was measured with the ZetaSizer (Nano-ZS90, Malvern Panalytical, Malvern, UK), starting at 0.025 mg/mL and ending at 1 mg/mL. The different samples were made using distilled water and loose, dry dust from the Cape Verde islands which had been collected several years prior. For the measurements, every sample was measured three times. After an equilibration time of 180 s, three runs were done with ten single measurements per run, each measurement lasting 10 s. The samples were measured with the same protocol and their concentration calculated according to the previously determined concentration curve. In order to measure the dust samples with the AFM (Molecular Force Probe 3D, Asylum Research, Santa Barbara,

USA), they needed to be fixed to microscope slides (R. Langenbrinck GmbH, Emmendingen, Germany). This was achieved by attaching double sided adhesive tape (Tesa, Norderstedt, Germany) to a slide and adding the dust solution on top of that. After drying, the sample was eligible for AFM measurements.

At first the topography of the samples was examined using the AC tapping mode, in which the cantilever of the AFM is oscillated at its resonance frequency to acquire a picture. For this the cantilever OMCL-AC160TS-R3 (Olympus, Shinjuku, Japan) was used. Of each sample several pictures were taken with different zoom levels ($50\,\mu m \times 50\,\mu m$, $5\,\mu m \times 5\,\mu m$, $1\,\mu m \times 1\,\mu m$) to better understand what differences or similarities there were between the dust particles. As a control measurement the adhesive tape surface was measured without dust.

To determine the adhesion forces of bacteria to the dust particles, *E. coli* bacteria of the PKL1162 strain were used, which fluoresce green. These *E. coli* bacteria are just a stand-in solution to allow a first test of the used method and assessment of attachment forces. The actual bacteria, that may be present in the dust samples, is analysed by a different group and can therefore be specifically used, once identification is complete.

The bacteria were fixed using paraformaldehyde (PFA) (Carl Roth, Karlsruhe, Germany) in a PBS buffer ($4\,\%$ solution). The PBS buffer contained $137\,mM$ NaCl, $2.7\,mM$ KCl, $10\,mM$ Na_2HPO_4 and $7.8\,mM$ KH_2PO_4 (Carl Roth, Karlsruhe, Germany). The *E. coli* were then washed three times to remove the PBS buffer and kept in distilled water. The bacteria were attached to the AFM cantilever MLCT-O10 (Bruker, Fällanden, Switzerland) using poly-L-lysine (PLL) (Sigma-Aldrich, St. Louis, USA). The cantilever was dipped into a $1\,mg/mL$ PLL solution for $2\,min$ and afterwards dried in air for $2\,min$. Then it was added to the bacteria solution for $2\,min$ and immediately used to measure force curves with the AFM.

For measurement of the force curves the contact mode was used in deionized water. At first, the cantilever was calibrated to determine the exact force constant to allow for precise results. As a control, measurements were made with a cantilever that was only coated with PLL without bacteria as well as with a bacteria coated cantilever on adhesive tape without a dust sample.

3   Results and Discussion

3.1   Measurement of Concentration Curve and Sample Concentration

In Fig. 1 the measured concentration curve can be seen. The measurements at the ZetaSizer showed that the samples were heterogeneous as they consisted of particles in many different sizes. This made an exact concentration determination difficult with this approach as ZetaSizer measurements are optimized for homogeneous samples. Nonetheless, the measurement data was used to determine the sam-

ple concentrations as a first estimate, as can be seen in Table 1.

The concentration of the samples is relatively low. This, on the one hand, may be due to minimal amounts of dust being gathered by the air filters (filters with a higher concentration also appeared darker). On the other hand, it is possible that the dust extraction via sonication isn't optimal and might be improved with other methods or buffer compositions.

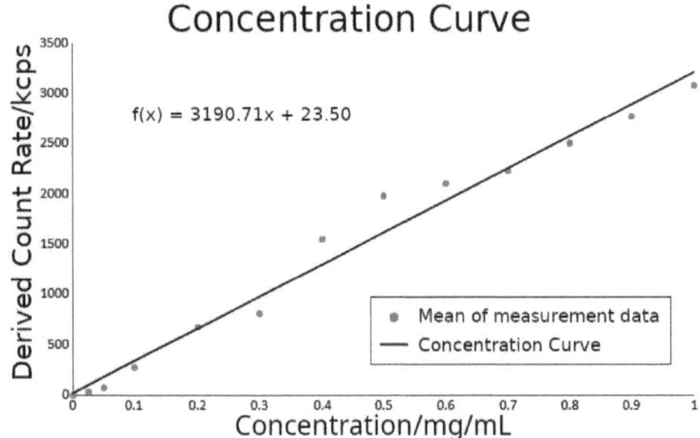

Figure 1: Concentration curve for determination of sample concentration measured at the ZetaSizer. The dots are the mean values of the measured data, the line is the standard curve given with the equation $f(x) = 3190.71x + 23.50$, which was used to determine the sample concentration.

Table 1: Sample Concentration

Sample	Derived Count Rate	Concentration
DR2	$1079.54\,kcps$	$0.331\,mg/mL$
DR8	$80.88\,kcps$	$0.018\,mg/mL$
DR11	$77.67\,kcps$	$0.017\,mg/mL$
DR17	$110.98\,kcps$	$0.027\,mg/mL$

3.2   Characterization of Dust Particles

It was possible to determine particles, that were prevalent in all samples. An example of these particles can be seen in Fig. 2, which showcases sample DR8.

The overview image Fig. 2 (a) clearly shows, that the samples were contaminated. The long strands, that appear in the image, are probably fibres from the air filter material, which were detached from the filter during the sonication process. It was impossible to fully remove these fibres, but it was easy to differentiate them from the other particles, which made further measurements possible.

Characterizing these particles in order to discern the amount of biological material requires an in-depth knowledge of the different particle classes and what their surface topography looks like in an AFM measurement. As a result, it was not possible to determine exactly how much biological material was contained within the samples or whether there perhaps was none at all. It was assumed that particles similar to Fig. 2 (b) and (c) were mineral dust particles.

One of the goals of the AFM measurements was, to investigate the topography of the dust particles and the biological material. This was, however, extremely difficult, as particles could not be discerned in the 50 μm x 50 μm overview images. Only upon zooming closer to the particles, they could be differentiated. Additionally, no obvious visual difference could be found between the particles from different days and different filter loads.

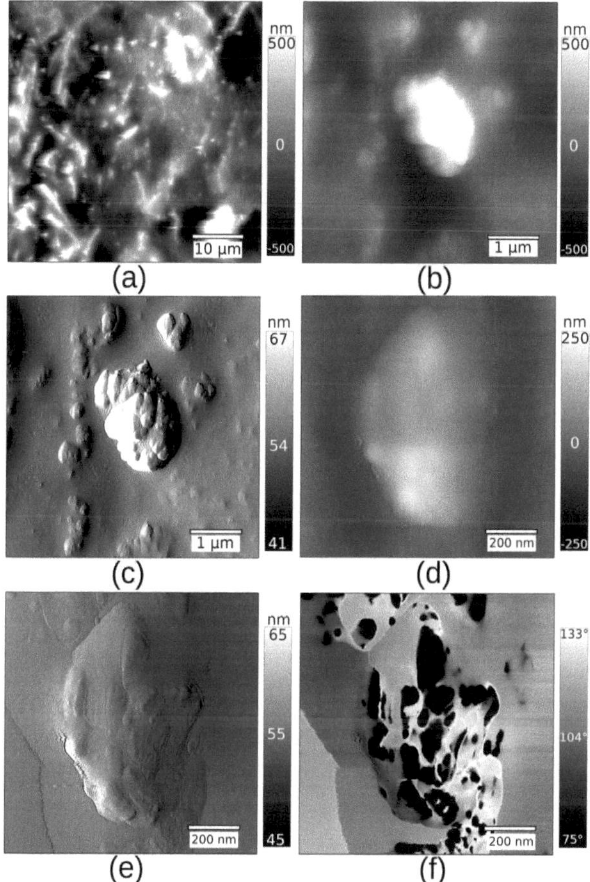

Figure 2: AFM measurements of DR8. (a) 50 μm x 50 μm overview image. Fibres and other particles are visible. (b) 5 μm x 5 μm zoom on several typical dust particles. (c) Amplitude image for better recognition of the structures of (b). (d) 1 μm x 1 μm zoom to show surface structures/domains. (e) Amplitude image of (d) shows structures better. (f) Phase image of (d). The domains have a different phase than the surrounding material.

In addition, it was found upon closer inspection, that certain particles' surfaces had different domains as can be seen in Fig. 2 (d)-(f). The different values in the phase image allude to a different degree of hardness on the particle surface.

3.3 Analysis of Adhesion Forces

Unfortunately, it was not possible to take enough measurements to statistically determine the binding strength of the *E. coli* bacteria to the dust, so that only a first qualitative analysis of the force curves could be carried out. When the cantilever is pulled off the sample, individual breaks appear in the form of steps in the black force curve, as can be seen in Fig. 3. The curves measured on dust samples were vastly different from the control measurements, which ensured that the correct measurement was performed.

These steps could be individual molecular bondings of the bacteria that detach from the surface of the dust. The binding strength of the individual bond breaks from 90 curves was determined and collected in a histogram (Fig. 4), which shows that there are two populations in binding strength: the first being around 0.06 nN and the second around 0.19 nN.

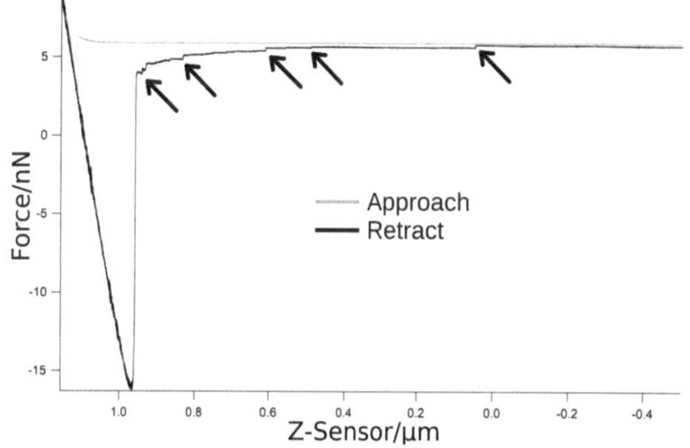

Figure 3: Force curve of *E. coli* bacteria on dust particles. The force is given in nN versus the distance to the sample in μm. The gray curve shows the approach of the cantilever to the sample and the black shows the retraction of the cantilever from the sample. Individual breaks can be clearly seen in the black curve to the right of the large downward peak, they are also indicated by black arrows. These seem to represent the breaking of molecular bindings as the bacteria detach from the dust surface.

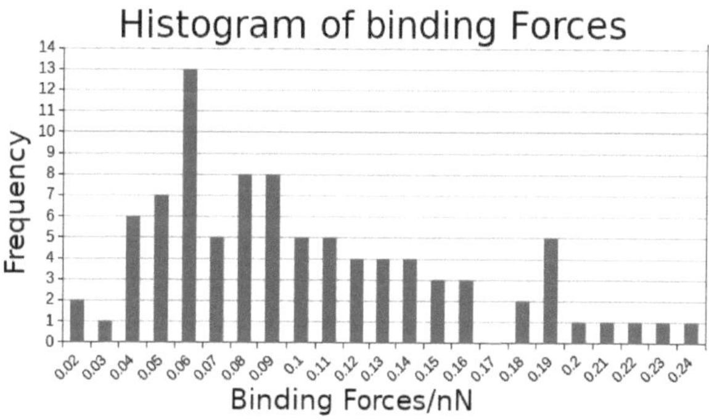

Figure 4: Histogram of the binding forces between *E. coli* bacteria and dust particles. Two populations can be seen around 0.06 nN and 0.19 nN. In total 90 molecular bond breaks from 19 force measurements were analysed.

These steps could be individual molecular bondings of the bacteria that detach from the surface of the dust. The binding strength of the individual bond breaks from 90 curves was determined and collected in a histogram (Fig. 4), which shows that there are two populations in binding strength: the first being around 0.06 nN and the second around 0.19 nN.

Taking these individual binding forces into consideration, it is possible that they lead to an agglomeration of bacteria and mineral dust particles. This could explain the transport mechanism of bacteria from the Sahara to the Cape Verde island within dust storms. However, further systematic measurements are necessary to come to a statistically sound evaluation.

4 Conclusion

In this work it was possible to extract Sahara mineral dust collected on the Cape Verde Islands from air filters and fix it for AFM measurements. The AFM cantilever was functionalized to enable measurements of adhesion forces of bacteria to the dust particles. A first estimate showed that *E. coli* bacteria were attached to the dust particles with adhesion forces around 0.06 nN or 0.19 nN.

This shows that it is possible for bacteria to be attached to dust particles and thus travel with dust storms over several miles from the Sahara desert to the Cape Verde Island. As a result the question arises, what influence bacteria from the Sahara can have in an area, it is not native to.

In the future more relevant samples for the project should be analysed according to the aforementioned procedure. Perhaps a further optimization of the extraction protocol could be useful, to allow for a higher sample concentration. Additionally, more force curves need to be measured for a statistically accurate result of the adhesion forces. Finally, a proper characterization of the particles seen in the AFM pictures should be done, which requires in depth knowledge of the surface topography of mineral dust, bacteria and other biological material.

As part of the DUSTRISK project other groups are analysing and characterizing the bacterial composition of the dust samples. So in the future it should be possible to use the exact bacteria that can be found in the samples instead of a stand-in *E. coli* strand for measurements. This way, more precise answers about the bacteria attachment can be made, which in turn will help better understand the bacteria's transportation method as well as the resulting health implications for the people of the Cape Verde islands, opening up new possibilities to improve their everyday lives.

Acknowledgement

This work has been carried out at the Research Center Borstel under the supervision of Christian Nehls and Thomas Gutsmann, both of which I would like to thank for their support and help during this project.

I'd also like to thank Kerstin Stephan (Research Center Borstel) for the preparation of the bacteria and EM samples, as well as Anna-Katharina Schmidt and Regina Scherließ (Christian-Albrechts-Universität of Kiel) for the execution of the EM measurements.

Author's Statement

All authors state no conflict of interest.

5 References

[1] Y. Shao, K.-H. Wyrwoll, A. Chappell, J. Huang, Z. Lin, G. H. McTainsh, M. Mikami, T. Y. Tanaka, X. Wangh, S. Yoon. *Dust cycle: An emerging core theme in Earth system science.* Aeolian Research, 2(4):181-204, 2011.

[2] M. Klose, Y. Shao, M. K. Karremann, A. H. Fink. *Sahel dust zone and synoptic background.* Geographical Research Letters, 37(9):L09802, 2010.

[3] P. N. Polymenakou. *Atmosphere: A Source of Pathogenic or Beneficial Microbes.* Atmosphere, 3(1):87-102, 2012.

[4] A. G. Cook, P. Weinstein, J. A. Centeno. *Health Effects of Natural Dust: Role of Trace Elements and Compounds.* Biological Trace Element Research, 103(1):1-15, 2005.

[5] X. Zhang, L. Zhao, D. Q. Tong, G. Wu, M. Dan, B. Teng. *Systematic Review of Global Desert Dust and Associated Human Health Effects.* Atmosphere, 7(12):158, 2016.

[6] R. Jaenicke. *Abundance of Cellular Material and Proteins in the Atmosphere.* Science, 308(5718):73, 2005.

[7] K. Schepanski, I. Tegen, A. Macke. *Saharan dust transport and deposition towards the tropical northern Atlantic.* Atmospheric Chemistry and Physics, 9(4):1173-1189, 2009.

[8] TROPOS: Leibniz Institute for Tropospheric Research. *Dustrisk.* https://www.tropos.de/forschung/grossprojekte-infrastruktur-technologie/verbundprojekte/dustrisk [Online; Accessed on 10.03.2022]

Development of a Low-Cost Process Chain for the Production of Microfluidic Structures by Additive Manufacturing

Martin Altenburger [1], Maik Rahlves [2], Ramtin Rahmanzadeh [3]

[1] Biophysics, Universität zu Lübeck, martin.altenburger@student.uni-luebeck.de
[2] Institute of Biomedical Optics, Universität zu Lübeck, maik.rahlves@uni-luebeck.de
[3] Institute of Biomedical Optics, Universität zu Lübeck, ramtin.rahmanzadeh@uni-luebeck.de

Abstract

Microfluidics is a commonly used technique in modern research and its use cases are continuously increasing. Finding a microfluidics system that suits the requirements of your project while not being too expensive can be quite challenging. Designing and manufacturing such a system is a challenge as well but possibly worth it in the end. In the project, which is being presented in this article, commercial microfluidic systems were analyzed and a more affordable custom system was designed. Once the the manufacturing process is finished, the system will be used to perform an experiment involving microfluidic chips. These are custom designed as well and are being produced using a 3D printer.

1   Introduction

There is a large variety of microfluidic systems, which are used for various applications, such as the study of antibiotic drug-resistant bacteria, transport of nanoparticles and observation of chemical reactions among many others [1]. One of the advantages of microfluidics is the resource friendly nature of these methods as only very small volumes in the microliter range are being used. In many cases, experiments are carried on microfluidic chips, which are made from polymers such as polymethyl methacrylate (PMMA), cyclo-olefin copolymer (COC) or Polydimethylsiloxane (PDMS) [2]. For mass manufacturing, microfluidic or even whole lab-on-chip (LOC) devices are made by cheap replication techniques such as thermal imprint or injection molding. Alternatively, if small series of prototypes are required, they can be manufactured using lithography or 3D printing. Especially during the design of such devices, the chip design needs to be modified iteratively until the desired properties are optimized. In this case, 3D printing allows maximum degree of freedom. After a prototype is manufactured, its hydrodynamic properties need to be evaluated. To pump fluids through the channels inside the chip, syringes or an air pressure system can be used.

This paper focuses on building a complete custom designed and manufactured microfluidic system and comparing it to commercial systems while also preparing for an experiment with vesicles containing porphyrins as a fluorescent dye.

2   Material and Methods

In this section, we will describe all technical components for our low-cost mircrofluiodic setup (Fig. 1). These include a microfluidic pump, the microfluidic chip as well as chemical components inside the chip.

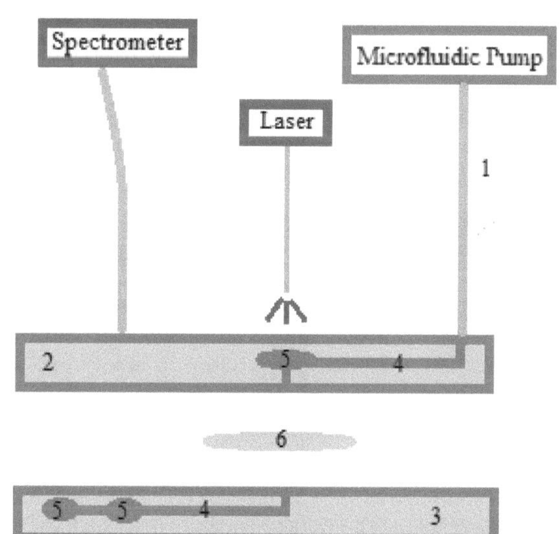

Figure 1: This sketch shows all components of the microfluidic setup. The fluid is pumped through the tubing (1) into the top half of the microfluidic chip (2). The top half is glued to the bottom half (3). Along the channel (4) there are three collection areas (5), each one fulfilling a different purpose. A membrane (6) is located between the two parts of the chip. The fiber of a spectrometer will be positioned over one of the collection areas in order to measure fluorescence during the experiment, which the chip is designed for (explained in 2.4).

2.1   Commercial Microfluidic Pump

Inspiration for the mechanism of the pump was taken from commercial microfluidic pumps (Fig. 2) [3]. The most important parameters are the size of the syringes, which can be used, the increments of the stepper motor and the pitch of the lead screw.

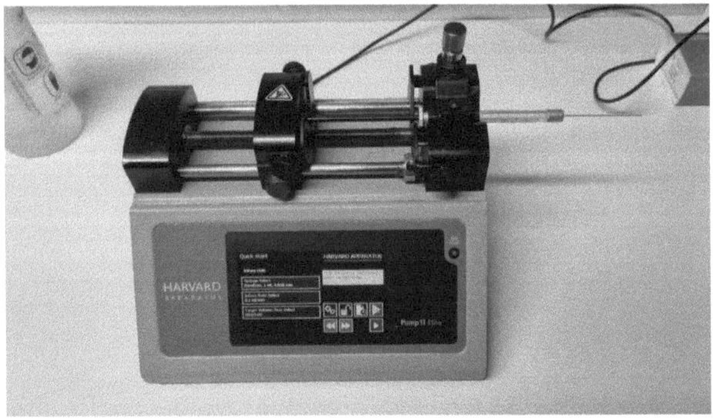

Figure 2: Commercial microfluidic pump (11 Elite, Harvard), that can be used with a large variety of syringes. The Hamilton syringe shown in this figure will also be used in the experiments with the custom system.

2.2   Custom Microfluidic Pump

Commercial systems, such as the Hamilton syringe pump, are extraordinarily expensive but cannot be programmed with complex temporal changes in the fluidic velocity profile. Thus, we opted for a custom built syringe pump, which will be shown in section 3.1. To control the stepper motor, an Arduino Uno in combination with the Adafruit Motorshield v2.3 is used. This presented itself as a simple solution for this exact problem.

2.3   Microfluidic Chip Fabrication

After designing the microfluidic chips in SolidWorks, they are being printed using the Anycubic Photon Mono X 4K 3D printer and Clear Resin from Formlabs. The printer works by submerging a metal plate in resin and then curing it layer by layer in certain areas by emitting UV light from a 4K display. The printed parts are then sticking to the metal plate and are ready to be separated from it. This is done using a spatula. After the printing process is finished, the parts have to be washed in ethanol and cured under UV light. The final step of the chip fabrication is gluing both parts of the chip together with the membrane in between. This can be done by applying a thin layer of resin onto the top side of the bottom half of the chip, while keeping the area for the membrane and the channel clean, and then placing the other half on top and applying moderate pressure before curing the layer of resin under UV light. Instead of the resin, cyanoacrylate or a different type of transparent superglue could possibly be used [4].

2.4   Microfluidic   Experiment   with   Porphyrins

Porphyrins will be used in the experiment the system is designed for. We will make use of their flourescent properties. The fluorescence intensity is highly dependent on the excitation wavelength [5]. This is very important, since the signal has to be strong enough to be detected after passing through a layer of the transparent chip material. Porphyrins consist of 4 pyrrole rings that are joined by methene bridges. The parent porphyrin is called porphin and different porphyrins are a result of substitution [6]. Before the experiment, the porphyrins will be located inside of vesicles provided by Ramtin Rahmanzadeh. The fluid containing the vesicles will be pumped through a translucent microbore tubing (Masterflex™ 06419-01). The tube is connected to the microfluidic chip by the tip of a dosing needle (Techcon Systems TE723050PK). In the first of three collection areas inside the chip, the vesicles will be held back by a membrane filter made by Avanti Polar Lipids. There they will be irradiated at a wavelength of around 460 nm, leading to the decay of the vesicular membrane. The porphyrins are small enough to fit through the pores of the filter (100 nm) and will flow into the bottom half of the chip where the second collection area is located. There they will be detected via flourescence spectroscopy. The third collection area functions as a reservoir for the fluid.

3   Results and Discussion

3.1   Pump System

The custom microfluidic pump (Fig. 3) consists of a stepper motor capable of 0.9° steps (RS PRO High Torque Hybrid Stepper Motor, Stock No: 535-0372), a lead screw with a pitch of 1.5 mm and a linear guideway made by HIWIN® (Typecode: MGN03C1R213Z0HM) as the main components. The screw is being held by two ball-bearings and is connected to the stepper motor via a claw clutch. The stepper motor is controlled using an Arduino Uno in combination with the Adafruit Motor Shield v2.3. The ball-bearings, the linear guideway and the stepper motor will be mounted onto a plate, which is yet to be manufactured. A 1 mL Hamilton syringe will be connected to the linear guideway in a similar way to the commercial pump (Fig. 2). The combination of 0.9° steps, a 1.5 mm pitch and a 1 mL Hamilton syringe allows for µL precision, as required.

3.2   Chip Design

The idea behind the chip design was described in section 2.4 and illustrated in Fig. 1. A first prototype has been printed (Fig. 4). The top half of the microfluidic chip is defective, as the design is not compatible with the way the 3D printer works (described in 2.3). Printing a thin layer is only possible, if the layer is attached to the metal plate. A new design was made to tackle this problem. The SolidWorks models are shown in Fig. 5-7. To keep the layer of material between

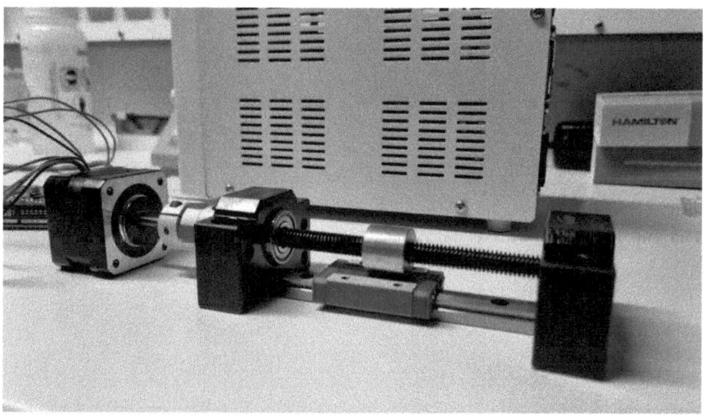

Figure 3: The stepper motor to the left is connected to the lead screw. Two ball bearings allow for minimal friction. The Hamilton Syringe will be connected to the block on the linear guideway between the ball bearings. The connection piece is yet to be manufactured.

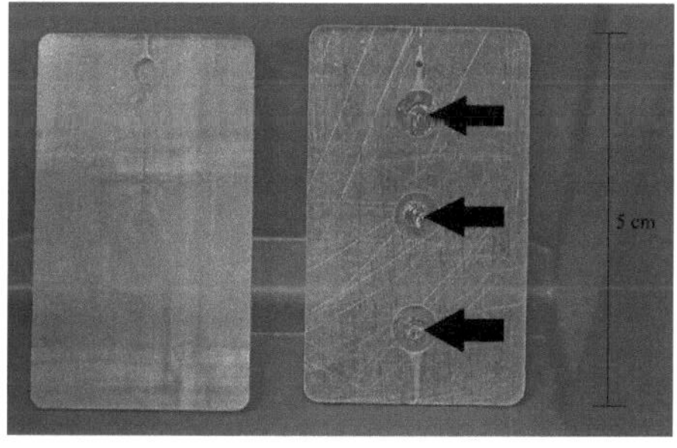

Figure 4: A thin layer in the top half of the chip (right side) could not be printed, which resulted in three holes, making the chip not suitable for any experiments or tests.

the channel and the spectrometer fiber as thin as possible, the location of the channel was moved to the inside of the top half of the chip. This uncovered another limitation. The resin cannot flow out of the channel quick enough before the next layer is printed, which results in the channel being blocked. Further adjustments at the level of the design have to be made, however, the process chain of designing and manufacturing the parts of the chips has been established, as well as methods to check the chips for their functionality. This is done using a microscope to take a closer look at the internal structures and the overall quality of the print.

4 Conclusion

A custom microfluidic pump has been designed and partially built and a process chain for the fabrication of microfluidic chips has been established. Chip designs are continuously being updated and tested. The next two steps of this project are finishing the pump by manufacturing the base plate and mounting the other parts onto it, as well as designing improved 3D models for the chip and testing them until one can be used for the experiment. After that, the experiment can be performed multiple times not only

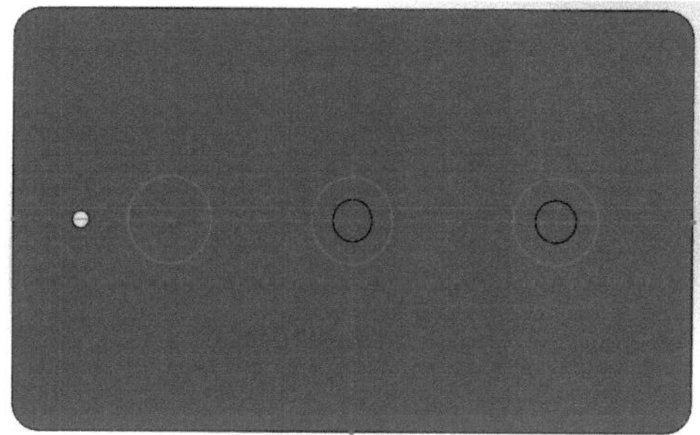

Figure 5: This is the top half of the chip viewed from below. It will be glued to the bottom half of the chip. To the left there is a visible hole where the tube will be connected to the chip. A channel reaching from the access hole to the hole in the center is located on the inside of this model and therefore not visible at this angle. In the center the fluid will be collected before passing through the membrane into the bottom half of the chip.

Figure 6: This is a cross section of the top half of the chip in the sagittal plane to show the channel from the access hole the the hole in the center.

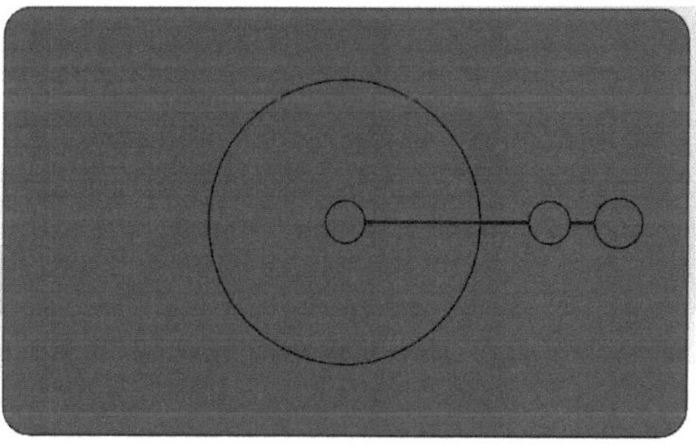

Figure 7: The model of the bottom half of the chip has a large circular area in the center where the membrane will be located. After passing through the membrane, the fluid will continue flowing through the channel and can be analyzed in the collection areas to the right.

using the custom system but also the commercial pump in order to compare both systems.

Acknowledgement

The work has been carried out at the Institute of Biomedical Optics and supervised by Maik Rahlves, Universität zu Lübeck. Assistance was provided by Ramtin Rahmanzadeh.

Author's Statement

Conflict of interest: Authors state no conflict of interest.

5 References

[1] Cheriyedath, Susha, *What is Microfluidics?*. News-Medical, 2019, viewed 17 January 2023, https://www.news-medical.net/life-sciences/What-is-Microfluidics.aspx.

[2] Bruijns, Veciana, Tiggelaar, Gardeniers, Han. (2019). Cyclic Olefin Copolymer Microfluidic Devices for Forensic Applications. Biosensors. 9. 10.3390/bios9030085.

[3] https://www.runzefluid.com/products/syringe-pump/

[4] https://all3dp.com/2/gluing-3d-printed-best-ways-bond-3d-prints/ viewed 18 January 2023

[5] Mahesh Uttamlal, A. Sheila Holmes-Smith, *The excitation wavelength dependent fluorescence of porphyrins* https://doi.org/10.1016/j.cplett.2008.02.012

[6] https://library.med.utah.edu/NetBiochem/hi2a.htm viewed 20 January 2023

Investigation of Sample Drift for Improved Recording of Single Molecule Time Traces at Low Temperatures (77 K)

Neele Rickert [1], Janosch Kappel [2], and Christian Hübner [3]

[1] Medical Engineering Science, Universität zu Lübeck, neele.rickert@student.uni-luebeck.de
[2] Institute of Physics, Universität zu Lübeck, kappel@physik.uni-luebeck.de
[3] Institute of Physics, Universität zu Lübeck, huebner@physik.uni-luebeck.de

Abstract

Single molecule spectroscopy plays an important role in science and medicine. It can provide more detailed information than conventional methods, in which ensembles of molecules are observed. When studying single molecules using a confocal fluorescence microscope, the observation time can be prolonged by cooling down the sample to low temperatures. The extended observation time allows an increase in detected photons. In this work, a custom-built fluorescence microscope is used to examine single molecules. For that, single perylen monoimide (PMI) molecules were frozen in a cryostat and observed with a confocal fluorescence microscope. During the measurements, problems occurred with the focusing of the samples, which could be minimized by an improved execution.

1   Introduction

In 1976, T. Hirschfeld performed the first successful single-molecule detection [1]. The key was to optimize the signal to noise ratio (SNR) by reducing the sample volume and thus reducing the background signal. Since then, single molecule spectroscopy by fluorescence has found multiple applications in science and medicine. Especially in analytical chemistry, the potential of single molecule applications, such as single-molecule bioaffinity assays or electrochemical or force based techniques, has become popular in recent years [2]. In general, fluorescence spectroscopy mostly deals with the investigation of molecule ensembles. Accordingly, the measurements provide an average value over the properties. In contrast, single molecule measurements, in which fluorophores or molecules labeled with fluorophores are examined individually, provide more detailed information [3]. The advantages of single molecule measurements include the elimination of the molecular synchronization step [4] that is necessary to assess dynamic kinetics when studying an ensemble. Furthermore, static and dynamic heterogeneities that may be lost when averaging values can be investigated by observing individual molecules. Among other things, blinking behavior of molecules based on their photophysics can be detected. Blinking behavior is seen when a fluorophore transitions between different states. It allows the study of rate processes and kinetics. For example, super-resolution localization microscopy takes advantage of the blinking behavior. However, if the molecular dynamics are exactly as long or longer than the observation time, a complete analysis of these dynamics is not possible [5]. Various methods already exist to ex-

tend this observation time, such as immobilization by gels [6] or increasing the excitation volume [7]. In this work, PMI molecules are immobilized by polymethyl methacrylate (PMMA) and used as samples. In order to reduce the interaction of the PMI molecules with their environment and thus increase the observation time, the PMI molecules are rapidly frozen. For rapid freezing, an evacuated custom built cryostat [5] is used, which is filled with liquid nitrogen.

The goal of this work is to study single molecules at low temperatures (77 K) in order to evaluate and optimize the cryostat setup and the performance of the measurements.

2   Material and Methods

In this section, the setup of the confocal microscope and the execution is explained, as well as the cryostat that is integrated into the setup. In the last subsection, the sample is introduced.

2.1   Setup of the confocal microscope

One of the advantages of confocal microscopy is the possibility to only illuminate a small volume to achieve the selection of a certain layer. This is realized by illuminating only a certain point at a time and by coinciding the illumination point and the observation focal point. However, illuminating a single point requires to scan the sample with the excitation laser spot to obtain a complete image. The optical setup used is shown schematically in Fig.1.

A diode laser (Oxxius LBX488-40) with a wavelength of 488 nm is used as an excitation light source, which is op-

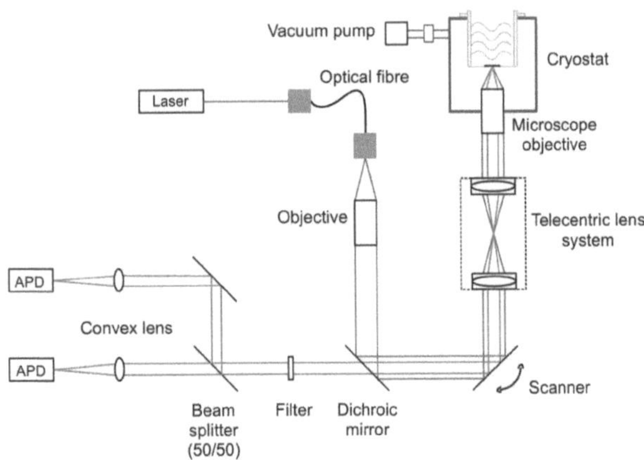

Figure 1: The laser generates excitation light with a wavelength of 488 nm, which is coupled into an optical fiber. After exiting the optical fibre, it is seen as a point source. Due to the occurring divergence of the beam, it is guided into a objective to collimate the excitation beam. The collimated excitation beam is then reflected by a dichroic mirror and the scanner into the telecentric lens system. From there, the excitation beam passes the objective of the microscope, is focused into the sample, and excites the fluorescent molecules in the sample. The emitted light takes the same path as the excitation beam, just in opposite direction, until it reaches the dichroic mirror. There it is not reflected, but can pass the dichroic mirror and is focused on two avalanche photodiodes (APD). To ensure that only the emission light reaches the detector, a filter is placed between the dichroic mirror and the APDs.

erated at different powers. First, the excitation light is coupled into an optical fiber (SMC-400Si, NA = 0.12, Schäfter & Kirchhoff) and the light exiting the fiber is considered as a point source. After leaving the fiber, the excitation beam diverges, therefore, it is collimated through an objective (4x CFI Plan Achromat, NA = 0.1, Nikon). The collimated laser beam now passes a dichroic mirror (Z488/633RPC, Chroma), which reflects the excitation beam onto a scanning unit (GVS212/M, Thorlabs). The scanning unit is driven via a galvanometer and deflects the laser horizontally and vertically. Then the excitation beam is directed into a telecentric lens system (tube lens with a focal length 20 cm), which generates an image of the scan mirrors in the back focal plane of the microscope objective. At the end, the beam passes the microscope objective (Nikon CFI Achromat 60X, NA = 0.8, WD = 0.3 mm), which is driven into the cryostat, and focuses the excitation beam into the sample. There, it excites the sample, which then emits fluorescent light. The emission light travels the same path as the excitation beam, just in opposite direction, until it reaches the dichroic mirror. Because the emission light has a longer wavelength due to the Stokes shift [8], it is not reflected but passes through the dichroic mirror. Since the dichroic mirror does not reflect 100 % of the excitation light, a filter (ET535/70m, Chroma) is placed in the emission beam path. The detection system consists of two avalanche photodiodes (APD) (SPCM-AQRH-14, Perkin Elmer), on to which the

emission light is split. For this purpose, the emission light is split by a beam splitter (50/50) and focused with lenses onto the detector surface of the APDs. The software that is used for data acquisition and to control the components of the microscope, e.g. laser and scanning unit, is implemented in LabVIEW 2020 (National Instruments, USA). The following describes how a measurement is performed. First, the focus is set to the upper cover glass side. This is done by a microscope fine drive, which can be used to manually adjust the height of the objective with micrometer precision. The concentration of PMI on the cover glass is so low that only a few individual molecules are visible when scanning an area of 10 µm x 10 µm. After the overview scan, the control software of the microscope setup is used to deflect the laser beam with the scanning unit, so that it reaches a single molecule. For this purpose, the corresponding molecule is marked over the image view in the control software. The laser is then switched on and the data acquisition is started. The photons of the emitted fluorescent light of the molecule reach the APDs and the arrival times are stored. A high resolution time-to-digital converter with a minimum time resolution of 5 ns is used (HRM-TDC, SensL). The detected photons per user-defined bintime are displayed as a time trace in the control software.

2.2 The cryostat

For measurements at low temperatures, an additional cryostat is required, which is integrated into the microscope setup, see top right in Fig.1. The cryostat is a cooling unit that allows to keep samples at a constant temperature for a long period of time. The cryostat consists of two vessels. One is a Dewar vessel, the other is a stainless steel cylinder. The Dewar vessel is placed in the stainless steel cylinder. Inside the Dewar vessel, the cover glass with the sample is placed, and fixed by a magnetic ring. Since the outer vessel is mechanically fixed to the stage of an inverted microscope (Nikon Eclipse TS100-F), the objective of the microscope can be moved up in order to place the excitation and detection focus inside the sample. For this purpose, both vessels have an opening at the bottom. Furthermore, a vacuum pump (Alcatel Pascal 1005) is connected so that the space between the inner and outer vessel is evacuated. This provides better thermal isolation. Vacuum grease and an O-ring are used to ensure tightness around the objective. During a measurement, the Dewar vessel is pressed into the steel cylinder by the atmospheric pressure, due to the vacuum in the cryostat. Liquid nitrogen is filled in from above for continuous cooling of the sample. Thus, the sample is cooled down to 77 K, which corresponds to the boiling temperature of liquid nitrogen.

2.3 The sample

PMI is a photoluminescent molecule that is well suited for single molecule spectroscopy because of its high thermal, chemical and photochemical stability. It consists of aromatic polycyclic hydrocarbons and an imide group. As with any fluorophore, the fluorescence is characterized by the conjugated π-electron system. The optical absorption spectrum of PMI ranges from 400 nm to 550 nm [9].

In this work, PMI was co-dissolved with PMMA in toluene and pipetted onto a rapidly rotating cover glass (spin coated). The toluene evaporates immediately, leaving a thin layer of PMMA with PMI molecules on the cover glass. The molecules are now immobilized by the PMMA. The cover glasses themselves were previously baked for several hours in an oven at 400 °C to remove impurities.

3   Results and Discussion

In order to be able to choose a suitable laser power to perform the experiments, measurements were first performed with 1 µW, 2 µW, 5 µW, 10 µW and 20 µW, both at 293 K and at 77 K. It showed, that at a laser power of 10 µW, the scans had a good SNR and it was possible to record blinking behavior. One of these time traces is shown in Fig.2. The data were analyzed and plotted by using Igor Pro 9 (Wavemetrics, USA).

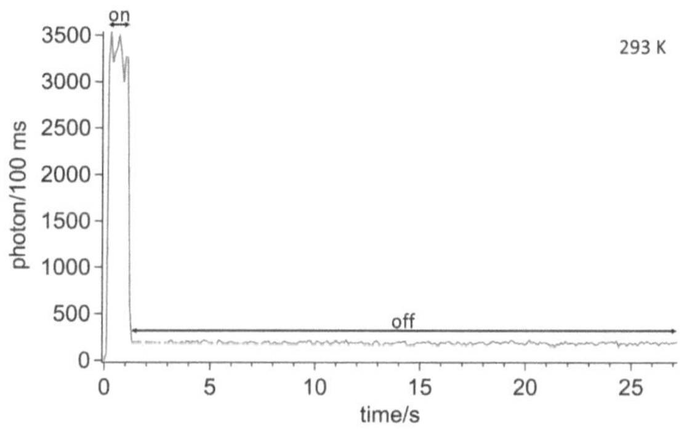

Figure 2: The time trace of a PMI molecule is recorded at room temperature, with an excitation laser power of 10 µW. At the start the molecule fluoresces, so the number of photons per 100 ms is high. In the short time where the number of photons is high, a slight drop can be seen before at 1.2 s the intensity drops almost vertically to below 500 photons per 100 ms.

In all graphs the number of photons per 100 ms (bintime) is plotted against the time in seconds. The time trace shown in Fig.2 was recorded using a excitation power of 10 µW. At the beginning the graph shows a very high number of photons per bin, which means that the molecule fluoresces. In the short time where the number of photons is high, a slight drop can be seen before at 1.2 s the intensity drops almost vertically to below 500 photons per 100 ms. So the survival time of the molecule is very short under these conditions and the slight decrease may indicate that the focus is shifting laterally and/or axially during the measurement. After 1.2 s the molecule does not emit fluorescence light anymore. Thus, a change of state of the PMI molecule is detected. The time from the beginning to the drop of the number of photons is called on state. Everything that is below the 500 photons per bin is called off state.

In general, problems have already occurred here, some of them aggravated during the measurements at 77 K. The manual marking of the molecule for the time trace was not very accurate, which partly lead to the fact that only the background noise was detected.

For measurements at 77 K often no time traces with blinking behavior could be recorded, but apparently only background noise. A possible cause is a drift of the excitation focus. This drift may be caused by thermal stress, when cooling with liquid nitrogen, and also by mechanical stress, caused by the vacuum. In the left column of Fig.4 it is clearly seen that the molecules are already outside the axial focus after 30 s. In addition, there is a lateral drift, which is probably responsible for the fact that, after imaging, the laser beam does not hit the molecule at all and thus only background noise is recorded. Although it was possible to record time traces where the blinking behavior could be observed, see Fig.3. The graph shows several on states and off states, but also a continuous decrease of the photon number due to the axial drift of the focus.

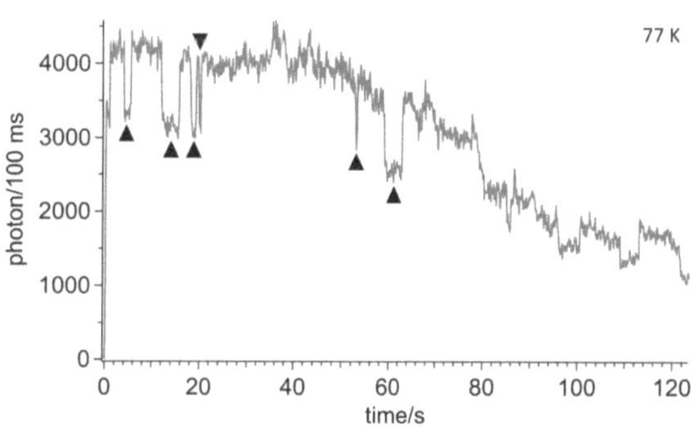

Figure 3: The time trace of a PMI molecule is recorded at 77 K (vacuum), with a laser power of 10 µW and a bintime of 100 ms. In the figure, the blinking behavior of the molecule can be seen, based on the changes between on states and off states. The off states in the first 70 s are marked by the black triangles. Furthermore, a slow decrease in the number of photons per bintime can be seen, which becomes stronger at 60 s. The decrease of the intensity indicates a possible focus drift.

In order to reduce this drift, a rest period was introduced after starting and evacuating the outer vessel. Also the time to cool down the cryostat was extended. In both cases, the rest period was 30 minutes to allow the pressure in the cryostat to reach a stable level. Due to the filling in of liquid nitrogen, the pressure changes strongly at first, which causes the microscope objective to move, since it is not completely in vacuum. By providing rest periods before the measurements, a significant improvement could be achieved, which is shown in Fig.4. This figure shows overview scans of size 10 µm x 10 µm. The left column shows measurements at 77 K without the described resting procedure and the right column shows cryostat measurements with rest periods. In both cases, an initial scan was started, followed by additional scans at 30 s intervals. As can be seen, in the measurement without rest periods, after 30 s all molecules are completely out of focus due to the strong drift. After another 30 s only a noisy image is visible. In stark contrast, in the measurement with rest periods before, all molecules only slowly lose their clear structure and intensity in the scans over time.

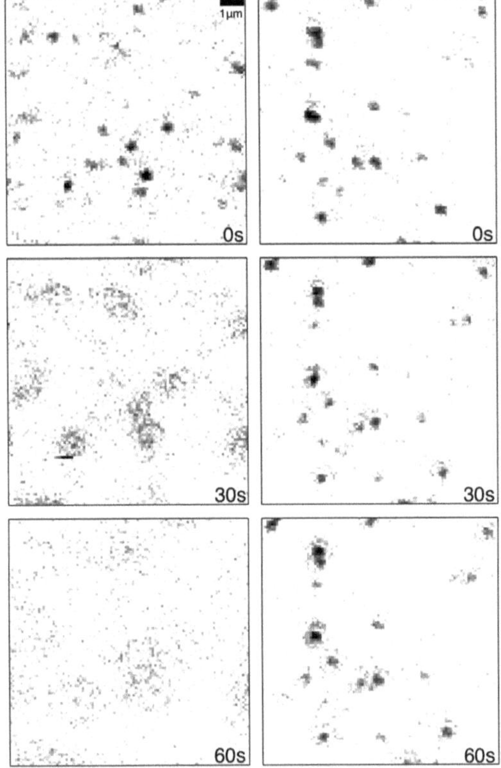

Figure 4: Overview scans of size 10 µm x 10 µm can be seen. The scans in the left column are from a cryostat measurement without rest periods and those in the right column are from a measurement with rest periods. In comparison, it can be seen that the molecules can still be identified after 60 s in the measurement with rest periods, while in the measurement without rest periods, the molecules can no longer be identified already after 30 s.

4   Conclusion

In conclusion, the survival time of the PMI is prolonged at 77 K, allowing the blinking behavior of the fluorescent molecules to be observed. However, the axial drift of the focus in particular makes it difficult to generate useful data. For this reason, 30 minutes rest periods have been introduced, which significantly reduce the drift.
It would be useful to find an automated solution that tracks all molecules and can subsequently determine the intensity maximum of a single molecule. Thus, it could be ensured that the single molecule is actually detected and counteract a possible lateral shift. Further work should focus on the automation of the tracking of all molecules and the tagging of a molecule for a time trace. For this purpose, a simplified form of orbital tracking [10] could be implemented in LabVIEW.

Acknowledgement

The work has been carried out and supervised by the Institute of Physics, Universität zu Lübeck.

Author's Statement

Conflict of interest: Authors state no conflict of interest.

5   References

[1] T. Hirschfeld, "Optical microscopic observation of single small molecules," *Applied Optics*, vol. 15, no. 12, p. 2965, dec 1976.

[2] Z. Farka, M. J. Mickert, M. Pastucha, Z. Mikušová, P. Skládal, and H. H. Gorris, "Fortschritte in der optischen Einzelmoleküldetektion: Auf dem Weg zu höchstempfindlichen Bioaffinitätsassays," *Angewandte Chemie*, vol. 132, no. 27, pp. 10 836–10 865, apr 2020.

[3] P. B. W. Intriago, "Einzelmolekülspektroskopie bei tiefen Temperaturen," Bachelor's thesis, Universität zu Lübeck, 2021.

[4] W. E. Moerner and D. P. Fromm, "Methods of single-molecule fluorescence spectroscopy and microscopy," *Review of Scientific Instruments*, vol. 74, no. 8, pp. 3597–3619, aug 2003.

[5] V. Hirschfeld, "Förster-Energietransfer an einzelnen Molekülen bei tiefen Temperaturen," Ph.D. dissertation, Universität zu Lübeck, 2011.

[6] R. M. Dickson, D. J. Norris, Y.-L. Tzeng, and W. E. Moerner, "Three-dimensional imaging of single molecules solvated in pores of poly(acrylamide) gels," *Science*, vol. 274, no. 5289, pp. 966–968, nov 1996.

[7] J. Widengren and R. Rigler, "Mechanisms of photobleaching investigated by fluorescence correlation spectroscopy," *Bioimaging*, vol. 4, no. 3, pp. 149–157, sep 1996.

[8] G. G. Stokes, "XXX. on the change of refrangibility of light," *Philosophical Transactions of the Royal Society of London*, vol. 142, pp. 463–562, dec 1852.

[9] R. Roy, A. Khan, O. Chatterjee, S. Bhunia, and A. L. Koner, "Perylene monoimide as a versatile fluoroprobe: The past, present, and future," *Organic Materials*, vol. 3, no. 03, pp. 417–454, jul 2021.

[10] K. Kis-Petikova and E. Gratton, "Distance measurement by circular scanning of the excitation beam in the two-photon microscope," *Microscopy Research and Technique*, vol. 63, no. 1, pp. 34–49, 2003.

11

Safety and Quality

Development and construction of a testing device for determining the tightness and verifying the durability of membranes

Franz Apel [1],
[1] Medical Engineering Science, Universität zu Lübeck, franz.apel@student.uni-luebeck.de

Abstract

In this work, the main objective is to develop a test rig capable of testing membranes, which are used in Anaesthesia devices, to 2.6 bar relative overpressure and -500 mbar relative underpressure. The motivation is to prove whether these membranes meet the requirements in a medical device for such applications and are therefore suitable for possible installation and thus meet the high standards of medical technology. It is important that a predefined pressure rise time is not exceeded in order to achieve the hardest and fastest possible pressure rise and thus a very high load on the membranes. The aim here is to check whether the membranes can withstand this stress by remaining leak-proof for the entire duration of the check. The test is carried out over 200,000 cycles at relative overpressure and 1000 cycles at relative underpressure. Between loads, the membranes are vented against the environment in order to exert as much stress as possible. The results are mainly defined by the leakage rate. This is decisive for whether the membranes are suitable for this stress. This then forms the conclusion, in that a statement can be made about the use of the membranes based on the evaluated results.

1 Introduction

When developing medical devices, it is particularly important that all installed components are absolutely safe and function in the appropriate and planned manner. After all, we trust these devices with the most important thing we have, our lives.

Of course, this also applies to the membranes that are important in this paper, which in this context means that the test specimens remain tight and survive the pressure shocks without damage. They are essential for the tightness within the airflow system of an Anaesthesia device.

The motivation for constructing and designing this test lies in the fact that only absolute safety and knowledge of the installed components will ensure that the medical device as a whole is absolutely safe and thus also guarantees functionality, which is especially in the medical part of the development very important. This is achieved through various types of tests, for example physical, chemical or other functional tests. In this testing device, the focus is on physical functionality and robustness against mechanical stress. Furthermore, the construction is developed by checking the tightness of the membrane in connection with the holder.

The assumption is that these membranes will be put under pressure and get vent against the environment about 100,000 times in their life as part of a medical device. In order to do this with a certainty of about 98%, about 200,000 test cycles are required for 30 test specimens. From these parameters it can be deduced that if all membranes pass the test without failure, they would be well suited for an application.

2 Requirements and Specifications

In this experimental trial, the aim is to build a test rig that tests these membranes for their tightness and mechanical robustness. The requirements for the test bench are to deliver reliable and reproducible results, which provide meaningful information about the behaviour and function of the membranes. The test stand should run as automatically as possible. Furthermore, it is important that the test stand is constructed in such a way that the membranes can be placed in a climatic cabinet in order to test temperature-dependent factors. Furthermore, it is a specification for the test stand that it is completely resistant to anaesthetics, so that it is possible to test the membranes used in anaesthesia in an narcotic environment.

3 Material and Methods

In this chapter the the set up and functionality of the test stand is described. In the process, all used materials are applied and interconnected through different methods, to build this test stand.

3.1 Experimental Setup

The pneumatic structure of this test stand is first shown in Figure 1 and thus includes all the installed components, which are explained below.
First of all, the membranes are required, whereby five test specimens are always used per set-up. It should be mentioned that two test benches are developed and these then

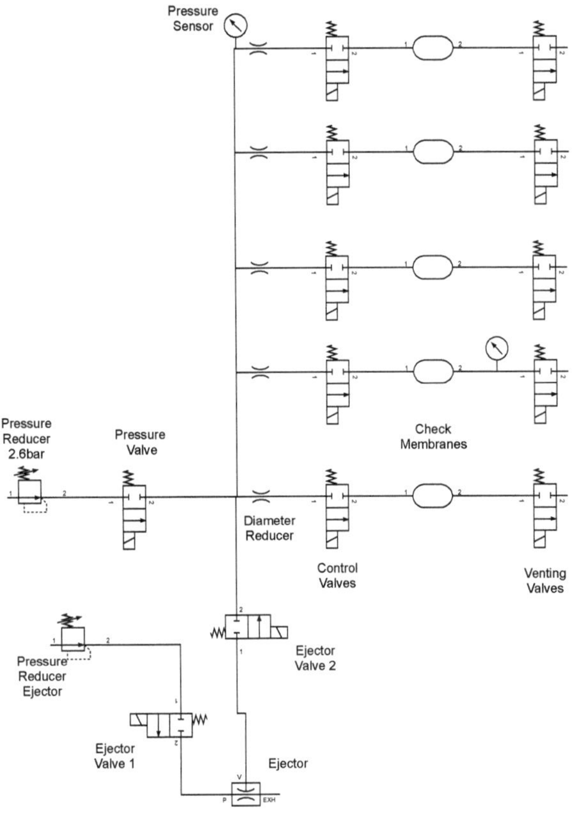

Figure 1: Pneumatic plan of the test.

carry out the required test three times with the five test specimens in each case, so that 30 membranes have been tested as a result. The membranes are inserted into the test block provided for this purpose, which is equipped with two pressure connections on the upper side, so that these can be used both for pressure them with $p_1 = 2.6\ bar$ relative overpressure and for vent against the environment. These are marked in the pneumatic plan by oval vessels and labelled "Check membranes".

To realise this, valves are required. Proportional valves are used, which hold in the open mode at an operating voltage of $U_{in} = 7\ V$, in order to generate as little heat as possible, but also to ensure sufficient flow. Proportional valves are also called control valves because they can assume any intermediate position, which in turn depends on the applied voltage [1] [2]. Since the valves are closed in the de-energised state, they are referred to as "normally closed" valves. The membrane is separated by a control valve, which ensures that the desired pressure is regularly applied, and the venting valve, which has the task of releasing the pressure to the environment after a pressure surge. To ensure that the volume between the control and venting valves, including the volume of the membrane, is exactly $V = 12\ ml$, so that the pressure rise time and thus the hardness of the pressure surge is the same as the conditions in the device. This is the same with the diameter, which determines the flow and is regulated to 1mm. This is realised by self-designed Diameter Reducer of the airflow, which thus

limit the flow to the membranes and can been seen in the pneumatic plan just before the control valves. This is a copper cylinder with G1/8 connections on both sides for the tube connections and an internal diameter of 1mm.

To realise the 2.6 bar relative overpressure, a pressure reducer is needed. This pressure is regulated by the pressure valve behind the reducer. This is in usually open to generate the pressure in the whole system, which causes it to heat up. In order to be able to monitor the pressures exactly and to make evaluations, pressure sensors are needed. In this case, the resolution of the pressure sensors is limited to 4 mbar, which is, however, sufficient for these dimensions and for this application. An ejector is used to generate the negative pressure. This works according to the Venturi principle, in that the compressed air is accelerated by a cross-sectional constriction in the Venturi nozzle, thereby creating a vacuum after the accelerated air has been released. This causes air to be subsequently pulled into the ejector, thus creating a relative negative pressure [3]. This is also supplied with compressed air via a second pressure reducer and generates a relative negative pressure. This pressure reducer is set to 2.3 bar, which ensures that a negative pressure of -500 mbar is generated in the ejector. Another factor is the temperature, as the test items and valves are placed in a climatic cabinet during the test or measurement and brought from 10°C to 40°C and back again in a 3-hour rhythm.

3.2 Algorithm

The algorithm written for this test experiment focuses on the efficient use of time and an optimal pressure rise time. For this an Arduino microcontroller was used. It is important to mention that it is not possible to rise the pressure for all five membranes at the same time with one pressure reducer, as this would make the volume too large and the pressure rise time too long. Therefore it is necessary to realise a sequence and a sequential switching of the valves.

At the beginning of each measurement, a leakage test is carried out. First, an offset leakage is determined that applies to the entire system without the test items. This ensures that the leak tightness of the entire test stand is guaranteed and checked. Then all test items are initially tested for leak tightness. For this purpose, the test items are pressurised to 2.6 bar and then the control and venting valves are closed. After a one-minute settling time, the prepressure is determined via the pressure sensor and a differential pressure is output after a two-minute test. Using this, a leakage value can be determined with $V = 12\ ml$

$$Q_L = \frac{\Delta P \cdot V \cdot 60}{\Delta t}, \qquad (1)$$

where Q_L is the leak rate in $[ml/min]$, ΔP is the pressure difference between the pressure at the beginning and after the check in $[mbar]$, V is the volume in $[ml]$ and Δt is the measured time in $[s]$ [4] [5].

Then the times where the membranes get the pressure are determined to ensure the best possible time management.

To do this, the time needed to bring the test volume, including membranes in the entire set-up, up to 2.6 bar is measured. This pressure rise time t_{rt} is important in order to be able to draw meaningful comparisons with the use in the medical device.

After the leak tests, the actual test begins by bringing pressure on all five membranes one after the other and releasing them again against the environment. This happens in parallel, so that when one valve is relieved, the next one is already letting the pressure to the membrane. Every 10,000 cycles, new leak tests are carried out in order to be able to make a statement about how the membranes behave over time and under increased cycle numbers. In addition, the tightness under different temperatures can be assessed.

After 200,00 cycles with overpressure, the pressure valve is closed and the ejector valves are opened. This causes compressed air to flow through the ejector and the negative pressure of -500 mbar is generated. The algorithm for applying the negative pressure is the same as for the positive pressure, so that it now runs through with a different number of cycles. Finally, a new leak test is carried out.

In order to obtain validated results of the leak test, a comparison measurement is carried out by hand both initially before the test and finally after the test.

4 Results and Discussion

This section presents the results that were obtained during the development of the test stand and serve to check whether this test stand is suitable for testing. In particular, the leak tests and the verification of whether the correct pressures are applied in the corresponding pressure rise time are essential to be examined.

4.1 Pressure Rise Time t_{rt}

In order to check the functionality of the test stand and thus the pressure values and pressure rise times, both overpressure and underpressure are recorded against time. This is shown in Figure 2 and 3.

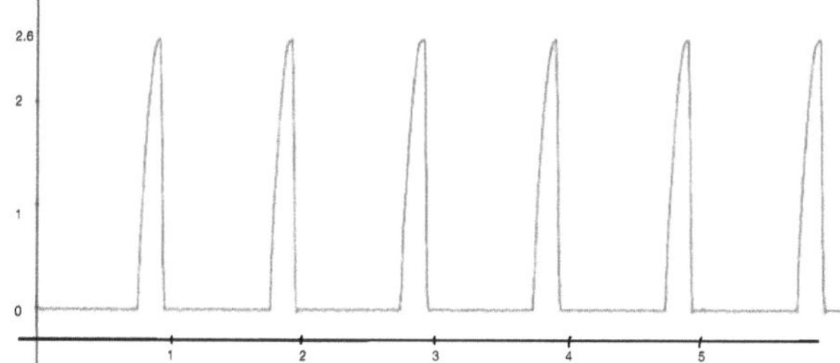

Figure 2: Overpressure graph of one out of five membranes. Y-axis shows the pressure in bar and the X-axis shows the time in seconds (exact times shown in Table 1).

For reasons of clarity, only one membrane out of five is shown. Figure 2 shows the overpressure, which rises to just over 2.6 bar, so that the desired pressure has been reached at the membrane. The other 4 membranes would be between the pressure peaks, so that the five membranes are always supplied with pressure one after the other.

Result of one cycle of a pressure of 2.6 bar	
time in [ms]	pressure in [mbar]
0	0
47	892
94	1692
139	2608
187	935
234	0

Table 1: Pressure and Time during one period of putting 2.6 bar pressure on a membrane

Table 1 shows the pressure rise times required for 2.6 bar relative pressure. It can be seen from this that the pressure rise time is about 140 ms. In total, a cycle with pressure increase and venting requires about 230 ms.

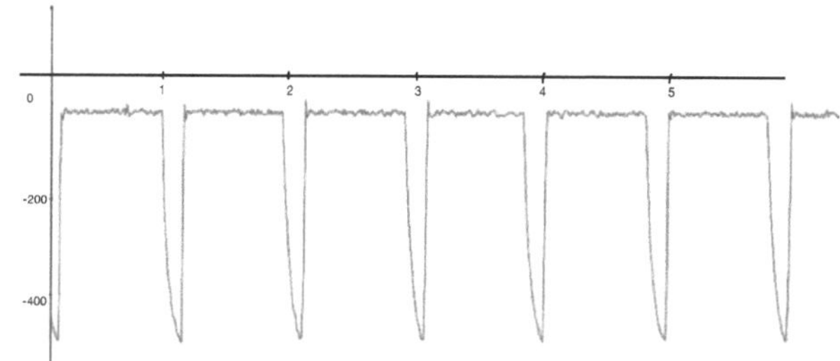

Figure 3: Underpressure graph of one out of five membranes. Y-axis shows the pressure in bar and the X-axis shows the time in seconds.

Figure 3 shows that the negative pressure of - 500 mbar is also applied to the membranes. Table 2 also shows the pressure rise times, which are also around 142 ms in the case of negative pressure. These measurement results are shown in Table 2. Overall, the duration of a cycle is also around 230 ms. For both positive and negative pressure, the pressure increase phase takes almost twice as long as the venting phase. It should be mentioned here that the pressure is set to -481 mbar as the minimum value, so that the pressure rise time can be increased more easily for further measurements.

One cycle of a underpressure of - 500 mbar	
time in [ms]	pressure in [mbar]
0	0
46	-264
94	-404
142	-481
187	-262
236	-13

Table 2: Pressure and Time during one period of putting - 500 mbar pressure on a membrane

4.2 Leaktest

In order to check whether the leak tests work in such a way that they provide reliable results, it is important to use comparative measurements. These are shown in Table 3. Leak tests were made for the system and for 2 membranes each before, during and after. These are compared with them being re-measured by hand. It can be clearly seen that these values correspond. It should be noted here that a leak test (in this order of magnitude) cannot agree in practice to the second decimal place, as this changes during a flow measurement even through slight heating or other minimal influences.

Leckage Test

Measurement	component	Leckage rate in [ml/min]
before	System	1.15
1	System	1.05
2	System	1.15
after (manual)	System	1.27
before	Membrane 1	0.29
1	Membrane 1	0.26
2	Membrane 1	0.26
after (manual)	Membrane 1	0.16
before	Membrane 2	0.26
1	Membrane 2	0.23
2	Membrane 2	0.23
after (manual)	Membrane 2	0.2

Table 3: Leckage test of 2 membranes during a test run and afterwards manual measurement to compare

5 Conclusion

Based on the results, it is possible to say that the test stand can be put into operation. The tests used to validate the test stand and prove that the test stand can deliver reliable results have been positive. The pressures are correct, the pressure rise times are in the ranges specified by the unit and the leak tests agree with the manual testing. Thus, it can be concluded that the test rig is suitable for a first test of the membranes, to get an impression, wether they could use in the medical device. Furthermore, it is possible to test other pneumatic components with this experimental set-up, easily and with little time expenditure. To do this, the software must be adapted and the components to be tested must be integrated into the pneumatic plan. This ensures that the test setup can also be used for other purposes.

It is generally very important that test equipment and general testing of specifically medical products are controlled down to the smallest detail. Both the testing itself and the tested devices must be absolutely safe and reliable. Therefore, it is all the more important to check exactly whether the results obtained are reliable and whether the exact way in which these values were generated can be traced. Fortunately, these important findings are precisely documented and also proven with every test, because not only the final result is decisive, but also the way to it and the equipment used for it are essential for assessment.

The test stand that has been created is therefore ready for use and sufficiently checked to be able to make a valid statement about the tested membranes. It is not only the tightness that is decisive, but also the temperature behaviour and endurance capacity of the membranes. This test is an example of the precision and conscientiousness with which the performance and safety of medical devices are worked on. These are tested to absolute satisfaction and reliability to ensure the best possible benefit for the patient, who, as mentioned at the introduction, entrusts their most important asset to these devices, their life.

Finally, now that it can be assumed that the test stand provides reliable and correct results, testing of membranes can take place. Of course, the resulting values must also be checked for correctness, but it is now possible and there is a tool with which various pneumatic components can be tested in the future.

Acknowledgement

The work has been carried out at Drägerwerk AG & Co. KGaA, Lübeck, in collaboration with Sven Pasdzior and supervised by Prof. Dr. Philipp Rostalski from the Institute of Electrical Engineering in Medicine, Universität zu Lübeck. I would also like to thank Carlotta Hennigs for her help and support.

Author's Statement

Conflict of interest: Authors state no conflict of interest.

6 References

[1] H. Watter, *Hydraulik und Pneumatik: Grundlagen und Übungen – Anwendungen und Simulation*, Springer, Wiesbaden, 2022

[2] N. Gebhardt, J. Weber *Hydraulik - Fluid Mechatronik: Grundlagen, Komponenten, Systeme, Messtechnik und virtuelles Engineering*, Springer, Berlin, 2020

[3] https://www.schmalz.com/de-de/vakuum-wissen/basiswissen/funktionsprinzipien-der-vakuum-erzeugung/; [last accessed: 2023/01/18]

[4] https://www.cetatest.com/fileadmin/pdf/daten-blatt_deutsch/Leckraten-Nomogramm_de.pdf; [last accessed: 2023/01/18]

[5] https://www.schweizer-fn.de/rohr/leckrate/leckrate.php#leckageart; [last accessed: 2023/01/18]

Development of a mechanical holder for laser drilling of diffusion membranes

Jan-Ole Knuth [1], Christopher Kren [2], Norbert Koop [3]

[1] Medical Engineering Science, Universität zu Lübeck, janole.knuth@student.uni-luebeck.de
[2] Medizinisches Laserzentrum Lübeck GmbH, christopher.kren@uni-luebeck.de
[3] Medizinisches Laserzentrum Lübeck GmbH, n.koop@uni-luebeck.de

Abstract

The "Medizinisches Laserzentrum Lübeck GmbH" is working on the optimisation of laser processes. In order to be able to statistically record fluctuations in the process parameters and their effect on the homogeneity of the lasered holes, recurring series of measurements have to be carried out. Therefore, a sensor holder was developed which securely fixes large numbers of membranes in position on the existing linear axes. Problems with the fitting and positioning of the membranes were noticed in a first version. Therefore, a second version was developed. Since the distance of the membrane to the laser focus is a critical process parameter, the height of the second version is adjustable. Also, the type of positioning was changed from stop bolts to a three-point support. To compare the two sensor holders, both were evaluated by height measurements using a confocal sensor. The height differences could be reduced by fine adjustment screws.

1 Introduction

Electrochemical gas sensors are used in many areas, including medicine, safety technology but also for monitoring air quality. With these sensors, the gas to be measured is not actively supplied. Rather, it reaches the measuring point through simple molecular movement. The measuring electrodes are preceded by a diffusion barrier to ensure a defined supply of the gas to be measured [1]. This diffusion barrier is realised by means of a microhole in a few 100 µm thick polymer membrane. The microhole is drilled by laser ablation [2] and has a diameter of 20-40 µm depending on the later application. The "Medizinisches Laserzentrum Lübeck GmbH" is working on the optimisation of laser processes for drilling holes in membranes. The membranes are processed here using an excimer laser with different configurations and parameter sets. Evaluation criteria of these holes are mainly geometry and oxygen diffusion. In order to be able to statistically record variations in the process parameters and their effect on the homogeneity of the lasered holes, recurring series of measurements with several hundred membranes must be carried out.This gave rise to the need to improve an existing set-up on which holes can be set individually by manual operation.

The aim of this project was the development of a mechanical holder that fixes large numbers of the respective membranes in a position-safe manner on the existing linear axes. Since the distance of the membranes to the laser focus is a crucial process parameter, the height variations of the membranes in relation to the laser focus should be minimised over the entire travel path of the axes. Furthermore, the laser process is controlled by an energy measurement below the membrane. The light passing through the resulting hole enables detection of the transmitted energy and can provide information on the hole geometry. An additional requirement was therefore that the design should enable energy measurement of each bore. A simple holder and an improved further development were evaluated and compared by height measurements using a confocal sensor.

2 Material and Methods

2.1 Membrane used

The membranes for which a holder was build in this project is internally identified as a 2in1 called electrode holder shown in Fig. 1. The 2in1 electrode holder is made of polypropylene. The membrane has a thickness of 200 µm and a radius of 0.52 mm.

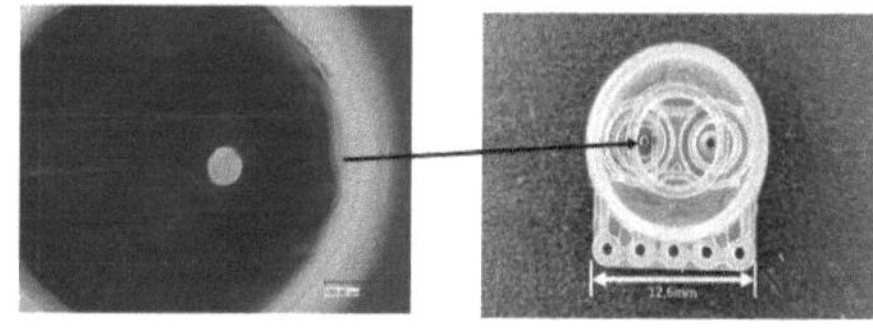

Figure 1: Frontal view of the electrode holder 2in1 (right) and a magnification (left) of the membrane, which appears black, with a microhole (small brighter circle)

2.2   Processing station: MicroMaster

Laser drilling is performed at a processing station using a UV excimer laser (wavelength= 193 nm) and a micrometer-accurate 3-axis system. The hole itself is created by masking the beam profile onto the membrane. By changing the mask and adjusting the distances of the imaging lenses, different hole diameters can be generated. The distances of the imaging lenses result from the imaging law (1) and the calculation of the magnification (2).

$$\frac{1}{f} = \frac{1}{g} + \frac{1}{b} \tag{1}$$

$$A = \frac{b}{g} \tag{2}$$

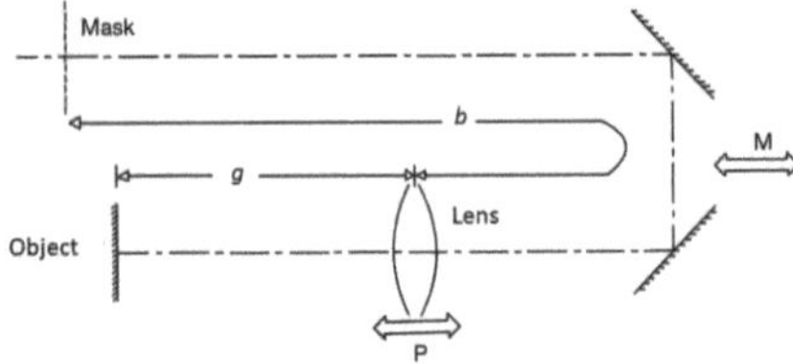

Figure 2: Sketch of the beam path in the MicroMaster, b: distance between lens and aperture; g: distance between lens and object; M: mobile mirror; P: projection lens [3]

2.3   Chromatic confocal sensor

The processing-related height fluctuations of the milled surfaces were measured using a confocal sensor. Table 1 lists the technical data of the chromatic confocal sensor. In chromatic confocal sensors, the height information is converted into colour information so that a mechanical Z-scan is no longer necessary. The conversion from height to colour information is done by an optical system with a well-defined longitudinal chromatic aberration (LCA). The LCA can be controlled in the design of optical systems by the dispersive properties of optical materials. The division of refractive power between refractive and diffractive components allows to design a system for a specific working distance and depth scanning range [4].

Table 1: Chromatic confocal sensor parameters

Parameter	
Model	CL4-MG35
Measuring range	4 mm
Working distance	16,5 mm
Numerical Aperture	0,32
Axial Resolution	0,66 µm
Lateral resolution	4,6 µm
Spot size	12,3 µm

2.4   Concept

To measure the pulse energy passing through a hole, a suitable energy sensor [5], is suspended between two plates. The lower plate serves as a base and is attached to the XY linear table of the MicroMaster. The upper plate is the receptacle for an exchangeable sensor holder.

3   Results and Discussion

3.1   Version A of the sensor holder

In this first version of the sensor holder, stop points are provided on the top plate to facilitate positioning. Fine positioning is then done with screws, as shown in Fig. 3. In the middle is a recess of 16x16 cm to measure the exit energy during the drilling process. The gap between the base plate and the upper plate for the energy sensor is enabled by cylindrical pins.

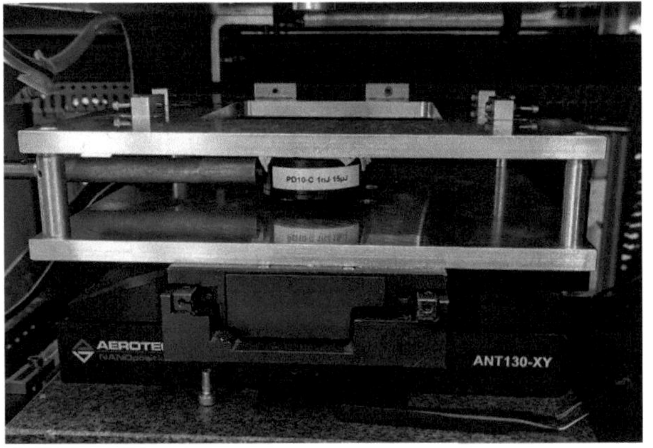

Figure 3: Built-in first version of the sensor holder in the MicroMaster

The sensor holder consists of a simple plate with 6x6 milled holes, which are suitable for the 2in1 electrode holders shown in Fig. 4. The milled holes were designed as a press fit, which has the advantage that the position of each membrane is clearly defined. The problem with this version is that the defined position of the membrane mentioned is only correct in theory. Due to the stop bolts, the sensor holder still has too many lines of freedom, which means that the approached positions do not correspond to the position of the membrane. In addition, the press fit has the disadvantage that a lot of pressure is necessary to place the 2in1 electrode holder.

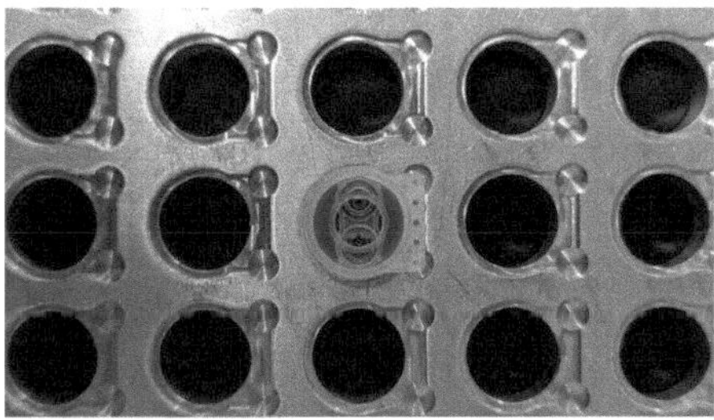

Figure 4: Magnified view of the milled holes for the 2in1 electrode holders and an inserted 2in1 electrode holder in the center

3.2 Version B of the sensor holder

Due to the negative aspects of the first version, a second version was designed. The construction of this version is shown in Fig. 5.

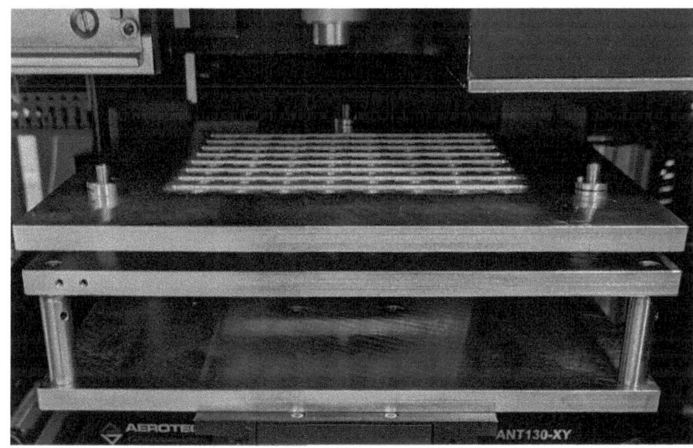

Figure 5: Built-in sensor holder version B, with guide corners at the rear left and right.

In order to improve possible differences in height or positioning, a three-point support with fine adjustment screws was used. The principle of the three-point support is shown in Fig. 6. In relation to the sensor holder, it means that three inserts must be inserted into the upper plate. The prism must be oriented to the ball socket.

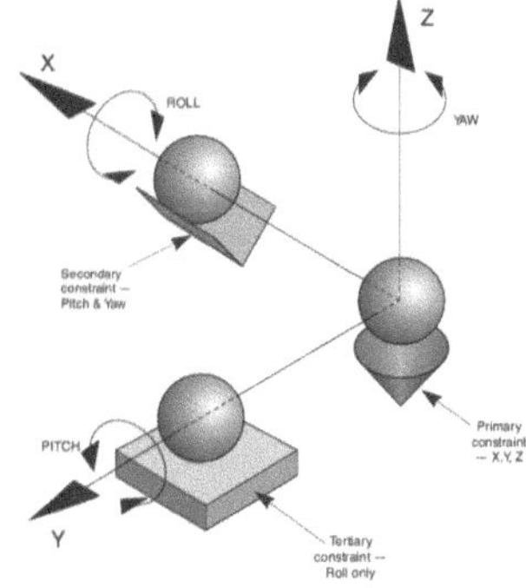

Figure 6: Principle of the three-point pad

For positioning assistance, two guide corners were printed Fig. 5, which should help to place the sensor holder more easily and quickly. In the second version, the milled holes were designed as a clearance fit with 0.5 mm clearance. This makes it easier to place the 2in1 electrode holder and also it is easier to remove it from the sensor holder. Furthermore, the size of the sensor holder was changed so that there is now room for 8x8 2in1 electrode holders.

3.3 Planarity comparison

To evaluate the planarity of the two sensor holders (version A and B), the distance from the sensor head to the surface was measured with a confocal sensor for each milling. For this purpose, the milling was scanned several times. Fig. 7 shows a sketch of this procedure. The measuring process was carried out as outlined in Fig. 7. Each cutout was scanned both in X and Y direction, using the XY linear table of the MicroMaster. The median (X_{1x1}) was determined from these measured values (X_1-X_n) to represent the milled out area (in the example the position 1x1). This was repeated for each milled area. The median is used because measurement inaccuracies and large jumps occur at the transition from the milled area to the borehole. In order to compare the medians with each other, they were scaled (3). Here the X_{nxn} stands for the median of a specific milled out area (N=1,2,3,4,5,6 for version A and N=1,2,3,4,5,6,7,8 for version B). The X_{min} and X_{max} stand for the largest and smallest median distance of the sensor holder.

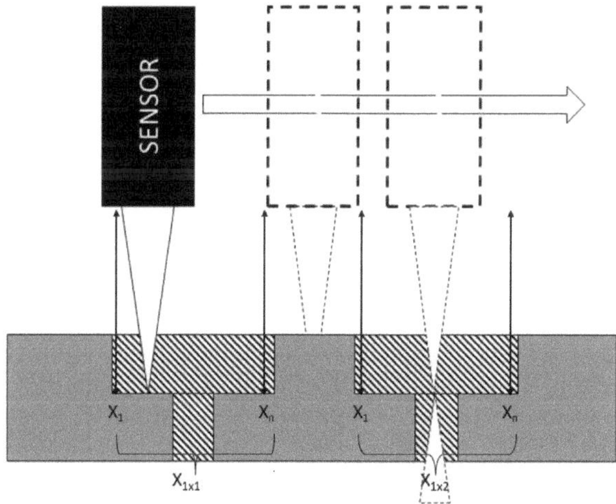

Figure 7: Sketched principle of confocal measurement

$$X_{scaled} = \frac{X_{nxn} - X_{min}}{X_{max} + X_{min}} \qquad (3)$$

According to this scaling principle, the lowest median of the sensor holder represents zero percentage and the highest median represents 100 percentage or zero and one. From this, the percentage deviation of the heights can be read off. The heat map in Fig. 8 represents the percentage deviation of the 6x6 boreholes in their elevation. The X-axis represents the rows of the sensor holder and the Y-axis the columns.

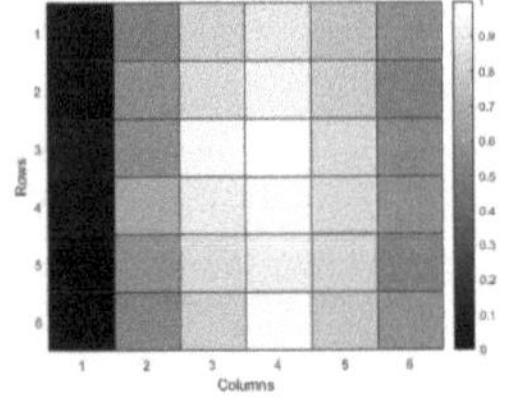

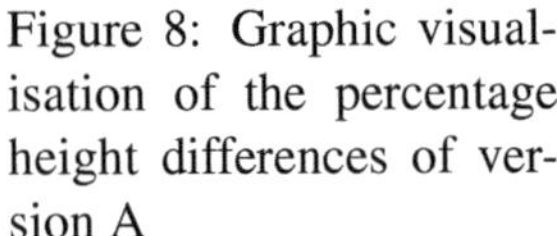

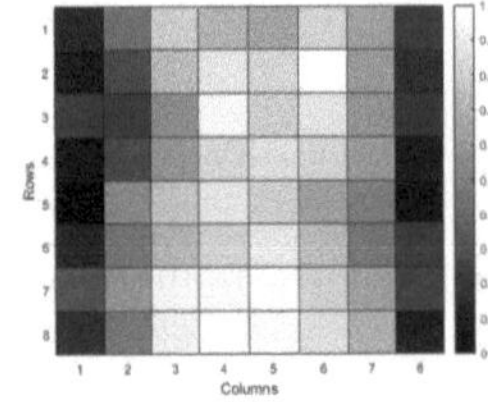

Figure 8: Graphic visualisation of the percentage height differences of version A

Figure 9: Graphic visualisation of the percentage height differences of version B

For comparison, the same measurement was done with sensor holder version B. In this case the fine adjustment screws were set before with the help of the confocal sensor so that the plate had the same distance to the measuring head at all four corners. The result is shown in Fig. 9 as a heat map. The X-axis represents the rows of the sensor holder and the Y-axis the columns. From the two heat maps it is possible to see that in version A the distance to the measuring head does not remain the same. Here you can see that the distance of the milled areas to the measuring head increases towards the centre. This is due to the milling, as more pressure is exerted on the centre of the plate when the plate is clamped by milling, resulting in a slight curvature. But even independent of this curvature, there is a difference in height between column one and column six. In version B, as can be seen in Fig. 9 this height difference could almost be eliminated by the fine adjustment screws. These height differences can also be seen in Fig. 10 by a box-plot diagram. Here the statistical distribution of the measured distances for each row of the sensor holder is plotted. This shows that the height differences of the second version Fig. 11 are smaller than those of the first version.

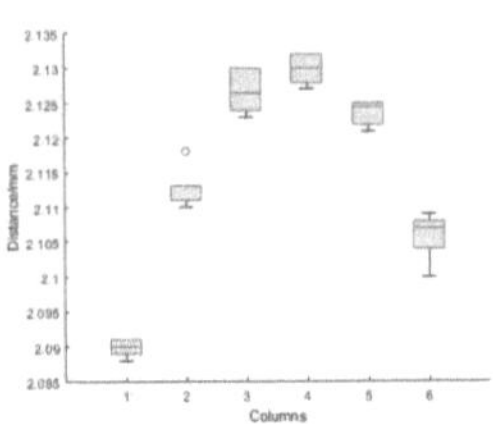

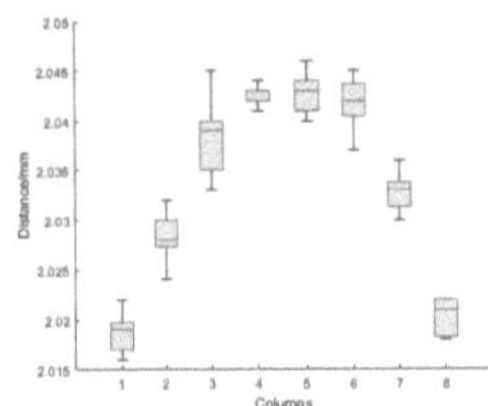

Figure 10: Statistical distribution of the measured distances for each row of the sensor holder version A

Figure 11: Statistical distribution of the measured distances for each row of the sensor holder version B

4   Conclusion

Version B of the sensor holder has the main advantages that it is easier to fit, the height differences can be compensated by means of fine adjustment screws and there is room for more electrode holders on it. In addition, the sensor holder clearly positioned by the three-point support. Due to the better planarity of version B, it should be possible to automatically drill through the membranes and to detect when the membrane is drilled through via the energy sensor.

5   Acknowledgement

The work was supervised by the "Medizinisches Laserzentrum Lübeck GmbH".

Author's Statement

Conflict of interest: Authors state no conflict of interest.

6   References

[1] C. O. Park and J.W. Fergus, N. Miura, J. Park and A. Choi, *Solid-state electrochemical gas sensors.* Available: https://doi.org/10.1007/s11581-008-0300-6 [last accessed on 2023-1-18].

[2] Y. Chen, H. Y. Zheng, T. K. S. Wong and S. C. Tam, *Excimer laser drilling of polymers.* https://doi.org/10.1117/12.280575 [last accessed on 2023-1-18].

[3] L. A. Rossa *Pulse energy on the outlet side as a control signal in the micro-drilling process.*

[4] C. Pruss, A. Ruprecht, K. Körner, W. Osten, P. Lücke *Diffractive Elements for Chromatic Confocal Sensors.* DGaO Proceedings, vol. 43, 2005 .

[5] Ophir® *PD10-C Datasheet.* Available: https://doi.org/10.1007/s11581-008-0300-6 [last accessed on 2023-1-18].

Automatic assignment of oregano species employing metabolomic fingerprints

Leif Tastesen [1], Friedemann Flügge [2], Ulrich Günther [3]

[1] Biophysics, Universität zu Lübeck, leif.tastesen@student.uni-luebeck.de
[2] LADR GmbH Medizinisches Versorgungszentrum Dr. Kramer Kollegen, Geesthacht, f.fluegge@ladr.de
[3] Institut für Chemie und Metabolomics, Universität zu Lübeck, ulrich.guenther@uni-luebeck.de

Abstract

Metabolomics deals with the entirety of molecules below a molecular weight of 1.5 kDa in a living organism. Nuclear magnetic resonance (NMR) is one of the main analytical techniques for the characterization of these metabolites. The NMR spectrum of a biofluid comprises information about all included metabolites and can be regarded as its metabolomic fingerprint. Principal component analysis (PCA) and fitting of Gaussian-mixture models allow the identification of spectral similarities and differences in reference data and the assignment of an unknown sample to one of the previously identified clusters. In this study, different extracts from different oregano species were used as references. The automated sample characterization presented in this paper can be used for quality control.

1   Introduction

Fraud in the herb and spices industry is a profitable but criminal activity. The market is growing because of the increasing demand. To be marketed as oregano, only impurities up to 2% are tolerated [1]. The number of publications on metabolomics by NMR is increasing. Compared to other methods like mass spectrometry (MS), the advantages are the high reproducibility and the noninvasive measurement, which allows different measurements with the same sample. The spectra are inherently quantitative because the metabolite concentration is directly proportional to the intensities and minimal sample preparation is required. The main disadvantage of NMR is the lower sensitivity compared to MS and thus a limited number of detectable metabolites. The detection depends on the spectral resolution, but it is usually limited to 200 metabolites [2].

Two-dimensional ^{1}H J-resolved (J-Res) NMR spectroscopy maintains the advantage that the intensity is proportional to the metabolite concentration, but with coupling in the second dimension, the signal overlap is reduced. This increases the metabolite specificity [3]. A J-Res is acquired in the magnitude mode, leading to completely in-phase signals which makes the automated processing easier [4].

A principal component analysis (PCA) can be done to extract information and reduce noise from data. The PCA is unsupervised. This reduced structure can reveal new information like the clustering of species. To reduce noise, the PCA reduces the basis of the data from the number of data points to a new set of orthogonal variables which are a linear combination of the original variables. The new variables are called principal components and are eigenvectors of the covariance matrix of the data matrix. The linear combination of the eigenvectors (loads) with the original variables creates the scores, which are the coordinates in the new basis. A singular value decomposition (SVD) can break down the data matrix into three parts, which contain all the information needed for a PCA [5].

A Gaussian-mixture model (GMM) can cluster data. A Gaussian-mixture model is created by the distribution of the data on each principal component. By combining multiple dimensions, a multidimensional distribution is created. This distribution can be modeled with a Gaussian function. Because the distribution has multiple points where data accumulates, the function has separated means. Each cluster has its weight according to the number of samples that accumulate around the mean. To create a normal distribution, the weights must add up to 1. Because of the change from one dimension of a normal Gaussian to a multiple-dimensional Gaussian the variance changes to a covariance matrix, to determine the shape of the fit. In this model, each data has a p-value for every cluster and can be assigned by choosing the maximum likelihood [6]. An assignment can be verified with univariate and multivariate verification.

Partial least square regression (PLS) analysis works similarly to a PCA but correlates two sets of data, where one dataset is dependent on the other. In contrast to a PCA, a PLS is a supervised method that can be employed to assess any additions in samples. The PLS decomposes both matrices as a product of common loadings, which serve as a new basis. In contrast to a PCA, the loadings in a PLS are not orthogonal. This analysis results in a prediction of the influential dataset [7].

2 Material and Methods

The data analysis software is implemented in Matlab (The MathWorks Inc., Massachusetts, USA). For this analysis, 534 J-Res spectra are used as a reference. 160 of these spectra contain additions. The spectra are read by the readspc-function. The Fourier-transformation, tilting and symmetrization are done by the xfb-function. After the J-Res is processed the calc_proj_ml-function does the projection for the resonances and the result can be further processed before the analysis is done. All these functions are from the NMRLab [8]. The symmetrization of the J-Res is accomplished by comparing the upper half and the lower half of the tilted spectra and comparing for each row of data which peak is closer to the center and this corresponding half is copied for the other half. This program can be employed to create a reference matrix consisting of spectra of different pure species and process a singular unknown spectrum and append it to the reference matrix. The reference is necessary to achieve a reliable assignment. The spectra are all baseline corrected and aligned. For the alignment first, the TMSP reference signal has to be aligned and subsequently, the whole spectra are scaled to the TMSP peak. Subsequently, the whole spectra get aligned.

Before the PCA can be applied, the spectra have to be scaled: First, the reference spectra are PQN scaled, Pareto scaled and median-centered. The scaling factors and centering values are later used for the test sample.

- Probabilistic quotient normalisation (PQN)
  The PQN scaling is used to normalize differences between samples that are caused by dilution effects. The scaling works by calculating a median spectrum with the median for each data point by using all reference spectra. Subsequently, the median of the quotients of a spectrum and median spectrum for each data point is used to normalize all data points of the spectrum [9].

- Pareto scaling
  For Pareto scaling, each data point is scaled by dividing by the square root of the standard deviations of the data points of all reference spectra [10].

- Median-centring
  A spectrum is median-centered by subtracting a median spectrum, which is calculated by using the median of each data point.

The PCA model is created by the reference spectra. In this study, the first six eigenvectors are used. After the model is created the test experiment is scaled and predicted, so it is projected on the new axis and thereby obtains new coordinates. In this new coordinate system, the data can be clustered by the GMM. This way the sample is assigned to a species if the p-value is greater than 0.001.

After the assignment to a reference cluster, an univariate and multivariate verification is necessary. For verification, only the data of the selected group is used. The univariate analysis implements a one-sided t-test for each data point and tests it for outliers. To compensate for multiple testing, the defined significance level ($\alpha = 0.01$) is divided by the number of data points. The multivariate analysis relies on Q-residual and Hotelling's T^2, which are both normalized by the 99% quantile. The Q-residual is the sum of all differences between the original data and the projected data calculated by the prediction. Hotelling's T^2 calculates in the scores space the distance of the test sample to the center of a PCA model, which is only created with the selected data. Subsequently, the ratio of possible additions is calculated if the univariate or multivariate verification shows too many deviations from the created model. Spectra of extracts from the following additions were included: *Myrtus communis*, *Olea europaea*, *Corylus avellana*, *Cistus creticus* and the species *Origanum majorana*. Numerically spiked data used for the PLS regression is created by picking a random spectrum from oregano and different additions and scaling it with a random concentration between 0 and 1 before adding them to one spiked sample. This is done 20001 times to create a whole matrix of spiked samples. All concentrations that are used for one spiked spectrum must add up to 1. To prevent the last addition from only getting a very low percentage assigned, only three of five additions are randomly selected for each spiked sample.

The spiked sample and concentrations are used for a partial least square (PLS) analysis. The PLS uses the information of the concentration and the spiked samples to create a model that can predict the test sample's concentration.[11]

3 Results and Discussion

To present the results, a sample with additions of marjoram and olive is used (Table 1). The species and the percentage of addition are known and therefore it is a suitable test for the program.

Table 1: Characteristics of the test sample

Test sample	
Species	Oregano
Origin	Turkish
Oregano	85%
Marjoram	5%
Olive	10%

The PCA and PLS are tested with the methods of the PLS_Toolbox (Eigenvector Research, Inc.) as a reference, therefore the same results are calculated. In this case, Turkish oregano is assigned with a p-value of 0.21, which is the correct assignment. The other species have a p-value below 0.001 (Fig. 1).

To illustrate the univariate analysis, the test spectrum is plotted on top of reference spectra in the background consisting of the data of the same species. The darker the background, the closer it is to the median of the reference samples. The positions which have a p-value below the threshold are marked (Fig. 2, 3). This univariate analysis marks 28 spots. This is expected as the additions should lead to different intensities at characteristic positions.

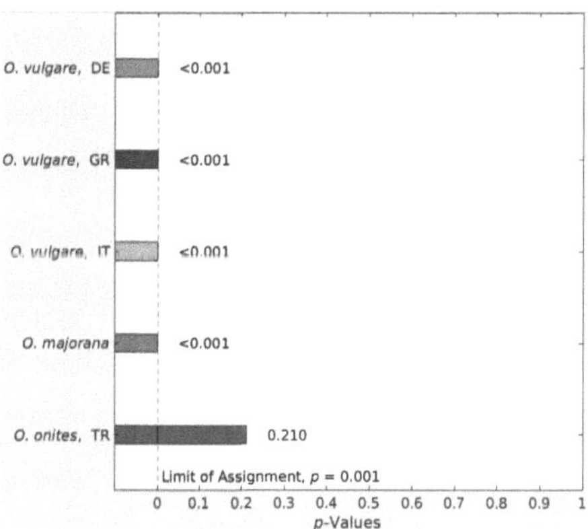

Figure 1: The p-values of the assignment are shown. The dotted line gives the minimum which is plotted. If the p-value lies below 0.001 the actual p-value is replaced with <0.001.

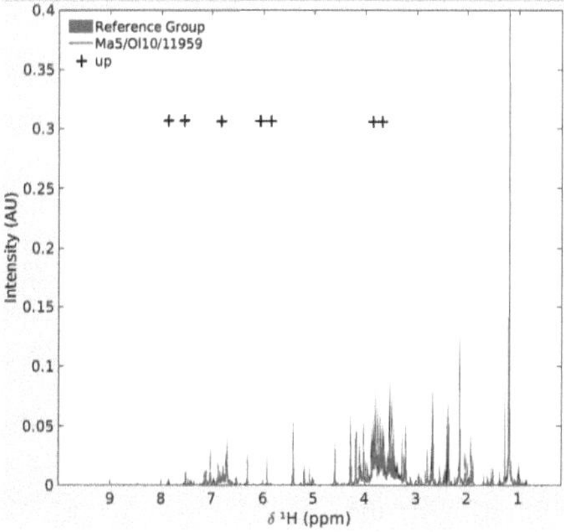

Figure 2: The plot shows a test sample (line) and a reference (black-grey background). To label outliers, crosses are plotted at the respective positions.

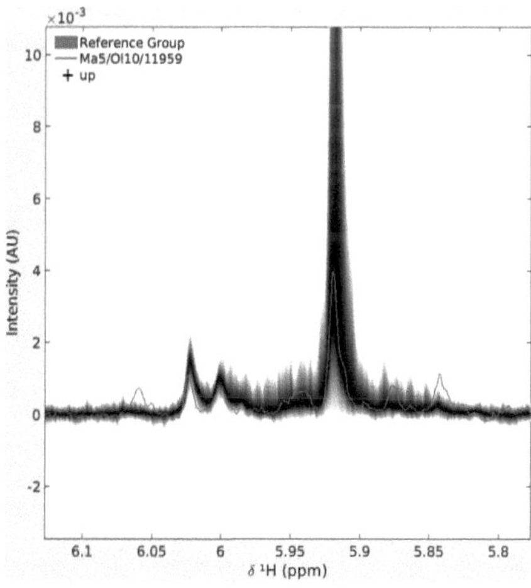

Figure 3: The plot shows a test sample (line) and a reference (black-grey background). It shows suspicious deviation from the reference.

The multivariate analysis is illustrated in a 2D-Plot, that shows Hotelling's T^2 vs. Q-residuals. Both quantities are normalized by their 99% confidence intervals (Fig. 4). If one of the statistical parameters is greater than one, the sample is defined as "off-model". Deviation in the univariate or multivariate verification triggers a calculation of additions. In the case of the test sample (Table 1), the Q-residuals are too high. Therefore, both univariate and multivariate analyses exhibit the case of a suspicious sample.

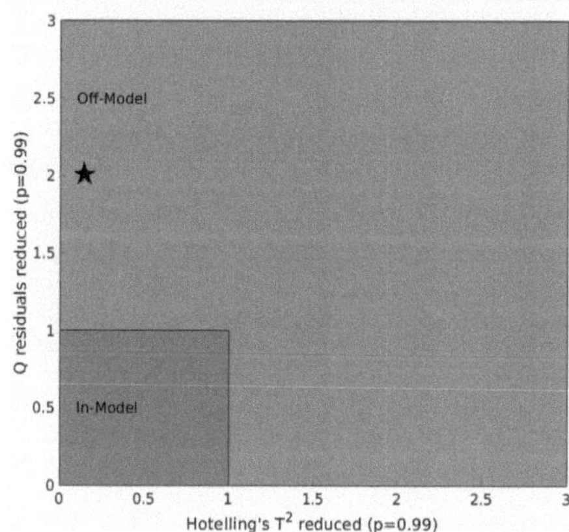

Figure 4: The star represents the Q-residuals and the Hotelling's T^2 of the test sample. If both parameters are less than one the sample is "in-model". A sample located in the "off-model" area indicates suspicious content.

The PLS model can be used to calculate the concentrations that were used to create the model at first. Therefore the model is created by concentrations of oregano and additions, the calculated concentration should match the concentrations of the spiked samples. To show this, a plot of the concentrations against the calculated concentrations can be displayed (Fig. 5).

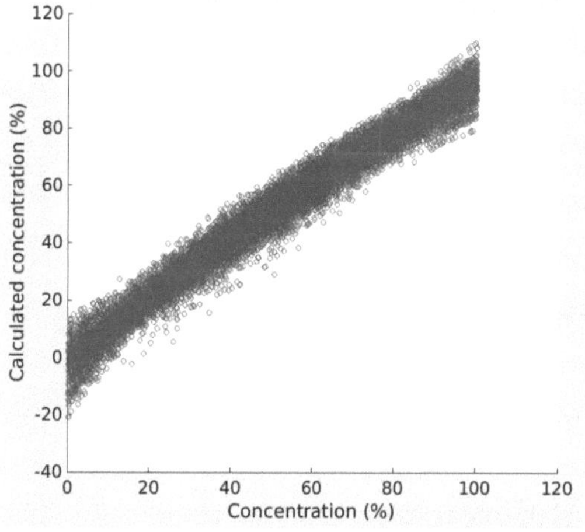

Figure 5: The figure shows the calculated concentrations of oregano against the real concentration of oregano.

Fig. 5 exhibits a linear plot meaning the calculated concentration correlates with the concentration of the simulated spiked samples. From this result, it can be concluded that the prediction is valid. Therefore this model can be used for calculating the concentration of the additions for the test sample. In this experiment, non-claimed supplements of

13.4% were estimated. So, there is a difference of 1.6% (Table 1) that can be tolerated. The total root mean square error of 160 measured spiked samples is 9.41% which is rather big and should be considered. It is worth mentioning that this large error is caused by some outliers and is not present throughout all spectra. The PLS itself has a reliable prediction with a root mean square error of 4.37% and an R-squared of 0.976 (Table 2).

Table 2: Errors of predicted additions and calibration data

Dataset (sample size)	RMS	R-squared
Spiked samples (160)	9.41%	0.54
Origanum majorana (50)	7.90%	0.64
Olea europaea (52)	9.18%	0.52
Calibration data (20001)	4.37%	0.98

Because of the large amount of randomized spiked samples, the PLS is highly reproducible.

4 Conclusion

As an analytical method to remove noise and extract information from data that can be used for clustering, the principal component analysis is suitable for analyzing NMR spectra of spices like oregano. The model must be verified afterwards, to check for additions. The partial least square analysis can calculate the additions in the case, that the model could not be verified, but this study has shown that the calculation has a rather big root mean square error of 9.41%, even if the calibration data can be predicted well. To reduce this error, it might help to examine the spectra that have a noticeably large error.

Acknowledgement

The work has been carried out at the institute of chemistry and metabolomics at the Universität zu Lübeck.

Author's Statement

Conflict of interest: Authors state no conflict of interest.

5 References

[1] Black, C., Haughey, S. A., Chevallier, O. P., Galvin-King, P., Elliott, C. T. (2016). A comprehensive strategy to detect the fraudulent adulteration of herbs: The oregano approach. Food Chemistry, 210, 551–557.

[2] Emwas, A. H., Roy, R., McKay, R. T., Tenori, L., Saccenti, E., Gowda, G. N., ... Wishart, D. S. (2019). NMR spectroscopy for metabolomics research. Metabolites, 9(7), 123.

[3] Ludwig, C., Viant, M. R. (2010). Two-dimensional J-resolved NMR spectroscopy: review of a key methodology in the metabolomics toolbox. Phytochemical Analysis: An International Journal of Plant Chemical and Biochemical Techniques, 21(1), 22-32.

[4] Baishya, B. (2022). Slice selective absorption-mode J-resolved NMR spectroscopy. Journal of Magnetic Resonance, 342, 107267.

[5] Kurita, T. (2019). Principal component analysis (PCA). Computer Vision: A Reference Guide, 1-4.

[6] Sahbi, H. (2008). A particular Gaussian mixture model for clustering and its application to image retrieval. Soft Computing, 12(7), 667-676.

[7] Abdi, H. (2003). Partial least square regression (PLS regression). Encyclopedia for research methods for the social sciences, 6(4), 792-795.

[8] Günther, U. L., Ludwig, C., Rüterjans, H. (2000). NMRLAB—advanced NMR data processing in Matlab. Journal of Magnetic Resonance, 145(2), 201-208.

[9] Kohl, S. M., Klein, M. S., Hochrein, J., Oefner, P. J., Spang, R., Gronwald, W. (2012). State-of-the art data normalization methods improve NMR-based metabolomic analysis. Metabolomics, 8, 146-160.

[10] Eriksson, L., Antti, H., Gottfries, J., Holmes, E., Johansson, E., Lindgren, F., ... Wold, S. (2004). Using chemometrics for navigating in the large data sets of genomics, proteomics, and metabonomics (gpm). Analytical and bioanalytical chemistry, 380, 419-429.

[11] Wold, S., Martens, H., Wold, H. (2006). The multivariate calibration problem in chemistry solved by the PLS method. In Matrix Pencils. Proceedings of a Conference Held at Pite Havsbad, Sweden, March 22–24, 1982, 286-293.

Improvement of the electro-magnetic brake for a medical supply system

Lucas Köllisch [1], Thomas Martin [2], Norbert Linz [3],

[1] Medical Engineering Science, Universität zu Lübeck, lucas.koellisch@student.uni-luebeck.de
[2] RnD Product Line Medical Supply Units, Drägerwerk AG Co. KGaA Lübeck, Thomas.martin@draeger.com
[3] Institute of Biomedical Optics, Universität zu Lübeck, norbert.linz@uni-luebeck.de

Abstract

In this study is the research for an improvement of an electro-magnetic brake utilized in a medical supply unit described. More and more costumers want to equip additional medical devices onto the medical supply systems. Therefore, the importance of this project is set through the continuously rising weights for supply systems. The data acquisition refers to the improvement of the friction force and the friction coefficient between bearing and brake. The results show that one simple solution is not sufficient. However, the combination of different modifications can lead to an improvement. In conclusion, it is possible to improve the braking torque of the electro-magnetic brake. Looking to the further future it could be considered to search for an other brake solution. Due to company secrecy, no quantitative measured values are published in the following study.

1   Introduction

Ceiling supply units allow hospital staff to move medical equipment (e.g., ventilators) around the room without much effort. To move the arms of the supply system the bearings are integrated. The brake is important to keep the supply system in the position the user want it to be. This will improve the staff's workplace [1]. In addition, a patient room

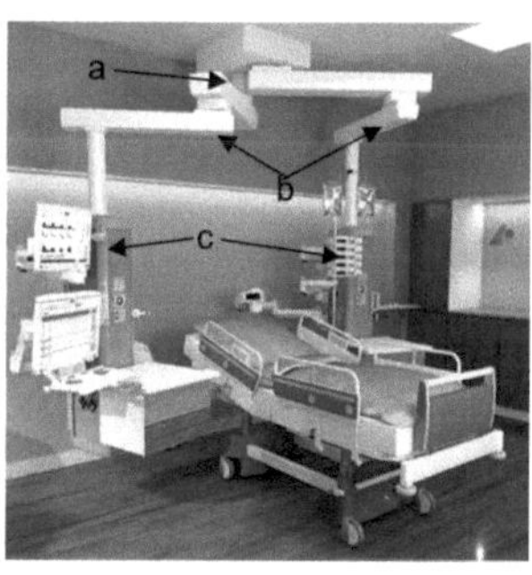

Figure 1: Ceiling supply unit in the patient's room [2]. a Ceiling bearing (no need for improvement), b Intermediate bearing (looking for improvement), c Column bearing (same brake as b)

or operating room is easier to clean because medical equipment has no contact points with the floor Fig. 1. The trend of medical ceiling supply units is developing in the direction of equipping more medical devices. This results in higher loads for this unit. The high load creates a bending of the support arm system, because each material has a certain bending. The higher the bending, the higher the potential torque. To compensate the increasing torque, the brake bearings require a higher braking torque. In this series of tests, the focus was on increasing the normal force F_N seen in Fig. 2 and improving the coefficients of friction. In this regard, tests are carried out to arrive at a development idea.

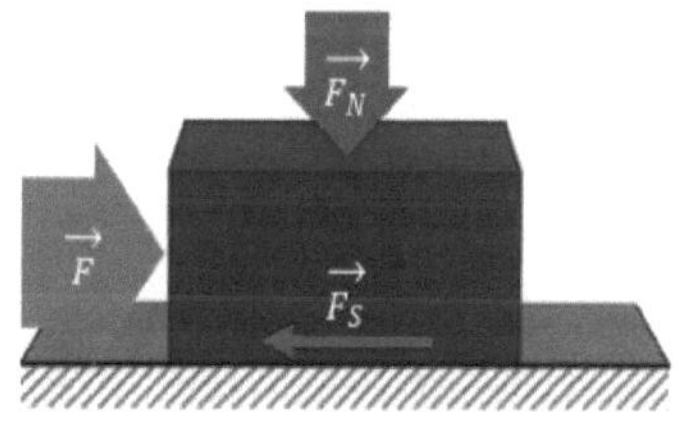

Figure 2: Representation of the effect of the normal force F_N [3]

The aim is an increase, in order to keep up with the progressive development for medical supply systems to fulfil the needs of customers. Due to company secrecy, no quantitative measured values are published in the following study.

2   Material and Methods

The Fig. 3 presents the construction of the bearing and shows every part that is needed for the testing. A spring f applies force to the brake shoes b to press the brake shoes against the bearing sleeve c. The magnetic drivers a consist of a coil, which is installed in the housing and an iron block for attaching the brake shoes. If the magnetic drivers are energized the coil generates a magnetic field and thus pulls the iron block into the housing. The brake is open because the brake shoes detach from the bearing sleeve. To grant safety the brake is closed when the magnetic drivers are not energized. The braking torque was determined by means of a test-setup shown in Fig. 4. With the Brake closed. This means that the magnetic drivers of the brake bearing are not energized. The brake shoes are connected to the bearing sleeve. Subsequently, the brake bearing is clamped so that the bearing sleeve can be moved with the help of a one-meter-long lever arm l seen in Fig 4. The applied force F_A is determined by a tension scale. By means of (1) the braking torque M can be calculated.

$$M = F_A * l. \tag{1}$$

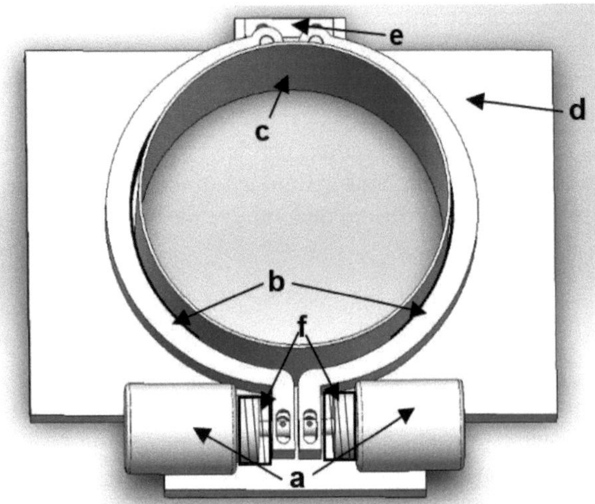

Figure 3: Electro-magnetic brake, a magnet drivers, b brake shoe with brake pads c bearing sleeve, d flange plate, e brake pad bearing, f spring

At the beginning, the basic braking torque must be determined, so that an improvement can be observed through various solutions. The following solutions are tested independent of each other to improve the braking torque.
1) The bearing points of the brake shoes are mounted on floating bearings to align the brake shoes convergently to the bearing sleeve. This is intended to compensate manufacturing tolerances. 2) Stronger magnetic drivers, these should increase the normal force and thus increase the braking force, will be presented in 3.1.2. 3) Modification of the bearing sleeve to improve the coefficients of friction. 4) Different brake pads have been used to improve the braking torque. In addition, the different brake pads should lead to an improvement in the locking behaviour. 5) "Miss-use"-tests are used to determine the wear behavior in the event of incorrect use. Furthermore, the brake is examined after about five days in the closed state with regard to its sticking behavior. This will not improve the braking torque but is important for the usability. Finally, it must be determined whether a possible change would affect the installation space and adjoining components.

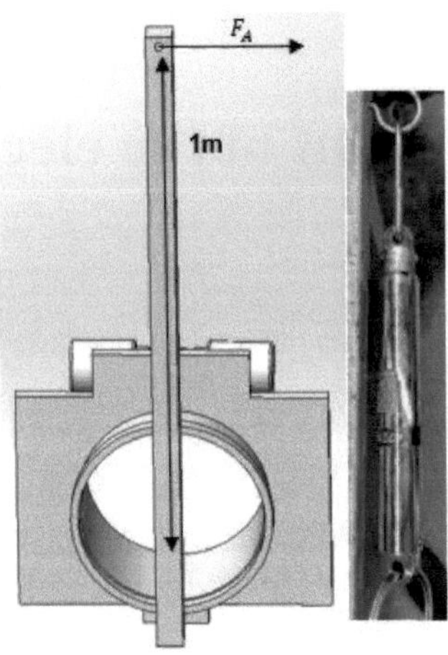

Figure 4: Right: Test setup for measuring braking torque with 1 meter lever arm, left: tension scale (connected to the end of the lever arm), F_A is the force which pulls the tension scale

3   Results and Discussion

3.1   Results

3.1.1   Modification of the bearing points

In order to improve the contact surface of the brake shoes, a floating bearing is being considered. As already described, the clearance of the bearing is intended to compensate for the manufacturing tolerance. The bearing points which are mounted to a floating bearing does not achieve a higher braking torque. But the advantage of this modification is a constant braking torque into both rotation directions. This means that the floating bearing in combination with further modifications of the electro-magnetic brake can be promising.

3.1.2   Increase of the normal force $\mathbf{F}_N$

Equation (2) shows the influence of the normal force on then friction force.

$$F_{FC} = \mu_{FC} * F_N. \tag{2}$$

The normal force can be increased by more powerful magnetic drivers. As it can be seen in Tab. 1. The medium-sized magnetic drivers led to a significant improvement of the braking torque. Due to the larger springs installed on the magnetic driver, which have a higher spring force. This leads to the increased normal force. The drawbacks behind larger magnetic drivers is the invasion of the existing installation space of the column seen in Fig. 1. An additional drawback is the increase of required electric power. Furthermore, the electrical power consumption needs a review. In addition, a new medical approval according to IEC 60601 [4] is required, as this results to the need of larger power supply units.

3.1.3 Improvement of friction coefficients

For this study we need the friction coefficient μ described in (2). In order to increase the coefficients of friction, roughening and smoothening of the bearing sleeve have been chosen in this project. However, both modifications show no significant improvement in braking torque.

Table 1: Results of the measurements of the braking torque in relation to the increase of the normal force

Modification	Result braking torque
floating bearing	constant braking torque
medium-sized driver	significant improvement
roughened bearing sleeve	no improvement
smoothed bearing sleeve	no improvement

3.1.4 Different brake pad hardness

Finally, the selection of the brake pad is considered. With rising normal force the soft material shows a higher wear behavior than the hard material.

However, soft materials have a higher coefficient of friction than hard ones [3]. For this reason different hardnesses are chosen. To temper a material means to heat it for a specific time at a specific temperature. This is simulating the ageing process. Which is modifying the characteristics of the materials [6]. Crosslinking substances are dissolved, which can otherwise lead to smearing. For the purpose of this project, brake pads of the following shore hardnesses are tested 40°-shore, 60°-shore, 60°-shore tempered and 70°-shore. The tempered shore and 70°-shore brake pads are the most promising. The tempered brake pad shows a significant improvement. Negative, however, is the sticking of the brake pad to the bearing sleeve. The softer brake pad (40°-shore) shows a good improvement, but this brake pad produces abrasion when used in a "Miss-Use"-case (3.1.5). This is not acceptable for a product in medical applications.

Table 2: Results of the measurements of the braking torque in relation to the increase of the normal force

Modification	Result braking torque
tempered	significant improvement
40°-Shore	good improvement,too much abrasion
60°-Shore	no improvement, brake pad destroyed
70°-Shore	significant improvement, fluctuations

The hardest brake pad tested (70°-shore) is the most promising. On the negative side, it is particularly dependent on the direction of rotation. This becomes clear in Tab. 2 by fluctuations and the large dispersion of the improvement.

3.1.5 "Miss-Use"-Tests

"Miss-use"-tests are used in the following to simulate incorrect use of the brake. For this purpose, the brake is used in the unpowered, closed initial position. Through findings from the field, it is known that the brake bearings are occasionally not used according to the instructions for use. In contrast to the measurement of the braking torque, the bearing sleeve is moved a total of 75 times at an angle of approx. 40. "Miss-Use"-tests are used in the following to simulate incorrect use of the brake. The brake is then disassembled to inspect the brake pads and the bearing sleeve for any abnormal wear. In the previous section, the behavior of the soft brake pad (40°-shore) was already mentioned. This left abrasion on the brake pad and a material film on the bearing sleeve seen in Fig. 5.

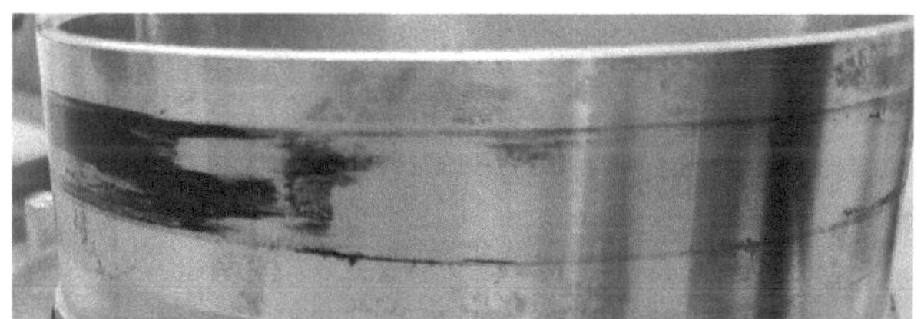

Figure 5: Film of material on the bearing sleeve

The harder brake pad (60°-shore) was destroyed by the "Miss-Use" test, so it is not compatible for further modification combinations. Whereas the 60°-shore tempered brake pad was neither destroyed nor produced any considerable abrasion. The used brake pads were then left glued to the bearing sleeve.

The duration was about five days until the brake was released again. The magnetic drivers are energized for this purpose. This ensures that the magnetic drivers can release the brake shoes from the bearing sleeve. The magnet drivers have been able to detach the brake pads from the bearing sleeve without any problems.

3.2 Discussion

The results of the performed test studies show that no modification is to be considered as a stand-alone solution. Furthermore, the modifications of the bearing sleeve as a solution approach are omitted . Changing the coefficients of friction through the brake pad is the most promising solution. However, this is even more effective in combination with an increase of the normal force and a floating bearing. In addition, the choice of hardness of the brake pad must be considered. If this is too soft, e.g., 40°Shore, abrasion occurs, and the brake pad is increasingly stuck to the bearing sleeve. If the brake pad is too hard, the braking torque decreases. With the additional difficulty here, the limited installation space, the size of the individual components must also be considered. The standards for medical devices are strict. Due to the installation in patient rooms and operating rooms, there is a special duty of care for the company. Which means that every aspect of the modifications must be tested and questioned.

4 Conclusion

By testing the different approaches already explained above, new modification variants have emerged. These need to be tested and evaluated. This includes testing brake pads with a shore hardness of 60° but differently tempered. This combined with floating bearing seems to be expedient. Adventitious it seems expedient to temper the brake pad material. The braking system in combination with the various influencing factors can be modified in a wide variety of ways. Nevertheless, it is difficult to find an improvement to the current variant. This realization emerges after the results. However, not purposeful variants and modifications resulted in new solution proposals. These can be evaluated in following tests.

Acknowledgement

This work was supervised by Dipl. Ing. Thomas Martin, M.Sc. Malte Hermann and Prof. rer. N. Linz. The work has been carried out at Dräger.

Author's Statement

Due to company secrecy, no quantitative measured values are published in the following study. Thomas Martin and Lucas Köllisch are working for Dräger. Norbert Linz has no conflict of interest.

5 References

[1] Reiling, Hughes, Murphy. Patient Safety and Quality: an evidence-based handbook for nurses. Chapter 28, The Impact of facility design on patient safety, 2008, https://www.ncbi.nlm.nih.gov/books/NBK2633/

[2] Dräger, Ambia short brochure, Dräger Ambia® Medical Supply Units, 2021, ambia-br-DMC-101147-en.pdf (draeger.com)[last accessed on 2023-01-03].

[3] M. Young, *The Technical Writer's Handbook*. University Science, Mill Valley, 1989.

[4] DIN-Deutsches Institut für Normung, Medizinische elektrische Geräte - Teil 1: Allgemeine Festlegungen für die Sicherheit einschließlich der wesentlichen Leistungsmerkmale, 2022, (https://www.din.de/de/mitwirken/normenausschuesse/dke/veroeffentlichungen/wdc-beuth:din21:357087758) [last accessed on 2023-01-03].

[5] B. Breuer and K. H. Bill, Bremsenhandbuch Grundlagen, Komponenten, Systeme, Fahrdynamik, Wiesbaden: Springer Verlag, 2017.

[6] G. Gottstein: Materialwissenschaft und Werkstofftechnik Physikalische Grundlagen. 4., neu bearb. Wiesbaden: Springer Verlag, 2014

Method for selection of a suitable level sensor for a coating station for injector systems

Eva Norkunas [1], Patrizia Plaskowski[2] and, Maria Henke [3]
[1] Medical Informatics, Universität zu Lübeck, eva.norkunas@student.uni-luebeck.de
[2] IOLUTION GmbH, plaskowski@iolution.com
[3] Institute for Robotics and Cognitive Systems, Universität zu Lübeck, henke@rob.uni-luebeck.de

Abstract

In cataract surgery, intraocular lenses are implanted into the eye with the help of injector systems. To perform an injection, injector tips are coated. For consistent application of the coating liquid with a robotic system, the liquid level has to be measured with a sensor. Various sensor principles exist for level sensors without a suitable selection procedure. For a systematic and structured selection, a method consisting of five steps is established. This includes a pre-selection of sensors and an integration of the requirements of the targeted application. With the use of the fluid specification and requirements for the system, the preselection is established. Subsequently, the requirements for the sensor are deduced. The application of the method to a robotic system led to the selection of an ultrasonic sensor. This method simplifies the selection of an application specific level sensor.

1 Introduction

Cataract is an eye disease that results in the clouding of the natural lens of the eye. With more than 800 million cataract treatments performed annually, these surgical procedures are among the most common worldwide. Treatment consists of implantation of an intraocular lens (IOL). Currently, there is no alternative treatment for this disease. The IOL is injected into the eye using an injector system. The coating of the injector tip plays a particularly important role. This enables the IOL to be injected through small incisions. Additionally, it greatly reduces friction between the IOL and the injector system. The coating process includes immersion in the coating liquid. For a regulated procedure, a controlled process of immersion is necessary. The accomplishment of this is possible by an automated process, using a robot system. This work is about the selection of a suitable level sensor for the coating liquid establishing a method that describes a systematic and structured selection. The selection of the sensor is made with consideration of the requirements of the robot system.

In this system, the injector tips are immersed in a coating liquid with the aid of the robot arm. For reproducible coating, it is necessary that the injector tips are immersed to as equal a depth as possible. A level sensor shall be used to control and regulate the immersion depth of the injector tips. There are different principles for sensors of level measurement. Each sensor model has its own advantages and disadvantages. In order to find the right sensor for a special application, a corresponding amount of time and research is to be expected. This is especially true for coating fluids, which should not come into contact with all materials due to their adhesive properties.

1.1 Level sensors

Level sensors are used to detect the level of liquids and bulk materials. The sensors can be divided into three categories and two measurement types, while the subdivision serves the purpose of categorizing the sensors in advance according to their measurement type. The categories include sensors that require contact with the medium (category 1), those that have contact with the container of the liquid (category 2) and those that measure contactless (category 3). Furthermore, the sensors are divided according to their measurement duration. There are continuously measuring level sensors and those which return the measuring signal at certain switching points. The classification can be seen in Table 1. In the following, the individual measuring principles are presented.

CATEGORY 1
Sensors that require contact with the medium include the hydrostatic, optical, conductivity, vibration, and float sensors.
Hydrostatic: The principle of hydrostatic is to measure the pressure of the fluid above the sensor.
Optical: This sensor uses the property of light. The difference between the refraction of light in a liquid compared to air is measured.
Conductivity: In this principle, resistance is measured

Table 1: Classification of the level sensors

		Continuous	Switching point
Contact with medium (Cat. 1)		Hydrostatic	Float
	Conductivity		Vibration
			Optical
			Conductivity
Contact with container (Cat. 2)		Capacitive	Capacitive
		Weight	
Contactless (Cat. 3)		Ultrasound	Ultrasound
		Radar	Radar

between two electrodes. If the electrodes are separated by air, no electric current is passed. If conductive liquid is present, a circuit is given and the sensor detects a liquid between the electrodes.

Vibration: The vibration sensor sends and receives vibrations. If the sensor is in contact with liquid, the received frequency is different from the resonant frequency.

Float: A float is an object with a lower density than the liquid. As a result, it floats on the surface. In conjunction with a sensor, the position of the object determines the level [2].

CATEGORY 2

Sensors that require contact with the container of the liquid include the capacitive and weight sensors. In this category, the sensors do not have contact with the liquid, but with the container.

Capacitive: The principle of capacitive level measurement is based on capacitance change. The capacitive sensor and the container form a capacitor. The capacitance depends on the amount of product in the tank.

Weight: The weight sensor measures the weight of the object and thus the level can be calculated [3].

CATEGORY 3

Sensors that neither require contact with the medium nor the tank include the ultrasonic and radar sensor.

Ultrasonic: Level measurement with an ultrasonic sensor works by sending and receiving ultrasonic waves. The measuring principle is based on the transit time calculation.

Radar: Radar measurement is based on the transit time measurement of the transmitted signal [4].

1.2 Sensor Selection method

Existing methods for the sensor selection are presented in [5] and [6]. These methods describe sensors for existing systems and IoT systems. Such sensors are not level sensors. Furthermore, they do not measure liquids.

2 Methods

In the following, a method was developed for the selection of a level sensor for a coating line for injector systems (Fig. 1). This method is inspired by the methods [5] and [6] through the step-by-step approach. In addition, this works shows that a method for the selection of a sensor is helpful.

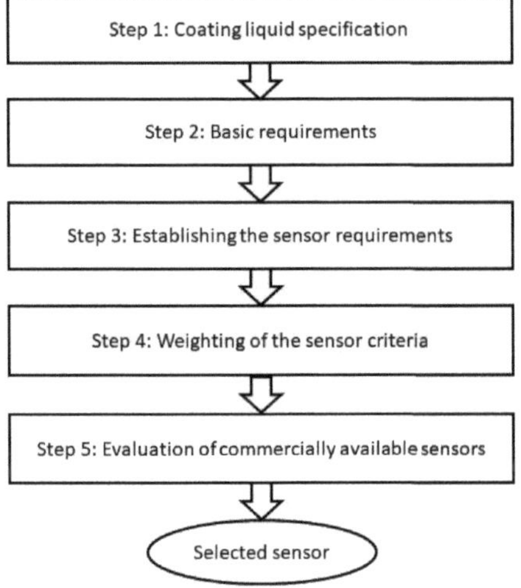

Figure 1: The five steps of sensor selection

Step 1: Coating liquid specification
The first step is the identification of the fluid to be detected, taking into account the requirements and specifications of the coating system. With regard to the equipment, the focus is on the method of application of the coating to the injector system. Included is the container of the coating fluid in terms of its construction, cleaning and filling. The specification of the fluid refers to its transparency, consistency, nature and reaction with other materials as well as other physical properties relevant for the respective measurement principle. This information is relevant to the interaction of the fluid with the sensor.

Step 2: Basic requirements
The listing of basic requirements for the level sensor is described below. Included is the influence of the liquid on objects that are in direct contact with the liquid.
The identification of requirements is performed using the information from step 1. The process of identifying the basic requirements can be seen in Fig. 2.
In the first section, using the information gathered from step 1 in relation to the specifications of the coating liquid, a direction is taken in the selection of the categories of sensors. It is decided whether there is a possibility that the sensor has contact with the liquid. In the next section, the evaluation of the equipment specification is considered. Based on this information, a further selection is made between the sensor categories. In the last section a selection of the type of measurement is made. It can be choosen between a switching point and a continuous measurement.

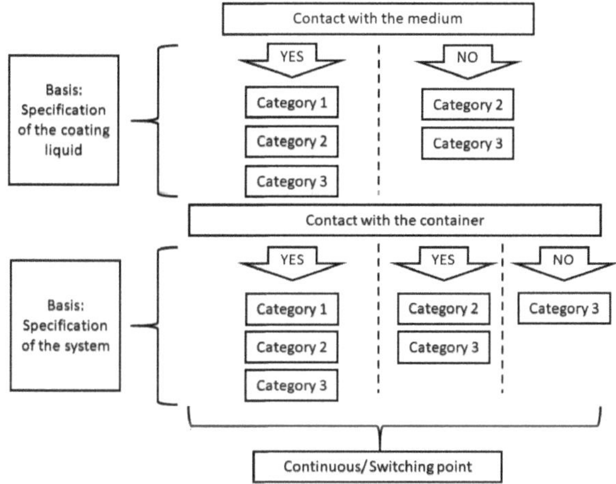

Figure 2: Process of identifying the basic requirements: Category 1: Contact with medium, Category 2: Contact with container, Category 3: Contactless

Step 3: Establishing the sensor requirements
In this step, the application-specific requirements for the level sensor are established. The list includes the functional, design and financial requirements related to the characteristics of the sensor. Some requirements do not have the same priority for the project as others. There are more important requirements, which have a great impact on the project, and less important requirements, which are not absolutely necessary. In this section, no distinction is made between primary and secondary requirements.

Step 4: Weighting of the sensor criteria
In this step, the sensor requirements are weighted. The distribution of the weights reflects the priorities and capacities of the project, related to the sensor.

Step 5: Evaluation of commercially available sensors
In this step, the selection of the level sensor is completed. The narrowing down of the possible sensor classes, definition and weighting of the sensor requirements serves as a basis for this step. Based on this, various sensors from different manufacturers are selected and compared. Only sensors that belong to the selected sensor class are considered.

Data relevant to the requirements from step 3 are collected for each sensor. The requirements are considered as criteria for a utility analysis. The evaluation with the weighted criteria supports the selection of a sensor for an individual adaptation to the targeted application of the robotic system. The selection is made considering the already pre-selected sensor categories and measurement types. The selected sensors receive for each criterion from the utility analysis an evaluation in how far they meet the criterion. The evaluation follows a point system between 1 and 3, where 1 indicates an insufficient fulfillment of the criterion and 3 a complete fulfillment. The points are multiplied by the weightings of the respective criteria. The sum of the points for the re-

spective sensor is the evaluation result. The highest score indicates the most suitable sensor for the application.

3   Results and Discussion

The application of the previously described method leads to the following results.

Step 1: The system dips injector tips into a basin containing a coating liquid. The basin is refilled manually and must be replaced regularly. The volume in the basin is severely limited. As a result, there is no space for a sensor in the basin.

The relevant information about the coating liquid for the selection of the sensor is as follows:
- The coating liquid is transparent, partially turbid.
- It consists of two components, primer and topcoat.
- The texture is adhesive and viscous.
- The curing of the coating can be completed in air.

Step 2: Following the principle from step 2 of the method, the most suitable sensor for the coating system is a sensor that measures the liquid without contact and does not require contact with the basin. A continuous measurement as well as a measurement at at least two switching points is suitable. These are sensors that do not require contact with the medium or the tank.

Step 3: The application-specific requirements are listed in Table 2 under "Step 3: Establishing the sensor requirements".

Step 4: The weighting of each criterion is distributed according to the relevance of the requirements. The weighting of the criteria of the plant can be seen in Table 2 under "Step 4: Weighting of the sensor criteria". Due to the limited space in the basin, a maximum of 10 of the injectors can be immersed in basins at the same time. The liquid level is slightly changed by an immersion process. This means that a sensor with a high accuracy is required for precise measurement. For this reason the criterion of the sensor accuracy belongs to the highest evaluated. The criteria with a weighting of 5 percent are weighted low because alternative solutions exist for these criteria. With constructive or electrotechnical measures, the non-fulfillment of the criteria can be compensated. The remaining weightings are distributed according to the requirements of the project.

Step 5: After step 3, the remaining category of sensors that can be considered for this installation is the third. This means the ultrasonic and radar sensor are available for selection. In advance, no radar sensors were included in the following evaluation. The reason is the big price difference between the two sensor principles. The radar sensors are five times more expensive. For this reason, only ultrasonic sensors were compared. There exist different ultrasonic sensors with different characteristics, from different manufacturers. In this step, the different sensors are compared and the relevant properties for the application are identified.

The number of selected comparison objects is based on the current offer of level sensors, as well as internal company

Table 2: Utility analysis

Step 3: Establishing the sensor requirements		Step 4: Weighting of the sensor criteria	Step 5: evaluation of commercially available sensors		
REQUIREMENT	**DESCRIPTION**	**Weighting [%]**	**SR04**	**UGT592**	**U500**
Trouble-free execution of the coating process	Does not interfere with the manipulator performing the process	10	3	3	3
Sensor accuracy	Sensor accuracy > 3mm	30	2	3	2
Signal transmission	Digital	10	1	3	3
Port	Direct, without additional components	5	2	3	3
Cleaning	Trouble-free cleaning of the tank	10	3	3	3
Sensor replacement	Easy	5	1	2	2
Size	Sensor size < 20 mm	10	2	3	3
Price	Possible low	20	3	2	1
		100	2,25	2,75	2,25

reasons, and is limited to the three sensors:
- Elec freaks Ultrasonic Ranging Module HC - SR04 [7]
- Ifm Ultrasonic UGT592 [8]
- Baumer Ultrasonic Distance Measuring Sensors U500 [9]

Table 2 shows the utility analysis for these sensors under "Step 5: evaluation of commercially available sensors". The distribution of the points is applied to the data of the individual sensors.

The method described in this paper allows a structured and systematic selection of a level sensor for coating plants. Through the five steps of the method, the potential sensors are subdivided according to the specific application. The result is a narrowing down of the possible sensor types and thus a reduction of the workload. The method is primarily independent of the currently available sensor types. The selected sensor for the coating plant is an ultrasonic sensor. This is able to measure without contact with the coating. Due to the low costs and a high measuring accuracy this sensor fits to the prioritized requirements. The small dimensions, as well as the distance of the measurement of the sensor, allow a flexible and space-saving installation of the sensor.

4 Conclusion

The method described in this paper leads to a simplified selection of a suitable level sensor. The application of the method to other coating liquids and for other systems is possible. The decision for a suitable sensor is strongly based on the function and the design of the robot system. It is possible to include other measurement principles if new measurement methods for level measurement are developed in the future. A next step with this method would be an adaptation to other sensors.

Acknowledgement

The work has been carried out at IOLUTION GmbH during a project internship, Hamburg and was supervised by the Institute for Robotics and Cognitive Systems, Universität zu Lübeck.

Author's Statement

Conflict of interest: Authors state no conflict of interest.

5 References

[1] T. Kohnen and O. K. Klaproth, *Intraokularlinsen für die mikroinzisionale Kataraktchirurgie"*. Der Ophthalmologe, 2010, pp. 127-135.

[2] H.-R. Tränkler, *Handbuch für Praxis und Wissenschaft*. Berlin: Springer, 2014.

[3] IBS, *Kapazitive Wegmesssysteme*. Available: https://www.ibspe.com/de/messsysteme [last accessed on 2022-12-13]

[4] O. Ahrens, *Mikrosystemtechnische Sensoren in relativ bewegten Systemen für die industrielle Anwendung*. Berlin: Logos Verlag, 2001.

[5] Löpelt, Martin, *Sensorauswahl für Bestandsanlagen*. Zeitschrift für wirtschaftlichen Fabrikbetrieb 114.5 (2019): 273-276.

[6] Hirayama, Masayuki, *Sensor Selection method for IoT systemsfocusing on embedded system requirements*. MATEC Web of Conferences. Vol. 59. EDP Sciences, 2016.

[7] Elec freaks, *Ultrasonic Ranging Module HC - SR04*. Available: https://cdn.sparkfun.com/datasheets [last accessed on 2022-01-06]

[8] ifm, *Ultraschallsensor UGT592*. Available: https://www.ifm.com/at/de/product/ [last accessed on 2022-01-06]

[9] Baumer, *Ultrasonic sensors U500 and UR18*. Available: https://www.baumer.com/medias [last accessed on 2022-01-06]

Integration and Restructuring of Existing Requirements of an Emergency Ventilator into a Model-based Requirements Management System Using SysML

Felix Herrmann[1], Mareike Wendebourg[2], Johannes Kreuzer[3]
[1] Medical Engineering Science, University of Lübeck, Felix.Herrmann@student.uni-luebeck.de
[2] Weinmann Emergency Medical Technology GmbH + Co. KG, M.Wendebourg@weinmann-emt.de
[3] Weinmann Emergency Medical Technology GmbH + Co. KG, J.Kreuzer@weinmann-emt.de

Abstract

Efficient requirements management provides the foundation for successful product development for medical devices, which is why it is useful to continuously develop the requirements management system. This applies even to the requirements management system used for devices on the market. With the help of the Systems Modeling Language (SysML), it is possible to replace an existing document-centric requirements management system and thus transfer requirements development to a model-based approach. In order to achieve a successful integration into the new approach, a structured insertion process has to be defined, which is oriented towards the available database of requirements. This work addresses the improvement of the requirements management of an emergency ventilator with the shift away from a document-centric to a model-based approach. The results show that most of the document-centric requirements could successfully pass through the defined integration process, thus laying the foundation for model-based requirements management.

1 Introduction

In modern system development, requirements form the basis of all development activities. Successful product development therefore depends on efficient management of these requirements. This fact is underlined by the CHAOS report of the Standish Group, which examines success and failure factors of software projects. The study from 1995 describes that incomplete requirements and specifications (13.10 %) are the main reason why software projects fail and changing requirements (11.80 %) are the third most common reason for a delayed or incomplete software project [1]. This fact has barely changed to this day. It has been shown that a transition from document-centric requirements management to a Model-Based Systems Engineering (MBSE) approach can help to minimise the risk factors mentioned above [2]. MBSE, unlike the document-centric method, is based on a database. This simplifies the tracking of changed and updated requirements in the system context, as continuous traceability is guaranteed. This work addresses the improvement of the requirements management of an emergency ventilator with the shift away from a document-centric to a model-based approach.

1.1 Current document-centric structure

The emergency ventilator defined by the requirements discussed in this paper is already on the market, but is still subject to software updates and product changes. In the cur-

rent situation, all the requirements are managed in two different documents. These documents contain requirements described at two different levels of detail which will be referred to as layers, as shown in Fig. 1. In the upper layer is the document "functional specification" in which all functional requirements are managed. The functional requirements define the fundamental functions of the ventilator, such as the different adjustable ventilation modes. The document "system specification", in which all system-specific requirements are managed, is located at the level below. A system-specific requirement describes the concrete technical implementation of a fundamental function. The test and thus the test cases of the requirements of both layers are arranged in the document "qualification program". A classification of layers does not take place at the corresponding test level. Within the documents, the individual specifications as well as the tests are presented in table form. Within these tables, all requirements are defined and managed with the associated links and the necessary data such as versioning. If a requirement is added or changed, it must be manually tracked whether this change also affects the linked documents.

1.2 SysML for MBSE

For the introduction of a model-based approach, a standardized modeling language is necessary. MBSE uses SysML, which is based on the Unified Modeling Language (UML). SysML extends UML, for example by introducing the re-

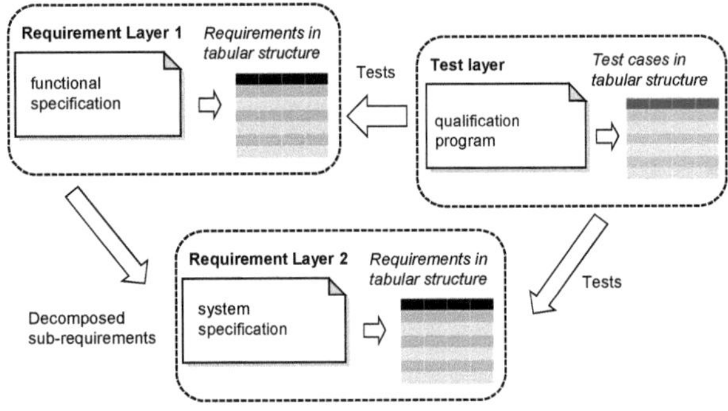

Figure 1: Structure of the document-centric requirements and test documents

quirements diagram and the requirements element. A standard SysML requirement element includes properties to specify its unique identifier and the requirement's textual content itself. Additional properties such as author, version, etc., can also be specified. Within the requirement diagram, requirement elements can be linked to other model elements such as test cases [3]. In addition, requirements can also be linked to each other, creating hierarchical structures of decomposed sub-requirements, as shown in an example in Fig. 2.

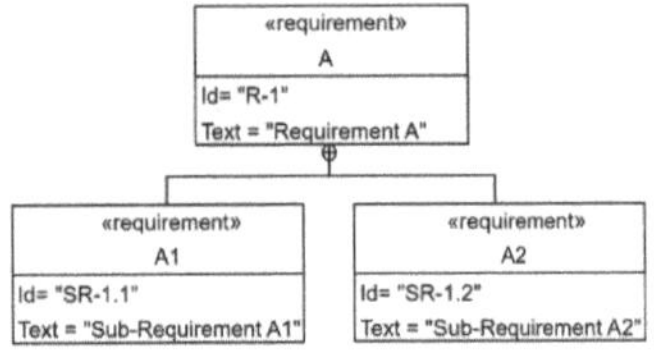

Figure 2: SysML diagramm with one parent and two sub-requirements. Figure modified from [4].

2 Material and Methods

This section first describes the model-based software tool for the implementation of the MBSE approach. Furthermore, the transition of the requirements into the software tool is described, which is divided into two steps. First, the document-centric requirements of both layers and the corresponding tests are transferred into the programme in their existing structure. After the creation of the SysML elements, the final integration and restructuring process is limited to the requirements elements. The complete application of the model-based approach to the test cases is not covered in this paper. Shortly before the integration process of the requirement elements is completed, the requirements pass through a restructuring process, which represents the second step. The completion of the restructuring process concludes the completion of the integration process.

2.1 Enterprise Architect

For the conversion to MBSE, a software tool that supports SysML is required. Enterprise Architect (EA) by SparxSys-

tems Ltd. is such a software modelling tool that uses UML modelling. The tool includes requirements management, which consequently supports SysML [5]. With EA, SysML elements such as requirement elements and requirements diagrams can be created and displayed graphically. The links to other elements are also made through the graphical interface. After the creation of a requirement element, all necessary information such as the ID or the requirement text as well as further information such as the time of creation or the author is shown. A traceability is also available, which shows all links to other elements such as sub-requirements or test cases, starting from the selected element. In addition, EA allows the user to structure elements in different layers.

2.2 Integration process

The integration process can be divided into four sections. These four sections are linked to the different statuses of the requirement elements in EA. The sections and their correspondig status are explained below using the ventilator color display requirements as an example. The scheme of the complete integration and restructuring process is shown in Fig. 5.

Draft

For each requirement from the two table-based requirements documents and for each corresponding test case, a SysML element is created in EA. During creation, the existing content of the elements is transferred and a new, appropriate ID is assigned.

Proposed

Each newly created requirement element undergoes a revision to integrate it into the context of the model-based system. As described in section 1.2, additional properties can be assigned to the requirement elements. In addition to this, further adjustments must be implemented. A summary of all necessary adjustment steps can be found in Table 1. For the test cases, this section is not executed. The status of the test cases remains in "Draft" status for the rest of the requirement integration process.

Table 1: Overview of the adjustment steps

Step	Type	Description
Content	Setting	Content of the requirement must be separated into title and description due to EA settings
Version	Property	Cumulative requirement version must be set
Traces	Setting	Traces to other SysML elements must be set
Author	Property	The responsible author of the requirement must be set

Approved

Before the requirement elements reach the "Approved" status, a review process is executed. All stakeholders of the requirement element must agree to the model-based and therefore updated variant of the requirement. After approval, the content of the requirement is fixed and may no longer be changed.

Released

During the transition from the "Approved" status to the "Released" status, the requirements are transferred into a refined layer structure. This includes the restructuring process, which is described in detail in the section 2.3. During restructuring, the requirement elements may be released in their new structure on a document basis. However, these documents are only used for official purposes and not for requirements management. Reaching the "Released" status completes the insertion process.

2.3 Restructuring process

The transfer of requirements management into a model-based approach would also be possible without a restructuring process. The reason for the further subdivision of the requirement layers is that the separation according to departments can be better guaranteed [6]. The two existing layers were further divided into a total of four layers, the lower two layers have an additional horizontal division. This is intended to improve responsibility for the different layers and, if applicable, their additional horizontal subdivision. This is to ensure that the responsibility for changes or updates of requirements in a layer is defined clearly. The updated layer structure is described in Fig. 3. The assign-

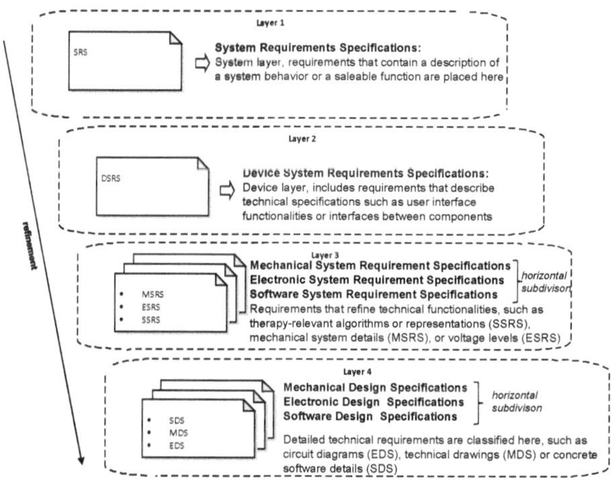

Figure 3: Restructured layer division

ment to a new layer is based on the content of the requirement. When a requirement is assigned to a new layer, the link to the new corresponding parent or sub-requirement is set as well.

2.4 Application of the model-based approach

Once the transfer process is defined, it has to be determined if all existing requirements can pass through this process successfully. If a requirement has reached the final status "Released", this requirement is listed as a "success". Otherwise, if the final status could not be achieved, the affected requirement is considered "challenged". A challenged requirement remains in its status and is marked with a flag indicating the reason.

3 Results and Discussion

3.1 Processability of the requirements

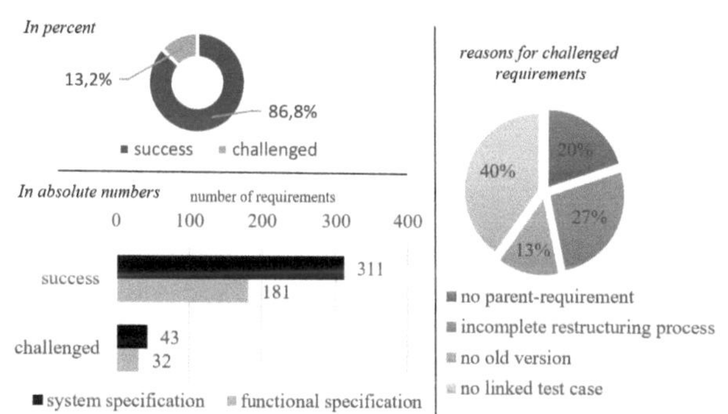

Figure 4: Summary of the process success

A total of 567 requirements had to pass through the process described above. Of these, 213 were functional specifications and 354 were system specifications. Of the functional specifications, 181 successfully passed, and of the system specifications, 311 passed. 32 functional requirements and 43 system requirements could not successfully complete the process and were therefore listed under "challenged" as shown in Fig. 4. There were several reasons why the transfer of some requirements was not completed successfully. The non-existence of a parent requirement affected 20 % of the requirements. This could only affect the system specifications, as a stand-alone requirement in a lower layer always requires a parent requirement in the layer above. An incomplete restructuring process affected 27 % of all requirements listed under "challenged". Due to the content of the requirements, no suitable layer could be found. In 13 % the cumulative version of the requirement was not noted in the document. Furthermore, 40 % of the challenged requirements had no existing link to a corresponding test case. As the evaluation of the test cases did not take place, this missing link was not repaired. This can be done by filling the missing information based on the redundant data in the test specification.

3.2 Discussion of results

A way could be found to incorporate most of the existing requirements of the emergency ventilator into the model-based approach. The reasons for an unsuccessful integration process resulted mainly from the incompleteness of the underlying database, which in some places did not fully correspond to the expected scope, caused by the historical context of the documents. However, by switching to the model-based approach, existing inconsistencies in the database could already be found and can be straightened out with help of the new system in the future. The defined implementation process nevertheless proves to be largely suitable, as indicated by the success rate of 86.8 %.

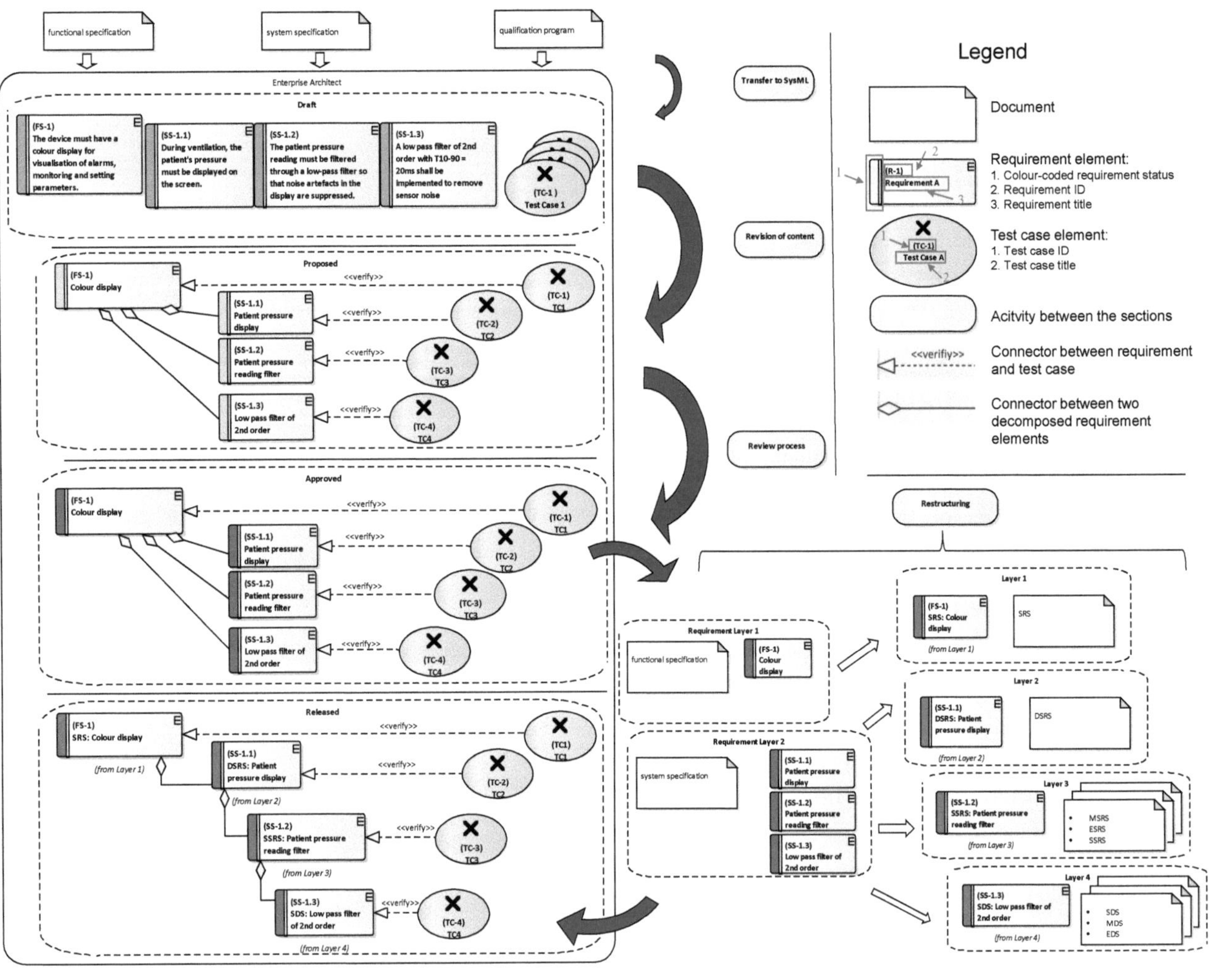

Figure 5: Scheme of the integration and restructuring process

4   Conclusion

The foundation for the transition to MBSE was successfully laid with the beginning of the integration of the requirements. Through a carefully defined integration process, the transition to a model-based approach can also succeed during ongoing device development. The next step towards model-based work would be to work through the requirements, which are marked with a "challenged" flag, and to further integrate the test cases and set up a change process. The new requirement management system should make it possible to minimise the risk factors mentioned above.

Acknowledgement

The work has been carried out at Weinmann Emergency Medical Technology GmbH + Co. KG and supervised by Prof. Dr. Thomas Gutsmann, Universität zu Lübeck.

Author's Statement

Conflict of interest: Authors state no conflict of interest.

5   References

[1] A. Hussain, E. Mkpojiogu, F. M. Kamal, *The Role of Requirements in the Success or Failure of Software Projects*, Universiti Utara Malaysia, Malaysia, 2016.

[2] D. Maeika, R. Butleris, *Integrating Security Requirements Engineering into MBSE: Profile and Guidelines*, Security and Communication Networks, Kaunas, Lithuania, 2020.

[3] O. Alt, *Integration textueller Anforderungen und Modell-basiertem Testen mit SysML*, Continental Division Chassis and Safety, Frankfurt, 2008.

[4] P. Roques, *Modeling Requirements with SysML*, Requirements Engineering Magazine, Karlsruhe, 2015.

[5] Sparx Systems, *Model Based Systems Engineering*, Sparx Systems Software User Guide, Creswick, 2019.

[6] M. d. S. Soares, J. Vrancken, *Framework for Multi-Layered Requirements Documentation and Analysis*, 2011 IEEE 35th Annual Computer Software and Applications Conference, Munich, 2011.

Influence of X-ray pulses on active electronic circuits

Florian Schmid [1], Saeed Milady [2]
[1] Department of Electrical Engineering and Computer Science, Technische Hochschule Lübeck - University of Applied Sciences, florian.schmid@stud.th-luebeck.de
[2] Department of Electrical Engineering and Computer Science, Technische Hochschule Lübeck - University of Applied Sciences, saeed.milady@th-luebeck.de

Abstract

In the field of explosive ordnance disposal, mobile X-ray systems are used nowadays. These systems are radiographing electronic circuits which contain semiconductors. This work aims to investigate whether and how this type of examination affects semiconductors. First, the basics of X-ray generation and its energy composition are discussed. Then the influences on semiconductors are listed, and possible ways to determine them are presented.

In conclusion, critical factors for the influence of X-rays on semiconductors could be found, and an evaluation of the impact could be made. It was found that in the case of explosive ordnance disposal, the influence can be neglected. However, this topic should be investigated further to understand this influence and the effects behind it. As a result of this, quantification of the impact would be possible.

1 Introduction

In the fields of public safety bomb disposal (PSBD), explosive ordnance disposal (EOD), and improvised explosive device disposal (IEDD), the use of highly mobile X-ray systems have gained more and more significance over the years. These systems are often used to radiograph potential threats containing semiconductors, especially in the case of PSBD- and IEDD missions. However, the influence of X-ray radiation on semiconductors is neglected in the daily work with these systems, but is there an influence, and if so, can it be neglected? This paper attempts to study the effect of X-rays on semiconductors in more detail and lay the groundwork for further investigations. As Complementary Metal−Oxide−Semiconductor (CMOS) is the semiconductor technology used in most of today's integrated circuits, the focus of this work will be on the influence of X-ray on CMOS devices.

The remainder of this paper is structured as follows. section 2 discusses the basic structure of X-ray tubes and their produced energy spectrum. Next, section 3 discusses the effects of X-rays on several MOS-based semiconductor devices. section 4 discusses a basic measurement method to measure the variation of MOS-transistors' threshold voltage after exposure to X-ray. The method's accuracy is then verified utilizing a simulation in section 5. The conclusion will follow in Sec. 6.

2 X-ray generation and spectrum

Portable X-ray systems consist of a source for X-ray radiation and a flat-panel detector that generates the images of the device under test (DUT) by converting X-ray radiation to visible light (with the help of a scintillator), which then gets processed by a standard image sensor. The luminosity value of the resulting greyscale image varies with the thickness and material type of the DUT. The X-ray radiation is produced with an X-ray tube, as shown in Figure 1. These tubes contain a vacuum, a heating coil (cathode), and a target anode.

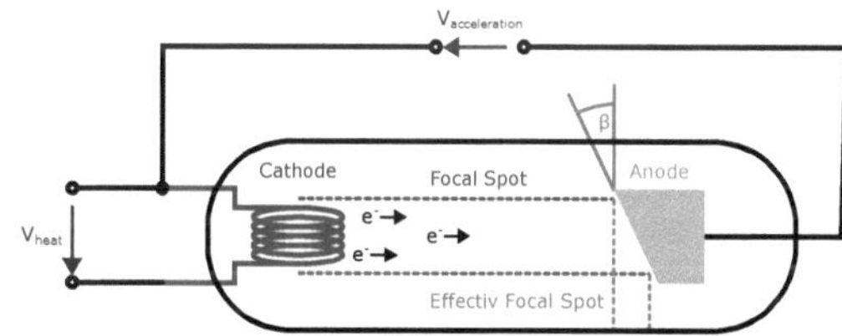

Figure 1: Basic structure of an X-ray tube.

A DC voltage $V_{acceleration}$ in the range of 150-450 kV is applied between the anode and the cathode. The heating coil emits electrons which are accelerated toward the anode. These energized electrons then hit the target anode made of tungsten (molybdenum or copper are also often used). This stream of electrons creates the focal spot of the X-ray tube. The number of electrons N which are getting accelerated, is given by (1):

$$N = \frac{I \cdot t}{e} \qquad (1)$$

where I is current, t is the exposure time and e is the elementary charge. The focal spot f then gets reduced by the angle of the anode to the effective focal spot $f_{eff.}$, which is given by (2):

$$f_{eff.} = f \cdot \tan(\beta) \qquad (2)$$

where β is the angle of the anode (see Figure 1). These electrons then get de-accelerated by hitting the atoms of the anode. A portion of the energy dissipated by this de-acceleration, equal to the kinetic energy loss of the electron through this collision, will be radiated as X-rays. The X-ray photon-generating effect is generally called the *bremsstrahlung* effect, a compound of the German *bremsen* meaning to brake, and *Strahlung* meaning radiation [1].

The spectrum can be calculated with the help of Kramer's law [2]:

$$\frac{dE}{d\lambda} = K \cdot I_h \cdot Z \cdot \frac{h}{c} \cdot (\frac{\lambda}{\lambda_{min}} - 1) \cdot \frac{1}{\lambda^3} \qquad (3)$$

where $E(\lambda)$ is the distribution of energy as a function of the wavelength λ, K is the Kramer's constant which can be experimentally determined, I_h is the current flowing through the cathode, Z is the atomic number of the anode material. λ_{min} is the minimal wavelength (corresponding to maximum photon energy) and is given by (4):

$$\lambda_{min} = \frac{h \cdot c}{e \cdot V} \qquad (4)$$

where h is the Planck's constant, c is the speed of light and V is equal to $V_{acceleration}$.

The energy spectrum for an X-ray source with an accelerating voltage of 370 kV, a current of 250 μA, and an anode made of tungsten has been calculated using (3). It has been depicted in Figure 2.[1] We should emphasize that the *characteristic* radiation, which consists of spikes in the spectrum, has not been shown here.

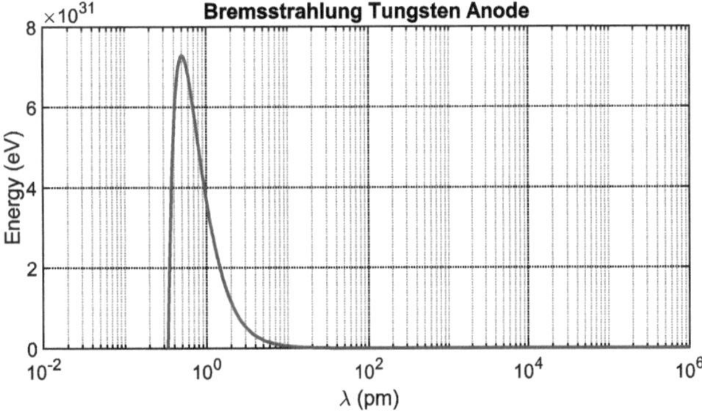

Figure 2: Calculated spectrum of an X-ray source at 370 keV and 250 μA without characteristic radiation and assuming $K = 1$.

3 Influence of X-ray radiation on semiconductors

The influences of X-ray radiation on semiconductors using CMOS technology have been extensively studied in many

---

[1]The Kramer's constant K 1 needs to be experimentally determined for the specific X-rays source. For this calculation, we have assumed for simplicity that K 1.

fields. For example, many works investigate X-ray radiation's long-term effects on integrated circuits' reliability. X-rays impinging the Silicon dioxide layer of semiconductors lead to the formation of oxide-trapped charges, and X-rays impinging the interface layers lead to so-called interface-trapped charges. These oxide charges influence the threshold voltage V_{th} and can result in the degradation in the mobility of the carriers [3]. Figure 3 shows the influence of a radiation dose on the threshold voltage variation on a MOS transistor which was irradiated at room temperature up to 10 Mrad (dose rate 10 Mrad/h) [4].

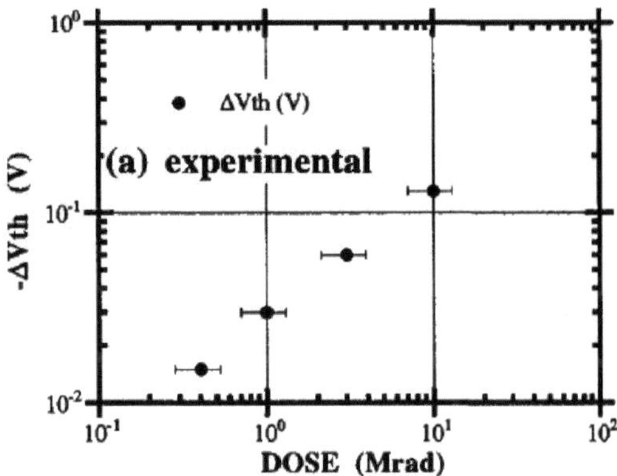

Figure 3: Threshold voltage shift vs. total dose of an MOS transistor. [4].

In an n-type metal-oxide-semiconductor (NMOS) device, the threshold voltage typically decreases, which results in an increase of drive and off-state (leakage) currents. In a p-type metal-oxide-semiconductor (PMOS) device, on the other hand, the threshold voltage increases (becoming more negative), resulting in decreasing of drive and off-state (leakage) currents.

X-rays can also affect flash memory cells, which are basically metal oxide semiconductors field-effect transistors (MOSFET) with an additional gate called a floating gate. This gate is located between the control gate and the substrate. The oxide layer between the control and floating gates is called the inter-poly-oxide. Tunnel oxide separates the floating gate from the substrate. Since the floating gate is surrounded by oxide, its charge remains trapped.

The total amount of variation of the threshold voltage ΔV_{th} is due to both charges trapped in the oxide, as well as the charges trapped at the interface of the oxide and semiconductor [5]. In general, this charge can be used to calculate the change in the threshold voltage by the following relation [6]:

$$\Delta V_{th} = -\frac{\Delta Q}{C_{ox}} \qquad (5)$$

where ΔQ is the charge density (total charge normalized to the gate area), and C_{ox} is the oxide capacitance. C_{ox} can be calculated by using (6):

$$C_{ox} = \varepsilon_{ox} \frac{A}{t_{ox}} \qquad (6)$$

where ε_{ox} is the permittivity of the dielectric which isolates the gate from the substrate of the transistor, A is the gate area, and t_{ox} is the oxide thickness.

As seen by (5), determining the total trapped charge is essential to determine the threshold voltage shift. However, the amount of the trapped charge can not easily be calculated. The influences of X-ray radiation on semiconductors are highly dependent on the exposure duration. With longer exposure times, the number of charges trapped in the oxide and interface layers is increasing [9]. In general, it can be said that the current flowing through the cathode of the X-ray tube, in combination with the time, controls the number of electrons that are accelerated, which has a direct effect on the intensity and the energy of the X-ray source (see (1) and (3)). As seen by (4), the accelerating voltage sets the minimal wavelength and the start of the X-ray spectrum. This area has the highest photon count with the most extensive energy in the bremsstrahlung (see Figure 2). With higher power, the penetration ability of the X-ray photons is increasing, which leads to a higher risk that semiconductors are getting more irradiated.

The die's physical dimensions (e.g., the thickness of gate oxide) of an integrated circuit play a major role in the influences of X-ray radiation because they influence the X-ray radiation's absorption and the build-up of trapped charges [9].

Due to the aforementioned complicated nature of this process, it is easier and more pragmatic to measure the threshold voltage shift directly rather than try to predict it theoretically. In the next section, a simple circuit is introduced for this purpose.

4   Experimental determination of V_{th}

In Figure 4, a simple circuit consisting of a diode-connected (gate and drain are shorted together) PMOS transistor and a constant current source is shown, which can be used to determine the variations of the threshold voltage [6].

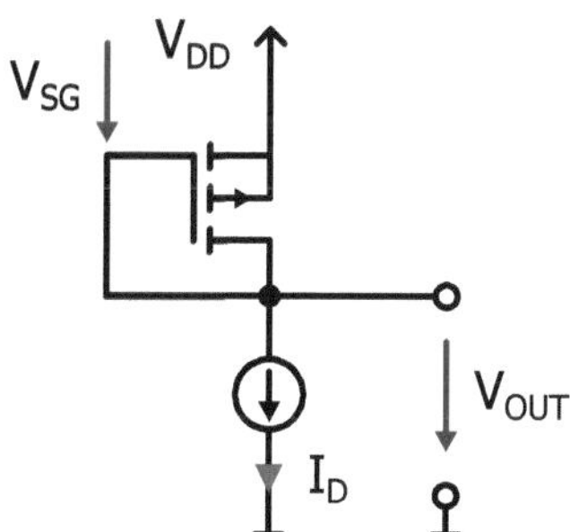

Figure 4: Circuit topology to determine the variations of V_{th}.

Assuming a level 1 MOS model and neglecting the channel length modulation, the drain current I_D of the PMOS transistor is given by [7]:

$$I_D = K_p(V_{SG} - |V_{th}|)^2 \qquad (7)$$

where K_p is a technology and geometry dependent parameter. $|V_{th}|$ can be calculated using (7) as:

$$|V_{th}| = V_{SG} - \sqrt{\frac{I_D}{K_p}} \qquad (8)$$

where $V_{SG} = V_{DD} - V_{Out}$ (see Figure 4), thus

$$|V_{th}| = V_{DD} - V_{out} - \sqrt{\frac{I_D}{K_p}} \qquad (9)$$

In (9) V_{DD} and I_D are constant circuit parameters. If we can, furthermore, assume that K_p will remain approximately unchanged after radiation[2], then we can determine the variation of the threshold:

$$\Delta|V_{th}| \approx -\Delta V_{out} \qquad (10)$$

Despite offering the most direct method for extracting V_{th}. In practice, short-channel effects (e.g., channel-length modulation, drain-induced barrier lowering, and carrier velocity saturation) can reduce the accuracy of this method [6].

5   Simulation of V_{th}

Circuit (SPICE) simulation using Orcad PSpice was performed to investigate whether the simplified assumptions used to derive (5) in the previous section might have a significant influence on the experimental determination of V_{th} variation or not. The circuit used for the simulation is shown in Figure 5. The supply voltage was chosen to be 12 V ($V_{DD} = 12V$).

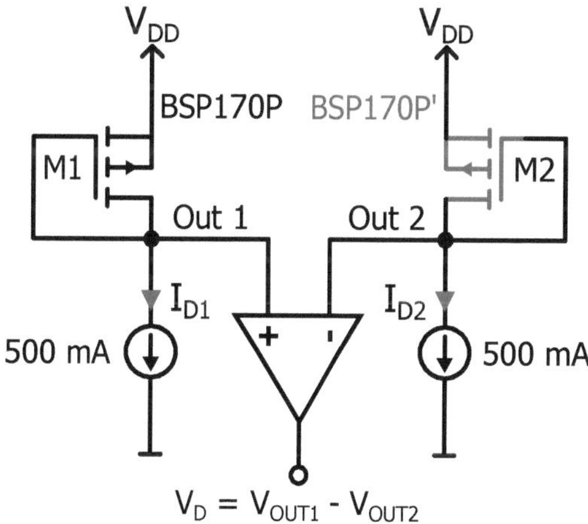

Figure 5: Simulation setup to study the second order effect of experimental determination of the threshold voltage variation.

---

[2] This assumption assumes implicitly that the mobility degradation of the carriers has a negligible effect than the threshold variation due to trapped charges.

The circuit contains two branches similar to the circuit shown in Figure 4. Both transistors are connected as a *MOS-diode* and biased by constant current sources $I_{D1} = I_{D2} = 500$ mA. A differential amplifier with a differential gain of 1 was used to directly measure the difference between the output voltages $V_D = V_{Out1} - V_{Out2}$, which would be ideally equal to the variation of the threshold according to (10).

For transistor M1 (in the left branch), the original manufacturer model, which is available by its manufacturer (Infineon), was used [8]. For transistor M2 (in the right branch), however, the V_{th_0} parameter of the model was varied from 10 mV to 110 mV in 10 mV steps to simulate the influence of X-rays. The simulation results are summarized in Table 1.

Real: $\Delta V_{th}/mV$	Calculated using accurate model: $\Delta V_{th}/mV$	Error/mV	$\Delta Q/nC$
10,00	9,978	-0,02	5,5
30,00	29,93	-0,07	16,4
50,00	49,88	-0,12	27,4
70,00	69,84	-0,16	38,4
90,00	89,79	-0,21	49,3
110,00	109,7	-0,30	60,2

Table 1: SPICE simulation results.

The first column shows the real change of the threshold voltage, the second column shows the measured value using the more realistic manufacturer model, the third column the absolute error between these two values is shown, and finally, the fourth column shows the calculated corresponding trapped charge due to radiation using (5). The comparison of the measured $\Delta V_{O\ T}$ and the actual change in V_{th} shows that, indeed, the neglection of the secondary effects results in minor errors (max. of 1 mV) in the determination of threshold voltage change by using this simple circuitry.

6   Summary and Conclusion

In summary, the basic of X-ray generation and its spectrum was reviewed in this paper. The main effect of radiation on semiconductors is the shift of the threshold voltage. This shift results from the formation of trapped charges in the oxide and interface layers of the semiconductors. The process of formation of these charges is complicated and depends apart from the energy spectrum of the X-ray on many parameters (like oxide thickness, and time of exposure). Finally, a simple measurement method was presented and analyzed using simplified assumptions (level 1 MOS model and neglecting the secondary short channel effects) to determine the threshold shift. It was shown using SPICE simulations, with more accurate MOS models, that the accuracy of the measurement method is acceptable (less than 1mV error).

In [6], this influence was defined as a sensitivity of 4 to 7,1 mV per Gy, depending on the MOSFET used. Compared to the dose of a 370 keV pulse X-ray tube at a distance of 30 cm, which is 51,398 μGy, the influence can be considered negligible if linearity of the sensitivity is assumed. Especially since the number of pulses from a pulsed X-ray tube in a counter IEDD mission averages around 50 pulses, equivalent to a dose of 2,57 mGy. The change in the threshold voltage by this dose would be between 10 to 18 μV. This amount can be considered harmless. The authors propose, as future work, to perform real measurements to validate these results. This quantization could also lead to applications such as the targeted irradiation of semiconductors to fine-tune the threshold voltage.

Acknowledgement

The work has been carried out at Technische Hochschule Lübeck - University of Applied Sciences.

Author's Statement

No conflicts of interest need to be disclosed.

7   References

[1] Wikipedia, "X-ray tube," 2023. [Online]. Available: https://en.wikipedia.org/wiki/X-ray_tube

[2] H. A. Kramers, "Xciii. on the theory of x-ray absorption and of the continuous x-ray spectrum," *The London, Edinburgh, and Dublin Philosophical Magazine and Journal of Science*, 1923.

[3] T. Oldham and F. McLean, "Total ionizing dose effects in mos oxides and devices," *IEEE Transactions on Nuclear Science*, 2003.

[4] N. T. Fourches, "Charging in gate oxide under irradiation: A numerical approach," *Journal of Applied Physics*, 2000.

[5] J. R. Schwank, M. R. Shaneyfelt, D. M. Fleetwood, J. A. Felix, P. E. Dodd, P. Paillet, and V. Ferlet-Cavrois, "Radiation effects in mos oxides," *IEEE Transactions on Nuclear Science*, 2008.

[6] O. F. Siebel, J. G. Pereira, M. C. Schneider, and C. Galup-Montoro, "A mosfet dosimeter built on an off-the-shelf component for in vivo radiotherapy applications," in *2014 IEEE 5th Latin American Symposium on Circuits and Systems*, 2014.

[7] B. Razavi, *Design of Analog CMOS Integrated Circuits*. McGraw-Hill, 2001.

[8] I. T. AG, "P-channel enhancement mode field-effect transistor (fet), -60 v, sot-223," 2023. [Online]. Available: https://www.infineon.com/cms/de/product/power/mosfet/small-signal-small-power/bsp170p/

[9] M. Alam, H. Shen, N. Asadizanjani, M. Tehranipoor, and D. Forte, "Impact of x-ray tomography on the reliability of integrated circuits," *IEEE Transactions on Device and Materials Reliability*, 2017.

Automated post-market surveillance of a microarray test system

Isabel Stephan [1], and Arne Schillert [2]

[1] Medical Informatics, Universität zu Lübeck, isabel.stephan@student.uni-luebeck.de
[2] EUROIMMUN Medizinische Labordiagnostika AG, a.schillert@euroimmun.de

Abstract

After being placed on the market, medical devices have to be verified regularly. The aim of this project is to develop an application that automates this post-market surveillance process for the microarray technology *EUROArray* developed by the company *EUROIMMUN*. By trying to align primer and probe sequences of the microarray system to all currently known DNA sequences, it can be determined whether the test system specifically detects all expected sequences. The alignment is performed by using the *Basic Local Sequence Alignment Search Tool*. Based on this information, statistical parameters such as sensitivity and specificity can be calculated. This automation is intended to replace the previously manual execution of the post-market surveillance, making the process more reproducible, saving time and expensive staff resources. Part of this project is the analysis and development of a suitable infrastructure as well as the development of a prototype.

1 Introduction

The *EUROArray* technology is a DNA-microarray system developed by the company EUROIMMUN AG. A microarray test is based on the amplification of defined gene segments by Polymerase Chain Reaction (PCR). Specifically designed DNA segments, so called primers, are used to determine the part of the sequence that should be amplified. The PCR-products are labeled with fluorescence tags. Subsequently, a hybridization reaction of the PCR products with probes on the microarray is initialized. Binding is measured by fluorescence signals generated at the microarray spots. Using the *EUROArray*, for example infectious diseases or disease-associated genetic traits can be specifically detected. [1]

As for all other medical devices, the functionality and quality of the *EUROArray* has to be verified regularly after being placed on the market. This process is called post-market surveillance (PMS). The Medical Device Regulation (MDR) and the In Vitro Diagnostic Regulation (IVDR) define post-market surveillance as followed:

„All activities carried out by the manufacturers in cooperation with other economic operators to institute and keep up to date a systematic procedure to proactively collect and review experience gained from their devices placed on the market, made available or put into service for the purpose of identifying any need to immediately apply any necessary corrective or preventive actions.“ [2]

The part of the PMS to which this project refers to has to be performed once a year for each developed test system. A test system is defined as the combination of a forward primer, a reverse primer and a probe. Currently, the PMS of the EUROArray is performed by domain experts in a mostly manual process.

The aim of the PMS process is to find out whether the test systems can still specifically detect the expected species although new DNA sequences were discovered during the year. In this way, it can be determined, for example, whether newly added subtypes are also detected by the test. To find this out, all currently known DNA sequences are tested to see if they would be detected by the test systems. This testing is simulated by performing an alignment between sequences of a DNA database and sequences of the test systems. By comparing the obtained detected sequences with those of species that the test system is desined for, one can calculate sensitivity and specificity.

Based on the current implementation of the EUROArray's PMS, this project will examine whether it is possible to make the entire process simpler, more efficient and more reproducible. For this purpose, the requirements for a possible application automating this process are defined at the beginning, followed by the development of a possible IT infrastructure and the implementation of a prototype.

2 Material and methods

2.1 Tools

2.1.1 Prototyping environment

A main component of this project is the development of a prototype. For this purpose, the programming language *R* is used. *R* is especially suitable for this project as it provides useful tools for data handling, statistics and bioinformatics.

For a convenient way to handle data, packages from the *tidyverse* [3], a collection of packages designed for data science, are used.

2.1.2 Remote processing

In this project, it is necessary to access remote servers as a computing and storage resource. For this purpose, an extra server has been set up by *EUROIMMUN* (further called *BLAST server*). It has a capacity of 256 CPUs and 251 gigabytes of RAM. The *R* package *batchtools* is used for interacting with this server. *batchtools* allows its user to run jobs asynchronically on a remote system. All relevant information, files and results of the computational jobs are stored in so called registries. This way, results can also be retrieved later. [4]

To make the remote access to external servers robust and reproducible, Docker is used. Docker is a containerization tool enabling the separation of applications from their infrastructure. Applications can thus be executed independently of the given infrastructure of a server in so-called docker containers, which contain everything necessary for the execution of the program. [5]

The communication with batchtool's batch system is managed via so-called cluster functions [4]. For this project a customized function that uses a modified docker image has been written.

For being able to apply a function over elements of a list when using *batchtools*, *batchtools* provides the function btlapply [4]. Using btlapply as a basis, a custom function is created. It manages the usage of functions over *batchtools*. This function contains in the first place btlapply's functionalities. Jobs can be created, submitted and the results can be collected and reduced. Additionally, it enables the use of an update parameter collecting the results from past registries if possible. This is especially useful in the development process. Furthermore, it exports all functions of the local *R* project using the batchExport [4] function provided by *batchtools*.

2.1.3 BLAST sequence alignment

To determine whether or not the developed EUROArray test systems are aligning to the expected sequences and whether unexpected sequences are being found, it is necessary to compare sequences with each other and quantify their similarity. A variety of different alignment algorithms exists for this purpose.

One of the most popular local sequence alignment tools is the *Basic Local Alignment Search Tool* (*BLAST*). It can be used via a web interface or via a command line tool. By comparing a users sequence query to sequences out of a database their similarity is determined. Different variants of *BLAST* exist. Here, the *blastn-short* program is used. It enables a comparison of a nucleotide sequence to nucleotide sequences in a database and is optimized for query sequences shorter than fifty bases. [6]

When determining the quality of matches, *BLAST* calculates and uses multiple statistical parameters. Table 1 displays the most important parameters.

Table 1: Statistical parameters used by BLAST. [6]

Parameter	Description
Raw-score	Sum of substitution scores, based on a substitution matrix and gap scores.
Bit-score	Derived from the *raw-score*. It takes into account the statistical properties of the scoring systems. Thereby, alignment scores from different searches can be compared.
Query coverage	The percentage of the query sequence aligning with the matching sequence.
E-value	Derived from the *bit-score*. It takes into account the probability that the match could be found just by chance. It is dependent on the size of the query sequence and the database.

All of the mentioned parameters except the *raw-score* are used in this project.

In addition to sequence alignment algorithms, *BLAST* provides biological sequence databases. As of February 4th, 2020, the *BLAST* databases are version 5. Since then, there are 22 sequence databases and one taxonomy database, providing additional taxonomy information. Every few month, the databases are updated with new entries. These databases are made available in a pre-formatted form allowing the user to directly use those databases for performing *BLAST* searches without having to convert it to an appropriate format beforehand. The databases are additionally provided in form of smaller-sized volumes. [7]

For this application the *nt* database containing partially non-redundant nucleotide sequences from all traditional divisions of GenBank, the European Molecular Biology Laboratory and the DNA Data Bank of Japan is used.

2.2 Previous approach

Previously, the PMS of the EUROArray test system has been performed by domain experts in a mostly manual process. This process is described in the following steps:

1. Sequences of forward primers, reverse primers and probes of all test systems (query sequences), are saved in separate *.fasta* files. *FASTA* is a data format designed for biological sequences.

2. The *blastn* command provided by *BLAST* is performed separately for each *.fasta* file. The following parameter options were used:

   - As alignment algorithm *blastn-short* was used.
   - The number of CPUs was set to 100.
   - A word-size of four bases was used.

- The e-value threshold was set to 1000

- A custom output format containing information about the query sequence, the matching sequence and statistical parameters signifying the quality of the hits was used.

3. The resulting output file was imported into *Excel* and the hits were filtered manually by the following criteria:

  - The length of of the aligned sequence should not deviate more than 10% from the query sequence length.

  - The *percentage identity* should be greater or equal to 95%.

  - The *query coverage* should be greater or equal to 95%.

  - Target sequences having an unspecific scientific name and synthetic constructs were excluded.

  - Cross-products, defined as a combination of a forward primer, a reverse primer and a probe from at least 2 different test systems binding the same target sequence, were marked separately. Those can be of special interest in case multiple test systems are used in the same microarray test.

  - Besides the cross products, only hits where both primers and the probe of one test system bind the same target sequence were maintained.

4. It was manually checked whether the scientific name of the target sequence of the obtained hits matches the expected scientific name of the test system. Sensitivity and specificity were calculated for each test system.

5. A final report containing the obtained sensitivity and specificity was generated.

3　Results and discussion

Based on the previous approach a prototype that automates this process is developed and implemented.

3.1　General idea

As input, query sequences of forward-primer, reverse-primer and probe per test system are expected. Additionally, the expected scientific names, that the test systems are designed for, should be given as input. Furthermore, the user should have the option to specify a *BLAST* database. Here, the *nt* database is used as default.

The general workflow for the development of the prototype can be structured into four parts:

1. Alignment of the query sequences to the sequences in the specified database using the *BLAST's blastn* command.

2. Filtering of the aligned sequences so that only plausible results are preserved.

3. Extraction of all database entries matching the expected scientific names.

4. Comparing the expected resuls to the obtained results. Statistical parameters such as sensitivity and specificity are calculated.

3.2　Analysis for an efficient use of *blastn* command

To enable a time efficient execution of *blastn* command when performing the first step of the workflow (see section 3.1) a run-time experiment is performed testing the following parameter:

- The number of query sequences.

- The number of CPUs used.

- Using the complete *nt* database in comparison to performing the *blastn* command on *nt* database volume chunks subsequently. The latter starts separate batchtools connections per volume chunk.

- Using a *.fasta* file containing all query sequences in comparison to performing the *blastn* command on separate *.fasta* files. The latter starts parallel running batchtools jobs.

Fig. 1 shows the results of the run time experiment. It can be seen that doubling the number of query sequences results roughly in a doubling of the run time. Increasing the number of used CPUs decreases the run time in general. The benefit for the run time by an increase in the number of CPUs is particularly large for time-consuming jobs. The increase in run time when using 15 query sequences between 120 and 150 CPUs is probably an outlier caused by a short-term overload of the *BLAST server's* computing capacity due to other applications running in parallel. Using the complete *nt* database for the alignment process decreases the run time as establishing several new connections to the *BLAST server* takes more time than reducing the sequence length in the chunks saves time. Furthermore, it can be seen that splitting the query sequences into separate *.fasta* files increases the run time. This is consistent with the information provided in the BLAST user manual, stating that BLAST works more efficiently if it scans the database once for multiple queries [6].
All in all, the fastest option is the combination of using the complete nt database with one .fasta input file as query in the alignment process together with the largest possible number of CPUs. Therefore, this option is used for the development of the prototype in this project.

3.3　Development of a prototype

The prototype is implemented according to the concept developed in section 3.1 together with the findings described in section 3.2. For the filtering of *blastn* results two additional filtering steps are added in addition to the filtering steps described in section 2.2:

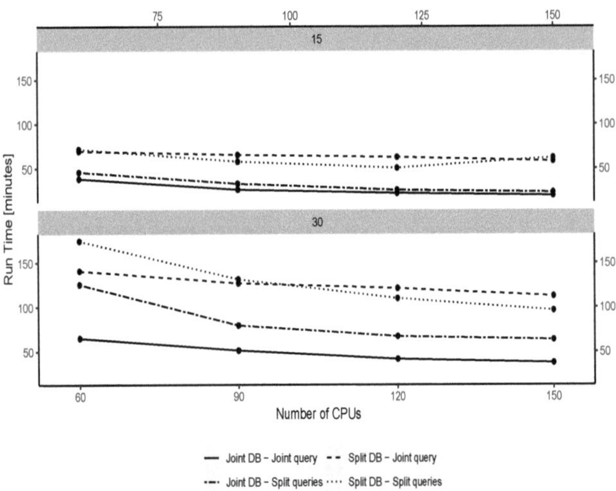

Figure 1: The lowest run time can be achieved by a combination of using the complete nt database with one *.fasta* input file as query together with the largest possible number of CPUs.

- Filtering for a realistic product length.

- Filtering for a realistic probe position in between both primers.

The resulting protoype is able to accept sequences for several test systems in combination with expected scientific names from a *.csv* file and perform all of the previously described steps automatically. As a result, the user obtains the determined sensitivities and specificities per test system.

For this prototype a run time analysis is being performed, whereby sequences of three microarray test systems against human alphaherpesvirus 1, human alphaherpesvirus 2 and human alphaherpesvirus 3 developed by *EUROIMMUN* are used as input. The results are displayed in Fig. 2. It can be seen, that performing the blastn command is the most time consuming step, followed by extracting the database information. In total, it takes less than half an hour for the whole analysis.

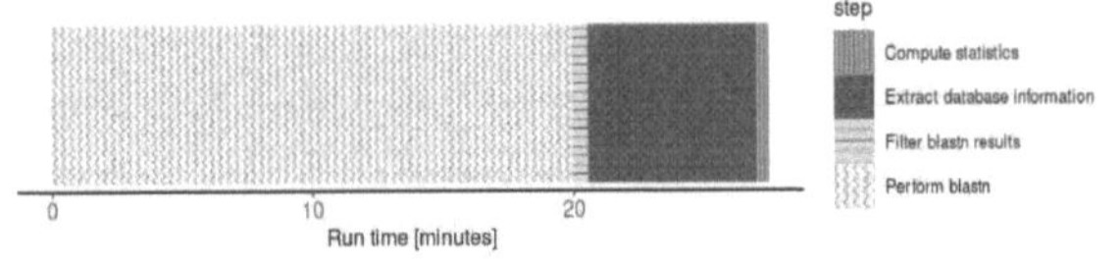

Figure 2: Performing the *blastn* command and extracting entries from the database are the most time consuming steps.

4   Conclusion

Aim of this project was to develop a proof of concept for an application that automates the PMS process of the *EUROArray* system. For this, a suitable infrastructure was set up. Furthermore, analyses of an efficient use of the BLAST software for this scenario were carried out. Finally, a functional prototype was developed following the manual steps. With the developed prototype, an input of three test species requires less than half an hour of evaluation time. Therefore, it can be said that it is possible to develop an application facilitating the PMS process of the EUROArray system, making the results more reproducible and reducing the time needed for the whole process substantially.

Acknowledgement

The work has been carried out at EUROIMMUN Medizinische Labordiagnostika AG and supervised by the Institute of Experimental Dermatology, Universität zu Lübeck.

Author's Statement

Arne Schillert is employed by EUROIMMUN Medizinische Labordiagnostika AG. Isabel Stephan is a master student at Universität zu Lübeck and receives financial support by EUROIMMUN Medizinische Labordiagnostika AG.

5   References

[1] EUROIMMUN AG, *Microarray*. Available: https://www.euroimmun.de/en/products/techniques/microarray/ [last accessed on 2022-12-24]

[2] Official Journal of the European Union, *REGULATION (EU) 2017/745 OF THE EUROPEAN PARLIAMENT AND OF THE COUNCIL of 5 April 2017 on medical devices, amending Directive 2001/83/EC, Regulation (EC) No 178/2002 and Regulation (EC) No 1223/2009 and repealing Council Directives 90/385/EEC and 93/42/EEC.* 2017.

[3] H. Wickham, *Tidyverse*. Available: https://www.tidyverse.org [last accessed on 2022-12-30]

[4] M. Lang and B. Bischl, *Batchtools*. Available: https://mllg.github.io/batchtools [last accessed on 2022-12-30]

[5] D. Merkel, *Docker: lightweight linux containers for consistent development and deployment* . Linux journal, vol. 2014, no. 239, pp. 2, 2014.

[6] National Center for Biotechnology Information (US), *BLASTo Command Line Applications User Manual.* 2008.

[7] National Center for Biotechnology Information (US), *The BLAST databases.* Available: https://ftp.ncbi.nlm.nih.gov/blast/documents/blastdb.html [last accessed on 2022-12-30]

Development and Implementation of Ground Control Station Functions for UAV Platforms

Mevluede Tigre

Robotics and Autonomous Systems, Universität zu Lübeck, mevluede.tigre@student.uni-luebeck.de

Abstract

The rising complexity of future scenarios requires higher autonomy in systems, leading aviation companies to develop new Unmanned Aerial Vehicles (UAVs) with cross-platform capabilities. A Ground Control Station (GCS) is needed to carry out missions and a common Graphical User Interface (GUI) is necessary for the interoperability of multiple vehicles [1]. In this project, the GUI was developed to monitor and control multi-UAV missions using the Robot Operation System (ROS2) network to communicate UAVs and GCS and use the User Datagram Protocol (UDP) network to stream the sensor data to the GUI. The project was tested in the Software in the Loop (SITL) and it was seen that it performed the desired tasks for GUI. Real-case testing will be conducted after obtaining permission from authorities.

1 Introduction

Unmanned Aerial Vehicles are revolutionizing the way both military and civilian operations are carried out. These vehicles offer a safe and efficient alternative to manned aircraft, as they can operate in hazardous conditions with higher degrees of autonomy. The cost-effectiveness of UAVs compared to manned aircraft has made them an attractive option for many organizations. With the continuous development of new types of UAVs, each with unique capabilities, the need for interoperability and ease of control by operators has become imperative. A Graphical User Interface can enhance the interoperability of these vehicles, while sensor data, camera footage, locations, etc., are transmitted to a Ground Control Station for operator monitoring and controlling of multiple vehicles by the operator.

The hexacopter drone platform focuses on using off-the-shelf components that have been integrated with easily prototyped mounting hardware to minimize overall costs. Since the chosen components keep payload mass and size requirements to a minimum, the UAV is based on a small quadrocopter design, measuring 40 x 40 x 15 cm in length, width, and height. The minimal design of drones keeps the platform mass at around 3 kg, leaving sufficient room for payloads of up to 2 kg. Depending on the takeoff weight, flight times range from 12 to 25 minutes. The main payload consists of a mono camera and an NVIDIA Jetson Nano as a mission computer [2].

1.1 Robot Operation System (ROS)

ROS2 is an upgraded version of the popular open-source software framework, ROS. It was developed for program-

ming and controlling robots and has improved the communication between robot components and between robots with its publish-subscribe architecture. The middleware used for communication in ROS2 is Data Distribution Service (DDS), which is designed for real-time data transmission in distributed environments. In ROS2, the basic architecture is composed of nodes, topics, and messages. Nodes can broadcast a message to a topic, and they can also follow a topic to receive messages. The messages are ROS2 data types used during the broadcast publishing and subscribing operations by topics [2]. In this project, ROS2 is utilized to control multiple drones and receive their sensor information, such as camera data. By using the communication framework and unified development environment provided by ROS2, it is possible to simplify the process of building and controlling advanced robotic systems. The ROS2 architecture, combined with the real-time data transmission capabilities of the DDS, allows for reliable and efficient communication between the drones and a central computer [2].

1.2 User Datagram Protocol (UDP)

The UDP [3] is a communication protocol used for transmitting data over networks. Unlike the Transmission Control Protocol (TCP), UDP does not provide guaranteed delivery of data or reliable communication. Instead, it is a fast and simple protocol that is best suited especially for video streaming. One of the key features of UDP is its low overhead, which makes it ideal for applications that require real-time communication, such as multimedia streaming [3]. In these applications, it is more important to have a fast and responsive communication channel than to ensure that every packet of data is delivered. This means that the sender is unaware of the receiver and does not perform a handshake before sending data, resulting in a fast and simple transmission process. UDP applications communicate through the use of datagrams, which contain the sender's address, which the server uses to send data to the correct client [3]. These datagrams are completely independent packets of information, allowing clients and servers to send and receive data without the need for a dedicated point-to-point channel. In the implementation of this project, several functions from the socket API were utilized to handle communication using the UDP that is shown in Fig. 1. The key functions used include *socket()*, *bind()*, *sendto()*, and *recvfrom()*.

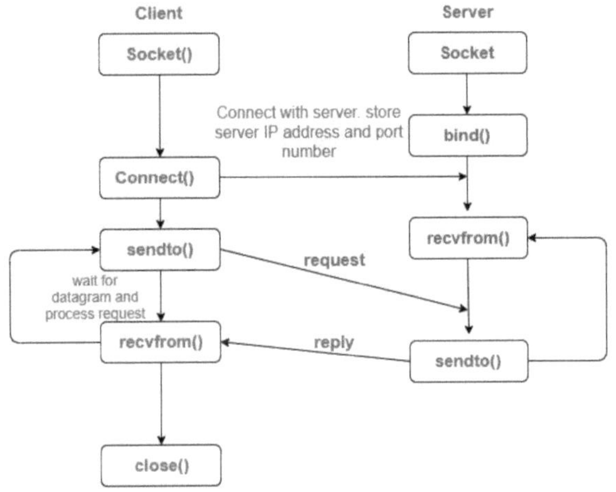

Figure 1: UDP Client-Server Connection [4]

1.3 Multi-Threading

Multi-threading is used in the project to handle multiple video streams from multiple drones effectively. By using multiple threads to retrieve the frames from the video streams, the GUI can avoid being stuck while reading the frames, which would cause latency in the video section. This multi-threading approach improves performance by alleviating the heavy I/O operations to separate threads, thus allowing the GUI to work smoothly and efficiently even when capturing multiple video streams. The implementation of multi-threading in the project uses a deque to handle retrieving the frames in parallel, thus reducing the latency and avoiding freezing of the GUI. Threads, allow multiple tasks to run concurrently within a single process. The basic structure of a thread includes a *start, run, sleep, wait* states as shown in Fig. 2 [5].

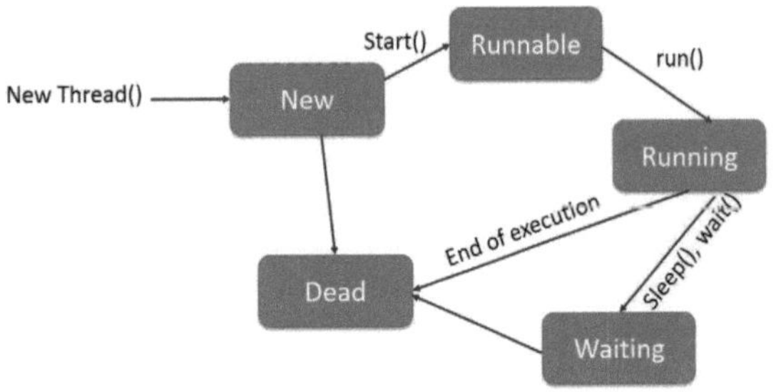

Figure 2: Life Cycle of a Thread [6]

2 Material and Methods

2.1 Implementation

In order to effectively control multiple drones simultaneously, Ground Control Station software was developed. The author designed several panels of the GUI as part of this project, including an Inspector Panel to observe the altitude and waypoints of each vehicle during flights, and a Camera Panel to increase the environmental awareness of the operator through the use of cameras mounted on each drone. Access to both panels is provided as an element of the toolbar that is located on the top of the GUI. In this section, the implementation of each panel will be explained in detail by referring to the panels that are shown in Fig. 3 and Fig. 4.

2.1.1 Inspector Panel

The inspector panel provides a centralized view of the real-time flight data for each drone, making it easy for the operator to monitor and control multiple UAVs at once. With the inspector panel, the operator can track the altitudes, waypoints, and flight paths of each drone, as well as the distances between each vehicle, without having to switch between different screens. This feature helps to reduce the workload and distractions for the operator, ensuring a more efficient and secure flight operation. The inspector panel that is shown in Fig. 3 can be accessed through the toolbar, providing quick and easy access to real-time flight data. This panel can also be used for the observation of the different types of sensors according to the will during the flight. Each sensor value is taken temporarily and dynamically it is shown on the panel. For the detail vision, it enables to the operator to zoom in or drag the panel.

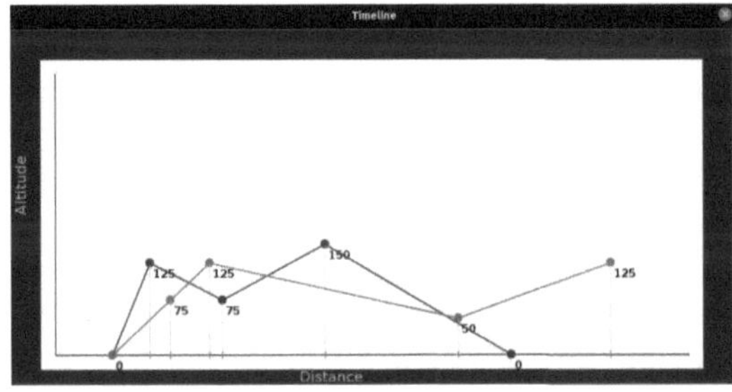

Figure 3: Inspector Panel : Points refer waypoints; values refer altitudes.

2.1.2 Camera Panel

The Camera Panel section in the toolbar menu serves as a graphical user interface for arranging the camera parameters and controlling the camera through the gimbal on a UAV. Besides that, the displays the camera's live stream as well as allows the operator to send commands to drones for various tasks such as orbiting around the target, approaching it, or moving away from a target that is remarked on the panel. The camera menu includes different elements that serve specific functions and are described in more detail in the Fig. 6 provided.

The ***Console*** is the main screen that appears when the Camera menu item is clicked. By default, the ***VideoStreams*** section is displayed. The ***CameraConfiguration*** opens when it is clicked, which is blank if there are no vehicles added to the map. For each added vehicle, a ***TaskPane*** is added to the container, displaying camera-related settings that can be adjusted. The ***CameraGimbalSettings*** section includes Network Settings, Display Settings, and limit values for the gimbal motors, which can be selected using a Combobox. The ***VideoStreamPanel*** displays the camera image from the drone and adds a ***VideoPanel*** for each attached vehicle. The *VideoPanel* displays the camera image and has a radio button, which when pressed, displays the camera image on a larger external panel called ***StreamingPanel***. To get the camera image, ***Camera*** class is also called as a thread and is where the camera image messages, which are taken from the drones, encoded to a packet and transferred over the UDP, are decoded into video. Moreover, ***CustomThread*** class allows using two different threads at the same time. ***CameraControlPanel*** is the external panel that opens when it is clicked the radio button on the *VideoPanel*. It consists of ***VideoDrawingPanel***, *StreamingPanel*, ***JStickArrow***, ***JStickSmall***, and ***LedStatusPanel***. The *VideoDrawingPanel* provides the ability to add target points. It has the same dimensions as the *StreamingPanel*. By clicking the left mouse button twice, the cursor appears, and the text on the upper left displays the pixel coordinates of the mouse position. To add or delete targets, bring the mouse to the desired point and right-click. A red dot will appear on the image when a target is added. To change the camera view, drag the mouse while pressing the mouse scroll button and adjust the gimbal motors' tilt and pan. This allows the movement of the camera within the motor's limits. The target points will also scroll with the image. Available actions include Follow, Orbit, Come Closer, and Get Away, accessible via a menu that appears upon right-clicking on the target point. The "Send Target" button is used to send target points to the UAV, after which all red dots on the *VideoDrawingPanel* will be cleared. Zooming in on the image can be done using the mouse scroll key, with the zoom level displayed on the left text on the panel. With the direction keys on the *JStickArrow*, the direction of the motors can be changed more precisely. This is the section that shows how far gimbal motors can be moved. The light-colored part on the circle is determined according to the minimum and maximum servo limits values in the tilt and padding areas under *CameraConfiguration*. Before the flight, the user is expected to determine these values. It is seen that the arrow position on *JStickSmall* changes when mouse dragging is done in the *StreamingPanel* or when the direction keys on *JStickArrow* are pressed.

2.2   Communication System

The camera image on the drone is taken over USB with the cam_pub file running in the mission control unit and

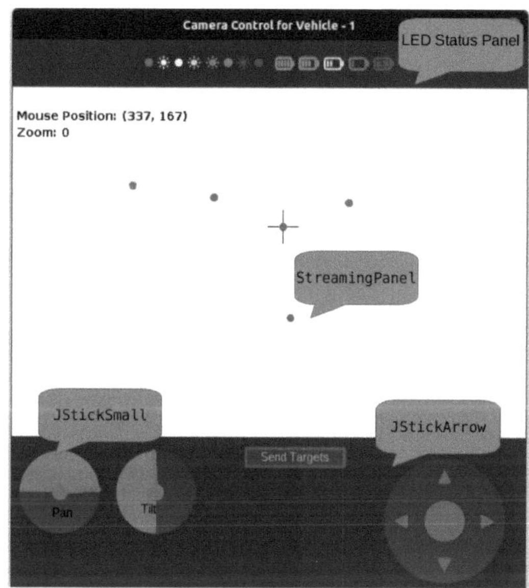

Figure 4: Camera Control Panel

published as a ROS2 message. The cam_sub node on the ground computer also receives this image message and converts this message into a datagram packet to send them over UDP protocol. Additionally, UDP network information regarding the IP address, port numbers, buffer size, etc. takes part in server_1 and server_2 files. cam_sub node uses the server information and streams the camera images to GUI part over UDP. Therefore, the message can also be received by the GUI. This whole process is explained in Fig. 5. Likewise, sensor messages are sent from the drone to the GUI in this way.

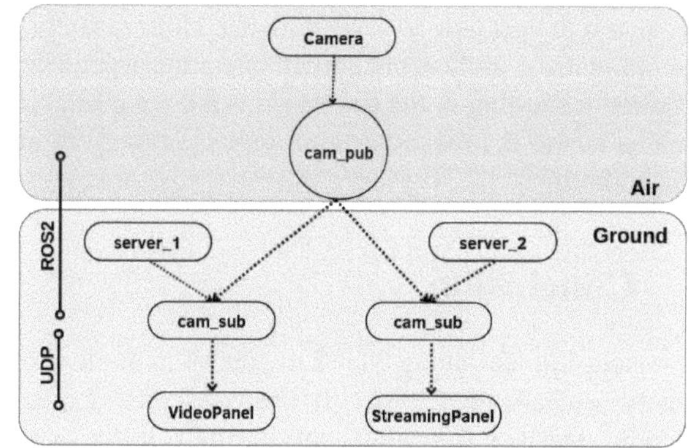

Figure 5: Communication between each UAV and GUI

3   Results

In this project, an interface that works in the Ground Control Station has been developed in order to track the movements of UAVs that can work collaboratively, observe the sensor data, and give a command for a certain task. This user interface is still under development, and only certain parts have been explained in this report. The parts described

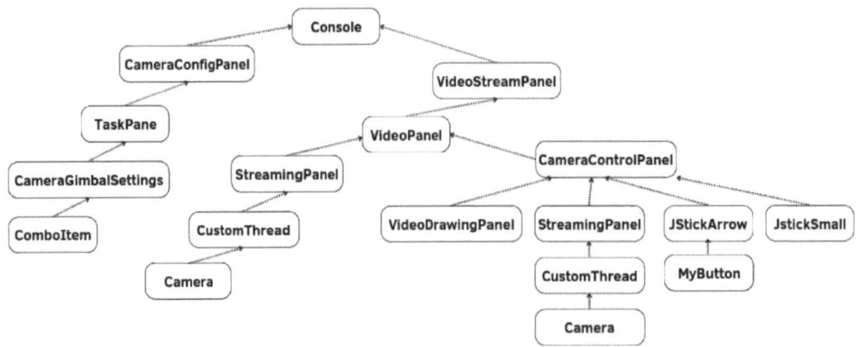

Figure 6: FlowChart of the classes for the Camera Panel: The direction of the arrow refers to the other class in which it is used.

have been tested in the STIL. For the camera section of the GUI, The recorded video was published using ROS2 and subscribed to it. The video was then streamed over UDP and viewed on the camera panels. Target points were added to the DrawingPanel and sent to the UAVs. The ROS2 topic was monitored to observe the pixel position of the target points. The inspector panel was tested by adding vehicles and defining paths using waypoints. It was seen that the panel dynamically changed based on the actions performed on the GUI. Mainly evaluation criteria of the GUI are being user-friendly of the GUI, effectively managing and monitoring multiple drones. GUI was tested by taking into account these criteria during the SITL test and it can be said that it was a success. With GUI, multiple drone values effectively got taken and the command messages to control the drones got sent to them. To provide the being user-friendly, commonly used mouse and keyboard commands are added on GUI and these features are tested by safety pilots in the office that is not get used to using our GUI. Unfortunately, the operational test could not be carried out as the dependencies required for testing in the real world is not yet available as well as due to the requirement of authorization from aviation authorities.

4   Conclusion

In conclusion, designing a GUI to control multiple drones can be a challenging task. It involves creating a user-friendly interface that allows users to effectively manage and monitor multiple drones simultaneously. The project described above showcases the implementation of such a GUI, with features such as observing sensor data, controlling the camera, and adding and sending target points information to the UAVs. While the test was carried out using a simulation environment, the potential for real-world applications is evident. However, there is still room for improvement and additional functionality to be added in the future. This can include object detection, target tracking, and target geo-localization to support the operator's awareness. With further improvements and considerations, such a GUI has the potential to revolutionize the way drone operations are managed and carried out.

Acknowledgement

The work has been carried out at Airbus and supervised by Jens Halbig and Prof. Dr. Georg Schildbach, Universität zu Lübeck.

Author's Statement

Conflict of interest: Authors state no conflict of interest.

5   References

[1] M. Pickard, P. Ludewig, J. Halbig, and B. Krach, "A multi-platform small scale drone demonstrator for technology maturation of next generation avionic functions," in *Software Engineering 2022 Workshops*, Gesellschaft für Informatik eV, 2022.

[2] S. Macenski, T. Foote, B. Gerkey, C. Lalancette, and W. Woodall, "Robot operating system 2: Design, architecture, and uses in the wild," *Science Robotics*, vol. 7, no. 6622, p. eabm6074, 2022.

[3] N. Ploplys and A. Alleyne, "Udp network communications for distributed wireless control," in *Proceedings of the 2003 American Control Conference, 2003.*, vol. 4, pp. 3335–3340 vol.4, 2003.

[4] Mohityadav, "Udp client server using connect." https://www.geeksforgeeks.org/udp-client-server-using-connect-c-implementation/, 2018.

[5] D. M. Tullsen, S. J. Eggers, and H. M. Levy, "Simultaneous multithreading: maximizing on-chip parallelism," in *25 years of the international symposia on Computer architecture (selected papers)*, pp. 533–544, 1998.

[6] tutorialspoint, "Java multithreading schematic picture." https://www.tutorialspoint.com/java/java_multithreading.htm, 2022.

A Touchpad as Replacement
for a Car's Steering Wheel Buttons
For the Control of an Infotainment System

Philip Bukowski [1], Ibrahim Awada [2] and Finn Jacobsen [3]

[1] Robotics and Autonomous Systems, Universität zu Lübeck, philip.bukowski@student.uni-luebeck.de
[2] Valeo, gestigon GmbH, ibrahim.awada@valeo.de
[3] Valeo, gestigon GmbH, finn.jacobsen@valeo.de

Abstract

As the automotive industry continues to expand the capabilities of car infotainment systems, drivers are becoming increasingly distracted when adjusting settings while driving. This project investigates the potential of a touchpad mounted on the steering wheel, utilizing simple touch gestures, as a more efficient alternative to buttons for controlling a car's infotainment system, and the design considerations necessary to enhance its usability. The touchpad, provided by Azoteq, was connected to an Arduino Nano microcontroller and the game engine Unity3D, which was used to implement basic infotainment system functions, such as navigation, media player, and climate control. The usability of the touchpad was evaluated through a survey of 11 participants. The results indicate that the majority of participants would likely adopt the use of a touchpad mounted on the steering wheel as a means of controlling their car's infotainment system.

1 Introduction

As car infotainment systems continue to expand in functionality, it becomes increasingly difficult for drivers to make simple adjustments while driving due to the limited number of buttons on the steering wheel. A touchpad mounted on the steering wheel allows for a wider range of adjustments to be made without removing the hands from the steering wheel or diverting the eyes from the road. This project aims to evaluate the usability of a steering wheel touchpad as a replacement for buttons in controlling a car's infotainment system. The goal is to determine if this new method of input improves the user experience and overall functionality of the system. The study will focus on various factors such as ease of use, accuracy, and user satisfaction. The findings of this project will provide valuable insights for the design and development of future steering wheel mounted touchpads and its corresponding infotainment system.

2 Material and Methods

The touchpad used in this project is IQS550EV02 trackpad module and evaluation board by Azoteq [3] mounted on the right side of a 15 inch racing steering wheel by HXYIYG [7] with a custom 3D printed mount. To connect the trackpad module with the game engine Unity3D, an Arduino Nano microcontroller [5] was used as a I2C master device to handle the communication between the touchpad and Unity3D [1] over an USB port. The user interface was animated using the DoTween library [4] for Unity3D.

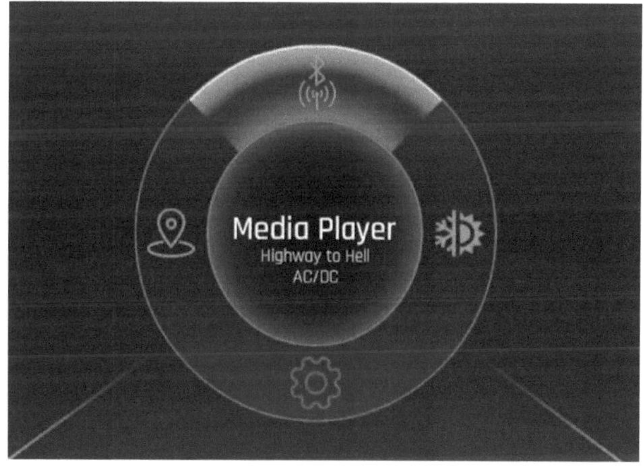

Figure 1: The figure shows the main menu with the media player page selected, displaying the page title and relevant information. Navigation options include swiping up for the media player, right for climate controls, down for settings, and left for the navigation page. However, it should be noted that the settings page was not implemented in this project due to time constraints and serves as a placeholder for future development.

A map was implemented using the MapBox API [6]. To be able to enter text a *$1 recognizer for user interface prototypes* [2] was used. The main issue with touchpads is the lack of precision in hitting specific points, leading to the implementation of a circular layout for the main menu as shown in figure 1. This allows for intuitive navigation by swiping in any direction in the center of the touchpad, while reserving the tangible edges for controls requiring sliders and corners for buttons. To return to the previous page the double tap gesture was chosen.

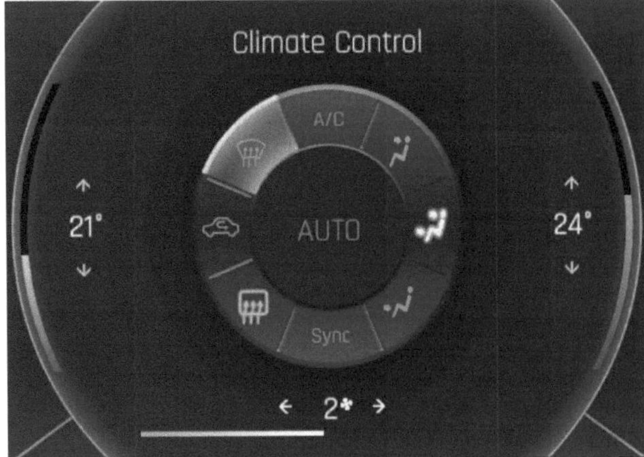

Figure 2: This figure shows the climate controls. With the driver and passenger temperature as well as the airflow intensity slider positioned at the left, right and bottom edges, respectively.

The above figure 2 shows the climate control page, which was designed similarly to the main menu, with switchable controls arranged in a circular layout. As with the main menu, settings are activated and deactivated by swiping in the center of the touchpad in the desired direction. The airflow speed, driver and passenger temperature sliders were positioned along the bottom, left, and right edges of the screen, respectively. This should indicate that the user is able to control the desired slider by swiping at the corresponding edge of the touchpad.

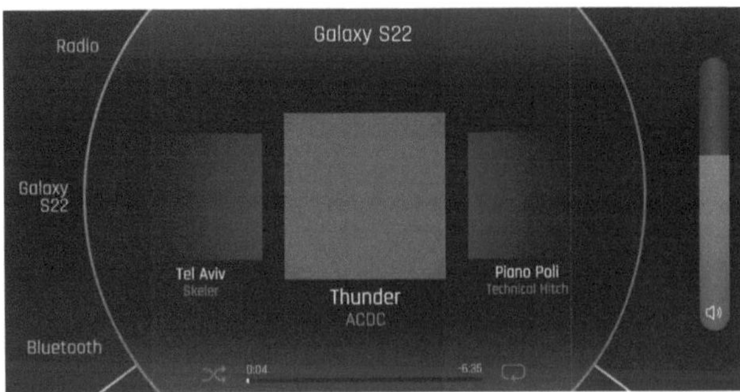

Figure 3: This figure depicts the media player interface. The left side displays labels for the current, next, and previous rows. The center highlights the currently active track of the connected Bluetooth device and shows the next and previous songs. Additional track information, such as song progress, can be found at the bottom of the screen. To control the volume a slider was added to the right side of the screen.

A grid layout was implemented for the media player (see figure 3), with each row representing a different type of audio source. In the beginning the first row displays place-

holder elements for different radio channels, while the second row displays available Bluetooth devices. Only one row is visible at a time and switching between rows is accomplished by swiping up or down and between elements in a row by swiping left or right. The selected element can be activated by simply tapping once. When activating a Bluetooth device the system plays a loading animation representing the connection process. After the animation is done a new row appears between the radio and Bluetooth sections displaying the currently playing track of the selected device. The active track can be paused and played by tapping once, as well as skipped by swiping left or right. With

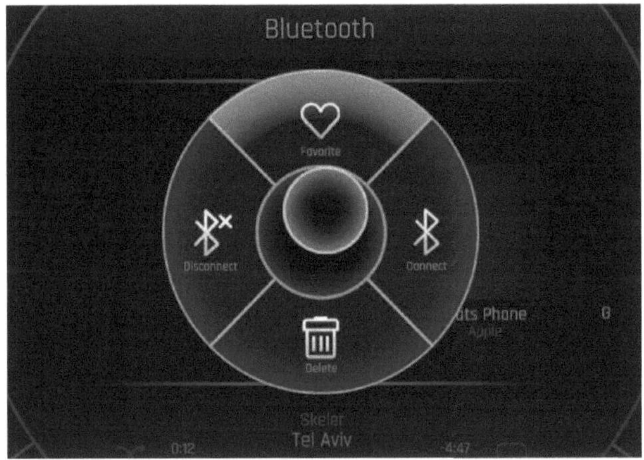

Figure 4: The figure illustrates the options menu accessed by holding a selected Bluetooth device. Navigation is achieved by swiping and releasing in the desired direction.

the use of a touch and hold gesture on a track or Bluetooth device, an options window pops up as illustrated in figure 4. The options are controlled similar to the main menu and climate controls by swiping in the desired direction. On the navigation page, only map movement and the ability to input letters in a textbox were implemented due to time constraints. When clicking on the textbox, a drawing region appears with buttons to delete and add spaces, allowing the user to input the address of the desired destination (see figure 5). An evaluation of the usability of the system was conducted by administering surveys to a sample group of 11 participants in order to gather their feedback and first impressions on the ease of use and functionality of the system. It has to be noted that the evaluation is the end of a first development iteration and serves as a guide for further improvements.

3 Results and Discussion

3.1 Questions before the test

Before showing the infotainment system to the participants, they were asked to rate their experience with touch controls on a scale from 1 (no experience) to 10 (expert level) and to specify the contexts in which they have used it. Figure 6 visualizes the results.

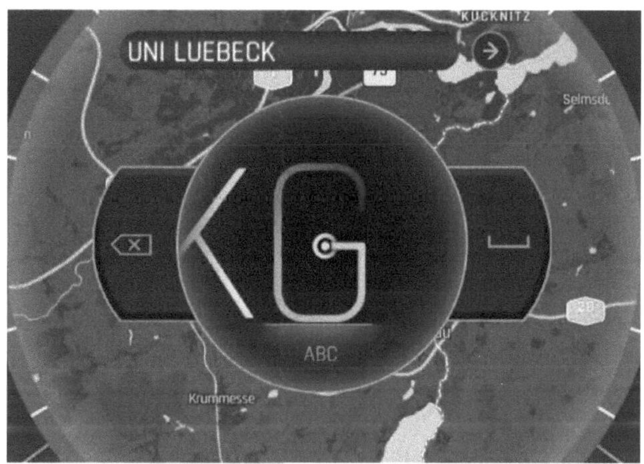

Figure 5: The figure illustrates the pop-up window for writing the goal address while navigating and is accessed by tapping the top edge of the touchpad. Users can write simple letters, and by tapping the left and right third of the touchpad, can delete and add spaces respectively.

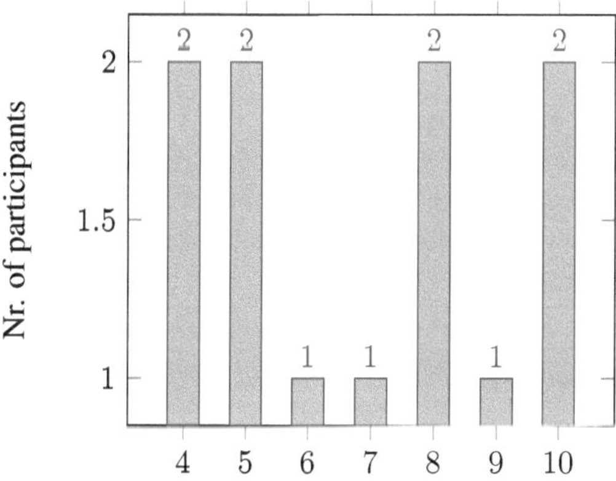

Figure 6: This figure displays the distribution of participants' self-assessed experience with touch control. With zero being no experience and ten representing expert level

The question whether they like touch control was answered by all 11 participants with *yes*. When asked, if they can imagine using touch control as a replacement for the steering wheel buttons for the control of the car's infotainment system, the first concerns become clear. The answers where the following:

- Yes (x2)

- Yes, but it might be too sensitive (x2)

- Yes, but I don't want to need to look to use it (x2)

- Yes, but I prefer buttons (x2)

- Yes, but not all buttons should be replaced (x2)

- No, I prefer buttons (x1)

3.2 Main Menu

After allowing participants to test the system independently, they were questioned about various aspects of the system, beginning with the main menu. When queried about their opinions on the main menu, six participants praised its minimalistic and intuitive design, while two preferred using tips instead of swipes to activate pages. Three individuals found the climate icon to be misleading and associated it with weather. All participants expressed approval of the double-click gesture for returning to previous pages, though two noted that it is a common activation gesture on computers.

3.3 Climate Control

When asked to adjust the passenger temperature to a specific value, eight out of eleven participants had no difficulty using the edge-swiping gesture, while three required guidance on how to operate the temperature sliders. One participant expressed concern that the temperature controls may be challenging to adjust while driving, and another noted that the controls felt slower than anticipated. When tasked with adjusting various climate settings, such as defrosting the windshield or heating only the leg room, five participants found the system to function as expected. Three noted that it takes some practice, but is easy to master, while others found it to be overly sensitive and distracting. One participant suggested the inclusion of a confirmation window to verify the intended setting.

3.4 Media Player

The usability of the media player was evaluated by tasking participants to connect to a Bluetooth device of their choice, skip the first track and test the pause and play functionality. Although the majority of participants were able to navigate the system as expected, three initially tried to play the next track by swiping right instead of left. Additionally, users noted that the volume slider is overly sensitive and should requires multiple strokes to reach maximum volume. The placement of the volume slider on the right was also criticized as it can be accidentally adjusted while driving. Furthermore, six users expressed a desire for the ability to quickly scroll in both horizontal and vertical directions using sliders positioned on the bottom and left edges, respectively.

3.5 Navigation

In evaluating the touchpad's writing capabilities, participants were tasked with setting a goal location. Shortcomings in the system became apparent, with some finding the drawing region too small, difficulty adjusting to the touchpad, and confusion with certain buttons. Two participants preferred one-stroke writing, while others required assistance with opening the window or identifying certain buttons. The results indicate that effective writing on a steering wheel-mounted touchpad requires utilizing the entire touchpad surface. Writing letters with one stroke is preferred as it allows for the letter recognition algorithm to process the drawing immediately after the user releases the touchpad, accommodating with users writing speed and time between strokes. The results also suggest the need for improved positioning of the delete and space buttons.

One participant proposed the inclusion of audible feedback to confirm the recognized letters, allowing for writing without diverting one's gaze from the road.

3.6 Questions after the Test

After all participants finished testing the infotainment system, they where asked what other parts of a car's infotainment system they can imagine to control with a steering wheel mounted touchpad. Three participants could imagine changing the car settings, like sound or ambient light. One user could also envision accepting an incoming call using the touchpad. Even though it is not part of a infotainment system three users also could imagine controlling drive assistance systems, like cruse control. Other ideas were, adjusting the mirrors, windows or even activating the turn signals. Considering the safety regulations these are also options worth exploring. Finally, participants were asked to rate their likelihood of using this type of interaction in a car on a scale of one to ten, with one indicating they were not likely to use it and ten indicating they were very likely to use it. The following figure illustrates the results.

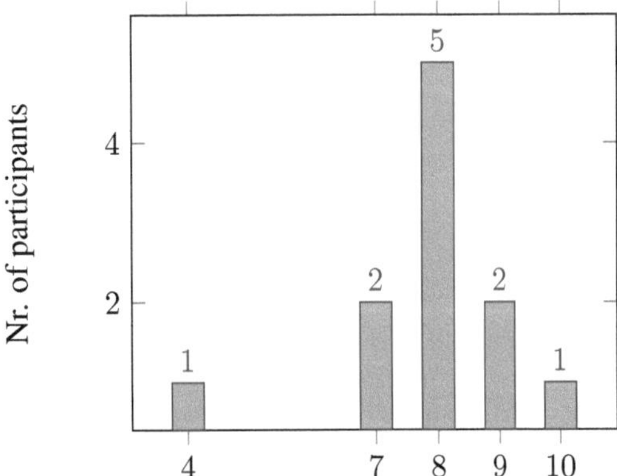

Figure 7: The figure illustrates that, even though this is the first development iteration, the majority of participants said they would likely adopt the use of a touchpad mounted on the steering wheel as a means of controlling their car's infotainment system.

Finally, the group was queried for suggestions to enhance the touchpad's usability. Ideas included labeling touch regions and incorporating raised sections and combining it with haptic feedback for improved functionality of the system.

4 Conclusion

The implementation of a touchpad as an alternative to steering wheel buttons offers increased control options for the driver, yet requires careful design considerations in the development of the corresponding infotainment system. One crucial aspect is the implementation of a secure unlocking mechanism to prevent accidental activation while driving and minimize distraction. Additionally, the system should prioritize simplicity and clarity in gesture design, enabling drivers to memorize short gesture sequences for adjusting settings without diverting their gaze from the road. Enhancing the touchpad's tactile feel through the use of elevated regions and haptic feedback can also improve usability and aid in quick and accurate navigation.

Acknowledgement

The work has been carried out at gestigon GmbH, Valeo and supervised by Prof. Dr.-Ing. Erhardt Barth of the Institute for Neuro- and Bioinformatics, Universität zu Lübeck.

Author's Statement

Conflict of interest: Authors state no conflict of interest. Informed consent: Informed consent has been obtained from all individuals included in this study.

5 References

[1] Haas, John K, *A history of the unity game engine.* Worcester Polytechnic Institute, 2014.

[2] Wobbrock, Jacob O and Wilson, Andrew D and Li, Yang, *Gestures without libraries, toolkits or training: a $1 recognizer for user interface prototypes.* Proceedings of the 20th annual ACM symposium on User interface software and technology, pp. 159–168, 2007

[3] Azoteq trackpad module with evaluation kit, *https://www.azoteq.com/product/iqs550-b000/.* [last accessed on 2023.01.19]

[4] DOTween Library for Unity3D, *http://dotween.demigiant.com/getstarted.php.* [last accessed on: 2023.01.19]

[5] Arduino IDE, *https://www.arduino.cc/.* [last accessed on: 2023.01.19]

[6] Mapbox, *https://www.mapbox.com/.* [last accessed on: 2023.01.19]

[7] Steering wheel by HXYIYG, *https://www.amazon.de/Sportlenkrad-Racing-Echtes-Drifting-Lenkrad/dp/B095M39WMJ.* [last accessed on: 2023.01.19]

12

Image Processing

Time-of-Flight Cameras for Medical Applications: A brief Review

Felicitas Brokmann [1]

[1] Medical Engineering Science, Universität zu Lübeck, felicitas.brokmann@student.uni-luebeck.de

Abstract

The acquisition of three-dimensional (3D) data and its processing in real time plays an important role in medicine. Time-of-Flight (ToF) cameras offer a fast and inexpensive way to capture not only two-dimensional (2D) color and depth images but also 3D point clouds. Such gain of information improves for example a precise monitoring of movements or detection and recognition of persons. This review surveys a selection of medical applications of ToF cameras and the related research. Insights into movement monitoring in radiotherapy, respiratory monitoring as well as detection and prediction of human poses are provided.

1 Introduction

The great potential of Time-of-Flight (ToF) cameras and their real time vision sensor for capturing depth images is evident in many fields, such as three-dimensional (3D) perception and computer vision, human-machine interaction and robotic navigation, and augmented reality [1]. By determining the phase shift between the emitted and reflected near infrared (IR) light, the ToF sensor calculates the distance of a scene for each pixel. A special advantage of the ToF imaging technique is the simultaneous capturing of the depth of the entire field of view. The quick generation of images is therefore particularly suitable for dynamic scenes. In addition, current ToF cameras are inexpensive in comparison to other 3D scanning methods such as laser devices while still exibiting accurate depth measurements in the range of mm $\sim$ cm. They are compact, reliable and enable both single and video capturing of depth data of the observed scene [2]. Due to the fact that the simultaneous acquisition of RGB and depth images already establishes a direct relationship between the two image informations, RGB-Depth (RGB-D) images can provide a gain in information regarding object positions in the scene, which can have a positive effect not only on applications such as object segmentation or recognition [1].

In the field of medicine, fast and accurate image acquisition is beneficial to continuously improve image-based diagnostic and therapeutic applications. Here, real-time images of the depth of scenes are mainly used for position recognition of persons [3] and motion detection or prediction [4], [5].

The purpose of this paper is to provide a brief overview of the applications of ToF cameras in a medical environment. The first part gives a summary of the basic principle of image acquisition of conventional ToF cameras. The second part presents a selection of applications relevant to the

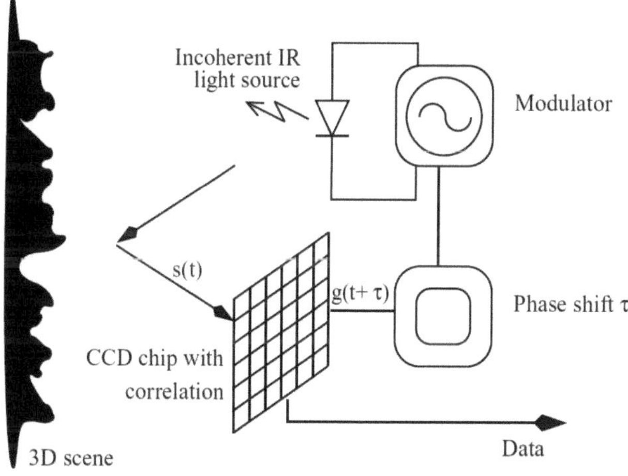

Figure 1: ToF imaging principle: Determination of the phase delay between the emitted and the detected IR signal [6].

clinic, as well as some related practical research examples.

2 ToF Imaging Principle

The acquisition of depth images with a ToF camera is based on the determination of the phase shift between an emitted near IR signal and an incident signal which results from the reflection of the emitted IR signal at the observed scene. Using a near IR light source enables the resolution of smaller details in the scene. The principle is illustrated in Fig. 1.

The correlation between emitted and incident signal is implemented directly on the ToF sensor, which consists of so-called *smart pixels* [2]. From this determined phase shift φ, the distance D of the reflecting scene can be calculated

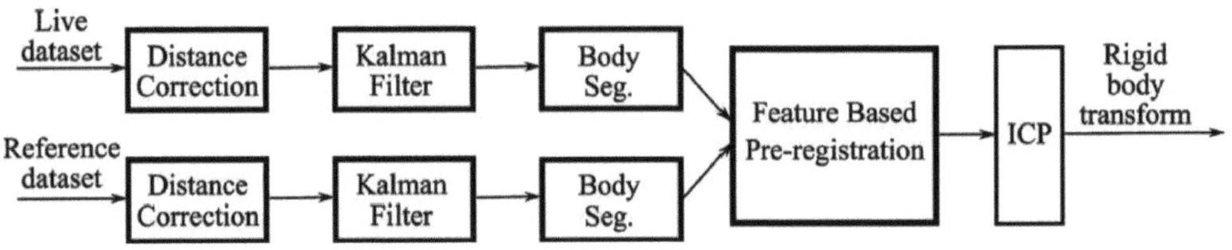

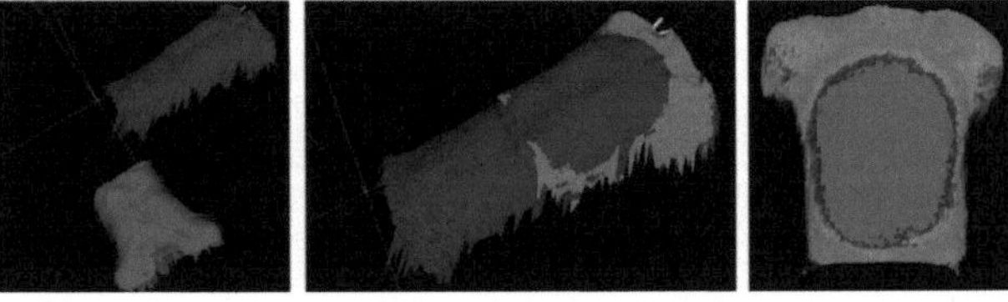

Figure 2: Processing pipeline of the registration framework for radiotherapy patient monitoring [4].

using

$$D = \frac{c}{2f} \frac{\varphi}{2\pi} \tag{1}$$

taking into account the speed of light c and the frequency f of the emitted IR signal. The maximum measurable depth d_{max} is given by

$$d_{max} = \frac{c}{2f} \tag{2}$$

and thus depends on the modulation frequency f of the emitted signal. TOF sensors are constantly evolving regarding the depth precision limitations but still suffer i.e. from distance errors which are related to integration-time of the sensor, temperature and the intensity of the emitted signal [6].

3   Medical Applications of ToF Camera Systems

Current research in the field of ToF camera applications in the clinical context includes monitoring patient position during radiotherapy, respiratory monitoring, and the pose estimation or prediction of medical staff in the operating room. These applications and their basic approaches and results will be discussed in more detail hereafter.

3.1   Radiotherapy monitoring

Monitoring the patient position in radiotherapy is of great importance for the outcome of the treatment. Correct positioning ensures delivery of the prescribed radiation dose to the tumor area as well as the protection of surrounding tissue from harmful radiation. Conventional approaches to image-based position monitoring consist of placing laser or adhesive markers on the patient's skin in combination with supplementary radiographic imaging. These approaches are not only limited by the number of markers on the patient and thus inadequate visualization of the treatment area. In addition, intrafractional radiographic imaging is associated with increased radiation exposure to the patient [7]. In this case, the application of the ToF technology could allow a fast and comparatively inexpensive imaging of the entire patient surface, however current laser based techniques like the systems from Vision RT are highly accurate and hard to beat. Nevertheless the ToF technology is suitable not only for an interfractional positioning of the patient but also to monitor the movement between radiation doses [4].
The potential accuracy of registering patient position in radiotherapy using real-time surface registration obtained by

Figure 3: Registration results of a thoracic deformation. Left: Untransformed live dataset and corresponding reference surface; Middle: Transformation of the live dataset and reference suface; Right: Distance map between both datasets after registration [4].

a ToF camera was investigated in [4]. Two ToF datasets of the upper body were acquired and registered: a reference dataset recorded before the first session and a live dataset acquired during each subsequent treatment session. The pipeline of the registration framework is shown in Fig. 2. Using custom-designed surface features, a pre-registration of both datasets was performed, followed by a more accurate registration using the iterative-closest-point algorithm. The visual results of the registration are shown in Fig. 3. The presented system achieved an accuracy of 1.62 ± 1.08 mm in the translational component and $0.07° \pm 0.05°$ in the rotational component. Besides that, it is characterized by a very short time delay between image acquisition and motion detection, which favors its suitability for motion detection. Further investigations were made in [7]. The authors proposed a stereo system consisting of two ToF cameras for daily positioning of patients during radiotherapy. By registering the recorded ToF data before the first fraction and after every subsequent fraction, a displacement was determined. This displacement was compared to the actual displacement of the treatment table which was estimated by conventional measurement methods. An error of the whole system of 1.5 ± 0.8 mm was indicated for the detection of displacement, which was considered acceptable for clinical application.

3.2   Breath monitoring

Applications of respiratory monitoring can not only be found in the screening of the population for pulmonary diseases, but also in gating control for radiologic imaging techniques or patient-ventilator sychronization during invasive or noninvasive mechanical ventilation [8]. Current standard of physiologic measuring of pulmonary function are spirometry devices which allow the user to asses static and

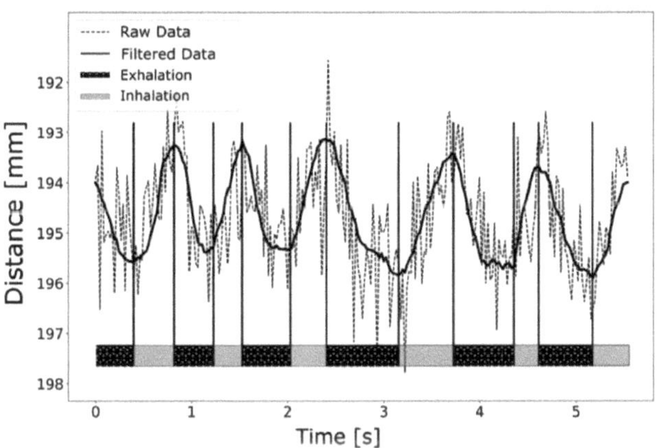

Figure 4: Respiration curve with breathing pattern of a preterm neonate, measured by a conventional ToF camera [5].

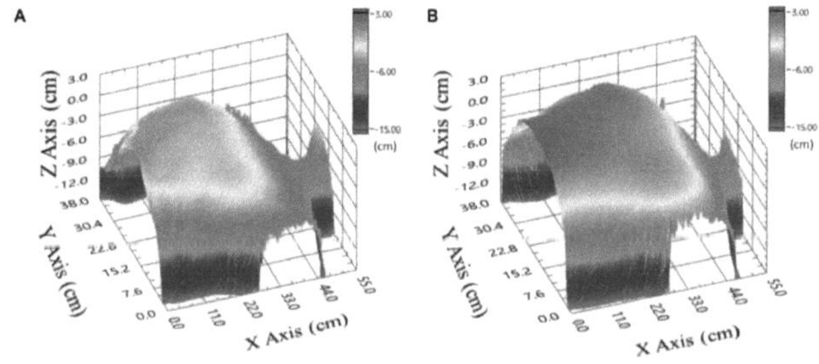

Figure 5: Three-dimensional images of the front thorax with neck and head at (A) maximum exhalation and (B) maximum inhalation [9].

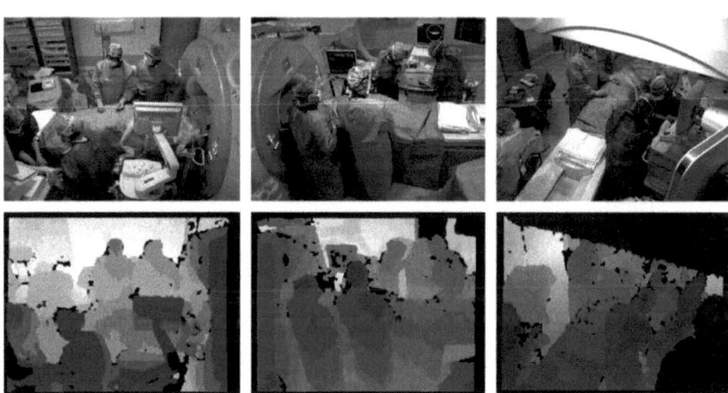

Figure 6: Corresponding pairs of RGB (top row) and depth (bottom row) images of the medical staff in the operating room [11].

dynamic breathing parameters via respiratory and volume flow. Although this technique is very accurate, there are some disadvantages especially regarding the handeling and usability at home. In contrast to that a monitoring of the patient's breathing by recording thoracical motion using ToF cameras can not only provide a noncontact measurement of respiratory volume but also provide a simple and inexpensive monitoring method for home use [9].

The feasibility of monitoring respiratory motion of newborns was demonstrated in [5]. For this purpose, simple ToF video recordings of the thorax of different newborns were taken. The analysis of the depth images over time resulted in the associated respiratory patterns which are shown in Fig. 4. Further analysis of these patterns allowed their classification into different categories such as forced breathing, sighing, apnea and crying. In addition to an analysis of the breathing pattern, [9] investigated the respiratory volume. The authors proposed a ToF data-based screening system to detect early airflow limitations at home. The principle is based on the acquisition of depth images of the patient's upper body. From these images, the thoracic region was subsequently extracted and a 3D moving image was generated. Examplary views of the generated 3D moving images are shown in Fig. 5. From this, the thoracic volume was then calculated and a volume-time curve was determined. The presented system achieved a sensitivity of 81% and a specificity of 90%, which the authors considered promising for the early detection of airflow limitations.

3.3 Pose estimation in the operating room

The detection and pose estimation of one or more persons in images and videos is a classical computer vision task. In the medical field, these tasks are for example suitable in the area of operating rooms or intensive care units. In these cases the tracking of people enables, amongst other things, a documentation of the clinical workflow [3] or a safe interaction of humans and robots in the operating room [10]. Operating rooms pose additional challenges for conventional computer vision systems. These highly special-

ized areas are characterized not only by visually complex scenes but also by adverse lighting conditions for recognition systems. There is usually a large number of clinical staff in the scene, working simultaneously on or near the operating table, partially obscuring it or being obscured by medical equipment. Further difficulties arise due to similar surfaces, wide surgical clothing and limited possibilities for camera positioning [11].

A growing number of current approaches are using Deep Learning methods to determine human poses in operating rooms [11], [3]. A first multi-view approach for person detection and pose estimation in a real clinical scenario without prior knowledge about the number of people present was developed by [11]. Body skeletons of the detected persons or body parts were extracted from multiple two-dimensional (2D) images acquired using a multiview system consisting of multiple RGB-D cameras. Fig. 6 shows the corresponding RGB-D images of their multiview dataset. By back-projecting the poses into three-dimensional space and merging different views paired with subsequent optimization, the body part positions of medical staff in the operating room were determined. The accuracy of the system was improved by including multiple viewpoints. The average body part localization accuracy of a system with three viewpoints was 15 ± 10 cm. A related but slightly different approach was proposed by [3]. The project also dealt with pose determination in 3D scenes of the operating room based on a network of several depth cameras. Input were the 2D depth images on which the joint posi-

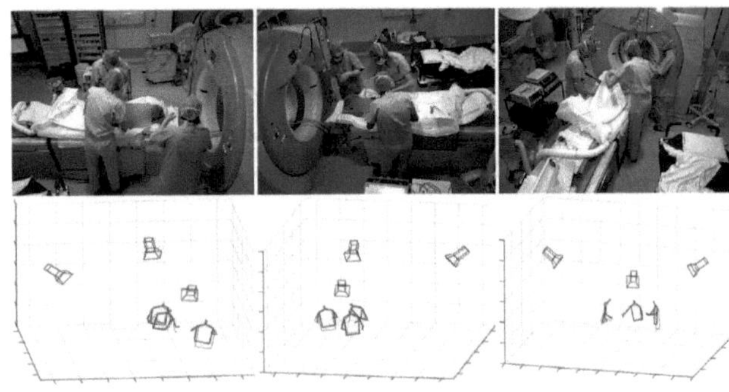

Figure 7: RGB images and views of the ground truth (green) and detected (red) 3D poses of the medical staff [3].

tions were determined. After fusing the recorded 2D scenes into a 3D point cloud, the final position of the joints was determined from the initially rough approximation using a pre-trained convolutional autoencoder. The results of the pose determination are shown in Fig. 7. The evaluation of accuracy was performed on an existing dataset and, as in [11], could be increased with an increasing number of viewpoints to a mean joint position localization accuracy of 7.1 ± 7.2 cm.

4 Conclusion

This paper provides a brief overview of selected applications of ToF camera data in the clinical practice. The strength of ToF camera systems lie in a fast recording of RGB-D data of the entire scene while ensuring an adequate accuracy. Nevertheless this accuracy is still lower than other vision sensors such as in laser devices or color cameras. In the medical field, the real-time acquisition of depth data as well as the inexpensive hardware of ToF cameras favor their use especially in diagnostic monitoring of patients. In radiotherapy, ToF camera-based monitoring systems are able to provide a cost-effective and sufficiently accurate alternative to conventional laser-based positioning systems. Further applications in the area of breath monitoring can not only record breathing patterns in real time by means of depth measurements but also the realization of a non-invasive measurement of the respiratory gas volume could be demonstrated. In addition to patient monitoring, recent deep learning-based approaches can be used to track the movements of medical staff in the operating room and thus evaluate and improve the workflow of clinical procedures. Future development opportunities in the field of clinical applications of ToF cameras could be systems that provide direct feedback for correction in addition to monitoring, i.e., motion detection especially in the radiology department.

Acknowledgement

The work has been carried out at the Institute of Neuro- and Bioinformatics, Universität zu Lübeck.

Author's Statement

Conflict of interest: The athor states no conflict of interest.

5   References

[1] Y. He and S. Chen, "Recent advances in 3d data acquisition and processing by time-of-flight camera," *IEEE Access*, vol. 7, pp. 12495–12510, 2019.

[2] D. Lefloch *et al.*, "Technical foundation and calibration methods for time-of-flight cameras," in *Time-of-Flight and Depth Imaging. Sensors, Algorithms, and Applications*, pp. 3–24, Springer, 2013.

[3] L. Hansen, M. Siebert, J. Diesel, and M. P. Heinrich, "Fusing information from multiple 2d depth cameras for 3d human pose estimation in the operating room," *International Journal of Computer Assisted Radiology and Surgery*, vol. 14, no. 11, pp. 1871–1879, 2019.

[4] S. Placht, J. Stancanello, C. Schaller, M. Balda, and E. Angelopoulou, "Fast time-of-flight camera based surface registration for radiotherapy patient positioning," *Medical Physics*, vol. 39, no. 1, pp. 4–17, 2012.

[5] F. C. Wiegandt *et al.*, "Detection of breathing movements of preterm neonates by recording their abdominal movements with a time-of-flight camera," *Pharmaceutics*, vol. 13, no. 5, p. 721, 2021.

[6] A. Kolb, E. Barth, R. Koch, and R. Larsen, "Time-of-flight cameras in computer graphics," in *Computer Graphics Forum*, vol. 29, pp. 141–159, Wiley Online Library, 2010.

[7] M. Gilles *et al.*, "Patient positioning in radiotherapy based on surface imaging using time of flight cameras," *Medical Physics*, vol. 43, no. 8Part1, pp. 4833–4841, 2016.

[8] C. Sharp *et al.*, "Toward respiratory assessment using depth measurements from a time-of-flight sensor," *Frontiers in Physiology*, vol. 8, p. 65, 2017.

[9] H. Takamoto *et al.*, "Development and clinical application of a novel non-contact early airflow limitation screening system using an infrared time-of-flight depth image sensor," *Frontiers in Physiology*, vol. 11, p. 552942, 2020.

[10] T. Beyl *et al.*, "Time-of-flight-assisted kinect camera-based people detection for intuitive human robot cooperation in the surgical operating room," *International Journal of Computer Assisted Radiology and Surgery*, vol. 11, pp. 1329–1345, 2016.

[11] A. Kadkhodamohammadi, A. Gangi, M. de Mathelin, and N. Padoy, "A multi-view rgb-d approach for human pose estimation in operating rooms," in *2017 IEEE Winter Conference on Applications of Computer Vision (WACV)*, pp. 363–372, IEEE, 2017.

Deep Regression as Initialization for 2D-3D Pelvis Registration

Friederike Katlun [1], Stephanie Häger [2], Annkristin Lange [2], and Jan H. Moltz [2]

[1] Medical Engineering Science, Universität zu Lübeck, friederike.katlun@student.uni-luebeck.de
[2] Fraunhofer Institute for Digital Medicine MEVIS, Lübeck/Bremen, stephanie.häger@mevis.fraunhofer.de

Abstract

The alignment of 2D intra-operative X-ray images with pre-operative 3D CT scans provides the foundation of image-guidance during orthopaedic surgeries. The 2D-3D registration typically used for this alignment is an ill-posed problem and requires proper initialization. In this paper, we propose a deep learning-based initialization approach. We compare and evaluate four different convolutional neural networks for deep regression to estimate the position of the intra-operative X-ray with respect to the CT data on a synthetic dataset. The first evaluations of the networks' performance are promising as the networks were able to predict a single rotational parameter with a deviation from the ground truth below $10°$ with an average runtime of 1 to 2 seconds. ResNet50 is the best network, it has the lowest deviation overall and the shortest runtime. The findings in this study indicate the substantial potential deep regression possesses when it comes to estimating positional parameters as a method of initialization for 2D-3D registration.

1 Introduction

Image-based guidance promotes great benefits for orthopaedic procedures, such as preoperative planning and modelling of the patients anatomical features, thus minimizing invasiveness and conserving surrounding tissues e.g. by enabling a more accurate screw placement [1]. Image registration is an important foundation of image guidance, especially, 2D-3D registration which aims to align data of different dimensionalities. Great solutions for this can be found in the literature [2]. Nonetheless, image registration is an ill-posed, non-convex problem requiring proper initialization. One possible method of initialization is the robust intensity-based initialization method (RobIn) which utilises a broad grid search [3]. In this paper, we propose a deep-learning-based approach for initializing the registration of an intra-operative 2D X-ray image from a C-arm device to a pre-operative 3D CT scan. The method we propose for the registration initialization is a deep regression using convolutional neural networks (CNNs). For the regression two types of CNNs generally used for classification are chosen, ResNets and DenseNets. ResNets employ the principle of residual learning, they have "shortcut connections" skipping one or more layers while performing identiy mappings and thus allowing deeper network architectures without increasing the training error; see [4] for details. DenseNets, on the other hand, combat the decrease in performance caused by naively increasing the depth of a CNN with dense blocks. Within each block, the current layer is connected to all its previous layers or in other words: the input of each layer is generated by concatenating all of the preceding layers [5]. In this work we compare two ResNet and two DenseNet architectures on a synthetic dataset. The aim of the deep re-

gression is to provide a starting point for a subsequent fine registration, as the one in [6].

2 Material and Methods

The dataset we use contains 90 pre-operative CTs of unfractured pelvises with expert segmentation sourced from CTPEL [7]. Since there is no corresponding X-ray data to the CT scans, the X-rays have to be simulated. The first step is creating digitally reconstructed radiographs (DRRs) [8]. Each DRR is generated with a projection geometry defined by eight parameters: two distances between the detector (D) and the source point (S) and projection center (P), respectively, three rotational angles (α, β, γ) of the central ray and three translation parameters (x,y,z) for the projection center. Visualization of the projection geometry is provided in Fig. 1. Assuming the X-Rays capture the whole pelvis, the three translational parameters are sufficiently estimated by the center of the 3D segmentation bounding box. As for the distances, it is assumed they can be read out from the X-ray device [3]. Therefore, we will focus on the initialization of the three rotational angles.

Before any training can take place the DRRs have to be created specifically for every angle that is to be estimated by the neural networks. For this the ground truth parameters are set as follows. Starting with the distances, the one from source to detector is set to 1200 mm, while the gap between detector and pelvis center is 450 mm. Additionally, each DRR is characterized by a set of rotational parameters $\eta = (\alpha, \beta, \gamma)$. According to literature [9] the rotational parameters are $\eta = (-125°, 0°, 180°)$ for the inlet images, $\eta = (-90°, 0°, 180°)$ for the AP images and

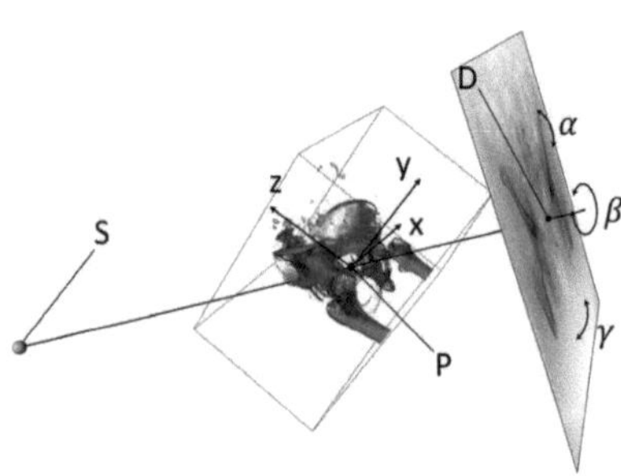

Figure 1: A square detector (D) parameterizes the DRRs in a plane, orthogonal to the central ray from the source (S) to the detector passing the bounding box center of the pelvis segmentation (P). P is defined by the translational parameters (x, y, z). The ray is defined by the Eulerian angles $\eta = (\alpha, \beta, \gamma)$ adhering to the coordinate system of the CT data centered at P.

$\eta = (-55°, 0°, 180°)$ for the outlet images. Fig. 2 provides an example for each view of the pelvis defined above. Our first target variable is the angle α. To start, DRRs of the 90 CT scans are generated. While generating the DRRs the angle α is consistently varied from $-130°$ to $-50°$ in $5°$ steps, keeping β and γ fixed at $0°$ and $180°$, respectively. Thus generating 17 DRRs ranging from inlet to outlet perspective for each patient, which provides a total set of 1,530 DRRs with known rotational parameters, we will call this dataset A in the following.

The second target variable is the angle γ. For the generation of DRRs in this case, α is set to $-90°$ and β again to $0°$. Now, for each pelvis the angle γ is varied from $90°$ to $270°$ in $5°$ steps. For each patient 37 DRRs are created for a total of 3,330 simulated X-ray images. We will call this dataset C in the following. Since we generated the DRRs knowing all defining parameters, the DRRs can be used as ground truth. To further simulate the appearance of X-ray images, all of the DRRs are cropped to a disc shape, typical for C-arm devices. Subsequently, the datasets A and C are split into a training, testing and validation set each, with the following ratios: 0.7, 0.1, 0.2. For the split, all DRRs of one patient are put together in one of the sets. The data split is kept exactly the same for all networks, so that every network is trained, validated and tested on the same patients to ensure comparability.

The specific architectures used in this paper are ResNet50, ResNet101, DenseNet169 and DenseNet201, the numbers at the end indicate the number of layers a network has. The decision to use these four architectures for the deep regression is based on preliminary experiments. Moreover, the preceding experiments confirmed the assumption that pre-trained networks would perform better, with lower training and validation loss, on the given data. The increase in performance when using pre-trained CNNs for the problem at hand can partly be attributed to the limited amount of data at disposal. As a conclusion, the regression task is performed with versions of ResNet50, ResNet101, DenseNet169 and DenseNet201, all pre-trained on ImageNet. However, to allow the usage of classification networks for a regression, the softmax layer at the end is replaced by a fully connected layer with linear activations. This so-called regression layer is always trained from scratch, even when pre-trained networks are employed [10].

3 Results and Discussion

In the following we conduct a feasibility study by training and testing four different CNNs for the regression of a single rotational parameter. Afterwards the results of the networks are evaluated and compared with each other to determine which one performs best on the given data.

3.1 Prediction of rotational parameter α

For the prediction of the rotational parameter α the four networks are trained on dataset A. To ensure comparability between the networks, the training parameters are kept as similar as possible for each architecture. Adam is chosen as the optimizer, the learning rate is set to 0.0001 and each network is trained for approximately five epochs, meaning the entire training set is passed five times through the network. Furthermore, the mean squared error (MSE) is used as loss function. Additional training parameters are listed in Table 1. The training batch size has to be reduced with increasing depth of the networks to avoid the GPU running out of memory during training.

Table 1: Overview of the CNNs' parameters while training to predict angle α including training batch size (TBS), validation batch size (VBS), the trainings duration (Time) and the best validation loss during training (Loss).

Architecture	TBS	VBS	Time	Loss
ResNet50	16	16	5 min	0.002
ResNet101	8	16	3 min	0.001
DenseNet169	8	16	6 min	0.001
DenseNet201	4	16	8 min	0.001

As shown in Table 1 both ResNets and DenseNets perform similarly during the training and validation process. Each training is completed in under 10 min, the ResNets are slightly faster because their computational costs are lower. In terms of best validation loss the networks have an MSE of 0.001, with exception of the ResNet50 having a loss of 0.002. To determine the accuracy of the trained CNNs, the best network - the network with the weights derived during the best validation iteration - is used on the testing data and the mean absolute error (MAE) between the ground truth of α and the predicted value is computed to evaluate each network's performance. The MAE was chosen as quality measure to show the difference between the prediction and the ground truth in degrees. For each choice of α from $-130°$ to $-50°$ in steps of $5°$, the MAE was calculated over all patients. Table 2 lists smallest, largest and averaged MAE for

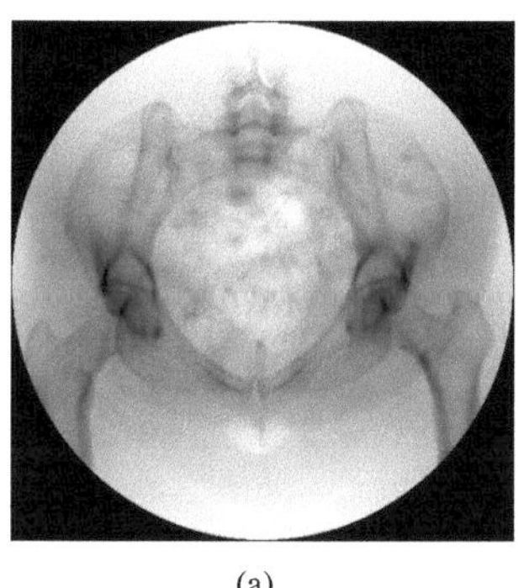
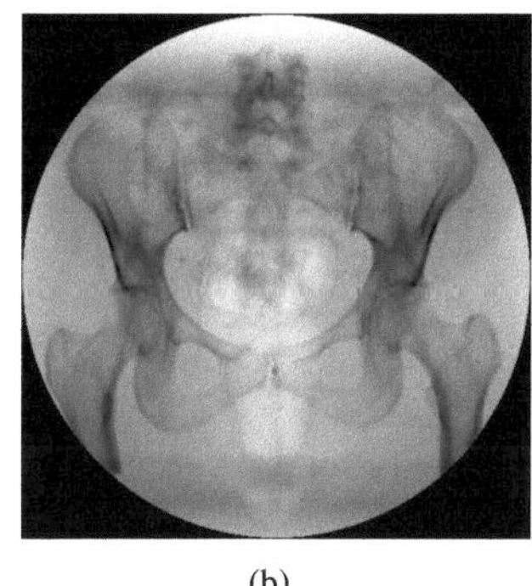
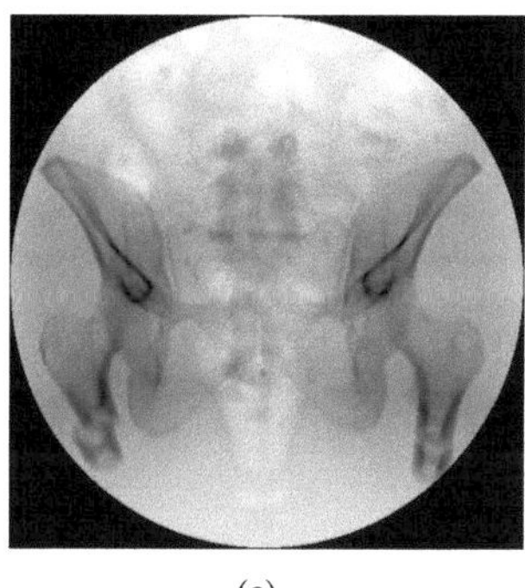

(a) (b) (c)

Figure 2: The figure shows three DRRs of the same pelvis after they are cropped to the typical disk shape of a C-arm X-ray. (a) is the inlet view, looking at the pelvis from above, (b) depicts the AP view, which is a frontal view of the pelvis and (c) shows he pelvis from the bottom, the outlet view.

each CNN, each averaged over all angles. It demonstrates

Table 2: Overview of the MAEs in ° for angle α.

Architecture	mean MAE	min. MAE	max. MAE
ResNet50	3.759	0.281	10.372
ResNet101	4.062	0.369	11.007
DenseNet169	4.234	0.342	12.147
DenseNet201	3.658	0.237	9.762

that the similar quality of the networks' performance during training translates into the testing.

With a deviation of around 4° for all four architectures a deep regression using each of the architectures above is a sufficient initialization for a subsequent registration. Only considering the preliminary results for predicting α the pre-trained DenseNet201 is the CNN with the best performance, having the lowest minimal, maximal and mean MAE of all the networks with ResNet50 as its runner-up. However, considering the time it takes to predict the angle for an unseen DRR, all four CNNs can predict α in a matter of two seconds, but ResNet50 is the fastest among them, taking one second, while the DenseNets take nearly two. The time the prediction needs increases with the networks depth.

3.2 Prediction of rotational parameter γ

In the next experiment, rotational parameter γ is the regression's target variable. The training and testing of the four CNNs is done on dataset C with the same training parameters as before. Table 3 depicts further parameters of the

Table 3: Overview of the CNNs' parameters while training to predict angle γ including training batch size (TBS), validation batch size (VBS), training duration (Time) and the best validation loss during training (Loss).

Architecture	TBS	VBS	Time	Loss
ResNet50	16	16	9 min	0.001
ResNet101	8	16	10 min	0.001
DenseNet169	8	16	12 min	0.001
DenseNet201	4	16	13 min	0.002

training for γ. It shows that the training of each architecture took slightly longer than before. This can be attributed to the increased amount of DRRs. The relationship of the networks' training duration amongst each other is similar to those of α, and increases with the networks' depth. The losses of the best validation iteration are also in the same scale as the ones above, with the exception that now DenseNet201 has the worst loss with 0.002 instead of ResNet50. This translates to the test results in Table 4. They

Table 4: Overview of the MAEs in ° for angle γ.

Architecture	mean MAE	min. MAE	max. MAE
ResNet50	7.145	0.426	20.877
ResNet101	7.152	0.418	22.204
DenseNet169	8.627	0.938	26.735
DenseNet201	9.041	0.513	25.038

show that Densenet201, previously the architecture with the highest accuracy, is now the one with the highest mean MAE and therefore has the worst performance. Again, all architectures perform similarly, the maximal difference of the mean MAEs is just under 2°. Still, focusing on the maximum MAE it becomes evident that the ResNets achieve a higher accuracy with their regression than the DenseNets. The ResNet50 beats the ResNet101 in terms of mean and maximal MAE by a small margin. The results in Table 4 have been calculated in the same manner as for α. See section 3.1 for details. The time each architecture needs to predict the angle γ for an unseen DRR is the same as before.

3.3 Discussion

Comparing the results of the two experiments, the MAE is higher for γ with a deviation of 7° to 9° compared to α with a deviation of 3° to 4°. In conclusion, the networks have more difficulties predicting γ than α. Taking the results of both angles into account, ResNet50 is a solid choice for the regression of the rotational parameters. It is faster than the DenseNets and achieves the best results for γ and the second best for α, despite having the worst validation loss for α, out of all tested architectures. ResNet50 is not only faster during training, it is also faster when predicting the angles for unseen DRRs.

In future work, we are going to perform the regression for the last rotational parameter β as well as testing the robustness of the networks in regards to noise, occlusions and real X-ray images. Additionally, the training and testing still has to be done for a multi-label regression, which allows to predict all the rotational parameters at the same time. Although the quality of regression achieved so far is sufficient there are some options to further enhance the performance of CNNs for this specific task. One option is to unfreeze the weights of the last convolutional blocks of each network, meaning: not only training the regression layer from scratch but also the weights of the last convolutional blocks. Another possibility lies in the usage of different loss functions. While the MSE achieves good results in our case, it may prove beneficial to test out other losses such as the MAE or L_2 loss. For details and examples on unfreezing convolutional blocks and usage of different losses see [10].

4 Conclusion

In this paper we propose a deep regression approach for parameter initialization for 2D-3D pelvis registration. First experiments show a mean deviation of only $4°$ to $7°$ in a single rotation parameter prediction. The regression seemingly performs worse than RobIn, which successfully estimates the rotational parameters with deviation below $3°$. However, the major advantage of the regression is its speed. Predicting the rotational angle of one rotational parameter for an image takes approximately one to two seconds, while RobIn needs several minutes for all three parameters. Nevertheless, it has to be taken into account that none of the networks have been tested for robustness. As of now, it is unclear how well the CNNs will perform, when they have to predict multiple angles at the same time or how fast they will be. In future work, we are going to test the robustness of the regression and extend the proposed method by a multi-label regression for all three angles. In conclusion,the preliminary findings show that deep regression is a promising approach for parameter initialization for 2D-3D pelvis registration.

Acknowledgement

The work has been carried out at Fraunhofer Institute for Digital Medicine MEVIS, Lübeck and supervised by Prof. Dr. Mattias Heinrich, Institute of Medical Informatics, Universität zu Lübeck. This work was funded by the German Federal Ministry for Economic Affairs and Climate Action (project KI-SIGS, funding code: 01MK20012Q).

Author's Statement

Conflict of interest: Authors state no conflict of interest.

5 References

[1] J. Kubicek, F. Tomanec, M. Cerny, D. Vilimek, M. Kalova, and D. Oczka, "Recent trends, technical concepts and components of computer-assisted orthopedic surgery systems: a comprehensive review," *Sensors*, vol. 19, no. 23, p. 5199, 2019.

[2] P. Markelj, D. Tomaževič, B. Likar, and F. Pernuš, "A review of 3d/2d registration methods for image-guided interventions," *Medical image analysis*, vol. 16, no. 3, pp. 642–661, 2012.

[3] S. Häger, A. Lange, S. Heldmann, J. Modersitzki, A. Petersik, M. Schröder, H. Gottschling, T. Lieth, E. Zähringer, and J. H. Moltz, "Robust intensity-based initialization for 2d-3d pelvis registration (robin)," in *Bildverarbeitung für die Medizin 2022*, K. Maier-Hein, T. M. Deserno, H. Handels, A. Maier, C. Palm, and T. Tolxdorff, Eds. Wiesbaden: Springer Fachmedien Wiesbaden, 2022, pp. 69–74.

[4] K. He, X. Zhang, S. Ren, and J. Sun, "Deep residual learning for image recognition," in *Proceedings of the IEEE conference on computer vision and pattern recognition*, 2016, pp. 770–778.

[5] Y. Zhou, Z. Li, H. Zhu, C. Chen, M. Gao, K. Xu, and J. Xu, "Holistic brain tumor screening and classification based on densenet and recurrent neural network," in *International MICCAI Brainlesion Workshop*. Springer, 2018, pp. 208–217.

[6] A. Lange and S. Heldmann, "Intensity-based 2d-3d registration using normalized gradient fields," in *Bildverarbeitung für die Medizin 2020*. Springer, 2020, pp. 163–168.

[7] C. Wang, B. Connolly, P. F. de Oliveira Lopes, A. F. Frangi, and Ö. Smedby, "Pelvis segmentation using multi-pass u-net and iterative shape estimation," in *International Workshop on Computational Methods and Clinical Applications in Musculoskeletal Imaging*. Springer, 2019, pp. 49–57.

[8] D. B. Russakoff, T. Rohlfing, J. R. Adler Jr, and C. R. Maurer Jr, "Intensity-based 2d-3d spine image registration incorporating a single fiducial marker1," *Academic radiology*, vol. 12, no. 1, pp. 37–50, 2005.

[9] A. Murphy. (2016) Reference articels: Pelvis (AP view) + Pelvis (inlet view) + Pelvis (outlet view)(accessed on 09.01.2023). [Online]. Available: https://radiopaedia.org/articles/44863;https://radiopaedia.org/articles/45242;https://radiopaedia.org/articles/45218

[10] S. Lathuilière, P. Mesejo, X. Alameda-Pineda, and R. Horaud, "A comprehensive analysis of deep regression," *IEEE transactions on pattern analysis and machine intelligence*, vol. 42, no. 9, pp. 2065–2081, 2019.

Investigation of Different Contrast Agents for Magnetic Resonance Imaging with Respect to their Relaxivity at Low Magnetic Field Strengths

Philipp Severin[1], Felix Kreis[2], Norbert Linz[3]

[1]Medical Engineering Science, Universitat zu Lubeck, philipp.severin@student.uni-luebeck.de
[2]Bayer AG Berlin, Head of Laboratory, High Field MR Imaging, felix.kreis@bayer.com
[3]Institute of Biomedical Optics, Universitat zu Lubeck, norbert.linz@uni-luebeck.de

Abstract

The aim of this study is to identify contrast agents (CA) which can generate a particularly high nuclear magnetic resonance (NMR) signal amplification at a low field strength and therefore produce a high Magnetic Resonance Imaging (MRI) signal at low field strengths. The motivation for this work, is the recent shift of interest into low-field MRI as a diagnostic and scientific tool [1]. Low-field MRI system scanner would lead to a reduction in cost and a higher accessibility for patients than scanners with a higher field strength. For this purpose, we have studied the behavior of 12 different CAs at low magnetic field-strengths. We used a special low field relaxometer which enabled us to measure at magnetic field-strength ranging from 0.23 mT to 0.47 T. We could demonstrate, that there is a large range in relaxivity between the investigated CAs at a low magnetic field strength and enough potential to justify further studies.

1 Introduction

For decades, CAs have been used with great success to increase the contrast of MR images, because they improve the capabilities of medical diagnostics. In approximately 30 % of all procedures that use MRI, CAs are used [2]. The imaging capabilities, enhanced by the use of CAs, are especially useful in the diagnostic of cardiovascular diseases, such as aortic aneurysms and cardiomyopathy [3], as well as a multitude of other diseases. The characteristic magnetic behavior of CAs depends on their pharmacokinetic and magnetic properties. There are also a multitude of surrounding parameters that influence the magnetic behavior of contrast agents including the field strength of the applied magnetic field or the surrounding temperature [4]. This necessitates that, during the relaxivity measurements, the CA samples are heated to 37°C to mimic in vivo conditions and obtain realistic results. During a scan, a patient or sample is placed in the magnetic field of the scanner. The strong field causes the magnetic dipoles inside the sample to align with the direction of the static magnetic field until they reach an equilibrium and form a net magnetization that depends on the strength of the field. The magnetic dipoles are then excited with a short, high frequency, on resonance pulse and align themselves perpendicular to the base magnetic field, which results in a net magnetization of the sample perpendicular to the base magnetic field. When perturbed in this way, relaxation drives the net magnetization back to the equilibrium state described by the Boltzmann distribution of energy states. This mechanism is called spin-lattice or T_1 relaxation and is facilitated by local field variations mainly caused by tumbling and rotation due to thermal motion of nearby magnetic dipoles. If the oscillation of a local field is in the range of the Larmor frequency, it will affect the reorientation of the magnetic moment under investigation and thereby, over a time span described by the T_1 relaxation time, restore the thermal equilibrium. Since CAs are magnetic dipoles, they accelerate the reorientation of the magnetic moments where they are present [5]. This shortens the T_1 relaxation time of dipoles in the vicinity of the contrast agents which increases their generated signal and leads to a better contrast in later MRI. In recent years there has been an increasing interest in MRI scanner utilizing weaker magnetic fields than the commonly used and widely available devices which operate at a static magnetic field at 1.5 T or above. There is a variety of reasons behind this. The most obvious reason is the price of a MR scanner which corresponds to roughly 1 million €/T [1]. On top of the initial procurement cost it is also expensive to operate, since skilled technical staff, high amounts of power and large dedicated spaces are necessary to operate the scanner. The magnet that is used in such a scanner also needs to be cooled down constantly with liquid helium, which in itself is expensive and a limited natural resource [1]. Low field strength MR scanners have the advantage of being smaller and potentially portable, making them practical in clinical conditions. This eliminates the requirement, of a separate room and shielding. The small size and a more open design would open access for treatment of patients that suffer from claustrophobia, since it would reduce feelings of being trapped in the otherwise tight scanner bore hole. Since a lot of diagnostic processes require the use of CAs, we need to investigate their behavior at low field strengths which is the main objective behind this study. For this purpose, we investigated a multitude of CAs, including discontinued, established, and novel CAs of Bayer AG. To determine if a CA is suitable at low magnetic field strengths it is necessary to determine the Spin-Lattice-Relaxation time (T_1) of the CA. The NMR signal is also influenced by the so-called Spin-Spin-Relaxation time (T_2). T_2 has influence on the relaxivity and subsequent on the quality of the resulting signal in MRI and must be investigated as well if we wish to use CAs for T_2 weighted images and/or estimate the effect on T_1 weighted images. This was not done in this study and should be a subject of a later study. To understand the measurements in this study it is important to understand that the term relaxivity is defined as the relaxation rate change per concentration of CA (slope of linear regression generated from a plot of the measured relaxation rates compared to the concentration of the CA in the solution) [2]. Therefore, it is necessary to first measure the relaxation times T_1 for at least two known concentrations (in this case water as our solution medium with a CA concentration of 0 mmol/L and with the CA at a nominal concentration of 1 mmol/L) of the compounds in the solution at the desired magnetic field strengths, from which we can then calculate the specific relaxivities. If this is done for several field strengths, we can create a Nuclear Magnetic Resonance Dispersion (NMRD) profile, which is essentially a plot of the specific relaxivities across the field strengths of the individual CAs.

2   Material and Methods

2.1   Compunds and dilution

A selection of 12 CAs was used in this study, all of which were diluted in distilled water which was further purified by a water purification system (Milli-Q IQ Ultrapure water purification system; Merk). The investigated CAs are listed in Table 1 together with their trade name or their internal identification number. Nine of these were based on superparamagnetic iron oxides (SPIOs) and three were based on gadolinium (Gd). Seven of the used CAs are currently commercially available, five are in different stages of development at Bayer AG. Due to the time consuming nature of the measurements, the measurements of each CA were limited to a nominal concentration of 1 mmol/L. Included in Table 1 are also the actual achieved concentrations that were used for the measurements and for the calculation of the relaxivity and their known particle size (Ps) for CAs with SPIOs. The actual concentrations of the metal in the solutions were measured with Inductively Coupled Plasma mass spectrometry (ICP-MS; Agilen Technologies 8900 triple Quad). The concertation determined by ICP-MS is differed from the nominal concentration due to pipetting and weighting inaccuracies as well as age related deviation of the labelled

Table 1: Investigated MRI CAs selected for low field relaxivity measurements and concentration

Tradename	Conc. in mmol/L	Comment
Feraheme	0.96	Fe, Ps 25nm
ZK186548	60.85	Fe
Supravist	1.32	Fe, Ps 22 nm
ZK93049	0.91	Fe
ZK183595	0.97	Fe
Resovist	1.03	Fe, Ps 70 nm
Endorem	0.98	Fe, Ps 75 nm
TOBY2831	1.15	Fe
TOBY2824-3-1	0.92	Fe
Primovist	60.87	Gd
Gadovist	1.01	Gd
Gadoquatrane	0.82	Gd

and actual concentration of the CA stock.

2.2   Measurements and relaxivity calculation

Measurements were performed using a SMARtracer fast field cycling NMR relaxometer (STELAR, MEDE (PV), Italy) for the proton Larmor frequency range from 0.01 MHz to 10 MHz in 40 steps, equally spaced on a logarithmic scale. The frequency range equals a magnetic field strength range from 0.23 mT to 0.23 T. To detect the signals, two different relaxometer pulse sequence programs for the measurements are used. At low magnetic fields, where the detection of the signal is very difficult, the SMARtracer uses a pre-polarized (PP) sequence. In this sequence the sample is first polarized in a higher magnetic field (10 MHz), the field is then switched to the desired measurement strength (0.01 MHz) so the sample can relax for a time τ in this field. The field is then switched the frequency at which the signal will be acquired (7.2 MHz) and the NMR signal is then recorded after a 90° pulse. Is the desired field strength high enough, a so called non-polarized (NP) sequence is used. The sequence follows the principle of the PP sequence, but the sample is not first polarized at a higher field but directly at the desired field strength for a time τ. Then again, the field is switch to the acquisition strength and the signal is recorded after a 90° pulse [6]. For each sample and field strength, the PP or NP sequence is repeated with different values of τ. Fitting an exponential recovery function to the resulting signal amplitudes corresponding to different τs allows determination of T_1. To measure the signal at 0.47 T, a high field relaxometer with a proton larmor frequency at 20 MHz (STELAR, MEDE (PV), Italy) was used. By combining the relaxometers we were able to cover a proton Larmor frequency range from 0.01 MHz to 20 MHz which is equivalent to a magnetic field range from 0.23 mT to 0.47 T. The T_1 time for of each contrast media (CM) solution was measured in 40 different equal steps from 0.23 mT to 0.23 T with the SMARtracer. For this, 1 mL of each CM solution was filled into a 10 mm x 220 mm flat bottom Fast Field Cycling Sample

Tube which was then placed into the probe of the SMAR-Tracer. With the build in software (Storm 2.0.18-FFC, STELAR, MEDE (PV), Italy) we determined the T_1 relaxation time at a given field strength for each probe. The polarization delay time between individual excitations was chosen at a value at least five times as long as the T_1 time of the first measurement before the automatic measurements continued. For the measurements at 0.47 T with the high field relaxometer, 300 µL of the investigated solution in a 5 mm diameter NMR tube were placed in the probe of the high field relaxometer. During the measurements, all samples were kept at a stable temperature of 37°C with the built-in variable temperature unit. This was also important since the temperature has a strong effect on the T_1 time of a protons [4]. After measuring the T_1 times at all frequencies, we calculated the corresponding relaxivities (r_1). For this we used the equations

$$\frac{1}{T_1} = \frac{1}{T_{1(0)}} + r_1 * [CM] \tag{1}$$

and

$$r_1 = \frac{(R_1 - R_{1(0)})}{[CM]} \tag{2}$$

In (1) T_1 is the measured longitudinal relaxation time of the compound with its given concentration $[CM]$. $T_{1(0)}$ in comparison is the longitudinal relaxation time of the solution (distilled water) without the CAs, which was also measured with the relaxometers. In (2) we convert the formula to calculate r_1. R is the relaxation rate which is equivalent to $1/T$. R_1 denotes the T_1 relaxation rate of the solution with the CA agent included and $R_{1(0)}$ the relaxation rate for the solution (water) without contrast agent [2].

3   Results and Discussion

The measurements revealed a significant range of relaxivities for the investigated contrast agents (CAs). CAs with superparamagnetic iron oxides (SPIOs) have significantly higher relaxivities in comparison to CAs which are based on gadolinium. The measured r_1 relaxivities of CAs based on SPIOs are shown in Fig. 1. CAs which are already established and in use show significantly higher relaxivities than substances that are not commercially available. Especially noteworthy is the significantly increase in relaxivity of Resovist at low-field strengths. The high-field values, shown in Fig. 1 were complemented from measurements performed by Rohrer and Matrin [2] for Primovist and Supravist (SHU555C). The high relaxivity in low-field strength correlate with an increase in particle size, for SPIOs.

Like the established SPIOs, CAs based Gd also show an increase in relaxivity at low-field conditions. Results for Gd based CAs are shown in Fig. 3. Despite the increase in relaxivity the overall ranking of the examined Gd-based CAs does not change compared to the relaxivity ranking in high-field environments, were Gadoquatrane does perform best followed by Primovist and GadoVist respectively. If

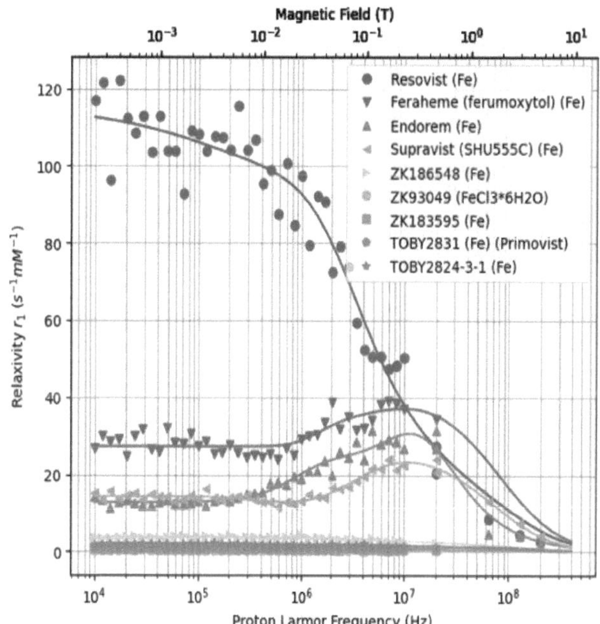

Figure 1: Result for r_1 relaxivity for CA with superparamagnetic iron oxides (SPIO). With corresponding field strenghts. Complemented with additional values for the high-field measurements from Rohrer and Martin [2] with fitted curve reference by Roch and Alain [7].

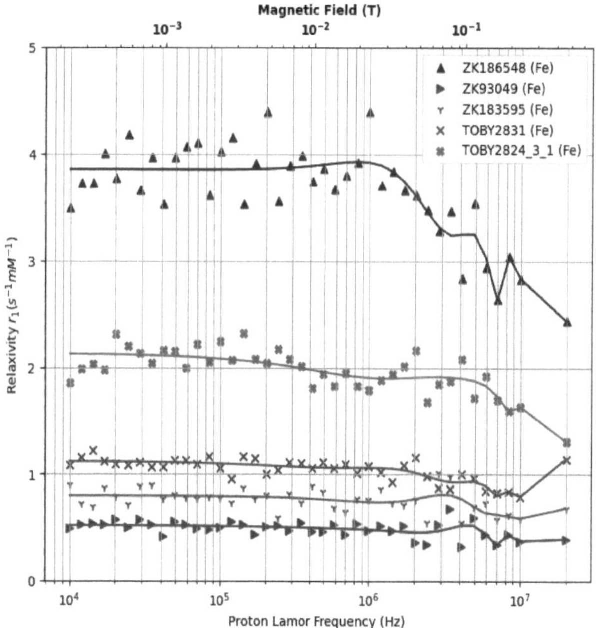

Figure 2: Result for r_1 relaxivity for CA with (SPIO) that are not commercially available. With corresponding field strenghts. With polynomial fit of the trendline.

we take a look at the plots in Fig. 3, we notice that the maximum of relaxivity is achieved at a low magnetic field strength for Gd based CAs. As shown in Fig. 1, some CA based on SPIOs (Feraheme, Endorem and Supravist) on the other hand displayed a local maximum at mid field strength.

The non commercially available CAs are shown separately in Fig. 2. We can see that the depicted CAs have a very low relaxivity and therefor offer almost no advantage for imaging compared to the established CAs with (SPIO).For comparison the relaxivity of pure water, in which we solved the CAs has a relaxivity ranging from 0.2 to 0.3 at 37°C. We were able to verify our methods by comparing the re-

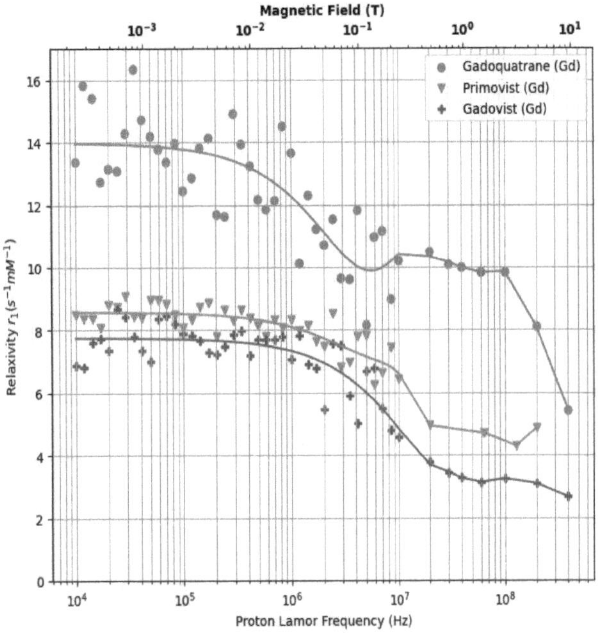

Figure 3: Result for r_1 relaxivity for Gadolinium based CAs. With corresponding field strengths. Complemented with additional values for high-field measurements from Rohrer and Martin [2] and Prof. Helm, Lausanne. With polynomial fit of the trendline.

sults from some of our measurements with the study of Rohrer [2], and measurements that were performed by Prof. Helm who conducted a study concerning the relaxivity of GadoVist and Gadoquatrane in the mid- to high-field magnetic field strength. The results of this study were supplemented and added in Fig. 3 for visualization of trend in high-field strenghts above 20 MHz.

4   Conclusion

In this study we investigated 12 contrast agents (CA) with different compounds, 9 with SPIOs and 3 with gadolinium to determine their respective relaxivity in water. We showed a strong relationship between the relaxivity of the investigated CAs and the magnetic field strength, low- and high-field. CAs that contain SPIOs have a significantly higher relaxivity, which correlates with their particle size, compared to the CAs based on Gd. The contrasts that could be achieved in MRI with CAs containing SPIOs at low field strengths is hard to predict, since the overall tissue relaxivity increases with decreasing magnetic field strength and the influences of T_2* effects are not fully known. There is more research needed of contrast medium in low field MRI

to make more accurate predictions on the effect of CAs. Especially the behavior of the examined CAs in human plasma and whole blood at low-field strengths should be subject to subsequent research.

Acknowledgement

This project has been carried out at Bayer AG Berlin, Radiology, Pharmaceuticals Lab High Field MR-Imaging and was supervised by Dr. Norbert Linz at the Institute of Biomedical Optics, Universität zu Lübeck. Thanks to Dr. Felix Kreis (Bayer AG, Berlin) for supervising this study and Prof. Helm (EPFL-SBISIC) for additional relaxation measurements.

Author's Statement

The author has no conflict of interest do declare. The submission is original work and is not under review at any other publication.

5   References

[1] M. Sarracanie and N. Salameh, *Low-Field MRI: How low can we go? A fresh view on an old debate.* Frontiers in Physics, vol. 8 no. 172, June 2020.

[2] M. Rohrer, H. Bauer, J. Mintorovitch, M. Requardt and H. Weinmann, *Comparison of magnetic properties of MRI contrast media solutions at different magnetic field strenghts.* In: Investigativ Radiology, vol. 40, no. 11, pp. 715-724, November 2005.

[3] J. van Zandwijk, F. Simonis, F.M. Heslinga, E. Hofmeijer, R. Geelkerken and B. ten Haken, *Comparing the signal enhancement of a gadolinium based and an iron-oxide based contrast agent in low-field MRI.* In POLS ONE, vol. 16, August 17, 2021.

[4] N. Bloembergen and L.O. Morgen, *Proton relaxation times in paramagnetic solutions. Effects of electron spin relaxation.* In: The Journal of chemical physics, vol. 34, pp. 843-850, 1961.

[5] F. Kreis *Development of magnetic resonance spectroscopic Imaging methodes to asses tumour metabolism* .University of Cambrideg, July 2019.

[6] User manual SMARtracer STELAR CE Directive 2006/42/CE, attachment I, p.tp 1.7.4 2019.

[7] A. Roch, R. N. Muller and P. Gillis, *Theory of proton relaxation induced by superparamagnetic particles.* In: The Journal of chemical physics, vol. 100, no. 11 pp. 5403-5411, 1999.

Heart rate estimation using Imaging Photoplethysmography

Sophie Wuthe [1], Mahdi Momeni [2], Michaela Bitten Mølmer [3,4], Emilie Löbner Svendsen [3,4], Mikkel Brabrand [4,5,6] Peter Biesenbach [7] and Daniel Teichmann [2]

[1] Biomedical Engineering, Luebeck University of Applied Sciences, sophie.wuthe@stud.th-luebeck.de

[2] SDU Health Informatics and Technology, The Maersk Mc-Kinney Moller Institute, University of Southern Denmark, Odense, Denmark, {mome,date}@mmmi.sdu.dk

[3] Faculty of Health Sciences, University of Southern Denmark, Odense, Denmark, {mimoe17,esven17}@student.sdu.dk

[4] Department of Emergency Medicine, Odense University Hospital, Odense, Denmark, mikkel.brabrand@rsyd.dk

[5] Department of Clinical Research, University of Southern Denmark, Odense, Denmark

[6] Accident and Emergency Medicine Academic Unit, Chinese University of Hong Kong, Hong Kong, China

[7] Department of Emergency Medicine, Hospital of South West Jutland, Esbjerg, Denmark, peter.biesenbach@rsyd.dk

Abstract

Imaging Photoplethysmography (IPPG) is a non-invasive method for heart rate (HR) estimation. The technique uses videos as an input and calculates the HR with several video processing steps. In the study, 18 subjects (average age 24 ± 2 years) were recorded while the participants laid in a bed and cold or warm fluid was infused into a vein. The recorded face was divided into five regions of interest: the forehead, both cheeks, the nose and the chin. For this paper, three video parts (beginning, middle, end) of four recordings were analysed. It was possible to detect the face, perform IPPG extraction and estimate the HR for all of them. The averaged HR values are in the range of possible HR values, from 62 to 90 beats per minute. A comparison with reference data remains part of future work to evaluate the quality of the achieved results.

1 Introduction

The measurement of human vital signs such as the heart rate (HR), body temperature, blood oxygen saturation and blood pressure, is part of many standard procedures in hospitals, medical practice and emergency care. They enable the evaluation of a person's physical state and make aware of potential medical conditions. Especially the monitoring of the HR can prevent cardiovascular adverse events via early detection of even minor abnormalities [1]. The electrocardiogram and photoplethysmography are standard tools for the measurement and monitoring of the HR but both techniques need to be in direct skin contact for accurate measurements. The implementation of Imaging Photoplethysmography (IPPG) enables the detection of the HR in a remote and contactless manner [2]. Non-contact measurement methods could improve the care of patients with sensitive skin as well as neonatal patients [3]. IPPG uses video recordings of a skin area as an input. Improvements in video processing enable the analysis of the videos where subtle skin color changes are detected in form of different pixel intensities [4]. Different methods have been developed to use the information in the Red-Green-Blue (RGB) color channels for the extraction of the IPPG signal. While the chosen method uses a combination of all three color channels, alternatively the difference of the green and red channel could have been used [2]. This study aims to create and test a workflow for the feasibility of HR estimation via IPPG video analysis of five facial regions of interest (ROIs).

2 Material and Methods

2.1 Study Description

For the generation of data, a study was carried out at Odense University Hospital. Besides the goal to gain new medical insights, the recording of video data was part of the study as well. This data was then used for analysis. The study consisted of two trial days. 18 healthy volunteers (15 female and 3 male), with an average age of 24 ± 2 years, were randomized to receive 30 ml/kg of Ringer's lactate either cold ($15°C$, $59°F$), or at body temperature ($37°C$, $98.6°F$) over a 30-minute interval. Core temperature, vital signs, blood tests, skin perfusion and subjects' discomfort were recorded over a 2-hour period with hospital equipment. After a minimum "washout period" of 24 hours, subjects were switched to receive infusion at the other aforementioned temperatures. The primary medical outcome of the study was to evaluate the increase in mean arterial pressure at 15 minutes after the fluid bolus. The secondary outcome was the time needed to return to baseline mean arterial pressure after infusion. While the subjects were in a supine position on the hospital bed, the video camera was recording videos of their face. In this paper, the results of three test subjects (two female and one male) in four sessions are evaluated. Cut-outs of about four minutes in the beginning, the middle and the end of the recording were analysed. Two sessions were performed with the infusion of cold fluid and two with warm fluid.

2.2   Experimental Setup

The RGB color videos were recorded with the FLIR Systems, GS3-U3-23S6C-C camera with an implemented Sony IMX174 CMOS sensor. The software for controlling and adjusting the parameters as well as the video recording can be downloaded from the FLIR website and is called Fly-Capture SDK. The camera was positioned at a distance of about 1.50 m from the subjects face and was then connected via USB 3.1 to a notebook computer (hp, 64-bit operating system, Windows 10 Enterprise). To ensure a stable frame rate, the computer was connected to the power supply of the hospital. In the FlyCapture software the following settings were adjusted: The automatic White Balance was turned off as well as the automatic adjustment of Sharpness and Saturation. The Exposure was manually set to 1.415 EV. Shutter and Gain were adjusted automatically. The frame rate was set to 35 frames per second (fps). The shutter in front of the window was closed and the indoor light was on. An additional light (LED daylight lamp) was positioned about 1.50 m above the subjects bed for additional illumination. For easier video processing the size of a video file was limited to 1500 MB. With the above mentioned frame rate, this resulted in a video length of 6 s.

2.3   Video and Signal Processing

For the video processing, the HR extraction and analysis of the signal, the MATLAB R2021a software was used. The total number of frames was determined by the program to create matrices corresponding to the lengths of the video samples that should be analysed. The individual RGB color videos were loaded into the program for the analysis. The first step was the recognition of the face and the detection of the ROIs. For this step the MATLAB toolbox „MTCNN Face Detection" [5] was used. This toolbox uses a deep-learning based face detection. The localization of facial landmarks (eyes, nose, left and right corner of the mouth) works with a model called „multi-task cascaded convolutional neural networks (MTCNNs)" [6]. Using the facial landmarks, the ROIs were manually determined. Therefore, the pixels above the right eye (left eye in the video) were determined as the forehead, the pixels next to the nose were used as the two cheeks and the nose itself and the pixels below the right corner of the mouth determined the chin. The information of the ROIs was saved in form of a box with the x- and y-coordinates of the upper left corner, the width and the height of the box. In Fig. 1 the ROIs are shown exemplary on a person's face.

Video frames, where the face could not be seen from the front were not used for analysis because the ROIs were not positioned in the subjects face anymore. For the evaluation, the distance between the subjects eyes was determined in the first video frame as a reference. For all following

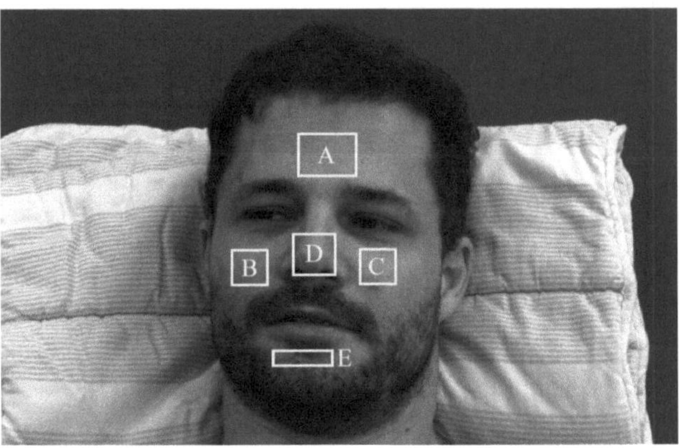

Figure 1: The considered ROIs (A-E) positioned on the face of a person.

frames this distance was calculated as well. If the face had shifted so much that the distance between the eyes was less than 70 % of the reference, the frame was discarded. For the evaluation of valid data from the video, a variable counted the discarded frames with 0 and usable frames with 1. The average value within each ROI was calculated for every frame. A new MATLAB file was generated that saved the following values: information of the boxes for the ROIs, reference distance between the eyes, distances between the eyes for each frame, overall number of discarded frames, frame number of each discarded frame, the valid data and the average pixel values for the ROIs in each color channel. Before the actual IPPG extraction, the valid data as well as the skipped frames were examined. It was determined that interpolation was only allowed for a maximum number of 15 skipped frames in a row. Due to a frame rate of 35 fps at the recordings and assuming that there was about one heart beat per second, it seemed appropriate to interpolate this number of frames with the previous valid value. The IPPG extraction was not performed if more than 15 frames were skipped in a row and if the number of valid frames between invalid frame sections was less than 381. The latter was due to the toolbox which only enabled an IPPG extraction for more than 381 samples in a row. For the estimation of the IPPG signal and the HR, the MATLAB toolbox „Imaging-photoplethysmogram-extraction-pulse-rate-estimation" [2][7][8] was used. The matrix of RGB average values was the input for the toolbox algorithm. The extraction of the IPPG signal included different IPPG pre- and postprocessing techniques [8]. The POS method was used which computes the IPPG signal using all three color channels [2]. For the HR estimation with the wavelet transform, the MATLAB toolbox used the IPPG signal as an input to search for values within the expected HR frequencies of humans (min. 0.5-0.7 Hz and max. 4.0 Hz). The HR was computed momentary for every step in time and as an averaged estimation in beats per minute (bpm). For this estimation a moving average filter was used. The number of samples averaged was half of the window used for the Fast Fourier Transform for the IPPG extraction [2][7][8] (here 1024 due to a sampling rate of 35 fps). As well as the IPPG extraction, the HR extraction was done for each ROI separately.

3 Results and Discussion

Using the toolbox for the IPPG extraction, it was possible to determine IPPG signals for all 12 cut-outs. Sometimes, depending on the distribution of the skipped frames in a row, the extraction was performed in different parts. Because of interpolation and the requirements for the IPPG extraction with the toolbox, the valid data after the IPPG extraction differed from the valid data after the face detection. The valid data after the face detection ranged from 90 % to 99 % (mean 96 ± 3 %). After the IPPG extraction the valid data was in the range of 84 % to 100 % (mean 95 ± 5 %). All percentages of valid data were high enough to take them into account for the analysis. As an example Fig. 2 shows the valid data after face detection (upper plot) and after IPPG extraction (lower plot). The valid data was set to one and the discarded data set to zero. In this case the percentage of valid data after face detection was about 90 % and after IPPG about 86 %.

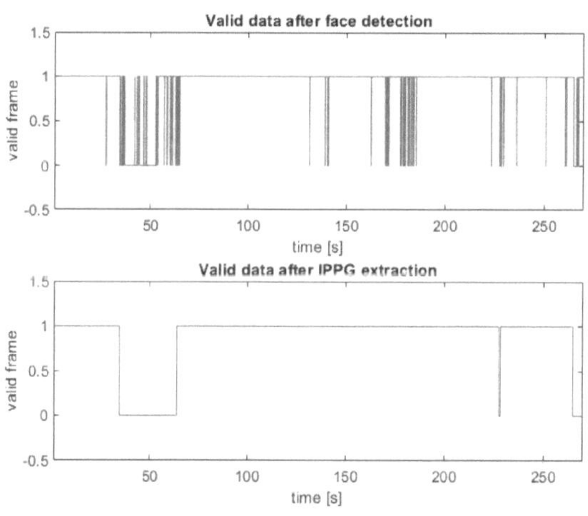

Figure 2: Valid data after face detection and valid data after IPPG extraction.

The extraction of the IPPG signal generated graphs like it is shown exemplary in Fig. 3. This signal could then be used for HR estimation. Table 1 shows the HR values for each ROI separately. Here it was noticeable that the determined HR values differed for the ROIs. As the light was not distributed equally over the subject's face, it is likely that this influenced the pixel intensities, which then had an impact on the HR estimation. For the momentary values, it could be noticed that the forehead region had a lower value than the other regions. However, comparing the estimated average values, all values for the ROIs were close together. The accuracy of the values was not always sufficient enough with a standard deviation of more than 10 %. For medical purposes, the precision in HR detection needs to have a standard deviation < 10 % [9].

For the determination of the average HR for each subject,

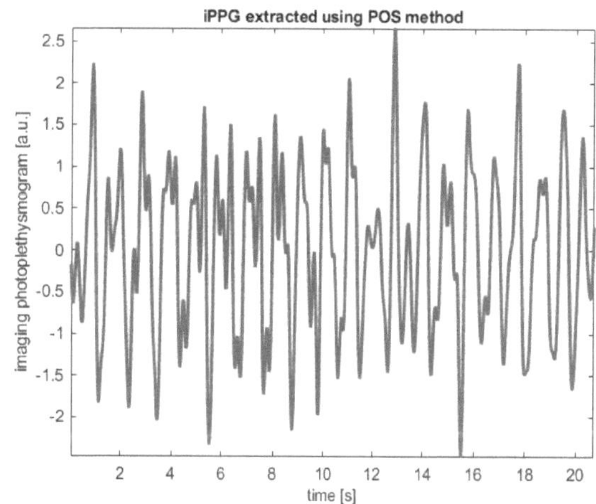

Figure 3: Extracted IPPG signal for the forehead region after using the POS method.

Table 1: Average values of the HR for each ROI

ROI	Momentary values	Estimated average
forehead (A)	78 ± 8 bpm	70 ± 7 bpm
left cheek (B)	83 ± 6 bpm	68 ± 5 bpm
right cheek (C)	86 ± 10 bpm	73 ± 9 bpm
nose (D)	85 ± 11 bpm	73 ± 7 bpm
chin (E)	87 ± 7 bpm	70 ± 7 bpm

it was averaged over all ROIs, as there is only one HR in a human, independent on the place where it was measured. Table 2 shows the results. It was noticeable that the estimated average values (62 - 81 bpm) were always significantly lower than the momentary values (72 - 90 bpm). This could be explained with the fact that the estimated average values were already averaged by the toolbox over a window of 512 samples (about 15 s). Therefore, outliers did not have such a big influence here. Hence, the estimated average values in Table 2 were good indicators for the change of the HR over time. Even though, the momentary values showed a slight trend in this regard as well, the values are expected to be more inaccurate.

Table 2: Average values of the HR for each subject

Subject_Cut-out	Momentary values	Estimated average
subject 1_01 cold	80 bpm	62 bpm
subject 1_02 cold	79 bpm	64 bpm
subject 1_03 cold	76 bpm	62 bpm
subject 2_01 warm	86 bpm	81 bpm
subject 2_02 warm	75 bpm	71 bpm
subject 2_03 warm	72 bpm	63 bpm
subject 3_01 cold	87 bpm	68 bpm
subject 3_02 cold	90 bpm	70 bpm
subject 3_03 cold	90 bpm	77 bpm
subject 3_01 warm	84 bpm	76 bpm
subject 3_02 warm	85 bpm	75 bpm
subject 3_03 warm	85 bpm	72 bpm

For the evaluation of the quality of the HR values by the IPPG method, it is necessary to compare the values with the reference data that was recorded with hospital equipment during the study. Unfortunately, these values were not available yet. Analysing the correlation between the fluid's temperature and the HR values estimated by using IPPG extraction, it could be said that no connection could be found in general, as the HR values for a certain temperature were not always higher or lower. Also for subject 3, who got cold and warm fluid inserted, it could not be said that the HR values for the insertion of cold fluid were significantly higher than the ones for the insertion of warm fluid. Furthermore, there was no evidence that the HR is going down or up during a session. Some sessions started with higher HR values then went down over time and some sessions resulted in higher HR values towards the end of the session. As the number of analysed subjects in this pilot study was not sufficient for general statements, the analysis of all subjects and considerable longer time periods (one hour or more) is necessary to determine, if the accuracy of the used method is insufficient in general and whether the other above mentioned issues are certainly true.

4   Conclusion

Overall the analysis of the few sessions showed that the face detection algorithm works accurately. The percentage of valid data for this step was high enough to enable an IPPG extraction for most of the samples. The estimated HR with the toolbox was in a suitable range. However, for a proper conclusion, it will be necessary to analyse the whole length of all video recordings. The generated data from the hospital can be used as reference data for a comparison and to determine how precisely the HR estimation with the MATLAB toolbox works. An analysis for every ROI separately can be useful to discover ideal light conditions. As there is data for every test subject with cold and warm fluid, these two recordings can be compared for just one subject but also for all subjects, as there might be significant differences in the HR depending on the temperature of the infused fluid. Furthermore, the MATLAB toolbox for the IPPG extraction offers other extraction methods than the POS method. It might be interesting to also use another method e.g. only the green channel for the IPPG extraction, to compare the results and find the best extraction method. Furthermore, it might be possible to give information about the blood perfusion within the ROIs. Here, a connection between the temperature of the infused fluid might be noticeable as well. Nevertheless, more research needs to be done and further improvement of video processing is necessary to implement IPPG as an accurate method for HR extraction in clinical use.

Acknowledgement

The work has been carried out at SDU Health Informatics and Technology, University of Southern Denmark and supervised by M. Ahlborg, The Fraunhofer Research Institution for Individualized and Cell-Based Medical Engineering, Luebeck, Germany.

Author's Statement

Authors state no conflict of interest. Informed consent has been given to all participants of this study.

5   References

[1] C. H. Cheng, K. L. Wong, J. W. Chin, T. T. Chan and R.H.Y. So, *Deep Learning Methods for Remote Heart Rate Measurement: A Review and Future Research Agenda.* In: Sensors 2021, 21, 6296. https://doi.org/10.3390/s21186296

[2] A. M. Unakafov et al. *Using imaging photoplethysmography for heart rate estimation in non-human primates.* In: PLoS ONE 13(8): e0202581, 2018. https://doi.org/10.1371/journal.pone.020258

[3] Jakob Emil Olsen *Camera Based Remote Photoplethysmography.* University of Southern Denmark – The Faculty of Engineering, report individual study activity, p. 1, 2021.

[4] Z. Marcinkevics et al. *Imaging photoplethysmography for clinical assessment of cutaneous microcirculation at two different depths.* In: J. Biomed. Opt. 21(3), 035005 (2016), doi: 10.1117/1. JBO.21.3.035005.

[5] Justin Pinkney *MTCNN Face Detection.* Available: https://github.com/matlab-deep-learning/mtcnn-face detection/releases/tag/v1.2.4 [last accessed on 2022-12-14]. GitHub, 2022.

[6] K. Zhang, Z. Zhang, Z. Li and Y. Qiao *Joint Face Detection and Alignment Using Multitask Cascaded Convolutional Networks.* In: IEEE Signal Processing Letters, vol. 23, no. 10, pp. 1499-1503, 2016, doi: 10.1109/LSP.2016.2603342

[7] A. M. Unakafov *Imaging photoplethysmogram extraction & pulse rate estimation.* Available: https://www.mathworks.com/matlabcentral/fileexchang e/67527 [last accessed on 2022-12-12]. MATLAB Central File Exchange, 2018.

[8] A. M. Unakafov *Pulse rate estimation using imaging photoplethysmography: generic framework and comparison of methods on a publicly available dataset.* In: Biomedical Physics & Engineering Express. 2018;4(4):045001. https://doi.org/10.1088%2F2057-1976%2Faabd09

[9] D. Hoevenaars et al. *Accuracy of Heart Rate Measurement by the Fitbit Charge 2 During Wheelchair Activities in People With Spinal Cord Injury: Instrument Validation Study.* In: JMIR Rehabil Assist Technol 2022;9(1):e27637, doi: 10.2196/27637

On-Screen Stitching Planner for X-Ray imaging
– Proof of Concept –

Tim Zarnekow [1] and Mathias Schlüter [2]
[1] Medical Engineering Science, Universität zu Lübeck, tim.zarnekow@student.uni-luebeck.de
[2] Philips Medical Systems - DMC, mathias.schlueter@philips.com

Abstract

Stitching acquisitions for X-ray images are uncomfortable to set up and provide the user with limited control over the partial images that are being acquired. In this paper we present a stitching planner that uses 3D Depth information to increase the ease of use for stitching acquisitions and allow for more flexibility in the settings of the individual partial images. The stitching planner is implemented on top of a tool designed for setting the collimation on a touchscreen for regular X-ray examinations. As of writing it supports the automatic calculation of all required information for a stitching procedure given a frame selected on the User Interface (UI), as well as selecting and displaying partial collimation regions. The implemented tool can already reduce discomfort during acquisition and with further work provide the user with more information and options then currently available in standard X-ray devices.

1   Introduction

X-ray images are limited in size by the detector used in the acquisition. For full length images of legs or spine multiple images need to be acquired and stitched together [1]. Setting up such an image is similar to a regular X-ray. Currently this requires the tube to be placed at the height level used during the examination and manually adjusting the collimation, using light to show the area that will be radiated. This means the user has to work at uncomfortable height level and with no information on the position of the partial images that are acquired. Furthermore, the body range to be examined is limited by the collimator opening. The use of 3D cameras to support radiographers is a recent development in the field of radiography systems [2].

This project is part of a proof of concept for a stitching planner. The stitching planner aims to make the acquisition process easier and more powerful by giving the user direct control of the partial image acquisition. There are 2 typical ways of creating the images required for stitching images. The first way is a single focus stitching. Here the tube remains at a single height and is only tilted to change the radiated area. The advantage of this procedure is, that there will be no parallax error. A disadvantage is an X-ray magnification of the anatomy and oblique X-ray paths, especially for large tube tilts. To minimize such errors, the tube is commonly positioned at a distance to keep tilting angles at a minimum.

The second method is parallel stitching, in which the images are taken parallel to the detector surface. Here detector and tube are moved in tandem. Advantage of this method is the ability to set the center beam in important spots like leg joints. Furthermore, the method can also be used in rooms with restricted space. A disadvantage of this method is an unavoidable parallax error, due to the shifting position of the tube. In this project the focus was on single focus stitching, but with easy adaptability for parallel stitching in mind, for future expansion.

2   Material and Methods

2.1   Data Acquisition

In order to test the implementation of the stitching planner UI, multiple video-sequences with 3D depth data were used. The sequences were acquired in house on a Philips Digital Diagnost C90 (DIDI C90). The sequences resembled typical acquisition set-up situations. These included single image acquisition, long length image acquisition, as well as sequences resembling a possible new workflow with the use of the stitching planner.

For the RGB image and depth data an Intel RealSense DepthCamera D435 is being used. The camera is mounted with a lateral displacement with regards to the X-ray source. The camera uses a standard RGB sensor for the color image and stereoscopic depth technology using an infra-red Projector for the depth data [3].

2.2   Projective Geometry

Projective geometry is a subsection of geometry which concerns itself with the geometric properties that are invariant with respect to projective transformations. For this project an important part is the change of perspective. The only data we have comes from a depth camera and we want to display the projected field centred in the collimation tube. In order to accurately display the selected field we have to shift the perspective from which we view the 3-Dimensional Information [4].

3 Implementation

The implementation of the stitching planner was built on top of an already existing tool for viewing the 3D Sequences recorded by the camera, as well as a system for on-screen collimation. The tool could be used to display points onto the image, that framed the area that will be radiated. With the depth information the points could be accurately displayed onto the 3D surface that was targeted. Integrated into the hardware the selected field could be sent to the machine and automatically change the collimator to the selected field size.

The system was limited in that it could only change the frame around the center point. Thus one would still have to change the height of the tube manually.

The main idea of the of 3D projection is a normalized point cloud in a distance of 1 m, that is calibrated for an accurate frame of the collimation. The point cloud consists of 3D Points whose x and y values span a frame of with a specified longitudinal and lateral length and the z value set to 1 m. The field size can be changed by adapting the total longitudinal or lateral length. There was also an offset from the center beam given, but in the existing implementation this value was always set to zero. The point cloud was then calculated onto the 3D surface given by the depth data through projective geometry. Important to keep in mind is that the depth data comes from the camera position, while the normalized field is determined in the tube position. Fig. 1 provides a visual representation of this idea.

3.1 Stitching Frame

The first step for the stitching planner was to make it possible for the stitching planner to move the upper or lower side separate from one another. The lateral sides remain movable in tandem, since for the stitching procedures the images are generally taken from top to bottom position. To make the frame edges move independently, it is detected at which side the frame is being selected and add the distance from the edge to the new indication position to the total vertical length. Further the center is moved by half the distance in the same direction. This way the side not being moved remains in its current position.

With the capability to select the frame freely in the vertical direction, the next step was to find the position for the stitching sequence. It is generally desired for single focus stitching to have symmetric tilting angles for the sequence. To find the desired height we find the projected point on the frame, that is closest to the tube in z-direction. We chose the closest point as it ensures, that a change of the tube height does not change the visual anatomy selected. Knowing the depth of that point as well as the total length of the longitudinal side of the frame and its offset from the center at the

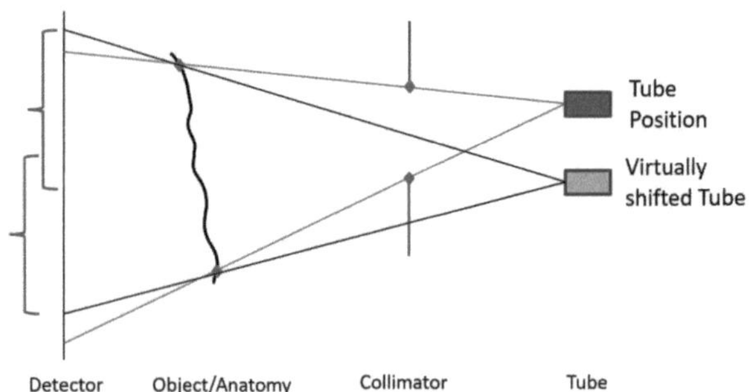

Figure 1: Illustration of the shift in tube position required for symmetric single focus stitching. The collimator lines represent the currently selected collimation in the current tube position at the normalized distance.

normalized distance we can use the intersecting line theorem and the current tube height to calculate the height of the point from the floor. Doing that for the upper and lower frame, as well as knowing the depth at which these points lie, we can now use the properties of similar triangles to determine the height needed for the tube to allow for symmetric acquisition.

In a similar fashion we implemented a function to lock in a selected field to allow the user to change the position of the tube whilst keeping the field on top of the targeted anatomy. The illustration in Fig. 1 shows that with a changed position of the tube we can keep the desired anatomy in the displayed frame. It is important to remember that on a three-dimensional object the radiated volume does change slightly with the changed position. Based on the change of the tube height, the vertical field length and offset are adapted to keep the frame on the same position in the object coordinates.

3.2 Partial Images

After implementation of the stitching frame we needed to calculate all necessary values for each partial image. This includes the detector position, tube position, tube tilt and collimation. To start we determine how many images are needed for the selected field. Since we are limited in size by the detector, we determine how much vertical space in the detector plane is needed, using the intersecting line theorem. We also need to account for an overlap between each image for the stitching algorithm to accurately combine the singular images. The standard overlap is at 45 mm, but we provide the user with a slider, that allows the user to change the value if wanted.

Given the overlap and detector space needed we can determine the minimum number of images required. With that number one can now calculate the maximum collimation at the detector plane. We can then determine the position of each collimation in the detector plane and calculate the tube tilt needed to orient the tube towards the position. Since the collimation in the detector plane remains at the same size, we must adapt the collimation at the system to make sure only the targeted area is radiated to reduce radiation for the

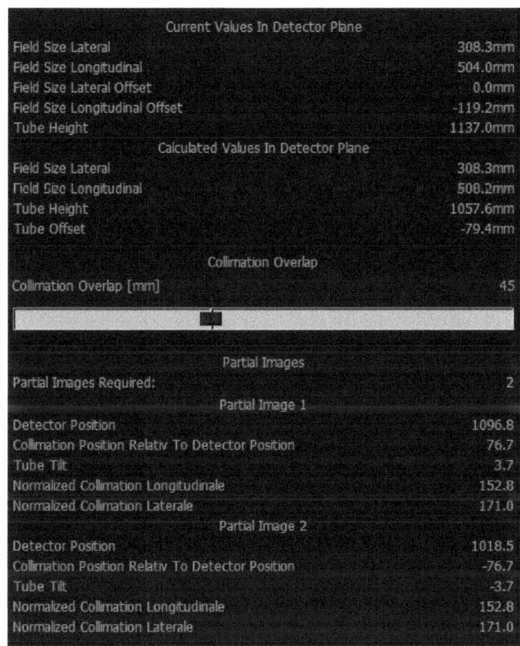

Figure 2: The collimation overlap slider at the standard 45 mm setting. Above and below the information that could be sent to the system to execute the stitching algorithm are displayed.

patient. For the detector positioning we determine it in a way, were the movement required for the detector is minimized. With this, all values required for the stitching algorithm are available. In Fig. 2 is displayed how these values are represented in the analysing tool used for this proof of concept. The values at the top refer to the overall stitching frame, whereas at the bottom the values needed for each individual image are shown.

3.3 Ray tracing

To display the virtual collimations we create multiple point-clouds for each individual collimation. We then use projective geometry to virtually place the X-ray tube at the position determined for the imaging process. Using the vector coordinates of the points from the virtual tube we can virtually project the rays outwards from the tube center, onto the surface given by the depth data [5].

3.4 Selection

For the display of the partial collimation overlay we chose to only display the points of the upper and lower edge to avoid cluttering the image with too many overlay points. With the edges displayed it can clearly be seen where the overlap of the images is. Since the stitching frame and the partial collimations are projected from different tube positions, the points of the upper and lower edge of the stitching frame can be slightly offset from their corresponding partial collimation edges. This is due to the perspective change and is expected. On the selected anatomy these offsets are fairly small, but increase when projected onto the background.

This difference can also be seen in Fig. 1 on the detector plane between shifted and current tube position.

To select an image, we also display a cross hair in the center of the image. The center is projected as the center beam onto of the object. This way it can also be used to quickly determine where the center beam is hitting the targeted area. The plus sign is based on the collimator coordinate system and equals 35 mm. Similarly, the indication point gets transformed into the collimator coordinates. This makes the selection robust against unintended behavior. When the selector is pressed all the points get shown on the screen over the stitching frame in red. The edges of the other partial images are removed only showing the selected partial collimation and the stitching frame.

3.5 Automatic Exposure Control

Automatic Exposure Control (AEC) chambers are designed to automatically terminate the X-ray device after a certain amount of radiation was received. They are important, as they provide consistent image exposure, even with changing anatomy. In order to work as intended they need to be covered by the anatomy that is being imaged and as such not all AEC chambers are required for every examination. When an image is selected, the chambers will be displayed and can be toggled on and off. This allows for easy control of AEC chamber selection and avoiding loss in image quality by errors due to wrongful selection of the chambers [6].

4 Results and Discussion

4.1 The Product

As a result of our work we have a stitching planner that allows the user to define an area for long length imaging. The system will automatically calculate the settings required for the stitching algorithm. The system will give the user the ability to see the individual sections that will be taken and adapt the stitching frame if vital parts are in the overlap regions. The user can also change the overlap. This can for example be useful on patients that have trouble to remain still to reduce the total number of images and thus the time required for acquisition. Further the user can select the AEC chambers for the singular images in order to make sure only the correct chambers are activated for the procedure, thus ensuring highly reliable image quality. In Fig. 3 the touchscreen interface is being shown with the central AEC chambers visible. Also seen are the collimation overlaps as well as the crosshairs used to select and show a singular collimation overlay.

4.2 Discussion

The product shows great promise, to be able to increase the comfort for radiographers when doing long length imaging. This is done by allowing the user to choose the desired anatomy at a height, which is comfortable for them. Being

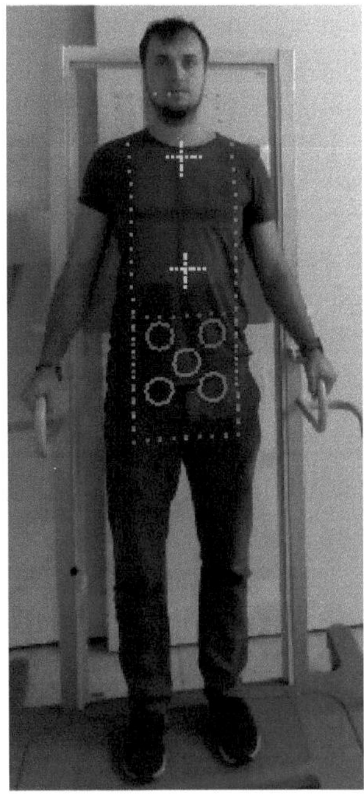

Figure 3: Image displaying the touchscreen-UI. The lowest image is selected, showing the selectable AEC Chambers. The other 2 center-beams are displayed as selectable crosshairs.

able to quickly adjust the AEC chambers for individual images can also be great for the workflow. Furthermore, the planner also allows for range selection outside of the examination room, as well the ability to make sure the patient has not changed position since positioning him in front of the detector. With this the reliability of imaging could also be improved. The ability to change the overlap can be used when right on the verge of needing one less image. By reducing the overlap slightly, the number of required images can be decreased, thus lowering the total time of acquisition.

As a proof of concept there are still a few limitations currently. With the focus being on single focus stitching, the functionality for parallel focus stitching has not yet been implemented. Further there have been singular points in the depth information, that were displayed much closer than supposed. This issue was very rare and did not occur on the more recent sequences, but it made us not choose the closest point, but instead one at the tenth percentile to avoid wrongful calculation of the partial collimations. Also, as of writing there is no hardware implementation. This means we could not test the setting of the field on the integrated touchscreen of the DiDi C90.

5   Conclusion

The stitching planner can improve the clinical workflow for stitching procedures. It can be used to reduce the discomforts for radiographers by allowing them to work at a height level that suits their needs. Further it can be used to control the positioning even outside the exam room and even make

changes. With the ability to see the partial collimations as well as the AEC chambers the correct positioning of patients and selection of stitching frame is easier than before. So even at the current stage of development the stitching planner shows great promise.

In time the planner can be further improved to provide radiographers with even more powerful tools to improve the image quality for their needs. For example, the ability to set points in leg joints to guarantee that the central beam of one partial radiation will be at that position ensuring the highest possible image quality where it is needed. Also, the ability to set the radiation values like X-ray tube current and voltage depending on the partial section is something that is of interest, to find out whether radiographers would like and use that amount of control. This could be used to adapt to changing physiology in different partial sections of the final image.

Acknowledgement

The work has been carried out at Philips Medical Systems - DMC and supervised by the Institute of Robotics, Universität zu Lübeck.

Author's Statement

Conflict of interest: Tim Zarnekow is an intern at Philips Medical Systems. Mathias Schlüter is an employee at Philips Medical Systems.

6   References

[1] A. Gooßen, M.Schlüter, T.Pralow and R. R. Grigat, *A Stitching Algorithm for automatic Registration of digital Radiographs.* In: International Conference Image Analysis and Recognition. Springer, Berlin, Heidelberg, pp. 854-862, 2008.

[2] K. Stephens, *FDA Clears Siemens Healthineers' YSIO X. pree Radiography System.* AXIS Imaging News, 2020.

[3] L. Keselman, J. Woodfill, A. Grunnet-Jepsen and A. Bhowmik, *Intel realsense stereoscopic depth Cameras.* In: Proceedings of the IEEE conference on computer vision and pattern recognition workshops. pp. 1-10, 2017

[4] C. R. Wylie, *Introduction to projective Geometry.* Courier Corporation, 2011.

[5] A. S. Glassner, *An Introduction to Ray Tracing.* Morgan Kaufmann, 1989.

[6] M. Söderberg, and M. Gunnarsson, *Automatic Exposure Control in computed Tomography–an Evaluation of Systems from different Manufacturers.* Acta radiologica 51.6: 625-634, 2010.

Methods for specular reflection reduction in eye images

Hanna Eilers [1], and Meik Frischke [2],

[1] Medical Engineering Science, Universität zu Lübeck, hanna.eilers@student.uni-luebeck.de
[2] Drägerwerk AG & Co. KGaA, Lübeck, meik.frischke@draeger.com

Abstract

In this paper, a method for pre-processing a dataset of eye images and removing reflections has been developed to solve problems in iris and pupil detection. Two approaches were analysed: First, an attempt was made to identify the reflection by determining contours in the image and then filling them in. In the second approach, the reflection was found by histogram analysis of the intensity values in the image. The area of the reflection found was extended and filled using OpenCV methods. Both algorithms were tested by applying them to test images and then comparing the results. In terms of reducing reflections, each algorithm was successful. The second approach produced better results for its intended purpose as a pre-processing stage for future work.

1 Introduction

Eye imaging offers a wide range of potential applications. For example, there is great interest in clear images for iris recognition. The iris, like a fingerprint, is unique to each person and can therefore be used to reliably identify a person. Another area of interest is pupil detection. Pupil detection can be used to control systems using the eyes. This can be helpful for a wide range of areas. One example is enabling accessibility options for people with disabilities who, for physical reasons, cannot use a keyboard or mouse.

Depending on the application of the images and the algorithm used, reflections in the eyes can lead to incorrect results. A reflection can be caused by frontal light in the room. This can be a lamp, a camera flash or a window.

Therefore it can be useful to produce images that are as clear as possible without reflections. But it is not always possible to create clear images, for example in unconstrained scenarios without illumination control. It may also be necessary to use existing images. Therefore, the aim of this work was to automatically retouch specular reflections in different images of eyes using an algorithm. To achieve this, two approaches to the algorithm were tested. The use of an algorithm makes it possible to process several images and to generalise the task, making manual processing redundant. It is therefore possible to consider this type of processing as a pre-processing step for other algorithms that require clear image files.

2 Material and Methods

2.1 Datasets

To develop an algorithm different images from two existing datasets were used and further images were taken indepen-

dently to test the algorithm.

The first dataset consists of portrait images of 16 people (StudentData). The images were taken with the camera of a OnePlus 8 Pro smartphone in different lighting conditions. The images were then cropped around the eyes. The dataset contains an equal number of images from the left and right eyes, and the images have different reflections in the eye area, as well as low contrast between the iris and pupil.

Selected images were also used from the Multimedia University Database 2 (MMU2), a public database of eye images [1]. It was published for iris recognition research. The dataset consists of 5 left and 5 right eye images from 100 individuals each. For this work, selected images were used, which were also cropped to the eye and scaled to 256×192 pixels (px). The images were taken under bright lighting and therefore contain only images with small pupils. In addition, there is usually a reflection around the pupil.

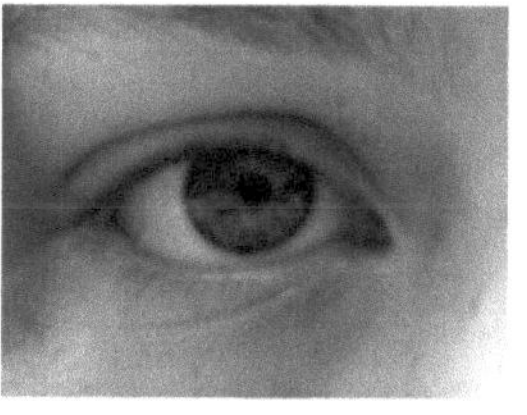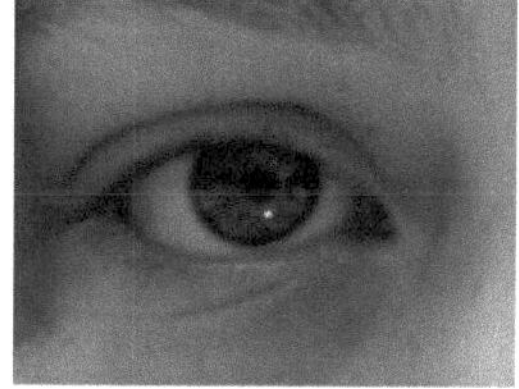

Figure 1: Images to test the algorithm; left: without reflection, right: with reflection

To test the algorithm, more photos were shot as well. The photos were taken with and without frontal light. No other changes were made to the external conditions in order to obtain images that were as identical as possible, differing only in that the images taken under the influence of light contained reflections. This resulted in a test data set of two

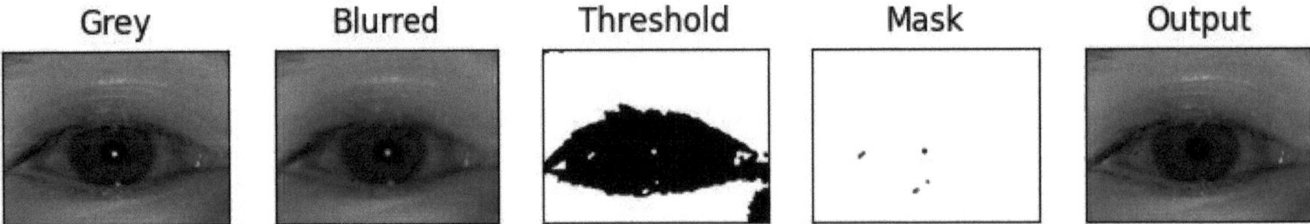

Figure 2: Intermediate results during the application of method 1; Grey: input image as greyscale image, Blurred: image after applying a Gaussian filter, Threshold: image after applying the threshold, Mask: mask after contours have been sorted out, Output: the resulting image.

eye images, one with and one without reflections. The images were cropped to the right and left eye. The resulting images are shown in Fig. 1.

After applying the algorithm developed in this work, a comparison can be made of how well the algorithm can remove the reflection and how much the images still differ before and after reflection reduction.

The other datasets, StudentData and MMU2, contain only images with reflections. However, since the comparison requires images that are as identical as possible, one with and one without reflections, the two datasets were not suitable for testing the algorithm. Furthermore, an independent dataset allows us to check whether the algorithm generalises sufficiently and works for images produced in different ways. The test data was taken with a digital camera and has a resolution of 685 × 516 px. After cropping, the images show a slightly larger section than the images from the MMU2 dataset.

2.2 Method

The aim of this work is to reduce specular reflections in the iris of eye images as well as possible. To achieve this goal, two simple approaches were tested.

The first approach is based on the work by Fuentes-Hurtado et al. [2]. The aim of the paper is to improve the segmentation of the iris using pre-processing steps. The input is a full portrait photo, not an image cropped to the eye, where facial features are first detected and the eye is extracted. This step is omitted in the current work because the input images are already cropped to the eye. Once the eye has been extracted, the Daugmans algorithm is applied to the dataset [3]. The Daugman Algorithm is an integrodifferential operator that finds the iris and pupil contours. In the mentioned paper it is used to perform a rough segmentation of the iris. This step is also omitted for this paper.

A similar procedure in the previous mentioned paper and in this work consists of applying a square Gaussian filter with a kernel size of 5x5 to the photographs after they have been converted to greyscale images to reduce noise. In addition, all images were reduced to 256×192 px to generate a uniform data set. In a second step, a threshold was applied to the images using Otsu's method, which is used to perform automatic image thresholding [4]. It separates pixel in foreground and background and is a way for binarization.

Next, the OpenCV method findContours is applied to the image. This method can be used to find continuous points of the same intensity or colour and can therefore be used for shape analysis [6]. The contours are analysed according to their size. The number of pixels of the contour must be within a certain range to be classified as a reflection. In addition, the roundness of the surface is determined as the ratio of the surface area to the circumference, as well as the position of the contour within the image. Only if the contour has a certain degree of roundness and lies within the selected area, it will be considered a reflection. If this is the case, the contour is transferred to a mask, initially with an intensity of 0.

The next step is to adjust the intensity of the contour in the mask by looking at the pixels surrounding each pixel of the contour and taking the average intensity of these pixels to determine the new intensity of the pixel in question. The exception is neighbouring pixels that are also in the contour. These are not included in the average intensity calculation. The mask is then applied to the original image. The different stages of this approach can be seen in Fig. 2.

For the second approach, the images were converted to greyscale images and an intensity histogram was constructed from the images. An example histogram is shown in Fig. 3. The bins of the histogram represents the number of pixel at a particular brightness level. A logarithmic scaling has been chosen to show the smallest changes. There is a small peak in the area of high intensities, which correlates with the expectation that specular reflections have the highest brightness in the cropped image.

To remove the reflection, the histogram is searched for all low points. The last low point is stored. As the reflection has the highest intensity in the image and can be seen as a rise in the histogram, the last low point separates the pixels belonging to the reflection and the remaining pixels from the image.

The last low point is set as the threshold and all pixels above this threshold are transferred into a mask for the image, as shown in Fig. 4 on the left. In the mask, all pixels below the threshold are initially given an intensity of 0 and all pixels above the threshold are given an intensity of 255.

When the mask is applied to the original image, the area of reflection is erased and appears as a black area in the im-

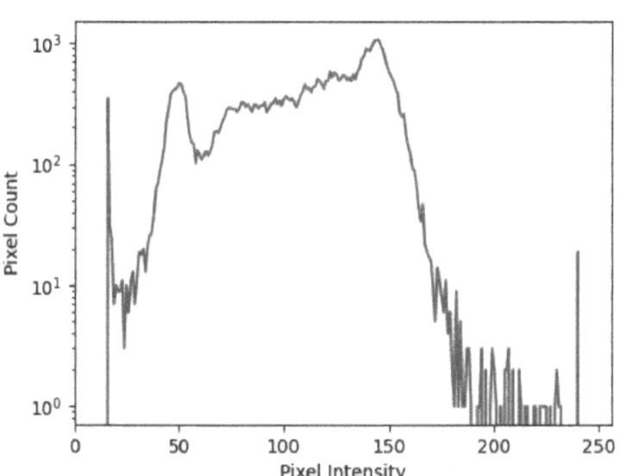

Figure 3: Intensity histogram of an example image from the MMU2 dataset

age. This can be seen in Fig. 4 on the right. Most of the reflection is blacked out. However, it is clear that not all of the reflection is detected and in particular the edge of the reflection remains visible. The edges of the reflections are therefore below the set threshold and are not retouched.

To improve this, the mask was enlarged using the OpenCV dilate method [7]. The method folds the mask with a previously defined kernel and calculates the maximal value in the kernel window area. This value is replaced at the centre kernel position in the mask. This maximisation operation causes bright areas within an image to grow, and the border areas around the mask are also added to the mask.

To fill the area in the original image in a reasonable way, the inpaint function was used [8]. This is an OpenCV method based on the Fast Marching Method by Alexandru Telea from 2004 [5]. The algorithm first fills the edge of the mask with pixels from the neighbourhood. The pixels are weighted according to their distance to the point to be filled.

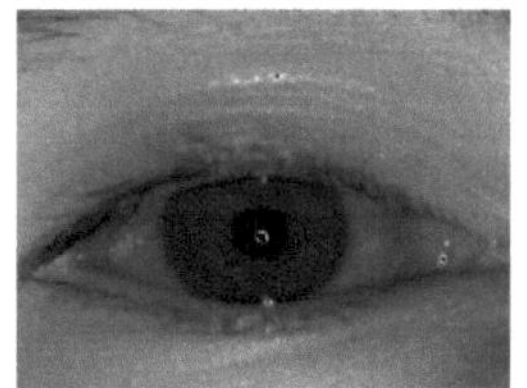

Figure 4: Intermediate results of variant 2; left: mask before using the dilate method, right: result of applying the mask without extending the mask with the dilate method

3 Results and Discussion

3.1 Result

A closer look reveals that the first method does not capture the entire reflection. A small bright ring remains. It can also be seen that several areas can be detected as reflections. This can also be seen in the resulting mask in figure 2. The reflections in the pupil area and in the lower iris are correctly detected and edited. Furthermore, it is par-

ticularly noticeable that a bright area on the sclera has also been retouched. With the second method, several areas in the image are detected and processed as reflections by the algorithm, as can be seen from the mask (see Fig. 4). The original image has several bright areas, which can all be interpreted as reflections. In addition, an area in the skin fold of the upper eyelid is also included in the mask. This is a false positive as it is intended to detect speculative reflections of the eyes.

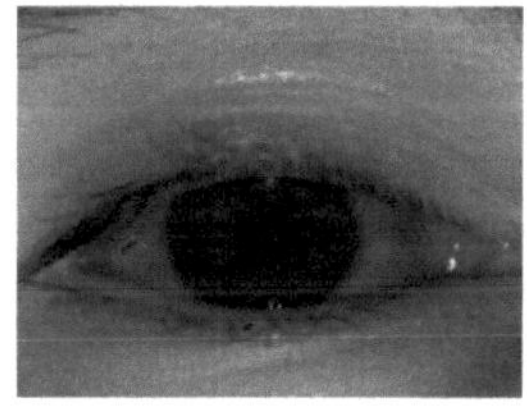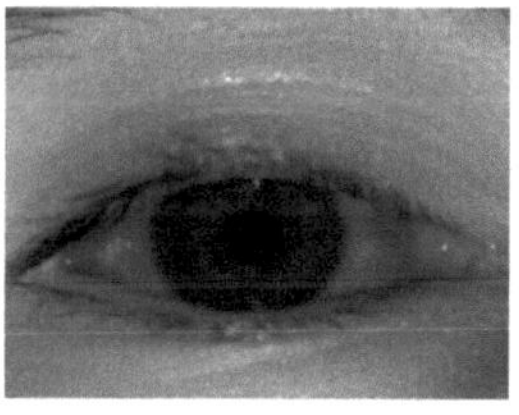

Figure 5: Results of the two approaches; left: Method 1 by determining the contours, Right: Method 2 via histogram analysis

Similar results are obtained by applying the algorithms to the test data images. Fig. 6 shows the result of method 1 on an image from the test data set. The comparison with the corresponding image without the reflection shows how well the algorithm removes the reflection. A comparison with the original images on the left is sufficient to determine where the reflection used to be. It takes a closer look to see that the area where the reflection was has a slightly too dark intensity. It is also noticeable that the area lacks texture. In addition another area at the edge of the eyelid has been detected as a reflection.

However, it is hard to notice any differences between the images.

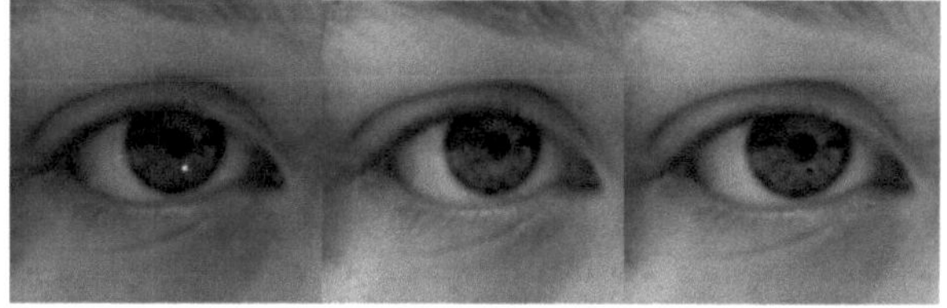

Figure 6: Left: image with reflection, Middle: Image without reflections, Right: Test data image originally with reflections, processed with the algorithm from method 1.

Better results can be seen in Fig. 7, which was obtained by applying the algorithm of method 2 to the test image. The reflection has been well retouched and there is hardly any difference to the test image without reflection. The areas that were mistakenly included in the mask and therefore processed in the image are also not visible.

It is also worth mentioning the applying of the algorithm to the StudentData. Here the image details are generally larger and a larger area of the face is visible. For example, there are images in the dataset where the subjects are wearing masks, and an area of the mask is still visible in the image

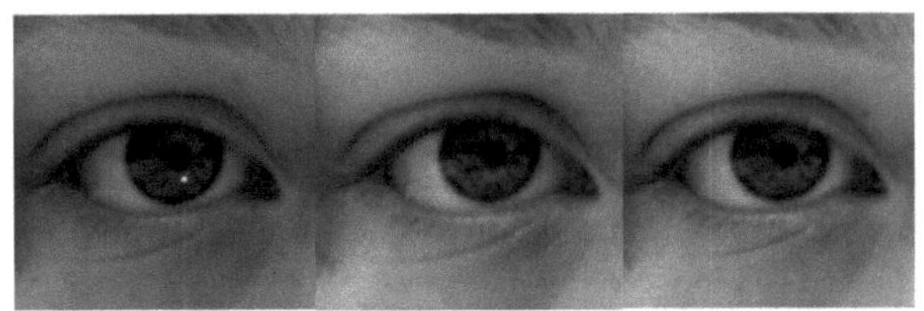

Figure 7: Left: Image with reflection, Middle: Image without reflections, Right: Test data image originally with reflections, processed with the algorithm from method 2.

detail. The masks have a high intensity and distort the determination of a correct threshold for method 2.

Problems with recognizing reflections in images also occur with method 1. Here the contours are sometimes not detected correctly and other areas are added to the reflection. This results in the contour being too large and excluded by the area and shape criteria.

3.2 Discussion

The results show that both methods are able to detect and process reflections. Method 2 gave better results in terms of retouching. It should be noted, however, that once the reflections had been detected using Method 1, the mask could have been expanded using the dilute function, and the inpaint function could have been used to fill the reflective area as well. Similarly good results can be expected for retouching. The test data showed that with this method the reflection is barely visible after processing.

In addition to the reflection, both methods incorrectly detect other areas as reflections. For method 1, further adjustments to the exclusion criteria for the contours could lead to better results. For example, it would be possible to restrict the coordinates in which the reflection is allowed to occur. However, this would further limit the application of the algorithm. The iris must not change position within the image section. The size of the reflection also limits the general application. The size of an outline that can be considered a reflection is determined by the number of pixels it covers. An image taken at a different distance may limit the application of the algorithm. However, better image quality has no effect as the number of pixels is fixed at 256x192 px at the start of the algorithm.

One problem with method 2 is that the last low point of the intensity histogram is always used to determine the threshold. Fluctuations in the intensity profile could lead to results that do not find the optimal threshold. Other criteria that adjust the choice of threshold may therefore give more stable results.

Filling in the reflective areas could also cause problems. Depending on the application for which the images are intended after processing, the changed texture of the iris due to the filling of the areas around the reflection could possibly lead to problems. Automatic filling could result in deformation of the iris and pupil, which could lead to incorrect results when determining the size of the pupil, for example.

4 Conclusion

Both methods are capable of detecting and retouching reflections. The second method, using histogram analysis, gave particularly good results. However, for use as a pre-processing stage for other algorithms, it might be advantageous to refine the threshold selection so that bright objects such as a mask or fluctuations in the histogram curve do not distort the result, making the application more stable.

Acknowledgement

The work has been carried out at Drägerwerk AG & Co. KGaA, Lübeck and supervised by Prof. Erhardt Barth, Institute of Neuro- and Bioinformatics, Universität zu Lübeck.

Author's Statement

Conflict of interest: Authors state no conflict of interest.

5 References

[1] Multimedia University, *Multimedia University iris database 2 (MMU2)*, 2006. Available: https://web.archive.org/web/20200721205358/https://andyzeng.github.io/irisrecognition

[2] F. Fuentes-Hurtado, V. Naranjo, J. A. Diego-Mas, and M. Alcañiz, *A hybrid method for accurate iris segmentation on at-a-distance visible-wavelength images*, 2019.

[3] J. Daugman, *High Confidence Recognition of Person by Rapid Video Analysis of Iris Texture*, 1995.

[4] N. Otsu, *A threshold selection method from gray level histograms*, 1979.

[5] A. Telea, *An Image Inpainting Technique Based on the Fast Marching Method*, 2004.

[6] Open Source Computer Vision, *Structural Analysis and Shape Descriptors*. Available: https://docs.opencv.org/4.7.0/d3/dc0/group__imgproc__shape.html#ga17ed9f5d79ae97bd4c7cf18403e1689a [last accessed on 2023-01-18].

[7] Open Source Computer Vision, *Image Filtering*. Available: https://docs.opencv.org/4.7.0/d4/d86/group__imgproc__filter.html#ga4ff0f3318642c4f469d0e11f242f3b6c [last accessed on 2023-01-18].

[8] Open Source Computer Vision, *Inpainting*. Available: https://docs.opencv.org/4.7.0/d7/d8b/group__photo__inpaint.html [last accessed on 2023-01-18].

Evaluation of an real-time object detector for traffic analysis

Ines Müller[1], Horst Hellbrück [2]

[1]Applied Information Technology, Technische Hochschule Lübeck, ines.mueller@stud.th-luebeck.de
[2]Technische Hochschule Lübeck, Department of Electrical Engineering and Computer Science, horst.hellbrueck@th-luebeck.de

Abstract

Smart cities are becoming more and more of a reality. An important component in the development of smart cities is automated traffic analysis. This involves the detection of traffic participants such as cars, bicycles, and pedestrians. For this purpose, the state-of-the-art real-time object detection system "You only look ones" (YOLO) is used in the evaluated application OpenDataCam. There are different network configurations that have been optimized for different targets. When using real-time object detectors, there are competing goals between accuracy and processing time. In traffic applications, where objects move quickly, the processing time is an important criterion. In this evaluation, YOLOv4 and YOLOv4-tiny were compared with the Common Objects in Context (COCO) data set in speed and accuracy. The result shows that YOLOv4 performs better than YOLOv4-tiny in object recognition, although YOLOv4-tiny performs better in terms of computational speed. YOLOv4 achieves a mean Average Precision (mAP) of 84%, and YOLOv4-tiny achieves a mAP of 49%. Nevertheless YOLOv4-tiny model is better suited for use in tracking due to its faster processing time (~18 FPS), while YOLOv4 has (~2 FPS) on Jetson Nano 4GB.

1   Introduction

In recent years, the number of transport users in cities has continued to increase [1]. This poses a challenge for smart cities in the realization of sustainability goals. Part of optimizing traffic involves analyzing and counting the number of road users. The investigated application OpenDataCam includes an AI-based real-time object recognizer to detect and track traffic participants [2]. A section of the user interface is shown in Fig. 1. The heatmap highlights the areas where the tracker's accuracy is less good. OpenData-Cam uses the neural network YOLO for object recognition. YOLO is written in Darknet [3], an open-source neural network framework written in C and Compute Unified Device Architecture (CUDA). It has been upgraded by continuous versions (YOLOv2, YOLOv3 and YOLOv4) [4]. YOLOv4-tiny was developed on the basis of YOLOv4 [5] but has a simplified network structure to reduce parameters, which makes it suitable for development on embedded devices. The more accurate the models work, the worse they are usually for use in a real-time application. In order to make object detection approaches comparable, uniform evaluation methods are needed. The most common metrics for evaluating an image classification problem are Precision, Recall, and Confusion Matrix. Since object recognition is not only about correctly classifying the object in the image but also about finding out where in the image it is located, Precision, Recall and Confusion Matrix are not sufficient. The most commonly used metric that takes this into account is mAP. In order to calculate this indicator, it is necessary to

have consistent information about the ground truth. For this purpose, the COCO dataset is used [6]. This paper is structured as follows. Section II gives an overview of the metrics used and the procedures for determining the results. Section III compares the calculated metrics in different categories of both models as well as the influence of the video quality. Section IV provides a summary of the results and an outlook for future work.

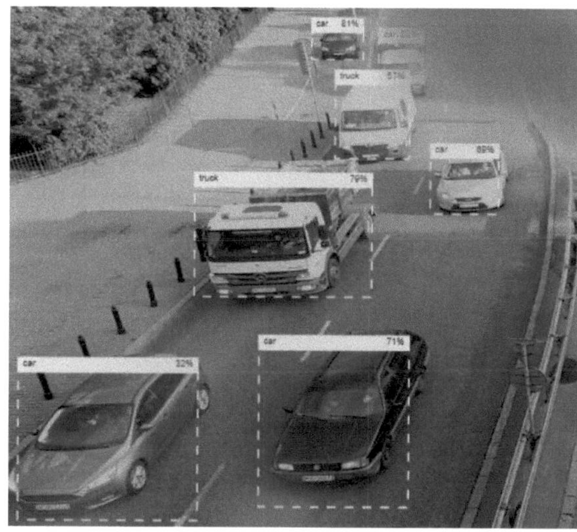

Figure 1: Exemplary object detection with the application

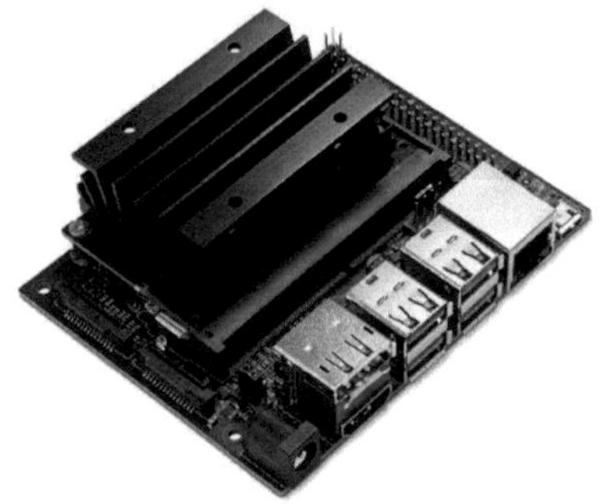

Figure 2: Jetson Nano 4GB from Nvidia [7]

2 Material and Methods

OpenDataCam runs on Linux and CUDA GPU-enabled hardware and is evaluated on Nvidia's Jetson Nano shown in Fig. 2. The Jetson Nano is a small but powerful computer for running neural networks in applications such as image classification, object recognition, and speech processing. To evaluate the application, a labeled ground truth with object class, size, and coordinates is necessary. The evaluation uses the COCO data set, which consists of everyday scene images labeled with 80 class bounding boxes (BB). The BB serves as the assumed ground truth (GT) for object classification and location. COCO also provides performance analysis metrics for object recognizers. The Intersection over Union (IoU) measures the overlap between the GT and predicted BB. An IoU value above 0.5 typically serves as the threshold for marking a recognition as true positive (TP). Fig. 3 illustrates an evaluation of an image with different IoU values. In both images, the presence of a bicycle is detected, with the predicted BB marked in blue and the GT marked in green. With an IoU of 0.5, the object in image 1 would be marked as false positive (FP), while in image 2, it would be marked as TP. Possible results of the evaluation are:

- True positive (TP): correctly predicted positive input sample as positive.

- False positive (FP): incorrectly predicted negative sample as positive.

- True negative (TN): correctly predicted negative sample as a negative.

- False negative (FN): incorrectly predicted positive sample as negative.

Fig. 4 shows the relationship of the possible outputs to each other. Precision is the ratio of correctly classified positive samples to the total number of samples classified as positive. Precision answers the question of how accurate the guesses were when the model guessed. Precision can be calculated as follows (1):

$$Precision = \frac{TP}{TP + FP} \quad (1)$$

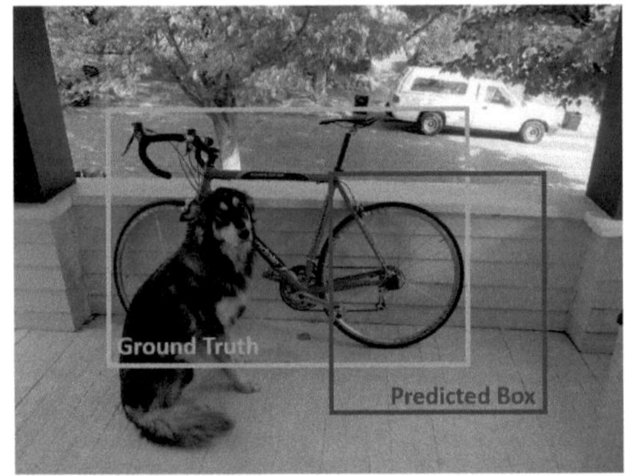

(a) FP because IoU < 0.5

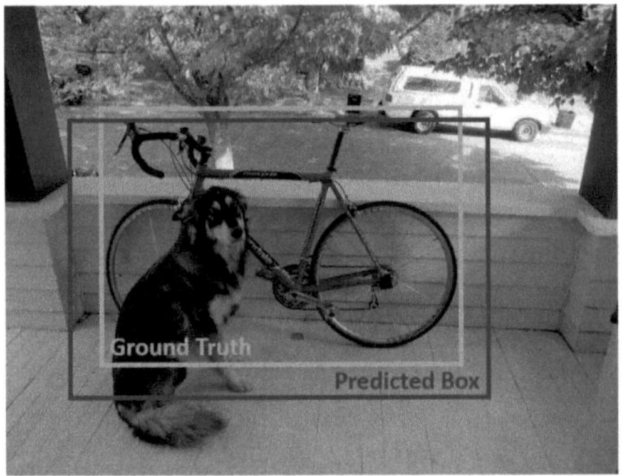

(b) TP because IoU > 0.5

Figure 3: Categorisation depending on the IoU [6]

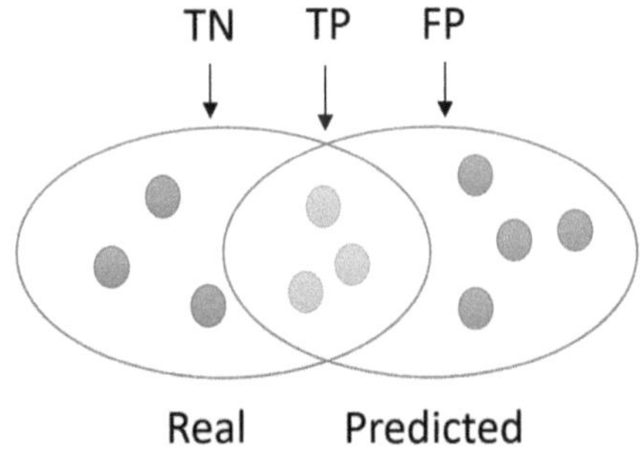

Figure 4: Shows the division into TP, TN, and FP

where TP+FP are the total predicted objects. Recall indicates whether the model guessed correctly every time it was asked to guess. The higher the hit rate, the more positive samples are recognized.

$$Recall = \frac{TP}{TP + FN} \quad (2)$$

where TP+FN are the set of truthful objects. If Precision and Recall are plotted against each other, the Precision-Recall curve is obtained. The area under this curve describes the average precision. This will be calculated for each class. To obtain the mean average precision, the APs of all classes (n) are averaged.

$$mAP = \frac{1}{|n|} \sum_{c=1}^{n} \frac{|TP_c|}{|FP_c| + |TP_c|} \qquad (3)$$

The mAP calculations are performed on the COCO data set, widely used as a standard for evaluating object detectors, with most research providing benchmarks using the recent COCO evaluations.

The COCO metric further breaks down the mAP for more comprehensive results. Using a single IoU threshold for evaluation may bias the metric and provide a lenient assessment of the model. To address this, COCO proposes an average mAP over 10 IoU thresholds ranging from 0.5 to 0.95 with a step size of 0.05 (AP@[0.5:0.05:0.95]). Averaging over IoUs rewards detectors with better localization. COCO contains more small objects than large objects, with 41% of the objects in the dataset being small (area < 322), 34% being medium-sized (area between 322 and 962), and 24% being large (area > 962). The area is measured as the number of pixels in the segmentation mask. AR in the evaluation stands for Average Recall and is given for the IoU=0.50:0.05:0.95 for small, medium, and large objects. In the second part of the evaluation, models are tested using traffic videos. To count objects in a video, the IoU of the objects is calculated between consecutive frames and assigned an ID if the IoU is above 0.05. False negative detections cause a track to stop immediately, and few missing detections result in a high number of ID switches, degrading track quality. Fig. 5 demonstrates how an object retains its ID and can be counted if detected in consecutive frames, highlighting the importance of fast frame processing for correct object counting. To determine object identity from one image to the other, the overlap areas of the detections between the images are compared [8].

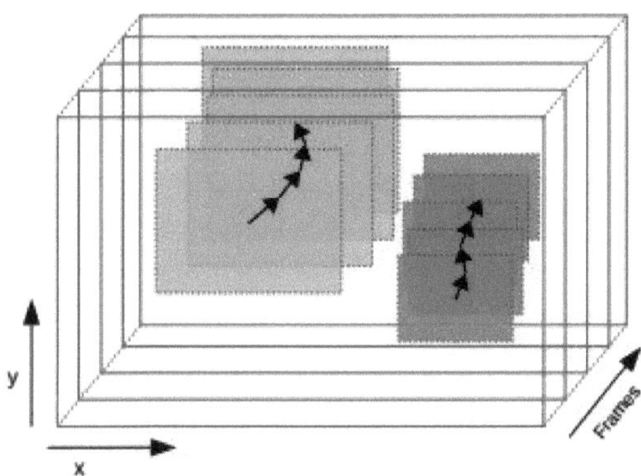

Figure 5: Moving objects keep their ID depending on the IoU for counting [8]

The traffic video data set compiles street records with varying object sizes, made at different times of day and weather conditions. During video analysis, we only consider the car category, as it holds the most significance for traffic analysis.

3 Results and Discussion

The results of the predicted objects with the coordinates, the width and height of the bounding box, and the class of the prediction were saved in a JSON file. With the help of another JSON file containing the ground truth of the bounding boxes, the results were evaluated in Python and the introduced metrics were calculated. Table 1 shows the results of the mentioned metrics for both models. With an IoU of 0.5, YOLOv4 achieves an mAP of 84% across all classes and YOLOv4-tiny achieves 49%. Cars are correctly detected by YOLOv4 with a mAP@IoU=.50 with 77%. YOLOv4-tiny achieved a mAP of 42%. In the individual classes, it is visible that cars and pedestrians are recognized better than bicycles. The object size has an important influence on the mAP. As a result, the lines for object tracking should always be set where the objects have the maximum size.

Table 1: Results all classes

	YOLOv4	YOLOv4-tiny
mAP@IoU=.50:.05:.95	0.620	0.285
mAP@IoU=.50	0.847	0.490
mAP_{small}	0.422	0.165
mAP_{medium}	0.662	0.323
mAP_{large}	0.770	0.458
AR_{small}	0.542	0.206
AR_{medium}	0.747	0.504
AR_{large}	0.833	0.631

Table 2: Results in class car

	YOLOv4	YOLOv4-tiny
mAP@IoU=.50:.05:.95	0.500	0.221
mAP@IoU=.50	0.769	0.421
mAP_{small}	0.393	0.106
mAP_{medium}	0.652	0.405
mAP_{large}	0.719	0.445
AR_{small}	0.549	0.179
AR_{medium}	0.766	0.588
AR_{large}	0.834	0.669

Table 3: Results in class person

	YOLOv4	YOLOv4-tiny
mAP@IoU=.50:.05:.95	0.584	0.334
mAP@IoU=.50	0.864	0.621
mAP_{small}	0.406	0.135
mAP_{medium}	0.658	0.438
mAP_{large}	0.739	0.517
AR_{small}	0.536	0.196
AR_{medium}	0.747	0.583
AR_{large}	0.819	0.678

In the second part of the study the traffic video dataset was used to compare the processing speeds of both models. YOLOv4 tiny processes the videos with a speed of $\sim$18FPS

Table 4: Results in class bicycle

	YOLOv4	YOLOv4-tiny
mAP@IoU=.50:.05:.95	0.414	0.166
mAP@IoU=.50	0.692	0.353
mAP_{small}	0.244	0.055
mAP_{medium}	0.501	0.228
mAP_{large}	0.669	0.362
AR_{small}	0.409	0.158
AR_{medium}	0.650	0.454
AR_{large}	0.798	0.600

Table 5: Comparison of average confindece

Video resolution	YOLOv4	YOLOv4-tiny
1280x720	74 %	59 %
854x480	74 %	59 %
426x240	74 %	59 %

on the Jetson Nano 4GB. YOLOv4 only achieves ∼2FPS. Furthermore, the influence of the video resolution on the average confidence of the models was examined. It became apparent that the average confidence remains largely constant up to 240p in the tested videos. In order to achieve a sufficiently good tracking accuracy for cars and moving objects, YOLO should run at least with 8-9 FPS [2]. This is why the YOLOv4-tiny model is more suitable for traffic counting applications in combination with the Jetson Nano.

4 Conclusion

This article investigates an application for monitoring and tracking traffic flow. For this purpose, two neural networks for object recognition are evaluated with the COCO data set. In addition, influences such as camera quality and processing speed were investigated. It was found that there are significant differences in the accuracy of object recognition between the two models. YOLOv4 performed better in terms of accuracy than the smaller model YOLOv4-tiny. YOLOv4 achieved a mAP@IoU=0.5 in the cars category of ∼77% on the Jetson Nano 4GB. YOLOv4-tiny only achieved a mAP@IoU=0.5 of ∼42%. In terms of processing speed, however, YOLOv4-tiny with ∼18 FPS performed significantly better than YOLOv4 with ∼2 FPS. However, for tracking objects at a fast speed, a fast processing speed is of great importance, as objects are only counted correctly if their IDs remain constant in the following frames. The YOLOv4-tiny model is therefore more suitable for use on a Jetson Nano. As inputs, video recordings with a resolution of up to 240p (426x240) are suitable. Of course, the object size of the cars under surveillance also plays a role here, which was not observed further in this study. Up to this resolution, the average confidence of the object recognizer is constant in the tested traffic videos. In summary, the application of a Jetson Nano with the YOLOv4-tiny model is suitable for use in traffic tracking in smart cities. Future work includes improving the performance and accuracy of the detection and tracking

algorithms. In principle, the application is already suitable for assessing the basic traffic development for individual regions and for planning traffic in a sustainable manner in the future.

Acknowledgement

This work was carried out at the CoSA Center of Excellence at the Technische Hochschule Lübeck - University of Applied Sciences. Thanks to Prof. Dr. Hellbrück for supervising the work.

Author's Statement

Conflict of interest: Authors state no conflict of interest.

5 References

[1] J. Barthélemy, N. Verstaevel, H. Forehead, and P. Perez, "Edge-computing video analytics for real-time traffic monitoring in a smart city," *Sensors*, vol. 19, no. 9, p. 2048, 2019.

[2] "GitHub OpenDataCam." https://github.com/opendatacam/opendatacam. Accessed: 2023-01-03.

[3] C.-Y. Wang, A. Bochkovskiy, and H.-Y. M. Liao, "Scaled-YOLOv4: Scaling cross stage partial network," in *Proceedings of the IEEE/CVF Conference on Computer Vision and Pattern Recognition (CVPR)*, pp. 13029–13038, June 2021.

[4] J. Lee and K.-i. Hwang, "Yolo with adaptive frame control for real-time object detection applications," *Multimedia Tools and Applications*, vol. 81, no. 25, pp. 36375–36396, 2022.

[5] A. Bochkovskiy, C.-Y. Wang, and H.-Y. M. Liao, "Yolov4: Optimal speed and accuracy of object detection," 2020.

[6] T.-Y. Lin, M. Maire, S. Belongie, L. Bourdev, R. Girshick, J. Hays, P. Perona, D. Ramanan, C. L. Zitnick, and P. Dollár, "Microsoft coco: Common objects in context," 2014.

[7] "NVIDIA Jetson Nano Developer Kit." https://developer.nvidia.com/embedded/jetson-nano-developer-kit. Accessed: 2022-11-24.

[8] E. Bochinski, T. Senst, and T. Sikora, "Extending iou based multi-object tracking by visual information," in *2018 15th IEEE International Conference on Advanced Video and Signal Based Surveillance (AVSS)*, pp. 1–6, 2018.

Automatic Detection of Changed Depth Camera Pose for Indoor Applications

Onurcan Köken [1]

[1] Robotics and Autonomous Systems, Universität zu Lübeck, onurcan.koeken@student.uni-luebeck.de

Abstract

Accurate and precise localization of a depth camera is critical for applications in medical imaging systems. To calibrate cameras and define their position in the world coordinate system, different types of calibration methods are used, such as chessboard pattern. However, in real-world scenarios, the camera may experience various disturbances, such as vibrations or accidental movements, which can cause the pose of the camera to deviate from its calibrated state. In this paper, an approach for detecting lost camera pose for depth camera systems is proposed. The approach is based on the usage of point clouds to estimate the normal vector of the floor with respect to the camera. Therefore, when the camera pose is drifted, the estimated plane equation of the ground changes. The results show that the proposed approach is able to detect that the camera position and orientation are changed.

1 Introduction

In 3D medical imaging systems, it is important to define the position and orientation of the camera in the world coordinate system. The process of those parameters is the calibration of the camera. There exist two main parameter types to transform a 2D image in pixels to a 3D point cloud in world coordinates, which are extrinsic and intrinsic parameters. Intrinsic parameters are used to map between camera coordinates and pixel coordinates, and extrinsic parameters are used to map between world coordinates and camera coordinates. In our application, it is assumed that intrinsic parameters are known, which are the optical center and focal length. Also, the calibration of a camera for extrinsic parameters, which are position and orientation, is determined before. Therefore, when the camera is drifted, its position and orientation change in world coordinates, but its intrinsic parameters remain the same.

The camera used in this project streams depth and grayscale near-infrared images, and the camera is assumed to be fixed while different non-moving objects are in various positions and orientations. However, when this single camera drifts and loses its position and orientation, it must be detected to avoid misguiding subsequent operations.

There exist several methods to handle the problem, such as keypoints matching [8], Inertial Measurement Unit (IMU) sensor usage [7], point cloud registration [4], etc. For the case of keypoints matching, two views are supposed to be compared in terms of detected keypoints, and then by using those matched keypoints, the Essential matrix can be detected [8] and can be used to determine the corresponding transformation matrix from the first fixed view to the second drifted view. However, the reason why it can not be

implemented is that the environment is dynamic, so objects are changing around the scene. Therefore, corresponding keypoints can not be matched. It should be also noted that they are not moving objects and the method is not a real-time application. As another method, an IMU sensor can be used to detect the instant movement of the camera, however it is assumed to use only computer vision methods, no additional devices. In terms of point cloud methods, a local registration method, which is Iterative Closest Point (ICP) [4], can be used to determine the transformation matrix between similar views. It is a powerful method to match point clouds, however it is not applicable to the dynamic environment. It matches the given two point clouds, therefore when objects are moved, it is even possible to mislead the estimation. Because it might result in the camera pose being lost, while in reality it is still calibrated well. In this research, we propose an algorithm to handle this problem based on the assumptions.

2 Material and Methods

As a setup, two depth cameras are used to demonstrate two views as a fixed camera view and a drifted camera view. Their intrinsic parameters are known, however extrinsic parameters are not used, instead the drifted camera is moved several times and tested. Therefore, the origin of each camera is set on the camera itself, instead of a single common origin of the world coordinate system. Additionally, to be able to process the point cloud processing methods, functions of open3d library [1] are used.

2.1   Denoising Point Cloud

Firstly, point cloud data is obtained from both cameras. However, in the scene there might be a window, mirror, or reflectors that might cause the points to distribute over further distances. Also, noisy measurements might occur during the operation. Therefore, denoising point cloud is first applied to remove unnecessary points and increase the processing performance.

One of the denoising methods is voxel downsampling. It uses a voxel grid, which is a set of small 3D boxes in space, to downsample the given point cloud uniformly over the space [1]. The voxel size is defined to create the voxel grid, as the size increases, the number of points in the cloud will be decreased. At the end of the process, a single point is left out of each small 3D box. Therefore, it is also important not to remove a high number of points, which might cause inaccurate processing in further steps.

After that, another denoising method, which is radius outlier removal, is applied. The method checks the number of neighbors around a point in a given sphere radius [1]. By using this method, several noisy points can be removed, but it is also important to tune the parameters of these functions.

2.2   Ground Detection

To extract a point set of the ground, the plane segmentation function of open3d library is used. It is based on Random Sample Consensus (RANSAC) [2], which can be used to detect a plane surface [3], [5]. There are 3 parameters to use the function, one of them is the distance threshold which checks the maximum distance of a point from the estimated plane. It should be selected carefully, because when it is set very low, it may not extract all the ground due to obstacles around the ground or noisy data can also cause this. For example, a set of points that are further away from the camera will be detected with higher error while a set of points that are near to the camera will be detected with lower error. Therefore, points of the ground dissipate as the distance to the camera increases. Another parameter is the number of randomly sampled points to estimate the plane, which can be at least 3 points. The limitation of this method stems from its random process, leading to incorrect detection of walls, grounds, or other surfaces. So, the number of points belonging to the ground is supposed to be high enough, otherwise it detects other objects. Lastly, there is a parameter to define the number of iterations to increase the robustness of the detection of the plane. A result of ground detection result can be seen in Fig. 1.

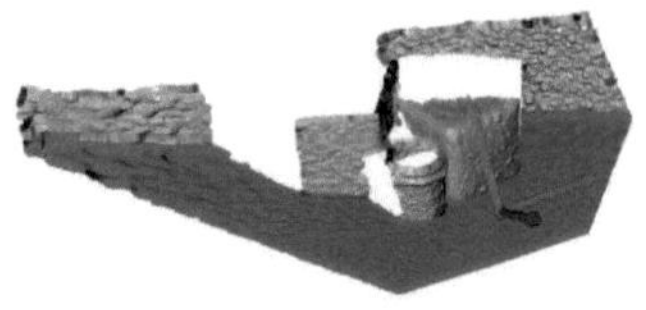

Figure 1: Given point cloud, red points are the result of successful ground detection, while gray points are the outliers

2.3   Evaluation Metrics

As a result of the ground detection method, a plane equation is obtained, which can be used to compare the plane equation of a fixed camera and the plane equation of drifted camera. To evaluate the results, evaluation metrics are used. Since our problem contains several assumptions, different metrics and equations are tested to compare estimated plane equations. The general plane equation is represented as $a\widehat{x} + b\widehat{y} + c\widehat{z} + d = 0$, where a, b, c and d are the constants, and $\widehat{x}, \widehat{y}, \widehat{z}$ are the axis.

The first metric is simply based on normalization of plane equations including the constant term of equations as it can be seen in (1).

$$q_1 = min(||\boldsymbol{w'_1} - \boldsymbol{w'_2}||, ||\boldsymbol{w'_1} + \boldsymbol{w'_2}||) \tag{1}$$

where

$$\boldsymbol{w'_{1,2}} = \frac{[\boldsymbol{w^T_{1,2}}, d_{1,2}]^T}{||[\boldsymbol{w^T_{1,2}}, d_{1,2}]^T||}$$

$$\boldsymbol{w_{1,2}} = a_{1,2}\widehat{x} + b_{1,2}\widehat{y} + c_{1,2}\widehat{z}$$

The second metric uses Cauchy-Schwarz inequality [6], which is based on the normal of the estimated plane normal and their inner products. It subtracts the constant terms d_1 and d_2 of plane equations as can be seen in (2).

$$q_2 = ||\boldsymbol{w_1}||||\boldsymbol{w_2}|| - |<\boldsymbol{w_1}, \boldsymbol{w_2}>| + |d_1 - d_2| \tag{2}$$

Since it is not easy to imagine plane equations and calculate corresponding metrics, a simple 3D visualization tool is built as can be seen in Fig. 2. So, by visualizing the estimated planes, it is easier to evaluate the behaviors of evaluation metrics.

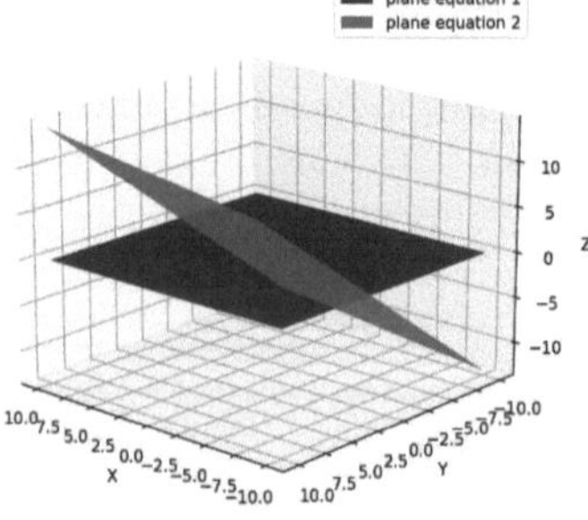

Figure 2: 3D plot of plane equation 1 in blue and plane equation 2 in red colors.

3   Results and Discussion

3.1   Denoising Point Cloud and Ground Detection

Firstly, denoising processes are applied on a point cloud that is obtained from a depth camera. The voxel size parameter is set to 0.02m as default in open3d. Since the ground detection method does not require high computation, it is not preferred to increase the voxel size and decrease the number of points in the cloud. This process performs uniformly over all the point clouds, so it does not remove a specific type of unnecessary points.

To remove outlier points, the radius outlier removal method is used. There exist two parameters, a minimum number of points in a sphere around a point and the radius of that sphere. In our application, number of points is set to 16 and radius is set to 0.15m, which are the suggested parameters by open3d. During the tests and demonstration, the environment is carefully selected so in most cases there is no window or a mirror. After denoising methods are applied, most of the outliers are removed and the points that contain the information of ground are extracted. In one of the experiments, single camera is fixed and number of objects on the ground is increased one by one from 0 to 5 objects. After a point cloud is read, voxel downsampling is the first step which removes significant amounts of points, around 80%, while in step 2 radius outlier removal is applied and removes a small number of points, around 2%. However, it is still important because it removes only the points that are noisy or further away from the camera. For all six cases, from 0 to 5 objects in the same camera view, the floor is extracted successfully. The last step is the estimated ground points, which get lower as the number of objects on the ground increases. The extracted ground with 5 objects case can be seen in Fig. 3 and the case where there is no object on the ground can be seen in Fig. 5.

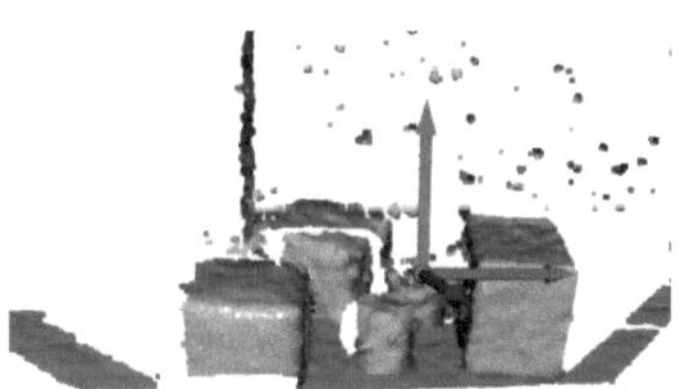

Figure 3: Ground detection while 5 objects on the ground

Parameter tuning is applied at the plane segmentation part since it is used to extract the plane equation of the floor. There are 3 parameters, which are distance threshold, number of randomly selected points, and number of iterations to estimate the plane equation every time. Due to random operation, it increases the possibility for a higher number of points, which sometimes causes wrong detection because the wall might be larger compared to the ground as it can be seen in Fig. 4. So, to handle this problem the normal vector of the estimated plane is used. Since it is already known that the origin is on the camera and the camera looks at the environment from a higher position with some angle. It is observed that scaling factor b of the y-axis is supposed to be higher than the threshold, which is set to 0.5. So firstly, the plane segmentation method runs and if the parameter b is not high enough, it removes the detected points, which is usually the surface of a wall. Then, the plane segmentation method runs again on the remaining data, until the scalar factor b of the y-axis is high enough as it can be seen in Fig. 5. Otherwise, it does not detect the ground, and only a small number of points remain. The points in red are detected by the method, while others are the outliers of point clouds.

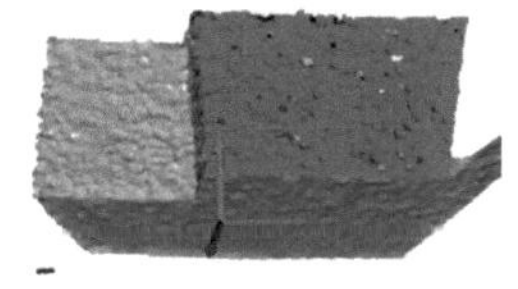 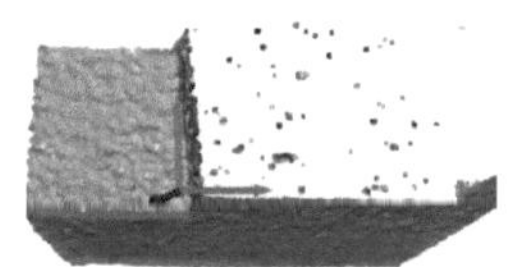

Figure 4: Wall detection instead of ground detection

Figure 5: Corrected ground detection

About the distance threshold parameter, it should be tuned so that the sampling of points is proper, otherwise it might cause a wrong estimation of the plane equation. It is set as 0.05m in our application which gives a proper ground extraction as it can be seen in Fig. 8. However, other parameters are also tested as it can be seen in Fig. 6 and Fig. 7. In one of the cases it under-samples the points belonging to ground with a lower distance threshold, while in another case it over-samples the points and both cases lead to wrong plane equation estimation.

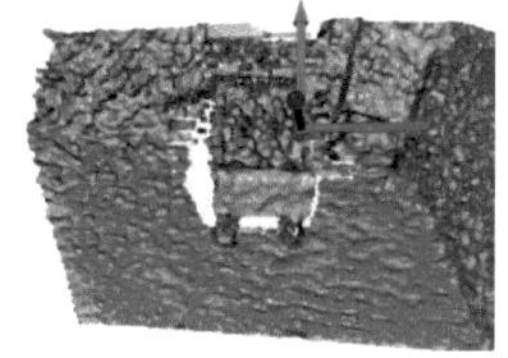 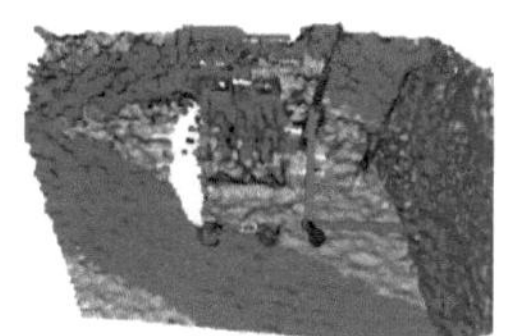

Figure 6: Ground detection result with 0.01m distance threshold, some of the points that belong to floor are not detected which are gray parts on the floor

Figure 7: Ground detection result with 0.3m distance threshold, red colored points represent the floor, while they actually do not only belong to the floor

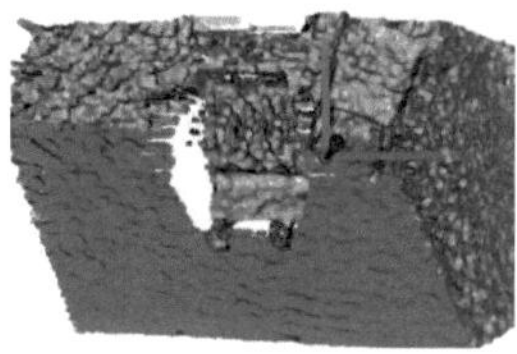

Figure 8: Successful ground detection result, points in red, with 0.05m distance threshold, gray points are the outliers

3.2 Comparing Estimated Plane Equations

In this case, one depth camera represents the fixed camera case and the second depth camera represents the drifted camera where the position and orientation are lost. Therefore, the ground truth is the plane equation of the fixed camera, while the method is applied on the second camera and metrics are compared. The origin is on the camera for both cases, so the extrinsic parameters of the first camera are not used to estimate if the camera calibration is lost, instead the estimated plane equation of the floor is used. In the experiment, the second camera is placed in several different positions and orientations to observe differences between estimated plane equation 1 and 2 which corresponds to fixed camera and drifted camera respectively.

As it can be seen in Table 1, plane equations for each camera are estimated by using ground detection method. The evaluation metric results (q_1 and q_2) are compared to observe which one is a better metric and to define a threshold. Therefore, at the end of the algorithm, it can be decided if the camera position and orientation are lost or not.

Table 1: Estimated plane equations for 3 different cases and corresponding evaluation metric results. For each case, the first plane equation belongs to the fixed camera.

	x-axis	y-axis	z-axis	d	q_1	q_2
case 1	0.00	0.90	0.44	1.03	0.0067	0.01
	0.00	0.89	0.45	1.04		
case 2	0.00	0.87	0.50	0.61	0.0815	0.0632
	0.08	0.86	0.50	0.55		
case 3	0.01	0.90	0.44	1.04	0.1160	0.0630
	0.01	0.96	0.29	0.99		

For case 1, cameras are only 3cm away from each other and look in the same direction. So, only the distance in the x-axis is changed slightly. However, for this case, it is also tested for 5cm, and 10cm differences. The orientation is increased up to $45°$ in the yaw-axis direction. Most of the estimated plane equations for case 1 are observed the same as it is shown in Table 1. For this case, the metrics can not be used to detect the difference because they give similar results also when the camera is not moved.

For case 2, the distance between cameras is increased by 36cm in the horizontal plane and the height of second camera is decreased by 7cm. It is rotated approximately $5°$ in the roll-axis and $2°$ in the pitch-axis. As a result of estimated planes and evaluation metrics, the difference is noticeable, and the pose change is detectable by both metrics. Lastly, for case 3, both distance and angles are increased dramatically by around 1.5m in the horizontal plane and the height of second camera is also increased by around 20cm. About the rotation, it is rotated around almost $90°$ in the yaw-axis. As a result, both metrics are increased, such that q_1 is increased more compared to q_2 metric. It should be also noticed that the difference in q_2 metric is quite low between case 2 and case 3. Therefore, q_1 is a better metric in this application, however for some cases, q_2 gives also good results and it is still possible to distinguish if the camera position and orientation are changed or not.

4 Conclusion

It is observed that the proposed method performs well to extract ground, while the plane equation is not that robust and accurate since it changes with each iteration. When the camera drifted slightly, case 1 in Table 1, the method does not perform well since the metrics do not change enough to set a threshold. However, when it is drifted dramatically, in cases 2 and 3, it detects that the camera pose is changed, where both metrics can be used. Therefore, the method can be applied in some cases but further methods can be combined with it so that small changes can be detected as well. Also, there must be further experiments to set precise thresholds for the metrics.

Acknowledgement

The work has been carried out at Drägerwerk AG Co. KGaA, Lübeck and supervised by Prof. Dr. Georg Schildbach, the Institute of Electrical Engineering in Medicine, Universität zu Lübeck.

Author's Statement

Conflict of interest: Authors state no conflict of interest.

5 References

[1] Q.-Y. Zhou, J. Park, and V. Koltun, "Open3D: A modern library for 3D data processing," *arXiv:1801.09847*, 2018.

[2] M. A. Fischler and R. C. Bolles, "Random sample consensus: A paradigm for model fitting with applications to image analysis and automated cartography," *Commun. ACM*, vol. 24, no. 6, p. 381–395, 1981. [Online]. Available: https://doi.org/10.1145/358669.358692 [last accessed on 2023-01-15].

[3] R. Schnabel, R. Wahl, and R. Klein, "Efficient ransac for point-cloud shape detection," *Computer Graphics Forum*, vol. 26, no. 2, pp. 214–226, 2007. [Online]. Available: https://onlinelibrary.wiley.com/doi/abs/10.1111/j.1467-8659.2007.01016.x [last accessed on 2023-01-15].

[4] S. M. Rusinkiewicz and M. Levoy, "Efficient variants of the icp algorithm," *Proceedings Third International Conference on 3-D Digital Imaging and Modeling*, pp. 145–152, 2001.

[5] R. Zeineldin and N. El-Fishawy, "A survey of ransac enhancements for plane detection in 3d point clouds," *Menoufia Journal of Electronic Engineering Research*, vol. 26, pp. 519–537, 07 2017.

[6] A.L. Cauchy, "Cours d'Analyse de l'Ecole Royale Polytechnique," Ire *Partie, Analyse Algebrique*, Paris, pp. 365-377, 1821.

[7] Y. Zhang, J. Tan, Z. Zeng, W. Liang and Y. Xia, "Monocular camera and IMU integration for indoor position estimation," *36th Annual International Conference of the IEEE Engineering in Medicine and Biology Society*, Chicago, IL, USA, pp. 1198-1201, 2014.

[8] J. Bian, R. Yang, Y. Liu, L. Zhang, M.-M. Cheng, I. Reid, and W. Wu, "MatchBench: An Evaluation of Feature Matchers," *arXiv:1808.02267*, 2018.

An approach to create 3D-models with voxel carving for a 3D scanning setup

Pia Lüdemann [1] and Gerrit Kolb [2]
[1] Robotics and Autonomous Systems, Universität zu Lübeck, pia.luedemann@student.uni-luebeck.de
[2] Vastly Underrated, Eichholz 52, 20459 Hamburg, gerrit.kolb@vastlyunderrated.com

Abstract

Despite the increasing popularity of 3D printing, 3D scanning remains a complex and expensive endeavor. In this research, we introduce a method for using a smartphone and a turntable to generate a 3D scan. We expand an existing laser scanning setup with another approach. It involves voxel carving and using and training *convolutional neural networks* (CNNs) to remove the turntable and background from the images. A key challenge is autonomously detecting the performance of the scan by utilizing multiple scores. They represent CNN accuracy, silhouette alignment, and a comparison with the laser scanning result. Our method provides a more accessible and cost-effective alternative for obtaining 3D scans.

1 Introduction

3D scanning has a lot of potential in terms of sustainability. With 3D scanners available to anyone, broken parts for non-working everyday objects can be scanned and printed rather than discarding the object or ordering a replacement, which may have to be shipped worldwide. Once 3D scanned, the models can be printed at the nearest available 3D printer, which have become more common over the years. The gaming industry is already using 3D scanning, allowing for the creation of more realistic and accurate in-game characters and environments. Being more cost-efficient provides more people with the possibility to easily create a virtual model. However, the concept has traditionally been the domain of specialized equipment, requiring the use of expensive scanners and complex software.

3D scanners in general capture the shape and appearance of a real-world object and create a point cloud. By connecting neighboring points with triangle-shaped surfaces, *meshes*, a point cloud with well-defined inner and outer areas can be easily converted to a 3D model. There are various types of 3D scanners, including *structured light scanners, laser scanners*, and *photogrammetry* scanners. Structured light scanners use a pattern of light and a camera to capture the shape of an object. Laser scanners use a laser and a camera or sensor to capture the reflected laser light, and photogrammetry scanners use multiple photographs to create a 3D point cloud [1]. 3D scanners are used in various fields such as manufacturing, engineering, design, and entertainment. They are useful for quickly and accurately capturing 3D data and creating digital copies of physical objects, as well as for tasks like 3D printing and visualization. However, 3D scanners can be expensive [2], especially when meeting high accuracy. They also require specialized software and expertise to operate.

With the rapid development of mobile phone technology, it has become more applicable to use smartphones for 3D scanning as well. In this paper, we expand a laser scanner infrastructure that enables the capture of a 3D scan with almost any smartphone camera, making 3D scanning available to a wide range of people, with a new scanning method. This expansion includes handling typical challenges to structured light scanning such as reflections, unstructured or bright surroundings, or objects made of glass.

2 Material

To create a complementary 3D Scanner technique to the existing laser scanner for smartphones, we use a variety of computer vision techniques and CNNs, which are described in the following.

The camera is an essential component in 3D modeling. It usually consists of a lens, an aperture, and a sensor. The *intrinsic* camera matrix describes how the parameters of these components can distort images. The *extrinsic* camera matrix describes the camera's position and orientation in 3D space. Together, these matrices can project 3D points onto the image plane and determine the camera's position, orientation, and distortion from an image [3]. An immensely popular 3D modeling approach in computer vision is photogrammetry [4]. It takes multiple pictures of an object from different viewpoints which are then processed by the algorithm to find the *key points*, meaning the most standout points in the picture, with *feature extraction*. Identical points will then be matched between the images to find the spatial relations between the images. From this, the 3D model can be built. But since this is a complex combination of algorithms and requires time to compute, another method is more applicable to our case. In contrast to photogrammetry, a simpler and faster approach to creating a point cloud from images is *voxel carving* [5]. Voxel carving starts with a virtual block, meaning a 3D space filled with points. We remove the background of the images of the object and map the silhouettes on the virtual block according to the extrinsic and intrinsic camera matrix. Everything that is not covered by the silhouette will be removed. Repeatedly doing this for every silhouette will result in a 3D point cloud of the object. One technique we employ in this project is CNN-based background removal. For voxel carving, we don't require raw images. Instead, we need the silhouette of the object to carve the model. Traditional methods for achieving this include using edge detection algorithms like Canny or the Sobel operator [6]. However, we can also use a CNN for a more modern approach. The U^2-*Net* [7] performs well on everyday objects and has been trained with an augmented version of the *DUTS-TR* data set [8]. We will also need to train a CNN by ourselves to segment the detected foreground. To model and train the network, we use the framework *PyTorch*.

3   Methods

3.1   Laser Scanning Method

To modify a common smartphone camera to a 3D scanner we need a simple setup of a turntable, a laser, and 3D printable parts. To scan an object, it has to be placed in the center of a turntable. The turntable gets augmented by a sleeve with a code for defining the rotational position of the turntable. The smartphone gets to be placed in front of the turntable such that the camera captures the whole turntable and the object. A laser from the right will project a red vertical line onto the object. The setup can be seen in Fig. 1 To record a scan, the turntable turns slowly with the laser

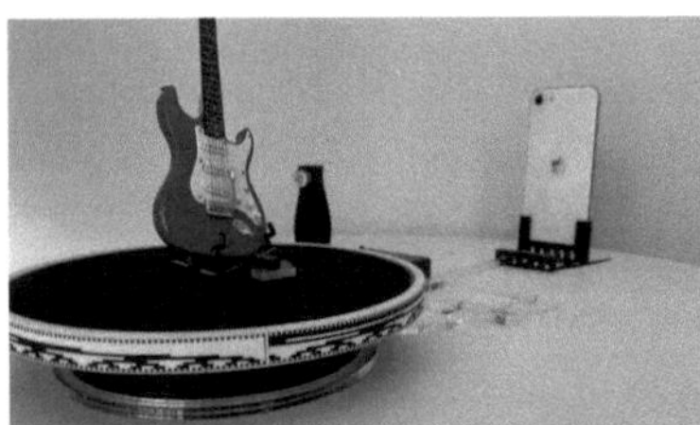

Figure 1: The setup of the Ascand. The laser projects a beam onto the turntable.

on while the phone records the video. To improve the colorization of the virtual 3D model, after one full rotation of the object, the laser has to be switched off to record another full rotation in the same video. This video can then be uploaded to the web application [9]to be processed by the algorithm. First, the video gets divided into images and sorted according to the encoded degree of rotation. The general pre-processing will then determine geometry information like the height and edge points of the turntable in the images. After this, the images with the laser get evaluated according to the deviation of the laser from its normal position without the object. The detected points get mapped

into the 3D space to create the point cloud. After the 3D coordinate system positions have been detected, the points get colorized. If available, the algorithm will take the pictures without the laser, maps them as close as possible to the points, and applies the color accordingly.

3.2   Voxel Carving Method

In some cases, like reflecting surfaces, laser scanning is not possible, so the task is to develop a suitable alternative. Voxel carving needs the silhouettes of the object from different angles to carve the 3D model. For this, we use the background removal capabilities of the U²-Net. The resulting images are shown in Fig. 6. In most cases, the turntable is detected as foreground. It is easier to segment the turntable from these pre-processed images rather than the full images required to fine-tune the given U²-Net. Therefore, we train a custom *turntable CNN* with PyTorch to segment the turntable in the next processing step. A data set of 187 images for training and 10 images for validation is created by segmenting the turntable from the images processed by the *background CNN*. We train a network with six layers and a learning rate of 0.0001 for about 600 epochs. The results are presented in Fig. 2. Because the data set is yet relatively small, we increase it to resume training for 200 epochs, with the results shown in Fig. 3. The dotted lines indicate the epochs where the validation results were acceptable, and the weights from these epochs are used for the turntable CNN in the next steps.

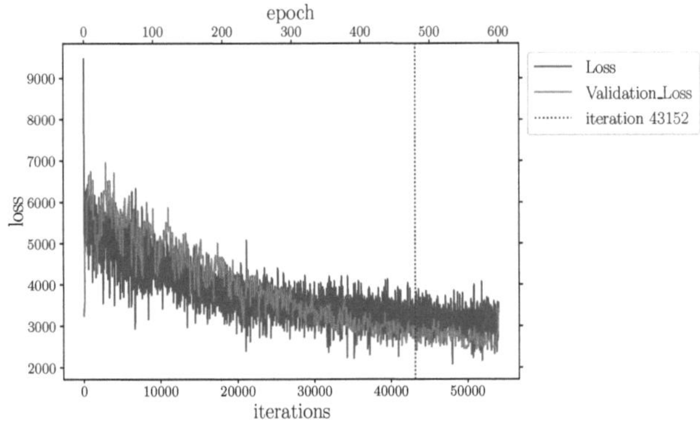

Figure 2: The loss function for the pre-training. The dotted line marks the iteration that has been used to resume the training in the next step because the result was the best one.

After the background removal, we use this CNN to remove the turntable. The next process evaluates the overall silhouette extraction by applying a grid to two sequential silhouettes and comparing matching grid pairs to detect differences. The rotation of the object will cause some differences, but by using a dynamic threshold that takes the degree of rotation into account, we can detect and remove outliers. This helps to get a general, measurable impression of how certain both CNNs were when removing the background and the turntable. If they are uncertain, there will be more movement on the edges of the object, which will be

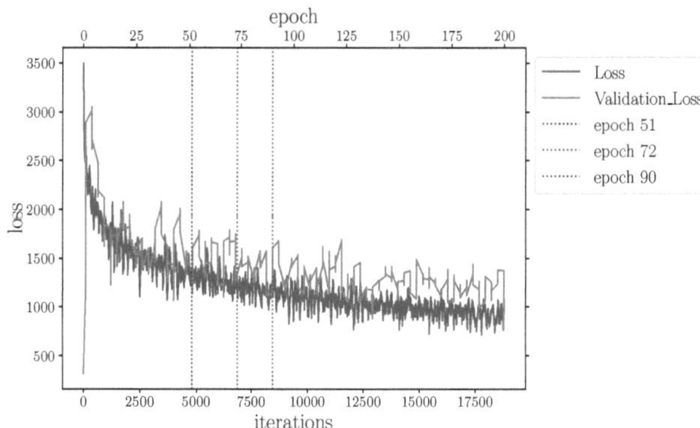

Figure 3: The loss function for the resumed training. The dotted lines mark the epochs with good results in the validation that can be used as weights for the turntable CNN.

detected by this algorithm. The remaining silhouettes are then processed using a voxel carving algorithm. A 3D point cloud representing the space above the turntable visible to the camera is created and rotated according to the degree of the image the silhouette belongs to. The silhouette is then projected onto the point cloud. Points that do not correspond to the silhouette are marked for removal. Points that have been marked frequently are removed, to reduce the influence of outliers. The remaining points are then colorized in a manner similar to the laser scanner approach. Finally, the inner points of the point cloud are removed by checking if they have neighboring points in every direction.

3.3 Rating

To compare the results of the laser and voxel scanning methods, multiple scores are used to estimate the performance of the voxel carving. The first score is the accuracy of the CNN, determined using the grid-motion-detection algorithm. It gives a clue about how easy the object was to detect for both CNNs. The second score is based on motion analysis. We extract the areas of differences between the raw images to create an estimated mask of where the object is likely to be. We then generate silhouettes of the 3D model from every rotational direction and merge them to create a motion mask for the model. Both masks are compared, resulting in the second score, determining whether the general shape is correct. Finally, we consider the results of the laser scanner. We find the nearest neighbors for each laser scanner point in the voxel carving result and compute the distances, ignoring the farthest 10 percent. The mean distance and the overall extent of the result are used to calculate the final score, which directly gives a relation between the two methods. Even if a simple approach may seem to be to compare the number of resulting points, it is not since there are various ways for both methods to fail, such that we can not simply define a measure for the relation of both amounts. Using these scores and manual evaluations of 293 test results, we create an *if-else structure* to assign a final grade to the resulting model.

4   Results and Discussion

Both the laser and voxel carving method can produce usable results under certain conditions, which Fig. 4 and Fig. 5 show. The input videos are bright, making it difficult for the laser method to detect the laser. This is one of the use cases where the voxel carving method is intended to complement the laser method. The two objects on the right show another use case with non-reflecting surfaces, like glass or slightly transparent silicone. The voxel carving, on the

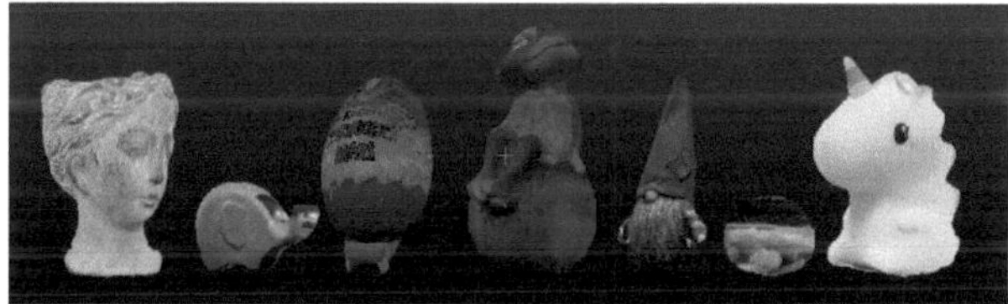

Figure 4: Resulting point clouds with the voxel carving method.

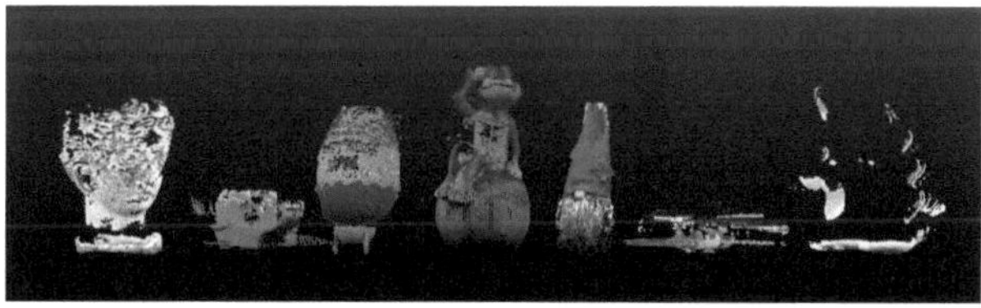

Figure 5: Resulting point clouds with the laser method. The videos are too bright for the laser, and many surfaces are reflecting or scattering. Therefore, we have problems like outliers and missing parts. Especially the flower in glass is highly challenging (object 6), as well as the semi-transparent silicone of the unicorn lamp (object 7).

other hand, struggles when the object has the same color as the turntable or background. It also has difficulty when the background is too close or chaotic, as the background CNN may detect parts of the background as the object. This issue can be addressed by focusing on the object and blurring the background in the video. It also helps to have a high contrast between the background and the object. On the contrary, the laser method is not affected by the color difference between the turntable, object, or background but may have difficulty with objects that are too large or too far away. It also has a higher resolution due to its algorithmic approach. To prepare the scanned models for 3D printing, a mesh is created by connecting the points to form continuous surfaces, which is straightforward for the voxel carving method but more challenging for the laser method due to many holes or missing points. Both methods have their specific challenges, but they complement each other well. We can use the automatic performance comparison to determine which one is better suited for a particular use case. If both results are applicable, the voxel result can be used to remove outliers produced by the laser method to have an overall high-resolution point cloud with minimal outliers.

It is worth exploring the possibility of further combining the results of both methods, like filling missing parts of the laser result with the voxel carving model. The voxel carving method has a major challenge in removing the background, including the turntable. The background removal CNN performs well, but the turntable removal CNN has room for improvement through further training, but the data set currently used is relatively small due to time limitations. Examples of the performance of the turntable CNN are presented in Fig. 6. We tried methods like *flood fill* to remove the turntable, but due to deviations like dust on the turntable, it did not outperform the CNN. It will also be necessary to further define the if-else structures parameter space for evaluation. Manually filling in gaps in the 3D parameter domain would be impractical due to the required time.

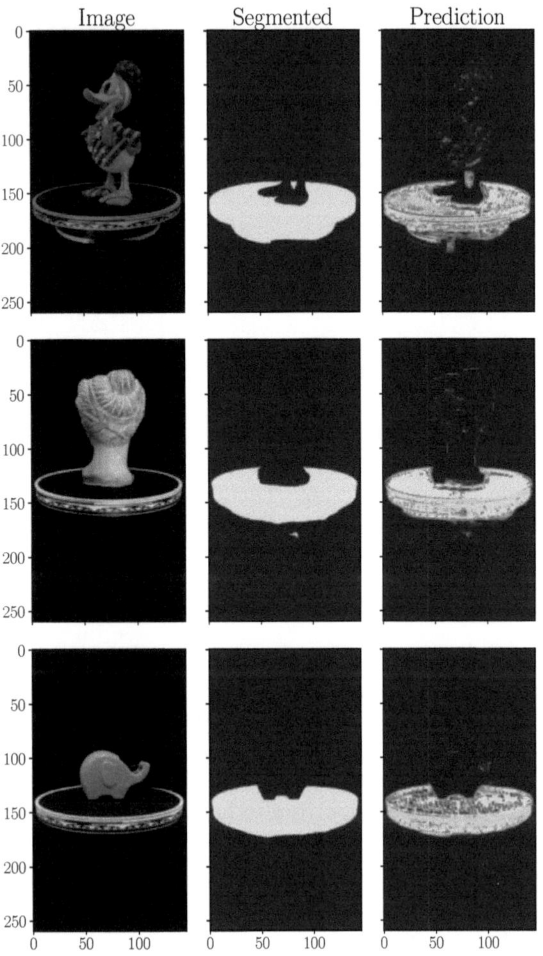

Figure 6: Performance of the turntable CNN. Left to right: Output image from the first CNN, manually segmented image, output image of the turntable CNN without threshold.

5   Conclusion

In conclusion, we found that both the laser and voxel carving approaches have their strengths and can be used effectively for different purposes. The laser method can create high-resolution scans when the video is relatively dark and the object fits on the small turntable. However, the voxel carving approach is more suitable for situations where the lighting conditions are suboptimal for the laser when scanning larger objects or objects with light-scattering surfaces. Overall, both methods are useful and can be effectively combined to achieve cost-effective 3D scanning with any smartphone and the presented setup.

Acknowledgement

The work has been carried out at Vastly Underrated in Hamburg and supervised by Prof. Dr.-Ing. Erhardt Barth, Institute for Neuro- and Bioinformatics, Universität zu Lübeck.

Author's Statement

Conflict of interest: Authors state no conflict of interest.

6   References

[1] M. Daneshmand et al., *3d Scanning: A comprehensive survey*. arXiv preprint arXiv:1801.08863, 2018.

[2] All3DP, *The best 3D scanners in 2023 – Buyer's guide*. Available: `https://all3dp.com/1/best-3d-scanner-diy-handheld-app-software/` [last accessed on 2023-01-12].

[3] M.A. Tehrani, T. Beeler and A. Grundhöfer, *A practical method for fully automatic intrinsic camera calibration using directionally encoded light*. In: 2017 IEEE Conference on Computer Vision and Pattern Recognition (CVPR), IEEE, 2017

[4] T. Schenk, *Introduction to photogrammetry*. The Ohio State University, Columbus 106, 2005

[5] M. Gaillard, C. Miao, J. C. Schnable and B. Benes, *Voxel carving-based 3D reconstruction of Sorghum identifies genetic determinants of light interception efficiency*. Plant direct 4.10, 2020

[6] D., Ziou and S. Tabbone, *Edge detection techniques-an overview*. In: Pattern Recognition and Image Analysis C/C of Raspoznavaniye Obrazov I Analiz Izobrazhenii, 8, 537-559, 1998

[7] X., Qin, et al., *U^2-Net: Going deeper with nested U-structure for salient object detection*. In: Pattern Recognition 106 107404, 2020

[8] L. Wang, et. al, *Learning to detect salient objects with image-level supervision*. In: Proceedings of the IEEE conference on computer vision and pattern recognition, 2017

[9] Web application of the Ascand, Available: `https://myascand.xplicator.com/en/app/dashboard`

Mapping and Navigation in agricultural fields using polytopes

Pranav Tej Gangavarapu [1], Ngoc Thinh Nguyen[2]
[1] Robotics and Autonomous Systems, Universität zu Lübeck, pranav.gangavarpu@student.uni-luebeck.de,
[2] Institute for Robotics and Cognitive Systems, Universität zu Lübeck, nguyen@rob.uni-luebeck.de

Abstract

This work addresses two major navigation problems: mapping and path planning. An advanced method for mapping and navigation using polytopes named *Navigation with polytopes*[1] is presented. First, the construction of a polytope map, which is a 2-D non-convex polytopic region decomposed into smaller connected polytopes (possibly with holes) from a standard gridmap, is presented. The next problem of finding a way within the polytope map is addressed by implementing a graph search algorithm that generates a sequence of connected polytopes from one point to another that ensures a safe traversable space for robots. This sequence can then be used to plan paths by interpolating curves and using various optimization methods. Finally, the algorithms are integrated into ROS (Robot Operating System) to be used as a global path planner.

1 Introduction

For academic and commercial applications, autonomous navigation using mobile robots is of tremendous interest to researchers [1–5]. For autonomous operations, there are certain important tasks like localization, path planning, motion control, mapping, etc. The path planning task plays an important role as it provides sequential movements for guiding the robot to a desired position. A global path planner has to be fed with information describing the environment. Most path planning approaches make use of discrete representations of the environment (e.g., occupancy grid maps) with traditional grid search methods like A*, Dijkstra, etc [3–5]. However, discrete representations of the environment are not accurate and the path obtained just from such grid maps and grid search methods is a linear piecewise path that is not feasible due to the lack of smoothness. This problem is usually countered by applying smoothing algorithms to the discrete path [4]. This points to an alternative line of research that involves directly using smooth interpolating curves like Bézier and B-spline curves. A continuous map can be used instead of discrete maps for representing the environment by using a so-called polytope map [1, 2]. Since the representation of the environment is continuous and divided into several polytopes, various optimization problems can be used with B-spline curves to plan a path within the polytope map. The basic idea is to create a safe polytopic region from starting point to a desired point and then place the control points of the curve within the safe polytopic region using optimization methods to obtain a short, continuous and safe path [1, 2] .The main content of this work is to describe the construction of the polytope map, finding of the sequence of polytopes required to traverse safely from the starting point to a desired point, ad-

dress some problems with the sequence of polytopes and integration of the algorithms that are published as a toolbox *Navigation with polytopes*[1] into ROS which can be used as a global path planner shown in Fig. 1.

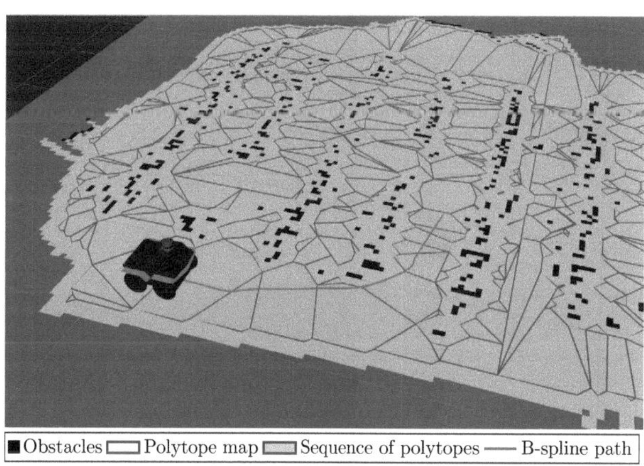

Figure 1: Illustration of the polytope map constructed from an agricultural field and sequence of polytopes from robot's position to a goal point in ROS visualized using Rviz.

2 Implementation and workflow

This section gives a brief introduction on the creation of a polytope map from a standard grid map and then finding a sequence of polytopes within this polytope map.

2.1 Problem definition

The work in this paper is based on previously published papers [1, 2], hence several notations and definitions are kept

---

[1]https://gitlab.rob.uni-luebeck.de/robPublic/
navigation_with_polytopes

the same for consistency. The first problem is obtaining a polytope map from a standard grid map. After obtaining a polytope map, the subproblem of the path planning problem is to determine the polytopes through which a path can be planned. The idea is to assume each of these polytopes as a node in a graph and the relation between them is defined by the sides of two successive polytopes. Then a graph search can be performed to obtain a set of sequential polytopes leading from one point to the other. The problem of determining the relation between two successive polytopes can be dealt using a geometric approach, which will be discussed in detail in this section.

2.2 Construction of polytope map

Definition 1 (Polytope map): A polytope map is defined as a list of connected 2-D convex polytopes with-in the free space of an environment.

$$\mathbb{P} = [\mathbb{P}_1, \mathbb{P}_2, ..., \mathbb{P}_n] \tag{1}$$

where $\mathbb{P}_1, \mathbb{P}_2, ..., \mathbb{P}_n$ are 2-D convex polytopes and n is the number of polytopes
A general convention of each polytope in polytope map is a list of ordered vertices:

$$\mathbb{P}_i = [V_1, ..., V_m] \; \forall i \in \{1, ..., n\} \tag{2}$$

where $V_1, ..V_m$ are vertices of a polytope. Each vertex is a pair of x,y coordinates w.r.t the grid map.

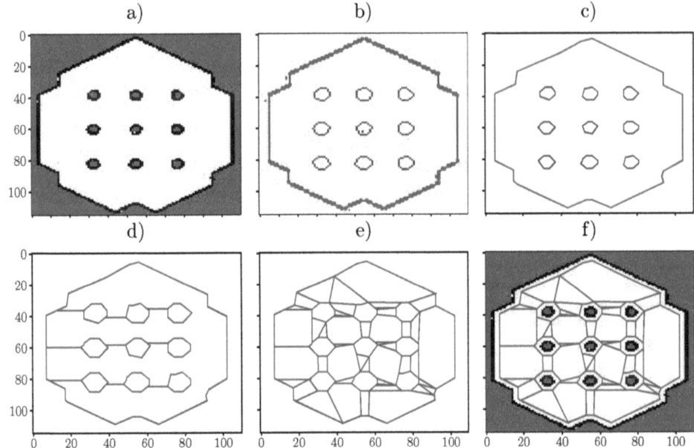

Figure 2: Illustration of sequential steps for construction of polytope map from grid map.

Such polytope map can be obtained from a standard grid map shown in Fig. 2a using the following sequential steps:

1. Extract the inner and outer boundaries of the complete map using the function *findContours* with the option RETR_EXTERNAL for external and RETR_LIST for internal obstacles from OpenCV toolbox[2] as shown in Fig. 2b.

2. Simplify the contours obtained using RDP(Ramer-Douglas-Peucker) algorithm[3] with two parameters

$\varepsilon_{rdp,o}$ for outer boundary and $\varepsilon_{rdp,i}$ for inner obstacles [6].

3. Shrink the outer boundary and enlarge the obstacles by a saftey offset o_p by using Gdspy toolbox[4] as shown in Fig. 2d.

4. Apply the Boolean operation to remove obstacles from the outer boundary polytope and Partition the obstacle-free polytope (possibly with holes) into connected polytopes by using Mark Bayazit's algorithm[5] as shown in Fig. 2e.

2.3 Sequence of polytopes

After obtaining a polytope map, a sequence of connected polytopes allowing safe travel from the initial point P_s to the final point P_f is obtained. The process for obtaining such a sequence will be explained in this section.

Definition 2 (Shared edge): A shared edge is defined as a pair of two common vertices of consecutive polytopes.

$$E_i = \mathbb{P}_i \cap \mathbb{P}_{i+1}, \; \forall \, i \in \{1, ..., n-1\}. \tag{3}$$

Definition 3 (Sequence of connected polytopes): Given two arbitrary points in the polytope map, a sequence of connected polytopes $\mathbb{S}$ is a list of connected polytopes from the initial point to the final point in which two consecutive polytopes share exactly one edge E_i as in (3). This will be referred as 'sequence' and the polytopes $\mathbb{P}$ that are defined in the sequence will be denoted with symbol 'S'..

$$\mathbb{S} = \{S_1, S_2, ..., S_q\}, \tag{4}$$

where q is the number of polytopes in a sequence. It is also straightforward to assume that initial point and final points belong to the first and last polytopes in the sequence respectively:

$$P_s \in S_1, \quad P_f \in S_q. \tag{5}$$

Definition 4 (Connections): Connections define relations between each polytope in a polytope map which can be defined as:

$$\mathbb{C} = [\mathbb{C}_1, ..., \mathbb{C}_n] \tag{6}$$

$$\mathbb{C}_i = \left[[\mathbb{P}_i \cap \mathbb{P}_i], [\mathbb{P}_i \cap \mathbb{P}_{i+1}], ..., [\mathbb{P}_i \cap \mathbb{P}_{i+n-1}]\right] \forall i \in n \tag{7}$$

where n is the total number of polytopes in polytope map.

Complete procedure of obtaining the sequence can be explained as follows:

1. First the polytopes S_1 and S_q will be initially identified using Shapely[6] package's function *polygon.contains(point)* for points P_s and P_f.

---

[2] https://opencv.org/
[3] https://github.com/biran0079/crdp
[4] https://github.com/heitzmann/gdspy
[5] https://github.com/wsilva32/poly_decomp.py
[6] https://github.com/shapely/shapely

2. All the connections(6) from each of the polytope to all the other polytopes are identified by checking the common vertices between two polytopes.

3. Only indices from each connection $\mathbb{C}_i$ where the intersection of two polytopes results in two vertices are chosen.

4. With the information from connections an adjacency graph is created through which graph search is performed to obtain the sequence.

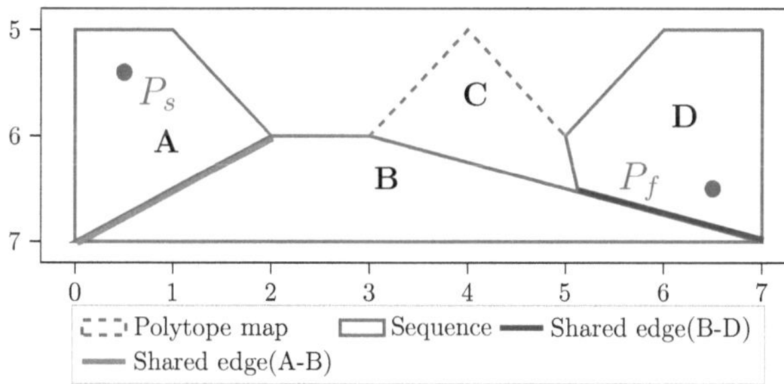

Figure 3: Illustration of a sample polytope map (gray) with four polytopes labeled with alphabets, initial and goal points (P_s, P_f) and the sequence of polytopes (green overlayed on the polytope map).

For example consider the polytopes for illustration from Fig. 3, if two points P_s=[0.5,5.4] and P_f=[6.5,6.5] are selected, first the polytope A and polytope D will be selected as S_1 and S_q. Then connections are identified and stored as a list with n lists each corresponding to each polytope, n being the number of polytopes $\mathbb{C} = [\mathbb{C}_A, \mathbb{C}_B, \mathbb{C}_C, \mathbb{C}_D]$. One connection corresponding to polytope A is given as below:

$$\mathbb{C}_A = \left[\left[A \cap A \right], \left[A \cap B \right], \left[A \cap C \right], \left[A \cap D \right] \right]$$

$$\mathbb{C}_A = \left[\underbrace{\left[[0,7], [2,6], [1,5], [0,5] \right]}_{len=4,\ index=0}, \underbrace{\left[[0,7], [2,6] \right]}_{len=2,\ index=1}, \right.$$

$$\left. \underbrace{[\ ]}_{len=0,\ index=2}, \underbrace{[\ ]}_{len=0,\ index=3} \right]$$

The list $\mathbb{C}_A$ shows the connection corresponding to polytope A. The terms *len*, *index* defines the length of the list and index of list in terms of programming language(python index starts from 0) respectively. In the list $\mathbb{C}_A$ the first list contains the common vertices of $A \cap A$ i.e all four vertices of A therefore the length is 4. The second list in $\mathbb{C}_A$ is $A \cap B$ i.e a list of two common vertices of A and B. The third list is $A \cap C$ which is an empty list suggesting that there are no common vertices. From this *len* information it can be easily determined whether two polytopes share exactly two edges. In the next step the indices of the list where *len=2* are extracted.

A graph can be created using this adjacency information which will be used to find the sequence. Sample graph

representation of the example given above is given as:

$$graph = \{0 : [1], \qquad\qquad = \{A : [B],$$
$$\qquad\quad 1 : [0,2,3], \qquad\qquad B : [A,C,D],$$
$$\qquad\quad 2 : [1,3], \qquad\qquad\quad C : [B,D],$$
$$\qquad\quad 3 : [2,1]\} \qquad\qquad D : [C,B]\}$$

Remark 1: For illustration purposes alphabets are used for labeling the polytopes. But actual graph would consist of the indices(of type int) as mentioned above.

Then the sequence of polytopes(plotted in green) making a possible way between S_1 and S_q (where q = 3 for number of polytopes in the sequence) is obtained in the form of indices (c.f. Remark 1) $[S_1, S_2, S_3] = [0,1.3]$= [A,B,D] by a standard graph search using the graph mentioned above. The lines plotted in orange and blue represent the shared edge as in (3) between A,B and B,D respectively.

3 Results and toolbox

The toolbox *Navigation with polytopes*[1] will be introduced in this section, along with the validation results for the aforementioned methods.Implementations of the algorithms discussed in the previous section, along with the reference path planning algorithms using B-spline curves from [1, 2] are made publicly available and maintained as *Navigation with polytopes*[1] toolbox. The toolbox can be used as a global path planner and is also compatible with ROS navigation tools. It provides a framework for the construction of a polytope map from a standard occupancy grid map, searching for an appropriate sequence of polytopes and finally planning a minimal-length path with different options on B-spline or Bézier characterizations. The repository can be further used for different research purposes.

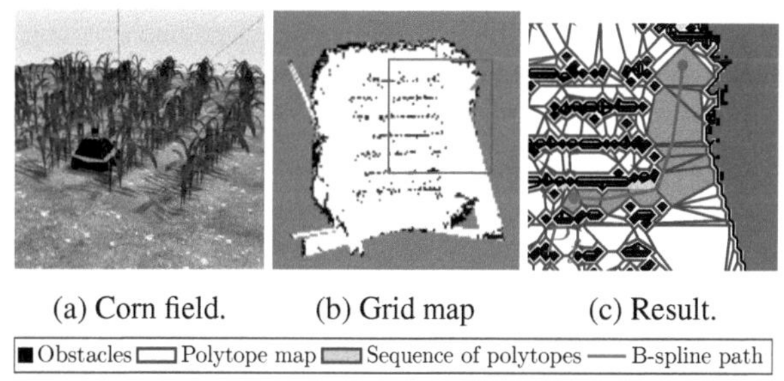

Figure 4: Figure depicting the corn field gazebo simulation, the grid map of the same field, and the sequence algorithm results plotted on a portion of the grid map (highlighted in red).

The algorithms discussed above are validated on a grid map shown in Fig. 4b obtained from a corn field simulation provided by Field Robot Event (FRE)[7] shown in Fig. 4a using ROS Gmapping package [7]. Fig. 4c illustrates the whole process where blue plot represents the polytope map

[7] https://github.com/FieldRobotEvent/virtual_maize_field

obatined using the steps mentioned in Section.2.2. For a given start(P_s) and final points(P_f) a sequence of polytopes (plotted in green) is obtained by using the approach mentioned in Section. 2.3. A path (plotted in red) can then be planned using path planning tools from the toolbox *Navigation with polytopes*[1].

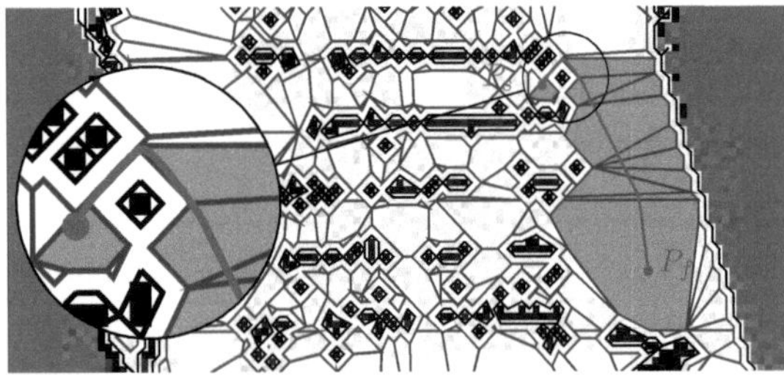

(a) Result of sequence neglecting robot size.

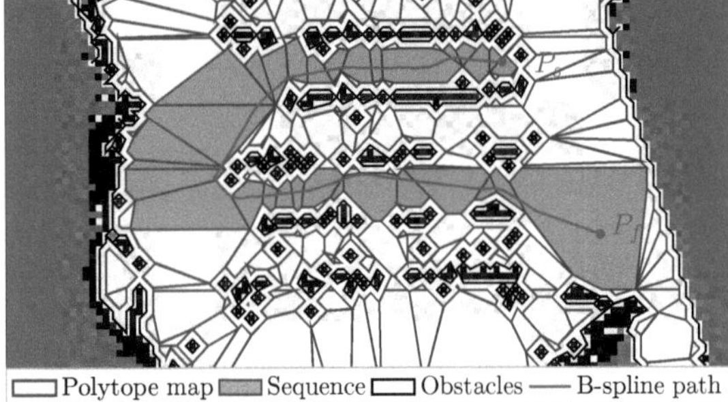

(b) Result of sequence considering robot size.

Figure 5: The sequence of polytopes depicting an infeasible path and its improvement after taking the robot's size into account illustrates the problem of robot size.

Agricultural fields are a very complex scenario for mapping due to several factors like surface unevenness, etc. The grid map of the field map is complex due to many individual obstacles (crops) in the field; likewise, the polytope map created is also very complex and contains very small polytopes possibly formed between two small, close obstacles. This type of problem can be seen in Fig. 5a, The result of just using the approach for sequence mentioned in Section 2.3 always tries to minimize length, but in this particular scenario (enlarged plot), the path planned is not feasible for the robot to move through. One way to solve this problem is to impose a constraint on the edge of the polytope to be greater or equal to the size of the robot (assuming a rectangular boundary that fits the robot) and that would result in a sequence as shown in Fig. 5b. Even though this sequence is not optimal, it is a safe path for the robot to move through.

4 Conclusion

In this work, an alternate line of research for mapping the environment using continuous maps is studied. The polytope map used in [1, 2] is one such continuous map that has been extensively studied and implemented for complex environments such as agricultural fields. A graph search-based approach is proposed to find a sequence of polytopes between two chosen polytopes in the polytope map for nav-

igation, ensuring a safe area for a robot to maneuver. A solution for preventing narrow passages within the polytope map is proposed that takes the robot's size into account to impose a constraint on the size of an edge of the polytope. Furthermore, the toolbox with all the implementations is integrated into ROS to be used as a global path planner. Future research will concentrate on improving sequence finding by accounting for the entire dimensions of the robot and adding a local planner and controller to the toolbox.

Acknowledgement

The work has been carried out at Institute for Robotics and Cognitive Systems, Universität zu Lübeck.

Author's Statement

Conflict of interest: Authors state no conflict of interest.

5 References

[1] N. T. Nguyen, P. T. Gangavarapu, A. Sahrhage, G. Schildbach, and F. Ernst, "Navigation with polytopes and b-spline path planner," *accepted for presentation and publication at 2023 IEEE International Conference on Robotics and Automation (ICRA), London, UK, 29 May – 2 June 2023.*

[2] N. T. Nguyen, L. Schilling, M. S. Angern, H. Hamann, F. Ernst, and G. Schildbach, "B-spline path planner for safe navigation of mobile robots," in *2021 IEEE/RSJ International Conference on Intelligent Robots and Systems (IROS)*. IEEE, 2021, pp. 339–345.

[3] P. Raja and S. Pugazhenthi, "Optimal path planning of mobile robots: A review," *International Journal of Physical Sciences*, vol. 7, no. 9, pp. 1314–1320, 2012.

[4] J. R. Sánchez-Ibáñez, C. J. Pérez-del Pulgar, and A. García-Cerezo, "Path planning for autonomous mobile robots: A review," *Sensors*, vol. 21, no. 23, 2021. [Online]. Available: https://www.mdpi.com/1424-8220/21/23/7898

[5] H.-y. Zhang, W.-m. Lin, and A.-x. Chen, "Path planning for the mobile robot: A review," *Symmetry*, vol. 10, no. 10, 2018. [Online]. Available: https://www.mdpi.com/2073-8994/10/10/450

[6] D. H. Douglas and T. K. Peucker, "Algorithms for the reduction of the number of points required to represent a digitized line or its caricature," *Cartographica: the international Journal for Geographic Information and Geovisualization*, vol. 10, no. 2, pp. 112–122, 1973.

[7] G. Grisetti, C. Stachniss, and W. Burgard, "Improved techniques for grid mapping with rao-blackwellized particle filters," *IEEE Transactions on Robotics*, vol. 23, no. 1, pp. 34–46, 2007.

13

Biomedical Optics

Image stitching of high-resolution optical coherence tomography en-face projections with an intensity-based and a feature-based approach

Gerrit Meußler [1], Hendrik Spahr [2], Timo Kepp [3], Léo Puyo [2], Clara Pfäffle [2], Jonas Franke [2] and Gereon Hüttmann [2, 4]

[1] Medical Engineering Science, Universität zu Lübeck, gerrit.meussler@student.uni-luebeck.de
[2] Universität zu Lübeck, Institute of Biomedical Optics, Center of Brain, Behavior and Metabolism,
    {he.spahr, leo.puyo, cl.pfaeffle, jon.franke and gereon.huettmann}@uni-luebeck.de
[3] Universität zu Lübeck, Institute of Medical Informatics, timo.kepp@uni-luebeck.de
[4] Medical Laser Center Lübeck GmbH

Abstract

Optical coherence tomography (OCT) is a non-invasive imaging technique, which is used to create 2D cross-sectional and 3D volume information of the retina. OCT systems that are currently in clinical use have high enough resolution to visualize photoreceptors in the retina. However, due to technical limitations, high-resolution imaging of the retina comes with the draw back of only imaging a very small field of view. We created a registration algorithm that stitches multiple en-face images of the retina together to create a high-resolution image with a larger field of view. The current algorithm only uses en-face projections, however we are able to restore the volumetric data after the computation. Here we compare a feature-based and an intensity-based image registration approach.

1 Introduction

Image registration is an important component for image analysis if valuable information is conveyed in more than one image [1]. A larger field of view combined with higher resolution could provide better detection of potential diseases and better treatment options.

The same applies in ophthalmology to OCT images of the retina, such as those obtained with the Heidelberg Engineering Spectralis OCT. Due to a technical limitation, it is not possible to acquire a large field of view with high resolution (i.e., densely scanned) with this device. Instead, a compromise between field of view and resolution must always be made. For certain applications, such as digital aberration correction, dense scanning of the retina is mandatory, which consequently severely limits the field of view. In order to still acquire high-resolution images over a large area of the retina, the complex volumetric OCT data must be acquired sequentially in small tiles and then be stitched together numerically. Several shorter measurements can also be beneficial for artifact reduction, as voluntary eye motions do not have to be suppressed for so long at a stretch, which would otherwise lead to motion artifacts.

For real-valued 2D data sets (i.e. classical images), a variety of existing tools and plugins for example for Matlab or ImageJ can be used. Since these are not applicable to complex-valued volumetric data, own algorithms were developed and evaluated in the context of this work.

2 Material and Methods

Registration methods that are based on pixel or voxel intensity are commonly known as *intensity-based approaches*, while those based on geometrical structures extracted from the image are known as *feature-based approaches* [2], [3]. Feature-based approaches typically provide excellent performance if there are sufficient reliable features in the images. In sparsely structured images or in images in which features cannot be reliably obtained intensity-based approaches might be the better alternative [2].

Since in [4] the image registration was done successfully with a feature-based approach, using the features extracted from retinal vessels, the assumption was, that the vessels found in the en-face projections would carry enough features to ensure a successful image registration. However, if the vessels do not carry enough features, because there are too few vessels or because the signal-to-noise ratio (SNR) is poor, intensity-based image alignment methods may be better suited for the task [2]. Prior to this work the phase correlation algorithm was used several times for correction of eye motion in our group. In comparison to the image registration in [4] the phase correlation algorithm does not use features in the registration process, instead it uses voxel intensity for image registration [2]. As both approaches are theoretically applicable to the task, the aim of this work was to find out which one leads to a better result. Thus, both algorithms were implemented and tested in Python.

2.1 Theory of the intensity-based approach

Our intensity-based algorithm uses a phase correlation for the image registration. The idea to use a phase correlation for image registration is based on the assumption that two images $I_i(\mathbf{x})$ and $I_j(\mathbf{x})$ contain nearly the same information except that $I_j(\mathbf{x})$ is shifted by $\Delta\mathbf{x}_{i,j}$, i.e. $I_j(\mathbf{x}) \approx I_i(\mathbf{x} - \Delta\mathbf{x}_{i,j})$. According to the Fourier-shift theorem, followed by the convolution theorem, the cross-correlation spectrum of both images $\tilde{\Gamma}_{cc}(\Delta\mathbf{x})$ can be calculated from the Fourier transforms $I_i(\mathbf{x})$ and $I_j(\mathbf{x})$ of the images [5]:

$$\tilde{\Gamma}_{cc}(\Delta\mathbf{x}) = \tilde{I}_i(\mathbf{k}) \cdot \tilde{I}_j(\mathbf{k})^* \approx |\tilde{I}_i(\mathbf{k})|^2 exp(-i\mathbf{k} \cdot \Delta\mathbf{x}_{i,j}). \quad (1)$$

Transforming the cross-correlation spectrum in (1) back into the spatial domain results in a delta peak $\delta(\mathbf{x} - \Delta\mathbf{x}_{i,j})$ folded with a point spread function (PSF), which is determined by the intensity of the spectrum $|\tilde{I}_i(\mathbf{k})|^2$ [6]. Since the intensity of the spectrum does not contain any information about the shift itself, this part of the cross-correlation is removed by a normalization in the frequency domain [5]:

$$\tilde{\Gamma}_{pcc}(\mathbf{k}) = \frac{\tilde{I}_i(\mathbf{k}) \cdot \tilde{I}_j(\mathbf{k})^*}{|\tilde{I}_i(\mathbf{k}) \cdot \tilde{I}_j(\mathbf{k})^*|} \approx exp(-i\mathbf{k} \cdot \Delta\mathbf{x}_{i,j}). \quad (2)$$

The correlation seen in (2) is called phase correlation, since only the phase of the cross correlation is remaining. The back transformation into position space of this phase can be used to correct the position of the two images in relation to each other. After the general registration with the phase correlation and the first correction step, which only involved a translation of one image towards the other, we did a non-rigid registration again based on a phase correlation.

For the non-rigid registration we performed the phase correlation on a grid of rectangular tiles of the image that only contain parts of the whole image. The non-rigid registration adds a certain amount of non-linearity which was necessary because of scanning aberrations and optical distortions of the OCT-system [5].

2.2 Theory of the feature-based approach

The feature-based algorithm implemented here uses the scale invariant feature transform (SIFT) algorithm for image registration. As a first step the scale-space image $L(\mathbf{x}, \sigma)$ is created by a convolution of the image $I(\mathbf{x})$ with a Gaussian function, with σ being a parameter used in the Gaussian function to define the width of the function. In the next step multiple Difference of Gaussian (DoG) images are computed by repeatedly taking the difference between scale-space images convolved with Gaussian functions with different k factors and the original scale-space image, as follows [7], [8]:

$$D(\mathbf{x}, \sigma) = L(\mathbf{x}, k\sigma) - L(\mathbf{x}, \sigma). \quad (3)$$

Each resulting image is down-sampled and this process is repeated. The extrema of the resulting images are detected by comparing the pixel values to its neighbours. Some of these candidate keypoints are removed by being classified as unstable. Unstable means that these extreme values are lower than a defined minimum contrast difference. In the next step a principal orientation is assigned to each keypoint location based on the directions of the local image gradients. To handle illumination differences information of neighbouring pixels is also used [7].

The keypoints found by SIFT are constant regarding scaling, rotation and intensity differences [8]. After the extraction of the SIFT interest points in the two overlapping images, the keypoints need to be matched. The matching is done via identifying the nearest neighbour from each keypoint descriptor based on Euclidean distance [7].

2.3 Preprocessing

A proper preprocessing, i.e. an adjustment of contrast, had a major impact on the performance of both algorithms. In fact both algorithms were not able to stitch images together without the adjustment of contrast, even though the images had an overlapping area of up to 90% and regions with big vessels which are typically rich of features to extract. Currently the preprocessing contains an adjustment of contrast of the images for both algorithms.

The preprocessing of the input images is an internal process, the stitching result only show the original images.

2.4 Image blending

Image blending is a process of blending the information of one image with a second image to generate a seamless image. Seams in stitching can be a result of general intensity differences in the images [9]. We use image blending at the overlapping area of the images. We use a 2D linear blending mask so that the information in the resulting image at the overlapping area is a combination of both images.

2.5 Data acquisition

The image data, which we used to generate the en-face projections, were taken from two different volunteers. All images were acquired with the Spectralis OCT from Heidelberg Engineering. The captured volumes were corrected by several correction algorithms to remove motion artifacts and encounter the curvature of the retina. These corrected volumes are used to extract the en-face projections. However, these projections are not free of artifacts. Common artifacts are black stripes from the left to the right and very bright areas at the edges of the projections, caused by motion of the patients retina during the measurement. The original en-face projections had a size of 1476x934 pixels. The size of the stitching result depends on the number of stitched images and the overlap area of the original en-face projections.

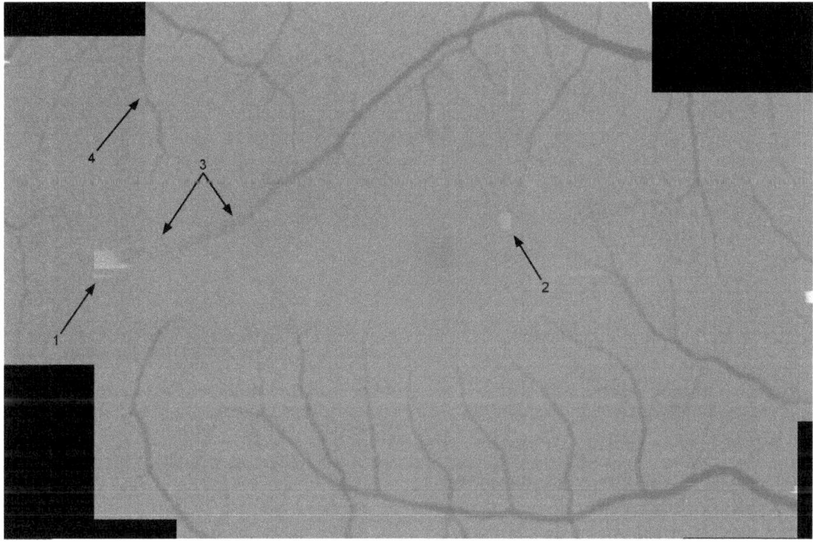

Figure 1: Stitching result from the intensity-based algorithm with movement artifacts at arrow 1 and 2, blurring at arrow 3 and seams at arrow 4. The final result consists of six individual partly overlapping en-face projections of one of the patients retinas.

3 Results and Discussion

3.1 The intensity-based algorithm

Fig. 1 shows the result of the intensity-based algorithm. The result consists of en-face projections of six individually taken, partly overlapping retinal OCT datasets. In Fig. 2 a scanning laser ophthalmoscope (SLO) image of a retina is shown. The presented section of the retina is roughly the same area section from which most of the en-face projections that were stitched in Fig. 1 originated from. Comparing Fig. 1 with Fig. 2 one can see that the stitching result resembles the vessel pattern of the SLO image. Comparing the vessel structure one might argue that the general stitching attempt was successful, in a sense that the general structure of the patients retina could be reconstructed and the field of view was expanded. The result of the intensity-based algorithm had a size of 2367x1527 pixels. The field of view has been increased by a factor of more than 2.5.

The very bright, white rectangles in Fig. 1, marked by arrow 1 and 2 are not fully corrected artifacts. Arrow 3 shows an imperfect matched vessel. Visible seams at which two or more images were connected are marked by arrow 4.

Besides these problems the intensity-based algorithm is quite tolerant regarding artifacts, as long as the overlapping area is big enough. Since every individual en-face image suffers from artifacts and from noise, these image artifacts sum up over multiple stitching processes. Especially areas that occur on several images blurred out due to imperfect registration and the summation of noise. The reason is that if the registration is not perfectly accurate vessels and photoreceptors are corrected to a slightly wrong position, leading to a blurring effect of edges. Nonetheless this algorithm was capable of stitching several individually taken en-face projections together in a row.

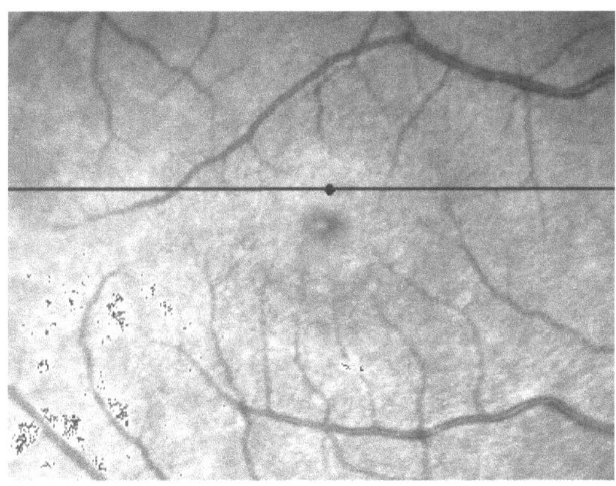

Figure 2: SLO image of one the volunteers retinas. The visible section of the retina is roughly the section from which most of the en-face projection originate from.

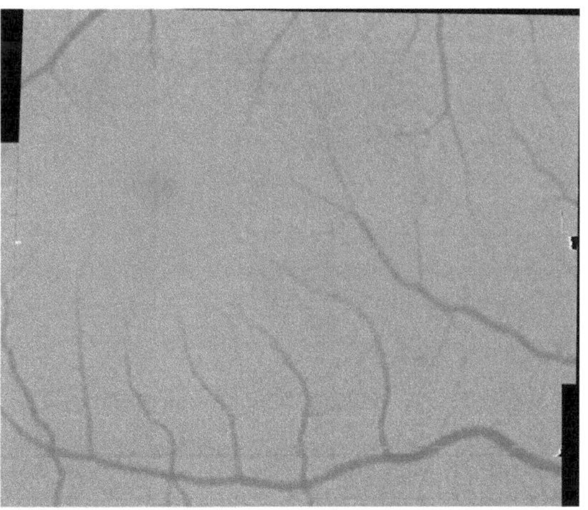

Figure 3: Stitching result from the feature-based algorithm. This image consist of two partly overlapping en-face projections.

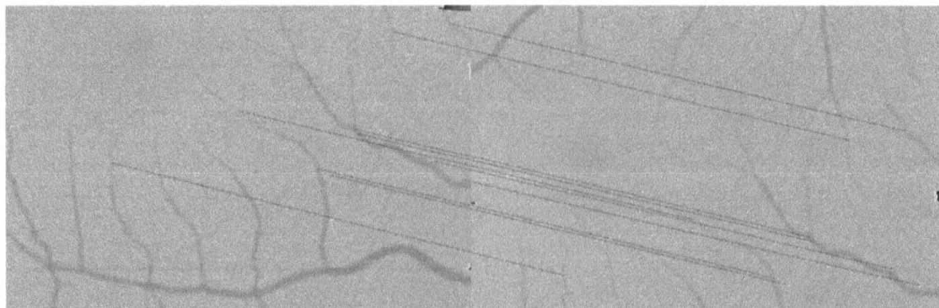

Figure 4: The two en-face projections side by side. The black lines between certain distinct points indicate the matched keypoints found by the SIFT algorithm.

3.2   The feature-based algorithm

Stitching results of two en-face projections generated with the feature-based algorithm can be seen in Fig. 3. In Fig. 4 the keypoint matches that were used in Fig. 3 can be seen. The keypoints are mostly between pixels at the edge or at least near bigger vessel structures. Comparing the image from Fig. 2 and the result of the feature-based algorithm in Fig. 3, it can be stated that the feature-based algorithm may also yield reasonable results. Images that lack collective features can not be stitched together, which is particularly problematic for the images we have taken, because there are no bigger vessels in the avascular zone around the makula. Also the motion artifacts seem to be a major problem for the feature-based algorithm, since artifacts tend to have similar characteristics as keypoints. For the feature-based algorithm one incorrectly matched keypoint could mean that two en-face projections are not stitchable. The summation of noise and artifacts due to stitching of multiple images in a row seem to be a bigger problem for this algorithm than for the intensity-based algorithm.

4   Conclusion

One intensity-based and one feature-based registration algorithms were implemented and their suitability for stitching complex OCT volumes was evaluated. In order to be able to apply existing algorithms such as a phase correlation or SIFT to this problem, the 3D data sets were first reduced to 2D image data by an en-face projection. After appropriate preprocessing of the data, the two registration algorithms were applied to the en-face datasets. Subsequently, the data sets were shifted accordingly and combined by linear blending. So far, the results have been evaluated purely qualitatively by visual inspection. The next step will be an objective, quantitative evaluation that assesses the performance of the different algorithms using manually set landmarks. Subsequently, the most suitable algorithm will be extended to be able to register and stitch 3D data sets as well.

Acknowledgement

This work has been carried out at the Center for Brain, Behavior and Metabolism and was supervised by the Institute of Biomedical Optics, Universität zu Lübeck. This work was funded by the Bundesministerium für Bildung und Forschung (13N15432) and Deutsche Forschungsgemeinschaft (HU 629-6-2).

Author's Statement

Authors state no conflict of interest.

5   References

[1] F. Oliveira and J. Tavares, *Medical image registration: A review*, Computer Methods in Biomechanics and Biomedical Engineering, pp. 73–93, 2014.

[2] G. Meneghetti, M. Danelljan, M. Felsberg and K. Nordberg *Image Alignment for Panorama Stitching in Sparsely Structured Environments*, Image Analysis, pp. 428–439, 2015.

[3] Z. Hossein-Nejad, H. Agahi and A. Mahmoodzadeh, *Image matching based on the adaptive redundant keypoint elimination method in the SIFT algorithm*, Pattern Analysis and Applications, pp. 669–683, 2020.

[4] R. Ramli, K. Hasikin, M. Idris, N. Karim and A. Wahab, *Fundus Image Registration Technique Based on Local Feature of Retinal Vessels*, Applied Sciences, 2021.

[5] C. Pfäffle, *Functional Imaging of Retinal Neurons*, Promotion at University of Lübeck, Lübeck, pp. 55–63, 2022.

[6] A. Eckstein, *Phase correlation processing for DPIV measurements*, Experiments in Fluids, pp. 485–500, 2008.

[7] A. Sima and S. Buckley, *Optimizing SIFT for Matching of Short Wave Infrared and Visible Wavelength Images*, Remote Sensing, pp. 2037–2056, 2013.

[8] H. Alberry, A. Hegazy, and G. Salama, *A fast SIFT based method for copy move forgery detection*, Future Computing and Informatics Journal, pp. 159–165, 2018.

[9] A. Zomet, A. Levin, S. Peleg and Y. Weiss, *Seamless image stitching by minimizing false edges*, IEEE Transactions on Image Processing, pp. 969–977, 2006.

Identification and Classification of Production-related Processing Defects in Welds in a Novel Large-format LASER Contour Welding Process for Multilayer Polymer Film Material

Justus Klinkforth [1], Michael Ahrens [2]

[1]Medical Engineering, Universität zu Lübeck, justus.klinkforth@student.uni-luebeck.de

[2] SURGITENT GmbH, ahrens@surgitent.com

Abstract

Scope of this project work, is the identification of methods for the improved detection and classification of defects in laser-induced welded on foils was accomplished. A wide variety of intended defects or deviations from the optimum weld seam due to different weld seam configurations were manufactured as test samples. These were tested for structural integrity according to the respective product standard using destructive testing methods. To reduce the loss of products and material costs, various imaging methods have been tested for the visualization of the welds and their defects. With additional information and further image processing steps, these should supplement or even replace the quality inspection. It turned out that the differential interference contrast provided the best results and the most practicable solution, to provided high resolution information about the weld seams.

1 Introduction

The quality analysis of polymer film and the control of sufficiently welded seams on multi-layer film is an essential part of the production of a number of medical devices. Therefore, it is necessary to prove and ensure a comprehensive, continuous quality assurance from the production of the extruded film material to the finished product. In the medical sector, heat-sealed films are used in a wide variety of applications. These include sterile packaging, infusion bags and storage technology. If the medical film meets the requirements, the welded seam is the final protective mechanism that prevents the penetration of micro-bacterial pathogens, viruses or particles. Contamination can have serious consequences for the patient or user. There are a number of guidelines and standards that ensure controlled quality assurance in medical technology. As a reference for this work, limit values and test methods of the standard EN ISO 13938-1 and EN 29073-3, which are summarized in EN13795, were used. These standards define applicable test methods, such as load capacity under tensile force or bursting pressure tests with the minimal values which have to be achieved. The methods require destructive testing of the welds and the product, which means an increased expenditure of raw materials and time.

At present, automated testing equipment is already in use in the production of film material, which very successfully detects control deviations in the manufacturing requirements and logs and evaluates them [1]. Transmittance or reflection measurements in bright or dark field configurations are used among others [1]. These techniques have been developed especially for flat films, tubular films or blown films with regular patterns and geometries [1]. Established testing is currently not suited to incorporate control of individual features such as freely defined welding patterns which in addition often have the side effects of wrinkling and shrinkage. However, other methods have also been tested which are not directly related to medical products, but which can be transferred to the problem of this paper. Among others, J.T. Johnson [2] lists real-time transmission densitometry, which can be used to determine film thickness via optical density. Cameras and image post-processing techniques, such as quantitative and statistical tools or neural networks and fuzzy logic, are used to acquire and post-process the data.

A similar technique also uses transmitted light, to detect defects in the form, inhomogeneities and holes [3]. If the film is homogeneously flat, the light will shine through material approximately unobstructed. This intensity was established as the baseline of the measurement data. Only in the case of defects such as inhomegineities is light increasingly scattered, resulting in a decrease in intensity at the detector. In the case of holes, a higher intensity is measured. This clear separation of events made it possible to identify whether and which types of defects were detected by simple threshold holding in the measurement data [3]. Among other things, the information content of optical coherence tomography (OCT) images was also assessed [4]. Measurements were performed on radiographic welded film samples. It was recognized that OCT is a potent imaging method to detect weld width, weld boundary representation, defects (air bubbles) and porosity in high resolution [4]. For samples of width 5 cm and length 20 cm, a full 3D scan was generated within 25 s. Similar results were also obtained by Shirazi et al. [5]. They checked for defect imageability via OCT volume images on LCD-like thin films. Here, it was particularly pointed out that even with good resolution, alignment of OCT optics is a critical factor. It was observed that under incorrect angles, strong reflections occurred and these produced double to multiple images in the images. Here, samples of a size 8x14 cm were measured within 38 s [5].

Other test methods such as measuring with terahertz radiation [6] or ultrasound [6], laser profilometry [2] or imaging with structured illumination [7] offer potential for detecting welds and defects, but were not reviewed within the scope of this work.

2 Material and Methods

For the selection of a potent method for the visualization of welded multi-layer films, potential methods were tested for their ability to detect welds and defects with their dimensions. The results were then compared with the outcome data of destructive tests (tensile force, burst pressure measurement). Requirements for the methods such as non-contact, fast measurement or imaging or displayability of the weld seams for highly transparent multi layer films and were selected by a literature research. The identified test methods included transmission measurements, OCT imaging and microscopic imaging in bright field configuration. In addition, the performance of phase contrast imaging and microscopic imaging with polarized light was tested on transparent films. For the tests, two types of films have been manufactured in two or three layers. Welding parameters were continuously adjusted to deliberately produce high, medium and low quality welds. Thus, 11 specimens were produced per film constellation, so that a total of 44 specimens were available for testing on the selected methods. In addition, for each specimen type, a portion of the weld seam was used for the evaluations of the tensile force and burst pressure measurements. In the case of three-ply welded films, the weld was tested between the top two films and with an additional sample between the bottom two films. This resulted in a total sample count of 176.

A Lambda 14 UV-VIS spectrophotometer (PerkinElmer LAS GmbH, Rodgau, Germany) was used for transmission measurement. For each type of foil, one layer was measured in the spectrum from 190 - 1100 nm. For this purpose, an insert with an integrating sphere was used to capture any light from the sample. The optical density D was caculated by the negative decadic logarithm of the transmissivity T_t which was calculated from the zero measurement of the light source ϕ_e and the transmitted light ϕ_i from the sample [2].

$$D = -log_{10}(T_t) = -log_{10}(\frac{\phi_e}{\phi_i}) \tag{1}$$

Two devices with different resolutions were used for OCT imaging Telesto® Series Spectral Domain OCT Imaging System and Ganymede Series Spectral Domain OCT Imaging System (Thorlabs GmbH, Bergkirchen, Germany) which had a central wavelength of 1300 nm and 930 nm respectively. Data acquisition and evaluation was done with ThorImage (Thorlabs, Bergkirchen, Germany) In the generated images, all detectable relevant structures such as weld width, defect size and irregularities were measured using the software's measurement tools. For each sample, the varying weld properties required the alignment to be changed to prevent imaging errors such as multiple images. A scan rate of 28 kHz and an A-scan average of 7 were used to provide a medium sensitivity. If the sensitivity was too high, artifacts were significantly increased due to strong reflections at the foil surfaces.

The ECLIPSE Ti microscope (Nikon Europe B.V. GmbH, Amstelveen, Netherlands) was used for imaging via bright field illumination. The Nis Elements program was used to control the microscope and acquire images. In order to display an area of the weld as large as possible on one image, serial images were combined to form an overall view. A lens with a magnification of 2 was used to display the weld seams, as well as an auto shutter to automatically adjust the exposure. The Nikon LWD 0.52 condenser module was used to select the aperture for exposure, such as a round aperture diaphragm for the brightfield images, or a ring aperture for phase contrast. On the condenser there is also a sliding element which can be used to select whether to image with a polarized or unpolarized light. For this series of experiments, imaging methods such as phase contrast, differential interference contrast (DIC), and pure brightfield illumination were examined. With sufficient image information, weld seams and defects were measured using a measuring tool from Nis Elements and compared with the measured values of the OCT images.

To make a valid statement about the real integrity of the weld seams, tensile force and burst pressure measurements have been performed. An FMT-310 (PPT GmbH & Co KG, t/a Alluris, Freiburg, Germany) was used for tensile force measurements and an Industrial seam testing station (PFAFF Industriesysteme und Maschinen GmbH, Kaiserslautern, Germany) was used to determine the burst pressure.

3 Results and Discussion

From the measurements, it became apparent that no relevant information about the film welds could be determined with the transmission measurement. The maximum overall optical density for both film types was 0.03842. It was suspected that there might be increased absorption outside the visible spectrum in the near infrared range. It was evident from the measurement data that only a slight increase in optical density prevailed with decrease in wavelength. Just fine differences for high transparent films cannot be detected with such a method.

In contrast, very good results could be achieved with OCT imaging. As shown in Fig.1, the weld seams are clearly visible. There are clear structures that can be assigned to the weld seam. Depending on the energy input into the film, elevations at the edges were also visible. Defects with the same cause were also clearly identifiable as bubbles and measurable by the images. It also turned out that the size of the defects (length and width) was not related to the depth of the bubbles in the films. The lower the applied welding power in the material, the smoother the welds were at the edge areas and the fewer defects were seen. In addition the width of the weld decreased as the absorbed energy decreased in width. In particular, limits were identified for three layers of the films where complete welding failed to occur.

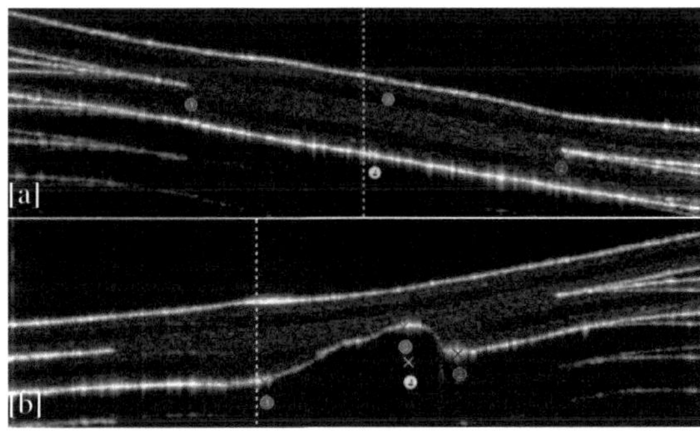

Figure 1: OCT can be used to image good [a] as well as welds with defects [b]. The colored markers and dashed line indicate the location for measurements of the weld seam. These are not relevant for this display.

Nevertheless, limits for imaging by OCT exist. Strong reflections at the interfaces between air and film material caused massive artifacts in some cases. Due to the highly variable geometries resulting from the shrinkage of the film, a clear image could only be generated after multiple adjustments. As already stated by K. Kim et al. [4] and M. Shirazi et al. [5], the evaluation of the data in 3D is very time-consuming, which is why volume images can not be generated in a reasonable time using this method.
When evaluating the results and generating images, it was clear that images of the welds cannot be generated using only bright field illumination. Even with different exposure times and reduction of the intensity of the light, it was only dimly recognizable that there was a change from non-welded to welded film. In contrast, in the images from the DIC as in Fig. 2 and phase contrast imaging as in Fig. 3, the welds can be seen in great detail. For the DIC images, the polarizer was rotated approximately $+10\,^\circ$, which allowed the contrast to be clearly detected due to path differences and birefringence of the material, from welded to non-welded film. The exact breakdown of the physical effects that led to this contrast were not investigated.
In the images, it was possible to identify not only the width of the weld seam, but also the concomitant effects of welding and defects (bubbles) of various sizes. In addition, it was noticed that with decreasing absorbed energy, not only the width of the weld decreased, but also the clear edges at the boundaries of the weld decreased. In addition, an increased variance in the width of the weld was noted.
In the images from phase contrast imaging, the weld seams could also be well visualized. Here, contours became visi-

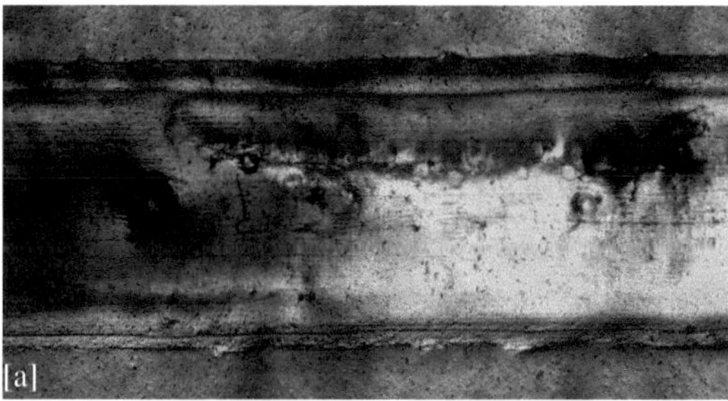
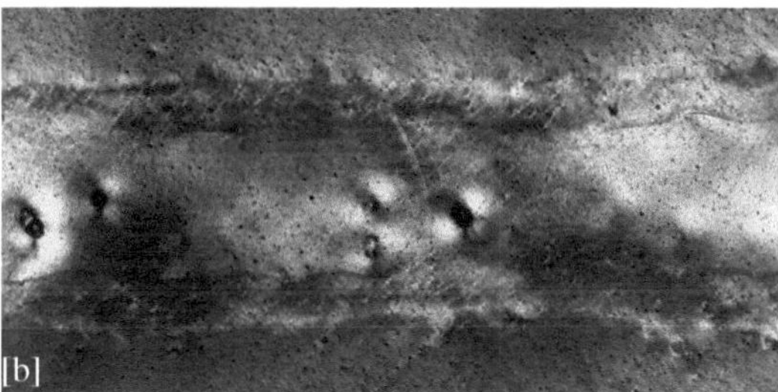

Figure 2: By DIC imaging a good contrast for identification of a good [a] and a bad weld [b] is created.

ble, in particular, due to the marking of the edges of the suture. The areas inside and outside the seams had the same appearance. In contrast to the images from DIC imaging, only defects that were more pronounced were visible in phase contrast. Basically, a kind of filtering of the extent of a defect would be possible via this method.

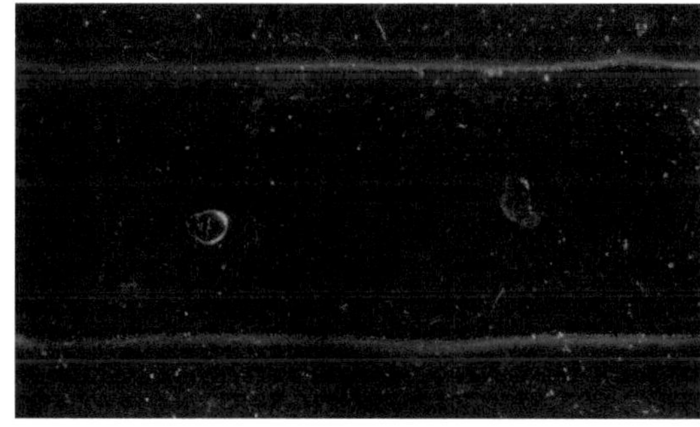

Figure 3: Weld edges and larger defects stand out brightly in phase contrast imaging.

In addition, it was noticed that with decreasing absorbed energy in the weld seams, in some cases the contours were not shown in the phase contrast display. This could be an indicator of a poor weld joint. Also, small bright spots were increasingly visible in the images. These are probably due to particle contamination of the film.
From the weld seam width data of the OCT and microscopic images, it was evident that there were only small deviations in the measured widths. Therefore, the measurements from the OCT and microscopic images were averaged for the representation of the seams width. These were plotted against the maximum tensile forces and burst pressures achieved in each case as Fig. 4 shows. In this figure, the results for both film types welded in two layers are shown. It can be seen that for the bursting pressure, as well as the tensile force,

the seam width for film type 1 above 800 μm shows a little difference in the integrity of the seam. Only below 800 μm does the strength of the welded joint decrease. Such a limit can also be seen for film type 2. Below a width of 1600 μm, the values drop sharply. For both films, the values belong to the worst settings of the laser for welding. There was not enough data available on these created measurements to cover the blind area to represent the transition from a good weld to a poor weld more accurately. These results only represent the integrity in terms of acting forces between the foils. For the general condition of the weld seams, the information from the images generated by the different methods has to be added.

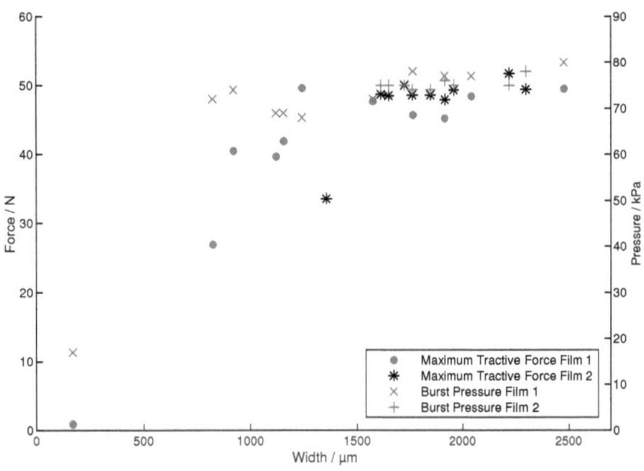

Figure 4: Context of measured weld seam widths, maximum tractive forces and burst pressures

From the results of the standard measurement procedures, it is now possible to define limits at which the weld seams meet the requirements of quality via width, appearance of the seam edges and defects.

4 Conclusion

From the achieved results, it is possible to image weld seams with high contrast, especially with DIC imaging, and that quality statement. It has been shown that different weld configurations can also be identified in the images of the welds and therefore can also be assessed in terms of their structural integrity.

This also applies to phase contrast imaging. Nevertheless, there are limitations with regards to the imageability of the various contours. Imaging via OCT devices are also suitable for imaging weld seams as well as defects, but are not practical for large areas due to the long scan time. No added value could be achieved from transmission measurement.

For future projects, collecting more data for each type of weld seam, should yield better comparative values to determine the statistics. With further image processing tools, automated evaluation of the images in the production process should also be possible.

Acknowledgement

The work was carried out by SURGITENT GmbH and supervised by the Institute of Biomedical Optics at the Universität zu Lübeck.

Author's Statement

Conflict of interest: J.K. and M.A. are employees of SURGITENT GmbH

5 References

[1] OCS Optical Control Systems GmbH. (2020, May) Bahninspektionssystem (FSP600). Company website. OCS Optical Control Systems GmbH. Wullener Feld 24, 58454 Witten, Germany. Last access: 28.01.2023. [Online]. Available: https://www.ocsgmbh.com/produkte/bahninspektionssystem-fsp600/

[2] J. T. Johnson, "Defect and Thickness Inspection System for Cast Thin Films Using Machine Vision ans Full-Fieldtransmission Densitometry," masters thesis, School of George W. Woodruff School of Mechanical Engineering, 2009.

[3] R. K. Krishnaswamy and J. D. Stark, "Continous Inspection of Optical Defects in Packaging Films," *Journal of Plastic Film and Sheeting*, vol. 16, no. 1, pp. 43–53, 2000.

[4] K. Kim, P. Kim, J. Lee, S. Kim, S. Park, S. H. Choi, J. Hwang, J. H. Lee, H. Lee, R. E. Wijesinghe, M. Jeon, and J. Kim, "Non-Destructive Identification of Weld-Boundary and Porosity Formation During Laser Transmission Welding by Using Optical Coherence Tomography," *IEEE Access*, vol. 6, pp. 76 768–76 775, 2018.

[5] M. Shirazi, K. Park, R. Wijesinghe, H. Jeong, S. Han, P. Kim, M. Jeon, and J. Kim, "Fast Industrial Inspection of Optical Thin Film Using Optical Coherence Tomography," *Sensors*, vol. 16, p. 1598, 2016.

[6] Y. Morita, A. Dobroiu, C. Otani, and K. Kawase, "A Real-Time Inspection System Using a Terahertz Technique to Detect Microleak Defects in the Seal of Flexible Plastic Packages," *Journal of Food Protection*, vol. 68, pp. 833–837, 2005.

[7] W. Michaeli, K. Berdel, and O. Osterbrink, "Real-Time Defect Detection in Transparent Multilayer Polymer Films Using Structured Illumination and 1D Filtering," in *SPIE Proceedings*, P. H. Lchmann, Ed., vol. 7389. SPIE, 2009.

Development of a 976 nm Ytterbium-fiber MOPA Laser

Kimberley Lynn Goodwin [1], Stefan Meyer [2], Florian Sommer [3], Tonio Franz Kutscher [4] and Sebastian Karpf [4]

[1] Medical Engineering Science, Universität zu Lübeck, kimberley.goodwin@student.uni-luebeck.de
[2] Medizinisches Laserzentrum Lübeck GmbH, s.meyer@uni-luebeck.de
[3] Leibniz Institute of Virology, Hamburg, f.sommer@uni-luebeck.de
[4] Institute of Biomedical Optics, Universität zu Lübeck, {t.kutscher, sebastian.karpf}@uni-luebeck.de

Abstract

Here, we present the development of a 976 nm laser with a *Master Oscillator Power Amplifier* (MOPA) architecture. This amplifier is being developed for later employment in *Spectro-temporal Laser Imaging by Diffractive Excitation* (SLIDE) microscopy of green fluorescing proteins for neuronal activity imaging. A big problem of using an *Ytterbium-Doped Fiber* (YDF) as the gain medium for amplification is the three-level nature of Ytterbium in the 976 nm range, resulting in high re-absorption of the signal light and strong *Amplified Spontaneous Emission* (ASE) background. To prevent this high re-absorption, the YDF needs to be optimized to be fully pumped and the fiber length needs to be carefully chosen. Therefore, the main focus was to determine an optimal fiber length for maximal amplification of the signal light. Around 11 W pulse peak power was achieved after the first amplification stage, using 30 ps pulses at 10 MHz repetition rate.

1 Introduction

Brain diseases, such as dementia, are becoming increasingly relevant as society ages. In order to further our understanding of neuronal diseases and to decipher the fundamental operation of the brain, a global research endeavour is trying to image inside the brain of rodent model systems using intravital optical imaging. The work horse for imaging neuronal activity *in vivo* is Two-Photon microscopy, employing *genetically encoded calcium ion* (Ca2+) *indicators* (GECIs), which can be targeted to specific cells and - more importantly - their fluorescence characteristics changes depending on the Ca2+ concentration. Since a change in concentration can be attributed to a change in neuron membrane potential, this provides information about the neuronal activity and can be used to trace neuron network activity and pinpoint processes in the brain [1].
Spectro-temporal Laser Imaging by Diffractive Excitation (SLIDE) as presented by S. Karpf [2] provides kHz frame rates, optimal for neuronal activity imaging. Up to now, SLIDE has only been implemented at 1060 nm, since it requires broadband fiber gain media. However, for imaging the mature green fluorescent GECI family of GCaMP, a SLIDE system at 976 nm is wanted.
Rare earth ytterbium-doped fiber amplifiers are particularly suited for generating and amplifying light in the range from 1030 nm to 1060 nm, but are only conditionally suitable for 976 nm, as this wavelength is strongly re-absorbed. This is due to three-level behaviour at 976 nm, whereas *ytterbium* (Yb) presents favorable four-level energy levels around 1060 nm [3].
As the SLIDE system is based on a *Master Oscillator Power Amplifier* (MOPA) using a *Fourier Domain Mode Locked* (FDML) laser as master light source [4], we will present the development of a novel 976 nm MOPA. If successful, this setup can then be upgraded by an FDML laser to enable SLIDE imaging at 976 nm.

2 Material and Methods

2.1 Master Oscillator Power Amplifier

The *Master Oscillator Power Amplifier* (MOPA) is a laser architecture employed to amplify light (typically pulsed) to high optical power levels. MOPAs comprise two main components: i) a seed laser source and ii) one or more amplifier stages. This multiple-stage amplifier configuration allows an easily controllable pulse width and pulse repetition rate by using low power Mach-Zehnder-based *Electro-Optical Modulators* (EOMs), while also providing high conversion efficiencies and excellent beam quality [5]. In order to amplify the seed light, active optical fiber amplifiers can be used. The fiber core of those active fibers is doped with rare earth ions such as Yb. The pump light will be absorbed by Yb, which is then excited into meta-stable states (relatively long upper state lifetime). The seed light is then amplified via stimulated emission, meaning that the light is emitted in the same mode as the seed light [3].

2.2 Amplification of 976 nm laser light

The absorption and emission spectra as shown in Fig. 1 demonstrate the three-level nature at 976 nm, where the high emission peak around 980 nm also leads to very strong absorption at the same wavelength. Therefore, the major challenge of a three-level laser is to ensure sufficient population inversion of the fiber gain media, so as to depopulate the ground state and thus shift the stimulated emission process in favour of a re-absorption process. A consequence of this strong pumping is a strong *Amplified Stimulated Emission* (ASE) background, which describes the light first emitted in all directions via spontaneous emission and then leads to stimulated emission if propagation occurs through a region with population inversion. In the modes of the optical fiber, ASE can thus gain significant power which may de-excite the stored power in the Yb ions and thus leads to lower available power for the signal light or may even destroy optical components if ASE pulses at very high peak powers occur. ASE can also lead to *gain saturation*, meaning that increasing the pump power will not significantly increase the signal gain as ASE gain increases. Therefore, ASE also significantly limits peak gain [3]. Here, ASE is occurring around 1030 nm, which corresponds to the second emission peak [6]. In this work, we employed a pump wavelength in the 920 nm absorption band, as shown in 1. This will be used for pumping the laser-active fiber for the 976 nm MOPA set-up described in the following.

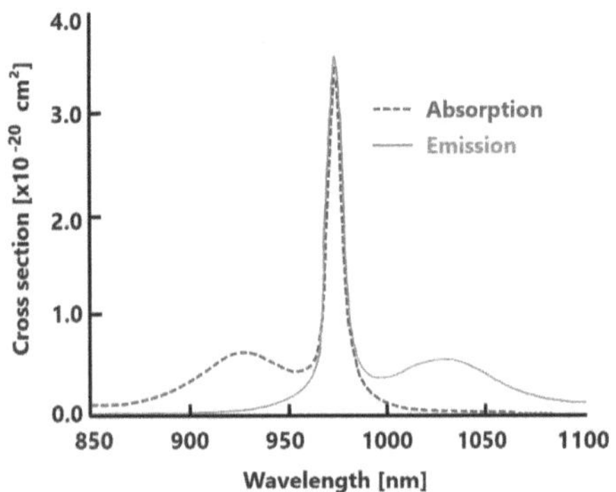

Figure 1: Absorption and emission spectra of a single-mode ytterbium-doped fiber. Graphic modified from [7].

2.3 Set-up of the 976 nm MOPA

In Fig. 2 the set-up of the 976 nm MOPA laser is shown. The seed pulse is generated with a 976 nm *single mode* (SM) butterfly laser diode (1999CVB 3CN01765JL, 3S-Photonics). This can later be replaced by an FDML for applications requiring wavelength-swept laser. The *continuous wave* (CW) diode is fed into an EOM (NIR-MX-LN-40, iXblue Photonics) which modulates the pulses. These are then fed into the first ytterbium amplification stage.
A 980 nm *Isolator* (Iso) (IO-F-780APC, Thorlabs Inc.) in the first amplifier stage is inserted to prevent any damage to the EOM and the seed diode from any reflections of the signal light, the residual pump light, or ASE. Downstream from the Iso, there is a 99:1 coupler, splitting the incoming light into two beams, one containing 99% of the light intensity and the other, also called *TAP*, accounts for 1% of the light intensity. The TAP is used to ensure regulation of the bias voltage of the EOM for maximum extinction in-between pulses [8]. The following YDF (YB1200-4/125,

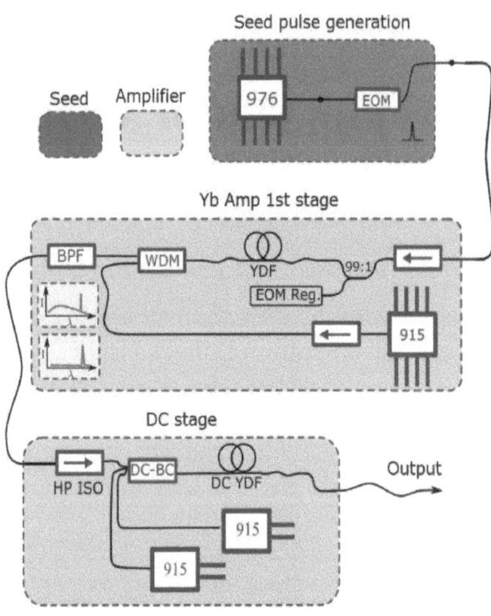

Figure 2: Set-up of the 976 nm MOPA laser. With a 976 nm laser diode and an EOM seed pulse are generated. In the first *YDF Amplifier* (YDFA) stage the YDF is pumped in backwards direction using a 915 nm laser diode. The DC stage is pumped with two multimode 915 nm diodes.

Thorlabs Inc.) is pumped in a backwards direction by a 915 nm single-mode butterfly diode (LLS-0153, Lumics), meaning that the pump light travels in the opposite direction to the signal light. By pumping backwards, the highest gain is directly at the output [3]. *Wavelength Division Multiplexers* (WDMs) are used to combine two single-mode signals with different wavelengths into one fiber, therefore they have a common port which directs both wavelengths and another port for each of the specified wavelengths. The WDM (WD9860AA, Thorlabs Inc.) is specified for 980 nm and 1060 nm but due to the *Fused Bionic Taper* (FBT) manufacturing method, the 1060 nm port also works for 915 nm and is used to feed the pump light into the YDF and separate the signal light. Instead of a 915 nm pump protector, a 980 nm Iso is used as these were confirmed to perform well also at 915 nm. The Iso is used to prevent damage to the pump diode by ASE light. The last part of the first amplifier stage is a 976 nm *Band Pass Filter* (BPF) to filter ASE light in order to exclusively feed the signal light into the second amplifier stage, otherwise the ASE would be amplified in the second stage and compete for the gain of signal light.
To obtain even higher gain in the second amplification stage, high pump power is required. Since high-power lasers often have low beam quality, there is a significant loss when launched into a single-mode fiber and the fiber can be destroyed due to high power pumped into the cladding. Therefore, for the second amplifier stage, a *double-clad* (DC) fiber (YB1200-10/125DC, Thorlabs Inc.) is used. As shown in Fig. 3, DC fibers have an additional pump cladding around the core. The refractive index of the core is higher than that of the pump cladding, therefore the signal light is still guided in single-mode or in only a few modes, while the pump light is introduced into the pump cladding

with a substantially higher diameter, which constitutes a *multi-mode* (MM) waveguide. In a DC-YDF, the core is ytterbium-doped and the pump cladding is undoped. Due to the multi-mode waveguide of the pump light, it also accesses the fiber core, where it can be absorbed. But as most of the pump light travels in the pump cladding, the overlap of the pump light with the fiber core is reduced [3]. Here, the DC-YDF will be pumped with two 915 nm multi-mode diodes (LU0915T090, Lumics). Depending on the usage of the laser or depending on whether another DC stage is necessary for further amplification, another BPF could be added to further filter ASE.

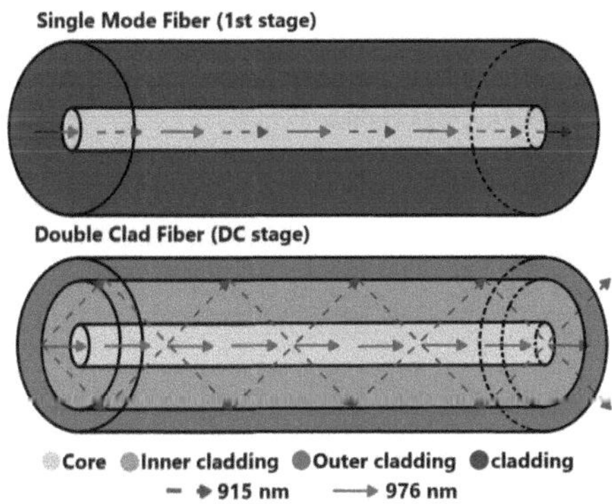

Figure 3: Single-mode fiber with a single cladding. Double-clad with additional inner cladding, with a lower refractive index than the fiber core, providing a multi-mode waveguide for 915 nm pump and single-mode waveguide for 976 nm signal light.

In this set-up, a *high-power Iso* (HP-ISO) is used to prevent reflections and residual pump light from accessing the first stage. The pump light is fed into the DC-YDF with a *double-clad beam combiner* (DC-BC).

2.4 Measurements

Due to the high absorption of the laser-active Yb ions at 976 nm, the YDF length for maximum peak power must be determined. As shown in Fig. 4, another WDM is added between the coupler of the EOM regulation and the YDF of the first amplification stage. The common port is attached to the YDF, the 980 nm port to the coupler and the 1060 nm port can then be used to measure the power through 915 nm. This is important to see whether the YDF is completely pumped. If the YDF is not fully pumped the signal light would be reabsorbed and mostly ASE will be emitted. Furthermore, we measured the time average power at the 980 nm port of the WDM downstream from the YDF, from which the maximum possible pulse peak power can be estimated in order to calculate how much the light needed to be attenuated in order not to exceed the limits of the *photodiode* (PD) (ET2030, Electro-Optics Technology, Inc.) used for measuring the actual pulse peak power. As the PD measures the power in terms of voltage in mV and peak power is then converted into mW using the formula

$$P_{peak} = C_{PD} * P_{PD} * A \tag{1}$$

where C_{PD} is the conversion factor of the PD, P_{PD} is the power measured with the PD in terms of voltage, and A corresponds to the attenuation of the couplers used.

In order to experimentally determine the optimal fiber length, the measurements were first made with a YDF length of 16 cm, which was then iteratively reduced centimeter by centimeter. The drive current of the seed laser was set to 200 mA in order to have smaller pulse peak power to avoid destroying the PD. The pump diode was operated at a maximum power of 600 mA.

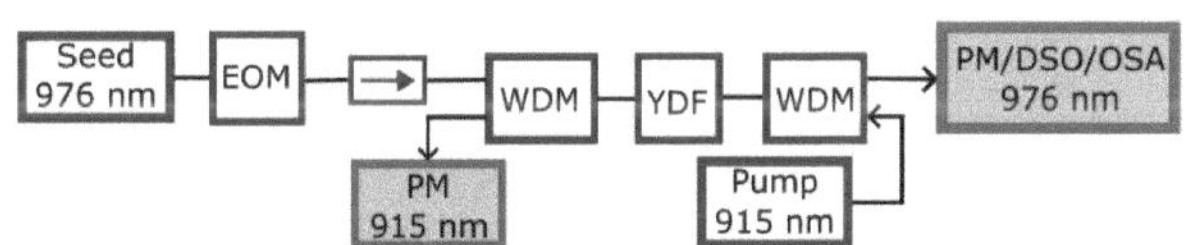

Figure 4: Schematic representation of the measurement setup, white: optical path, grey: measurement devices.

3 Results and Discussion

The power of the 915 nm single-mode butterfly diode at 600 mA was measured to be 345.1 mW. After the Iso, 206 mW pump power is fed into the YDF, which corresponds to a loss of 2 dB on account of the Iso. The seed diode at 200 mA measures 20.12 mW downstream from the Iso. In Fig. 5, the residual pump power, the time average power of the signal light as well as the pulse peak power are plotted against the length of the fiber.

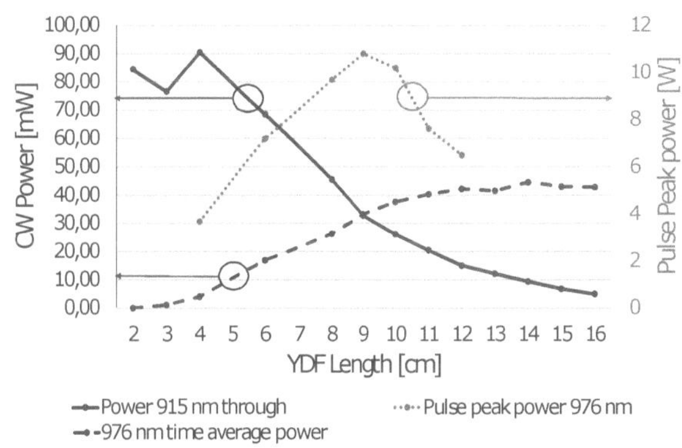

Figure 5: Power measurement for the first core pumped ytterbium amplifier stage over different YDF lengths.

At first, the residual 915 nm pump power decrease is virtually linear, but at 9 cm the rate of decrease starts to slow down. The peak at the beginning of the curve is probably due to measuring errors.

It is reasonable to assume that the power decrease is linear to the length of the fiber. However, with longer fiber lengths, more ASE is produced around 1030 nm, which is not completely filtered out by the second WDM in the measurement set-up, and therefore a higher value is measured. The 976 nm time average power increase is linear until it reaches a nearly steady state at 12 cm fiber length.

Measuring the pulse peak power, no pulse peaks for YDF lengths under 4 cm and over 12 cm could be detected by the PD. Because of the limited bandwidth of the PD, the peak visible on the oscilloscope showed about 3 times lower power than the real peak power of the 30 ps pulse. Additionally, to accurately determine the actual peak power, the high amount of ASE must also be considered. The maximum is visible at 9 cm which corresponds to the point where the slope of the residual pump power changes.

This could indicate that 9 cm corresponds to the length at which the YDF is fully pumped. For shorter fibers, the gain potential is not fully exploited as it increases with longer fibers. In longer YDF, the fiber is not fully pumped, therefore in the first few centimetres, the signal input light is absorbed, which facilitates ASE. Therefore, we measure more backward ASE at the 915 nm port and the gradient of the 915 nm power decreases. Furthermore, the forward ASE experiences strong reinforcement as there is less 976 nm signal light to be amplified, therefore the 976 nm time average power still increases but the pulse peak power drops. By comparing the spectrum for 9 cm and 16 cm in Fig. 6, it can be seen that for higher YDF length the peak at 976 nm is lower, while the ASE around 1030 nm increases. The 980 nm port of the WDM has no loss for 980 nm but for the ASE which is around 1030 nm there is, according to the datasheet, about 5 dB loss. Therefore the actual generated ASE is about 3.3 times higher than the measured value.

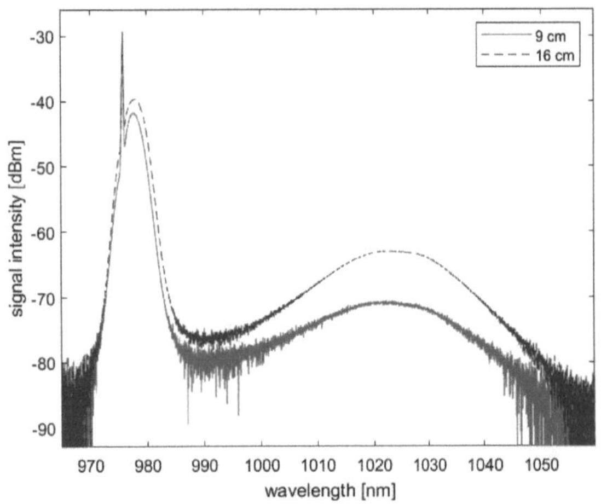

Figure 6: Spectrum of the first amplifier stage for 9 cm and 16 cm YDF length. ASE around 1030 nm significantly increases with longer fiber length.

A pulse peak power of 11 W was achieved, but the measured values can only be evaluated semi-quantitatively, as the PD employed has a longer rise time than the optical pulses. Therefore, the determined peak power of 11 W is only used as an approximation of the actual value.

4   Conclusion & Outlook

We were able to show that it is possible to reach around 11 W with the first core pumped ytterbium amplifier stage with a YDF length of 9 cm. In the next step, we will characterize the first amplifier stage with a 9 cm long YDF by measuring the time average power, the peak power and the emission spectra. Most important here is the evaluation of the peak power. In the following we will set up the DC Stage as described in 2.3. Here, the peak power for different DC-YDF lengths will be evaluated to determine the optimal DC-YDF length for maximum gain.

Furthermore, we will build a 976 nm FDML in order to use this as a seed laser for the MOPA (FDML-MOPA configuration), as already presented by S. Karpf [4], which can then be used for an 976 nm SLIDE system to image neuronal activity based on two-photon excitation of GECIs.

Acknowledgement

The work has been carried out in the research group of Prof. Dr. Sebastian Karpf under supervision of Stefan Meyer and Florian Sommer at the Institute of Biomedical Optics, Universität zu Lübeck.

Author's Statement

Conflict of interest: Authors state no conflict of interest.

5   References

[1] C. Grienberger and A. Konnerth, *"Imaging calcium in neurons"*, Neuron, 73, 862-885, 2012.

[2] S. Karpf, et al.*"Spectro-temporal encoded multiphoton microscopy and fluorescence lifetime imaging at kilohertz frame-rates"*, Nature Communications, 11, 2062, 2020.

[3] R. Paschotta, *Fiber amplifier*. Available: https://www. rp-photonics.com/tutorial_fiber_amplifiers.html [last accessed on 2023-01-09].

[4] S. Karpf and B. Jalali, *Fourier-domain mode-locked laser combined with a master-oscillator power amplifier architecture*, Optics Letters, 44, 1952-1955, 2019.

[5] R. Paschotta, *Master oscillator power amplifier*. Available: https://www.rp-photonics.com/master_ oscillator_power_amplifier.html [last accessed on 2023-01-09].

[6] P. Dupriez et al., *High average power, high repetition rate, picosecond pulsed fiber master oscillator power amplifier source seeded by a gain-switched laser diode at 1060 nm*, IEEE Photonics Technology Letters, vol. 18, no. 9, pp. 1013-1015, May 1, 2006, doi: 10.1109/LPT.2006.873486.

[7] M. R. A. Moghaddam, S. W. Harun and H. Ahmad(2012). *Comparison between Analytical Solution and Experimental Setup of a Short Long Ytterbium Doped Fiber Laser*. Optics and Photonics Journal. 2. 65-72. 10.4236/opj.2012.22010.

[8] S. Meyer, T. Kutscher, P. Lamminger, M. Wiggert and S. Karpf, *Development and evaluation of an Arduino based EOM Regulation*, Student Conference Proceedings 2022, ISBN ISBN-13: 978-3945954676

Simultaneous microbubble detection by optical coherence tomography and optoacoustics for selective retina therapy

Leonie Hoffmann [1,2], Christian Burri [2,3], Simon Salzmann [2], Mylène Amstutz [2], Christoph Meier [2], and Ralf Brinkmann [4,5]

[1] Medical Engineering Science, Universität zu Lübeck, DE-23562 Lübeck, Germany,

leonie.hoffmann@student.uni-luebeck.de

[2] Bern University of Applied Sciences, HuCE optoLab, BFH-TI, CH-2501 Biel, Switzerland

[3] Biomedical Photonics Group, Institute of Applied Physics (IAP), Universtity of Bern, CH-3012 Bern, Switzerland

[4] Institute of Biomedical Optics, Universität zu Lübeck, DE-23562 Lübeck, Germany

[5] Medical Laser Center Lübeck, DE-23562 Lübeck, Germany

Abstract

Selective retina therapy (SRT) is an emerging method to treat retinal diseases which are associated with a disfunction of the retinal pigment epithelium (RPE). The aim of the treatment is a selective damage of the RPE while sparing the neural retina. The main challenge is treatment energy dosing due to local variations in pigmentation. To measure successful irradiation, microbubble formation (MBF) can be detected as optoacoustics (OA) transients and optical coherence tomography (OCT) signal washouts. In this work, time resolved OCT M-Scan and OA were used simultaneous to investigate the relationship between washouts visible in OCT and MBF. Five ex-vivo porcine RPE-choroid-sclera explants were treated with single laser pulses between $6\,\mu$s and $20\,\mu$s (wavelength: 532 nm, spot size: $100\,\mu$m x $100\,\mu$m). The lesions were quantified with a calcein-AM staining after treatment. The results indicate that OCT signal washout correlate with optoacoustically detected MBF.

1 Introduction

1.1 Selective retina therapy

Selective retina therapy (SRT) is a retinal laser treatment which aims to selectively destroy cells of the RPE without affecting the neuronal retina [1]. The key concept of SRT is using microsecond laser pulses shorter than the thermal confinement time which induce microbubbles at the RPE-melanosomes to destroy the RPE-cells and stimulate the regeneration [1], [2]. The RPE wound will be closed with the neighbouring cells through migration and proliferation [1]. SRT proved to be beneficial in diseases associated with RPE dysfunction, such as diabetic macular edema or central serous retinopathy [2]. A laser in the green spectral range is suitable, due to the high absorption of green light in the RPE-melanosomes (20 - 80 % of the incoming light) [1]. It should be treated close above the microbubble threshold to reduce the risk of overtreatment [3]. The main problem is the local variation in pigmentation and an individual transparency of the eye media and lens, which requires varying pulse energies [3].

1.2 Techniques to detect microbubbles

In order to still be able to treat reliably in the optimal treatment window, various methods for detecting MBF have been developed.

1.2.1 Optical coherence tomography

One technique is spectral-domain OCT, whereby backscattered light from the eye is interfered with reference light and evaluated with a spectrometer. It is assumed that a change in reflectivity of the tissue results in a signal change in time-resolved A-scans (M-scans) [5].

1.2.2 Optoacoustics

Another technique is OA, which is independent of light scattering and detects the acoustic wave generated from the MBF [3].

In this study we investigated tissue changes by OCT and OA simultaneously to obtain a relation between an OCT washout in a M-Scan and an optoacoustically measured transient.

2 Material and Methods

2.1 Experimental setup

A previously built SRT test bench was used and extended with a two dimensional scanner and a telescope in the sample arm based on the Spectralis Centaurus system. The SRT test bench consists of an experimental SRT laser (modified MERILAS 532 shortpulse, Meridian, Thun, CH) and emits at a wavelength of 532 nm. To achieve a top hat profile a multimode square core fibre (LEONI Fiber Optics, DE) with a core diameter of $50\,\mu m \times 50\,\mu m$ and a numerical aperture of 0.1 was used. The SRT laser beam is coaxially aligned to an OCT system using a collimator (60FC-SMA-0-A15-01, Schäfter & Kirchhoff, Hamburg, DE) and a dicromatic mirror (T610lpxr, Chroma Technology, Bellows Falls, US). The OCT system consists of the laser source (EXS210022-03, SN: 1141117, Exalos, Schlieren, CH), which emits at a central wavelength of 840 nm with a bandwidth of 48.6 nm, a spectrometer and an interferometer built by HuCE optoLab.

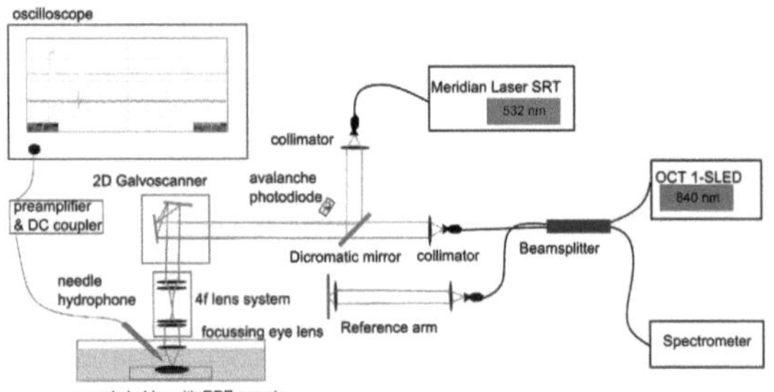

Figure 1: The modified SRT test bench is shown, in which the SRT laser (532 nm) is focused on the sample and provides the SRT effect. For focusing, the lens is used after the 4f-system. The pattern is applied by changing the position of the scanner mirrors. The mircobubble detection is realized on the one hand by the needle hydrophone, whose signal is measured on the oscilloscope. On the other hand with a spectral-domain OCT, where the superposition of the backscattered light from the sample and reference arms are detected by a camera in the spectrometer.

A two-dimensional scanner (GVS002, Thorlabs, Newton, New Jersey, US) and telescope were integrated into the sample arm. The scanner is used to generate a B-scan (cross-sectional view) over the RPE sample to bring the sample into the focus of the two aligned laser beams and to apply the pattern. Additionally the scanner is used to apply a treatment pattern onto the sample. Between the telescope and the sample a focusing lens with a focal distance of 17.5 mm is used to focus the laser beams onto the sample. In order to detect tissue changes a needle hydrophone (NH2000, Presision Acoustics, Dorset, UK) is placed about 2 mm away from the treated spot. The measured amplitude is preamplified (DC Coupler with Power Suppy, SN: DCPS0310, Presision Acoustics) and aquired with an oscilloscope (Wavepro 760Zi, LeCroy, SN: 49501, New York, US). To trigger the OA signal logging synchronously to the treatment laser pulse, an avalanche photodiode (APD110A2/M, SN: M0027914, Thorlabs, New Jersey, US) is placed above the dichromatic mirror detecting scattering light from the treatment laser pulse. The telescope consists of a 4f-lens system and is designed with four achromatic lenses (VIS-NIR coated achromatic lenses, Edmundoptics Inc, Barrington, US). The first two lenses have a focal length of 120 mm. The third lens has a focal length of 100 mm and the last lens has a focal length of 40 mm. The telescope was simulated

with Zemax and a distance was calculated between the two lens packages in order to collimate the aligned laser beams after the telescope. Both the calculation and the experimental measurement using the beam diameter after the telescope gave a distance between the lens packages of about 75 mm, which was found to be optimal. The telescope can be used to correct possible ametropia of the whole porcine eyes in different experiments.

2.2 Tissue preparation

For the experiments fresh porcine eyes were used. They were collected at a local slaughterhouse and were used within five hours post-mortem. The posterior part of the

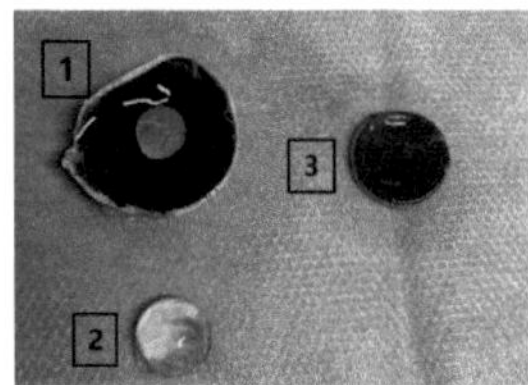

Figure 2: Part of the tissue preparation is shown, after the eye was cut in half and the anterior part of the eye (1) and the lens (2) were removed. The retina-RPE-choroid-sclera explant (3) is used for the experiments after removing the retina.

porcine eye was used. The eye was first cut in half and the anterior part with the lens were removed. Subsequently a round piece in the visual streak was cut out, seen in Fig. 6 (3). After that the vitreous body and the retina were removed carefully, the RPE-choroid-sclera explant was retained in a moveable explant holder and placed in the cuvette filled with water. The lens of the eye is simulated with a glass lens with a focal distance of 17 mm, shown in Fig. 1.

2.3 OCT and OA recording and processing

The treatment software recording the OCT signal was provided. An A-scan rate of 76923 Hz with an integration time of 12.3 μs was used. The OCT laser source was set so that a power of 850 μW reached the sample. OCT processing

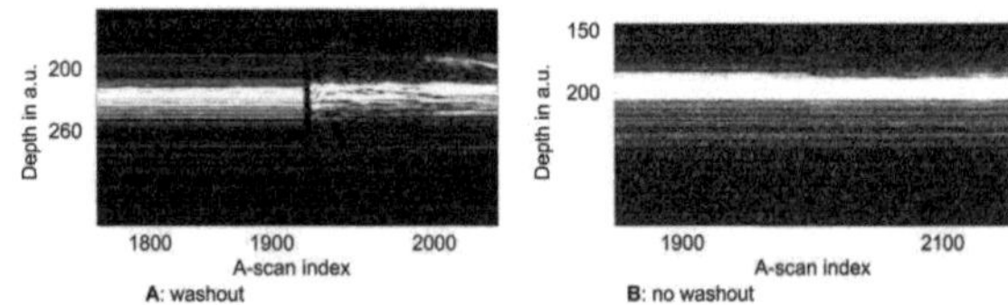

Figure 3: In A ($8\,\mu s$, $66\,\mu J$) an OCT signal washout in a M-scan is shown. In B ($20\,\mu s$, $32\,\mu J$) no OCT signal washout is shown. A signal washout was defined as a signal loss over the RPE layer over one or more rows.

included DC removal, dispersion correction, windowing, remap, and Fourier transformation. A signal washout was defined if one or more rows in an OCT M-scan at the RPE layer showed a signal loss, shown in Fig. 3 on the left side. The needle hydrophone to detect the acoustic waves was placed near the treated spot on the RPE-explant. The detected acoustic wave was synchronized with the laser pulse. A time resolution of 20 μs/div was chosen to record 200 μs, with a sampling rate of 50 MS/s. This sampling rate was chosen because the hydrophone has a frequency band of 0,1 MHz to 10 MHz. According to Nyquist the sampling rate needs to be at least twice as high as the highest frequency in the signal. Five porcine eyes were treated. If

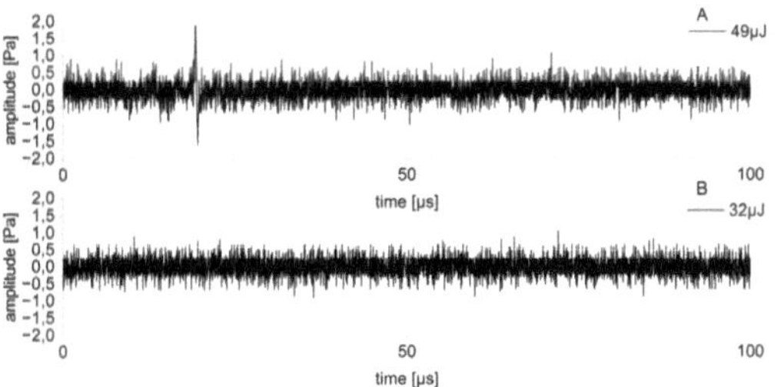

Figure 4: In the two graphs two measured signals are shown, where in (A) a transient, defined as an OA signal and in B a noise signal, defined as no OA signal is shown.

a transient could be separated by eye from the noise level, it was defined as an OA signal, shown in Fig. 4. The hydrophone has a sensitivity of 3,5 V/MPa.

2.4 Experimental process

After tissue preparation the sample was placed in the sample holder underneath the setup, shown in Fig. 1. Subsequently the pattern was applied. An irradiated sample is shown in Fig. 6. Marker lesions were placed for orientation

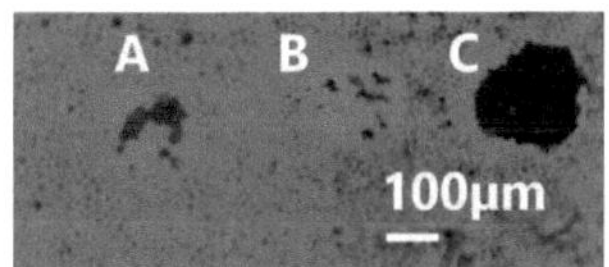

Figure 5: A (8 μs, 49 μJ) and B (20 μs, 66 μJ) are defined as no lesion, even though hyperfluorescence or a lesion consisting of a small cluster of cells can be seen. In C (20 μs, 83 μJ) a lesion is shown.

on the sample, for which the pulse duration was set to 20 μs and the pulse energy to the maximum of 270 μJ. Each row was irradiated with a single pulse and a different pulse duration increasing from top to bottom (6 μs to 20 μs). The pulse energy is increasing from left to right (15 μJ to 100 μJ) and the radiant exposure increased from 150 mJ/cm² to 1000 mJ/cm², calculated with the spot size on the explant of A = 100 × 100 μm² and the applied energy. Comparable radiation exposures were reported by Burri et al. (135 mJ/cm² to 1354 mJ/cm²) [5]. After every laser pulse the triggered signal on the oscilloscope was saved. When the pattern was finished the sample was stained with Calcein AM for 30 minutes. The sample was obtained under the fluorescence microscope (Axio Lab.A1, Carl Zeiss, Oberkochen,

Germany) using a microscope camera (Gryphax Progres, Jenoptik, Jena, Germany) [4]. If the treated tissue showed a cluster of dead cells larger than 50 % of the spot size (100 μm x 100 μm), it was evaluated as lesion (C, Fig. 5) and noted as a 1 (Fig. 6). Otherwise it was evaluated as no lesion (0 in Fig. 6).

3   Results and Discussion

3.1   Results

In Fig. 6 the applied pattern on the RPE-explant is shown. The lesions are mostly larger than the spot size. With the chosen energy it indicates a suprathreshold treatment.

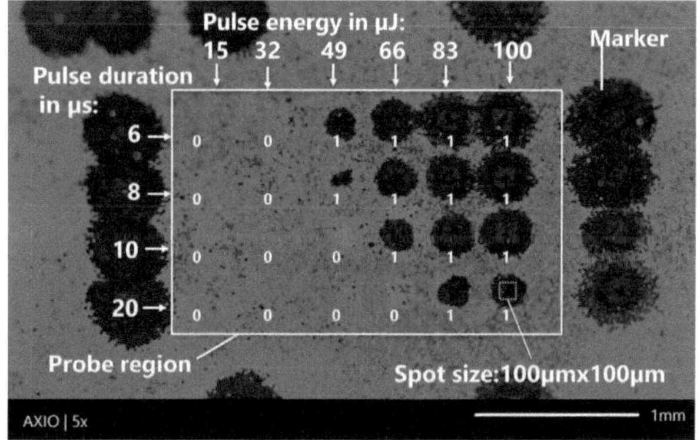

Figure 6: With a magnification of factor five the applied pattern on the RPE-explant under the fluorescence microscope is seen. Additionally the spot size is shown as a dotted square in the right corner of the probe zone. With 0 and 1 the lesions were defined for the probit analysis.

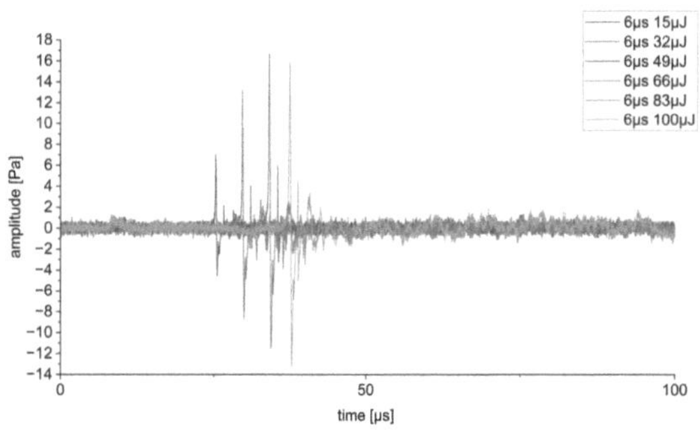

Figure 7: The graph displays OA pressure waves for an treatment with a pulse duration of 6 μs and different pulse energies (15 μJ to 100 μJ).

There are spots that show hyperfluorescence. This result is not analysed in this work, but will be evaluated in the future. For a pulse duration of 6 μs the OA pressure waves are shown in Fig. 7. With rising pulse energy the amplitude of the signal is increasing. The pattern was applied by moving the mirrors in the scanner and therefore the laser beam was moved over the sample. This results in different distances between the needle hydrophone and the treated spot.

Is the distance larger, the pressure waves need longer to be detected from the needle hydrophone. The ED values are displayed in Fig. 8. Mostly the ED50$_{OA}$ values are larger than the ED50$_{Calcein}$ values for a pulse duration of 6 μs and 20 μs. Comparing OCT and OA, OCT always detects a signal washout at less pulse energy than OA detects a pressure wave. Added to that, OCT detects a signal washout even if no lesion greater than 50 % of the spot size was seen in the Calcein AM staining.

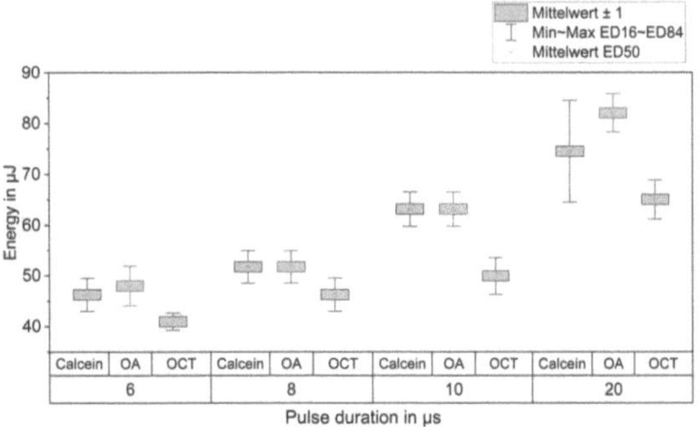

Figure 8: The graph displays the ED16/50/84 values for the probit analysis of the Caclein AM staining (grey), the OA transient detection by eye (red) and the OCT signal washout detection by eye (blue). The OCT signal washout detection detects a washout at less pulse energy than a lesion >50 % of the treated spot size in the Calcein AM staining.

3.2   Discussion

The experiments indicate that OCT signal washout correlate with optoacoustically detected MBF. For further experiments the energy range should be adjusted. With smaller energy steps the damage threshold and the beginning of MBF could be evaluated in more detail. The bigger lesions result due to lateral heat diffusion. Added to that the pattern could be applied by moving the sample, so that the distance between treated spot and needle hydrophone would be constant in the future. The needle hydrophone is very sensitive to direction. Over the measuring range, the needle hydrophone has a mean effective radius of approximately 1 mm. Due to the setup, the hydrophone had to be placed at an angle, so that the optimum sensitivity of the hydrophone was certainly not optimally used. This could be a reason why OA detects pressure waves at higher pulse energies than OCT detects a signal washout. The OA pressure waves should be filtered as shown by Seifert et al. [3]. It was assumed that an OA transient indicated a MBF if the amplitude could be separated by eye from the noise level. For evaluating if this assumption is correct further experiments by applying more than one pulse onto the same spot could be done. For further analysis the OCT signal washout could be detected with the OCT algorithm published in [5]. A reason why OA detects pressure waves at higher pulse energies than OCT could be either that OA is less sensitive or as mentioned before the orientation of the needle hydrophone could be improved. Especially at a pulse duration of 20 μs

the difference can be seen. In [6] it was shown that the quantity of dead cells associated with cavitation decreases with a longer pulse duration. For a pulse duration of 20 μs Lee et al. [6] observed that only 65 % of dead cells were associated with cavitation. That could be another reason why OA detects microbubbles only at higher pulse energies when a pulse duration of 20 μs was used.

4   Conclusion

Our experiments show that it is possible to detect microbubbles simultaneously with OCT and OA. It was further shown that OCT detects a signal washout at lower pulse energies than OA detects a microbubble with a needle hydrophone. However, this needs to be investigated in more detail with adjusted parameters, a fixed distance between hydrophone and the treated spot and an optimized orientation of the needle hydrophone.

Acknowledgement

The work has been carried out at Bern University of Applied Sciences, Biel, Switzerland and was supervised by the Institute of Biomedical Optics, University of Lübeck, Lübeck, Germany.

Author's Statement

Conflict of interest: Authors state no conflict of interest.

5   References

[1] R. Brinkmann et al., *Selektive Retina-Therapie.* In Ophthalmologe, Springer Medizin Verlag, 2006.

[2] A. Hutfilz, C. Burri, D. Theisen-Kunde, C. Meier and R. Brinkmann, *Ex-vivo investigation of different µs laser pulse durations for selective retina therapy.* In Proc. of SPIE, Vol. 11079, 2019.

[3] E. Seifert et al., *Algorithms for optoacoustically controlled selective retina therapy.* In Photoacoustics 25, Elsevier, 2022.

[4] M. Amstutz, *Dynamic OCT signal loss in microsecond microsurgery.* Master Thesis, Bern University of Applied Sciences, 2022.

[5] C. Burri et al., *Dynamic OCT Signal Loss for Determining RPE Radiant Exposure Damage Thresholds in Microsecond Laser Microsurgery.* In Applied Science, 11, 5535, 2021.

[6] H. Lee, C. Alt, C. Pitsillides and C. Lin, *Optical detection of intracellular cavitation during selective laser targeting of the retinal pigment epithelium: dependence of cell death mechanism on pulse duration.* In Journal of Biomedical Optics, Vol. 12(6), 064034, 2007.

Design of low cost thermal and UV nanoimprint devices

Nikolay Tesmer [1], Maik Rahlves [2]
[1] Medical Engineering Science, Universität zu Lübeck, nikolay.tesmer@student.uni-luebeck.de
[2] Institute for Biomedical Optics, Universität zu Lübeck, maik.rahlves@uni-luebeck.de

Abstract

Optical microstructures made from polymers are important components in fields such as biomedical imaging and biosensors. Methods to replicate such structures include thermal nanoimprint lithography (T-NIL) and UV nanoimprint lithography (UV-NIL). In this work, we report on the development of two low cost devices to produce optical microstructures using both NIL methods. The first device is capable of fabrication of large area structures from thermoplastic polymers such as sensor networks. The second device imprints silicone based stamps into UV-curable resin using the UV-NIL approach. Additionally, preliminary imprinting results are shown to indicate the general feasibility of the designed systems. The presented devices are going to be constructed and tested for their specific task which will be subject to future work.

1 Introduction

Microoptical components made from polymers are nowadays of high importance in various fields such as biomedical imaging, biosensors or communication technology. Such components include for example diffractive structures like gratings with structure sizes in the nanometer range that control the phase, amplitude or state of polarization of light [1]. Furthermore, the semiconductor industry uses nanometer structures on wafers to design precisely patterned thin films of suitable materials to protect these patterned areas during subsequent etching or deposition. These fabrication techniques, however, require high precision and therefore cost intense machines. The price range goes from tens of thousand to several hundred thousand dollars depending on the features of the machine which limit their use in smaller research labs. That is why this work focus on designing and constructing low budget devices to produce such structures using NIL which is often distinguished in thermal nanoimprint lithography (T-NIL) and ultraviolet nanoimprint lithography (UV-NIL) [2].

T-NIL, also called hot embossing, uses heat and pressure to mold a master structure into a thermoplastic such as polymethyl metacrylate (PMMA). Here, the polymer has to be heated over its specific glass transition temperature in order to be molded into the desired shape by an imprinting mold. Therefore, the polymer is heated up and subsequently being pressed in a mold with a defined pressure. After that, the mold can be separated from the polymer after it has cooled down to a specific demolding temperature and adopted the shape of the mold. This is a crucial step, because inadequate separations most likely lead to defects in the imprinted structure [3]. The expansion and shrinking of the components due to the change of temperature is also a factor that impacts the quality of the results [3]. Nevertheless,

T-NIL is able to produce structures with a resolution of tens of nanometers [4].

In comparison, UV-NIL is a method that imprints a structure into a fluid resin. This is achieved by pressing a mold into a UV-curable resin and subsequently exposing it to UV-light. The UV-light causes crosslinking between the molecules in the resin and, therefore, change the characteristic of the material such as its hardness [5]. UV-NIL can operate with low stamp pressures under 1 bar at room temperature due to the use of specific UV-curable resins that have a low viscosity [6] as well as soft, elastic stamps often made of polydimethysiloxane (PDMS) [7]. As a result, UV-NIL does not need constant energy for heating cycles and requires no cooling time before separation. In addition, the resin can generally be molded fast because the low viscosity of the resin allows it to easily adapt the molds shape [8]. One factor that affects the production time is the curing time, which depends on the thickness of the produced structure as well as on the specific resin and the power of the UV-LED. With UV-NIL it is possible to produce feature heights over 1 μm [2] with an achievable resolution of sub 25 nm [9]. All in all, fast printing times and low energy usage enables UV-NIL to be highly suitable for cost efficient high throughput production. That is why it is widely used in the industry with different imprint contact procedures such as plate-to-plate (P2P), roll-to-plate (R2P) or roll-to-roll (R2R) [8]. In R2R, the contact between resin and a mold is made by rolls while one contains the mold and the other holds the substrate. The rolls are in permanent contact with the resin while being illuminated by UV-light at the point of contact. The molded structure is demolded and transported through the rotation of the rolls. This production process is a continuous motion which is favorable for industrial large scale production but it has some complex challenges such as an integrated continuous resist coating mechanism [8]. That is why the basic stamping mechanism of P2P illustrated in Fig. 1 is more suitable for the low cost approach in this project.

The following sections provide an insight in the current state of the project by presenting the developed designs for P2P T-NIL and UV-NIL systems. In addition, requirements and difficulties in designing such devices are evaluated and preliminary results of a reduced, simplified system are presented to verify the theoretical feasibility of this approaches.

2 Material and Methods

The systems designed within this work focus on plate-to-plate imprinting using T-NIL and UV-NIL with the intention to combine these two approaches in one system in the future. T-NIL is intended to be used to fabricate large area microstructured substrates while UV-NIL will be used to create local sensor structures on the substrate such as grating based refractive index sensors which may be used to detect various biomarkers when functionalized by, e.g., antibodies.

2.1 T-NIL Design

The developed design for the T-NIL system can be seen in Fig. 2. It consists of a thermal press with a height of 325 mm and a width of 300 mm. The basic construction is based on three solid 300x300 mm and 15 mm thick aluminum plates, each having four holes where guiding rods are located. The guiding rods provide stability and are shaped in a way that the top and bottom plates can be fixed in position using threaded nuts whereas the plate in the middle is movable due to sliding bearings. A hydraulic press with a pressure gauge is placed underneath the middle stage to generate the needed pressure for the imprinting process. As the used hydraulic system can theoretically generate a pressure up to 700 bar, the material has to have specific strength and grade for safety reasons. Therefore, the guiding rods are made of hardened stainless steel with an M12 thread at each end while the threaded nuts have the tensile strength class of 12 which can theoretically jointly withstand the maximal pressure of the hydraulic press. The aluminum plates are a special alloy of aluminum, magnesium, copper, and lead (AlMgCuPb) while being thick enough to withstand the generated force without showing permanent deformation. For the application of T-NIL, the stamp with a diameter up to 120 mm can be mounted at the upper heating plate while the polymer can be placed on top of the heating plate on the middle stage. The heating unit consists of heating cartridges with a combined power output up to 1600 watts to heat the polymer above its glass transition temperature.

2.2 UV-NIL Design

The mobile design for the UV-NIL system is illustrated in Fig. 3. It has a height of around 130 mm, a width of 90 mm

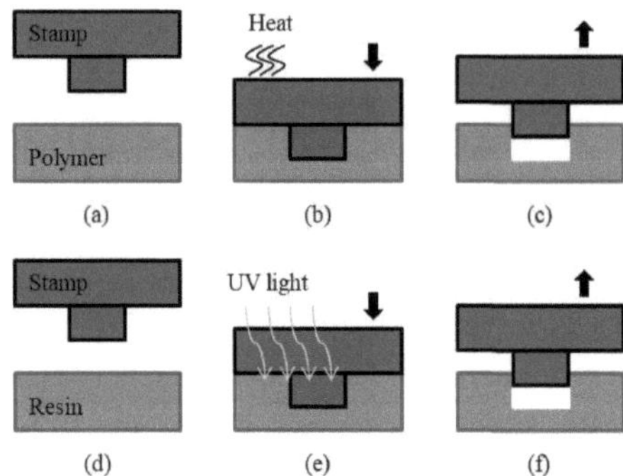

Figure 1: Basic principle of plate-to-plate nanoimprint lithography with T-NIL (a-c) at the top and UV-NIL (d-f) at the bottom half. (a) shows the stamp and the polymer which is imprinted in (b) using heat and pressure. (c) shows the demolding process and the imprinted structure after a sufficient cooling time. (d) shows the stamp and the resin that is imprinted in (e) using low pressure and UV-light to cure the resin that is done prior to the demolding in (f).

and a depth of 50 mm and can be mounted on a gantry with high precision axes to allow to position the UV-NIL head with respect to a substrate. Its function is to automatically press the stage with the UV-LED and the stamp onto a photoresin that has to be placed at the desired location underneath the stamp. The stamp is mounted under the movable stage while the UV-LED is located over the stamp. The LED is able to expose the resin due to a recess in the stage and the transparency for the UV wavelength of the PDMS stamp material. The vertical movement of the stage which is mounted to a linear guide is generated with an electric motor that is controlled by an Arduino microcontroller and attached to a bevel gear at the top of the system. This bevel gear is clamped on a threaded rod which moves the stage by the rotation through a threaded nut which is attached to the stage. Therefore, the stage can be moved by around 2.6 μm with the smallest step size of 0.225 degree of the electric motor in combination with the 4:1 transmission of the bevel gear and the thread pitch of 3 mm on the threaded rod.

3 Results and Discussion

The devices were constructed but not fully assembled and ready to be tested at the time of the paper submission due to supply bottlenecks and extended production time for custom made parts. To demonstrate the general feasibility of our approach, we restrict ourselves to results obtained during preliminary experiments prior to the construction of the devices. During the preliminary experiments, a grating with grid spacing of 10 μm made from BK7 glass was replicated in PDMS (Sylgard 184). The stamp was produced by casting liquid PDMS onto the BK7 grating and placing it into a desiccator to remove the air trapped inside the PDMS prior to position it on a heating plate for the hardening phase. Subsequently, the PDMS copy was used as UV-NIL mold by pressing it onto UV-curing adhesive (Norland NOA 61).

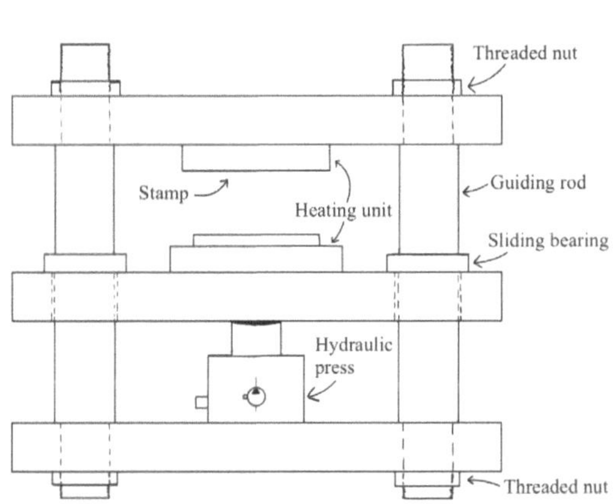

Figure 2: A side view of the designed T-NIL system. It consists of three aluminum plates with 300x300 mm with four holes with each holding a 325 mm guiding rod. The plates at the bottom and top are fixated using threaded nuts while the middle plate is movable due to sliding bearings. The middle plate holds a heating plate and can be pressed against the stamp at the top using the hydraulic press underneath.

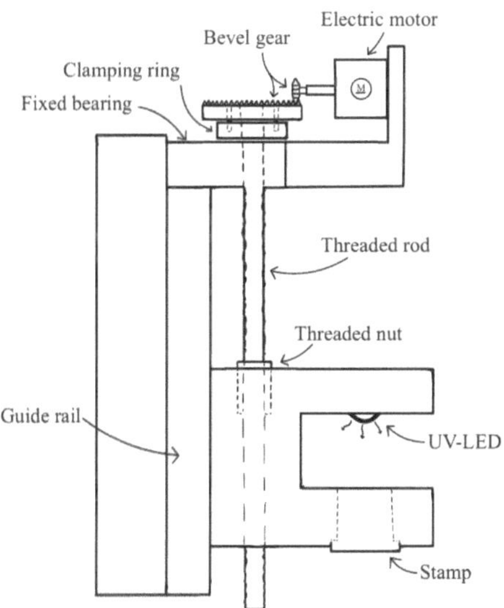

Figure 3: An illustration of the designed UV-NIL system. It consists of at an electric motor attached to a bevel gear which is clamped to a threaded rod and held in place by a fixed bearing. The threaded rod moves the stage containing a UV-light and a stamp holder through the rotation in a threaded nut which is attached to the stage.

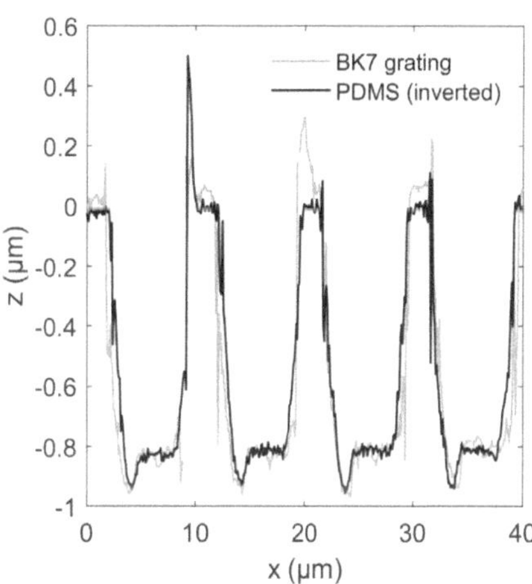

Figure 4: Measured side profile of the original grating on BK7 glass and the inverted PDMS stamp recorded with a Keyence VK9600 confocal microscope.

For that, the photresist was placed between the stamp and a glass plate. A mass of 500 g was used as pressure by placing it on the glass while illuminating the vented photoresist by high power UV-LEDs.

Fig. 4 shows a profile of the grating on BK7 glass and the inverted profile of the stamp made from PDMS recorded with a Keyence VK 9600 confocal microscope. The result of the stamping process was recorded with the same microscope and is presented in Fig. 5. The results shows that the imprinted structure has some imperfections such as slightly tilted grids as well as marginally different grating heights which led to a imperfect diffraction pattern. This could originate in an uneven stamping surface, wrong stamping pressure and particles between stamp and resin. Nevertheless, the results indicate, that the designed nanoimprint systems should be able to provide sufficient results when this issues are addressed. Hence, the designed P2P nanoimprint devices indeed require high precision in its movable parts as well as a favorable dust free working environment. As a consequence, the mechanical components that influence the movement of the stages have to be as smooth and precise as possible in order to produce the best results which is one of the most challenging aspect of development.

For future work, an additional feature for the UV-NIL system could be a magnifying camera to precisely place the sample at the desired place. This can be crucial, if, for example, multiple microstructures are going to be combined which requires a precise positioning of the stamp. For repeatable results, a force sensor could be installed to the system. But the placement of this sensor is not so trivial as it should not block the UV-light nor have an impact on the angle of the stamp which is a problem that can be addressed in further development.

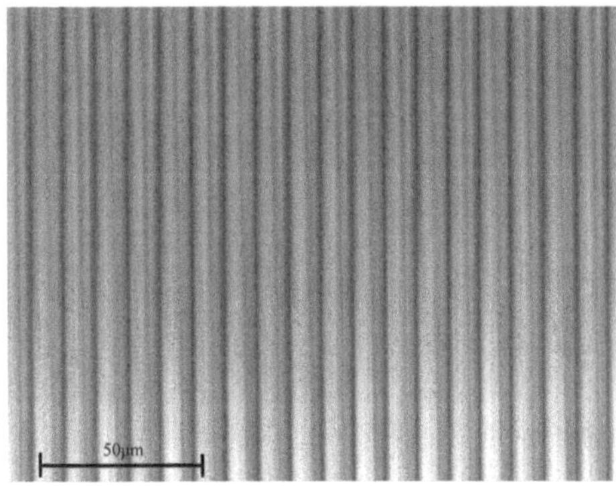

Figure 5: Imprinted grating in the cured Norland NOA 61 photoresist recorded by a Keyence VK9600 confocal microscope.

4   Conclusion

This work presents two low cost designs for the imprinting techniques T-NIL and UV-NIL. The T-NIL is intended to be used to replicate large area microstructured polymers up to diameters of 4". The UV-NIL consists of a small movable head which can be moved in the vertical direction using a stepper motor. It is designed for being mounted on a high precision gantry platform and allows to fabricate small area microstructures at defined position on a substrate. The applicability of the process was demonstrated during preliminary results where a grating with a pitch of 10 μm was replicated in UV-curing adhesive which indicated that the designed system should provide sufficient results. Future work will include the assembly and test of the designed systems while one could also try implementing a tracking system with a magnifying camera for the UV-NIL device.

Acknowledgement

The work has been carried out at institute for Biomedical Optics at the Universität zu Lübeck and was supervised by Prof. Dr. -Ing. Maik Rahlves.

Author's Statement

Conflict of interest: Authors state no conflict of interest.

5   References

[1] J. Turunen, *Diffraction Theory of Microrelief Gratings.* In: Micro-Optics: Elements, systems and applications, Taylor & Francis Ltd, London, pp. 31–52, 1997.

[2] H. Zappe, *Fundamentals of Micro-Optics.* Cambridge University Press, Cambridge, 2010.

[3] Y. Hirai, S. Yoshida and N. Takagi, *Defect analysis in thermal nanoimprint lithography.* Journal of Vacuum Science Technology, vol. 21, 2765, 2003.

[4] L.J Heyderman, H. Schift, C. David, J. Gobrecht and T. Schweizer, *Flow behaviour of thin polymer films used for hot embossing lithography.* Microelectronic Engineering, vol. 54, no. 3, pp. 229–245, 2000.

[5] V. Shukla, M. Bajpai, D.K. Singh, M. Singh and R. Shukla, *Review of basic chemistry of UV-curing technology.* Pigment & Resin Technology, vol. 33, no. 5, pp. 272–279, 2004.

[6] U. Plachetka, M. Bender, A. Fuchs, B. Vratzov, T. Glinsner, F. Lindner, and H. Kurz, *Wafer scale patterning by soft UV-Nanoimprint Lithography.* Microelectronic Engineering, vol. 73–74, pp. 167–171, 2004.

[7] T. Handte, N. Scheller, L. Dittrich, M. W. Thesen, M. Messerschmidt and S. Sinzinger, *Manufacturing of nanostructures with high aspect ratios using soft UV-nanoimprint lithography with bi- and trilayer resist systems.* Micro and Nano Engineering, vol. 14, 100106, 2022.

[8] N. Kooy, K. Mohamed, L. T. Pin and O. S. Guan, *A review of roll to roll nanoimprint lithography.* Nanoscale research letters, vol. 9, pp. 320–333, 2014.

[9] S. Y. Chou, P. R. Krauss and P. J. Renstrom, *Nanoimprint lithography.* Journal of Vacuum Science Technology B, vol. 14, pp.4129–4133, 1996.

Visualization of Intraocular Lenses Edge Roughness

Laura Zarbuch [1], Johanna Dinkel [2], and Niklas Damm [3]

[1] Medical Engineering Science, Universität zu Lübeck, laura.zarbuch@student.uni-luebeck.de
[2] Medical Engineering Science, Universität Stuttgart
[3] Carl Zeiss Meditec AG

Abstract

Cataract operation belongs to the most practiced surgery in the world, whereby the natural opaque lens in the eye is replaced by an artificial intraocular lens (IOL). Thereby, the IOL's rotational stability is an important parameter, in particular for toric IOLs. It is already proved that a high roughness of the IOL's surface influences the stability in a desired way. Therefore, in this work there shall be visually investigated if the roughness can be increased by variating the manufacturing parameters. Two groups of IOLs were used, whereby in group A different materials for manufacturing were provided and in group B the milling parameter was changed. Under a microscope, the IOL's edges were imaged and compared to each other. Objective roughness measurements supported the image evaluation. As a result, there was a difference in the visual impression by comparing the roughness of both materials. Considering the distinct milling parameters, no variation could be observed. Also the roughness measurements showed no statistical significance.

1 Introduction

1.1 Cataract Surgery

Cataract is the medical term for an eye disease which is indicated by the lens's opacity. Typically, the visual acuity is decreased, the impression of contrast and colors is reduced, and glare sensitivity develops. If there is no treatment, the cataract will finally lead to blindness. The general therapy is an operation in which the natural lens is replaced by an artificial so-called intraocular lens (IOL). This operation belongs to the most practiced surgery in the world [1].

There are different techniques used for cataract surgery. Today, the extracapsular cataract extraction (ECCE) in combination with phacoemulsification is the most applied method. ECCE means that the posterior capsular bag remains where the IOL is inserted after the natural opaque lens is removed [1].

After the patient's eye is locally anesthetized, the surgeon makes a small incision of less than 3 mm between cornea and sclera. A circular cut by a cannula or micro forceps opens the anterior capsular bag. Subsequently, the phacoemulsification follows, which guarantees the micro incision surgery. The lens is fragmented by an instrument emitting an ultrasonic frequency, while it simultaneously aspirates the pieces of the lens tissue. In the end, only the posterior capsular bag remains [1]. For several steps as for incisions, capsulotomy, and phacoemulsification a femtosecond laser can be used, too [2].

The inserted IOL consists of two main parts: the optic and the haptic, whereby the haptic can be typically designed as C-loop or as plate. It is folded and placed in the eye with the help of an injector. There, the IOL unfolds again and the haptic supports the optical part with the help of the posterior capsular bag. In this way, the optic keeps its central position in the optical path. The capsule bag will contract and cling to the IOL, which primarily happens in the first three months after surgery [1], [3].

1.2 Stabilization in Position

The IOL's refractive power is calculated before the cataract surgery, based on individual eye parameters of the patient. One of these parameters includes the IOL's position inside the patient's eye. Keeping this position stable in the capsule bag is important for the optical function of the IOL [6].

Besides decentration and tilt, an axial shift along the optical axis is a possible instability. The IOL's axis position affects the calculation of the IOL's refractive power and therefore the axial shift influences the surgery's outcome in a negative way. Another critical factor is the rotational stability, in particular for toric IOLs compensating an astigmatism. If the displacement exceeds a certain tolerance, an additional surgery procedure might be necessary for correction [6].

How much the rotation of a toric IOL impacts the correction of an astigmatism as well as possible causes and preventions have been investigated in several studies. It has been discovered that a rotation of $10°$ already decreases the correction by 1/3 to 1/4. For a rotation of $30°$ the postoperative astigmatism is stronger than the preoperative one. If the rotation is higher than $30°$, the astigmatism will be even stronger postoperatively. Accordingly, a rotational stability is desired [3]-[5].

There are a lot of aspects influencing the rotation of an IOL. The postoperative contraction of the capsular bag is assumed to be the main reason. But if there are injuries of the capsular bag during the operation or if the viscoelastic is not completely removed after IOL insertion, instability may occur, too. Also the intraocular pressure of the patient can influence the rotation [3], [5].

Furthermore, an impact due to different haptic designs is possible. Warlo, Krummenauer, and Dick performed a study related to the rotation of IOLs with a C-loop haptic in comparison to a Z-haptic design. With respect to a rotation of less than 10° no statistical significance was given [3]. In an analysis by Cabeza-Gil and Calvo it has been shown that a plate haptic design deforms the capsaular bag significantly in comparison to a C-loop design. Consequently, the rotation stability is higher for the plate haptic than for the C-loop haptic. But in exchange for less rotation, the axial shift is stronger [6].

Vandekerckhove compared the rotational stability between IOLs being identical in haptic shape and manufactured of the same material. The difference between the groups of this study was the optical part of the IOL. For one group monofocal IOLs were inserted, meanwhile for the other group trifocal IOLs were used. As a result, the trifocal IOLs showed less rotation in comparison to the monofocal IOLs. Vandekerckhove assumes that the distinct results with respect to rotation are caused by different surfaces of the IOLs' optics. The trifocal lenses had diffractive rings which provide surface roughness. In contrast, the monofocal lenses had a smooth surface. The concomitant friction, and therefore a surface's roughness, seems to be responsible for the rotational stability, in particular for the time shortly after the surgery before the capsular bag contracts [5].

In Vandekerckhove's study the surface roughness of the IOL was induced by a component being necessary for the desired optical imaging. But there are also surfaces outside of the optical path, e.g., the edges, where different roughness values can be induced. In this work, the IOLs' edge roughness shall be imaged. The use of different materials and variating milling parameters for the production of the IOL indicate individual visual impressions of the IOLs' surfaces, which shall be compared to each other.

2   Material and Methods

The difference in surface roughness of IOLs' edge shall be imaged. To do so, hydrophobic IOLs with C-loop haptic design were used. The lenses were manufactured by Carl Zeiss Meditec AG and delivered in two groups A and B.

The provided IOLs of group A were manufactured of two different materials under same conditions. The delivery was split in 5 trays per material, whereby the respective trays were consistently filled over time. In this way an undesired variety in production may be detected. From each tray two IOLs were picked and numbered in chronological order. Thus, for each material 10 IOLs were chosen.

The trays of group B were also consistently filled over time but only two trays were used for transportation. In both trays the lenses were made of the identical material but the milling parameter (MP) varies from tray 1 to tray 2, whereby MP 1 includes a higher number of rotations per

minute during the milling process than MP 2. During the imaging process of the IOLs from group A it was noticed that 5 lenses per material would have been sufficient. For group B, thus for imaging 5 lenses were extracted from each tray.

All selected IOLs were positioned under a microscope with the help of a tweezer. The microscope was an *Axio Zoom.V16 zoom microscope system* in camera mode with the installed camera *Axiocam 305 color*. For the illumination flexible arms were used in addition to the system. The lens used was the *Plan Apo Z: 0.5x0.125* with a free working distance of 114 mm. The possible magnification was in the range from 3.5x to 56x.

The parameters for the photos were set in the software *Zen-Core 3.4* and can be seen in Table 1.

Table 1: Parameters being set for the microscope for imaging of the IOL's haptic or optic edge, which are distinctly selectable. EDoF stands for Extended Depth of Focus and is a microscope's focus stacking function.

Parameter	Haptic edge	Optic edge
Magnification	50x	50x
Relative aperture	60 %	100 %
Illumination time	700 ms	660 ms
Itensity	120 %	110%
EDoF	Yes	Yes

Both edges were imaged by using the Extended Depth of Focus (EDoF). In a normal image, there is a defined depth of focus. Due to the EDoF function the area in which the sharp image is selectable. *ZenCore* recognizes in which area the image would be sharp in case of a normal image and determines the number of images which is needed to cover the defined area. The microscope's lens acts in corresponding steps along the z-axis and all images are combined to a single one by the software. The object of interest is completely sharp in the image.

In our investigation, after all images were generated, the images were cut equally and positioned next to each other. Thereby, the timeline of production was considered.

The optical impression of the IOLs' surfaces was supported by objective measurements. The evaluation of R_z- and S_z-value was performed (Fig. 1).

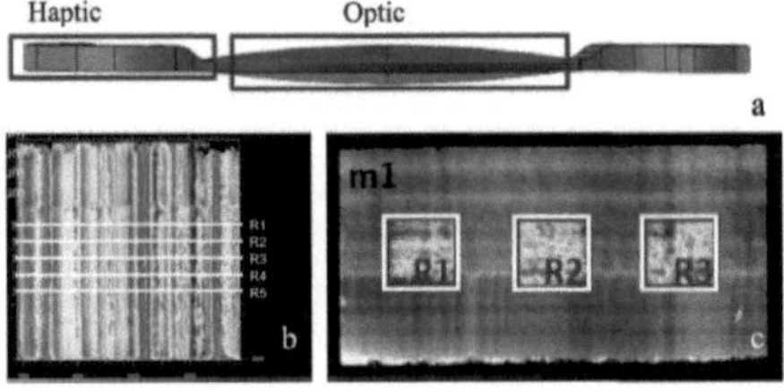

Figure 1: *a)* An IOL's top view with the positiong of roughness measurement *a)* lines related to R_z respectively *b)* areas related to S_z.

R_z is the mean roughness depth and represents the roughness of a line. It is divided into five subsections. In every section R_i, the difference from the highest to the lowest point is determined, and R_z is calculated as the mean of the five heights, as in (1).

$$R_z = \frac{1}{5} \sum_{i=1}^{5} R_i.$$ (1)

The line lay parallel to the edges' structure so that the measurements do not follow the preferred direction caused by the milling process. Because R_z represents the roughness of a single line, in addition the difference between the highest S_p and lowest S_v point of an area S_z was also determined, as in (2). In order to represent this area, 5 lines were included. In this way, a general impression of the lens's edge was generated in comparison to only one line, characterized by R_z.

$$S_z = S_p - S_v$$ (2)

These two values were measured for the haptic and the optic of six lenses in each case: In group A for both materials and in group B for the different milling parameters. The number of chosen lenses was arbitrary set. As null hypothesis we assume that there is no difference between both sample groups so that the value for the hypothesis is 0. The results were checked with regard to statistical significance by performing an one-tailed t-test, whereby the p-value for actual statistical significance was set to $p \leq 0.05$. Due to the low number of observations, the distribution of the roughness values is assumed to be normal.

3   Results

For the visual comparison of the haptics' edges from group A, only 5 of 10 images were included in Fig. 2. Because there were only 5 lenses per tray from group B, a clear layout of the images is guaranteed.
For each box the manufacturing material and milling parameter were constant. In Fig. 2 the IOLs' haptic edges of material 1 (Fig. 2a), material 2 (Fig. 2b), with milling parameter 1 (Fig. 2c), and milling parameter 2 (Fig. 2d) are contrasted. Thereby, the timeline of production is considered inside the respective boxes.

Table 2: Mean values for R_z and S_z for respective two sample groups and the corresponding p-values. For encoding: *group (A/B) - parameter of interest (material M/milling parameter MP) - IOL component (haptic H/optic O)*

Parameter	R_z	P - R_z	S_z	P - S_z
A - M1 - H	0,698 μm	0,002	2,860 μm	0,223
A - M2 - H	0,537 μm		2,445 μm	
A - M1 - O	0,702 μm	0,004	2,647 μm	0,052
A - M2 - O	0,589 μm		2,098 μm	
B - MP1 - H	0,555 μm	0,430	2,386 μm	0,428
B - MP2 - H	0,550 μm		2,341 μm	
B - MP1 - O	0,644 μm	0,304	2,155 μm	0,433
B - MP2 - O	0,622 μm		2,122 μm	

Because the impression of the optic edges' images is quite similar to the images related to the haptic, only one image is exemplarily shown for material 1 (Fig. 2e), material 2 (Fig. 2f), with milling parameter 1 (Fig. 2g), and milling parameter 2 (Fig. 2h).
The roughness values R_z and S_z were calculated for the respective sample groups within each group A and B. The mean values for both parameters were determined, whereby 6 lenses were selected. Besides, the p-values for the t-tests corresponding to the single comparisons were provided. A summary of the results is shown in Table 2.

4   Discussion

In general, an artifact in the images occurs near a particularly high roughness, which is caused by the use of the EDoF function of the microscope. Mostly, this type of artifact could be reduced by adapting the aperture or decreasing the range of the sharp area in the image. Consequently, the number of single images for the complete EDoF image is lower and a reduction in sensitivity to vibrations and high roughnesses is realized.
Also the illumination was not as constant as desired but the repositioning of illumination arms was performed as much as possible.
With respect to the haptics of the IOLs delivered in group A, it could be observed that the impression of the surface is constant over time for both materials (Fig. 2a,b). The same result was available for the IOLs' optic edges, although the edges were more narrow, which led to a more complicated evaluation of the surface. What it looks like for the optic is exemplarily presented in Fig. 2e,f. Comparing the IOLs' haptic edges of material 1 with those of material 2, there seems to be a little higher roughness for material 1. The measured values support this litte disparity. The mean R_z-value of IOLs of material 1 with 0,698 μm shows a little increase in comparison to 0,537 μm of material 2. For the optic, a similar gap in R_z-values between both materials could be recognized (Table 2). By single consideration of the R_z, the p-value calculated was 0.002 for the haptic respectively 0.004 for the optic. As these values were below 0.05, significance regarding this aspect was given. In contrast, evaluating the S_z-values, there was also an increase from 2,445 μm for material 2 to 2,860 μm for material 1, which is not of statistical significant. Considering both factors together, a lack of statistical significance can be concluded.
By inspection of the images related to IOLs which are manufactured with MP 1 and MP 2, neither for the haptic nor for the optic edge a difference in surface treatment is apparent (Fig. 2c,d,g,h). A look at the objective measurements shows that the R_z-values 0,555 μm for MP 1 and 0,550 μm for MP 2 related to the haptic respectively 0,644 μm for MP 1 and 0,622 μm for MP 2 are quite similar. The same is demonstrated by the S_z-values where 2,386 μm and 2,341 μm in case of the haptic or 2,155 μm and 2,122 μm in case of the optic are not significantly different.
To sum up, the visualization of the edge roughness met the results of the objective measurements. Although there seemed to be a variation in roughness between both mate-

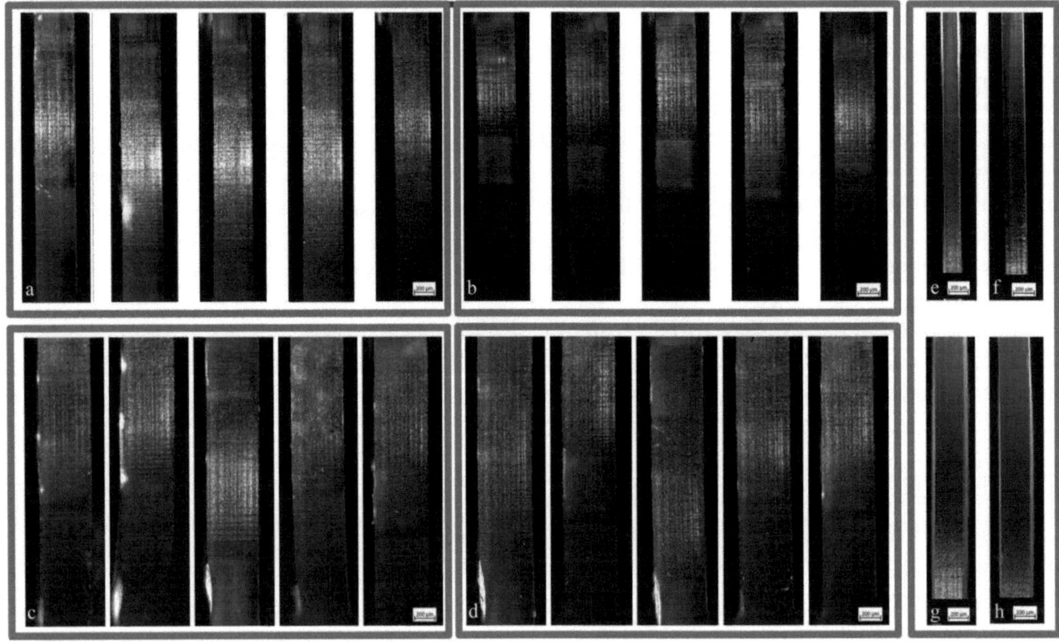

Figure 2: Comparison of IOLs' haptic and optic edges under the *Axio Zoom.V16* with a magnification of the factor 50. Regarding to the haptic, five images were chosen with respect to each scenario, considering the timeline. For the optic, one representing image in each case was chosen. Following matches hold: *a)* A - M1 - H, *b)* A - M2 - H, *c)* B - MP1 - H, *d)* B - MP2 - H, *e)* A - M1 - O, *f)* A - M2 - O, *g)* B - MP1 - O, and *h)* B - MP2 - O. For encoding: *group (A/B) - parameter of interest (material M/milling parameter MP) - IOL component (haptic H/optic O)*

rials, no significance could be proven. Also the t-test for different surface treatments in manufacturing did not result in statistical significance. Thus, these results do not meet the expectations.

5   Conclusion

The comparison of both materials shows a little difference in visual impression of the surface roughness. Considering the distinct milling parameters, no variation between both IOL groups could be observed. Altogether, neither for different materials nor for distinct milling parameters statistical significance was given.

Acknowledgement

The work has been carried out at Carl Zeiss Meditec AG, and supervised by Prof. Dr. rer. nat. Gereon Hüttmann, Institute of Biomedical Optics, Universität zu Lübeck.

Author's Statement

Conflict of interest: Authors state no conflict of interest.

6   References

[1] F. Grehn, *Linsentrübung (Katarakt, grauer Star)*. In: Augenheilkunde, Springer, Heidelberg, pp. 162–178, 2006.

[2] H. S. Uy, K. Edwards and N. Curtis, *Femtosecond phacoemulsification: the business and the medicine*. In: Current opinion in ophthalmology, Vol. 23, pp. 33-39, 2012.

[3] I. Warlo, F. Krummenauer and H. B. Dick, *Rotationsstabilität monofokaler Intraokularlinsen mit C-Haptik versus Z-Haptik nach Kataraktchirurgie*. In: Der Ophthalmologe, Vol. 102, pp. 987-992, 2005.

[4] G. Gerten, A. Michels and A. Olmes, *Torische Intraokularlinsen - Klinische Ergebnisse und Rotationsstabilität*. In: Der Ophthalmologe, Vol. 98, pp. 715-720, 2001.

[5] K. Vandekerckhove, *Rotational Stability of Monofocal and Trifocal Intraocular Toric Lenses With Identical Design and Material but Different Surface Treatment*. In: Journal of Refractive Surgery, Vol. 34, pp. 84-97, 2018.

[6] I. Cabeza-Gil and B. Calvo, *Predicting the biomechanical stability of IOLs inside the postcataract capsular bag with a finite element model*. In: Computer Methods and Programs in Biomedicine, Vol. 221, 106868, 2022. Available: https://doi.org/10.1016/j.cmpb.2022.106868 [last accessed on 2022-11-01]

Tomographic Flow Cytometry using SLIDE Two-Photon Microscopy

Matthea Thielking [1], Florian Sommer [2], Christian Stock [3], and Sebastian Karpf [3]

[1] Medical Engineering Science, Universität zu Lübeck, matthea.thielking@student.uni-luebeck.de

[2] Leibniz Institute of Virology, Hamburg, florian.sommer@student.uni-luebeck.de

[3] Institute of Biomedical Optics, Universität zu Lübeck, {ch.stock, sebastian.karpf}@uni-luebeck.de

Abstract

This paper presents three-dimensional tomographic cellular imaging in a microfluidic setting. To obtain three-dimensional images of cells at sub-cellular resolution, nonlinear two-photon imaging is employed to achieve optical sectioning, yielding tomographic imaging of cells in motion. As imaging setup, we applied a high-speed technology called Spectro-Temporal Laser-Imaging by Diffracted Excitation (SLIDE). To realize tomographic acquisition, a custom microfluidic flow chip was designed to achieve a flow direction perpendicular to the imaging plane. As the cells move through the focal region of the excitation laser, they are excited layer-by-layer with SLIDE two-photon microscopy (TPM), leading to three-dimensional imaging coverage. We present high-resolution tomographic imaging of Euglena gracilis microalgae. The recorded data is processed to three-dimensional representations. Additional segmentation and quantitative analysis of these tomographic cell images provide novel insights into biomedical studies of large, heterogeneous cell populations and can be applied to biomedical analysis of liquid biopsies and various therapeutic applications.

1　Introduction

Flow cytometry is a well established technique to study high numbers of cells at high throughput for biomedical diagnostics, development of therapeutic agents or even basic biology studies [1] [2]. For this purpose, cells are suspended in liquid and sent through a microfluidic channel where the cells are irradiated by a laser. Typically, several detection channels are acquired based on forward and sidewards scattered light and fluorescence labelling. The signals are then used to generate scatter plots visualising size, granularity and molecule-specific labelling [3].

In the present work we want to provide a new tool for high-throughput flow cytometry which not only generates basic laser interaction contrast but rather records a high-resolution microscopic image of the cells in flow. Here, we combine homebuilt microfluidic flow cytometry with the high-speed two-photon technology, called Spectro-Temporal Laser-Imaging by Diffracted Excitation (SLIDE). This method allows the generation of fluorescence images at kilohertz frame-rate, which enables precise, blur-free imaging of cells even at high flow rates [4]. Here we want to go one step further and not only record a two-dimensional image of the cells in flow but rather harness the inherently high three-dimensional resolution of two-photon microscopy (TPM) and record three-dimensional acquisition of cells at high, sub-cellular resolution. We term this technique tomographic flow cytometry (TFC).

In TFC, the cells are recorded layer by layer upon movement in a microfluidic stream and later reconstructed into three-dimensional volumetric images. These cell recordings will provide a range of detailed information about the cellular constituents like the shape of the nucleus, mitochondria counts, the cytoskeleton etc. and can be used to study protein expression and protein interactions within a cell at high resolution and single molecule sensitivity. Furthermore, due to the non-linearity of the SLIDE excitation, imaging is not limited to single cells but also cell organoids or even smaller tissue fragments can be tomographically imaged to also record the three-dimensional morphology and thus the tissue context, at high throughput of up to 4000 events per second.

In the following, we will describe the development of the TFC SLIDE system together with the custom development of a TFC flow chip. The imaging optics and the data processing and segmentation used to study the cells in tomographic flow imaging are also described in the following.

2　Material and Methods

2.1　Flow cytometry and SLIDE

In typical flow cytometry, cells are focused in an enveloping stream and are then individually passing a measurement point where they are exposed to a laser beam. In order to enable a single-cell-based analysis it is crucial that at a given time only a single cell is present in the focal point of the laser beam as the single-pixel detection does not permit spatial distinction of various scatterers or fluorescence emitters [3]. Due to this requirement, this method is limited in the cell throughput. This can be alleviated using imaging methods, where also several cells can be present at once in the recorded area. In addition, more detailed information about the cells can be obtained with imaging methods, such as information about the cell structure and morphology [5].

To obtain fluorescence images of a sample, it must first be excited. A common method to excite a plane by means of a laser is to use two mechanical deflections such as galvanometric mirrors. These mechanically moving mirrors, however, are inertia-limited in their scanning speeds to rates of typically less than 10.000 lines per second. The SLIDE technology overcomes these limitations by using the novel spectro-temporal laser-scanning mechanism which can reach orders of magnitude faster scanning speeds. To this end, a swept source laser is pulse modulated and directed onto a grating, producing the spectro-temporal line scan, where each imaging pixel is addressed by a unique time and unique spectrally encoded position. The various wavelengths of the excitation laser beam impinge on the grating, which causes each wavelength to be diffracted at a different angle. In this way, an excitation line is formed without using a mechanical deflection. For y-axis scanning only one additional galvanometric mirror is needed to create an excitation plane [4].

After fluorescence excitation, the signal is detected on a highly sensitive hybrid photodetector (HPD) and the images are generated after digitization of the time-trace using a fast analog-to-digital converter (ADC) at 4 Gsamples/s. This high bandwidth enables generation of fluorescence images of 4 kHz frame-rate.

2.2 Principle and imaging setup

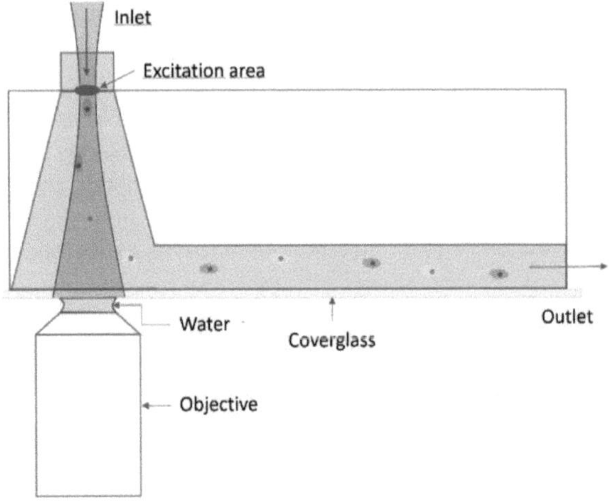

Figure 1: Schematic principle of the imaging setup.

The principle of TFC is shown in Fig. 1. The observed cells within a fluid sample flow along the optical axis, perpendicular to the image plane of the objective and after bending before the microscope coverslip leave the chip horizontally. The excitation laser beam is focused into the fluid stream such that the imaging plane is in an area of axial flow direction. Thus, tomographic acquisition stems from a two-dimensional image scan provided by SLIDE. The third dimension is scanned by the microfluidic flow of the cells. As they move through the excitation plane, they are excited and recorded layer by layer. The high three-dimensional resolution and the excitation only in the imaging plane is achieved through the nonlinearity of the multiphoton excitation by SLIDE [6]. Each layer of the cells is sequentially excited at 4000 fps.

2.2.1 Flow chip

For TFC, a flow chip needs to be designed that allows i) imaging a plane perpendicular to the flow direction, ii) a flow cross-section similar to the image plane area (100 x 100 µm2) and iii) high optical quality to achieve a high-quality focal spot in the imaging plane even when using high Numerical Aperture (NA) microscope objectives with long working distances. Further, laminar flow needs to be ensured to prevent tumbling of cells or tissue fragments upon transversing the imaging plane. A CAD construction of the final chip with connected tubing and cover glass is shown in Fig. 2.

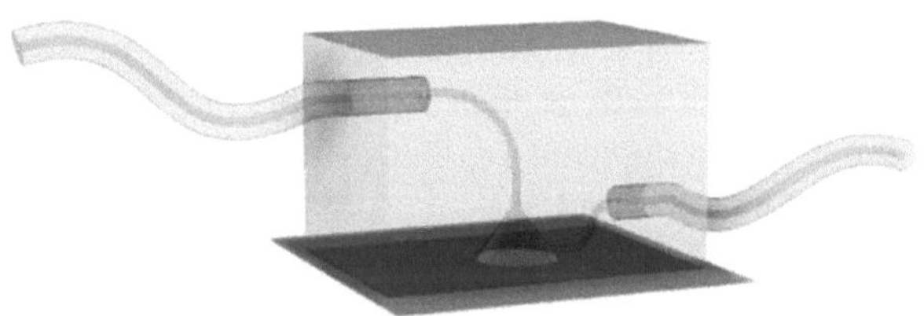

Figure 2: CAD construction of the flow chip, view from the side including cover glass at the bottom of the chip and tubes on its side. Inside the chip the channels and the cone-shaped opening can be seen under which the objective will be placed.

For compact design and to accommodate the microscope condenser lens, the tube inlet is planned on the side, from where the liquid enters the chip through a channel that runs in an arc until it points vertically downwards and opens in the cone-shaped cavity. This opening is implemented at the bottom of the chip so that the exciting laser beam reaches the sample completely.

The imaging itself takes place at the point where the fluid flows from a channel into the cone, so that the cells can be viewed in a fluid stream that is as laminar as possible. At this taper position, it can be ensured that the entire sample flows through this location. The chamber height of this opening has to be compatible with the used objective in terms of its working distance. A cover glass is attached at the bottom of the chip to seal the chip and to ensure high optical quality of the excitation beam entering the flow channel. After passing the cone-shaped opening the sample flows out of the chip at its side into another tube. To move the fluid uniformly through the chip, an automatic syringe pump (Harvard Elite) is used to continuously pump a defined volume per time unit.

2.2.2 Image acquisition and processing

Euglena gracilis microalgae were used as cell sample for the creation of three-dimensional cell images with SLIDE. Due to the contained chlorophyll, their chloroplasts are autofluorescent at the employed two-photon excitation wavelength of 1060 nm (emission around 700 nm), which makes them well suited for fluorescence imaging without additional staining. To generate three-dimensional images of Euglena gracilis cells, a suitable parameter for the volume displacement of the syringe pump must be determined. This value affects the rate at which the cells flow through the focal area. For the first proof of concept of this technique, a flow rate of 10-30 µl/min is chosen to preserve a well-proportioned distance between the individual tomographic layers.

While the cells flow through the focal area of the chip, they are excited by the laser, which leads them to fluorescence emission. The Nikon objective used for this purpose is a 40x water immersion objective with an NA of 0.8. The working distance of 3.5 mm is sufficient for reaching the imaging location in the chip. The excitation power on the sample is about 200 mW (peak power 35 W). The raw data of the emitted fluorescence light recorded with an HPD is converted into an image stack file with ICY, an open-source image processing program. The stack files can be imported in various other programs, where the subsequent image processing to three-dimensional images as well as the segmentation and analysis can be realized. For this purpose Imaris was used in the following, which is a microscopy image analysis software.

3   Results and Discussion

3.1   Flow chip

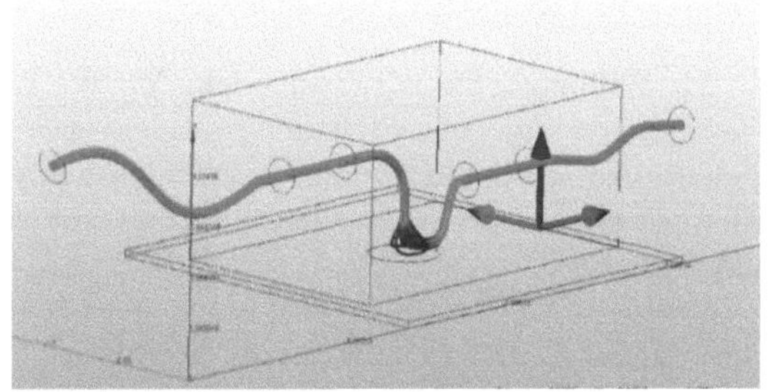

Figure 3: Result of the flow simulation of the flow chip, representation of particle traces.

Based on the construction of the chip, a flow simulation can be performed to analyse the behaviour of the fluid in the channels and the cone-shaped chamber. For this purpose, the Autodesk CFD simulation program was used. The result of this simulation is shown in Fig. 3, where particle tracks are visualized to illustrate the flow behaviour. These run from the tube inlet on the left, through the chip and the cone shaped chamber to the tube outlet on the right.

Since no turbulence occurred during this simulation of the fluid behaviour, a laminar flow profile is assumed. Based on this result, the flow chip is manufactured using a high resolution Stereo-lithography (SLA) printer (Photon Mono 4K, Anycubic). This is a fast and reproducible way to manufacture customized flow chips. A transparent resin is used for the chip fabrication in order to prevent heat-up due to light absorption. The clear design further allows to determine the exact imaging location of the channel opening during transmission observation. The result of the SLA printed flow chip is shown in Fig. 4. The dimensions of the chip are 20 x 8 x 8 mm and the channel width is approx. 200 µm.

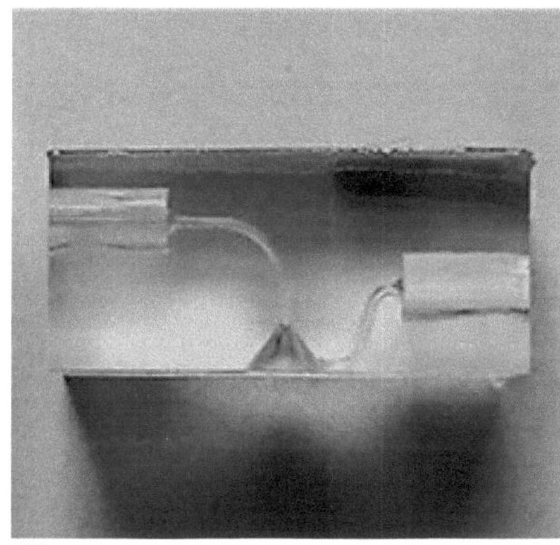

Figure 4: Image of the final flow chip printed using an SLA printer. View from the side. Due to the transparent resin, the channels inside the chip are visible.

3.2   Image processing

The result of the three-dimensional reconstructed tomographic images of Euglena gracilis cells created with Imaris are shown in Fig. 5. Pictured is an approx. 0.5 s long section of the result of a data recording. The field-of-view of the excited region is about 100 x 100 µm2. The z-axis can be interpreted as a time axis since only one defined area, as shown in Fig. 1, is recorded over a defined period of time. Based on the cell reconstructions, a surface-based segmentation is applied to identify the individual cells, on which further processing can be based. This allows initial analyses, regarding the volume of the cells, to be performed. The additional recording of the arrival time of the cells allows the identification and assignment of determined properties to the individual cells and could permit filtering or sorting of cells in a future application.

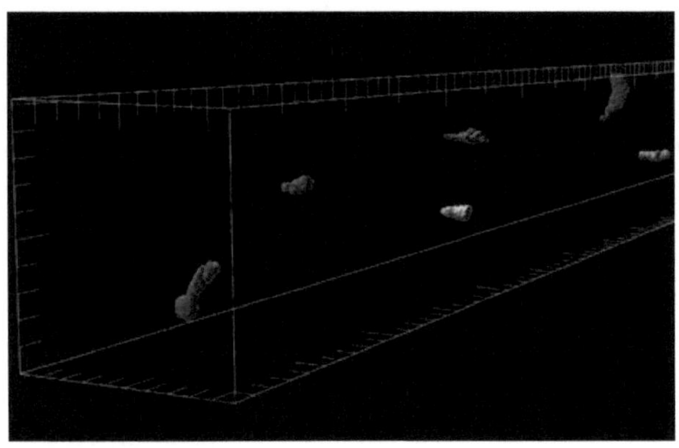

Figure 5: Three-dimensional representation of the layer-by-layer recorded Euglena gracilis cells, segmented to individual micro algae.

Furthermore, a distinction can be made between the different fluorescent regions of individual cells based on the acquired cell images. Fig. 6 shows the segmentation of an Euglena gracilis micro algae to their chloroplasts-regions which was created in Imaris. The "Split touching objects" function was used for this purpose, which separates the individual brightness areas from each other.

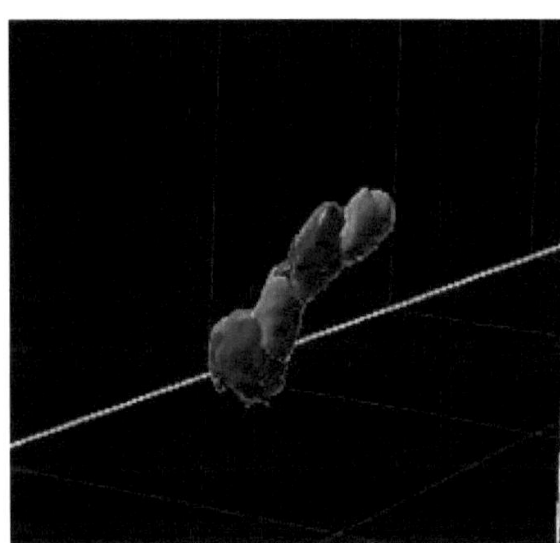

Figure 6: One single recorded Euglena gracilis micro algae, reconstructed to a three-dimensional representation and segmented to its individual chloroplast regions.

4   Conclusion

In this work a flow chip was developed with which flow cytometric imaging can be realized using two-photon SLIDE microscopy. The flow chip enables the recording of a fluid stream in a defined area over a specifiable period of time, allowing tomographic fluorescence images to be created. The acquired data can be processed to three-dimensional volume reconstructions with a high spatial resolution of the cells under consideration. Even the individual chloroplasts of recorded Euglena gracilis cells are identifiable and could further be processed and analysed.

TFC with SLIDE microscopy provides a great basis for further studies. An exemplary application of this imaging method is due to the high excitation depth of TPM, the imaging of larger and more complex cells, such as cell clusters or tumour spheroids, which is to be validated in a subsequent process. Another further development that can build on the present work is the automatic recognition and evaluation of the recorded cell data. With real-time recognition of different cell cultures, this new technique holds the potential to also be supplemented with cell sorting which could enable a large field of further applications.

Acknowledgement

The work has been carried out at the Institute of Biomedical Optic, Universität zu Lübeck under the supervision of Prof. Dr. Sebastian Karpf, Florian Sommer and Christian Stock.

Author's Statement

Conflict of interest: Authors state no conflict of interest.

5   References

[1] A. M. Gressner and T. Arndt, *Lexikon der Medizinischen Laboratoriumsdiagnostik.* Springer-Verlag GmbH Deutschland, 2019.

[2] G. Freer and L. Rindi, "Intracellular cytokine detection by fluorescence-activated flow cytometry: Basic principles and recent advances," *Methods*, vol. 61, pp. 30–38, 2013. [Online]. Available: https://www.sciencedirect.com/science/article/pii/S1046202313001047

[3] H. Chmiel, *Bioprozesstechnik.* Spektrum Akademischer Verlag, 2011.

[4] S. Karpf, C. Riche, D. Di Carlo, A. Goel, W. Zeiger, A. Suresh, C. Portera-Cailliau, and B. Jalali, "Spectrotemporal encoded multiphoton microscopy and fluorescence lifetime imaging at kilohertz frame-rates," *Nature Communications*, vol. 11, p. 2062, 04 2020.

[5] N. S. Barteneva, E. Fasler-Kan, and I. A. Vorobjev, "Imaging flow cytometry: Coping with heterogeneity in biological systems," *Journal of Histochemistry & Cytochemistry*, vol. 60, no. 10, pp. 723–733, 2012, pMID: 22740345. [Online]. Available: https://doi.org/10.1369/0022155412453052

[6] R. M. Williams, D. W. Piston, and W. W. Webb, "Two-photon molecular excitation provides intrinsic 3-dimensional resolution for laser-based microscopy and microphotochemistry," *The FASEB Journal*, vol. 8, pp. 804–813, 1994.

Experimental determination of the quantum efficiency of CMOS cameras

Nathalie Beutel [1], Frank Wienhausen [2], Dirk Stroeker [3] and Natalia Kowalczyk [4]

[1] Medical Engineering Science, Universität zu Lübeck, nathalie.beutel@student.uni-luebeck.de
[2] Evident Technology Center Europe, Hardware Development, Frank.Wienhausen@evidentscientific.com
[3] Evident Technology Center Europe, Hardware Development, Dirk.Stroeker@evidentscientific.com
[4] Evident Technology Center Europe, Hardware Development, Natalia.Kowalczyk@evidentscientific.com

Abstract

Scientific cameras are often employed in recording very low-light levels and thus high sensitivity is of utmost importance. Especially the spectral quantum efficiency is responsible for the signal quality. The measurement setup presented in this paper is intended to experimentally determine the quantum efficiency of CMOS cameras. The measurement setup for this purpose consists of a light source, a filter wheel, a monochromator, a power meter and a spectrometer. The quality of the results depends on the stability of the light source and the calibration of the monochromator. To determine the quantum efficiency of the cameras, the accumulated response signal of the incoming light is set in relation to the respective energy (photon number), measured by a power meter, for small spectral bandwidth. For the DP23M monochrome camera, the measurements result in a maximum quantum efficiency of 83 % at $\lambda = 460$ nm. For longer wavelengths, the quantum efficiency decreases.

1 Introduction

Especially for the application of the more advanced fluorescence microscopy it is mandatory to use cameras with a high signal to noise ratio for the wavelength of the used fluorescence. Thus, beside the noise level, the sensitivity of the camera for respective wavelength is of main interest. The quantum efficiency measurement result of a camera provides this information. A company bringing professional microscopy cameras into the market is highly interested in providing such data to their customers. This paper will describe in detail such a measurement setup. The current state of research is that quantum efficiency measurement provides reproducible results for monochrome cameras.

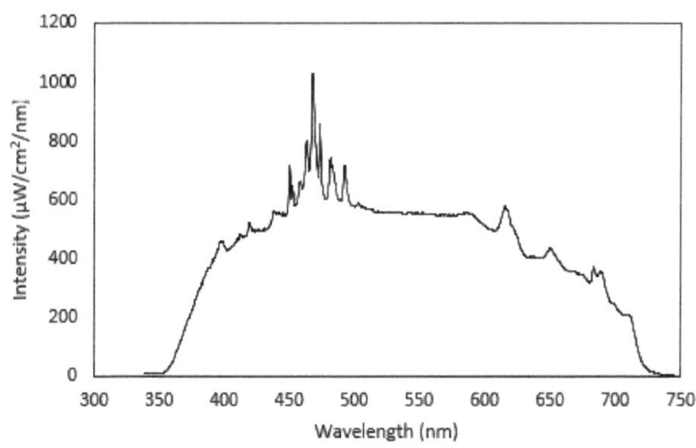

Figure 1: Spectrum of the MT20 lightsource

2 Material and Methods

2.1 Measurement setup and components

The measurement setup consists of an MT20 xenon short-arc lamp (Evident Technology Center Europe GmbH), an M150 monochromator (Solar Laser Systems), a power meter (Coherent, Inc. - Deutschland GmbH) and an AvaSpec spectrometer (Avantes B.V.). The light source has a broad spectrum and an 8-position filter wheel [1]. The spectrum of the lightsource is shown in Fig. 1. The monochromator isolates a narrow wavelength range from the broad spectrum of the light source using a grating. The incident light passes through the entrance slit onto a concave mirror. This creates a parallel beam which is reflected by the grating. Constructive and destructive interference occurs. The angle between the beam and the surface normal of the grating determines which wavelengths are constructively superimposed and which destructive interfere. Therefore, by changing the angle, the wavelength of the band-pass can be changed. A second concave mirror focuses the light onto the focal plane [2]. An M150 monochromator spectrograph was used in the measurement setup, which is schematically shown in Fig. 2. It has one input port and two output ports. The input slit is automated and the opening width of the slit can be controlled by software or manually. A port switcher allows manual switching between the output ports. The axial and lateral outputs operate alternately. Actuating the switcher moves a folding mirror that directs light to the lateral output. The monochromator has two different gratings. One is a 1200 LP/mm grating and the second is a 900 LP/mm grating [3]. In this setup the 1200 LP/mm grating is used. A spectrometer breaks down the measured light beam into its spectral characteristics. The spectrometer used in this setup is the AvaSpec spectrometer. It uses a CMOS sensor as a detector and covers the wavelength range of $\lambda_{\text{range}} = 200\,\text{nm} - 1100\,\text{nm}$ [4]. The light source, the monochromator and the spectrometer are connected by optical fibers. The optical fiber is used in combination with a diffuser to which the spectrometer is calibrated in terms of area and angle.

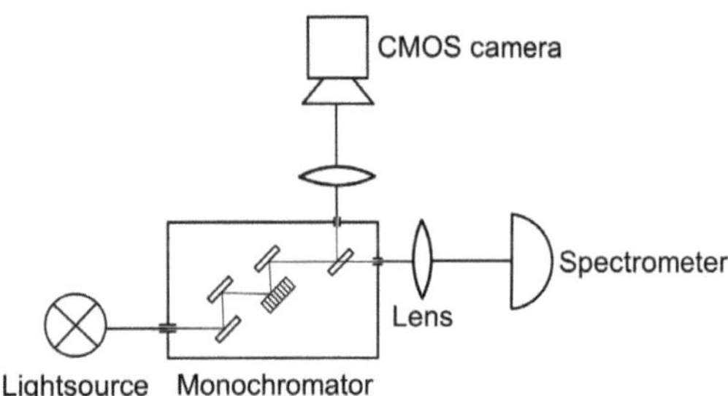

Figure 2: Measurement setup

The Camera makes use of an objective lens to focus the incident light to create an image on the sensor wall. In digital cameras, the image is generated on an electronic sensor. Both CCD chips and CMOS chips are used as image sensors. They consist of an array of photodiodes, also called pixels, providing the lateral resolution of the image. When light hits such a photodiode, it releases electrons by means of the photo effect, which are then collected, summed, read out, and digitized using an analog-to-digital converter. The photodiode continues to collect photons until the pixel is saturated or the electrons are read out at the end of the chosen exposure time [5]. CMOS cameras are investigated in this setup. A measurement system is called linear if the digitized measurement signal is linear. Small nonlinearitys are negligible to a certain degree [6]. The CMOS cameras used in this setup are largely linear. The results of a linearity test of the DP23M camera are shown in Fig. 3. The spectral sensitivity of CMOS cameras reaches from the visible to the infrared range. In the green range $\lambda_{\text{range}} = 480\,\text{nm} - 560\,\text{nm}$, modern sensors are most sensitive. The quantum efficiency is the ratio between the number of emitted electrons to the average number of incoming photons. So it indicates how many photons of a given wavelength are converted into electrons (as a percentage) [7]. The maximum of the quantum efficiency is expected to be in the range of $\lambda_{\text{max}} = 460\,\text{nm} - 500\,\text{nm}$. A tunable light source is required for investigating the quantum efficiency of cameras at different wavelengths. This is done by measuring the ratio of the charge carriers (electrons) generated in a material to the number of photons incident on its surface, at a given exposure time [8]. The pixel is irradiated with light of a known wavelength and the electrical output signal is measured.

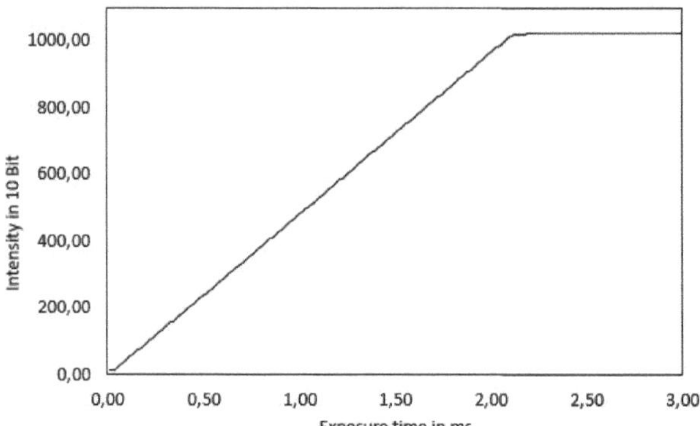

Figure 3: Linearity of the DP23M camera

To measure the quantum efficiency for as many colors of the spectrum as possible, the wavelength is changed in small steps. In this measurement the wavelength was changed in steps of $\Delta\lambda = 20\,\text{nm}$, by adjusting the angle of the grating in the monochromator.

2.2 Raw Data and reference values

To have the entire light as the reference value, it is coupled into the optical fiber as completely as possible. For this purpose, it is focused with lenses to the fiber incoupling surface, respecting the total reflection angle. Unlike the setup shown in Figure 2, the reference value is measured at the same monochromator output to which the camera is connected. This is for the reason that the two outputs show too large differences, which become larger with increasing wavelength. To capture the cameras raw data, the camera is placed behind the lateral output of the monochromator so that the CMOS sensor is illuminated. The raw data images can be captured by software. Then the intensity values are summed up over all pixels. This yields to the total signal intensity in the camera caused by the incident light. Exposure times are selected so that the maximum intensity values are just below saturation. In addition, a dark image is taken to eliminate possible artificial signal offset often present in raw data images.

2.3 Quantum efficiency calculation

To calculate the quantum efficiency for a given wavelength, the ratio between the total number of incoming photons and the counted free electrons is formed. The total number of incident electrons can be calculated as follows:

$$N_{\text{Photon}} = \frac{P \cdot t \cdot \lambda}{h \cdot c}. \qquad (1)$$

Where P is the measured intensity at the power meter, λ is the wavelength, t is the exposure time of the camera, h is the Planck constant, and c is the speed of light. The total intensity for each image captured by the camera is calculated using software. The background intensity is subtracted from the total intensity to obtain the signal in the image. The signal is given in Digital Units. For the DP23M camera, one Digital Unit corresponds to 2.891 electrons [9], so the signal is multiplied by this factor.

The quantum efficiency (QE) corresponds to the ratio of the free electrons and the number of detected photons:

$$QE = \frac{N_{\text{electron}}}{N_{\text{photon}}}. \qquad (2)$$

3 Results and Discussion

3.1 Characterization of the light source

For a precise measurement, it is important to know the stability of the light source. The results, evaluated with the spectrometer, show that the light source needs about $t_{\text{start}} \approx 15\,\text{min}$ after its start until sufficient stability of the power output is reached. The output behaviour of the light source after start is shown in Fig. 4.

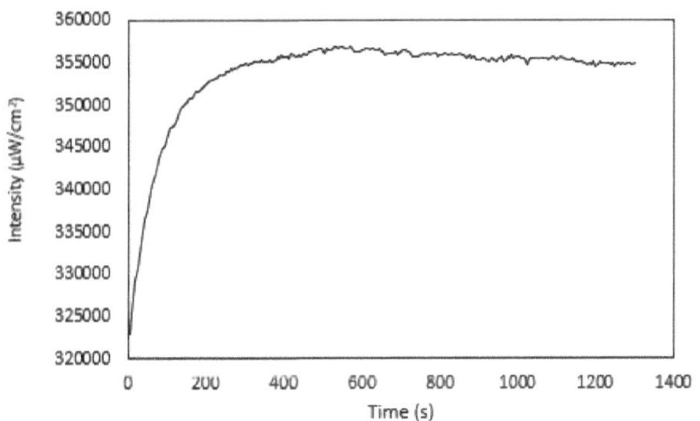

Figure 4: Output power behavior of the light source after start.

3.2 Characterization of the monochromator

Further, the monochromator was characterized in terms of resolution and sensitivity. If the entrance and exit slits are enlarged, more light can pass through the slit and the intensity of the signal becomes higher. But due to increasing diffraction effects the spectral resolution decreases. The spectrometer signal is a peak with a width of $\Delta\lambda \approx 7\,\text{nm}$, as average for all wavelength. Fig. 5 shows the output at $\lambda = 500\,\text{nm}$.

When the monochromator outputs a wavelength longer than $\lambda_{\text{threshold}} = 640\,\text{nm}$, the second diffraction order becomes visible in the spectrum. Therefore, a long-pass filter GG 435 can be used to filter out the second diffraction order.

3.3 Reference values

The power values can be measured with the power meter for the different wavelengths at a distance of $\Delta\lambda = 20\,\text{nm}$. They are shown in Fig. 6.

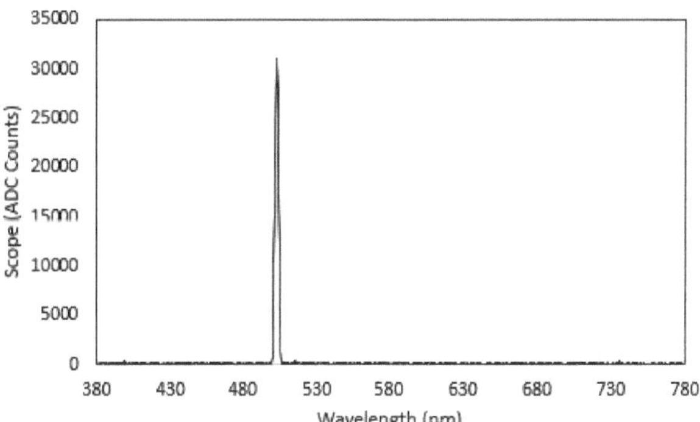

Figure 5: Spectrometer output at $\lambda = 500\,\text{nm}$.

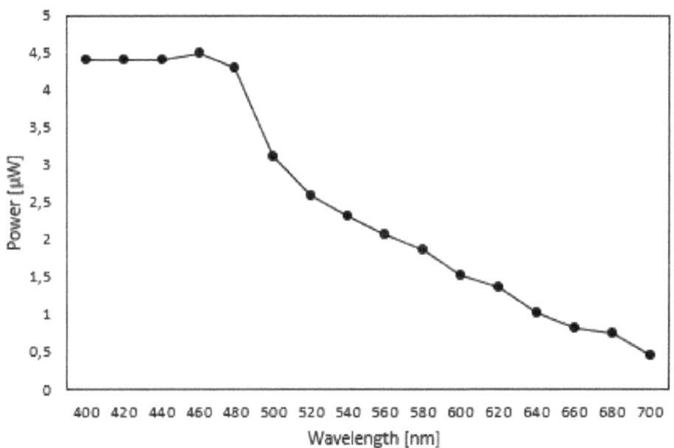

Figure 6: Measured power at different wavelength

3.4 Raw data

Table 1 shows the measurement results from the DP23M camera. Fig. 7 shows the raw data image of the DP23M camera at $\lambda = 480\,\text{nm}$ and $t_{\text{exp}} = 0,85\,\text{ms}$ exposure time rotated 90 degrees. The DP23M is a monochrome camera, so the image is shown in grayscale. To determine the quantum efficiency of the camera, the ratio between the intensity values of the camera (in Digital Units) and the corresponding light intensity is calculated.

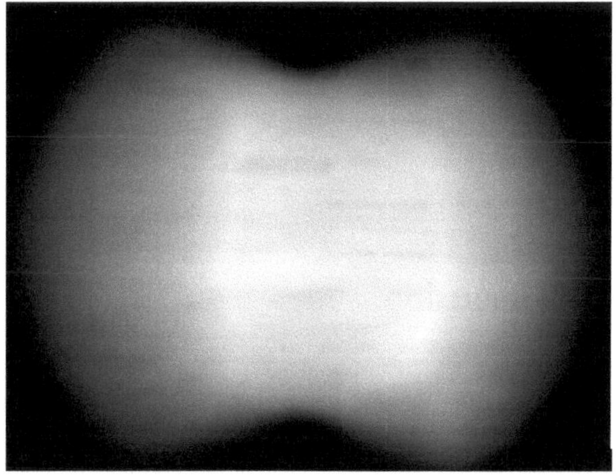

Figure 7: Raw data image.

3.5   Quantum efficiency

Using the calculation described in chapter 2.3, the quantum efficiency can then be calculated for each wavelength. The results are shown in Table 1. As can be seen in Fig. 8, the quantum efficiency of the DP23M camera in the visible range is between 43 % and 83 % . The camera is most sensitive at $\lambda = 460$ nm. For longer wavelengths the quantum efficiency decreases. Why the quantum efficiency collapses slightly at $\lambda = 480$ nm is unclear. A possible reason could be interfering light on the camera.

Table 1: Measurements and quantum efficiency

wavelength [nm]	N_{photon}	N_{electron}	QE [%]
400	9,740E+09	7,654E+09	78,5393
420	9,303E+09	7,631E+09	82,0243
440	9,746E+09	8,007E+09	82,1589
460	8,858E+09	7,376E+09	83,2730
480	8,832E+09	7,103E+09	80,4248
500	9,363E+09	7,685E+09	82,0782
520	9,492E+10	7,654E+09	80,6420
540	9,419E+09	7,350E+09	78,0346
560	9,920E+09	7,406E+09	74,6588
580	1,080E+10	7,494E+09	69,3679
600	1,109E+10	7,293E+09	65,7539
620	1,283E+10	7,444E+09	58,0260
640	1,315E+10	7,284E+09	55,4106
660	1,292E+10	6,876E+09	53,2283
680	1,463E+10	6,733E+09	46,0102
700	1,410E+10	6,538E+09	42,9747

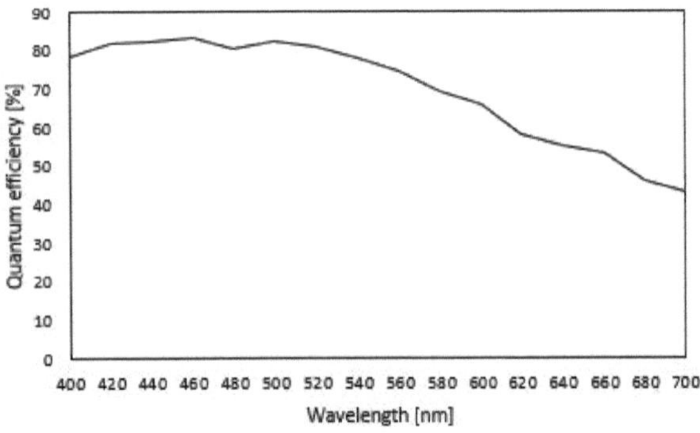

Figure 8: Quantum efficiency of the DP23M camera.

4   Conclusion

In this project, a measurement setup was realized which allows the measurement of the quantum efficiency of CMOS cameras. The measurement setup consists of a broadband light source with filter wheel, a monochromator, a power meter and a spectrometer. After the setup was installed, a characterization with regard to the stability of the light source as well as the resolution and sensitivity of the monochromator was performed. For this purpose, a spectrometer was used to image the output of the monochromator. Using lenses, the light was focused and the absolute intensity was measured with a power meter. Finally, the camera sensor was illuminated, images were taken, and the total intensity of all pixels was calculated. A dark image was also subtracted. From these measurements, the quantum efficiency of the DP23M monochrome camera could be calculated in wavelength steps of $\Delta\lambda = 20$ nm. The measurements showed a maximum quantum efficiency of 83 % at $\lambda = 460$ nm. For longer wavelengths, the quantum efficiency decreases. In the near future, the measurement setup will be improved with regard to its stability. In addition, achromatic lenses can be used to reduce chromatic aberrations. The measurement setup will also be better shielded from interfering light to further ensure that only light from the light source is detected.

Acknowledgement

The work has been carried out at Evident Technology Center Europe GmbH in Münster and supervised by the Institute of Biomedical Optics, Universität zu Lübeck.

Author's Statement

Conflict of interest: Authors state no conflict of interest.

5   References

[1] Olympus Corporation, URL: MT20-E | Olympus LS URL: *olympus-lifescience.com*

[2] IR-Gerätetechnik-ChemgaPedia, Monochromatoren, URL: *http://www.chemgapedia.de/*

[3] M150 Multi-Purpose Compact Monochromator and Spectrograph *User's Manual*

[4] AvantesB.V., URL: *https://www.avantes.com/products/-spectrometers/starline/avaspec-uls2048cl-evo/*

[5] Wolfgang Paech, *CMOS- und CCD SENSOREN - Technik und technische Daten mit ihren jeweiligen Vor- und Nachteilen im Vergleich*, Baader Planetarium (2020)

[6] James R. Janesick, *DN to [lambda]*, Chapter 7: Non-linearity, SPIE Press, 2007

[7] STEMMER IMAGING, Spektrale Empfindlichkeit, URL: *https://www.stemmer-imaging.com/de-de/grundlagen/spektrale-empfindlichkeit/*

[8] L.Classen, *The mdom- a multi-pmt digital optical module for the icecube gen2 neutrino telescope*, Doktorarbeit, Münster, Feb.2017

[9] IDS, U3-3880CP-M-GL Rev.2.2, 4104340807, July 26, 2022

Combination of 3D Imaging Methods with an Endoscope

Paula Belén Wessling Intriago [1],
[1] Medical Engineering Science, Universität zu Lübeck, paula.wesslingintriago@student.uni-luebeck.de

Abstract

The advantages of 3D imaging technologies in combination with endoscopy, especially laparoscopy, are supported by several comparative studies. However, the use of 3D imaging technologies such as Fourier lightfield microscopy (FLMic) or the use of a liquid lens (LL) are not a standard in endoscopy. This article describes an attempt to combine these technologies with endoscopy. To explore the utility of combining an FLMic or LL with endoscopes it is necessary to characterize the parameters of the endoscopes. This paper attempts to do so using a reverse engineering approach. The process provided insights into the optics of the endoscope used that could be applicable to rigid endoscopes in general. In summary, the combination of 3D imaging requires a deeper understanding of the optical behavior of endoscopes, perhaps even a different design of the endoscope.

1 Introduction

3D imaging systems are already used in laparoscopy, although not commonly. Several clinical and comparative studies demonstrate that 3D imaging systems have significant advantages over 2D laparoscopic imaging systems in terms of a lower surgical error rate and a shorter learning curve for learning surgeons [2]-[3]. It is suggested, that it is due to the improved depth perception and accuracy during surgery, that 3D viewing offers [1]. Endoscopes used in diagnostics rarely use 3D Imaging technologies, but could also benefit from 3D imaging systems, especially, if depth information could also be acquired through the usage of depth reconstruction algorithms. This may be useful to assess the dimensions of certain post-operative resections. In this work, a combination of 3D imaging technologies with endoscopy systems is attempted.

1.1 The Fourier Lightfield Microsope

Typically, 3D imaging is based on scanning methods, such as confocal microscopy. In these cases, the 3D image is not acquired in a single shot but is reconstructed computationally after a stack of 2D images is acquired from different sections of the sample. The sequential scanning of each image slows down the acquisition and can cause errors due to vibrations of the mechanically moving scanner. The Fourier Lightfield Microscope (FLMic) enables the acquisition of the information required for 3D reconstruction in a single image, using a micro lens array (MLA). Each lens of the array captures a 2D image of the 3D scene, but from a different perspective in a single shot and therefore the MLA collects spatial and angular information from 3D microscopic specimens with a single image. Computational post-processing with conventional algorithms of this information enables 3D reconstruction of the sample. The

FLMic was developed by the Department of Optics at the University of Valencia and is a new configuration of the Integral microscope (IMic) [5]. The MLA is not placed in the image plane,like in the IMic, but at the aperture stop (AS) of the microscope objective (MO). A telecentric relay system is used to conjugate the MLA to the AS of the MO. The telecentric relay system consists of two afocally coupled converging lenses (RL1 and RL2 in Fig.1) with a field stop (FS) in their common focal plane. This system increases the spatial resolution by a factor of 1.4 and increases the depth of field compared to the previous IMic system [4],[5].

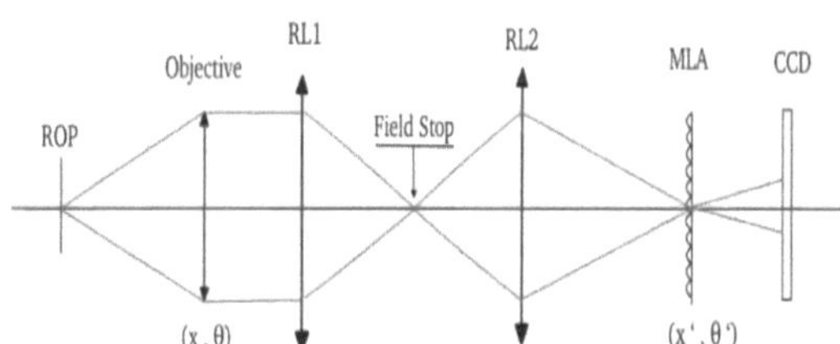

Figure 1: Optical schematic of the FIMic. Here, the aperture stop of the microscope objective is accessed using a telecentric relay system consisting of two converging relay lenses RL1 and RL2. The reference object plane (ROP) must be defined because there is no single object plane in a 3D scene. The ROP is located in the central region of the 3D scene

1.2 The Liquid Lens

By inserting a liquid lens (LL) into the optical imaging system used, the focus can be changed electronically without affecting speed or image quality. The focal length, and therefore the optical performance, of a lens depends on the refractive index associated with the material of the lens and on its radius of curvature. The optical power of a LL can be changed by manipulating a voltage of up to 70 V between two ring electrodes around the LL. This voltage modulation changes the radius of curvature of the transparent liquid inside the lens, spatially distributing the molecules and thus spatially distributing the refractive indices [6]. The modulation occurs over a time range of milliseconds. Variable focal length allows reconstruction of 3D images by capturing elemental images in different image planes. The depth information corresponding to each pixel of the elementary images can be calculated.

2 Material and Methods

2.1 The Endoscope

The endoscope used in the setup is a laparoscope of the model Flexi-lux 4 from the brand Schölly. It has a diameter of 10 mm and a working length of 344 mm. It has a wide-angle field of view and a direction of view of 0 degrees. Other optical parameters are not provided by the manufacturer for reasons of confidentiality. A laser was used to guide the light through the endoscope. The laser from Oxxius produces a light of 488nm with variable intensity. Further elements used were lenses of different fixed focal lengths, a CMOS camera as a sensor of the model DFM 37UX250-ML with a pixel size of 3.45 μm x 3.45 μm. To understand the optical function of the endoscope, different approaches were taken with different setups and objectives.

2.2 Detection of Overlapping Planes

The laser required for the experiments was collimated through a lens of 75 mm. Collimation was performed using a shear plate. To identify the focal plane, different auxiliary lenses, e.g. L_1 in Fig. 2 with known focal lengths were placed in front of the distal end of the endoscope. In addition, a sensor focused to infinity was placed behind the auxiliary lens. This sensor consisted of a sensor placed in the back focal plane of a second lens L_2. In this configuration, shown in Fig. 2, the objective was, by moving the auxiliary lens, to detect the focused beam on the sensor as soon as the front focal plane of the auxiliary lens intersected with the rear focal plane of the objective of the endoscope.

2.3 Measurement of Focal Length and Magnification

A further experiment consisted in finding out the focal length of the endoscope, as well as the magnification of the system. This required inserting diffused light from an LED through the proximal end and detect it with the sensor at the distal end. The LED used for illumination, was a 3-channel PWM LED power source, powered at 300 mA and 3 W from IBM. Using a LED instead of a Laser was a challenging task, as it became more difficult to align the

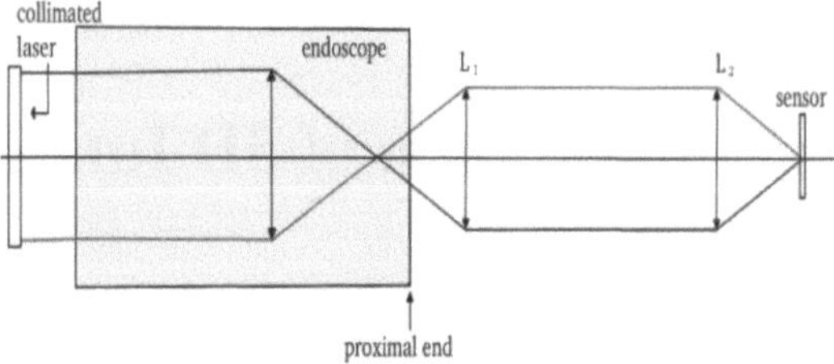

Figure 2: Setup used for detecting overlapping planes. The experiment was performed with a variety of different focal lengths for L_1. L_1 is shifted axially on the optical bench. A focus appears on the sensor as soon as the front focal plane of the auxiliary lens intersects the rear focal plane of the endoscopes objective.

system to produce an image on the sensor distal to the entrance pupil, since it was so small. Before the measurements could be performed, the right position for the auxiliary lens had to be located using the configuration shown in Fig. 3. For this purpose, a collimated laser with a lens of 75 mm was placed 1mm from the proximal end of the endoscope and a sensor was focused to infinity using a lens with a focal length of 100 mm. An auxiliary lens with focal length f_{aux}= 100 mm was placed so that a focused laser bundle appeared on the sensor, which is approximately 8 cm from the distal tip of the endoscope. For the measurements, the laser was replaced by the IBM LED illuminator, and a Siemens Star (with 36 segments) from Edmund Optics was used as the object. Part of the Siemens Star appeared as an image on the sensor and was used for further calculations. Fig. 4 illustrates the described setup. To calculate the magnification, it was necessary to measure the image size, which, as explained earlier, was a fraction of the siemens star. The image size was measured using the IMAGE J program. Knowing the magnification, the focal length f could be calculated by rearranging the magnification equation for afocal systems shown in (1). f_1 and f_1 beeing the focal lengths of the two lenses that form an afocal system.

$$ M = \frac{f_2}{f_1} \tag{1} $$

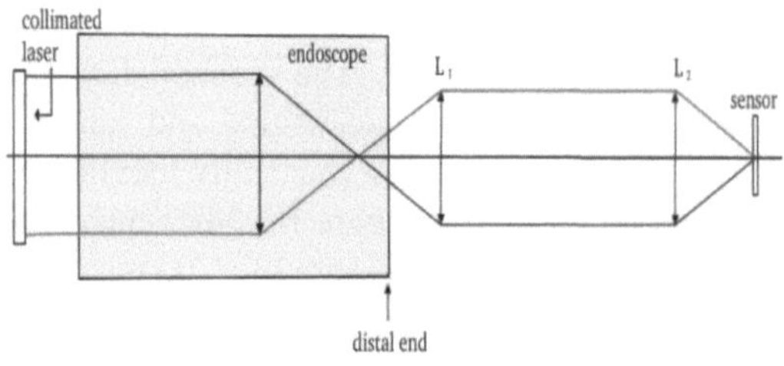

Figure 3: Setup to select the localization for L1. It is similar to the configuration described in Fig.2, only that the endoscope is inverted.

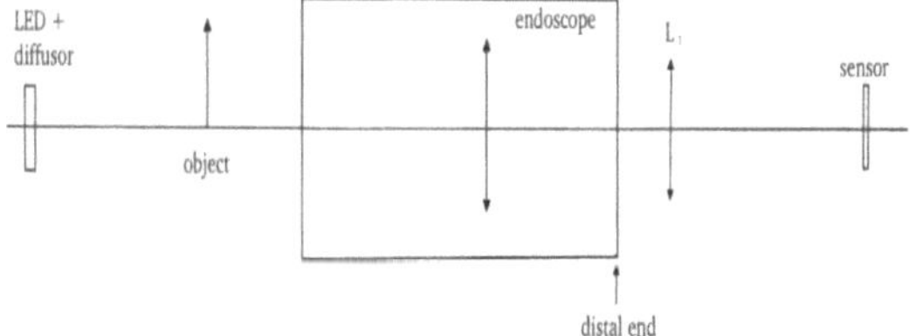

Figure 4: Setup to measure the focal length and the magnification of the system.

2.4 Calculation of Resolution

A USAF 1951 plate was used as the object, and it was placed at 1 mm from the distal tip of the endoscope. The liquid lens was placed 1mm from the proximal end. The sensor was placed behind the LL and moved axially. The voltage applied to the lens varied. The LED powered at 300 mA and 3 W from IBM was used as illumination. A USAF 1951 chart serves to measure resolution. The chart is divided into "groups" of 6 "elements" each. Resolution ρ_{obj} was calculated through the formula:

$$\rho_{obj} = \frac{\frac{32000}{2\,(\,6+\,group)}}{(2^{\frac{1}{6}})(element-1)}\,\mu m \qquad (2)$$

3 Results and Discussion

In order to take images with the FLMic it is very important to work with instruments with a localized aperture stop. This is not the case with the used endoscope. After trials of implementing the FLMic concept to the system, no promising results could be found. Instead, the project was shifted towards the implementation of a LL that can be used to obtain different captures of different depths with the endoscope, which enables the possibility for application of depth algorithms.

3.1 Reverse-Engineering-Method for Characterization of the Endoscope

When analyzing the endoscope with the initial setup described in section 2.2, the goal was to find the focal plane of the endoscope lens using different auxiliary lenses with different focal lengths. By moving the auxiliary lens axially, it was aimed to find the configuration where the focal point of the auxiliary lens overlapped with the focal point of the endoscope. The desired configuration would be detected when a focused focal point appeared on the sensor. This configuration did not provide the expected results. Various focal lengths ranging from 50 mm to 400 mm, longer than the endoscope itself, were used. Since the focal plane of the endoscope did not appear to exist, the next step was to measure the focal length and the magnification of the endoscope. For this experiment, the setup in Section 2.3 was used. Here, the difficulty was aligning the system so that an image could be transmitted through the endoscope. The

system was aligned once an image of the exit pupil of the proximal end was detected on the sensor. Once the system was aligned, a USAF Siemens Star was placed in front of the proximal end of the endoscope. Because the field of view was extremely small, only a small portion of the Siemens Star could be seen. A small circle on the sides of the chart was chosen for display as represented in Fig. 5. Axially moving the USAF chart did not change the image or the image size. With an image of the imaged circle, the magnification m of the endoscope can be measured. The diameter of the imaged circle in the object space is 1.7 mm. The diameter of the image was calculated with the help of the program IMAGE J. With this program it is possible to measure the number of pixels in an image. The average of all measurements was 29 pixels. Considering that the sensor used has a pixel size of 3.45 µm, the image diameter can be calculated to be 100.05 µm. The image size divided by the object size results in a magnification of m = 0.0588. Considering the equation for magnification in afocal systems, the effective focal length of the endoscope f_{LAP} can be determined:

$$f_{LAP} = -\frac{f_{aux}}{m} = -\frac{100\ mm}{0.0588} = -1724.13\ mm, \qquad (3)$$

where f_{aux} is the focal length of the selected auxiliary lens.

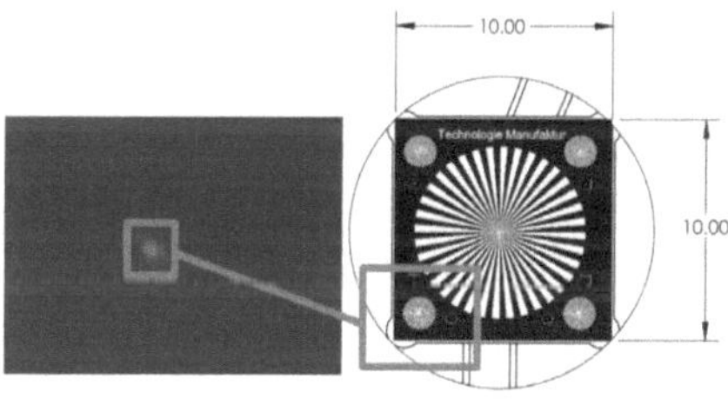

Figure 5: Here the image (left) of the small circle of the Siemens Star (right) that was chosen to perform the measurements.

3.2 Combination of the Liquid Lens with the Endoscope

First, the functionality of the LL and its compatibility with the endoscope was evaluated. For this purpose, the measurements were performed to confirm that the behavior of the LL indicated in the data sheet was also true under laboratory conditions. At lower voltages, the images were of very low quality, so only values above 62 V were considered. 70 V is the maximum permissible voltage. The LL was placed in front of the proximal end of the endoscope, to perform resolution measurements. A sensor was placed in front of the liquid lens. The object that was to be imaged was placed 0.1 cm from the distal end of the endoscope. The object , a USAF Chart 1951, was illuminated using the integrated illumination system of the endoscope. The USAF Chart 1951 was used as the object to measure the resolution of the new system at various optical powers of the lens. Images were acquired by operating the LL with volt-ages ranging from 63 V to 70 V. Table 1 shows the average of the resolutions measured at 8 different voltages. As can be seen in Table 1, the resolution did not vary significantly when using the LL at different optical powers. However, there appears to be a trend toward lower resolution at higher voltages on the lens. The calculated values for resolution depend on the sensor used and may change when other sensors are used.

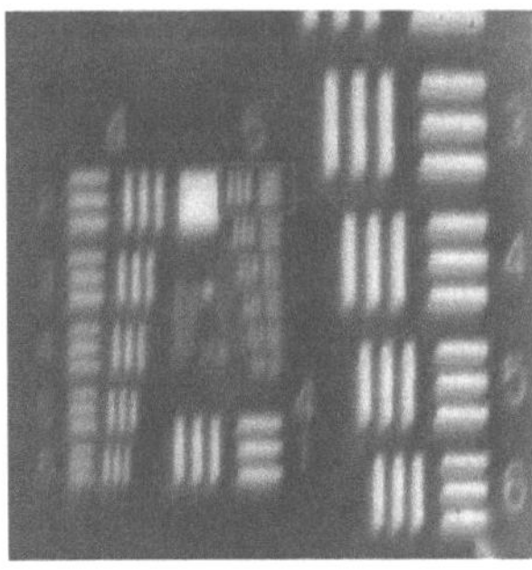

Figure 6: This is an example of an image taken at 70 V. The smallest resolvable distances are in the first element of group 5 (marked red).

Table 1: Resolution of the combined system at different voltages

Voltage (V)	Resolution (μm)
63	12.4
64	11
65	11
66	11
67	12.4
68	12.4
69	15.6
70	15.6

4   Conclusion

The goal of combining FLMic with endoscopy was desirable because of the advantage of single-shot imaging, which allows rapid imaging of dynamic probes. The economic efficiency of using an MLA instead of other costly 3D imaging techniques was also an advantage. However, the combination requires a deeper understanding of the optical behavior of endoscopes, perhaps even a different design of the endoscope, to make the AS accessible. The attempted combination with the liquid lens must be processed with a reconstruction algorithm for 3D visualization. The reconstruction algorithms are not fast enough to be used in surgical procedures where real-time visualization is required. However, the use of a LL could be a useful tool in diagnosis when a specific depth measurement is required, and real-time 3D display is not necessary. Nevertheless, the process provided an opportunity to learn about the optics of the endoscope used that may be applicable to other rigid endoscopes in general. Several observations of the results from

Section 3.1 indicate that the endoscope behaves in a nearly afocal manner. The name "afocal" implies a system without focus or with a focal plane at infinity. The endoscope does not appear to have a localizable focal plane, which is a characteristic of afocal systems. Another indication that the laparoscope behaves nearly afocal is the fact that the focal length f_{LAP} of the endoscope is 1724.13 mm, which is close to infinity in the dimensions of conventional optics. Another argument in favor of afocal behavior is that the magnification is independent of the position of the object, which is the case for the magnification of afocal systems, which can be seen in (1) . In summary, the endoscope's optical behaviour can be described as an inverted Galilean telescope.

Acknowledgement

The work has been carried out at the Department of Optics, University of Valencia and supervised by Prof. Dr. sebastian Karpf, Institut für Biomedizinische Optik, Universität zu Lübeck.

Author's Statement

Conflict of interest: Authors state no conflict of interest.

5   References

[1] S. Kong et al, *Comparison of two- and three-dimensional camera systems in laparoscopic performance: a novel 3D system with one camera.* Surg Endosc 24(5):1132-43, 2010.

[2] A. Buia, F. Stockhausen, N. Filmann, E. Hanisch, *3D vs. 2D imaging in laparoscopic surgery an advantage? Results of standardised black box training in laparoscopic surgery* In: Langenbecks Archives, Surg.9. Epub 402(1):167-171., 2017.

[3] A. Ghedi et al, 3D vs 2D laparoscopic sys-tems: Devel-opment of a performance quantitative validation model. In: Annual International Conference of the IEEE Engineering in Medicine and Biology Society (EMBC), Milan, 6884–6887, 2015.

[4] M. Martínez-Corral, B. Javidi, *Fundamentals of 3D imaging and displays: a tuto-rial on integral imaging, light-field, and plenoptic systems* In: Optica, Advances in Optics and Photonics, Vol. 10, Issue 3, pp. 512-566, 2018

[5] A. Llavador, J. Sola-Pikabea, G. Saavedra, B. Javidi, M. Martínez-Corral, Resolution improvements in integral microscopy with Fourier plane recording In: Optics Express, 24(18),pp. 20792–7, 2016.

[6] Edmund Optics,"Liquid Lens Basics",edmundoptics.eu.,https://www.edmund-optics.eu/knowledge-center/application-notes/imaging/introduction-to-liquid-lenses/

Shifted Excitation Raman Difference Spectroscopy for the Investigation of Fluorescent Animal Bones

Renée Busch [1,2], Kay Sowoidnich [2], Lara Sophie Theurer [2], André Müller [2], Martin Maiwald [2] and Bernd Sumpf [2]

[1]Medical Engineering Science, Universität zu Lübeck, renee.busch@student.uni-luebeck.de

[2]Ferdinand-Braun-Institut, Leibniz-Institut für Höchstfrequenztechnik, Berlin, {kay.sowoidnich, larasophie.theurer, andre.mueller, martin.maiwald, bernd.sumpf}@fbh-berlin.de

Abstract

Raman spectroscopy is a valuable tool for chemical analysis and well-suited for biological material but interfering backgrounds can pose a major challenge. Bone is one prominent example of biological tissue and molecule-specific bone analysis has many implications, e.g. in medicine, animal health and forensics. To remove fluorescence and other background interferences a combined approach of shifted excitation Raman difference spectroscopy (SERDS) and long-wavelength excitation was applied. An in-house-developed distributed-Bragg-reflector ridge waveguide (DBR-RW) diode laser emitting at 830.18 nm and 830.98 nm served as excitation light source. Pork metacarpal bones and chicken thigh bones were investigated exemplarily using 35 mW optical power at the sample and 10×5 s recording time. The mineral-to-collagen ratio calculated from the SERDS spectra enabled a clear distinction between these two bone types. This paper demonstrates the suitability of SERDS at 830 nm excitation to study bone composition and lays the foundation for further research.

1   Introduction

Raman spectroscopy is an established molecule-specific technique for the chemical analysis of samples. Since water is a weak Raman scatterer in the fingerprint region, the technique is well-suited for biological samples [1] and has the advantages of no need for sample preparation and being non-destructive. Raman signals are inherently weak and, in the case of fluorescent samples, can be almost completely obscured by the fluorescence background. Bone which is a composite material made up of organic (mainly collagen) and mineral (mainly apatite) components is one prominent example of a highly fluorescent biological sample. Molecule-specific bone analysis has many implications, e.g. in medicine, animal health and forensics.

Several methods for fluorescence rejection have already been developed [1]. A method to reject not only fluorescence in bone samples but also other background interference (e.g. ambient lights and fixed-pattern noise arising from CCD detectors), is shifted excitation Raman difference spectroscopy (SERDS) [2]. This method applies two slightly shifted laser wavelengths and exploits that the Raman signals follow the wavelength shift, while fluorescence and other interfering contributions remain unaffected. This allows the undesired background to be removed by subtracting the two recorded spectra. In this way the SERDS difference spectrum is obtained. The derivative-shaped difference spectrum is then integrated to obtain a SERDS spectrum in conventional form.

SERDS requires a laser that can emit at two slightly shifted wavelengths with the necessary spectral spacing which should be similar to the full-width at half-maximum of the Raman bands [1]. If the wavelength shift chosen for SERDS is too small, intensity is lost through the subtraction as Raman signals excited at both wavelengths will be subtracted from each other. However, if the shift is too large, the spectral resolution is reduced [3]. Dual-wavelength diode lasers are well-suited and have already been used as excitation light sources for SERDS [3].

In this work, a compact 830 nm DBR-RW single diode laser [4] with implemented heaters to adjust the emission wavelength is used to investigate bone samples from two selected animal species with SERDS. Pork metacarpal and chicken thigh bones were exemplarily selected as test samples for our study. An excitation wavelength of 830 nm is particularly suitable for biological samples due to the spectral range of low absorption in biological tissue [5], also the fluorescence intensity generally decreases with increasing wavelength. To the best of our knowledge, this is the first time that the combination of excitation at 830 nm and SERDS is assessed as effective technique for fluorescence removal in fluorescent animal bone specimens.

2   Material and Methods

Laser: For this work, a DBR-RW diode laser is used, which emits at 830 nm. At an operation point of 83 mA injection current the laser reaches an optical output power of 44 mW, has a peak wavelength of 830.18 nm and a measured spectral width of 0.02 nm (Fig. 1) at full-width at half-maximum, limited by the spectral resolution of the spec-

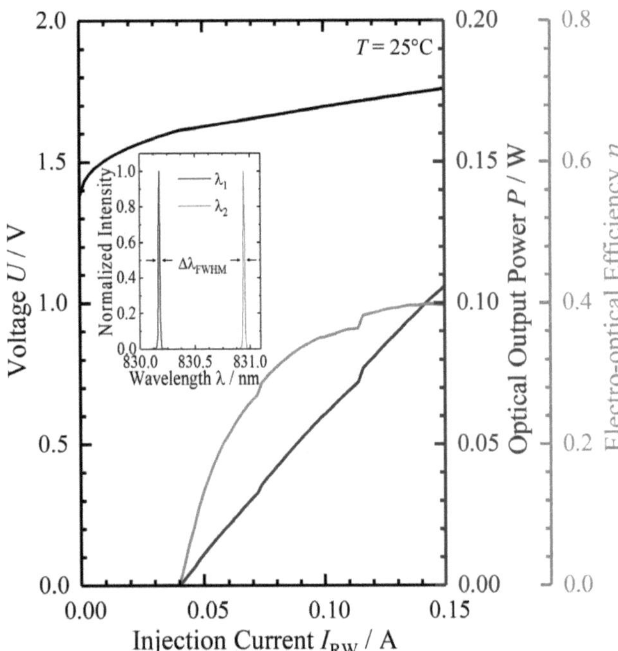

Figure 1: Laser characteristics including voltage, optical output power and electro-optical efficiency at injection currents from 0 mA to 150 mA and intensity-normalized laser emission spectra at $\lambda_1 = 830.18$ nm and $\lambda_2 = 830.98$ nm, both with a spectral width of $\Delta\lambda_{FWHM} = 0.02$ nm.

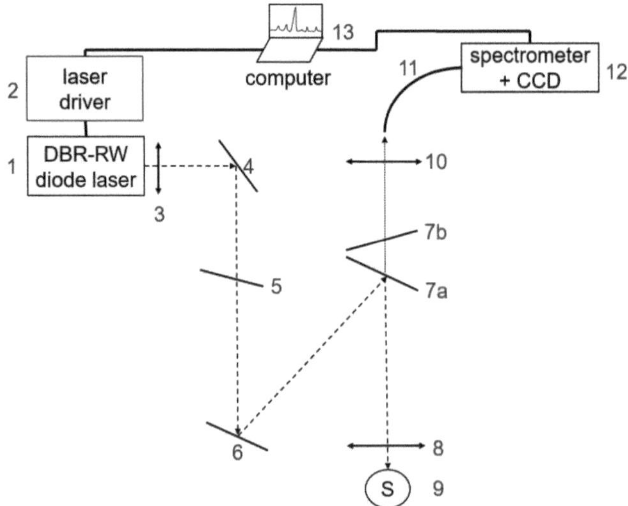

Figure 2: Scheme of SERDS setup. DBR-RW diode laser (1), laser driver (2), aspheric lenses (3: $f = 8$ mm, $\varnothing = 12.24$ mm, 8: $f = 19$ mm, $\varnothing = 25$ mm), mirrors (4, 6), bandpass filter (5), Raman long-pass edge filters (7a, 7b), bone sample (9), achromatic lens (10: $f = 60$ mm, $\varnothing = 25$ mm), multimode optical fibre (11), spectrometer with CCD detector (12), computer (13).

trometer. In order to achieve a wavelength tuning, the wavelength selected by the grating is shifted by Joule heating using the implemented heaters. A spectral tuning of up to 1.29 nm at a maximum specified heater current of 300 mA can be achieved. The narrow spectral emission is retained for the entire operation range. This tuning range allows free adjustment of the excitation wavelength for the experiment. In our study heating currents of 0 mA and 250 mA are applied to shift the spectrum by $12\,\mathrm{cm}^{-1}$ which corresponds to 0.8 nm. To obtain the same optical power at sample location (35 mW), the injection current is adjusted to 108 mA for the heater current of 250 mA.

Setup: Fig. 2 shows a scheme of the experimental setup. The diverging output beam of the DBR-RW diode laser (1) at 830 nm, which is controlled by the laser driver (2) is collimated using an aspheric lens (3) with $f = 8$ mm. A bandpass filter (5) from Semrock is used to remove amplified spontaneous emission. Two mirrors (4,6) and a long-pass edge filter (EF, 7a) from Semrock direct the emission light to an aspheric lens (8) with $f = 19$ mm, which focuses the beam on the sample (9). The 180°-backscattered light is collected by the same lens and is directed to two long-pass EFs (7a, 7b). Here, the laser light and the inelastically scattered anti-Stokes shifted light (at shorter wavelengths compared to the excitation wavelength) are reflected. The Stokes-shifted light (at longer wavelengths compared to the excitation wavelength) passes the EFs and an achromatic lens (10) with $f = 60$ mm couples the light into a multimode optical fibre (11) with a $200\,\mu$m core diameter and a numerical aperture of NA = 0.22. The fibre is connected to

a spectrometer HyperFlux U1 from Tornado Spectral Systems with attached CCD camera (12). The operating temperature of the CCD camera is $T_{CCD} = -10\,°$C and the dispersed light is focused onto it. The spectral resolution is $8\,\mathrm{cm}^{-1}$. A computer (13) is connected to the CCD camera and the laser driver to synchronize the alternating laser emission with the spectral acquisition. In-house developed software was used for setup control and data handling.

Sample material and data analysis: Pork metacarpal bones and chicken thigh bones were provided by the Research Institute for Farm Animal Biology (FBN). Each bone was cleaned of surrounding soft tissue before Raman spectroscopic measurements. The samples were probed at 20 different positions and 10 spectra were recorded and averaged for each measurement spot. Thereby, 200 single SERDS spectra from 20 sample positions per bone type were obtained. The optical power at the sample location was 35 mW and the measurement time used for each of the two excitation wavelengths was 10×5 s. SERDS spectra were calculated using an in-house developed reconstruction method as outlined in our previous publication [6].

3   Results and Discussion

Despite the long excitation wavelength of 830 nm, the Raman spectra displayed in Fig. 3a (based on a measurement on a chicken thigh bone) show a distinct fluorescence background. Although the main peak at 957 cm^{-1} attributed to the symmetrical phosphate stretching vibration is visible in the Raman spectrum, many of the smaller peaks are superimposed by fluorescence. From the Raman spectrum alone it is difficult to identify which features are Raman signals

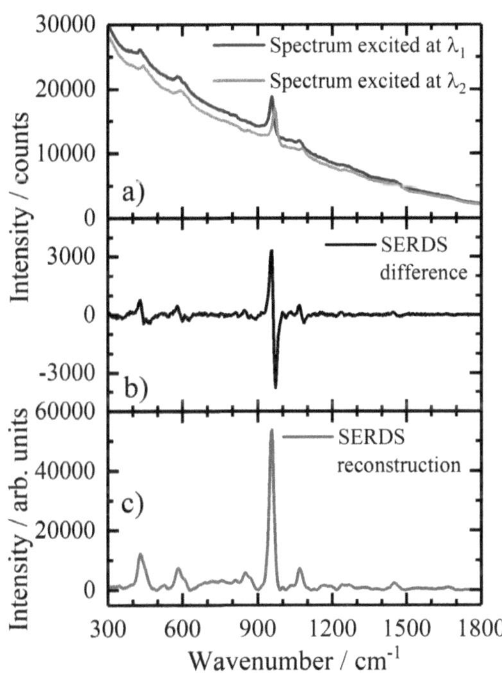

Figure 3: (a) Average of 10 Raman spectra excited at $\lambda_1 = 830.18$ nm and $\lambda_2 = 830.98$ nm, (b) SERDS difference spectrum and (c) corresponding reconstructed SERDS spectrum obtained from 1 measurement position from chicken thigh bone.

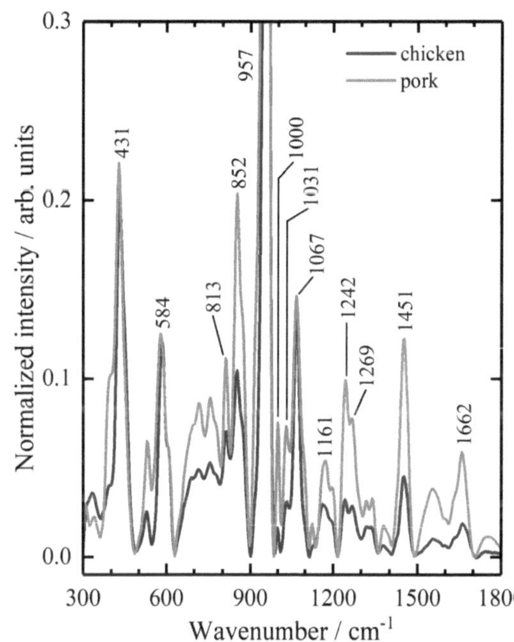

Figure 4: Comparison between reconstructed SERDS spectra from chicken thigh bones and pork metacarpal bones normalized to their maximum intensity at 957 cm^{-1}, labels indicate characteristic bone Raman signals identified with the literature [7].

and which are background interferences. The SERDS difference spectrum (Fig. 3b) is calculated by subtracting the two Raman spectra recorded at the two excitation wavelengths. By using SERDS, the fluorescence background can already be removed in the difference spectrum. The difference spectrum shows a derivative-like shape and can be converted into a SERDS spectrum in conventional form by numerical integration. This reconstructed SERDS spectrum is displayed in Fig. 3c.

For a comparison between the chicken thigh bones and the pork metacarpal bones the average reconstructed SERDS spectra obtained from all 20 measurement positions are presented in Fig. 4. In order to achieve better comparability the spectra of the bones are normalized to the highest mineral peak, the symmetric phosphate stretching vibration at 957 cm^{-1}. Because of that it is the difference in organic content (collagen) that is evident. So the positions of mineral and organic components can be recognized by the differences in the peak height of chicken and pork. In the investigated spectral range the reconstructed SERDS spectrum enables the identification of the strongest characteristic Raman bands and also of weak Raman bands like the phenylalanine signal at 1000 cm^{-1}. The characteristic bone signals determined and their corresponding vibrational assignment based on data compiled in the literature [7] are given in Table 1.

To evaluate the observed differences between the two bone types in more detail and to quantify the compositional variations of the bone samples, a well-established Raman signal

Table 1: Raman bands identified in the SERDS spectra of chicken thigh bones and pork metacarpal bones and assignment of vibrational modes according to data compiled in the literature [7]. Stretching vibration (ν), deformation vibration (δ).

Wavenumber /cm^{-1}	Vibrational assignment	Bone component
431	ν_2 PO$_4^{3-}$	Apatite
584	ν_4 PO$_4^{3-}$	Apatite
813	ν C-C	Collagen
852	ν C-C	Collagen
957	ν_1 PO$_4^{3-}$	Apatite
1000	Phe ν CC ring	Collagen
1031	ν_3 PO$_4^{3-}$	Apatite
1067	ν_1 CO$_3^{2-}$, ν_3 PO$_4^{3-}$	Apatite
1161	ν CH$_2$	Collagen
1242	Amide III	Collagen
1269	Amide III	Collagen
1451	δ CH$_2$	Collagen
1662	Amide I	Collagen

intensity ratio [8] was taken. The intensity of the symmetric phosphate stretching vibration at 957 cm^{-1} divided by the intensity of the CH$_2$ deformation band at 1451 cm^{-1} was calculated giving the mineral-to-collagen (mineralization) ratio. The mineral-to-collagen ratio is exemplarily presented in Fig. 5 and shows that chicken thigh bones have a significantly higher mineral-to-collagen ratio (22.3 ± 3.0) compared to pork metacarpal bones (8.4 ± 2.0) (given as mean value ± standard deviation). Mineralization ratios found for chicken thigh bones are on average 2.7 times greater than the values calculated for pork metacarpal. This ratio can thus be used as a simple way to distinguish between the two investigated bone types.

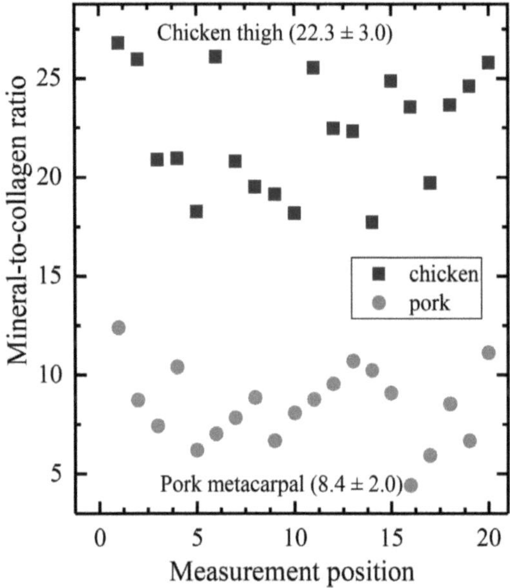

Figure 5: Mineral-to-collagen ratio calculated from 20 individual measurement positions from pork metacarpal bones and chicken thigh bones. Values in parenthesis give mean value ± standard deviation.

4 Conclusion

A combined approach of SERDS and 830 nm excitation wavelength was used to probe highly fluorescent bone samples. During the investigations, the optical power at sample location was 35 mW and the measurement time was 10×5 s. Pork metacarpal bones and chicken thigh bones were examined as examples. An effective separation of the Raman signals from the fluorescence background was achieved in all cases. In addition, differences in the composition of the different bones were visible. Calculations of peak ratios for quantification were performed. Based on the mineral-to-collagen ratio, it was possible to distinguish between the two bone types. This represents an important basis for further investigations, which can address other influencing factors for bone composition, such as age, sex, bone type or feeding.

This study demonstrated the ability of SERDS at 830 nm excitation for an effective fluorescence removal in the case of bone as selected biological material. In that way, SERDS has a great potential for numerous other analytical Raman applications which were limited by the fluorescence issue up to now, for example, investigation of various natural compounds, medical diagnostics, and forensics.

Acknowledgement

The work has been carried out at Ferdinand-Braun-Institut, Leibniz-Institut für Höchstfrequenztechnik, Berlin and supervised by Prof. Dr. Sebastian Karpf, Institut of Biomedical Optics, Universität zu Lübeck. We would like to thank Maria Krichler (Ferdinand-Braun-Institut, Leibniz-Institut für Höchstfrequenztechnik) for developing the software used to control the experimental setup and Dr. Michael Oster (Research Institute for Farm Animal Biology, Dummerstorf) for preparing and providing the bone samples.

Author's Statement

The Authors state no conflict of interest.

5 References

[1] D. Wei, S. Chen, and Q. Liu, 'Review of Fluorescence Suppression Techniques in Raman Spectroscopy', Applied Spectroscopy Reviews, vol. 50, no. 5, pp. 387–406, May 2015.

[2] A. P. Shreve, N. J. Cherepy, and R. A. Mathies, 'Effective Rejection of Fluorescence Interference in Raman Spectroscopy Using a Shifted Excitation Difference Technique', Applied Spectroscopy, vol. 46, no. 4, pp. 707–711, Apr. 1992.

[3] M. Maiwald, B. Sumpf, and G. Tränkle, 'Rapid and adjustable shifted excitation Raman difference spectroscopy using a dual-wavelength diode laser at 785 nm', Journal of Raman Spectroscopy, vol. 49, no. 11, pp. 1765–1775, Nov. 2018.

[4] R. D. Diehl, Ed., High-power diode lasers: fundamentals, technology, applications. Berlin; New York Springer: 2000.

[5] L. T. Kerr, H. J. Byrne, and B. M. Hennelly, 'Optimal choice of sample substrate and laser wavelength for Raman spectroscopic analysis of biological specimen', Analytical Methods, vol. 7, no. 12, pp. 5041–5052, Jun. 2015.

[6] K. Sowoidnich, S. Vogel, M. Maiwald, and B. Sumpf, 'Determination of Soil Constituents Using Shifted Excitation Raman Difference Spectroscopy', Applied Spectroscopy, vol. 76, no. 6, pp. 712–722, Jun. 2022.

[7] K. Sowoidnich and H.-D. Kronfeldt, 'Fluorescence Rejection by Shifted Excitation Raman Difference Spectroscopy at Multiple Wavelengths for the Investigation of Biological Samples', ISRN Spectroscopy, vol. 2012, Article ID 256326, pp. 1–11, Aug. 2012.

[8] A. J. Makowski, C. A. Patil, A. Mahadevan-Jansen, and J. S. Nyman, 'Polarization control of Raman spectroscopy optimizes the assessment of bone tissue', Journal of Biomedical Optics, vol. 18, no. 5, p. 055005, May 2013.

Infinite Science
Publishing